FRENCH'S INDEX OF DIFFERENTIAL DIAGNOSIS

French's Index of

EDITED BY

F. Dudley Hart MD, FRCP

Physician, Westminster Hospital, London

Differential Diagnosis

ELEVENTH EDITION

With eight hundred and eight illustrations
of which two hundred and eighty
are in colour

BRISTOL
JOHN WRIGHT & SONS LTD.
1979

British Library Cataloguing in Publication Data
French, Herbert
    French's index of differential diagnosis. — 11th ed
    1. Diagnosis, Differential
    I. Hart, Francis Dudley   II. Index of differential
    diagnosis
    616.07′5′03   RC71.5

ISBN 0 7236 0490 8

First Edition, March 1912
Reprinted October 1912 and September 1913
Second Edition, Revised and Enlarged, March 1917
Third Edition, with additional Illustrations, December 1917
Reprinted August 1918, June 1919, February 1920, February 1921, and May 1922
Fourth Edition, thoroughly Revised and Enlarged, with many additional Illustrations, September 1928
Reprinted July 1929
Fifth Edition, fully Revised, with additional Illustrations, January 1936
Reprinted February 1938
Sixth Edition, fully Revised, with additional Illustrations, April 1945
Reprinted April 1947 and September 1948
Seventh Edition, completely Revised, January 1954
Eighth Edition, completely Revised, with many new Illustrations, June 1960
Ninth Edition, completely Revised, with many new Illustrations, April 1967
Tenth Edition, completely Revised, with many new Illustrations, June 1973
Eleventh Edition, completely Revised, with many new Illustrations, May 1979
Reprinted January 1982

Printed in Great Britain by John Wright & Sons (Printing) Ltd., at The Stonebridge Press, Bristol BS4 5NU

Preface to the Eleventh Edition

SINCE THE TENTH EDITION of this book there have been several changes in authorship. Mr. Miles Foxen has largely rewritten the sections dealing with disorders of ear, nose, and throat, replacing Mr. Philip Reading. Professor Malcolm Milne and Dr. Joan Zilva have written new sections to replace those previously contributed by Professor Noel Maclagan. Dr. E. C. Huskisson has contributed two new sections on pain and lethargy, two of the commonest of all complaints. Professor Guy Scadding has contributed a useful new section on the patient who presents with no signs or symptoms but with an abnormal or odd chest X-ray necessitating correct and critical interpretation. Many new illustrations have been added and many old favourites removed, but some are so excellent in illustrating disorders now rare in this country that I have retained several, such as *Fig.* 472 on p. 467, always a favourite of mine!

In clinical medicine sins of omission are more common than sins of commission. It is the disorders one does not think of and the conditions one forgets that lead to misdiagnosis or no diagnosis. This book aims to help the clinician to be sure that he has considered all the disorders that might lie behind his patient's particular symptoms or physical signs. In these days when there is a tendency (in hospitals other than our own, of course) for ward rounds to be sometimes recitals of biochemical, haematological, and radiological findings, the patient's bedclothes unruffled, and the patient a silent witness, the importance of signs and symptoms cannot be overemphasized. I said in my Preface to the Tenth Edition that I hoped this book had retained its usefulness for the practising clinician, and it seemed clear from its popularity that it had. I only hope that this Eleventh Edition will prove as popular as its predecessors.

Many sections have been changed considerably in the light of recent discoveries and changes in attitudes to old problems. But signs and symptoms of disease remain remarkably constant over the years, and though certain disorders, such as tuberculosis, syphilis, and rheumatic fever, may be less evident today in our own and some other countries, in many parts of the world they remain a common and constant public health and diagnostic problem which can be transported, as can any infectious disease, to our shores overnight by modern air services. This fact, and the fact that modern therapeutics has changed the face of medicine very considerably, largely eliminating certain disorders in some countries, suppressing others (and thereby making diagnosis sometimes more difficult) and in some cases producing new syndromes, though in general benefiting mankind enormously, has often added considerably to the difficulties of differential diagnosis and has often extended the range of disorders that one has to consider in any individual case.

I would like to acknowledge advice and assistance from Dr. Basil Strickland and Dr. Joe Gleeson and from Professor M. H. Lessof and Professor Ariel Lant.

I must thank, once again, my secretary, Mrs. Valerie Mayblatt, the staff of John Wright & Sons and, of course, the most noble, hardworked and highly co-operative contributors. With such colleagues and publishers team work is a joy and the production of a new Edition of French's Index a most pleasant and exciting experience!

F. DUDLEY HART

March, 1979

Preface to the First Edition

THIS BOOK is a treatise on the application of differential diagnosis to all the main signs and symptoms of disease. It aims at being of practical utility to medical men whenever difficulty arises in deciding the precise cause of any particular symptom of which a patient may complain. It covers the whole ground of medicine, surgery, gynaecology, ophthalmology, dermatology, and neurology.

Whatever the disease from which a patient is suffering, the importance of diagnosing it as early as possible can hardly be over-rated. The present volume deals with diagnosis from a standpoint which is different from that of most textbooks, having been written in response to requests for an *Index of Diagnosis* as a companion to the publishers' *Index of Treatment*, issued in 1907. The book is an index in the sense that its articles on the various symptoms are arranged in alphabetical order; at the same time it is a work upon differential diagnosis in that it discusses the methods of distinguishing between the various diseases in which each individual symptom may be observed. Whilst the body of the book thus deals with *symptoms*, the general index at the end gathers these together under the headings of the various *diseases* in which they occur.

The Editor lays particular stress upon the importance of using these two parts of the book together. Unless reference is made freely to the general index, the reader may miss a number of the places in which is discussed the diagnosis of the disease with which he has to deal; for while each *symptom* is considered but once, each *disease* is likely to come up for discussion under the heading of each of its more important symptoms.

The guiding principle throughout has been to suppose that a particular symptom attracts special notice in a given case, and that the diagnosis has to be established by differentiating between the various diseases to which this symptom may be due. One of many difficulties arising during the construction of the work was that of deciding where to draw the line as regards symptoms themselves. The exclusion of many borderline headings such as 'Dullness at the base of one lung', 'Inability to breathe through the nose', and various signs such as Romberg's, Stellwag's, von Graefe's, and so forth, may perhaps seem arbitrary; but reference to the minor symptoms and physical signs which have not been thought sufficiently important to merit separate articles will be found in the general index at the end of the volume.

Treatment, pathology, and prognosis are not dealt with except in so far as they may bear upon differential diagnosis—the employment of salicylates, for instance, in distinguishing acute rheumatic from other forms of arthritis; the use of the microscope in distinguishing malignant neoplasms from inflammatory or other tumours; the value of the lapse of time in distinguishing between tuberculous and meningococcal meningitis.

Coloured plates and other illustrations have been introduced freely wherever it was thought they might be helpful in diagnosis. Most of them are original, but a few are reproduced from other sources, and thanks are due to the authors and publishers who have kindly lent them.

So far as the Editor is aware, although there exist indexes of symptoms, and medical works in which various maladies are discussed in alphabetical order, the present Index of Differential Diagnosis of Main Symptoms is unique in medical literature. It rests with the medical profession to decide whether it strikes the mark at which it aims. There must be room for improvement in many respects notwithstanding the great amount of time and labour that have been bestowed upon it.

However this may be, the work undoubtedly owes much of what value it possesses to the suggestions and kindly help of the many contributors who have assisted in its making; and to the practitioners and the authorities of various institutions who have generously lent the material for many of the illustrations. Indeed, it is difficult to see how the book could have been produced in its present completeness without their willing collaboration: to all of them the Editor tenders his sincere thanks.

HERBERT FRENCH
62 *Wimpole Street, London, W.*1
March 1912

List of Contributors and their Subjects

R. G. Beard, MA, MB, M.CHIR, FRCS
Consultant Surgeon, Guy's Hospital and St Olave's Hospital, London

P. M. F. Bishop, BA, DM(OXON), FRCP, FRCOG
Endocrinologist Emeritus, Guy's Hospital; Consultant Endocrinologist, Chelsea Hospital for Women; lately Senior Lecturer in Endocrinology, Institute of Obstetrics and Gynaecology, Royal Postgraduate Medical School, London; lately Senior Lecturer in Applied Physiology, Guy's Hospital Medical School, London

Harold Ellis, MCH(OXF), FRCS(ENG)
Professor of Surgery, Westminster Hospital Medical School, London

Peter R. Fleming, MD(LOND), FRCP

Senior Lecturer in Medicine, Westminster Medical School, London; Consultant Physician, Westminster Hospital, London

E. H. Miles Foxen, FRCS, DLO

Consultant Surgeon, Department of Otolaryngology, Westminster Hospital, Westminster Children's Hospital, Chelsea Hospital for Women, and Queen Charlotte's Maternity Hospital, London

F. Dudley Hart, MD, FRCP

Consulting Physician, Chelsea Hospital for Women, The Hospital of St John and St Elizabeth and Westminster Hospital, London

Edward C. Huskisson, BSC, MD, MRCP

Senior Lecturer and Consultant Physician, St Bartholomew's and St Leonard's Hospitals, London

T. L. T. Lewis, FRCS, FRCOG

Obstetric and Gynaecological Surgeon, Guy's Hospital; Surgeon, Chelsea Hospital for Women; Obstetric Surgeon, Queen Charlotte's Maternity Hospital, London

I. C. K. Mackenzie, TD, MD, FRCP

Physician to the Department of Nervous Diseases, Guy's Hospital, London; Consultant Neurologist to West Kent General Hospital, Maidstone

Malcolm D. Milne, BSC, MD, FRCP, MRCS, FRS

Professor of Medicine at Westminster Hospital Medical School, London

T. A. J. Prankerd, MD(LOND), FRCP

Professor of Clinical Haematology, University College Hospital Medical School; Honorary Consultant Physician, University College Hospital, London

Peter D. Samman, MD, FRCP

Physician, Dermatology Department, Westminster Hospital, London; Physician, St John's Hospital for Diseases of the Skin, London

J. G. Scadding, MD, FRCP

Emeritus Professor of Medicine, University of London; Honorary Consulting Physician, Brompton Hospital and Hammersmith Hospital, London

W. H. Trethowan, CBE, MB, BCHIR(CAMB), FRCP, FRACP, FRC PSYCH, FRANZCP

Professor of Psychiatry, University of Birmingham; Honorary Consultant Psychiatrist, United Birmingham Hospitals

P. D. Trevor-Roper, MD(CAMB), FRCS

Consultant Ophthalmic Surgeon, Westminster Hospital; Moorfields Eye Hospital and King Edward VII Hospital

Christopher Wastell, MS(LOND), FRCS(ENG)

Reader and Honorary Consultant Surgeon, Westminster Hospital and Medical School, London

Joan F. Zilva, BSC, MD, FRCP, FRCPATH, DCC(BIOCHEM)

Reader and Honorary Consultant in Chemical Pathology, Westminster Hospital and Medical School, London

FRENCH'S INDEX OF
DIFFERENTIAL DIAGNOSIS

ABDOMEN, RIGIDITY OF

Rigidity of the abdomen is a sign of the utmost importance, since in most cases it indicates serious intra-abdominal mischief requiring immediate operation. It is the expression of a state of tonic contraction in the muscles of the abdominal wall. The responsible stimulus may be in the brain or basal ganglia, or in the territory of the six lower dorsal nerves which supply the abdominal wall,

after patient persuasion; a request to take a few deep breaths, or to draw their knees up and keep their mouths open, will often help. During this preliminary examination one hand, well warmed, may be laid gently on the abdomen and passed over its surface with a light touch that cannot possibly hurt; this manoeuvre will help to allay the patient's anxiety still further and give the examiner an idea of the extent, intensity, and constancy of the rigidity which he must later investigate in more detail.

Site of Stimulus	Causative Agent	Characters of Rigidity
Cerebral cortex or basal ganglia	Nervousness, anticipation of pain, cold	Affects the whole abdominal wall; varies in intensity, can be abolished by appropriate means
Dorsal nerve-trunks	Pleurisy; infections of the chest wall	Limited to one side of abdomen. Varies in extent and degree
Nerve-endings in abdominal wall	Injury or infection of muscles	Limited to injured or infected segment
Nerve-endings in peritoneum	Irritation by any foreign substance: infection, chemical irritant, or blood.	Degree varies with nature of irritant and suddenness with which stimulus has arrived. Extent corresponds to area of peritoneum involved. Both degree and extent remain approximately constant during the period of examination.

but not in the visceral sensory fibres of the sympathetic system. The extent of the rigidity will depend on the number of nerves involved, and its degree on the nature and duration of the stimulus. The analysis above and on the following page may be considered.

The patient should be examined lying on the back with the whole abdomen and lower thorax exposed, but the shoulders and legs well covered. The room must be warm. The examiner, seated on a level with the patient, should first watch the abdomen to see whether it moves with respiration or not, and whether one part moves more than another; at the same time he may observe other things which will help in the diagnosis, such as asymmetry of the two sides, local swelling, or the movement of coils of bowel. While watching and later when examining he should engage the patient in conversation, encouraging him to talk in order to allay nervousness and to remove any part of the rigidity which is due to voluntary contraction. Some nervous patients, especially if the room is cold, hold their abdomen intensely rigid, and can be induced to relax only

For more exact examination the observer should sit at the patient's side facing his head, and place both hands on the abdomen, examining comparable areas on both sides simultaneously, and taking in turn the epigastrium, right and left hypochondrium, umbilical region, both flanks as far back as the erector spinae (for the rigidity of a retrocaecal appendix may only affect the posterior part of the abdominal wall), the hypochondrium, and both iliac fossae. First, the whole hand should be applied with light pressure; next, the fingers held flat should be pressed more firmly to estimate the extent of the rigidity and to discover deep tenderness; lastly, detailed examination may be made in suspected areas with the firm pressure of one or two fingers. Evidence is not complete without a search for skin hyperaesthesia, and without percussion and auscultation. A rectal examination is indispensable.

After a leisurely examination with warm hands in a warm room, during which the physician has also been able to sum up the patient, his temperament, and whether he is really ill or not, the rigidity of anxiety or cold will have been dispelled or recognized. The abdominal rigidity due to a lesion in the chest or chest wall usually involves a wide area limited to one side—a distribution most unusual with intra-abdominal mischief, which, if it has spread widely but not everywhere, tends to be limited to the upper or lower half. The extent and degree of rigidity in chest affections also vary widely during examination. Other things such as a flushed face, rapid respiration, movement of the alae nasi, or a temperature of more than 102° F., may suggest that the lesion is not abdominal, and a friction rub may be felt or heard in the chest.

Auscultation and rectal examination dispel any remaining doubts, for in chest conditions peristaltic sounds remain normal, and there is no tenderness in Douglas's pouch. Examination of the blood may show a high leucocytosis, up to 30,000 or 40,000, whereas in peritonitis the count is seldom over 12,000.

Injuries of the abdominal wall, particularly those caused by run-over accidents, lead to very marked rigidity of the injured segment. Here the rigidity is not necessary to establish a diagnosis, for the injury is already known, but its degree and extent should be carefully noted. There must always be a doubt as to whether abdominal viscera are damaged as well as the walls, and this point can only be settled by careful observation. The patient is put to bed and kept warm, the pulse is charted every quarter of an hour, and the abdomen is re-examined from time to time. In the case of a mere contusion collapse will soon disappear, the abdomen will become less rigid, and the pulse-rate will fall. If the contents of a viscus have escaped, rigidity will extend beyond the area of the damaged muscles, and the signs of peritonitis will develop rapidly. If there is internal bleeding the mucous surfaces will become pale, the skin cold and clammy, and the pulse small and frequent, while the haemoglobin estimates will show a progressive drop. In case of doubt an exploratory laparotomy should not be delayed.

PERITONITIS

The commonest and the most important cause of general abdominal rigidity is peritonitis, and it is a safe rule when meeting true rigidity to diagnose peritonitis till it can be excluded. Actually rigidity means no more than that the peritoneum lining the abdominal cavity is in contact with something differing from the smooth surfaces which are its normal environment. The *presence of rigidity* therefore announces a change in the coelomic cavity that is probably infective in origin. When gall-stone colic is followed by rigidity of the right rectus, it means, not only that a stone is blocking the cystic duct, but that the pent-up bile is infected and the wall of the gall-bladder inflamed. Intestinal obstruction of mechanical origin (such as that due to a gall-stone impacted in the ileum) gives colic referred to the umbilicus, but no guarding of the muscles; local rigidity accompanying the clinical picture of intestinal obstruction indicates that there is also a local inflammatory focus such as a strangulated loop of bowel, while a more diffuse rigidity suggests changes such as a thrombosis of the superior mesenteric artery, affecting a large segment of bowel. In appendicitis, rigidity denotes that infection has spread beyond the coats of the appendix.

The *degree of rigidity* varies with the nature of the irritant, the rapidity with which the peritoneum is attacked, and the area involved. At one extreme is the rigidity of a duodenal perforation, where the abdomen is suddenly flooded with a digestive fluid. Here the whole abdominal wall is fixed in a contraction that can best be described as board-like: there is no respiratory movement, and no yielding to the firmest pressure. At the other extreme is the quiet postoperative peritonitis that may follow any abdominal operation, where an organism of low virulence invades a peritoneal cavity already roughened by recent handling; there is perhaps only a slightly increased resistance when the hands are pressed on the abdomen. Perforation of gastric or duodenal ulcer produces the most intense rigidity; the escape of pancreatic enzyme in acute pancreatitis leads to less; escape of other sterile fluids, urine for instance, or blood, still less. Bacterial invasion of the peritoneum produces marked rigidity. When the infection is sudden and diffuse, as in perforation of the ileum or bursting of an appendix abscess, the protective reaction is more intense than in a blood-borne peritonitis, but seldom reaches the extreme degree seen in a duodenal perforation. A streptococcal peritonitis gives more rigidity than a pneumococcal one, a tuberculous one very little. The degree of muscle contraction also alters during the development of a case. The board-like abdominal wall of a perforation is considerably softer after three or four hours when the peritoneum has recovered from the shock of the first insult. The slight resistance apparent when sterile urine escapes from a ruptured bladder rapidly increases as infection supervenes.

The *extent of the rigidity* usually corresponds to the area of peritoneum affected. The whole abdomen may be rigid, the upper or lower part only, one side, or a restricted part. Total rigidity should mean a total peritonitis, but because the peritoneum reacts immediately to invasion by forming adhesions which localize the mischief, a general peritonitis is only seen when an irritant or infected fluid is suddenly discharged in large quantities—as in duodenal perforation, pancreatitis, or the bursting of a large abscess or distended viscus—or when the infection is brought by the blood-stream and reaches all parts simultaneously. Occasionally, particularly in children, the reaction to a sudden infection may be very excessive and the muscles contract over a wide area in response to a purely local infection, for instance of the appendix, but this exaggerated response rapidly disappears. Conversely the aged, with atrophic abdominal muscles, may exhibit only slight rigidity, even in generalized peritonitis. Local peritonitis starts around some site of infection, and as it spreads is guided by certain peritoneal watersheds, of which the most important is the attachment of the great omentum to the transverse colon, dividing the abdomen into supra- and infra-colic compartments: rigidity accompanies the infection. Thus localized rigidity is found over any inflamed organ, and as the infection and the guarding spread, they tend to involve the upper or the lower half of the abdomen as a whole. When we have mapped out the extent of the rigidity, we should, from a knowledge of the organs at that site and of the watersheds that guide the spread of infection, be able, in conjunction with the history, to make a diagnosis.

The influence of natural subdivisions in guiding intraperitoneal extension must always be taken into account. Infections in the right supra-colic compartment tend to pass down between the ascending colon and the right abdominal wall, while one in the pelvis is guided by the pelvic mesocolon to the left side of the abdomen as it ascends. Thus rigidity in the right iliac fossa may indicate a leaking duodenal ulcer, and in the left may be due to a pelvic appendix.

Since the diagnosis of peritonitis in most cases means immediate operation, every endeavour must be made to confirm the diagnosis, particularly by the simple tests of percussion, auscultation, and rectal examination. Percussion may reveal the outline of some dilated hollow organ, such as the caecum; it may disclose free gas escaped from a perforation as a shifting circle of resonance or a tympanitic note where liver dullness should be; it may map out an abnormal area of dullness where there is an abscess or a collection of blood; or it may indicate free fluid in the peritoneum. Auscultation is even more important, for with infection peristalsis ceases: in a normal abdomen peristaltic sounds can be heard every four to ten seconds; in obstruction they are increased in loudness, pitch, and frequency, in peritonitis there is complete silence over the infected area. Rectal examination nearly always reveals tenderness when there is intra-abdominal infection, even if it is distant and localized.

Other signs must be mentioned: the patient lies still, sometimes with the knees drawn up, and resists interference. The abdomen gradually becomes distended, tense, and tympanitic. The tongue is brown and dry. Vomiting is to be expected at the onset of any abdominal catastrophe, but, except in intestinal obstruction, it usually ceases; with advancing peritonitis it reappears, and the vomit becomes first bile-stained, later brownish and faecal smelling, and is allowed to dribble from the corner of the mouth in contrast to the projectile vomiting of obstruction. There may be diarrhoea at first, but constipation soon succeeds it. The temperature tends to fall; the pulse is small and rapid, rising progressively. In late stages the sunken cheeks, wide eyes, and anxious expression of the patient form a characteristic feature—the Hippocratic facies.

These signs are indications of a peritonitis discovered too late, and the heralds of approaching death. Abdominal rigidity, abdominal silence, rectal tenderness, and a rising pulse are a tetrad that call for immediate definitive treatment.

A more detailed diagnosis is usually possible when the history and other signs are taken together, but a consideration of all the alternatives is out of the question in this section. Abdominal paracentesis with a fine needle is widely practised but experience shows that this can be dangerous, even fatal, in intestinal obstruction. A list of the more common conditions associated with rigidity may, however, help the inquiry:

STOMACH OR DUODENUM:
Perforation of peptic ulcer.

GALL-BLADDER:
Acute cholecystitis
Rupture of gall-bladder.

PANCREAS:
Acute pancreatitis.

SMALL INTESTINE:
Strangulation of a loop
Perforation of a typhoid ulcer
Thrombosis or embolus of superior mesenteric artery
Strangulation, perforation, or inflammation of Meckel's diverticulum.

LARGE INTESTINE:
Appendicitis
Volvulus
Diverticulitis with perforation or pericolitis.

PERITONEUM:
Acute blood-borne peritonitis:
Streptococcal
Pneumococcal
Gonococcal.

FEMALE GENERATIVE ORGANS:
Twisted ovarian cyst
Ruptured ectopic gestation
Acute salpingitis
Torsion or red degeneration of fibroid
Perforation of uterus or posterior fornix in attempted abortion.

Perforation of a peptic ulcer is characterized by the most sudden onset, the worst agony, and the most extreme abdominal rigidity that the physician is ever likely to see. Immediately afterwards the patient is motionless and speechless, in a state of obvious collapse. A few hours later pain, rigidity, and shock have all diminished, and only the dramatic history and persistent rectal tenderness may remain to indicate the seriousness of the condition.

Acute pancreatitis is seldom accompanied by the severe pain described in textbooks, or indeed by pain as bad as that of gall-stone colic. The abdominal rigidity is more marked in the upper abdomen but is not profound. On the other hand, the patient shows a degree of toxaemia out of all proportion to the physical signs in the abdomen. The diagnosis is confirmed by a rise in the serum amylase to values of over 800 units per cent.

A *ruptured ectopic gestation* may simulate a lower abdominal peritonitis, but the signs of bleeding predominate and rigidity is not well marked. Auscultation often reveals very active harsh peristaltic sounds. If the patient is a woman of child-bearing age who is known to have missed a period, the onset of abdominal pain and pallor suggest the diagnosis. The extent of blood-loss will be indicated by a haemoglobin estimation, and extravasated blood will be felt in the pelvis, together with acute tenderness on vaginal and rectal examinations.

Blue discoloration of the skin around the umbilicus, Cullen's sign, may be associated with rigidity. This discoloration is due to extravasated blood coming forwards from the retroperitoneal space. The sign is seen in ruptured kidney, leaking abdominal aneurysm, and acute pancreatitis. Occasionally it is seen in ruptured ectopic gestation, when the blood gains entry to the subperitoneal space through the broad ligament. Although pancreatitis may produce this sign, it is more common to see a green discoloration in the loins (Grey Turner's sign).

R. G. Beard.

ABDOMINAL PAIN, ACUTE, LOCALIZED: 'COLIC'

'Colic', strictly speaking, should be employed only in the case of paroxysmal abdominal pain but is a word used loosely to include any extreme abdominal pain of a griping type due to intense and maintained contractions of the non-striped muscles in disease of various abdominal viscera. The causes may be summarized as follows:

1. Biliary. Due to:

Stone in the gall-bladder
Stone in the cystic duct
Stone in the common bile-duct
Stone in a hepatic duct
Acute or subacute cholecystitis
Acute inflammation of the larger bile-ducts
Carcinoma of the gall-bladder
Carcinoma of the cystic duct
Carcinoma of the common bile-duct
Carcinoma of ampulla of Vater
Carcinoma of the duodenum
Secondary carcinoma of the portal lymph-nodes
Secondary sarcoma of the portal lymph-nodes
Lymphadenoma of the portal lymph-nodes
Tuberculosis of the portal lymph-nodes
Syphilitic enlargement of the portal lymph-nodes
Chronic pancreatitis
Carcinoma of the head of the pancreas
After injury, with haemorrhage into the portal fissure

2. Renal. Due to:

Stone in the kidney
Mobile kidney (Dietl's crises)
Blood-clot passing from the kidney: after injury; after renal infarction, as in infective endocarditis;

from blood diseases as leukaemia, scurvy, purpura; from tubercle; from growth
Hydronephrosis
Pyonephrosis
Pyelonephritis
Tuberculosis
Carcinoma
Sarcoma
Rhabdomyoma
After pyelography

3. Ureteric. Due to:

Stone in the ureter
Blood-clot
Acute ureteritis
After instrumentation (ureteric catheterization)
From obstruction to the ureter by adjacent tuberculous or calcareous lymph-node
Obstruction by adjacent retroperitoneal tumours, e.g., lymphosarcoma

4. Vesical. Due to:

Stone in the bladder
Acute cystitis
Chronic cystitis
Foreign body in the bladder
After instrumentation
Blood-clot in the bladder
Tubercle of the bladder
Villous tumour of the bladder
Carcinoma of the bladder
Invasion of the bladder by carcinoma or sarcoma from without, e.g., from carcinoma of the uterus, carcinoma of the rectum, or carcinoma of the pelvic colon
Irritation of the bladder by adjacent inflammation, e.g., appendicitis, parametritis, pelvic abscess, perirectal abscess, pyosalpinx
Bilharziasis

5. Pancreatic. Due to:

Stone in pancreatic duct
Chronic pancreatitis
Acute haemorrhagic pancreatitis
Carcinoma of ampulla of Vater
Carcinoma of duodenum
Gall-stone impacted in ampulla of Vater
Injury
Diabetes mellitus, especially when coma is impending

6. Appendicular. Due to:

Faecal concretion within the appendix
Foreign body in the appendix
Inflammation of the lymph-nodes adjacent to appendix
Acute appendicitis
Tuberculous appendix
Carcinoma of appendix

7. Fallopian Tube. Due to:

Salpingitis
Pyosalpinx
Ectopic pregnancy
Tuberculous iliac lymph-nodes
Adhesions

8. Uterine. Due to:

Dysmenorrhoea (q.v.)
Displacement
Endometritis
Injury
Instrumentation

Ergot
Retained products of conception
Carcinoma
Sarcoma
Tuberculosis
Labour
Chorion-epithelioma

9. Central Nervous System. Due to:

Tabetic crises (gastric, intestinal, biliary, renal, rectal)
Acute infective meningitis
Benign lymphocytic meningitis
Subarachnoid haemorrhage
Posterior nerve root pain from prolapsed inter-vertebral disk, collapsed vertebra
Neurosis
Hysteria

10. Gastric. Due to:

Indigestible food
Gastric ulcer
Carcinoma
Duodenal ulcer
Alcoholic gastritis
Pyloric stenosis
Haemorrhage into mucosa, e.g., in acute infections; in blood diseases such as leukaemia, Henoch's purpura
Irritant poisons
Hiatus hernia

11. Intestinal. Due to:

Acute intestinal indigestion
Lead poisoning
Carcinoma
Diverticulitis
Hirschsprung's disease
Obstructed or strangulated hernia
Partial volvulus of intestine
Intussusception: (a) Acute; (b) Chronic
Colitis, whether simple or ulcerative
Dysentery
Cholera
Enteritis
Regional ileitis (Crohn's disease)
Tuberculous ulceration
Haemorrhage into the bowel wall from: injury, Henoch's purpura, blood diseases such as pernicious anaemia, leukaemia, scurvy, purpura
Ileocaecal kinking
Overloaded caecum
Chronic failure to evacuate contents of colon
Impacted faeces
Superior mesenteric artery syndrome (intestinal angina)
Obstruction by orange-pith or melon-seeds
Obstruction by adhesions
Sigmoid volvulus
The over-action of purgatives especially aloes, colocynth, calomel, castor oil, croton oil, jalap, podophyllin, phenolphthalein, senna, cascara sagrada, rhubarb
Impacted gall-stones
Abdominal migraine
Abdominal epilepsy
Porphyria (see p. 807)
The Peutz-Jeghers syndrome

12. Infections. Due to:

Measles
Mumps
Streptococcal tonsillitis

13. Aorta. Due to:

Ruptured aneurysm

14. Ovary. Due to:

Twisted ovarian cyst
Endometriosis
Ovulation (*Mittelschmerz*)

15. Peritoneum. Due to:

Peritonitis due to perforated peptic ulcer, spread of infection from inflamed intraperitoneal organ or external trauma
Perforation of intestine by foreign body, e.g., fish-bone
Torsion of appendix epiploicae
Tuberculous peritonitis

16. Splenic. Due to:

Infarction
Spontaneous rupture as in infective mononucleosis and malaria
Trauma

17. Hepatic. Due to:

Infective hepatitis
Congestive cardiac failure
Malignant disease, primary or secondary
Trauma

18. Referred. From:

Heart
Pericardium
Pleura
Dorsal spine

When confronted with a patient with severe abdominal pain, an early consideration is to decide whether or not a laparotomy is required. This decision will be arrived at by consideration of the history, clinical examination, and relevant special tests.

While the clinical history normally reflects the nature of the pathological process, it is generally true that severe abdominal disease presents as a distinct episode with a relatively short history. Some idea as to the presence or otherwise of true colic can be gained from the attitude of the patient. If, when the pain is present, the patient finds it difficult to lie still and is constantly moving in an attempt to find a comfortable position, the diagnosis is probably one of colic. Alternatively, if the patient lies still and movement is resisted the more likely diagnosis is one of intraperitoneal inflammatory disease, in which any movement tends to produce contact between the inflamed surfaces of the peritoneum. Most patients who require urgent laparotomy look ill.

CONDITIONS REQUIRING URGENT LAPAROTOMY:

1. Inflammatory diseases
    Acute appendicitis
    Perforation:
        Gastric ulcer
        Duodenal ulcer
        Carcinoma of the stomach
        Small bowel (typhoid)
        Large bowel (foreign body)
    Failure to localize
        Cholecystitis
        Diverticulitis (of colon, Meckel's)

2. Haemorrhage
   Ruptured ectopic pregnancy
   Ruptured aortic aneurysm
   Massive bleeding from duodenal or gastric ulcer

3. Trauma
   Damage to viscus:
   Spleen
   Kidney
   Liver
   Intestine
   Gall-bladder

4. Obstruction, with or without strangulation
   Dynamic, e.g., by peritoneal band
   Adynamic, e.g., mesenteric vascular occlusion

5. Pelvic
   Twisted ovarian cyst
   Twisted uterine fibroid.

Of this list it will be noted that there is only one condition which presents with true colic, that is dynamic intestinal obstruction. Great care is required in making the diagnosis in a patient with severe pain in the abdomen at the extremes of life. Young children may present with abdominal pain and on examination have all the appearance of an intra-abdominal catastrophe when they suffer from no more than tonsillitis.

Old people may have relatively few abdominal signs in the presence of severe peritonitis. Some of the points to pay particular attention to when examining a patient are as follows:

CONDITION OF THE ABDOMEN AND ITS WALL. The patient must be placed in a good light and lie supine. The entire surface of the abdomen is uncovered from the nipples to the knees.

Movement. If the abdomen does not move with respiration there may be underlying peritonitis.

Contour. Abdominal distension is present in intestinal obstruction. If the obstruction is of the small bowel the distension is central and dilated loops of small bowel may give a 'ladder pattern' and peristalsis within them may be visible. If the obstruction is of the colon the distension is of the flanks; the caecum may be observed as a bulge in the right iliac fossa. Gastric distension in pyloric stenosis may be seen in the epigastrium and gastric peristaltic waves may be seen in the thin patient. Retraction of the abdomen may occur in acute peritonitis and the abdomen assumes a scaphoid appearance following perforation of a duodenal ulcer.

Guarding. A voluntary contraction of the abdominal wall on palpation betokens underlying inflammatory disease. It may also reflect apprehension.

Tenderness. A sensation of pain on palpation indicates an underlying inflammatory condition, although renal and biliary colic are also associated with some tenderness.

Rigidity. Rigidity is indicated by an involuntary tightness of the abdominal wall and has the same implication as tenderness. It may be generalized or localized, situated over one particular organ, as for example in acute cholecystitis.

Rebound Tenderness. Rebound tenderness is present when there is an area of peritonitis.

Percussion. A diminished percussion note indicates the presence of intraperitoneal fluid. This is confirmed by eliciting the sign of 'shifting dullness'. In this case the edge of the dull area changes position when the patient lies first on one side and then on the other.

A resonant percussion note indicates underlying gas. A resonant, distended abdomen is found in obstruction. It is occasionally possible to detect a band of resonance above the liver in a perforated duodenal ulcer.

Bowel-sounds may be present or absent. If absent, the small intestine has been paralysed, the condition being known as 'paralytic ileus'. If the bowel-sounds have a particular 'tinkling' quality, this is caused by dilatation such as occurs proximal to an obstruction. If obstruction has been present for some length of time the bowel-sounds may be audible without a stethoscope (borborygmi).

EXAMINATION OF THE HERNIAL ORIFICES. It is extremely important when examining the abdomen in any patient to examine the inguinal regions. A strangulated femoral or inguinal hernia may occasionally present with severe vomiting and a minimum of pain in the inguinal region. Obturator and retroperitoneal herniae are often impossible to recognize until laparotomy.

TREND. One of the important aspects in the assessment of the acute abdomen is the establishment of trend. In particular the physical signs previously mentioned must be elicited from time to time when the diagnosis is not known. Increasing pain, tenderness, guarding, or rigidity indicate that the condition is worsening. Extension of an area of tenderness associated with developing rebound tenderness indicates a failure of localization of the underlying inflammatory condition. Increasing distension in a patient with intestinal obstruction means that the obstruction has not been relieved.

Of considerable use in establishing trend is the observation and recording of the objective physical signs. By far the most important of these is the pulse. If the pulse is taken every hour and if it rises this is a clear indication of a worsening condition. It will be expected, for example, that a patient with acute cholecystitis being treated conservatively with bed-rest, analgesics, antibiotics, and intravenous fluids, admitted with a high pulse-rate in the region of 100, will improve from admission so that the rate steadily falls from the admission point, providing that the inflammation in the gall-bladder remains localized.

The temperature is of rather variable significance since in some conditions it is either normal or even subnormal. Typically in acute appendicitis the temperature is not raised. In some old patients with quite severe peritonitis the temperature is either normal or only slightly raised. Extremely high temperatures, occasionally associated with a rigor, are suggestive of hepatic or renal infection. A swinging pyrexia which becomes raised each evening and falls to the normal level the following morning indicates the presence of pus.

VOMITING. This is an extremely common symptom with all gastro-intestinal conditions. All cases of intestinal obstruction have some associated vomiting sooner or later; in general the higher the obstruction and the younger the patient, the sooner the vomiting is experienced. This symptom is also present in intraperitoneal inflammatory conditions and it is extremely unusual to find appendicitis in the absence of at least one bout of vomiting. Generally, the more persistent the vomiting the more ready should one be to perform a laparotomy.

THE FACIES OF THE PATIENT. As previously mentioned patients with serious abdominal disease look ill. An extreme example of this is provided by the Hippocratic facies, in which the cheeks are sunken and the face is drawn, in terminal generalized peritonitis.

THE BOWELS. The presence of diarrhoea or constipation is often of considerable significance. In intestinal obstruction classically there is absolute constipation, that is the patient passes neither flatus nor faeces. If the obstruction is of acute onset it is often found that the patient passes one or perhaps two stools, thus emptying the alimentary canal distal to the obstruction. Two enemas will then produce no faeces and the symptoms and signs of intestinal obstruction will persist.

THE URINE. The presence of blood, albumin, pus, or bile may help to distinguish a renal or biliary colic from peritoneal inflammation. In obscure cases of abdominal pain the urine should be examined for porphyrins to exclude porphyria, particularly when the attack appears to have been precipitated by barbiturates. Frequency of micturition will occur, together with dysuria, in a urinary-tract infection.

An absence of urine or oliguria (less than 400 ml. urine per 24 hours) should first of all be confirmed by catheterization. If no urine is found in the bladder then the patient must be treated as for renal failure.

THE SKIN. The skin may be pale if the patient is anaemic. This can obviously occur when there has been some long-standing bleeding condition into the gastro-intestinal tract. Biliary colic, with a stone impacted at the lower end of the common bile-duct, may be associated with jaundice and there is often associated itching. In this case scratch marks are often to be seen on the surface of the skin. In very ill patients who are dehydrated the skin is usually lax. Care has to be taken in interpreting this, however, because the skin of many older patients is also lax. In hypovolaemic states such as in extreme dehydration skin perfusion is reduced. In this case the skin is not only pale but cold and clammy by virtue of secretion of sweat in response to a raised level of circulating adrenaline and noradrenaline. Failure of the peripheral circulation in the ill patient is of bad prognostic significance.

RECTAL AND VAGINAL EXAMINATION. Rectal examination is essential in all patients with abdominal pain. In intestinal obstruction the rectum has a characteristic 'ballooned' feel. It is occasionally possible to feel a tender swelling in the pelvis in peritonitis. It is possible to examine the female pelvic organs by this route.

VASCULAR LESIONS. Acute mesenteric vascular occlusion is difficult to diagnose. Usually it is of vague onset and eventually gives rise to the signs of dynamic intestinal obstruction. The danger lies in the fact that the symptoms may be of slow onset, and the gangrenous bowel may ultimately perforate. Superior mesenteric artery stenosis gives rise to the syndrome known as 'intestinal angina'. The features of this are: abdominal pain which may appear to be colicky in nature, appearing after a meal, associated with diarrhoea, a positive occult blood, and weight-loss.

Aneurysms of the aorta may enlarge and be painful, or even rupture. There is usually severe abdominal pain together with the symptoms and signs of profound shock. The femoral pulses may be absent.

Dissecting aneurysm of the aorta is unusual in the abdomen, more commonly starting in the ascending thoracic aorta. When in the abdomen the symptomatology is similar to rupture of an aortic aneurysm.

When faced with a patient with severe abdominal pain the main decision that must be taken is whether to perform a laparotomy or not. If the patient appears to be ill but laparotomy is not indicated then careful assessment of the trend of the patient's condition has to be made. If he becomes worse then laparotomy may have to be performed.

C. Wastell.

ABDOMINAL PAIN (GENERAL)

(*See also* ABDOMINAL PAIN, ACUTE, LOCALIZED, p. 4.)

Most abdominal pain is localized, for example, that due to a renal stone or biliary stone, acute appendicitis, peptic ulceration, and so on. There are, however, a number of causes of generalized abdominal pain, the commonest of which is peritonitis.

Acute General Peritonitis. Peritonitis must be secondary to some lesion which enables some clue in the history to suggest the initiating disease. Thus the patient with established peritonitis may give a history of onset which indicates acute appendicitis or salpingitis as the source of origin. Where the onset of peritonitis is sudden, one should suspect an acute perforation of a hollow viscus. The early features depend on the severity and the extent of the peritonitis. Pain is always severe and typically the patient lies still on its account, in contrast with the restlessness of a patient with abdominal colic. An extensive peritonitis which involves the abdominal aspect of the diaphragm may be accompanied by shoulder-tip pain. Vomiting often occurs early in the course of the disease. The patient is obviously ill and the temperature frequently elevated. If initially the peritoneal exudate is not purulent, the temperature may be normal. It is a good aphorism concerning the two common causes of this condition that peritonitis due to appendicitis is usually accompanied by a temperature above 100° F. (38° C.), whereas the temperature in peritonitis due to a perforation of a peptic ulcer seldom reaches this level. The pulse is often raised and tends to increase from hour to hour. Examination of the abdomen demonstrates tenderness, which may be localized to the affected area or is generalized if the peritoneal cavity is extensively involved. There is marked guarding, which again may be localized or generalized, and rebound tenderness is present. The abdomen is silent on auscultation, although sometimes the transmitted sounds of the heart-beat and respiration may be detected. Rectally, there is tenderness of the pelvic peritoneum. As the disease progresses, the abdomen becomes distended, signs of free fluid may be detected, the pulse becomes more rapid and feeble. Vomiting is now effortless and faeculent, and the patient, still conscious and mentally alert, demonstrates the Hippocratic facies with sunken eyes, pale, cold, and sweating skin, and cyanosis of the extremities.

X-ray of the abdomen in the erect position may reveal free subdiaphragmatic gas in peritonitis due to hollow viscus perforation (e.g., perforated peptic ulcer), but its absence by no means excludes the diagnosis.

The main differential diagnoses are the colics of intestinal obstruction or of ureteric or biliary stone. Intraperitoneal haemorrhage, acute pancreatitis, dissection or leakage of an aortic aneurysm, or a basal pneumonia are also important differential diagnoses.

Tuberculous Peritonitis. In Great Britain this is now a rare disease. Usually there is a feeling of heaviness rather than acute pain. The onset of symptoms is gradual, with abdominal distension, the presence of fluid within the peritoneal cavity, and often the presence of a puckered, thickened omentum, which forms a tumour lying transversely across the middle of the abdomen.

Intestinal Colic. (*See* ABDOMINAL PAIN.)

Intestinal Obstruction. This is a common cause of generalized abdominal pain. In peritonitis there is no periodic rhythm, whereas waves of pain interspersed with periods of complete relief or only a dull ache are typical of obstruction. In contrast to the patients with peritonitis who wish to remain completely still, the victim of intestinal obstruction is restless and rolls about with the spasms of the colic. Usually there are the accompaniments of progressive abdominal distension, absolute constipation, progressive vomiting, which becomes faeculent, and the presence of noisy bowel sounds on auscultation. X-rays of the abdomen almost invariably reveal multiple fluid levels on the erect film together with distended loops of gas-filled bowel which are obvious on the supine radiograph.

Lead Colic may cause extremely severe attacks of general abdominal pain. There may be preceding anorexia, constipation, and vague abdominal discomfort. The severe pain is usually situated in the lower abdomen radiating to both groins and may sometimes be associated with wrist-drop (due to peripheral neuritis) and occasionally with lead encephalopathy. There may be a blue 'lead line' on the gums if oral sepsis is present, due to the precipitation of lead sulphide. Frequently there is a normocytic hypochromic anaemia with stippling of the red cells (punctate basophilia). Inquiry about the patient's occupation may well be the first clue to the diagnosis. Other signs of lead poisoning are considered on p. 169.

Gastric Crises may cause general abdominal pain. The patient has other evidence of tabes dorsalis, with Argyll Robertson pupils, optic atrophy and ptosis, loss of deep sensation (absence of pain on testicular compression or squeezing the tendo Achillis), and loss of ankle- and knee-jerks. The pain is severe and lasts for many hours or even days. There may be accompanying vomiting and there may also be rigidity of the abdominal wall. The visceral crisis may be the sole manifestation of tabes. The mere fact that a patient has tabes dorsalis does not, of course, mean that his abdominal pain must necessarily be a gastric crisis. The author has repaired a perforated duodenal ulcer in a patient with all the classic features of well-documented tabes dorsalis.

Abdominal Angina occurs in elderly patients as a result of progressive atheromatous narrowing of the superior mesenteric artery. Colicky attacks of central abdominal pain occur after meals and this is followed by diarrhoea. Complete occlusion with infarction of the intestine is often preceded by attacks of this nature.

Functional Abdominal Pain. One of the most difficult problems is the patient, female more often than male, who presents with severe chronic generalized abdominal pains in whom all clinical, laboratory and radiological tests are negative. Inquiry will often reveal features of depression or the presence of some precipitating factor producing an anxiety state. In some cases the abdomen is covered with scars of previous laparotomies at which various organs have been reposited, non-essential viscera removed, and real or imaginary adhesions divided. Some of these patients prove to be drug addicts, others are frank hysterics, others seek the security of the hospital environment, but in still others the aetiology remains mysterious. This forms one type of the so-called 'Munchausen syndrome', described by the late Dr. Richard Asher.

Abdominal Pains in General Disease. Acute abdominal pain may occur in a number of medical conditions not already considered. These include sudden and severe pain complicating malignant malaria, familial Mediterranean fever, and cholera, or may accompany uncontrolled diabetes with ketosis, that rare condition porphyria (*see* p. 807), and any of the blood dyscrasias; the best example is Henoch's purpura in children. Bouts of abdominal pain may occur in the hypercalcaemia of hyperparathyroidism.

Harold Ellis.

ABDOMINAL SWELLING

This may be acute or chronic, general or local, and caused by abdominal accumulations that are either gaseous, liquid, or solid. They may arise in the abdominal cavity itself or in the abdominal wall.

I. SWELLINGS IN THE ABDOMINAL WALL

Swellings situated in the abdominal wall itself can be recognized by their superficial position, by their adherence to the skin, subcutaneous fascia or muscles, or by their failure to follow the movements of the viscera immediately underlying the abdominal wall (*Fig.* 1). It may be impossible to differentiate, for obvious reasons, an intra-abdominal mass that has become attached to the

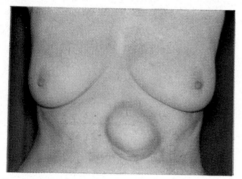

Fig. 1. Large subcutaneous lipoma in the epigastrium. This moved freely on the abdominal wall even when the underlying muscles were tightly contracted.

abdominal parietes either as an inflammatory or malignant process. A simple test which should be applied to all abdominal masses is to ask the patient to raise either his legs or shoulders from the couch. This procedure tightens the abdominal muscles; if the lump is intraperitoneal it disappears, but if it is situated in the abdominal wall itself it persists.

Inflammatory swelling of the abdominal wall most commonly complicates a laparotomy incision and the diagnosis is obvious. A superficial cellulitis may complicate infection of a small abrasion or hair-follicle infection. Inflammation of the abdominal wall may be secondary to an extension of an intraperitoneal abscess, particularly an appendix abscess in the right iliac fossa or, on the left side, a paracolic abscess in relation to diverticular disease of the sigmoid colon or to perforation of a carcinoma of the large bowel.

Inflammatory swelling of the umbilicus in newborn infants is rare except in primitive communities where the cord is not divided with the niceties of modern aseptic practice. Suppuration at the umbilicus in adults is not uncommon if the navel is deep and narrow.

A tender haematoma in the lower abdomen may result from rupture of the rectus abdominis muscle or tearing of the inferior epigastric artery which may occur as the result of a violent cough.

Tumours of the abdominal wall are usually subcutaneous lipomas. These may be multiple and may be a feature of Dercum's disease (adiposis dolorosa). Lipomas should be carefully differentiated from irreducible umbilical or epigastric herniae containing omentum.

A desmoid tumour may arise in the lower part of the abdominal wall and occasionally malignant fibrosarcomas or melanomas may be encountered. A neoplastic deposit may occasionally be palpated at the umbilicus and represents a transcoelomic seeding, usually from a carcinoma of the stomach or large bowel.

II. GENERAL ABDOMINAL SWELLINGS

Every medical student knows the mnemonic of the five causes of gross generalized swelling of the abdomen: Fat, Fluid, Flatus, Faeces, and Foetus.

In *obesity* the abdomen may swell either in consequence of the deposit of fat in the abdominal wall itself or as the result of adipose tissue in the mesentery, the omentum, and in the extraperitoneal layer. In very obese persons it is rarely possible to diagnose the exact nature of an intra-abdominal mass by the usual clinical methods. Indeed, tumours of quite remarkable size, including the full-term foetus, may remain occult to even the most careful examiner.

Distension of the intestines with gas occurs in *intestinal obstruction* and is particularly marked in cases of volvulus of the sigmoid colon, chronic large bowel obstruction, and megacolon. It also occurs in paralytic ileus and its diagnosis is discussed under METEORISM (p. 529). The whole of the abdomen, or, in special cases, some part of it, is distended and gives on percussion a highly resonant or tympanitic note. The outlines of the gas-distended viscera are often visible; loops of dilated small bowel, one above the other, may produce a characteristic 'ladder pattern'. The increased size of the inflated intestine may produce displacement of the other viscera; the dome of the diaphragm is pushed up into the chest, shifting the apex beat of the heart upwards. The liver is similarly displaced. The distended *stomach* may occasionally be gross enough all but to fill the abdomen in very advanced cases of pyloric stenosis and in acute gastric dilatation.

The diagnosis of the various causes producing an accumulation of liquid in the peritoneal cavity is given under the heading of ASCITES (p. 75).

In severe cases of *chronic constipation*, abdominal distension may result from accumulation of faeces in the large intestine, particularly where megacolon exists. The scybala may be felt, usually soft and plastic in the region of the ascending colon, and hard and nodular in the descending and sigmoid colon. Rectal examination often reveals an enormous accumulation of faeces. In some cases of tuberculous peritonitis, semisolid inflammatory masses may bring about a general swelling of the abdomen. The diagnosis is discussed under ASCITES (p. 75). General swelling of the abdomen may occur in *malignant*

1*

disease involving the peritoneum due to the growth of numerous secondary nodules in addition to a concomitant ascites. *Pseudomyxoma peritonei* may follow rupture of a pseudomucinous cystadenoma of the ovary or of a mucocele of the appendix. The whole abdominal cavity becomes distended with gelatinous material.

III. LOCAL INTRA-ABDOMINAL SWELLINGS

These may be due to some general cause or to a mass arising in a specific viscus.

1. Due to General Causes. Causes which ordinarily produce general swelling of the abdomen may sometimes give rise to only a local swelling. Thus with *encysted ascites* left after an acute diffuse peritonitis or accompanying tuberculous peritonitis, an accumulation of fluid

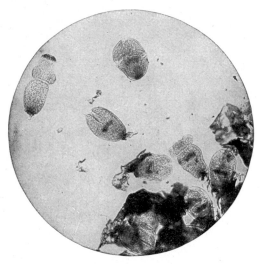

Fig. 2. Scolices of *Taenia echinococcus* in fluid from a hydatid cyst. In some, the hooklets are seen as a ring on the free extremity; in others the ring is invaginated. (× 30.)

bounded by adhesions between the adjacent viscera may be found in any part of the peritoneal cavity, most often in the flanks or pelvis. A reliable history may be a clue to the nature of such a mass although its cause may not be revealed until a laparotomy has been performed.

Abdominal swellings may occur in *tuberculous peritonitis* resulting from the rolled-up matted and infiltrated omentum, doughy masses of adherent intestine, or enlarged tuberculous mesenteric lymph-nodes. The amount of ascites in such cases varies considerably from a gross degree to almost complete absence (the obliterative form). Discovery of a tuberculous focus elsewhere in the body is support for the diagnosis.

Hydatid cysts may occur in any part of the abdominal cavity. They are usually single. The liver, particularly the right lobe, is the most common situation; more rarely the spleen, omentum, mesentery, or peritoneum. The cyst grows slowly and is spherical except in so far as it

is moulded by the pressure of adjacent structures. It contains a clear fluid in which may be found hooklets, scolices (*Figs.* 2, 3), and secondary or daughter cysts detached from the walls of the parent cyst. Unless large enough to cause mechanical pressure, the single hydatid cyst gives rise to little pain or indeed to any complaint of any kind. It may produce a smooth, rounded, tense bulging of the overlying abdominal wall, it is dull on percussion, and it may yield a 'hydatid thrill' as may any other cyst; this thrill is the vibratory sensation experienced by the rest of the hand when, with the whole hand laid flat over the tumour, a central finger is percussed. Occasionally there may be pain and fever due to inflammation within these cysts, and rupture into the peritoneal cavity may cause a severe anaphylactic reaction. Rupture of a hydatid cyst of the liver into a bile-duct may cause jaundice due to biliary

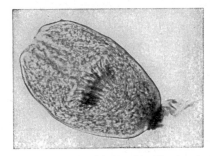

Fig. 3. A single scolex with ring of hooklets invaginated. (× 120.)

Figs. 2 and 3 from photographs by Sir William Lister from a specimen belonging to Dr. Louis Werner, of Dublin.)

obstruction by daughter cysts. Hydatid disease is rare except in countries where the inhabitants live in close association with dogs that are the hosts of *Taenia echinococcus* (Australasia, South America, Greece, Cyprus, and, in the British Isles, North Wales). About one-quarter of patients demonstrate eosinophilia and about half show a positive Casoni test, a weal and flare of over 2 cm. diameter appearing within half an hour of an intradermal injection of hydatid fluid. A complement fixation test gives a higher degree of accuracy but it is not always positive. X-rays of the abdomen may reveal calcification of the cyst wall in long-standing cases.

Any part of the abdomen may swell from the formation of *an abscess*. A subphrenic abscess following a general peritonitis is occasionally large enough to produce an upper abdominal swelling. The patient is usually seriously ill with a swinging fever, rapid pulse, leucocytosis, and all the general manifestations of toxaemia. However, in this antibiotic era, more and more examples are being seen of a more insidious and chronic progress of the disease, with onset delayed weeks or even many months after the initial peritoneal infection. X-ray examination together with screening of the diaphragms is extremely useful and at least 90 per cent of patients with subphrenic infection have some abnormality on this investigation. On the affected side the diaphragm is raised and its sharp definition is lost. Its mobility on screening is diminished or absent. There is frequently a pleural effusion, collapse of the lung base, or evidence of pneumonitis. About 25 per cent of patients have gas below the diaphragm, frequently associated with a fluid level. This gas is usually derived from a perforated abdominal viscus but occasionally is formed by gas-producing organisms. On the left side, gas under the diaphragm may be confused with the gastric bubble. An important differential feature is that the gas shadow of the stomach rarely reaches the lateral abdominal wall, but if there is doubt, a mouthful of barium is given in order to demarcate the stomach.

Pus may localize in either the right or left paracolic gutter or iliac fossa. On the right side this commonly follows a ruptured appendix or occasionally a perforated duodenal ulcer. On the left, a perforation of an inflamed diverticulum or carcinoma of the sigmoid colon is the usual cause. A large pelvic abscess frequently extends above the pubis or into one or other iliac fossa from the pelvis and can be palpated abdominally as well as on pelvic or rectal examination. About

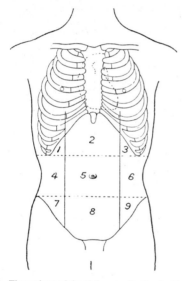

Fig. 4. The regions of the abdomen; for the significance of the numerals, see the adjoining table.

75 per cent result from gangrenous appendicitis and the rest follow gynaecological infections, pelvic surgery, or any general peritonitis.

2. The Regional Diagnosis of Local Abdominal Swellings. For clinical purposes the abdomen may be subdivided into nine regions by two vertical lines drawn upwards from the mid-inguinal point midway between the anterior superior iliac spine and the symphysis pubis, and by two horizontal lines, the upper one passing through the lowest points of the tenth ribs (the subcostal

line), the other drawn at the highest points of the iliac crests. (*Fig.* 4.)

The three median areas thus mapped out are named, from above downwards, the epigastric, umbilical, and hypogastric (or suprapubic) regions; the six lateral areas are, from above downwards, the right and left hypochondriac, lumbar, and iliac regions.

The viscera, or portions of viscera, commonly situated in the areas thus demarcated are given in the accompanying table.

THE NORMAL CONTENTS OF THE ABDOMINAL REGIONS

1. Right Hypochondriac	2. Epigastric
Liver Gall-bladder Hepatic flexure of colon Right kidney Right suprarenal gland	Liver Stomach and pylorus Transverse colon Omentum Pancreas Duodenum Kidneys Suprarenal glands Aorta Lymph-nodes
3. Left Hypochondriac	**4. Right Lumbar**
Liver Stomach Splenic flexure of colon Spleen Tail of pancreas Left kidney Left suprarenal gland	Riedel's lobe of the liver Ascending colon Small intestine Right kidney
5. Umbilical	**6. Left Lumbar**
Stomach Duodenum Transverse colon Omentum Urachus Small intestine Kidneys Aorta Lymph-nodes	Descending colon Small intestine Left kidney
7. Right Iliac Fossa	**8. Hypogastric**
Caecum Vermiform appendix Lymph-nodes	Small intestine Sigmoid flexure Distended bladder Urachus Enlarged uterus and adnexa
9. Left Iliac Fossa	
Sigmoid flexure Lymph-nodes	

The abdominal swellings that may be felt in and about these nine regions, excluding the tumours situated in the abdominal wall itself that have already been described, are as follows:

A. RIGHT HYPOCHONDRIAC REGION. Most tumours in this area are connected with the liver or gall-bladder and their differential diagnosis is discussed under LIVER, ENLARGEMENT OF (p. 503) and GALL-BLADDER ENLARGEMENT (p. 311).

A mistake easily made is to regard the firm and rounded swelling produced by the upper segment of the right rectus abdominis muscle, especially in a well-developed subject, as a tumour of the liver or gall-bladder.

Tumours in connexion with the hepatic flexure of the colon, scyballous collections in the hepatic flexure region, or the head of an intussusception may present as masses in this area.

B. EPIGASTRIC REGION. Enlargements of the *liver* may be felt in this area, and indeed it is common to feel the normal liver in this region, especially in infants and in adults with an acute costal angle. The dilated *stomach* produced by pyloric stenosis in either children or adults may present as a visible swelling demonstrating waves of peristalsis travelling from left to right. A succussion splash

Swellings in connexion with the *omentum* may be due to tuberculous peritonitis or, more commonly, due to infiltration with secondary malignant deposits.

Swellings arising from the *pancreas* push forward from the depths of the abdominal cavity towards the epigastric and the upper part and umbilical areas, and present themselves as vaguely palpable deeply seated masses. They have the stomach, or the stomach and colon, in front of them and are fixed to the posterior abdominal wall, thus moving but little on respiration. They may transmit a non-expansile pulsation from the subjacent aorta. Unless extremely large such swellings are resonant on percussion, due to the overlying air-filled gut. A pancreatic swelling may be carcinomatous, in which case wasting, anaemia, and jaundice are likely to be observed. There may be clay-coloured stools and dark urine and it is important to note that frequently the onset of jaundice is preceded by deeply placed abdominal pain, or pain in the back. Glycosuria of recent origin in an elderly patient also raises suspicion of a pancreatic carcinoma. In about half the patients with jaundice due to carcinomatous obstruction the gall-bladder is palpably

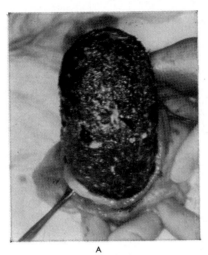

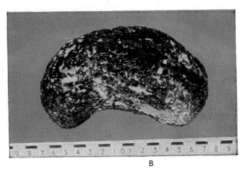

Fig. 5. Gastric hairball. This formed a large, mobile epigastric mass in a young married woman with long hair. A, shows the mass being removed at gastrotomy. B, Demonstrates the specimen.

is usually elicited. Tumours of the stomach, apart from malignant growth, are rare. At the turn of this century a hair ball or trichobezoar was frequently encountered as an epigastric mass in hysterical girls who chewed and swallowed their hair, which then formed an exact mould of the stomach. Hairballs are only rarely encountered in these days and modern textbooks hardly mention them; however, as fashions and hair styles change they may reappear on the clinical scene. (*Fig.* 5). Other foreign bodies are sometimes ingested by mental defectives and form a palpable mass. In congenital pyloric stenosis a tumour the size of a small marble is palpable at the right border of the right rectus.

The *transverse colon* usually passes across the upper part of the umbilical area and may be palpated when it is the site of a carcinoma, when it is impacted with faeces, or when it is distended by a large-bowel obstruction placed distal to it.

distended (Courvoisier's law). Occasionally the mass may result from chronic pancreatitis; the swollen pancreas of acute pancreatitis has only exceptionally been palpated before laparotomy.

Pancreatic cysts are the pancreatic swellings which are most commonly palpable. Only 20 per cent are true cysts; these are either single or multiple retention cysts which usually result from chronic pancreatitis, neoplastic cysts (cystadenoma and cystadenocarcinoma), and the rare congenital polycystic disease of the pancreas and hydatid cyst of the pancreas. Far more often the cysts are not in the pancreas itself but comprise a collection of fluid sealed off in the lesser sac due to closure of the foramen of Winslow (pseudocyst of the pancreas). This may occur after trauma to the pancreas, following acute pancreatitis, or, less commonly, resulting from perforation of a posterior gastric ulcer. They may reach an enormous size and fill the whole upper part of the abdomen.

Retroperitoneal cysts are rare. The majority arise from remnants of the mesonephric (Wolffian) duct and occur in adult women. Others are teratomatous, lymphangiomatous, or dermoids.

Retroperitoneal tumours (apart from those arising in the pancreas, suprarenal, or kidney) originate in the mesenchymal tissues, the sympathetic nerves, and the para-aortic lymph-nodes.

Swellings in connexion with the *duodenum* are excessively rare. They may result from an inflammatory mass developing around a penetrating duodenal ulcer or be due to a duodenal malignant tumour, but the latter is a pathological curiosity. Those in connexion with the *kidneys* and *suprarenal glands* are found in the epigastrium only if very large. Their diagnosis is considered below.

Enlargement of the *spleen* may bring its notched anterior edge into the epigastric area; a splenic swelling always lies in contact with the anterior wall of the abdomen (*see* SPLEEN, ENLARGEMENT OF, p. 746).

Lymph-nodes, which are numerous in the para-aortic retroperitoneal tissues and in the mesentery, may become palpable in reticuloses, tuberculous peritonitis, or malignant disease as nodulated chains or masses.

C. LEFT HYPOCHONDRIAC REGION. An abnormal lobe or a tumour in the left lobe of the *liver* may appear as a superficial tumour in this area.

Much of the *stomach* normally lies in the left hypochondrium; the diagnosis of gastric swelling has been considered above and a gastric tumour is commonly felt in this region. On physical signs alone it must be differentiated from a swelling of the adjoining *spleen*. A barium-meal X-ray examination helps considerably in differentiating between a gastric and a splenic swelling.

The diagnosis of a tumour of the splenic flexure of the *colon*, whether scybalous or malignant, is arrived at in the same way as a case of a tumour of the hepatic flexure or transverse colon (*see* (A) and (B)).

The diagnosis of the various causes of enlargement of the *spleen* is discussed under SPLEEN, ENLARGEMENT OF (p. 746). The distinguishing features are that it comes down from under the left costal margin in direct contact with the anterior abdominal wall (and is therefore dull on percussion), descends on inspiration, has a smooth surface, and a notch may be palpable on its inner margin. A splenic swelling may be identified on a plain X-ray of the abdomen and differentiated from a renal mass by means of pyelography. A barium-meal examination may show displacement and indentation of the adjacent stomach.

Tumours of the *pancreas* may project into the left hypochondrium as may retroperitoneal tumours and cysts (*see* (B)).

Tumours of the left *kidney* and *suprarenal gland* have the stomach and colon in front of them and therefore, unless extremely large, are resonant on percussion. Since they arise in the loin, these masses can usually be balloted by bimanual palpation.

D. RIGHT LUMBAR REGION. Occasionally a congenital projection of the *liver*, known as Riedel's lobe, may appear as a superficial tumour continuous with the liver above it in this zone. It may be mistaken for a dilated gall-bladder.

The *ascending colon* may be palpable due to contained faecal masses, owing to thickening as a result of long-standing colitis, Crohn's disease, or hyperplastic tuberculosis, or due to malignant disease.

The ascending colon can be felt in acute or chronic *ileocaecal and ileocolic intussusception* as a sausage-shaped tumour, at first situated in the right flank, then moving across the abdomen above the umbilicus and finally down the left flank into the pelvis. The vast majority of these cases occur in infants or young children commonly aged between 3 and 12 months. Boys are affected twice as often as girls. The history is of paroxysms of abdominal colic typified by screaming and pallor. There is vomiting and usually the passage of blood and mucus per rectum, giving the characteristic 'red-currant-jelly stool'. Rectal examination nearly always reveals this typical feature and rarely the tip of the intussusception can be felt. In infants there is usually no obvious cause, but the mesenteric lymph-nodes in these cases are invariably enlarged. In adults a polyp, carcinoma, or an inverted Meckel's diverticulum may form the apex of the intussusception.

Tumours in connexion with the *right kidney* and *suprarenal gland* usually appear deep down in this region, having the ascending colon and small intestine in front of them. They can be lifted forwards *en masse* from behind by a hand placed at the back of the loin and thus palpated bimanually. For their diagnosis *see* KIDNEY, ENLARGEMENT OF (p. 470). The lower pole of the right kidney can be felt in many normal persons on deep abdominal palpation, especially in thin females. When abnormally low and mobile, the whole of the otherwise normal kidney may be palpable. Its shape and consistency are characteristic. Renal swellings move on respiration and, unless very large, are resonant on percussion due to the anteriorly related gut. However, Riedel's lobe of the liver, an enlarged gall-bladder, masses in the ascending colon, and secondary deposits in the omentum have all been mistaken for it, although they are all more superficially placed and lie in contact with the anterior abdominal wall. Other wandering masses, e.g., those arising from the ovary, Fallopian tube, and mesentery, as well as hydatid cysts, are all liable to the same error of identification.

E. THE UMBILICAL REGION. The grossly dilated *stomach* resulting from long-standing pyloric obstruction may occupy the umbilical region; indeed it may descend below it down into the pelvis.

Tumours in connexion with the *transverse colon* have been considered in (B) and (D) above.

Tumours in connexion with the *omentum* are common in this region; those arising from the *small intestine* are much rarer, although the thickened small bowel in Crohn's disease may form a palpable mass.

Swellings arising from the *kidneys, suprarenals, pancreas, retroperitoneal tissues, para-aortic glands*, and *mesentery* may all present themselves in the deeper parts of the umbilical region, usually as more or less fixed masses arising from or connected with the posterior wall of the abdomen.

The *aorta* bifurcates half an inch below and to the left of the umbilicus (at the level of the 4th lumbar vertebra). In thin patients, pulsation of the aorta can often be felt and indeed seen in this region and may lead to the incorrect diagnosis of an abdominal aneurysm. Careful examination, however, will show that this pulsation is no more than a throbbing, an up-and-down movement, and is not laterally expansile. Aneurysm of the abdominal aorta forms an expansile mass situated above the umbilicus itself and may be accompanied by pain in the back from erosion of the bodies of the lumbar vertebrae. Often X-rays of the abdomen in such cases will reveal calcification in the aneurysmal wall.

F. LEFT LUMBAR REGION. An enlarged *spleen* (*see* (C)) may protrude into this area. It forms a firm mass in contact with the abdominal wall and its dullness to percussion continues with its thoracic dullness which extends back up into the axilla along the line of the 9th or 10th ribs. Tumours in connexion with the *right kidney*, the *right suprarenal gland*, and the *descending colon* give similar features to those considered in (C) above.

G. RIGHT ILIAC FOSSA. An inflammatory mass in this region is most commonly associated with an *appendix abscess*. Less commonly there may be a *paracaecal abscess* in relation to a perforated carcinoma of the caecum or a solitary caecal benign ulcer. A *pyosalpinx* may result from salpingitis and, rarely, inflammatory swellings may arise in connexion with suppurating *iliac lymph-nodes* or a *psoas abscess*.

An important differential diagnosis is between an appendix mass and a carcinoma of the caecum. Usually in the former there is a preceding episode of an acute abdominal pain, typical of appendicitis, with fever and leucocytosis. The inflammatory mass subsides progressively over two or three weeks and the occult blood-test in the stools is negative. A carcinoma of the caecum may be suspected if there is a preceding history of bowel disturbance in a middle-aged or elderly patient, if the mass fails to resolve rapidly, and if the occult blood-test in the stools is repeatedly positive. If there is any clinical doubt, a barium-enema X-ray examination should be carried out and, if necessary, resort made to laparotomy.

It is not at all rare for a soft 'squelchy' caecum to be palpable in a perfectly normal thin, usually female, subject.

Occasionally a grossly distended *gall-bladder* may project down as far as the right iliac fossa and a low-lying *kidney* may form a palpable mass in this region. An *ovarian* tumour or cyst or a pedunculated *fibroid* of the uterus may project into this area.

H. HYPOGASTRIC REGION. The commonest mass to be felt in this region is the distended *bladder*. This may reach as high as, or slightly above, the umbilicus. Not uncommonly this midline structure tilts over to one or other side. A distended bladder has been tapped as ascites, operated upon as an ovarian cyst or fibroid, or mistaken for the pregnant uterus. No diagnostic opinion should be advanced, and no operative procedure undertaken respecting a tumour in this situation, until the bladder has been emptied, either by voluntary micturition or by the passing of a catheter.

Abdominal swellings arising from the *uterus, ovaries, Fallopian tubes*, and *uterine ligaments* may all rise up out of the pelvis and present themselves as swellings in this region; as they grow larger they may be spread into any part of the abdomen. While they remain comparatively small and are manifestedly connected with some intrapelvic organ, their origin is not difficult to determine (*see* PELVIC SWELLING, p. 626). However, when they have extended into the abdomen or have acquired a long pedicle, or have become fixed by adhesions to some distant part of the abdominal wall or to some other viscus, these pelvic tumours may give rise to signs and symptoms which bear no relation to pelvic disease. In such cases they may only be correctly diagnosed at laparotomy. The discerning clinician will always remember the possibility of pregnancy in every female patient between the menarche and menopause.

Tumours of ileal Crohn's disease arising in the *small intestine* may be felt in the hypogastric area.

The *urachus* is a fibrous cord running in the middle line in front of the peritoneum from the fundus of the bladder to the umbilicus. Occasionally it becomes the seat of cyst formation, more often in women than in men. The urachal cyst is a rounded tumour lying between the umbilicus and the pubic symphysis, which occasionally becomes infected.

I. LEFT ILIAC FOSSA. The *pelvic colon* can often be felt in normal subjects as a tube-like cord either when empty and in spasm or else when distended with faecal masses. This region is a common site for carcinoma of the colon and there are usually symptoms of chronic intestinal obstruction, or bowel disturbance with the passage of blood and mucus in the stools. It is clinically impossible to differentiate between such a mass and that associated with diverticular disease of the sigmoid colon. Similarly a para-colic abscess in this region may equally well be associated with suppuration of an inflamed colonic diverticulum or a perforating carcinoma. Rarely such an abscess may be due to perforation of the tip of a long *appendix* passing over the left iliac fossa, or as an extreme rarity due to local perforation of a left-sided appendix in transposition of the viscera. The diagnosis would be suggested by finding the cardiac apex beat to lie on the *right* side.   *Harold Ellis.*

ACROPARAESTHESIAE

Acroparaesthesiae is the name given to un-comfortable tingling in the extremities. At one time the term implied that there were no signs of nervous or vascular disease but identical symptoms may occur in early polyneuritis or subacute combined degeneration of the cord. Cervical ribs or fibrous bands may also give rise to peripheral tingling by compressing the neurovascular bundle behind the clavicle. Another form, also confined to the hands, occurs predominantly in women and is due to compression of the median nerve in the carpal tunnel (p. 595). In this syndrome the little finger may also be involved in the tingling.

Ian Mackenzie.

ALOPECIA

There are many causes of alopecia or baldness and the extent may range from a few isolated patches in the scalp to universal loss of hair from the whole body. Classification may be based on the extent of hair loss and the presence or absence of scarring; there is, however, inevitably some overlap in the groups.

1. Patchy Hairfall without Scarring:
   a. Alopecia areata.
   b. Ringworm (common types).
   c. Secondary to trauma:
      Hair dressing.
      Marginal alopecia.
      Use of curlers.
      Trichotillomania.
      Rubbing of the scalp in infancy.
   d. Secondary syphilis.

2. Patchy Hairfall with Scarring:
   a. Ringworm (less common types).
   b. Folliculitis decalvans.
   c. Pseudo-pelade (lichen planus).
   d. Secondary to other skin diseases:
      Lupus vulgaris.
      Lupus erythematosus, systemic and discoid.
      Localized scleroderma, especially *coup de sabre* type.

3. Diffuse Hairfall without Scarring:
   a. Male pattern alopecia.
   b. Diffuse hairfall of young women.
   c. Senile alopecia.
   d. Ectodermal defects.
   e. Pili torti.
   f. Monilethrix.
   g. Alopecia totalis and universalis (variants of alopecia areata).
   h. Secondary to infection.
   i. Endocrine causes.
   j. Drugs and ionizing radiation.
   k. Systemic lupus erythematosus.

4. Diffuse Hairfall with Scarring:
   X-ray atrophy.

1. Patchy Hairfall without Scarring. *Alopecia areata* (*Fig.* 6) is a common condition of unknown aetiology; familial cases occur occasionally. Although some cases seem to be related to anxiety or recent shock, in the great majority of cases no such cause can be incriminated. It may be considered among the auto-immune diseases of organ-specific type. The incidence of thyroid disorders and of vitiligo in patients with alopecia areata is significantly greater than in control subjects. It may start in childhood or at any later period of life, and shows a marked tendency to recurrence. It shows up by the presence of completely bald patches without scales but with short stumpy hairs most often found around the edge of the patch; these are known as 'exclamation mark' (!) hairs because they are thinner near the scalp than distally. Their presence indicates that the condition is still active as also does the presence of loose hairs around the patch. The condition may be limited to one or two patches in the scalp, or it may extend to the beard, eyebrows and eyelashes, or to all hairs on the body. Except in very long-standing cases the hair follicles are present and in most cases the hair regrows satisfactorily, starting in the centre of the patch and progressing to the periphery. Additional areas may form whilst the first patches are clearing so that complete resolution is unlikely to occur in less than six months. Often the early hairs to return are white but the natural colour soon returns in most cases, although occasionally permanent white patches remain. When the beard is involved complete resolution is much less likely and universal alopecia is often permanent. The most important differential diagnosis is from ringworm and pseudo-pelade. Alopecia areata is common in mongols, and it may also be part of the Voigt-Koyanagi syndrome, a rare disorder, other features being uveitis, deafness, leuchotrichia (especially white eyelashes), and patches of vitiligo.

Ringworm. The common types of ringworm of the scalp due to microsporon infections produce patches on the scalp which are not completely bald but are covered with short, broken-off, lifeless hairs and the areas are covered with scales (*Fig.* 7). Diagnosis is confirmed by finding fungal spores and hyphae in the affected hairs or scales. The affected hair fluoresces a green colour under filtered ultra-violet light (Wood's light). The hair regrows when the infection comes under control. These cases are almost confined to childhood.

Trauma as a Cause of Patchy Hairfall. As a result of overheating or the use of too strong chemicals during permanent waving the hair may become brittle and break off. In Negresses a similar effect is produced by attempts at straightening the hair. These cases may involve a few small patches or the whole scalp and the diagnosis is readily confirmed from the history. Regrowth is usually complete.

Marginal Alopecia. This is a form of baldness affecting the margins of the scalp as the result of continual traction in certain types of hair fashion, e.g., the ponytail. There may be some inflammation of the follicles and in these cases complete regrowth is unlikely, although scarring if it occurs is minimal. Diagnosis is from alopecia areata affecting the scalp margin, a not un-common occurrence.

The use of curlers in hairdressing may be responsible for patches of baldness over the vertex of the scalp exactly corresponding to areas where pressure is exerted by the curlers. In the early stages the process is reversible, but after a time there may be some scarring and the condition will then become permanent. A very similar condition is seen in Negro children as a result of tight curling practised in some communities.

Trichotillomania: This is a condition most often occurring in children, usually highly neurotic children. The hair is pulled out by the individual and this gives a rather bizarre appearance of hairs broken off at various levels. It is usually

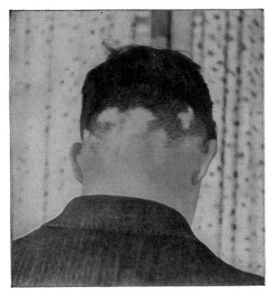

Fig. 6. Alopecia areata.

easily diagnosed and can be confirmed by the parent observing the child carefully, especially during periods of stress.

Rubbing the scalp on the pillow will very often produce patches of alopecia of the fine hair on the scalps of infants. The hair regrows when it becomes stronger or when the habit ceases.

Secondary Syphilis is a rare cause of alopecia. The baldness is never complete and the patches are often described as of moth-eaten appearance because of their irregular shape and variations in length of the hairs over the patch. Regrowth is complete in most cases when the disease comes under control.

2. Patchy Hairfall with Scarring. The rarer forms of *ringworm* of the scalp, especially those producing kerion formation (usually of animal origin) and also favus (*Fig.* 8), not infrequently result in permanent hairfall with scarring. Although commonest in childhood, these infections may occur in adults. Diagnosis is

confirmed by finding fungus present during the active phase. Several hairs should be examined as only a minority may be infected, although all in the area are loosened.

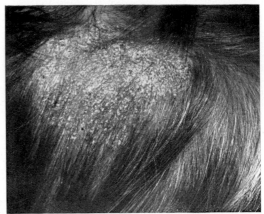

Fig. 7. Tinea capitis. (*St. John's Hospital.*)

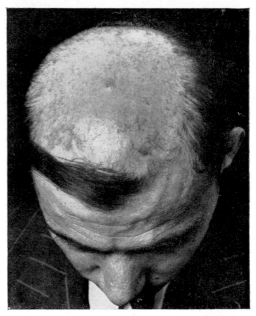

Fig. 8. Scarring of the scalp with consequent baldness as the result of a severe attack of favus when a child. Note atrophy and destruction of the hair follicles. The residual hairs on the affected area are kept clipped for cosmetic reasons. (*Dr. Peter Hansell.*)

Folliculitis Decalvans. There is considerable dispute about this entity, which is now relatively rare. A low-grade chronic infection gives rise to patches of scarring alopecia. The only evidence of active infection is usually at the margin of the patch. It is almost certainly a staphylococcal infection and its decrease in incidence corresponds to the use of antibiotics in treatment. Lupoid sycosis

(*Fig.* 9) is a more active variant of the same condition and usually begins with a chronic sycosis barbae and progresses relentlessly, ultimately producing large areas of baldness in the scalp. Diagnosis is from ringworm and pseudo-pelade.

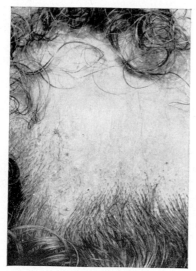

Fig. 9. Lupoid sycosis. (*St. John's Hospital.*)

Pseudo-pelade. Pelade is the French word for alopecia areata, so this represents pseudo-alopecia areata. Quite small patches of complete baldness (*Fig.* 10) appear scattered over the

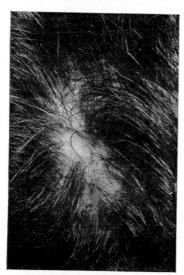

Fig. 10. Pseudo-pelade. (*Dr. Peter Hansell.*)

scalp, with atrophy of the hair follicles. There is usually no preceding evidence of disease of the scalp and no active folliculitis. In many cases, however, there is evidence of lichen planus else-where on the body or a recent history of lichen

planus. It seems probable, therefore, that pseudo-pelade is usually a manifestation of lichen planus, the hair follicles being destroyed by the infiltrate penetrating deeply around them, even though it may produce no overt signs on the surface of the scalp during the period of activity. The condition is usually progressive for a few months or a few years and then becomes static. The hair never regrows. This condition has often been mistaken for folliculitis decalvans, but it seems certain that the two conditions are quite distinct.

Scarring Secondary to Other Skin Diseases. When lupus vulgaris, lupus erythematosus (*Fig.* 11), or localized scleroderma, especially the *coup de sabre* type (*Fig.* 12), occur in the scalp they may all produce permanent alopecia with scarring of the involved areas.

3. Diffuse Hairfall without Scarring. *Male pattern alopecia* is the commonest form of hairfall. Although normally not apparent until middle age, many cases start much earlier and they may be well developed by the late teens. It begins with a recession on both sides of the frontal area and extends to involve the whole of the vertex. In

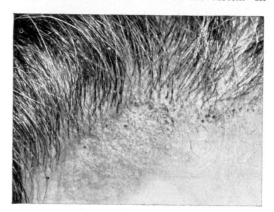

Fig. 11. Edge of a patch of lupus erythematosus affecting the scalp. Note complete atrophy of the scalp towards the centre with scaliness, and horny plugging of the follicles in the active edge. (*Dr. Peter Hansell.*)

the fully developed cases only a fringe of hair remains around the sides and the occiput. The affected area is shiny but the hair follicles are intact. The cause is unknown but there is an undoubted familial tendency to the condition. No treatment is of any value in arresting the progress or of restoring the hair, although many claims of success are made by trichologists. Any improvement which does occur during treatment is the result of discouragement of overactive massage by the patient himself which may at times exaggerate the condition by rubbing off hairs which have not yet fallen. Diagnosis is usually obvious but alopecia areata must be excluded.

Diffuse Hairfall of Young Women. This is a condition which appears to have increased greatly in recent years. Whether this is a real increase or is due to the fact that people are now more conscious of their hair than previously cannot be said with any certainty. The hair is lost over the vertex of the scalp progressively and usually by the time the patient reports almost half of the hair has been lost from the affected area. In a minority of cases there are tiny atrophic patches scattered over the scalp, patches which are much smaller than those in pseudo-pelade. The cause remains obscure but modern hairdressing fashions are sometimes incriminated, including the use of detergent shampoos. The

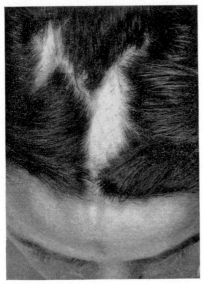

Fig. 12. Scleroderma: *coup-de-sabre*. (*Dr. Peter Hansell*.)

prognosis is usually poor but some hair may regrow. A diffuse form of alopecia areata and hairfall following pregnancy may produce the same appearance but the hair will regrow in these cases. In *telogen effusion* many hairs enter the resting phase at the same time and are shed some 3 months later. This may be due to physical or psychological factors. The hair usually regrows satisfactorily.

Senile Alopecia. In both men and women much of the scalp hair is likely to be lost in old age.

Ectodermal Defects. There are a number of congenital abnormalities associated with defects of the nails and diffuse alopecia and in some cases other ectodermal defects including anhidrosis. All are rare.

Pili Torti. This is a rare congenital abnormality in which the hairs are twisted through 180 degrees. The hairs are dull and lustreless and easily broken, giving the appearance of diffuse alopecia. Clinically it is very similar to monilethrix but can be distinguished by microscopic examination of the hairs.

Monilethrix (*Fig.* 13). This is also a rare congenital anomaly in which the hairs show regular periodic constrictions and tend to break at the

constrictions. Both pili torti and monilethrix appear to be primary diseases of the hair follicles, and both are usually inherited as autosomal dominant conditions.

Alopecia Totalis and Universalis. These are variants of alopecia areata, already described.

Secondary to Infection. Any infection accompanied by pyrexia of 103 degrees or over may produce a temporary diffuse hairfall. Typhoid is especially liable to produce this effect.

Endocrine Factors. In myxoedema diffuse alopecia is an important symptom. In addition to the scalp the outer one-third of the eyebrows may be affected. In conditions producing symptoms of Cushing's disease there is often a diffuse alopecia of the scalp accompanied by increased growth of hair in other areas.

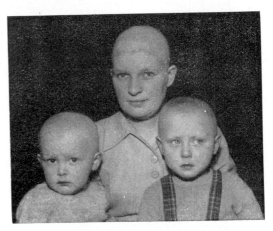

Fig. 13. Monilethrix in a mother and two daughters.

Drugs. Thallium acetate will produce hairfall of a type closely resembling severe male pattern alopecia, the hair on the neck and sides of the scalp being unaffected. At one time thallium was used to induce hairfall for the treatment of tinea capitis. The dosage required was near the limit of tolerance and this treatment has now been abandoned.

Some of the drugs used in the treatment of malignant disease produce extensive alopecia in the dose required for treatment. This is especially true of cyclophosphamide (endoxana). Heparin may also cause alopecia.

Ionizing Radiation. For many years X-ray epilation was the standard treatment for ringworm of the scalp. If the dose is correct (about 400 r) hair falls after about two weeks and starts to regrow 4–6 weeks later. Any dose above 400 r given in a single application will cause hairfall. Permanent loss is likely if the dose is double this figure.

Systemic Lupus Erythematosus. In this condition alopecia is a common and characteristic finding, being circumscribed or patchy, with or without an associated skin lesion. Where discoid lesions are present, alopecia is often also present at the same sites. Alopecia may be diffuse but does not progress to complete baldness and is reversible, though often recovery is very slow.

4. Diffuse Hairfall with Scarring. *X-ray atrophy* (*Fig.* 14) is the only important member of this group. Almost every case is the result of X-rays used in the treatment of ringworm of the scalp in childhood. Doses greatly in excess of the therapeutic level will cause the hair to fall and never regrow. Pigmentation, telangiectasia, scarring, and later keratoses and epitheliomata (basal and squamous) develop insidiously over a period

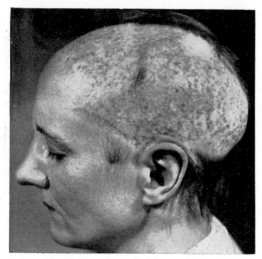

Fig. 14. Destruction of the scalp caused by an overdose of X-rays for the treatment of ringworm when a child. Note atrophy, telangiectasia, and patches of brown pigmentation. (*Dr. Peter Hansell.*)

of many years. A dose of X-ray only slightly excessive will cause the hair to fall and regrowth may be complete, but after a period of years (sometimes over 20 years) the hair falls again and the damage caused by the X-rays becomes visible.

The only treatment for this condition is the supply of wigs to conceal the defect and more radical treatment if malignancy occurs.

P. D. Samman.

AMENORRHOEA

The age at which menstruation first appears is variable, being influenced by climatic and racial peculiarities; in England about thirteen years may be taken as the average. About one girl in a hundred does not menstruate until the age of sixteen years and it is usual to wait until then before becoming concerned. When the menstrual flow has not become established it is usual to speak of primary amenorrhoea, while premature cessation of the flow after it has once been regularly established is known as secondary amenorrhoea. From the table of the causes of

amenorrhoea below it will be seen that some of them must of necessity give rise to the primary variety, while others more commonly produce the secondary. In investigating a case one should ascertain first whether the condition is primary or secondary, and next whether it is real or only apparent. The latter condition, known as *cryptomenorrhoea*, implies that the menstrual flow takes place but is unable to escape externally because there is some closure of a part of the genital canal. The congenital form of cryptomenorrhoea is the only variety met with commonly, acquired closure of a part of the genital canal being very rare. Stenosis of the vagina may result from injury or infection, but a small sinus is usually left which suffices for the escape of the menstrual fluid. We are led to suspect cryptomenorrhoea when the patient volunteers the statement that she has pelvic pain, headache, and possibly vomiting, of monthly occurrence—in fact the usual menstrual symptoms, unaccompanied by any visible flow. Secondary sexual development is normal. A not uncommon deciding symptom is the occurrence of acute retention of urine, the result of elongation and stretching of the urethra by a haematocolpos. A physical examination should be made, including abdominal palpation, inspection of the vulva, and a recto-abdominal bimanual examination. The common form is that in which the lower end of the vagina is imperforate, the hymen usually being visible on the outer side of the occluding membrane through which a dark blue cystic swelling protrudes. The complete examination will reveal a fluctuating swelling reaching from the vulva to the pelvic brim, above which the uterus can often be palpated and moved about. Distension of the vagina or *haematocolpos* is complete in this case, but may be partial where the lower part of the vagina is absent, and then is likely to be accompanied by distension of the uterus (haematometra) and haematosalpinx. It is important to make out whether the uterus and Fallopian tubes are distended with menstrual products along with the distended vagina, for in the presence of haematosalpinges the uterus and tubes may take longer to recover following surgical drainage. Congenital absence of the vagina can only be inferred from local physical examination. Since the vulva is normally formed and a slight depression is present, only a careful examination, if necessary under anaesthesia, will reveal absence of the vagina. Very often the patient only presents at the time of marriage, complaining of dyspareunia. Complete absence of the vagina is nearly always associated with absence also of the uterus which means that amenorrhoea will be permanent and there is no hope of child-bearing.

Acquired cryptomenorrhoea produces the same symptoms and requires the same kind of investigation as the congenital cases. Acquired closure of the vagina following the vaginitis of specific fevers may occur in infancy, and then produces primary amenorrhoea.

Causes of Apparent Amenorrhoea:

CONGENITAL:
  Imperforate vagina
  Imperforate hymen
  Absence of the vagina
  Imperforate cervix
  Double uterus with retention
  Haematocolpos
  Haematometra
  Haematosalpinx.

ACQUIRED:
  Closure of the Vagina:
    Due to specific fevers
    Due to injury
  Closure of the Cervix:
    Due to injury
    Following operations.

Causes of Real Amenorrhoea:

PHYSIOLOGICAL:
  Before puberty
  After the menopause
  During pregnancy
  During lactation.

PATHOLOGICAL:
  Generative System:
    Congenital absence of uterus
    Congenital absence of ovaries (rare)
    Uterine hypoplasia of infantile type
    Uterine hypoplasia of adult type
    Ovarian agenesis
    Gonadal dysgenesis (Turner's syndrome)
    Destruction of both ovaries by double ovarian
      growths, pelvic inflammation, operation,
      irradiation
    Hysterectomy
  Circulatory System:
    Anaemia
    Leukaemia
    Hodgkin's disease
  Wasting Diseases:
    Malignant growths
    Tubercle
    Prolonged suppuration
    Diabetes
    Late stages of nephritis
    Late stages of some forms of heart disease
    Late stage of cirrhosis of the liver
  Nervous System:
    Imbecility
    Cretinism
    Various forms of insanity
    Cold just before or during menstruation
    Suggestion—fear of pregnancy (pseudocyesis)
    Anorexia nervosa
  Altered Internal Secretions:
    Primary hypothalamic-pituitary failure
    Following oral contraceptives
    Anterior pituitary failure (Simmonds's disease)
    Absence of ovarian hormones
    Certain rare functioning tumours of the ovary:
      arrhenoblastoma; granulosa-cell tumour
    Stein-Leventhal syndrome (polycystic ovary)
    Myxoedema
    Addison's disease
    Thyrotoxicosis
    Adrenal hyperplasia
    Adrenal cortical tumours
    Acromegaly
    Obesity

Dystrophia adiposo-genitalis (Fröhlich's syn-
  drome)
Change of habits and environment causing emo-
  tional strain
Climatic changes
Dietetic deficiencies, the result of attempts to slim
Toxic:
  After specific fevers
  Chronic poisoning by lead, mercury, morphine,
    alcohol.

Real amenorrhoea may be: (1) Primary with delayed onset; (2) Primary and permanent; (3) Secondary. If menstruation has once been established regularly, it is clear that there cannot be any serious congenital anomaly of the generative system; the uterus and ovaries must at least have been present and functioning. We must then make a systematic examination of the generative, circulatory, nervous, and ductless-gland systems, in order to learn by a process of exclusion which group of causes we have to deal with. If, however, the amenorrhoea is primary and real, that is, the patient has no symptoms, our examination must first be directed towards finding out whether the essential organs, namely uterus and ovaries, are present, and are normal in size and shape as far as a bimanual examination can ascertain. If necessary, an anaesthetic may be given for this purpose. In doubtful cases laparoscopy with ovarian biopsy may be helpful.

Certain rare inter-sex cases may present with primary amenorrhoea. They include Turner's syndrome (gonadal dysgenesis) in which there is also dwarfism, web-neck, cubitus valgus, and an XO sex-chromosome pattern; testicular feminization (which is in reality androgen insensitivity) in which the form is female with well-developed breasts but absent or sparse pubic and axillary hair and the gonad, which may be found in the groin or in the abdomen, is a testicle that should be removed because of the risk of malignancy; and ovarian dysgenesis in which there are streak ovaries, an infantile uterus, and absent secondary sexual characteristics. (*Figs.* 15–18.) In these cases a buccal smear for sex chromatin and a chromosome analysis on a sample of peripheral blood are indicated. In ovarian dysgenesis there is a chromatin negative smear but only 45 chromosomes, a single X chromosome (XO); in testicular feminization the smear is also chromatin negative but there are 46 chromosomes, XY. Gonadal biopsy is also helpful in diagnosis. When the secondary sexual development is absent or very poor and there is no chromosome abnormality, further investigation becomes necessary. This includes assay of gonadotrophin and adrenal excretion and of thyroid function.

Apart from congenital anomalies remarkably few lesions of the generative organs produce amenorrhoea; only those diseases which destroy both ovaries completely or render the uterus functionless can cause amenorrhoea, and under this heading we find only bilateral malignant ovarian growths and complete removal of the endometrium by too vigorous curetting. A tumour destroying one ovary has no effect on menstruation, provided the other is present and functioning. The presence of two tumours in the abdomen symmetrically arranged with regard to the uterus will sometimes permit of the diagnosis of double ovarian destruction if there is amenorrhoea in addition, especially in the case of malignant growths, but commonly one tumour is much larger than the other and the double nature of the lesion cannot be established until the abdomen is opened. The common benign tumours, cystic adenomata, even if bilateral, do not destroy the ovarian tissue and consequently do not produce amenorrhoea. On

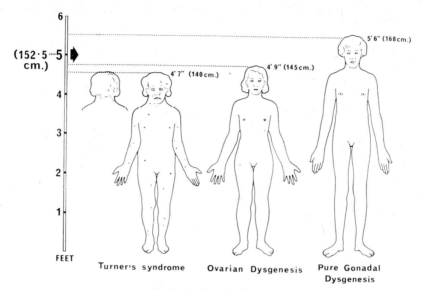

Turner's syndrome   Ovarian Dysgenesis   Pure Gonadal Dysgenesis

Fig. 15. *Professor Paul Polani.*

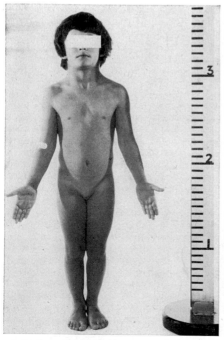

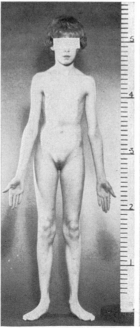

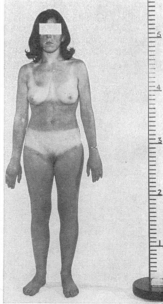

Fig. 16. Turner's syndrome. (*Professor Paul Polani.*)   *Fig.* 17. Pure gonadal dysgenesis. (*Professor Paul Polani.*)   *Fig.* 18. Testicular feminization. (*Professor Paul Polani.*)

rare occasions bilateral fibromata of the ovaries may destroy all ovarian tissue and therefore be the cause of amenorrhoea.

In the absence of the above-mentioned gross lesions, which are rare causes of amenorrhoea, most cases, other than those due to pregnancy, will be found to be the result of deficient secretion of gonadotrophins by the anterior pituitary body or failure of the ovaries to secrete oestrogen and progesterone (ovarian failure). Pituitary failure may be due to a tumour but is more commonly due to inhibition of hypothalamic releasing factor from extreme loss of weight as the result of severe dieting or anorexia nervosa, from emotional disturbances, or from taking the combined oestrogen–progestogen contraceptive pill. The thyroid, or more rarely the adrenal glands, may be at fault. In some cases the evidence of the failure of certain glands is clear, in others it is difficult to be sure. Such investigations as endometrial biopsy, blood and urine hormone estimations, basal temperature charts, vaginal smear tests, the basal metabolic rate estimation, sugar tolerance tests, and X-ray examination of the pituitary fossa may all be useful in determining the main gland at fault. The details of the estimations are dealt with elsewhere.

Gonadotrophin estimations in the urine indicate premature ovarian failure when the gonadotrophins (particularly F.S.H.) reach menopausal levels. If gonadotrophin excretion is low or normal, the ovaries are probably still responsive and induction of ovulation is likely to be successful. Although severe loss of weight is associated with amenorrhoea, young women who are subjected to emotional strain may suffer temporarily from amenorrhoea and suddenly gain in weight. Women who have long intervals between periods (oligomenorrhoea) from puberty are particularly liable to have prolonged amenorrhoea, and therefore inability to conceive, when they stop taking the contraceptive pill, which, for them, is contra-indicated (post-pill amenorrhoea).

Amenorrhoea may be associated with galactorrhoea. Typically the syndrome occurs post-partum but it may follow the contraceptive pill or arise without any apparent cause. Raised serum prolactin levels are found probably because of a lowered secretion by the hypothalamus of prolactin-inhibiting factor.

Simmonds' disease (or Sheehan's syndrome) is a rare cause of pituitary failure. It commonly follows very severe post-partum haemorrhage causing necrosis of most of the anterior pituitary gland through venous thrombosis. It is accompanied by failure of lactation, loss of body hair, wasting and lowered basal metabolism, and the periods fail to be re-established.

An arrhenoblastoma is a very rare ovarian tumour causing virilism in the female, often a young adult woman. In addition to amenorrhoea and atrophy of the breasts, there is growth of hair on the face, chest, and abdomen, deepening of the voice and enlargement of the clitoris. 17-Ketosteroid excretion is normal. Granulosa cell tumours of the ovary secrete oestrogen which gives rise to bouts of amenorrhoea interspersed with prolonged irregular vaginal bleeding.

The various disorders of the circulatory, nervous, and other systems that may be associated with amenorrhoea are discussed under the headings of other symptoms. With regard to pregnancy, which is the commonest of all causes of secondary amenorrhoea, it may be formulated as an axiom that an otherwise healthy woman who has had perfectly regular menstruation is probably pregnant if she suddenly gets amenorrhoea. Nevertheless, the presence of pregnancy must never be assumed without careful consideration of the history, combined with a complete physical examination. The diagnosis of pregnancy is made upon a complex of symptoms rather than upon any one; but the combination of amenorrhoea, secretion to be squeezed from the breasts, morning sickness, vaginal discoloration, and uterine enlargement, can only mean pregnancy in the majority of cases; the addition of foetal movements and the foetal heart-sounds makes the diagnosis absolute. Immunological pregnancy tests and ultrasound examination are helpful when the diagnosis is in doubt.

T. L. T. Lewis.

AMINO-ACIDURIA

Although microscopic examination of the urine deposit may occasionally show crystals of leucine and tyrosine (usually in cases of acute liver atrophy) urine amino-acids are now demonstrated by *paper chromatography*, a procedure which has expanded enormously the significance of this observation. By routine methods normal urine usually shows small amounts of five amino-acids (glycine, glutamine, alanine, serine, and histidine), whereas in pathological states other single amino-acids, or groups of up to fifteen amino-acids, may be excreted in excess.

Two general classes of amino-aciduria are recognized, the *overflow* and the *renal* type. In the former the excretion is caused by high blood levels due to some metabolic abnormality, while in the latter the renal tubules fail to reabsorb one or more of the amino-acids normally present in the blood. The main types of amino-aciduria are listed in the Table opposite on which the following comments may be made.

In liver disease this organ may fail to deaminate amino-acids effectively so that a large number may appear in the urine. This is particularly noticeable in severe chronic liver disease and the appearance of visible crystals of leucine and tyrosine is a bad prognostic sign. The other examples of overflow amino-aciduria are all concerned with specific metabolic blocks due to the absence of individual enzymes. These rare conditions are congenital and are usually associated

CAUSES OF AMINO-ACIDURIA

CONDITION	ACIDS EXCRETED	CLINICAL MANIFESTATIONS
	Overflow types	
Liver damage ..	Many	Gross liver disease
Phenylketonuria ..	Phenylalanine. Phenylpyruvic acid	Mental deficiency
Citrullinuria ..	Citrulline	Mental deficiency
Cystathioninuria ..	Cystathionine	Mental deficiency
Arginosuccinuria ..	Arginosuccinic	Mental deficiency
Maple syrup disease ..	Valine. Leucine. Isoleucine ..	Mental deficiency. Hypertonicity of muscle. Characteristic urine smell
Histidinuria	Histidine	None or speech defect
Tyrosinaemia	Tyrosine	Hepatic cirrhosis. Mental deficiency
Homocystinuria ..	Homocystine	Mental deficiency
Prolinuria	Glycine. Proline. Hydroxyproline ..	Mental deficiency or normal
	Renal types	
Cystinuria	Cystine. Ornithine. Arginine. Lysine	Renal calculi
Hartnup disease ..	Many mono-amino-monocarboxylic acids (e.g., tryptophane)	Pellagra
Fanconi syndrome ..	Many	Resistant rickets. Acidosis. Cystinosis
Wilson's disease ..	Many	Hepatic cirrhosis. Neurological symptoms (tremor, etc.)
Galactosaemia ..	Many	Failure to thrive. Hepatomegaly. Cataracts

with severe mental deficiency. Phenylketonuria (q.v. p. 643) has perhaps attracted most attention on account of its greater ease of detection. The urine gives a transient green colour when ferric chloride solution is added, and a convenient test paper ('Phenstix') is available; the reaction is due to phenylpyruvic acid. Maple syrup disease is readily detected by the characteristic urine smell. The list given is not complete as many similar but very rare syndromes are still being discovered.

The renal amino-acidurias fall roughly into two classes. In cystinuria (q.v.) and in Hartnup disease there is a selective failure of tubular reabsorption of a limited group to related amino-acids. In the former symptomatology is entirely due to the renal calculi (cystine), while in the latter the pellagra-like symptoms are due to tryptophane deficiency and are therefore accentuated by a poor diet. The remaining examples of amino-aciduria are those in which a generalized tubular damage is present so that a large number of amino-acids appear in the urine.

'Fanconi syndrome' is a term indicating any condition in which there is widespread damage to the proximal renal tubules as shown by renal amino-aciduria, renal glycosuria, and increased phosphate and urate clearances causing abnormally low serum phosphate and urate concentrations. Cystinosis (Lignac-Fanconi disease) is a congenital disorder of childhood with widespread deposits of cystine in the tissues accompanied by severe rickets resistant to vitamin D and by acidosis; the tubular reabsorption of glucose, phosphate, and bicarbonate is defective as well as that of amino-acids. Deposits of cystine in the renal cortex usually cause chronic renal failure in adolescence. Treatment may be either by continued intermittent haemodialysis or by renal transplantation. A less severe inherited disease may present in adult life as osteomalacia with acidosis and a similar condition may be acquired, e.g., after heavy metal poisoning and occasionally in nephrosis. Wilson's disease and galactosaemia are special cases since, although the conditions are inherited, the tubular damage is a secondary manifestation due to the toxic effects of copper and galactose-*l*-phosphate respectively. As indicated in the table the clinical manifestations of these various conditions are quite different.

M. D. Milne.

AMNESIA (LOSS OF MEMORY)

The transcendent role of memory in mental development and human evolution requires no emphasis. Without it there is no capacity to learn, to calculate, or to speak. The process of memorization depends in the first place on attention, which focuses the mind on the matter to be remembered; consequently amnesia will result if attention is diverted by other preoccupations as in anxiety states, psychotic conditions, and lack of interest. Secondly, memory depends on the integrity of certain portions of the cerebral cortex, notably the parieto-occipital area, the temporal lobe, and the hippocampus, for it is in these areas that most memories are stored. Thirdly, memory may be affected by a reduced power to recall the stored material, which cannot readily be brought into consciousness; this occurs in mental fatigue, toxaemia, and anxiety states.

Mental fatigue, psychoneurosis, drug intoxication, closed head injuries, and generalized infections and degenerations of the brain, usually depress memory in all its modalities. Localized cortical lesions, on the other hand, may cause loss of particular units of memory; thus a lesion of the posterior portion of the left parietal lobe may, in right-handed persons, cause loss of visual memories—familiar faces are no longer recognized, although they are clearly seen; the significance of written speech is not appreciated; the meaning of pictures is lost, spatial relationships and distances between external objects are not understood, so that the patient may collide with things that he can quite clearly see. Similarly disease of the temporal lobe of the dominant hemisphere (the left in right-handed persons) may cause loss of auditory memories, so that noises and speech are heard but their meaning is not understood. A lesion of the parietal lobe immediately behind the post-central convolution may interfere with the recognition of objects placed in the hand, although sensation is not grossly impaired. This condition, known as 'astereognosis', is found equally in disease of both hemispheres.

It is clear that memory is a function of more than one portion of the brain, and that it is necessary to carry out formal tests of all its aspects in order to come to a correct conclusion as to the severity and form of amnesia in a given case, and in particular to determine whether loss of memory is limited to a single group of sensory experiences or is part of a more generalized depression of memory as a whole.

Toxaemia. In the acute intoxications of *severe infections* (typhoid, streptococcal septicaemia, pneumonia), cerebral functions may be depressed and chaotic. Attention suffers, and on recovery there may be little or no memory of the events during the illness. The same applies to endogenous intoxications such as *uraemia* and *diabetic coma*, and to drug intoxications such as *alcoholism, opium poisoning*, and *barbiturate addiction*. Chronic alcoholism is sometimes responsible for a particular form of memory disorder known as *Korsakow's syndrome*, a condition in which there is loss of memory for recent events, disorientation for time and place, and a remarkable capacity to fill in the memory blanks with a plausible account of events and activities which have not actually occurred. So natural may be the patient's manner that an observer may not realize that the patient is confabulating. It can occur in less marked degree in other intoxications, both chemical and bacterial.

Diseases of the Brain. Inflammatory disease of the brain will affect memory in greater or lesser degree, according to its severity and location. In *cerebrospinal fever* there is usually some degree of amnesia for the period of illness. It can be followed by a general impairment of memory which may persist throughout life, and thus interferes with the capacity to recall former memories and the ability to retain new ideas. The blunting of the ability to remember may, in conjunction with the impairment of other intellectual functions, considerably reduce the efficiency of the patient. This unhappy sequel of meningitis is not seen when the disease is cut short by the prompt use of modern antibiotics. The after-effects of other forms of meningitis are similar.

Suppurative encephalitis and *cerebral abscess*, being more localized, are less likely to cause permanent impairment of memory. The *encephalomyelitis* which occasionally follows the specific fevers of childhood is rarely followed by permanent intellectual changes.

General paralysis of the insane and *cerebral malaria* are familiar examples of infective disease in which the capacity to remember is impaired during the active phase of the disease.

Cerebral tumours, especially widely infiltrating gliomata, sometimes cause intellectual loss, including a reduction of memory for recent events. When located in the parietal or temporal lobes, the memory loss may be confined to visual or auditory impressions. When intracranial pressure is raised, memory shares in the general depression of intellectual acuity.

Degenerative diseases of the brain such as *Huntington's chorea, hepatolenticular degeneration, Pick's disease, Alzheimer's disease, and cerebral arteriosclerosis* are commonly accompanied by a generalized loss of memory for recent events coupled with other features of intellectual deterioration. Of these, cerebral arteriosclerosis is the most common. As age advances, the capacity to absorb and retain new facts is progressively reduced; the impressions are shallow and are easily lost. Consequently while past memories survive, recent ones are less easily retained.

Brain Injury. Severe blows to the head produce a temporary amnesia, followed in a few cases by a permanent impairment of memory for day-to-day events. The immediate result of a severe head injury is unconsciousness, lasting minutes, hours, or even weeks. When consciousness is recovered it is usually found that there is a retrograde amnesia, extending over minutes or hours preceding the accident. The duration of this retrograde amnesia is not a reliable guide to the severity of the injury, whereas the post-traumatic amnesia is of considerable value in this respect. This post-traumatic amnesia lasts longer than the apparent unconsciousness of the patient; indeed the patient may at one stage appear to be fully conscious and capable of conversing and carrying out ordinary activities, yet these activities may not be recalled when recovery is complete. It is the duration of the post-traumatic amnesia which affords the best guide to the severity of the cerebral injury. After recovery, memory is often impaired, the patient being forgetful and therefore inefficient in his daily tasks. Considerable degrees of improvement are to be expected over a period of two to three years after the injury, but if there is any residual defect after this period has elapsed it is likely to be permanent.

Gunshot wounds and other penetrating injuries may or may not be associated with concussion and unconsciousness. If there has been no loss of consciousness there may be no residual memory defect unless there has been focal destruction of the temporal or parieto-occipital lobes. If this has occurred, there may be a loss of specific modalities of memory without any generalized depression of this all-important function.

Epilepsy. Amnesia is an important feature of the epileptic seizure. In petit mal the break in consciousness is so transitory that the continuity of memory is hardly impaired at all. When consciousness is lost, however, whether there is a convulsion or not, there is a true amnesia lasting for a few minutes. Rarely a fit is followed by post-epileptic automatism, comparable to the automatism that sometimes occurs after recovery of consciousness after a head injury, during which the patient carries out a series of seemingly conscious actions which are often bizarre and out of character and of which he has no memory on recovery. Post-epileptic automatism seldom lasts more than one or two hours, in contrast to the sustained amnesias of hysterical subjects. Sometimes an epileptic attack may be represented simply by a period of amnesia during which time the patient may appear outwardly normal. At other times a period of amnesia may be preceded by smacking of the lips and champing movements and the behaviour of the patient during the period of amnesia may be quite odd and consist, for example, of undressing or in the performance of useless repetitive movements or actions. Between fits memory is usually good, but when fits are frequent there is some degree of mental deterioration to which repeated minor head injuries, anoxia in convulsions, or drugs, contribute their share.

Neurosis and Psychosis

In *anxiety states*, mental fatigue resulting from emotional stress interferes with the capacity to attend and to memorize. Consequently there is forgetfulness, and inability to recall past events.

In *hysteria*, the emotional conflict can have a similar effect on immediate memory; the forgetfulness thus engendered suggests to the patient that he is losing his memory, and since this is usually an acceptable state of affairs to the hysteric, it rapidly develops into a complete amnesia for past events. In such a case the patient may spend a period of days, or even weeks, doing irresponsible things of which he later professes no memory, e.g., a soldier may leave camp without leave and spend several days wandering about before giving himself up to the police. This type of hysterical fugue differs from epileptic automatism in that it serves some purpose; moreover, memory for the events during the fugue can usually be restored under hypnosis or narcosis. In the depressive phase of *depressive psychosis* attention is impaired and mental activity is slowed, with the result that memory for recent and past events may be temporarily inhibited. In *mania*, on the other hand, memory is sometimes abnormally acute. In *schizophrenic states* memory may be well preserved, but preoccupation with fantasies and hallucinations is apt to engross the attention of the patient to the exclusion of events around him, and memory for such events is liable to suffer. Nevertheless it is extraordinary how much a catatonic schizophrenic will remember after he has been sunk in reverie for a considerable time.

Ian Mackenzie.

ANAEMIA

Anaemia literally means lack of blood. The term as used, however, has no reference to the total volume of blood in the circulation; it refers simply to a reduction of the quantity or quality of the red cells: a patient with anaemia is one in whom the concentration of the haemoglobin in the blood is below normal. Most often a significant reduction in the haemoglobin is associated with reduction in the number of red cells per c.mm. of blood, but the red cells may be normal in number and the amount of haemoglobin in each cell reduced. In certain types of anaemia there is an associated abnormality in the white cells or leucocytes. The examination of the white cells is thus often of great value in the differential diagnosis of the anaemias.

The normal red-cell count may be taken as about 5 million per c.mm. irrespective of sex. Actually the *average* figure is higher for males and slightly lower for females (*see table below*).

Determination of haemoglobin (Hb) concentration has in the past been very inaccurate because of the different scales in use. The normal is now taken as 14·6 g. per 100 ml., disregarding the sex differences (male average 16 g.; female average 14 g.). To calculate Hb percentage from grammes per millilitre, multiply by 7.

Estimation of haemoglobin is most accurately and quickly performed by the use of a photoelectric colorimeter. For a physician unlikely to possess the apparatus other more simple colorimeters are available (e.g., M.R.C. Grey-wedge). These colorimeters rely on comparing the colour of oxyhaemoglobin or its cyanide derivatives with standards of the same colour. The number of red cells in the peripheral blood can be counted by means of a haemocytometer (counting chamber), the counting being done by eye, or by means of an electronic particle counter, in which the counting is done electronically, when each red cell produces a change in current flow as it passes through a narrow aperture separating two electrodes. This is much more accurate.

The haemoglobin and red cells in anaemia are not necessarily reduced in the same proportion; in fact the relation between the haemoglobin percentage and the red-cell count is of importance in distinguishing between the different types of anaemia. In much the largest group of the anaemias, such as those due to a deficiency of iron, the haemoglobin is usually reduced to a much greater extent than the red cells; in another group, due to marrow hypoplasia, the haemoglobin and red cells tend to be reduced about equally; while in a third group, of which pernicious anaemia is characteristic, the reduction in cell count is generally more marked than is the reduction in haemoglobin percentage because

The Normal Blood Count*
(The ranges of the normal cellular components of the peripheral blood)

		MALES	FEMALES
Haemoglobin		14–18 g. per cent	12·5–16·5 g. per cent
	Infants (at birth)	13·5–19·5 g. per cent	
	1-year-olds	10·5–12·5 g. per cent	
Red-cell count		4·5–6·5 millions per c.mm.	4·0–5·0 millions per c.mm.
	Infants (at birth)	5·5–6·5 millions per c.mm.	
	1-year-olds	4·0–5·0 millions per c.mm.	
Packed-cell volume		40–52 per cent	39–47 per cent
	Infants (at birth)	45–60 per cent	
	1-year-olds	35–40 per cent	
Total red-cell mass		25–35 ml. per kg. body-weight	
M.C.H.C.		32 36 per cent	
M.C.V.		78–96 μ^3	
M.C.H.		28–31 $\mu\mu$g.	
White-cell count		4·0–10·0 × 10³ per c.mm.	
	Neutrophils	3·0–6·0 × 10³ per c.mm.	
	Eosinophils	0·5–2·5 × 10³ per c.mm.	
	Basophils	0–1·0 × 10³ per c.mm.	
	Lymphocytes	1·0–3·0 × 10³ per c.mm.	
	Monocytes	1·5–4·0 × 10³ per c.mm.	
Platelets		1·5–5·0 × 10³ per c.mm.	

* S.I. units. The standard international units for haematology have not necessitated a change in individual values and these are as follows:

Haemoglobin:	g./dl. (decilitre)	M.C.H.C.:	g./dl.
Red cell count:	× 10¹²/l. (litre)	M.C.V.:	fl.
P.C.V.:	0·40–0·52 l./l.	White cell count:	× 10⁹/l.
M.C.H.:	pg. (picogrammes)	Platelets:	× 10⁹/l.

the red cells are larger than normal. The relation between the two can be expressed quantitatively by means of the *colour index*, which is the haemoglobin as a percentage of normal divided by the red-cell count as a percentage of normal. In a patient in whom the haemoglobin concentration is reduced to a greater extent than the red-cell concentration the colour index will be less than 1·0 as it is in iron-deficiency anaemia. A colour index greater than 1·0 suggests that there are fewer red cells containing a greater concentration of haemoglobin such as occurs in one of the megaloblastic anaemias. Anaemia with a colour index of approximately 1·0 suggests that there is an equal reduction in haemoglobin and red-cell concentration, as may occur from marrow hypoplasia. This simple assessment of anaemia may still be of value but it is more usual nowadays to calculate certain red-cell indices which are derived from the haemoglobin concentration, the red-cell count, and the packed-cell volume (haematocrit) of the peripheral blood. The packed-cell volume represents the percentage red-cell composition of whole blood after centrifuging a column of blood to a constant volume of cells. From these measurements the following indices can be calculated:

1. Mean corpuscular volume (M.C.V.) equals P.C.V. (per cent)/R.B.C. (10⁶ per c.mm.) × 10, normally 85–95 μ^3.

2. Mean corpuscular haemoglobin concentration equals Hb (g. per cent)/P.C.V. (per cent), normally 32–36 per cent.

3. Mean corpuscular haemoglobin (M.C.H.) equals Hb (g. per cent) per R.B.C. (10⁶ per c.mm.), normally 28–31 $\mu\mu$g.

In *absolute* values the colour index is represented by the Mean Corpuscular Haemoglobin (M.C.H.).

Modern electronic cell-counters do not actually measure the P.C.V. but compute indirectly from the red-cell count and the M.C.V. which are measured directly. The red-cell count measured electronically is usually of greater accuracy than when measured manually, while the P.C.V. is more prone to variations. The practical result is that the M.C.H. becomes a more reliable index of hypochromia than the M.C.H.C. with electronic counting, the reverse being the case with manual counting.

These indices only give mean values for certain red-cell measurements in the peripheral blood. They tell one nothing about the variation that occurs from cell to cell. To appreciate the variations from cell to cell a smear of blood must be stained and examined microscopically. In this way variations in shape, size, and haemoglobin concentration can be assessed and interpreted.

Various terms are in general use to classify anaemias in terms of their average cell size and average cell haemoglobin concentration. An anaemia is said to be *macrocytic, normocytic,* or *microcytic* according as the average cell size is above normal, normal, or below normal. Again, an anaemia is said to be *hyperchromic, normochromic,* or *hypochromic* according to whether the mean cell haemoglobin concentration is above normal, normal, or below normal. By using such a system it is possible very often to obtain a short cut to the type of anaemia present (*see* p. 39).

The normal amount of haemoglobin and number of red cells in the peripheral blood are the result of a balance between the production and destruction of these components. Any decrease in production of haemoglobin or red cells will inevitably lead to anaemia, while any increase in destruction (or increase of blood-loss) may lead to anaemia. It is, however, possible for the production of haemoglobin and red cells to be increased by the bone-marrow and this is a normal compensatory mechanism which occurs when there is increased destruction or increased blood-loss; this compensatory mechanism is brought into play through the hormone erythropoietin. Provided the requirements for erythropoiesis can be fully met the bone-marrow can increase its output of red cells some tenfold. This means that there can be a considerable reduction in red-cell life span, or loss of red cells from the body, without the development of anaemia at all.

A logical approach to the cause of anaemia would first involve estimating the rate of blood production or the rate of destruction and these parameters can be measured accurately by the use of radio-isotopes. However, in clinical practice time does not usually permit the use of such involved procedures as these, and it is necessary to obtain a crude assessment by some other means. Two important tests, the reticulocyte count and the serum bilirubin, are very valuable in assessing alterations in the balance between production and destruction of red cells. A reticulocyte is a young red cell which has lost its nucleus but still contains some nucleic acid remnants; it is the final stage of maturation before the mature erythrocyte. If the bone-marrow activity increases there is an increased production of reticulocytes and these appear in increased numbers in the peripheral blood. It is now known that there is a direct correlation between the reticulocyte count and bone-marrow activity. Reticulocytes are usually counted in the peripheral blood as a percentage of normal red cells and if the latter are reduced it is important to correct the reticulocyte percentage for the appropriate reduction in red-cell count (or packed-cell volume). Normally the reticulocyte concentration is between 0·5 and 2 per cent of the total red cells.

The serum bilirubin is a less sensitive measurement of red-cell destruction in the body since the concentration in the serum is both a function of its rate of production and the capacity of the liver to remove it. In haemolytic disease the serum bilirubin is of the unconjugated type. It is clear, therefore, that an increase in reticulocyte count in the peripheral blood suggests that the bone-marrow is overactive and this is likely to be because there is increased destruction of red cells or their loss from the body. If the serum bilirubin is also raised and unconjugated, then haemolysis is the probable disorder. A reduction in reticulocyte count is more difficult to assess because of the low concentration present in the normal individual. However, by the use of a reticulocyte count, the serum bilirubin concentration, and the detection of blood-loss in the stools or elsewhere, it is usually possible to obtain a dynamic assessment of the cause of anaemia.

Symptoms of Anaemia. Certain symptoms are common to all forms of anaemia such as lassitude, shortness of breath, and often palpitation and tachycardia on exertion. Swelling around the ankles above the upper margin of the shoes may occur in chronic anaemia, as also dizziness or faintness on standing. Pallor can be deceptive. Many persons look almost white although their blood is not necessarily abnormal; the distribution of the cutaneous capillaries may be such that the superficial skin has little, if any, of the normal colour of blood, and yet the individual may not have any diminution in his haemoglobin percentage. Pallor is common in night workers and in those who work underground. In most cases where the skin is very white one can avoid a mistaken diagnosis of anaemia by examining the colour of the mucous membranes, the inner part of the lower eyelid, the lips, the inside of the mouth, and the nail-beds. If any doubt remains the haemoglobin concentration should be estimated. If the haemoglobin is found to be appreciably below normal the next step is to discover the type and cause of the anaemia.

When the haemoglobin falls, anginal pain may be experienced on effort indistinguishable in type from that of coronary disease, especially in those patients with asymptomatic coronary disease. The occurrence of the symptoms of anaemia in any particular individual varies greatly with the level of haemoglobin and the two frequently do not correlate. This is because two methods of compensation may operate in the body in the presence of any anaemia. In the first place, the cardiac output is increased and results in a hyper-kinetic type of circulation, the blood-flow through the peripheral tissues being increased and delivering more oxygen per unit of time. In the second place, in some anaemias there is a shift of the oxygen-association curve of haemoglobin in the cells so that more oxygen may be released to the tissues at a particular level of tissue-oxygen tension. Thus a patient with pernicious anaemia with a haemoglobin of 30 per cent or even less may be able to walk slowly without dyspnoea or other symptoms, whereas sudden loss of blood or any other cause of acute anaemia will produce severe symptoms at a haemoglobin level of 60–70 per cent. The slower the onset of anaemia the less marked the symptoms tend to be.

Purpura and retinal haemorrhages may be detected in chronic severe anaemia.

Acute severe anaemia, particularly when due to haemorrhage, is characterized by thirst, dry tongue, pallor, subnormal temperature, extreme restlessness, coldness, sweating, tachycardia, rapid and shallow breathing, faintness, and even loss of consciousness. Blurring of vision arises in severe bleeding, notably in the elderly in whom blindness may partially persist.

Examination of the Blood. A sample of blood is most conveniently obtained either by finger-prick or by venepuncture. The sample is then analysed for haemoglobin concentration, red-cell count, and packed-cell volume, and from these measurements the three indices already discussed are calculated. A total white-cell count is made and a peripheral blood-film prepared on a glass slide. This film should be not more than one cell thick and is prepared by spreading a drop of blood slowly over a grease-free glass slide; the film is then stained with one of the Romanowsky stains. On this film the appearance of the red cells can be noted and a differential white-cell count can be made. Because there is a tendency for neutrophils to congregate at the margins of the film and lymphocytes to spread themselves more evenly over the whole film it is important that all areas of the blood-smear should be counted in order to arrive at a correct differential count. During the differential white-cell count the presence of any abnormal cells should be noted and the distribution of platelets also observed. It may even be possible to make a crude assessment of their numbers from their distribution on the film. If there is any reason to suspect that they are present in pathological numbers then a platelet count should also be performed on the blood sample. This count will also be relevant if the patient complains of any symptoms suggesting a bleeding tendency and it should always be performed in all patients who are anaemic.

Blood Grouping. When a blood transfusion is to be performed, it is necessary to make certain that the donor's blood is compatible with that of the patient, otherwise grave consequences may follow. Two agglutinogens (antigens) A and B occur in human red cells and two agglutinins (antibodies) α and β in human serum. Since cells containing A are agglutinated by serum containing α, and cells containing B are agglutinated by serum containing β, it follows that neither A and α together, nor B and β together, can occur in the blood of a given individual. It is found that the vast majority of individuals can be classed in one of four groups numbered as follows: Group I containing A and B only; Group II containing A and β only; Group III containing α and B only; and Group IV containing α and β only. The four groups are also named in accordance with the cell agglutinogens they contain: I is AB, II is A, III is B, IV is O (neither A nor B). The great danger of a transfusion lies in the possible agglutination of the cells. Generally, however, one is only concerned with the agglutination of the *donor's cells* by the *recipient's blood*, because when the donor's blood enters the recipient's circulation it becomes so diluted that the converse reaction is unlikely to occur. Thus in addition to being able to give a patient blood from a donor of the same group as himself, one can give Group O blood (which contains no agglutinogens) to patients of *any*

group, and one can give patients of Group AB (which contains no agglutinins) blood from donors of *any* group. Individuals of Group O are known as 'universal donors', and individuals of Group AB are known as 'universal recipients'.

Although much use is made of universal donors when it is impossible to wait for the full grouping and cross-matching of a patient's blood, it should be remembered that there are hazards in using O Group in this way as it may contain a potent anti-A haemolysin which can lyse the recipient's cells. In most centres Group O patients with this type of haemolysin are screened off and are not used as blood donors.

The group of an individual is easily determined by testing his cells against stock sera of Groups A and B. A drop of blood obtained from his finger is mixed with about twenty times its volume of normal saline. A drop of this cell suspension is then placed upon each of two clean microscope slides marked respectively A and B. To the drop on slide A is added a drop of the stock A serum, and to the drop on slide B is added a drop of stock B serum. Care must be taken to use a clean pipette for each manœuvre, so that one serum does not become contaminated with the other. If agglutination is going to occur, it usually does so within a few minutes; but the speed of the reaction depends on the state of the stock sera, and no reading should be taken as finally negative until half an hour has elapsed. By rocking the slides gently one not only hastens agglutination but also tends to prevent false agglutination due to rouleaux formation. If the individual is of Group O no agglutination will be seen on either slide; if of Group AB, there will be agglutination on both slides; if of Group A, there will be agglutination on slide B but not on slide A, and if of Group B there will be agglutination on slide A but not on slide B.

It is usual when blood-grouping patients to determine both the antigen on their cells by the use of sera of known groups, and the antibody in their plasma by the use of cells of known groups, and then to cross-check to make sure that these match. When testing a large number of Group-A donors with anti-A sera it is sometimes found that a proportion of them agglutinate poorly or fail to do so with a particular serum. It is known that this is due to the fact that there are two sorts of A cells often called A_1 and A_2 and that some anti-A sera react only with A_1 cells. About 25 per cent of Group-A patients are Group A_2; occasionally Group-A_2 patients who have been transfused develop an anti-A antibody and may appear incompatible with some Group-A cells. From the blood-transfusion point of view once a patient's blood and a suitable donor have been selected it is important to make sure that the serum of the patient is compatible with the donor's cells and this is done by cross-matching. To do this the two components are incubated together at 37° C. in saline and also with the addition of albumin, agglutination is looked for, and in addition the donor's cells are tested for adsorbed antibody after incubation with the patient's plasma by means of the Coombs' test. If all these tests are compatible then the blood is suitable for transfusion.

The technique of blood grouping is sometimes complicated by the phenomenon of cold agglutination, but the agglutination can be prevented by carrying out the test at 37° C. The phenomenon, which occurs to a minor degree in many normal people, may be much exaggerated in a number of diverse conditions, including virus pneumonia, trypanosomiasis, cirrhosis of the liver, and some haemolytic anaemias. Usually it is only a laboratory finding, but rarely the titre of the agglutinins is so high that agglutination leading to haemolysis occurs *in vivo* and the patient suffers from attacks of haemoglobinuria.

RHESUS FACTOR. The discovery that the red cells of 85 per cent of white people are agglutinated by animal sera prepared against the cells of the Rhesus monkey, while those of the remaining 15 per cent are not so agglutinated, has explained the occurrence of serious transfusion reactions in spite of the blood used being perfectly compatible as far as the AB agglutinogens were concerned; it also explains the group of haemolytic diseases of the newborn known as erythroblastosis foetalis. The people whose cells react with the Rhesus serum are Rhesus (or Rh)-positive, those who do not react are Rhesus (or Rh)-negative. If a Rh-negative individual receives a transfusion of Rh-positive blood he is liable to develop antibodies which will destroy any Rh-positive cells given at a subsequent transfusion. The reaction at the second transfusion is usually absent or mild, but at later transfusions it becomes increasingly severe or even fatal. Some Rh-negative people fail to develop such antibodies and so may survive with impunity an unlimited number of Rh-positive transfusions; but the possibility of reactions occurring cannot be eliminated, and a Rh-negative individual must be given Rh-negative blood whenever possible. With Rh-negative women the risk of serious reactions is much greater. If such a woman marries a Rh-positive husband and becomes pregnant with a Rh-positive foetus, she is liable to develop antibodies against the Rh-positive cells of the foetus. A single subsequent Rh-positive transfusion is then capable of producing a serious or even fatal reaction. Apart from any transfusion, the antibodies formed in the mother against the Rh-positive foetal cells are likely to destroy the foetal cells and give rise to erythroblastosis foetalis in one or other of its forms. Usually when this happens, the first pregnancy is normal and the disease appears only in the second, third, or fourth; the first infant to be affected may survive, but subsequent ones will probably die shortly after birth, be born dead, or be prematurely expelled as a macerated foetus. If, on the other hand, this same woman had, prior to her pregnancy, been sensitized by even a single Rh-positive blood transfusion, then her first infant

might have been affected with a serious or even fatal form of erythroblastosis foetalis. Thus by transfusing a Rh-negative female, even in infancy, with Rh-positive blood one may be jeopardizing her chance of bearing a healthy infant in later life. Therefore prior to transfusion, Rh grouping must be done as well as AB grouping; and every individual who is Rh-negative must be given Rh-negative blood of the appropriate AB group. In an emergency when no Rh-negative blood is available it would be permissible to give Rh-positive blood but only in the following circumstances: (1) in the case of a male provided he has never received a previous transfusion; and (2) in the case of a female provided she has passed the child-bearing age, has never had a child or a miscarriage, and has never received a previous transfusion.

The Rh-negative quality of blood (denoted by rh) does not imply merely the absence of the Rh-positive quality (denoted by Rh), for the rh quality is also capable of producing antibodies against the cells containing it. The Rh factor is determined by two genes, Rh and rh; and every individual possesses either two Rh genes, or two rh genes, or one Rh and one rh gene, the two being situated on separate chromosomes. There are thus three types of individual: the homozygous Rh-positive (Rh Rh), the heterozygous Rh-positive (Rh rh), and the homozygous Rh-negative (rh rh). The Rhesus group of a child is determined by his parents, the offspring receiving one gene from each parent. This matter is clearly of importance in considering the future outlook for the parents when a Rh-negative mother has already had an infant with erythroblastosis foetalis: if the father is homozygous Rh-positive all future pregnancies are bound to result in the disease; but if he is heterozygous Rh-positive, there is an even chance that any particular future pregnancy may result in the birth of a healthy infant.

In man, as opposed to the Rhesus monkey, the matter is further complicated by the fact that the gene on each of the two chromosomes is in reality a complex of three genes. The three genes represent three different Rh antigens, each of which can occur in at least two alternative forms. They are C or c, D or d, and E or e. Thus the three genes on each chromosome may occur in any of the eight following combinations: CDe, cDE, CDE, cDe, Cde, cdE, CdE, and cde. Now the first three and the last of these combinations occur much more frequently than the other four; and as a result of this, and of the fact that D is of all the six antigens the one most liable to produce antibodies, it so happens that the vast majority of transfusion reactions and cases of erythroblastosis foetalis are the result of the formation of antibodies of type anti-D. It is therefore customary to limit the Rh-positive group to those individuals who possess the antigen D; and to include in the Rh-negative group not only the pure Rh-negative type, in which the antigens cde occur on both chromosomes, but also the three rare types which, while not possessing the antigen D, do possess the antigens C or E or both. For this purpose it is sufficient to group the cells of the individual against anti-D serum, a procedure which can be carried out by the majority of laboratories if supplied with a few millilitres of venous blood that has been allowed to clot in a clean tube. Occasionally, and more particularly in cases of erythroblastosis foetalis, it is desirable to make a more detailed study of the Rhesus type or to investigate the presence of antibodies in the serum. Samples will then have to be sent to one of the special laboratories where the often rare antisera required for the purpose are alone available.

PATERNITY EXCLUSION TESTS. Since the agglutinogens A and B are inherited as Mendelian dominants, blood-grouping tests may be of value in proving that a man is not the father of a given child, but it is only in a certain proportion of cases that the test is of help; in no circumstances does it prove that the man *is* the father of the child. In addition to the four common AB groups and the eight Rhesus groups there are now known to be two additional subgroups of A, three groups dependent on the so-called M and N agglutinogens, and many others. By combining all these different groups it is possible to distinguish a great number of varieties of human blood. If the complete procedure was practicable it would not only be possible on the one hand to exclude paternity in a very high percentage of cases, but also on the other to add considerable weight to the evidence that the man *was* the father. Owing, however, to the labour involved and to the many technical difficulties, as well as to the extreme rarity of many of the anti-sera required, such detailed grouping of blood has in general to be confined to those criminal cases in which it might be of supreme importance to the evidence.

The Erythrocyte Sedimentation-rate (E.S.R.: B.S.R.). If a tube of blood containing some anticoagulant is allowed to stand, the red cells slowly settle to the bottom, leaving a clear layer of plasma on top. The rate of sedimentation naturally depends on the technique employed; but if this is standardized, the rate is remarkably constant in healthy individuals. The rate is increased in certain pathological conditions and in pregnancy, and to a slight extent at the time of menstruation. The factors responsible for increasing the rate are not fully understood; but it seems that the most frequent and important of them is an increase in the fibrinogen or globulins in the blood. There is an increased sedimentation-rate whenever there is tissue breakdown: with infective, toxic, or neoplastic processes, and to some extent after operations and fractures of bone.

The rate, moreover, may be regarded as a measure of the activity or extensiveness of the underlying pathological process. Chronic anaemia itself does not produce a high sedimentation-rate, in fact it is usually normal in iron-deficiency anaemia; but if for any reason, such as a growth or an infection, the sedimentation-rate is increased, then the anaemia will have the effect of exaggerating that increase to an extent which is dependent upon the degree to which the cells are reduced. One of the most convenient methods to use is that of Westergren: 0·4 ml. of a 3·8 per cent solution of sodium citrate is mixed with 1·6 ml. of venous blood. The mixture is immediately transferred to a tube and thoroughly mixed by gentle agitation, and then sucked up into the Westergren tube as far as the zero mark. This tube is 2·5 mm. in internal diameter and is graduated in millimetres (not cubic millimetres); the graduations mark the distance from the tip of the pipette, and the zero mark, towards the upper end of the pipette, is exactly 200 mm. from the tip. After introducing the blood, the pipette is placed vertically in a stand, its tip being pressed well into a soft piece of rubber (to prevent the blood escaping) by the pressure of a spring cap on its upper end. The time is noted when it is placed in position, and after the lapse of an hour the level of the upper end of the column of red cells is read off from the graduations. In health the fall in one hour should not exceed about 7 mm. in men, or 10 mm. in women who are not pregnant or near a menstrual period. A fall of 15 mm. in the first hour is definitely pathological; and in some conditions there may be a fall of 100 mm. or more in the first hour even in the absence of anaemia, notably in acute rheumatoid arthritis, myelomatosis, collagen diseases, and in the presence of cold agglutinins. The E.S.R. is usually reduced by the presence of heart failure, dehydration, or polycythaemia.

One of the values of the sedimentation-rate lies in the indication it gives of the *progress* of a patient suffering from such chronic diseases as tuberculosis, rheumatoid arthritis, or nephritis, and in its ability to detect early any recurrence of these conditions. But it is also of value in diagnosis: in distinguishing organic from functional disease; in deciding whether a patient may have a chronic infection or malignant disease, or in deciding whether a child said to be suffering from 'growing pains' is not in reality suffering from rheumatic fever.

Too much reliance must not be placed on the E.S.R. as a diagnostic aid. When raised it points to the possibility of organic disease. It may be normal, however (inexplicably), in a minority of chronic infections and even in the presence of metastases especially from prostatic carcinoma.

In assessing the significance of a high sedimentation-rate one must bear in mind that it may be exaggerated by any anaemia present, especially if the anaemia be acute.

One can apply suitable corrections to the E.S.R. in the presence of anaemia but these, which are dependent on the red-cell count, ignore the effect of red cell-size and deformation and are not of very much value.

CLASSIFICATION OF THE ANAEMIAS

An Aetiological Classification of the Anaemias:

1. Due to acute blood-loss.
2. Due to defective erythropoiesis (dyserythropoietic)
   Deficiencies of
   Iron
   Vitamin B_{12}
   Folic acid
   Vitamin C
   Thalassaemia
   Sideroblastic anaemias
3. Due to bone-marrow failure (hypoplastic or aplastic)
   Malignant disease
   Leukaemia and lymphoma
   Chronic renal failure
   Chronic infection
   Collagen diseases
   Chronic liver disease
   Endocrine deficiencies
   Chemical poisons and drugs
   Irradiation
   Idiopathic
   Congenital
4. Due to increased blood destruction (haemolysis)
   Abnormalities of the red cell
   Hereditary spherocytosis
   Hereditary non-spherocytic anaemias
   Red-cell-enzyme deficiencies
   Haemoglobinopathies
   Paroxysmal nocturnal haemoglobinuria
   Abnormalities of red-cell environment
   Immune lysis
   Non-immune lysis

The above classification is based on aetiology and is not of great value as a basis for reaching a diagnosis. In clinical practice a system is required through which a diagnosis can be reached from the changes found in the peripheral blood; such a classification is based mainly on the haemoglobin content of the red cells and any change in their average size. The changes observed provide a lead to possible causes of anaemia, but usually several possible causes are suggested and then additional tests are required to differentiate these.

Changes in the Red Cells common to Most Severe Anaemias. In most severe anaemias certain striking alterations occur in the appearance of the red cells. Though in themselves such changes are not in general pathognomonic of any particular type of anaemia, they give important information as to the condition of the marrow function and frequently assist in leading us to a precise diagnosis. These changes are as follows:

1. HYPOCHROMIA. This term refers to a deficiency of haemoglobin within the red cells, and can be detected in a stained blood-film as a pallor extending from the centre of the cell outwards. It is expressed quantitatively by the M.C.H.C. which falls below 32 per cent, by the M.C.H. which is less than 29 μμg., or by the colour index which is less than 1·0. Hypochromia is almost always a result of iron deficiency and less commonly a deficit in haemoglobin synthesis as a result of thalassaemia or one of the sideroblastic anaemias.

2. MICROCYTOSIS AND MACROCYTOSIS. These terms refer respectively to a diminution or an increase in the size and volume of the red cells. The changes can be appreciated to some extent in a stained smear of blood but are expressed quantitatively by the M.C.V. which falls below 82 μ³ in the first instance and increases above 92 μ³ in the second. Microcytosis is a common accompaniment of hypochromia, most often when it is due to iron deficiency. Macrocytosis is associated with many clinical states, particularly vitamin-B_{12} and folic acid deficiency and some haemolytic anaemias. Reticulocytes, being larger than mature red cells, produce a macrocytosis when present in sufficient numbers.

3. ANISOCYTOSIS. Increased irregularity in the *sizes* of the cells. Normally, though there is some irregularity in the sizes of the cells, the great majority approach closely the average diameter of about 7·2 μ (*Fig.* 20), but often in severe anaemia the irregularity is very striking owing to a large excess of small cells (microcytes) and of large cells (macrocytes) (*Fig.* 21).

4. POIKILOCYTOSIS. Increased irregularity in the *shapes* of the cells. Normally the red cells are approximately circular; but when poikilocytosis is marked they may appear oval or pear-shaped or have the form of a torpedo or an hour-glass (*Fig.* 24). One must not mistake for poikilocytosis, crenated cells (*Fig.* 23) or cells that have become polygonal through mutual moulding when fixed in too close apposition with one another (*Fig.* 22). Poikilocytosis is common in anaemias due to defective erythropoiesis.

5. POLYCHROMASIA. Irregularity in the *colour* of the cells. In some anaemias some of the red cells have a slightly violet or bluish tint instead of a uniform pink (*Fig.* 28). Such cells when stained supravitally are found to be reticulocytes (*Fig.* 27); however, all reticulocytes do not appear as polychromatic cells in the Romanowsky-stained film.

6. STIPPLED CELLS—PUNCTATE BASOPHILIA. Such cells appear like ordinary red cells except for the presence of minute dark-staining particles, like fine pepper, scattered through their cytoplasm (*Fig.* 28). The cytoplasm itself may stain normally or may show any degree of polychromasia. All stippled cells, like all polychromatic cells, appear similar to reticulocytes when stained supravitally. Generally, stippled cells are numerous only when anaemia is severe; but in lead poisoning they may be seen in large numbers even when anaemia is mild or absent, and, moreover, the stippling tends to be coarser than that in anaemia generally.

7. NUCLEAR REMNANTS. These are occasionally found in the red cells and take one of two forms: the *Cabot ring* stains a deep purple and appears as a loop arranged more or less circularly or as a figure-of-8; *Howell-Jolly bodies* consist of one, two, or sometimes more deep-purple-staining, sharply defined, round dots of varying size (*Fig.* 26). Both types may be found in any severe anaemia; but Howell-Jolly bodies almost invariably appear in large numbers immediately after

splenectomy, and may persist as a prominent feature for years. Large and numerous Howell-Jolly bodies are associated with splenic atrophy.

8. TARGET CELLS. These are abnormally thin cells often bowl-shaped. In stained smears the haemoglobin appears to be arranged as a central disk and also as a peripheral ring, thus giving a resemblance to a target. They occur in severe iron-deficiency anaemia and strikingly in thalassaemia (*Fig.* 19).

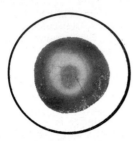

Fig. 19. Target cell showing central and peripheral accumulations of haemoglobin. (*Drawing by Miss G. Sanders.*)

9. SPHEROCYTES. These are cells in which the diameter : thickness ratio is decreased, and they appear in the stained film as dense cells usually reduced in diameter. These cells show increased osmotic fragility and are found mainly in hereditary spherocytosis and in the presence of a circulating red-cell antibody.

Normal red cells may be suspended in solutions of buffered saline of which the concentration has been reduced from the isotonic level of 0·9 per cent to 0·45 per cent before appreciable haemolysis appears. In anaemia generally the fragility is diminished, but in hereditary spherocytosis it is always increased if not with fresh cells then after blood has undergone sterile incubation for 24 hours. Sometimes the increase is great and haemolysis may appear in a saline concentration of 0·8 per cent, but sometimes the increase is only slight. The fragility may also be increased in cases of acquired haemolytic anaemia but when that is so the red cells will give a positive direct Coombs' test which will distinguish this condition from hereditary spherocytosis.

10. INCLUSION BODIES. These are not usually apparent in Romanowsky-stained smears but can be demonstrated with methyl violet and cresyl blue stains. They appear to be denatured fragments of haemoglobin and may be present in red cells in the haemoglobinopathies and glucose-6-phosphate dehydrogenase deficiency and are produced by a variety of drugs and chemical agents.

11. SICKLE CELLS. These cells are characteristic of the presence of haemoglobin-S in the red cells. They occur frequently in the peripheral blood when the Hb-S concentration of the cells is greater than 60 per cent but much less frequently if the concentration is below this. However, sickling may readily be produced in all Hb-S-containing cells if the concentration exceeds 40

per cent by the reduction of the haemoglobin. This is readily accomplished by the addition of 1 per cent sodium metabisulphite to the blood. Completely sickled cells occur with high concentrations of Hb-S while with the lower concentrations sickling is only partial, and the red cells are likened to the appearance of holly leaves.

12. RETICULOCYTOSIS. Normally the reticulocytes do not exceed more than 1–2 per cent of the red cells, but in haemolytic anaemias or in the presence of chronic blood-loss they may be increased to between 5 and 40 per cent. The absolute number of reticulocytes in the peripheral blood is a direct reflection of the increase in erythropoietic activity of the bone-marrow above normal. In routine practice, however, it is tedious to count absolute numbers of reticulocytes and the numbers are usually expressed as a percentage of the red cells present. It is obvious, therefore, that the reticulocyte count may be artificially raised if the red-cell count is reduced, and the percentage of reticulocytes should therefore be corrected for any change in the packed-cell volume of the peripheral blood. Apart from haemolysis and chronic blood-loss the reticulocytes also increase in the peripheral blood when bone-marrow activity is increased in response to some therapeutic agent. The rise in the reticulocyte count then occurs before any rise in haemoglobin can be appreciated and it is therefore an early sign of the effectiveness of treatment. The reticulocyte count is one of the most valuable tests in an analysis of anaemia, a high count indicating increased erythropoietic activity in response to haemolysis or blood-loss, whereas a low reticulocyte count suggests that the cause of the anaemia is diminished production of red cells. The reticulocyte count thus helps to resolve the question of which side of the steady-state balance between the production and destruction of red cells is disturbed. From the appearance of the peripheral blood and the measurements that have been discussed it is possible to classify anaemias according to the size and haemoglobin content of circulating red cells.

13. PRIMITIVE RED CELLS. Primitive precursors of red cells and white cells are normally only seen in the bone-marrow but occasionally the red-cell precursors occur in the blood in the newborn infant. Either or both types of cells make their appearance in the peripheral blood in certain pathological conditions when the blood-picture is known as leuco-erythroblastic or myelophthisic. This picture is important to recognize as it usually results from some mechanical damage to the bone-marrow such as may occur in secondary carcinomatosis, leukaemia, and myelofibrosis. Occasionally during the response to severe anaemia primitive red cells appear in the peripheral blood, and likewise in response to severe infection primitive white cells may appear in the peripheral blood.

RED-CELL MATURATION. The mature red cell represents the culmination of the processes of cell division and maturation which begins with the primitive undifferentiated stem-cell of the bone-marrow. This cell is multipotent and may differentiate into any of the cells formed in the bone-marrow. Its differentiation into red-cell precursors and the rate control of this process is a result of the production of the hormone erythropoietin which appears to be formed in the kidney. Excess of this hormone can usually be demonstrated in most patients who are anaemic, but not those who have renal failure from chronic nephritis. The various stages of development of the cell precursors in the bone-marrow can be differentiated according to their staining characteristics. The earliest cell is large, with bright blue-staining cytoplasm and with a large nucleus in which the chromatin structure is very finely stippled and which may contain one or more nucleoli. As the cell matures it tends to shrink in size, while the cytoplasm gradually loses its basophilic staining properties, and after passing through a series of intermediate violet stages, becomes frankly pink, like the fully mature red cell. This is due to the formation of haemoglobin. The primitive nucleus also tends to get smaller, so that it comes to occupy less and less of the cell; at the same time the nucleoli disappear, and the nuclear chromatin, at first so delicate, begins to form clumps of increasing coarseness. These clumps by coalescing gradually become larger and less numerous, until finally they merge into a single solid-looking, structureless mass, the *pyknotic* nucleus, which is the final stage before its extrusion from the cell. The precursors of the mature red cells found in the bone-marrow are known as *normoblasts* and are differentiated into pronormoblasts and early, middle, and late types according to the features described above. In certain types of anaemia due to vitamin-B_{12} or folic acid deficiency an abnormality of red-cell maturation occurs, when the cells are known as *megaloblasts*. This disturbance is essentially one of nucleic acid synthesis and as a result the nucleus contains less stainable material (RNA), the megaloblast appears as a cell in which nuclear maturation and formation is deficient, yet maturation of the rest of the cell—that is the formation of haemoglobin in the cytoplasm—has occurred normally.

The Significance of Red-cell Changes in Diagnosis. The morphological abnormalities described above enable us to make certain general deductions as to the state of the marrow function and sometimes more specific deductions as to the nature of the anaemia. In general, irregularities in the size, shape, and staining of the red cells, a moderate increase in reticulocytes, and the appearance of a few late type erythroblasts are indicative of a purely physiological response on the part of the marrow to repair the anaemic state. With a normal marrow function these features tend to vary with the severity of the anaemia. Their absence, or existence in only moderate degree, when anaemia is severe suggests an aplasia of the marrow or some depression of its function. Thus in anaemia associated with long-continued

infection or toxaemia (e.g., rheumatoid arthritis, chronic infection) the marrow response may be poorly developed, indicating depressed function. In aplastic anaemia the response may be practically absent, so that one finds the remarkable combination of extreme anaemia with a practically normal-looking blood-film. On the other hand, the presence of the more primitive types of nucleated red cells, often in association with an extreme degree of the above marrow reaction, suggests some fundamental disturbance of the marrow rather than a simple physiological response, e.g., chronic myelogenous or acute leukaemia, or carcinomatosis of the skeleton. There are, however, certain particular combinations of the above responses that are more or less pathognomonic of a disease. An obvious excess of macrocytes, often with a tendency to an elliptical shape, together with nucleated red cells of various types, suggests pernicious anaemia. The striking appearance of a minority of large, deeply staining cells of uniform size and shape, standing out against a background of a majority of small, pale cells of irregular size and shape, is characteristic of the recovery stage of an iron-deficiency or post-haemorrhagic anaemia. It is often seen during the spontaneous recovery from the latter condition and is then of considerable diagnostic value. As it invariably occurs after about the seventh day of the successful treatment with iron of an iron-deficiency anaemia, it serves as a therapeutic test of the correctness of the diagnosis, or if that is not in doubt, as an indication of the efficacy of the iron preparation being administered.

Normal Varieties of White Cells. Variations in the total white-cell count and in the relative numbers of the different types of white cells normally found in the blood often assist in differential diagnosis. The total count varies considerably between individuals and in the same individual even in the course of the day. The normal limits may be taken as 5000 and 10,000 per c.mm. There are five main varieties of normal white cell: (1) Polymorphonuclear neutrophil granulocyte—55–65 per cent; (2) Polymorphonuclear eosinophil granulocyte—0·5–3·0 per cent; (3) Polymorphonuclear basophil granulocyte—0·25–1·0 per cent; (4) Small and large lymphocytes—20–35 per cent; (5) Monocytes, or large mononuclear cells—5–10 per cent. It is common practice to express the numbers of different white cells in the peripheral blood as percentages but this can be very misleading and the numbers should always be converted into absolute numbers for comparison. Thus a patient with a total white-cell count of 2000 per c.mm. with 70 per cent lymphocytes does not have a lymphocytosis but rather a neutropenia.

The different types of white cells have different functions. Granulocytes are phagocytic cells and the granules are really lysozomes containing a variety of digestive enzymes. These enzymes either digest organic matter engulfed by the cells, or they are liberated following lysis of the cells in the tissue spaces. Monocytes are also

2

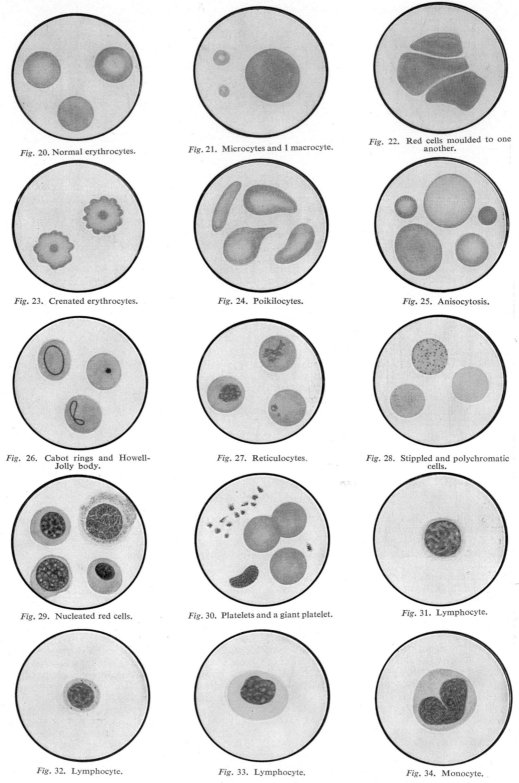

Fig. 20. Normal erythrocytes.

Fig. 21. Microcytes and 1 macrocyte.

Fig. 22. Red cells moulded to one another.

Fig. 23. Crenated erythrocytes.

Fig. 24. Poikilocytes.

Fig. 25. Anisocytosis.

Fig. 26. Cabot rings and Howell-Jolly body.

Fig. 27. Reticulocytes.

Fig. 28. Stippled and polychromatic cells.

Fig. 29. Nucleated red cells.

Fig. 30. Platelets and a giant platelet.

Fig. 31. Lymphocyte.

Fig. 32. Lymphocyte.

Fig. 33. Lymphocyte.

Fig. 34. Monocyte.

Figs. 20–34. RED AND WHITE BLOOD-CELLS AS SEEN UNDER AN OIL-IMMERSION LENS.
(The blood-films were stained with Leishman's stain.)

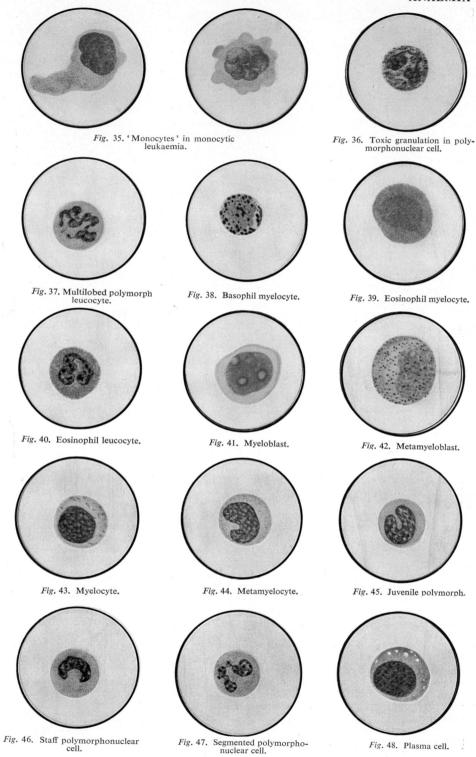

Fig. 35. 'Monocytes' in monocytic leukaemia.

Fig. 36. Toxic granulation in polymorphonuclear cell.

Fig. 37. Multilobed polymorph leucocyte.

Fig. 38. Basophil myelocyte.

Fig. 39. Eosinophil myelocyte.

Fig. 40. Eosinophil leucocyte.

Fig. 41. Myeloblast.

Fig. 42. Metamyeloblast.

Fig. 43. Myelocyte.

Fig. 44. Metamyelocyte.

Fig. 45. Juvenile polymorph.

Fig. 46. Staff polymorphonuclear cell.

Fig. 47. Segmented polymorphonuclear cell.

Fig. 48. Plasma cell.

Figs. 35–48. WHITE BLOOD-CELLS AS SEEN UNDER AN OIL-IMMERSION LENS.
(The blood-films were stained with Leishman's stain.)

phagocytic but leave the blood-stream and migrate through the tissues, a phenomenon not shown by granulocytes. Lymphocytes, on the other hand, are non-phagocytic but are responsible for the production of antibodies, and for gathering the information that leads to the appropriate production of an antibody in the lymph-glands. Whereas granulocytes only survive 4 or 5 days in the circulation lymphocytes may pass in and out of the circulation and live for several months or years. The appearances with Romanowsky's stain are:

1. *Neutrophil granulocytes* have a deep blue, compact nucleus, which is generally multilobed but sometimes single-lobed and S-, T-, or C-shaped, and pinkish-violet cytoplasm with fine brownish granules (*Figs.* 37, 45, 47).

2. *Eosinophil granulocytes* have a nucleus similar to the above cells but most often bilobed, and much coarser granules, which tend to fill the cytoplasm completely, are uniform in size, round in shape, and stain anywhere between a pale pink and a pillar-box red (*Fig.* 40).

3. *Basophil granulocytes* have a nucleus similar to those of the above cells, but generally both nucleus and cytoplasm are largely obscured by numerous dark-blue-staining granules which vary greatly in size (*Fig.* 38).

4. *Lymphocytes* have dark-blue-staining nuclei which may be round, oval, or more or less notched, in which the chromatin has a coarse, 'lumpy' arrangement. The cytoplasm stains sky-blue, and though generally free from granules may contain a few coarse red granules (*Fig.* 31). The small lymphocyte has relatively little cytoplasm (*Fig.* 32); the large lymphocyte has a larger nucleus and relatively more cytoplasm (*Fig.* 33).

5. *Monocytes* may superficially resemble large lymphocytes. The nucleus, however, is usually kidney-shaped, and the chromatin structure is more delicate. The cytoplasm stains steel-blue, appears excessively thin and finely spongy (*Fig.* 34). Most often there are no visible granules, but occasionally one can make out numerous extremely fine reddish granules.

In most cases in making a differential count there is no point in differentiating between large and small lymphocytes. Normally the small forms considerably outnumber the large. As far as possible one should distinguish between monocytes and large lymphocytes, but one often comes across individual cells in which this distinction is impossible. The normal percentages of the five types of white cells given above apply to the adult, but minor variations outside those limits need not by themselves be of pathological significance. In infants after the first few days of life the lymphocyte and polymorphonuclear neutrophil percentages become practically the reverse of what they are in the adult: lymphocytes up to 60 per cent, polymorphonuclear neutrophils about 25 per cent. The change from the infantile to the adult type of differential count is gradual and very variable in its rate: sometimes the adult count is found in comparatively young infants,

sometimes the infantile type of count may persist more or less markedly till puberty or even later, and this last is more likely to happen in females than in males.

Apart from the various types of leukaemia, in which there may be an increase in the total white-cell count (*leucocytosis*) of enormous proportion, there are numerous conditions in which a more moderate increase occurs. Though this subject is considered elsewhere (*see* LEUCOCYTOSIS, p. 493) it is necessary to mention a few points in the present connexion. A leucocytosis is most often the result of an increase in the numbers of the polymorphonuclear neutrophil cells; and this occurs in the majority of acute infections, and sometimes in toxaemias and new growths and after an acute haemorrhage. A leucocytosis due to an increase in the numbers of lymphocytes (*lymphocytosis*), apart from that normally found in infants, may occur in whooping-cough, rubella, tuberculosis, syphilis, and particularly in infectious mononucleosis, and usually in the convalescent stage of any infection. An increase in eosinophils, which is seldom large enough to produce a significant increase in the total white-cell count, may occur in most parasitic diseases, in diseases involving the skin, in allergic conditions like asthma, angioneurotic oedema, serum sickness, during liver therapy in pernicious anaemia, and sometimes in Hodgkin's disease. A diminution of the total white-cell count (*leucopenia*) is almost invariably the result of a gross reduction in the numbers of polymorphonuclear neutrophil cells. This occurs regularly in typhoid fever and occasionally in overwhelmingly severe infections of a type which normally produces a neutrophil leucocytosis. It most often occurs in an extreme degree in blood diseases such as aplastic anaemia, whether idiopathic or secondary, in acute leukaemia, whether the total white count be high or reduced, and in agranulocytosis, due to various drugs which have a selective effect on the granulocyte-producing elements of the marrow. In a lesser degree it is a useful diagnostic point in pernicious anaemia and Banti's syndrome.

Abnormal Varieties of White Cells. Whereas the above five types are the only kinds of white cells normally found in the circulating blood, other types may make their appearance under certain conditions. The most important of these are *myelocytes* and *myeloblasts*, which are both precursors of the granulocytes and normally only found in the marrow.

MYELOCYTES. It is generally accepted that the single-lobed polymorphonuclear cells are in a slightly earlier developmental stage than the fully matured multilobed polymorphonuclear cells. As one passes back through more primitive stages the nucleus grows fatter, becoming in turn sausage-shaped, kidney-shaped, deeply indented, and, still earlier, oval or round; at the same time its chromatin becomes less compact and its staining less dense. The cytoplasm meanwhile tends slightly to change its colour from less of a pink-violet to more of a muddy-violet; but the granules remain as before, neutrophil, eosinophil (*Fig.* 39), or basophil according to the type of cell. In a still earlier stage the cytoplasm loses all its pinkish tint and becomes frankly blue, while the three specific types of granules tend to become replaced by non-specific bright-red granules. The typical myelocyte may be taken as a cell with round or oval nucleus, with cytoplasm which is more pink than blue and which still retains its specifically staining granules (*Fig.* 39). The later cell, with more or less kidney-shaped nucleus, may be called a late myelocyte or *metamyelocyte* (*Fig.* 44); while the earlier cell, with frankly blue cytoplasm and red granules, may be called a *promyelocyte*.

MYELOBLASTS. These cells, though precursors of all the granulocytes including the myelocytes, are themselves non-granular. With their clear blue cytoplasm and finely reticulated nucleus they are immediately distinguishable from the more mature cells in the series, but on the other hand they are liable to be confounded with lymphocytes and monocytes. From these two cells, however, they can usually be distinguished by the finer and more homogeneous reticulation of the nucleus and by the presence frequently within the nucleus of one or more lighter-staining, egg-shaped areas (*nucleoli*), demarcated from the rest of the nucleus by a definite condensation of the chromatin (*Fig.* 41).

The primitive granulocytes occur in excessive numbers in chronic myelogenous leukaemia and acute leukaemia; but they may be sufficiently numerous to complicate the diagnosis both in carcinomatosis of the skeleton and in pernicious anaemia. One may also see moderate numbers of myelocytes and even a few myeloblasts in very severe infections. In infancy, however, both with anaemias and with infections, all these cells occur much more commonly; one must therefore be extremely cautious in attaching any grave prognostic significance to their appearance in the blood of young children.

OTHER ABNORMAL WHITE CELLS. Three other types of abnormal cells remain to be mentioned. The *lymphoblast*, or primitive lymphocyte, closely resembles the myeloblast; but the internal structure of the nucleus is somewhat coarser, and the nucleoli are demarcated by a much heavier chromatin condensation. A small percentage of lymphoblasts are occasionally seen in chronic lymphatic leukaemia; and a greater number in acute lymphatic leukaemia. In young children with a lymphocytosis a few may occur without particular significance. They, or cells indistinguishable from them, may be quite numerous in glandular fever. In infectious mononucleosis several types of morphological abnormality may be found in the lymphocytes. Sometimes they closely resemble lymphoblasts but more commonly their cytoplasm stains deeply and their nuclear pattern is coarse and segmented; the cells resemble abnormal monocytes. The *monoblast* also closely resembles the myeloblast; but the nucleus instead of being round may be kidney-shaped or convoluted, and the cytoplasm may

contain very fine reddish granules and show pseudopodia (*Fig.* 35). Some authorities regard this cell as quite distinct from the myeloblast; others regard it as an abnormal variety of myeloblast. It is found in large numbers, together with cells resembling more or less normal monocytes, in certain cases of acute leukaemia which are sometimes distinguished as 'monocytic leukaemia'. The *plasma cell* has an extremely deep-blue cytoplasm often with peripheral vacuoles, and a nucleus with coarse structure which is usually eccentric (*Fig.* 48). An occasional plasma cell may appear in normal blood, and they tend to be more frequent whenever there is a lymphocytosis. Plasma cells, or cells closely resembling them, may occur in the peripheral blood in rubella, infectious mononucleosis, and the earlier stages of infective hepatitis. In myelomatosis, abnormal types of plasma cells are usually found in great numbers in the marrow. Most of these so-called 'myeloma cells' are distinguishable from ordinary plasma cells; they exhibit certain features not usually found in normal plasma cells: large variations in size and shape, a tendency to occur in sheets or close groups, the possession of multiple nuclei, and the presence in their cytoplasm of what look like clear spherical globules, pink or blue in colour, known as 'Russell bodies'. When some of these features are present, and especially when the cells are very numerous, a diagnosis of myelomatosis is practically certain. However, plasma cells may comprise as much as 5–20 per cent of the marrow cells in many other conditions, such as chronic infections and secondary carcinomatosis, and in diseases where the serum gamma-globulin is increased, as in systemic lupus erythematosus.

THE L.E. CELL PHENOMENON. By suitable techniques this phenomenon can be demonstrated in the marrow or peripheral blood of most patients suffering from systemic lupus erythematosus. The characteristic appearance is a circular homogeneous mass of basophilic material (probably a lysed polymorph or lymphocyte nucleus) with the stretched-out nucleus of one or more polymorphs plastered round its circumference (*Fig.* 49). The finding is a valuable aid in the diagnosis of systemic lupus erythematosus.

Sampling and Examination of the Bone-marrow. Examination of the bone-marrow is of very great importance in the diagnosis of blood diseases. It may be sampled in one of two ways: either by aspiration of material through a needle which is inserted into the medullary cavity of a bone, or by biopsy of a solid piece of compact and cancellous bone. The bone-marrow aspirate obtained is prepared as a smear on a glass slide, while the biopsy requires decalcification before sectioning. The aspirate is stained with Romanowsky stains, whereas the biopsy is usually stained by ordinary histological methods. It may be valuable when aspirating bone-marrow to add a small amount of heparin and to centrifuge the material into a plug which can also be sectioned. The importance of this plug and of biopsy material is that an impression can be gained of the architecture of the bone-marrow which is not apparent in a smear and may be disorganized in certain diseases. Bone-marrow aspirations are usually made through the sternum, iliac crest, or vertebral spines, whereas a biopsy is usually obtained either by a trephine, or surgically, from the iliac crest. Bleeding is not usually a hazard unless the patient

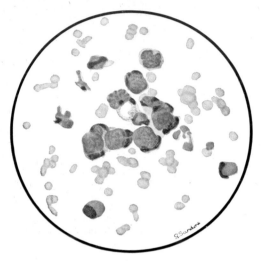

Fig. 49. The lupus erythematosus (L.E.) or Hargraves cell, showing oval inclusion bodies displacing neutrophil nuclei to periphery. (*Drawing by Miss G. Sanders.*)

has thrombocytopenia or some other haemorrhagic conditions. Films from the marrow sample are made in exactly the same way as blood-films; and it is equally important to make the films thin if one is going to obtain unshrunken and properly stained cells. To the naked eye a marrow film has a very characteristic appearance: it is obviously greasy. This point may be most useful; for if on examination one finds it to contain very few nucleated cells, the question arises as to whether the case is one of aplastic anaemia or whether the sample is of blood instead of marrow; the greasy appearance of the film may help to settle the matter.

The composition of normal marrow varies within wide limits. Here we need give only a few approximate figures which will suffice for the recognition of those conditions in which the marrow shows gross variations from the normal. The white cells are usually between three and eight times as numerous as the erythroblasts. Of the white cells, neutrophil granulocytes and their precursors form about 85 per cent, lymphocytes seldom exceed 15 per cent, while eosinophilic granulocytes are generally between 1 and 6 per cent, monocytes around 2 per cent, and basophilic granulocytes fewer than 1 per cent. In the neutrophil granulocyte series the most numerous cells are the polymorphonuclear cells and the metamyelocytes, while the most primitive type,

the myeloblast, forms generally less than 1 per cent of the total white count. Among the erythroblasts the large majority are of late type, while the remainder, with the exception of less than 1 per cent which are of the earliest type, are of intermediate type. Finally the megakaryocyte, from which thrombocytes are probably derived, and which is a very large cell with numerous deeply staining and overlapping nuclei, constitutes from 0·1 to 1 per cent of the nucleated cells.

Aspiration of the bone-marrow is liable to certain artefacts, as the tip of the needle may on occasions be in a sinusoid and predominantly blood only is aspirated. It is therefore not always possible to be certain about the degree of cellularity of the bone-marrow; in assessing this a biopsy specimen is more valuable. Certain points are looked for when examining a bone-marrow smear. First, the cellularity of the bone-marrow; secondly, whether there is a predominance of one type of marrow cell; thirdly, whether the maturation of the different types of marrow cells is occurring normally; and fourthly, whether any abnormal cells are present. The cellularity of the marrow is decreased in hypoplastic and aplastic anaemias whereas in all other types of anaemias it is increased either as a result of effective or ineffective erythropoiesis. The cellularity of the marrow may also be increased when one type of cell predominates to the exclusion of the others, as occurs in the leukaemias, myelomatosis, and secondary carcinomatosis. The ratio of erythroid to myeloid cells (normally 1 : 3) may be assessed and found of value in diagnosing hypoplasia of one cellular element of the marrow provided there is no reason to suspect that other elements are abnormal.

Examination of the marrow is usually of value in the following conditions:

1. The megaloblastic anaemias: The marrow in these anaemias is usually very cellular and there is a predominance of erythropoietic cells. Erythropoiesis is, however, largely ineffective. The important change is in the character of the red-cell precursors which in varying numbers appear as megaloblasts.

2. In acute leukaemia the normal elements of the marrow are largely, and often almost completely, replaced by either myeloblasts, monoblasts, or lymphoblasts. Since this is equally the case when the condition is completely aleukaemic as regards the blood, this finding is often a most important aid to the diagnosis.

3. In chronic lymphatic leukaemia the marrow contains a large number of lymphocytes as compared with the normal upper limit of about 15 per cent. This is of diagnostic value when, as quite often happens in this condition, the total white count is only slightly raised and there is but a moderate lymphocytosis.

4. In chronic myeloid leukaemia the marrow is extremely cellular with a predominance of myelocytes, metamyelocytes, and mature granulocytes. There is usually only a slight increase in myeloblasts. Culture and analysis of the marrow

will reveal the presence of a Philadelphia chromosome.

5. In aplastic anaemia one characteristically finds a film containing extremely few nucleated cells which give a differential count practically identical with that of the blood. The greasy appearance of the film to the naked eye will, however, make it clear that one has in fact obtained a true sample of marrow. In order to be sure that a hypocellular marrow is not the result of an artefact a biopsy should also be obtained.

6. Abnormal cells may be found in the marrow smear. Myeloma cells, deposits of secondary carcinoma and Gaucher cells, and occasionally Reed-Sternberg cells may provide valuable diagnostic evidence. In myelomatosis the presence of abnormal cells is usually striking when they constitute some 10–60 per cent of the marrow elements. Rarely there is only a small percentage of such cells or the disease may be focal and none is seen.

7. In thrombocytopenia examination of the marrow will reveal the presence or deficiency of megakaryocytes, and demonstrate any abnormality of their morphology. Clinical interpretation of these changes is uncertain.

8. The bone-marrow may be stained for iron and in certain types of anaemia sideroblasts may be seen. Sideroblasts are nucleated red cells with iron granules arranged around the nucleus, and they may occur secondary to malignant disease and infections or as a primary condition which is sometimes responsive to piridoxin.

Apart from the confirmation or exclusion of the above conditions, the examination and interpretation of the marrow picture are unlikely to serve any useful purpose except in very expert hands. However, a sternal puncture should be performed in all obscure anaemias, leucopenias, and thrombocytopenias, as in a considerable proportion of such cases one of the above diseases will be found to be responsible.

Clinical Classification of Anaemia. The important diagnostic criteria in this classification are the haemoglobin concentration in the red cells, their size, and the presence or absence of reticulocytosis.

HYPOCHROMIC. NORMOCYTIC/MICROCYTIC:
  Iron deficiency
  Thalassaemia
  Sideroblastic anaemias
  Chronic infections

NORMOCHROMIC. NORMOCYTIC:
  Without reticulocytosis:
    Bone-marrow failure
  With reticulocytosis:
    Blood-loss
    Haemolysis

NORMOCHROMIC. MACROCYTIC:
  Without reticulocytosis:
    Vitamin-B_{12} deficiency
    Folic acid deficiency
    Vitamin-C deficiency
    Thyroid deficiency

    Bone-marrow failure (occasionally)
    Chronic liver disease
  With reticulocytosis:
    Haemolysis
    Chronic liver disease

HYPOCHROMIC. MACROCYTIC:
  Combined deficiencies of iron and/or vitamin B_{12} and folic acid.

LEUCOERYTHROBLASTIC

We now pass on to consider the classes of anaemia, grouped according to the blood-pictures they present.

A. HYPOCHROMIC ANAEMIAS

1. Iron-deficiency anaemia (+ post-haemorrhagic anaemias).

2. Thalassaemia.

3. Sideroblastic anaemias.

4. Chronic infection (*see* p. 43).

The essential feature of this group of anaemias is the hypochromia in the peripheral blood-film. Red-cell indices show a low M.C.H.C. (<32 per cent) and colour index, and the size of the red cells may vary but tends to be microcytic. The haemoglobin concentration in the peripheral blood is always reduced but the red-cell count is often normal or only slightly reduced unless the anaemia is severe. Target cells are often seen in the peripheral blood-smear; in iron deficiency, however, they are few in number whilst in thalassaemia they are plentiful. Iron deficiency is by far the commonest of this group of anaemias and in practice makes up 90 per cent of all anaemic patients in the United Kingdom. Failure of patients with a hypochromic anaemia to respond to iron suggests that they are either bleeding or that they are suffering from one of the other two alternative diagnoses; in this respect a serum iron estimation may be of value in arriving at a diagnosis, as it is always low and the transferrin undersaturated in iron-deficiency anaemia.

1. Iron-deficiency and Post-haemorrhagic Anaemias. Blood-loss leads to anaemia when the rate of loss outstrips the capacity of the bone-marrow to replace the deficient cells or when iron deficiency supervenes as a result of a more chronic form of loss. After a sudden large loss of blood, e.g., as a result of injury, or of haematemesis or haemoptysis, there may be no immediate change in the blood. The passage of fluid from the tissues into the circulation to restore the original blood-volume, with the consequent dilution of the blood, takes time; it may require one to two days for the dilution to reach a maximum, and for the red cells and haemoglobin to drop to their lowest levels. After this the red-cell count and haemoglobin percentage start to rise, but since the haemoglobin is replaced more slowly than the red cells, the former lags behind the latter. Immediately following an acute haemorrhage the red-cell count and haemoglobin estimation do not, therefore, afford a measure of the blood-loss, which has to be assessed on general clinical grounds or by blood-volume measurements. The patient presents the symptoms described on page 27. Following on an acute haemorrhage there is generally a leucocytosis, up to about 20,000 per c.mm., with an increased percentage of polynuclear cells and some immature forms.

In cases of chronic haemorrhage, as in bleeding from a chronic gastric or duodenal ulcer or from carcinoma of the stomach, frequent nose-bleeds, piles, or menorrhagia, iron deficiency results. It is common in infestation with *Ankylostoma duodenale*. On the whole the more severe the bleeding and the longer it has continued, the more pronounced will be the anaemia.

In many *post-haemorrhagic anaemias* the occurrence of haemorrhage may be immediately obvious from the history, e.g., bleeding piles, nose-bleeds,

symptom in diaphragmatic hernia and carcinoma of the caecum. It may arise from a growth of the rectum or colon, or from an ulcerative colitis. It occurs in patients with a gastric or a duodenal ulcer, with a carcinoma of the stomach, as the result of prolonged consumption of aspirin, or with oesophageal varices in association with cirrhosis of the liver. In such cases there may be HAEMATEMESIS (p. 329), MELAENA (p. 523), or occult blood in the stools.

A common and often undiagnosed cause of hypochromic anaemia is diaphragmatic hernia which may give rise to repeated blood-loss, usually small, but sometimes severe. The anaemia is commoner in para-oesophageal hernia than in hiatus hernia and is commoner in middle-aged women than in men. Heartburn may provide the clue to the hiatal variety, but there may be no

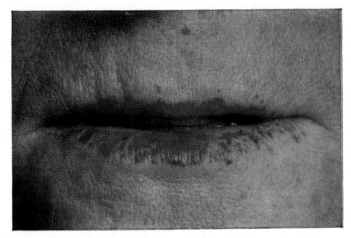

Fig. 50. The lips in telangiectasis. (*Dr. R. G. Ollerenshaw, Manchester Royal Infirmary.*

excessive menstruation, haemoptysis, haematemesis, melaena, or post-partum haemorrhage. In many cases, however, the fact that haemorrhage has occurred is by no means obvious from the history, and it is only from a study of the blood-picture that an anaemia of haemorrhagic type is suggested. To confirm this, and to discover the site of the bleeding, a very thorough investigation may be required. A patient with bleeding piles often underestimates the significance of the blood-loss and may not even mention them unless specifically questioned; yet the piles may be the sole cause of the anaemia. Women may fail to mention that they suffer from excessive menstruation, for the simple reason that it has continued so long that they do not realize it is abnormal. In essential thrombocytopenic purpura the anaemia may be severe and yet the purpura may never have been noticed; and here the difficulty may be increased by the purpura being temporarily absent at the time of the physician's examination.

A frequent cause of severe anaemia is bleeding from the alimentary tract. It may be the presenting

localizing symptom of the former type. X-ray examination is an essential study of the digestive tract in all obscure cases of hypochromic anaemia.

Haemophilia and *Christmas disease* must also be remembered as possible causes of anaemia. The origin of the blood-loss is usually obvious as it is generally due to injury or to a tooth extraction. But the discovery of the underlying blood condition depends on finding a history of excessive bleeding from cuts and scratches and of bleeding into joints on slight trauma; a family history of such symptoms occurring only in the males; and an association of a prolonged clotting-time with a normal bleeding-time. Another cause of severe anaemia is the rare disease *hereditary telangiectasia* (*Fig.* 50) (*see* ANGIOMA, p. 59). The telangiectases, which may bleed copiously when situated only in such obscure sites as the back of the nose, the stomach, or the intestine, render the diagnosis difficult.

Apart from bleeding, other causes of iron deficiency are inadequate dietary intake and deficient absorption. Inadequate dietary intake is common in areas of poverty and malnutrition and results when the intake is less than about 10 mg. a day in women and 5 mg. daily in men. Normally, 10–30 per cent of the intake is absorbed depending on whether a state of iron deficiency exists or not, but in some diseases absorption is permanently impaired. This is likely to occur in the malabsorption syndromes, particularly those that result from non-tropical sprue with gluten sensitivity and other causes of steatorrhoea. All types of iron-deficiency anaemias show similar types of blood-picture, but in the presence of chronic haemorrhage, providing the deficiency of iron is not too severe, reticulocytosis is a common feature; this is absent in other types of

that the hypochlorhydria contributes to the latter situation. It is most important in hypochromic anaemia in middle age to exclude a gastro-intestinal neoplasm.

The symptoms of iron-deficiency anaemia can often be traced back over several years. Dyspnoea and tiredness are common. Glossitis is frequent: at first the tongue is red, later it becomes smooth, flabby, and pale (*Fig.* 52); but actual soreness and pain are not nearly so common as in pernicious anaemia. Dysphagia occurs in some cases, constituting the *Plummer-Vinson syndrome* (anaemia, dysphagia, and glossitis). A characteristic but rare finding is a flattening or

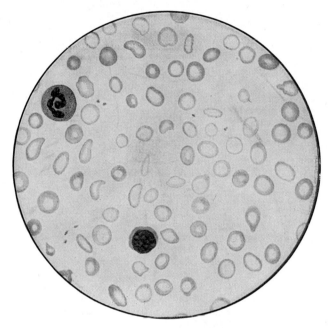

Fig. 51. Blood-film in iron-deficiency anaemia. Note the pale centre of the red cells, anisocytosis, and poikilocytosis.

iron deficiency until after some form of iron therapy has been given.

Iron-deficiency anaemia, as a result of inadequate diet or inadequate absorption, also occurs in infancy, in pregnancy, following gastro-intestinal operations, in association with gastro-intestinal fistulae, in idiopathic steatorrhoea, and occasionally in tropical sprue. (*Fig.* 51.)

Iron-deficiency anaemia is sometimes seen in middle-aged women in whom no obvious site of bleeding is found. This condition has received the name of *idiopathic hypochromic anaemia* and has been attributed to the presence of achlorhydria, which is thought to interfere with iron absorption. There is some doubt about the significance of the lack of gastric acid in the cause of this type of anaemia and it is probable that the anaemia results more often from an occult form of blood-loss which is associated with a failure of the normal augmentation of iron absorption that occurs in iron-deficiency states. It is possible

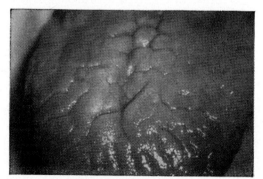

Fig. 52. The tongue in iron-deficiency anaemia. (*Professor Martin Rushton.*)

actual concavity of the finger-nails, which are brittle and tend to split longitudinally—*koilonychia*. A mild degree of splenomegaly is occasionally found. A reliable early sign in confirming the diagnosis, and in indicating the efficacy of the iron preparation used, is the appearance, within a few days, of a reticulocytosis, or of the new normal red cells: these stand out in the films as large, deeply staining cells of uniform shape and size, in striking contrast against the background of smaller and paler poikilocytes. The haemoglobin may be expected to rise at an average rate of about 1 per cent a day. Sternal puncture, which is seldom necessary in this condition, may show a great increase above normal of the proportion of nucleated red cells to white cells, the increase being mainly in respect of the late type nucleated cells.

CHLOROSIS, which was once common, is now rare. It constituted a severe iron-deficiency anaemia occurring in young women which was probably a result partly of inadequate dietary intake and partly of excessive iron loss from menstruation.

An iron-deficiency anaemia may also coexist with anaemias due to other causes such as pernicious anaemia.

2. Thalassaemia. This condition used to be known as 'Mediterranean anaemia' or 'Cooley's anaemia' and is basically an inherited disorder of haemoglobin synthesis. In addition to this defect there is also a mild haemolytic process and the serum bilirubin is commonly raised. However, the excess bilirubin is derived more from ineffective erythropoiesis in the bone-marrow than from lysis of mature red cells in the circulation. The full disease only appears in homozygous individuals, heterozygous persons carrying the trait. However, there is some degree of clinical variation in the disease state, and it is common to separate three clinical types of thalassaemia; the minor form or trait in heterozygous individuals, and the major form and an intermediate form which differ in severity and occur in homozygotes. The disorder is widespread throughout the world although particularly common in the Mediterranean races.

Thalassaemia Major. This produces severe anaemia which appears in an affected child about 9 months after birth. The commonest form involves a failure to synthesize the β-chains of adult haemoglobin, and as soon as haemoglobin-F synthesis decreases after birth so anaemia becomes apparent. An analogous form in which there is a failure to synthesize the α-chains of haemoglobin is probably not compatible with life in homozygous individuals. The anaemia of β-thalassaemia is severe and individuals show certain striking clinical features: their facies are often mongoloid in appearance due to an increase in the medulla of the maxillary bones which elevates the outer eyelids, a thickening of the vault of the skull leads to a turret-shaped head, and splenomegaly and hepatomegaly are usually marked. Extensive hyperplasia of the bone-marrow and extramedullary erythropoiesis are responsible for the bony changes and the hepatosplenomegaly respectively. X-rays of bones show characteristic changes: the long bones show rarefaction and disorganized architecture in many sites, and the skull shows curious radiating spicules in the vault. The peripheral blood-count is characteristic. There is a severe anaemia with marked hypochromia, some microcytosis, and many target cells in the peripheral blood-smear; in addition nucleated red-cell precursors are usually present in moderate numbers. The serum bilirubin is moderately raised by the presence of increased unconjugated pigment; the serum iron is usually raised and the transferrin 180 per cent or more saturated. The diagnosis can be established by demonstrating an excess of foetal haemoglobin in the individual's red cells by electrophoresis. The bone-marrow in thalassaemia major is very cellular, containing very many erythrocytic precursors, amongst which sideroblasts are usually numerous.

Thalassaemia Minor. This is the trait form of the condition and can affect either the synthesis of α- or β-chains of haemoglobin. β-Thalassaemia minor is a very mild condition in which there is only minimal anaemia and mild hypochromia but it is important in differential diagnosis from mild iron-deficiency anaemia, from which it can be differentiated by the serum iron which is normal, and by haemoglobin electrophoresis in which an excess of haemoglobin-A_2 is found. There is no hepatosplenomegaly. It is well to remember that iron deficiency can complicate thalassaemia minor. α-Thalassaemia minor is a slightly more severe condition than the β-form and a moderate anaemia usually exists. Diagnosis can be made by finding haemoglobin-H (β_4) in the red cells on electrophoresis, whilst in infancy an excess of haemoglobin-Barts (γ_4) is usually found. Mild hypochromia is present in the peripheral blood with occasional target cells, and inclusion bodies may be seen in the red cells on supravital staining. α-Thalassaemia major seems to be incompatible with life.

None of the thalassaemic states responds to iron or any other form of treatment. Occasionally in thalassaemia major the spleen may get very large and a functional state of hypersplenism occurs which responds to some extent to splenectomy. However, as a rule this operation is not of value. Thalassaemia major may be complicated by haemochromatosis, which arises partly as a result of the excessive iron absorption that occurs in any chronic anaemia and partly as a result of repeated blood transfusions.

3. Sideroblastic Anaemias. This heading describes a group of anaemias in which hypochromia is the predominant finding in the peripheral blood although a dimorphic picture is common, some cells being fully haemoglobinized. In the bone-marrow the characteristic finding is an excess of erythrocytic precursors many of which show sideroblastic granules on staining for iron. This syndrome includes a number of different conditions which may be inherited or acquired. The acquired forms usually complicate malignant disease, especially the leukaemias, myeloid metaplasia, chronic infections, and collagen diseases, and also the administration of isonicotinic acid hydrazide (isoniazid; INH) in tuberculosis therapy. Inherited forms include thalassaemia and a rare type which can be differentiated by having normal haemoglobins on electrophoresis. In all these conditions the serum iron is raised and the transferrin nearly or fully saturated. In some, the sideroblastic granules appear to arrange themselves in rings around the nuclei of the erythrocyte precursors; and it is sometimes thought that the types showing these 'ring sideroblasts' are particularly likely to respond to pyridoxin therapy.

B. NORMOCHROMIC, NORMOCYTIC ANAEMIAS

In this group of anaemias the red-cell indices are usually within normal limits although the mean corpuscular haemoglobin concentration may be decreased and the red cells then appear hypochromic. This blood-picture may therefore mimic the hypochromic blood-pictures described previously but the changes are less marked and the red cells are normocytic. In addition the serum iron is not decreased and is usually within normal limits. The anaemias of this group are a result of a number of factors which tend to produce bone-marrow hypoplasia but which particularly affect the red-cell precursors. The diseases which cause these changes in the bone-marrow are as follows:

1. INFECTION. The following infections may produce this type of anaemia:

Bacterial endocarditis (especially when subacute)
Tuberculosis
Chronic pyogenic infections in the bone, lungs, and kidneys
Chronic pyelonephritis
Secondary syphilis
Chronic rheumatic heart disease.

Usually the infections causing this type of anaemia are obvious, and the finding of the anaemia is a secondary feature to the causal condition.

In *chronic infections* and '*toxaemias*' and in *neoplastic disease*, anaemia is often severe and occasionally the presenting symptom. It is often normocytic but may be normochromic or hypochromic. It is possible that the anaemia is largely due to some toxic inhibition of the marrow function, but blood-loss and iron deficiency may occur. Of the infections one may mention colitis, particularly ulcerative colitis and tropical dysentery, in which much blood may be lost from the bowel; chronic pelvic infections; psoas abscess; sinusitis; secondarily infected tuberculosis with cavitation; bronchiectasis; lung abscess; the late stages of syphilis in adults, or congenital syphilis in children, and rheumatic fever. With a long-standing *empyema* there is usually severe anaemia; the anaemia may develop remarkably quickly, and increasing pallor after the crisis of lobar pneumonia or in connexion with bronchopneumonia not infrequently suggests the presence of an empyema. Chronic sepsis may produce *amyloid*

disease, which is itself associated with a progressive and often extreme anaemia.

In *infective* or *bacterial endocarditis* (see FEVER, PROLONGED, p. 287) there is a progressive and ultimately severe anaemia, which may occasionally predominate to such an extent as to obscure the diagnosis. More often, however, the anaemia helps in distinguishing the conditions from other forms of valvular heart disease, in which anaemia does not ordinarily occur. It is often difficult to distinguish a heart case without infective endocarditis from one in which infective endocarditis has supervened; but the *occurrence of a progressive anaemia should always arouse suspicion*.

In most *acute infections*, apart from those described in which a definite haemolytic anaemia is produced, the course of the disease is usually not long enough to cause any significant degree of anaemia. Exceptions to this rule include: puerperal septicaemia and other septicaemias due to a haemolytic streptococcus, in which a profound anaemia, partly haemolytic in nature, may develop very rapidly; typhoid fever with or without intestinal haemorrhage; acute rheumatism when it runs a prolonged course; and sometimes small-pox and the severer forms of scarlet fever. In cholera extreme dehydration tends to produce an apparent polycythaemia, but during convalescence when fluid returns to the circulation an anaemic state supervenes.

2. COLLAGEN DISEASES. Rheumatoid arthritis, polyarteritis nodosa, and diffuse lupus erythromatosus are disorders which are commonly accompanied by this type of anaemia.

3. MALIGNANCY. The anaemia of cancer may be profound and may result either from chronic blood-loss which leads to the hypochromic anaemia of iron deficiency, or from bone-marrow depression, producing the type of anaemia under consideration. A third type of anaemia may occur in widespread cancer, leucoerythroblastic anaemia (see below), when the bone-marrow is infiltrated. Any type of malignancy may produce a normochromic, normocytic anaemia and the malignant process may or may not be widespread. The anaemia presumably results from some toxic factor produced by the malignant cells which causes erythropoietic hypoplasia. Although the hypoplasia most commonly affects the red-cell precursors it may on occasions affect white-cell and platelet production also, and a pancytopenia may result. Like other forms of malignancy the reticuloses such as Hodgkin's disease and lymphosarcoma tend to produce this type of anaemia. One special tumour, however, thymoma, is responsible for a form of chronic anaemia in which the white cells and platelets never appear to be involved.

Some forms of *cancer* produce the most profound anaemia, others produce no anaemia at all. We have seen how metastatic carcinoma of the skeleton occasionally produces leucoerythroblastic anaemia (p. 54), but it occasionally gives rise to severe anaemia without the appearance of immature red and white cells, and it often leaves the blood-picture entirely unchanged. Those carcinomata which ulcerate and cause much bleeding naturally result in profound anaemia, but occasionally there may be a progressive anaemia with a carcinoma when there is no discoverable bleeding; and this is particularly so when there are widespread metastatic deposits even though the skeleton is not involved. Presumably the cause in such cases is some toxic depression of marrow function. In malignant disease generally the sedimentation-rate of the red cells is usually raised; there is often a leucocytosis due to an increase in polymorphonuclear cells; and there is occasionally a considerable degree of pyrexia. The growths that are most prone to produce severe anaemia are those of the alimentary canal, particularly of

4. CHRONIC LIVER DISEASE. Cirrhosis of the liver may be associated with anaemia of several types. Chronic blood-loss from oesophageal varices can produce iron deficiency, chronic alcoholism may result in folate deficiency with a macrocytic anaemia, whilst a normochromic normocytic anaemia also commonly occurs.

Cirrhosis of the liver sooner or later leads to anaemia, although in the earlier stages the alcoholic patient may have no anaemia but rather a rubicund complexion. The diagnosis usually depends on the history and clinical findings, and on the occurrence of HAEMATEMESIS (p. 329), ASCITES (p. 75), and a slight degree of JAUNDICE (p. 433). The patients often have some evening pyrexia. The skin tends to be pigmented; and the facies, with its sallow pallor and diffuse but

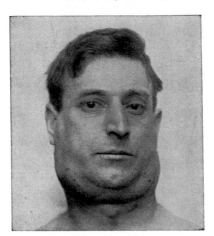

Fig. 53. Hodgkin's disease simulating Mikulicz's syndrome.

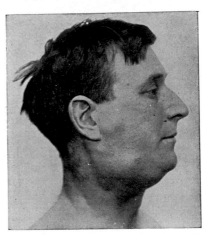

Fig. 54. The same patient as in Fig. 53 seen in profile.

the stomach. Sometimes the only symptoms are those of the anaemia; but usually the diagnosis of carcinoma of the stomach is suggested by the history. The anaemia is usually hypochromic, due to bleeding from the growth, but a megaloblastic anaemia may be superimposed and give rise to a mixed blood-picture. In most cases the growth will be found on X-ray examination. *Lymphosarcoma* (*see* LYMPH NODE ENLARGEMENT, p. 513) must be mentioned, as it may produce a blood-picture which is indistinguishable from that of chronic lymphatic leukaemia; but in the majority of the cases there are no blood changes except anaemia.

Hodgkin's disease (*Figs.* 53, 54) produces no characteristic blood changes; but a blood examination is always called for in view of the generalized LYMPH NODE ENLARGEMENT (p. 513) and the enlargement of the spleen (p. 746). In the later stages anaemia develops and may become extreme, and there is then usually a marked polymorphonuclear leucocytosis. Only a small proportion of the cases show an eosinophilia, but occasionally this may reach a high level, and when present in an early stage may be helpful in the diagnosis.

rather uneven pale-brown pigmentation and numerous fine telangiectases (spider naevi), is very characteristic. The anaemia complicating cirrhosis of the liver may be due to several factors. Folate deficiency (mainly dietary in origin) may produce a macrocytic picture, whilst in acute alcoholism the anaemia is usually normocytic and may be haemolytic. A reticulocytosis may indicate chronic bleeding from oesophageal varices, when there will also be hypochromia, or the presence of a haemolytic condition. A mild degree of haemolysis often accompanies chronic liver disease but on occasions may become marked (especially if there is jaundice, Zieve's syndrome) and may be accompanied by a positive antiglobulin test. Congestive splenomegaly may be associated with chronic bleeding from varices or with a state of hypersplenism (Banti's disease) when red cells, white cells, or platelets, or all of them (pancytopenia), are destroyed within the spleen. In the earlier stages it can only be diagnosed by a process of exclusion, by ruling out such conditions as Hodgkin's disease, pernicious anaemia, the leukaemias, acholuric jaundice, essential thrombocytopenia, malaria, and other infections, and by a splenic venogram.

In children the diagnosis may be extremely difficult owing to the still more numerous causes of splenomegaly and anaemia. *Gaucher's disease*, which is most common in Ashkenazic Jews and is usually first seen in children, may be associated with hypersplenism, and frequently with an expanded plasma volume. A definite diagnosis can only be made by splenic or sternal puncture and the discovery thereby of the typical Gaucher cells. *Leishmaniasis* (*kala-azar*) may also produce an extreme degree of splenomegaly. There is usually an irregular fever, leucopenia, and anaemia. The diagnosis depends on finding the protozoa, *Leishmania donovani*, in cells obtained by sternal or splenic puncture.

5. ENDOCRINE DEFICIENCY. Deficient secretion of the thyroid, pituitary, and adrenal glands are all associated with anaemia. In the case of thyroid deficiency the anaemia may be macrocytic and a definite statistical association exists between thyroid disease and pernicious anaemia. These anaemias tend to improve wi.h treatment of the glandular deficiency.

6. CHRONIC RENAL FAILURE. The anaemia of chronic renal disease is probably due to defective production of erythropoietin as a result of destruction of the renal substance; it may occur in any type of chronic bilateral renal disease and usually appears when renal function is sufficiently reduced to raise the blood-urea persistently above 100 mg. per 100 ml. It is commonly overlooked as a cause of anaemia because there may be no other clinical features present to suggest the renal background. However, if the uraemia is severe and chronic then other features of renal failure such as acidosis, purpura in the absence of thrombocytopenia, and the foetor of uraemia may be present.

In *chronic nephritis* anaemia is very variable. It may occur in the nephrotic variety, but often despite the whiteness of the person there is surprisingly little anaemia. Severe anaemia is more frequent in the late stages of nephritis when there is gross nitrogen retention. This may be accompanied by purpura, which usually takes the form of numerous large ecchymoses; but the platelets are not reduced, which suggests that the cause may be some toxic effect on the capillary walls.

7. CHEMICAL AGENTS AND IONIZING RADIATION. Many chemicals and drugs may act as bone-marrow poisons and affect one or more components of cell proliferation in the bone-marrow, resulting in anaemia, leucopenia, or thrombocytopenia, or all three deficiencies together. Some chemical agents act as marrow poisons in all individuals and then the effect on the bone-marrow is usually dose dependent; other agents act only on the marrows of susceptible patients, and the effect is then not dose dependent and some form of idiosyncrasy must therefore exist. The following table shows some of the agents which produce bone-marrow failure selectively or generally. Excessive radiation also damages the bone-marrow but in a selective fashion first

depleting the lymphocytes, then the platelets, the granulocytes, and finally the red cells; this effect is dependent on the dosage of the irradiation received.

The bone-marrow in all these conditions appears hypoplastic, or even aplastic, on biopsy, the deficiency affecting one type or more of cell precursor.

CHEMICAL AGENTS INDUCING BONE-MARROW FAILURE

1. Invariable toxic action on all marrows, if the dose is sufficient:

Benzene	Antimetabolites (6-mer-
Nitrogen mustards	captopnrine, etc.)
Urethane	

2. Variable toxic action on bone-marrow probably due to idiosyncrasy:

Chloramphenicol★	Trinitrotoluene
Tetracycline	Dinitrophenol★
Sulphonamides	DDT
Streptomycin	Phenylene diamine (hair
Phenylbutazone★	dyes)★
Oxyphenbutazone★	Carbon tetrachloride★
Perchlorates★	Mepacrine
Chlorpromazine	Gold salts★
Troxidone★	Mercury salts★
Carbimazole★	Lead salts
Meprobamate	Organic arsenicals
Phenytoin	Bismuth salts★

★ Compounds associated with fairly frequent reports of bone-marrow damage.

8. IDIOPATHIC APLASTIC ANAEMIA. When this condition affects erythropoiesis in children it is known as 'erythrogenesis imperfecta' (the Diamond-Blackfan syndrome), while another form presenting with pancytopaenia in association with a group of congenital abnormalities is known as the 'Fanconi syndrome'. It is important in children and adults to exclude all the known causes for bone-marrow hypoplasia before a diagnosis of the idiopathic condition can be made as a result of exclusion.

Idiopathic aplastic anaemia is a severe anaemia in which there is little or no evidence of red-cell regeneration, associated with variable thrombocytopenia and polymorphonuclear leucopenia, and due to the normal marrow being more or less completely replaced by a pale, fatty material. Even in extreme cases, however, a few islands of normal marrow are usually to be found in some bone in the body. Typically the anaemia is normochromic, there is little or no irregularity in the size, shape, and staining of the red cells, reticulocytes are scarce or absent, and no normoblasts are present. The striking feature is that, despite the severe anaemia, the red cells in the stained film appear practically normal. The symptoms are those due to the anaemia; when the platelets are low there may be purpura and haemorrhages; and when the polymorphonuclear cells are greatly reduced, as often happens, there may be necrotic lesions of the mouth and throat. The anaemia is further distinguished by its failure to respond to any anti-anaemia drug and, most important of all, by the persistent drop in red cells and haemoglobin after they have been raised to an approximately normal level by a series of blood transfusions.

The condition is usually fatal, but presumably when the marrow is hypoplastic rather than aplastic the patient can be kept alive indefinitely by repeated transfusions; and sometimes the hypoplasia has apparently been temporary and the patient has ultimately recovered. The chances of recovery are much greater when the marrow hypoplasia is secondary to one of the causes already listed: they depend on the early diagnosis of an aplastic type of anaemia and on the timely recognition of the underlying cause of the aplasia. The differential diagnosis of the idiopathic form of the disease is simplified if we appreciate its relationship to agranulocytic angina and essential thrombocytopenia. In *agranulocytic angina* (*see* LEUCOPENIA, p. 495) the granulocytes are completely, or almost completely, absent from the blood, but there is no anaemia and no thrombocytopenia. In essential thrombocytopenia there is no reduction in granulocytes and the anaemia is hypochromic and merely secondary to the blood-loss due to the purpura. In idiopathic aplastic anaemia all three elements of the marrow are affected, though usually it is not until a late stage of the disease that the platelets and granulocytes reach those extremely low levels at which severe bleeding and stomatitis appear. Occasionally, however, these symptoms antedate those of anaemia. Cases occur illustrating all sorts of combinations of red-cell hypoplasia, thrombocytopenia, and granulocytopenia, in varying degrees of severity. Occasionally the course of the disease has been indistinguishable both clinically and haematologically from that of idiopathic aplastic anaemia, and yet the bone-marrow has been found to be very hyperplastic, showing a great increase in the proportion of nucleated red cells of all types. This condition often appears to be preleukaemic.

C. MACROCYTIC ANAEMIAS

In these anaemias the essential feature is an increase in red-cell volume and diameter. The cells may or may not also be hypochromic, depending on whether iron deficiency is an associated feature or not, and there is usually considerable anisocytosis and poikilocytosis. Only in the haemolytic group is the reticulocyte count increased before the onset of any treatment. The following conditions are associated with macrocytic anaemia:

1. Vitamin-B_{12} deficiency.
2. Folic acid deficiency.
3. Vitamin-C deficiency.
4. Hypothyroidism.
5. Haemolytic anaemias (*see below*).

Vitamin-B_{12} Deficiency. The commonest cause of this deficiency is pernicious anaemia in which the deficiency results from a failure of the stomach to secrete intrinsic factor. The cause of this failure remains unknown and in the adult is associated with total gastric atrophy and a failure

to secrete hydrochloric acid and pepsin. In children a very rare deficiency of vitamin B_{12} (juvenile pernicious anaemia) results from a failure of intrinsic-factor production but there is no associated deficiency of acid or pepsin. The relationship between these disorders is not clear. Vitamin-B_{12} deficiency may also be a result of dietary lack and occurs in very strict vegetarians and in the tropics (tropical macrocytic anaemia). Total gastrectomy and occasionally partial gastrectomy (if extensive) may lead to vitamin-B_{12} deficiency and anaemia, which may occasionally occur in the malabsorption syndromes especially when affecting the terminal ileum (regional ileitis) where the vitamin is absorbed. The fish tapeworm (*Diphylobothrium*) may also result in this deficiency because of its high avidity for the vitamin. The normal level of vitamin B_{12} in the serum is 150–600 μμg. per ml. and anaemia does not usually result until the concentration has fallen below 100 μμg. per ml.

PERNICIOUS ANAEMIA (Addison's Anaemia; Biermer's Anaemia) is a disease in adults, of insidious onset, characterized by progressive pallor, weakness, and tiredness, and frequently by symptoms referable to the alimentary system, such as soreness of the tongue, loss of taste, anorexia, nausea, abdominal pain, and diarrhoea. There is moderate but not excessive loss of weight. Frequently there is pyrexia. Usually the patient does not seek advice until the anaemia is far advanced, when the diagnosis is generally straightforward; but even in the early stages the blood-picture is often characteristic. In advanced stages other symptoms due to the anaemia include shortness of breath, headache, palpitations, oedema of the ankles, and anginal pains. Often, though not invariably, the skin has a definite lemon-yellow colour and the conjunctivae have an icteric tinge. The symptoms referable to the alimentary system may have been present for a long time and are commonly periodic in nature. In an early phase the tongue may be sore and look raw and red; later it becomes smooth, pale, and flabby, while ulcers and fissures may appear. This Hunter's or Moeller's glossitis may even arise with subacute combined degeneration of the cord before any blood changes (*Fig.* 781, p. 798). In all cases there is a histamine-fast achylia gastrica. Often the spleen is moderately enlarged.

Pernicious anaemia is not infrequently complicated by subacute combined degeneration of the spinal cord and sometimes there may be considerable mental disturbance. Though occasionally the symptoms of subacute combined degeneration of the cord may develop side by side with those of pernicious anaemia, it is much more usual for one of the two conditions to be well advanced before symptoms of the other become prominent. The commonest neurological symptoms are 'pins and needles' or numbness in the extremities, but these may be due to the anaemia *per se* or to peripheral neuritis, which is commonly found in association with the cord diseases, and not necessarily to the cord lesions. More definite neurological signs, such as loss of vibration sense, alterations in reflexes, weakness, or spasticity, are seen much less commonly in cases starting as pernicious anaemia since the advent of liver therapy; for in such cases, if properly controlled by treatment, the progress of the nervous disease is also arrested.

The essential peculiarity of the blood-picture is the increased red-cell diameter and increased mean cell volume. Because of the macrocytosis the reduction in red-cell count is proportionally greater than the reduction in haemoglobin concentration. Stained films (*Fig.* 55) may show gross anisocytosis with an obvious excess of

The final confirmation of the correctness of the diagnosis depends on the response of the patient to injections of vitamin B_{12} (hydroxo- or cyanocobalamin). The first indication is a rise in the reticulocytes which should reach a maximum figure after an interval of about six days. The height of the maximum response depends on the initial level of the red count, and should be 55 per cent for an initial red count of 0·5 million; 35 per cent for 1 million; 20 per cent for 1·5 million; 15 per cent for 2 million, and so on. As the reticulocyte percentage begins to fall, the total red-cell count and haemoglobin start to rise; and this should continue uninterruptedly

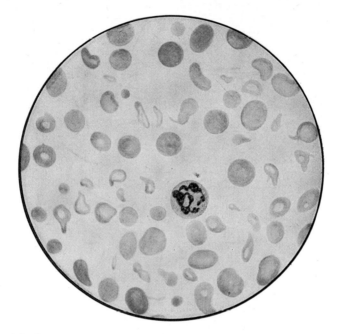

Fig. 55. Part of a blood-film from a case of severe pernicious anaemia, showing poikilocytes, microcytes, macrocytes, a nucleated red cell, and a polymorphonuclear cell with complex lobulation.

large cells which may tend to be definitely oval; in addition there may be numerous cells of grossly irregular shape. Polychromatic and stippled cells are present, but the reticulocytes seldom exceed 2 or 3 per cent of the red cells except during treatment. Nucleated red cells of all types are occasionally seen. The more mature types of these cells with pink cytoplasm, which may contain either comparatively mature compact nuclei or less mature large nuclei with open structure, also tend like the non-nucleated cells to be larger than usual. There is often a mild neutropenia. Some of these cells are unusually big and have nuclei with exceptionally large numbers of lobes which are often arranged radially like the petals of a flower (*Fig.* 55). There are occasionally a few myelocytes and rarely earlier forms. The platelets are typically diminished but seldom to a marked extent, and rarely a general haemorrhagic tendency may be present.

until the normal levels are reached. Moreover, as the normal levels are approached all the abnormal characteristics of the blood should gradually disappear.

It is important to confirm the diagnosis without waiting the six days for the reticulocyte response, and a sternal puncture should be performed before giving the first injection of B_{12}. In pernicious anaemia the marrow shows an enormous increase not only in the proportion of nucleated red cells to white cells, but also in the number of the most primitive type of nucleated red cells: large cells with deep blue cytoplasm and large nuclei with very fine chromatin structure, the so-called 'megaloblast'. The serum vitamin-B_{12} concentration is always less than 100 $\mu\mu$g. per ml. The marrow changes, the low serum vitamin B_{12}, and the histamine-fast achlorhydria confirm the diagnosis of pernicious anaemia. Occasionally if the diagnosis is in doubt it can be proved by demonstrating a failure to absorb radioactive vitamin B_{12} except in the presence of intrinsic factor (Schilling test). An interesting finding in the serum of about 70 per cent of patients with pernicious anaemia is the presence of organ-specific antibodies active against gastric parietal and thyroid cells; their significance is not yet understood. The blood-picture may be very closely simulated by a number of other conditions, and in particular by acute aleukaemic leukaemia, aplastic anaemia, and myelomatosis, each of which has a characteristic marrow picture of its own. The characteristics of the bone-marrow in pernicious anaemia completely disappear from the marrow within 24 hours of giving a single injection of liver or vitamin B_{12}. Unless, therefore, the puncture is done in the first instance, it will be of no help in confirming the diagnosis.

There are certain circumstances which may give rise to difficulties in the diagnosis of pernicious anaemia. If a physician is unaware that the patient consulting him has a few days earlier received an injection of liver or vitamin B_{12}, he might quite reasonably misinterpret the reticulocyte response due to the liver as the reticulocytosis of a haemolytic anaemia. If he is aware of this possibility he can distinguish between the two by repeating the examination a week later: the therapeutic reticulocytosis will by then have disappeared, that due to haemolytic disease will have persisted. During the therapeutic reticulocytosis of pernicious anaemia there may be poured out into the blood numbers not only of nucleated red cells but also of primitive granulocytes, and these latter may persist for several days and give a picture suggestive of myelogenous leukaemia. The question also arises in a patient who has previously been diagnosed as suffering from pernicious anaemia and has since been treated as such, whether in fact he or she ever had the disease. If the patient has been receiving adequate treatment the blood-picture will in either case be normal and of no help in the decision. A test-meal should be done and if free acid is present the original diagnosis was almost certainly in error. If treatment is stopped a year or two must elapse before the blood-picture returns to its original abnormal state, but a Schilling test will be abnormal even though treatment is continued. In this test radioactive vitamin B_{12} is given by mouth and simultaneously ordinary vitamin B_{12} is injected muscularly. If a significant amount of radioactive material can subsequently be detected in the urine it can safely be concluded that the patient is not suffering from pernicious anaemia. When anaemia is slight and the blood shows only minor variations from the normal, the diagnosis of pernicious anaemia is not always easy, e.g., in very early cases, cases almost but not completely controlled by treatment, and some cases in which subacute combined degeneration of the cord is the prominent feature. Difficulty may also arise when the macrocytic anaemia is secondary to a gross interference with absorption, as occurs sometimes in carcinoma of the stomach, after gastro-intestinal operations, in patients with gastro-intestinal fistulae, and in infestation with *Diphyllobothrium latum*. In such instances a Schilling test performed with and without an intrinsic-factor preparation is very helpful. Occasionally the peripheral blood-picture in vitamin-B_{12} deficiency is also hypochromic when there is also iron deficiency. This does not arise often but may do so if there is a bleeding lesion in the gastro-intestinal tract such as a gastric carcinoma.

Folic Acid Deficiency. We now come to an anaemia which as regards the blood and marrow pictures is very similar to pernicious anaemia but which nevertheless fails to respond to B_{12} but responds fully to folic acid. This anaemia is most frequently found in association with profound disturbances in intestinal absorption, as in sprue, idiopathic steatorrhoea, and jejunal diverticulosis. It is common in pregnancy, especially with twins when the demand for folic acid exceeds the dietary supply. It also occurs in extreme dietary deficiency as in tropical macrocytic anaemia. In recent years it has been described in patients under treatment with phenytoin (Epanutin) for the control of epilepsy and during the administration of folic acid antagonists such as amethrotrexate and pyrimethamine, phenytoin, and occasionally barbiturates. Rarely the folic acid deficiency appears to be but part of a more general deficiency so that the patient requires treatment with B_{12}, folic acid, and iron. Folic acid deficiency is common in chronic alcoholism and may complicate haemolytic anaemias and leukaemias when there is an increased demand. Clinically there are two points which may help in distinguishing a folic deficiency from pernicious anaemia: (1) the presence of free hydrochloric acid in the stomach while excluding pernicious anaemia is quite compatible with a folic acid deficiency; and (2) subacute combined degeneration of the cord while frequently associated with vitamin-B_{12} deficiency never occurs with folic acid deficiency. However, the crucial tests in the differential diagnosis of the two conditions are the serum levels of the respective vitamins and their therapeutic effects. One first gives an injection of B_{12}, and if the patient has pernicious anaemia a full reticulocyte response will occur, but if he has folic acid deficiency there will be no response. In this latter contingency one next gives folic acid by mouth, and if there is a folic acid deficiency there will be a full reticulocyte response. But it is of prime importance never to treat an anaemia with folic acid until one has proved that it is not pernicious anaemia. For in pernicious anaemia folic acid will produce a reticulocyte response and cure the anaemia as efficiently as B_{12}, but it will have no effect in preventing the subsequent development of subacute combined degeneration of the cord. In fact if pernicious anaemia is treated with folic acid the last state of the patient will be worse than the first. It must be remembered in carrying out these tests that if the patient happens to have at the time an incidental infection the reticulocyte response both to B_{12} and folic acid may be partly or wholly obliterated.

Scurvy in its fully developed form is characterized by tenderness of the bones due to subperiosteal haemorrhages, oozing of blood from swollen, spongy gums, and anaemia which is often severe. There may also be generalized bleeding from the mucous membranes and extensive purpura and ecchymoses. In the olden days it was common among mariners; but now in civilized countries, under normal conditions, it is rare except among infants and the aged. It is due to a lack of vitamin C as a result of an insufficiency of fresh food, particularly of fruit and vegetables, in the diet. *Infantile scurvy*, or *Barlow's disease*, was prone to occur in infants fed exclusively on boiled or pasteurized milk or patent foods, and usually appears in the latter half of the first year; it is exceptional in breast-fed infants. There is tenderness chiefly of the legs and the child cries when handled. In the more severe forms there is definite swelling over the bones and tenderness is extreme, so that the child lies motionless and screams out on the slightest touch. The temperature may reach 102° F. or 103° F. (39° C.), and anaemia may be profound. The gums are not usually affected unless the teeth have erupted or are about to erupt. Anaemia is usually normochromic and normocytic but may be macrocytic. If the bone-marrow appears megaloblastic, it is likely that folic acid deficiency coexists. The platelets are not grossly diminished, thus serving to distinguish the condition from essential thrombocytopenic purpura and acute leukaemia. In the absence of haemorrhages diagnosis may be assisted by finding the capillary resistance test to be positive. A blood-pressure armlet is wrapped round the upper arm and the pressure raised to a level half-way between the systolic and diastolic pressures, and kept there for five minutes. The pressure is then released; and if the test is positive numerous purpuric spots will appear on the arm distal to the armlet. The other conditions in which it may be diminished are thrombocytopenic purpura, other forms of purpura, and certain of the eruptive fevers. The way in which the patient rapidly improves under treatment with vitamin C finally clinches the diagnosis. It must be remembered, however, that infantile scurvy is often associated with rickets, and that both conditions will then require treatment.

Myxoedema is much commoner in women than in men; it usually develops slowly, but occasionally acute myxoedema leading to coma and death arises. Milder phases (hypothyroidism) are often overlooked and mistaken for middle-age fatigue or anaemia. But when advanced, the clinical picture is characteristic. The skin of the face, neck, hands, and lower limbs is most affected (*see* FACIES, ABNORMALITIES OF, p. 273). The typical spade-like shape of the hand is due to a general broadening of it and to a thickening of the fingers (*Fig.* 56). The pallor, with yellow tinge, and against this the bright malar flush stands out strikingly (*Fig.* 290, p. 273). The skin is dry and sometimes rough, and the hair tends to fall out over the forehead, at the nape of the neck, and in the outer third of the eyebrows. Constipation, achlorhydria, and loss of appetite

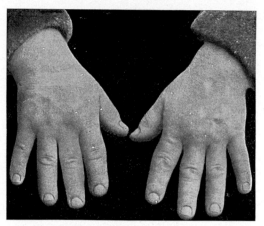

Fig. 56. Hands of a patient suffering from myxoedema, illustrating the swelling of the soft parts, the broadening of the fingers, and their consequent stumpy or podgy appearance.

are common. The expression is dull, bodily movements, speech, and mental processes are slow. Speech is further hampered by thickening of the tongue, and the voice is deep or gruff. Deafness is common and the sense of smell may be lost. Apart from the mental slowness, the patient may be irritable or suspicious and suffer from delusions and hallucinations. The pulse is slow and the temperature tends to be subnormal. There is often increase in weight; the patient may feel intensely cold, even in warm weather; symptoms are much exaggerated during cold weather. The basal metabolic rate is greatly lowered, and may be 40 per cent below normal and the serum cholesterol raised (N 154–260 mg. per ml.). The I^{131} uptake is low (N 20–50 per cent); the protein bound iodine (P.B.I) is low (N 3·5–8 μg. per 100 ml.). Examination of the blood generally reveals a moderate or even severe degree of anaemia, which may be macrocytic in type. It responds well to treatment with thyroid. Myxoedema is most frequently confused with post-menopausal obesity and psychoneurosis, nephrosis, or anaemia. Slow relaxation of the knee- and ankle-jerk (*snaky response*) is very strongly suggestive of myxoedema and thus helpful in differential diagnosis (*see* VOLKMANN'S REFLEX, p. 179). Sometimes anaemia overshadows the rest of the picture, and pernicious anaemia is suggested by the yellow tint, the malar flush, and the macrocytosis. There is an increased coincidence of hypothyroidism and pernicious anaemia, and in both organ-specific antibodies to thyroid and gastric mucosa may coexist.

D. ANAEMIAS WITH RETICULO-CYTOSIS

If a reticulocyte count is done as part of the routine blood-count of all doubtful anaemias, then a group emerges which is usually normo-chromic and normocytic, but occasionally macro-cytic, and in which the reticulocyte count is raised. The anaemias in this group are the result of either chronic blood-loss, in which case there is usually hypochromia and a low serum iron, or of haemolysis, when hypochromia is almost always absent (cf. paroxysmal nocturnal haemoglobinuria) and the serum iron raised. The haemolytic anaemias will be considered here.

Haemolytic anaemias result from the destruction of red cells within the body and typically result in pallor with an icteric tinge of the skin and conjunctiva. Apart from the reticulocytosis in the peripheral blood there is also an increased turnover of bile-pigment so that often the unconjugated serum bilirubin is raised and there is an increase in the excretion of urobilinogen in the urine and stercobilinogen in the faeces. Thus the patient appears jaundiced and has dark urine and dark stools. If the haemolysis is very acute there may also be haemoglobinuria (see p. 350) and there may be methaemalbuminaemia, which can be detected by Schumm's test. Haemolytic anaemia also leads to a depletion of serum haptoglobins. A classification of haemolytic anaemias is shown below.

HAEMOLYTIC ANAEMIAS

Due to Abnormalities of the Red Cell:
Hereditary spherocytosis
Hereditary non-spherocytic anaemias
    Elliptocytosis
    Acanthocytosis
    Stomatocytosis
    Red-cell enzyme deficiencies

Glycolytic
{ Hexokinase
  Phosphoglyceratekinase
  Pyruvic kinase

Oxidative
{ Glucose-6-phosphate dehydrogenase
  Reduced glutathione deficiency
  Glutathione reductase deficiency

Haemoglobinopathies
    S, C, D, E,
    Unstable haemoglobins
Paroxysmal nocturnal haemoglobinuria.

Due to Abnormalities of Red-cell Environment:
Immune
    Incompatible blood transfusion
    Haemolytic disease of newborn
    Auto-immune haemolytic anaemia
    Paroxysmal cold haemoglobinuria
Non-immune
    Chemical poisons (lead, benzene, phenylhydrazine, chlorates, sulphonamides, arsenic, phenothiazines)
    Bacterial and parasitic infections, snake-bites
    Chronic disease (malignancy, liver disease, collagen disease, uraemia)
    Lederer's anaemia
    Micro-angiopathic (defibrination syndrome).

1. Hereditary Spherocytosis (Congenital Haemolytic Anaemia; Familial Acholuric Jaundice) (p. 434) is a disease in which there occurs chronic haemolysis accompanied by jaundice, and in which in most cases there is splenomegaly.

Anaemia is usually present but in some patients compensation for the shortened red-cell survival by the bone-marrow is so adequate that no anaemia occurs.

Chronic ulceration of the legs occurs in some of the cases. The disease is inherited as a dominant condition from either parent. Usually a family history can be obtained: but since the anaemia and jaundice vary enormously in severity in different patients and may be so mild as to pass unnoticed, a failure to obtain a family history does not exclude the condition. There are certain characteristic abnormalities of the red cells that are pathognomonic, and these are occasionally present in some of the members of an affected family in whom all symptoms and clinical signs are missing. Moreover, only a proportion of the children of an affected parent will inherit the condition. The characteristic abnormality of the red cells, spherocytes, is an increase in their thickness in proportion to their diameter; they tend to be more nearly globular than the normal red cell, which is a comparatively thin biconcave disk. The cell *diameter* is usually diminished; but owing to the increased thickness of the cells their *volume* may be normal. The mean corpuscular haemoglobin concentration is usually raised, and there is a mixture of normal cells and smaller cells which stain deeply; the appearances in stained films are also usually characteristic: a practical absence of poikilocytes, and marked polychromasia with an exceptionally high reticulocytosis—20 per cent and often much higher, depending on the severity of the anaemia—with very few stippled cells, which distinguish it from the reticulocytosis of lead poisoning. In severe cases nucleated red cells may appear, sometimes in large numbers; there may also be considerable leucocytosis.

Although affected patients have a chronic haemolytic anaemia this is sometimes subject to acute exacerbations. The sudden fall in haemoglobin concentration which results may be due to an increase in the haemolytic process, or more commonly to a temporary aplasia of the bone-marrow which is thought to result from a deficiency of folic acid. These episodes are known as 'crises' and are either haemolytic or aplastic in type. Most, and probably all, cases of this condition show an increased fragility of the red cells to hypotonic solutions of saline (see p. 32). But sometimes this increase in fragility is only brought out by prior incubation of the patient's blood under sterile conditions for 24 hours. As would be expected in a haemolytic anaemia, the van den Bergh reaction gives a negative direct and a positive indirect result; but if there is an obstructive jaundice due to gall-stones—an occasional complication—there will also be a positive direct reaction. After splenectomy, which almost invariably leads to a complete disappearance of the anaemia, the jaundice, and the ulceration of the legs, the characteristic abnormalities of the red cells seem to remain essentially unchanged.

There are a few conditions which are liable to be mistaken for familial acholuric jaundice. Certain acquired haemolytic anaemias, acute and subacute, due to the presence of circulating antibodies, may show the same morphological features of the red cells as well as an increased fragility. But they can readily be distinguished by their red cells giving a positive direct Coombs' test—a test which is almost invariably negative in familial acholuric jaundice.

2. Sickle-cell Anaemia predominantly occurs in Negroes and is characterized by a tendency of the red cells to assume a sickle shape. It is a familial disease inherited as an autosomal recessive. Members of a family may therefore be heterozygotes, in which case they show only the trait condition, or homozygotes when they show the complete disease. The disorder is due to the inheritance of an abnormal haemoglobin molecule, the abnormality residing in one of the amino-acids in the β-polypeptide chain. This abnormality results in a tendency for the haemoglobin molecules to pack together forming crystals, when in a reduced state. Deformity of the red cells which results leads to their destruction within the circulation and at the same time blockage of small blood-vessels occurs. In the homozygous individual the process of sickling goes on continuously but is subject to episodes of acute acceleration when extensive capillary blockage may occur with resulting infarction of tissue and a considerable increase in the haemolytic rate. These episodes are known as 'crises'.

The anaemia is haemolytic and associated with jaundice, and both anaemia and jaundice may show repeated exacerbations; ulceration of the legs occurs frequently, and the spleen is usually enlarged in children, but as a result of progressive infarction it is not palpable in the adult. During a crisis there may be acute abdominal and back pain and also pain in the muscles of the thigh; there is fever and a rapid fall in haemoglobin. Between the episodes of acute crises joint pains are common, especially swelling and pain in the phalanges (dactylitis). The peripheral blood typically shows a high reticulocyte count, and in the homozygous individual some sickled cells are usually apparent; there may also be a moderate number of normoblasts, and during crises a leucocytosis. The red-cell fragility is normal. The diagnosis can be made by producing sickling by the addition of a reducing agent (1 per cent sodium metabisulphite) to a sample of peripheral blood; sickling occurs within a few minutes and can be seen readily under the microscope. Confirmation of the presence of haemoglobin-S can be obtained by electrophoresis of the haemoglobin when the quantity of the abnormal haemoglobin can be assessed. In homozygous individuals about 95 per cent of the haemoglobin is haemoglobin-S whereas in the heterozygote only 40–50 per cent is haemoglobin-S. The heterozygous individual has no symptoms and is not usually appreciably anaemic because haemolysis only occurs under exceptional situations. These circumstances are usually brought about by the presence of anoxia such as may occur with acute pneumonia or during high-altitude flights; a mild crisis may then occur with tissue infarction, often in the spleen, and the development of anaemia. The incidence of the trait is about 5–10 per cent amongst the general Negro population, but varies in different countries; about 1 per cent have sickle-cell disease. There is evidence which suggests that the presence of Hb-S in the red cells protects the individual to some extent against malaria.

Most of the many other haemoglobin variants do not produce haemolytic disease although the globin moiety may differ chemically from Hb-A. Haemoglobins C, D, and E occur rarely in Negro and Eastern races and may result in haemolysis and moderate anaemia in homozygotes. Some haemoglobin variants (Zürich, Hammersmith, Koln, etc.) show an inherent instability and denature spontaneously in the red cell, resulting in the formation of many intracellular Heinz bodies, haemolysis, and persistent moderate to severe anaemia. These abnormal haemoglobins can be detected by *in vitro* stability tests to heat, etc., and by electrophoresis.

3. Red-cell Enzyme Deficiencies. A number of inherited metabolic defects occur in the red cell and some of these are associated with shortened cell survival and a haemolytic anaemia results. The two most common defects involve the intracellular enzymes glucose-6-phosphate dehydrogenase (G-6-PD) and pyruvic kinase, and of the two the former is very much more common.

Deficiency of G-6-PD is common among the Mediterranean races and Negroes with an incidence varying from 5 to 20 per cent in different localities; its inheritance is sex-linked. The enzyme deficiency only predisposes to haemolysis in the presence of certain drugs and chemical agents (*see Table below*) which produce oxidative denaturation of haemoglobin in the cell. The enzyme deficiency results in a lack of protection against these processes. Affected males, and to a less extent affected females, may develop an acute haemolytic episode after taking one of the agents listed in the Table. There is often haemoglobinuria and marked anaemia developing rapidly with a reticulocytosis a few days later. Jaundice is common. The haemolysis is self-limiting once the most susceptible (the older) cells have been destroyed, and the remaining cells are not susceptible until they have undergone further ageing over several weeks. The patient recovers after about 10 days, the haemoglobin slowly rises to normal, and the reticulocytosis subsides, even if the offending drug is continued. In between haemolytic episodes, which may be frequent or only occur once or twice in a lifetime, the individual is well and not anaemic. Ingestion of fava beans (favism) produces one form of this type of anaemia. There are no specific changes in the peripheral blood other than reticulocytosis, but Heinz bodies may be produced in the patient's red cells by incubating blood with acetylphenylhydrazine. Estimation of the red-cell G-6-PD activity is reduced, although immediately following a haemolytic episode it may be normal because of the increased enzyme activity present in reticulocytes. The hemizygous male has much lower enzyme activities than the heterozygous female.

CHEMICAL AGENTS REPORTED TO CAUSE HAEMOLYSIS IN PATIENTS WITH GLUCOSE-6-PHOSPHATE-DEHYDRO- GENASE DEFICIENCY

8-aminoquinolines	Primaquine
	Pamaquine
	Pentaquine
Sulphonamides	Sulphanilamide
	Sulphamethoxypridazine
	Salicylazosulphapyridine
	Sulphacetamide
Sulphones	Sulphoxone
	Thiazosulphone
Nitrofurans	Nitrofurantoin
	Nitrofurazone

Acetylphenylhydrazine	Methylene blue
Fava bean	Ascorbic acid
Antipyrine	Naphthalene derivatives
Paraminosalicylic acid	Quinidine
Amidopyrine	Probenecid
Acetophenetidin	Trinitrotoluene
Acetanilide	
Acetylsalicylic acid	

Pyruvic kinase deficiency is a much rarer disorder found mainly in North Caucasians resulting in a congenital type of haemolytic anaemia in homozygous individuals. Haemolysis is continuous throughout life, anaemia moderately severe, without specific features in the peripheral blood other than the reduced enzyme activity.

4. Auto-immune Haemolytic Anaemia. These haemolytic anaemias result from the presence of an antibody in the patient's plasma which reacts with their red cells and leads to agglutination within the circulation and subsequent red-cell destruction. The antibody is an auto-antibody and will usually react with all human red cells. Occasionally it shows certain types of specificity, usually to one of the Rh antigens (especially 'e'). The antibody present is usually one of two types depending on the temperature at which it reacts. The warm antibody is usually an IgG and occasionally IgA and reacts at temperatures over 20° C. whilst the cold antibody is always an IgM. These antibodies are agglutinins but occasionally a cold haemolysin is found (see PAROXYSMAL COLD HAEMOGLOBINURIA, p. 350). The cause of the production of the antibody may not be known when the condition is termed 'idiopathic', but in many instances the antibody complicates the presence of some other disease which may be a collagen disease such as systemic lupus erythematosus (SLE), or a reticulosis such as lymphasarcoma, or chronic lymphatic leukaemia. It may also follow the administration of drugs such as methyldopa and penicillin. The cold

type of antibody may complicate mycoplasma infection of the lung.

CAUSES OF IMMUNE HAEMOLYTIC ANAEMIA:
  Incompatible transfusion
  Haemolytic disease of newborn
  Autoimmune
    Idiopathic
    Lymphoma
    S.L.E.
    Autoimmune diseases
      Myxoedema
      Hepatitis
      Rheumatoid arthritis
      Myasthenia gravis
      Colitis
  Drug-induced
    Methyldopa
    Chlordiazepoxide
    Quinine
    P.A.S.
    I.N.A.H.
    Sulphonamides
    Phenacetin
    Penicillin
    Chlorpromazine

The haemolytic anaemia which results is very variable in its severity and may occasionally be subject to episodes of acute exacerbation. Reticulocytosis is usually marked and spherocytes may be visible in the peripheral blood and some red-cell fragmentation may also be seen. The diagnosis is made by the presence of a positive Coombs' test which detects antibody either in the patient's red cells or in the patient's plasma. Splenomegaly is frequently found in affected individuals. The presence of cold antibody is often associated with the occurrence of Raynaud's phenomenon, but anaemia may not be marked. When present it is not usually responsive to treatment whereas the anaemia from the warm-type antibody usually responds to the administration of adrenal cortical steroids or splenectomy.

Other forms of immune haemolytic anaemia may complicate the administration of an incompatible blood transfusion as when the donor's cells are incompatible with the recipient's plasma antibody. Immune haemolysis is also found in haemolytic disease of the newborn when the presence of an Rh antigen in the foetus, which is absent in the mother, leads to the formation of an antibody in the maternal circulation against the foetal antigen. Depending on the amount of antibody formed by the mother and the ease with which it crosses the placenta, so there may result death of the foetus in utero, or the birth of an anaemic, jaundiced infant with moderate to severe haemolytic disease. The peripheral blood of affected infants shows reticulocytosis and numerous primitive red cells which give a positive Coombs' test. Immunization of the mother against the foetal antigen, which is inherited from the father, usually occurs only after repeated pregnancies so that the disease is not seen in the first-born but only in later children. If steps are taken to eliminate foetal red cells from the maternal circulation after the first labour, which can be done by the injection of an anti-Rh antibody, evidence suggests that the disease can be prevented in subsequent pregnancies. Affected infants may die unless treated by exchange transfusion.

5. Non-immune Haemolytic Anaemias. The *acute haemolytic anaemia of Lederer* is not a specific condition. As a diagnostic title it may be used to describe haemolytic anaemias of unclassified origin. The essential features are often a rapidly increasing anaemia associated with a slight or moderate icteric tinge and more or less pyrexia. The onset is usually fairly sudden; and the symptoms, apart from those due to the anaemia, which may be severe, include rigors, headache, backache, vomiting, diarrhoea, paralyses, and coma. Rarely there may be haemoglobinuria. Though the mortality is high in untreated cases, a few recover spontaneously within a few weeks. Transfusion, repeated if necessary, occasionally results in a dramatic recovery, but more often there is only a transient improvement in the anaemia. Splenectomy is sometimes beneficial; but cortisone, given in sufficiently large doses, may control the haemolytic process. There is a high and often extreme reticulocytosis, perhaps 50 per cent or more, and late type nucleated red cells may be numerous. There is generally quite a high leucocytosis and primitive granulocytes may be present. The fragility may be increased, in which case the red cells will show the morphological features found in familial acholuric jaundice—confusion with which will be avoided by the absence of family history or history of previous attacks.

Paroxysmal haemoglobinuria and *nocturnal haemoglobinuria* may cause anaemia (*see* HAEMO-GLOBINURIA). Apart from malaria and Oroya fever, the only infection that definitely produces a haemolytic anaemia is that due to *Clostridium welchii* (*gas gangrene*). Extreme anaemia may develop in a few hours, and there may be deep jaundice. The leucocytosis may be as high as 50,000 per c.mm., and there are large numbers of reticulocytes, nucleated red cells, and primitive granulocytes. The diagnosis is made by finding the organism in direct smears from the wound, and by culturing it from the site of infection and from the blood. Many drugs and poisons besides lead may produce a haemolytic anaemia (*see* HAEMO-GLOBINURIA, p. 350). Most of these do so only if given in very large doses when other symptoms of their poisoning overshadow those of the anaemia. Others, like *benzol* and the *sulphonamides*, more frequently produce a different type of blood disorder, and only rarely in individuals with some special idiosyncrasy give rise to a haemolytic anaemia. Individual susceptibility seems also to play a part in the acute haemolysis which may result from the use in malaria of the drug *pamaquin*. The most important drug capable of producing intravascular haemolysis, and one which can be relied upon to do so, is *phenylhydrazine hydrochloride*, which was used for this express

purpose in the treatment of polycythaemia rubra vera. An acute haemolytic anaemia also results from the bites of certain snakes, and from the ingestion of the fava bean. This last condition, known as *favism*, is most frequently seen in southern Italy and Sicily. (*See* G-6-PD DEFICIENCY.)

Malaria is described under FEVER, PROLONGED, p. 287.

Oroya fever, due to infection with *Bartonella bacilliformis*, occurs in the Andes. After three weeks' incubation there is irregular fever with headache, malaise, bone and joint pains, and later anaemia and jaundice. There is enlargement of the spleen, liver, and lymph-nodes. A considerable proportion of the severer cases end fatally. The picture is that of a haemolytic anaemia, except that there is usually a macrocytosis and a colour index above 1·0. In addition, the rod-shaped organism is to be found in the blood-films.

Lead poisoning is now a rarity and a detailed description is no longer called for. The best known features are: a blue line on the gums, which a lens shows to be composed of discrete dots; constipation; colic; various paralyses, particularly wrist-drop; optic neuritis; and in late stages arterial and chronic renal disease. In very acute lead poisoning, such as may occur in workers with lead tetra-ethyl (used in the preparation of 'ethyl' petrol), a lead encephalopathy may develop with acute mania, convulsions, and coma. The pallor of the patient is out of proportion to the degree of anaemia and is typically of an ashen-grey hue. The haemoglobin is seldom reduced below 7 g. per 100 ml.; but the striking feature of the blood is the presence of stippled cells in numbers out of all proportion to the severity of the anaemia. Further, the granules in some of the cells often tend to be unusually large. Reticulocytes are even more numerous than the stippled cells; and their numbers remain raised after the stippled cells have disappeared. A reticulocytosis is thus a more delicate though a less characteristic indication of lead absorption than is the presence of stippled cells. Reticulocytes and stippled cells are signs of *recent* lead absorption. They are thus almost invariably found in association with the abdominal symptoms. But with an acute encephalitis the blood changes may not have time to appear. Evidence of a minor degree of lead absorption, such as may be found in almost all lead workers, is not necessarily an indication of lead poisoning. Thus a count of 5 or even 10 stippled cells in every 10,000 red cells is to be expected in a lead worker, especially if he is new to the work; but when the count exceeds 10 per 10,000 red cells one should regard the degree of absorption as being outside the limits of safety. A still more sensitive test for recent lead absorption is the spectroscopic detection of porphyrins in the urine. They persist long after stippled cells have disappeared and reticulocytes have dropped to normal. Three unusual sources of lead poisoning merit special mention—the use of grease-paint by actors; cigar-making, during which cigars are cut on plates that contain lead; and electrolysis of water-pipes owing to deficiencies in adjacent electric wires.

PARASITIC INFECTIONS ASSOCIATED WITH EOSINO-PHILIA. Most of the parasites which affect man produce little or no anaemia; but many of them give rise to a striking increase in the number of eosinophil leucocytes in the blood. They are discussed under EOSINOPHILIA.

BLOOD-BORNE PARASITES ASSOCIATED WITH ANAEMIA. The four commonest diseases in man in which parasites are present in the blood are: filariasis, malaria, trypanosomiasis, and relapsing fever. In all these there may be much destruction of red cells with consequent anaemia. History of residence in a tropical country where such disease is endemic suggests the diagnosis, and examination of the blood, fresh or in films, may be confirmative. The last three diseases are described under PYREXIA, PROLONGED.

Filariasis may be latent for a long time before it produces symptoms. Its best-known effects are elephantiasis of the legs or external genitalia (*Fig.* 712, p. 711) with or without chyluria. It occurs in many parts of the tropics, particularly in some of the Pacific Islands, such as Fiji. The elephantiasis and chyluria are due to the mechanical obstruction of the pelvic and abdominal lymphatics by the mature worms. The blood exhibits more or less anaemia of the hypochromic type, with a varying degree of eosinophilia, whilst at certain times of the day or night the peripheral blood also contains the long and narrow microfilariae. There are different varieties of the organism, but they cannot be easily distinguished by the appearance of their microfilariae. Without stressing generic differences, it is important that in most cases they are to be found in the peripheral blood only at night (*Filaria bancrofti, Microfilaria nocturna*); during the day they seem to retire to the larger arteries and lungs; there are other cases, however, in which the microfilariae, very similar in appearance, occur in the peripheral blood in the daytime (*Microfilaria loa*); while yet others show no periodicity and microfilariae are present in the blood both night and day. The microfilariae have an average measurement of 300 μ in length and 7 μ in breadth, and they stain by Leishman's method. They may be found in the blood of patients who have returned to England after contracting the disease abroad.

E. LEUCOERYTHROBLASTIC ANAEMIA

Leucoerythroblastic anaemia results either from acute marrow stress (haemolysis, blood-loss, or infection) or some destructive, usually malignant, disease involving the bone-marrow. Much the commonest of these is metastatic carcinoma of the bone-marrow; the others are *leukaemia, lymphoma, myelomatosis* (*Kahler's disease*), *myelosclerosis*, and *marble-bone disease of Albers-Schönberg*. The anaemia is not necessarily severe; the striking features are the presence of nucleated red cells, and a moderate leucocytosis with immature granulocytes. Occasionally the nucleated red cells outnumber the total number of white cells. Rarely the number of primitive granulocytes may be large enough to suggest chronic myelogenous leukaemia. The peripheral blood is usually normocytic and normochromic but occasionally macrocytic. Platelets may be unaffected, but often they are reduced. When the condition is caused by carcinomatosis of the bones the dominant clinical picture is most often that of the primary or of the metastatic growth. In the latter case there may be pain, tenderness, or fractures of the bones, or neurological symptoms due to involvement of the spine with pressure on the cord or nerve-roots. In a few cases the only symptoms may be those of severe anaemia; and occasionally this anaemia may progress rapidly. Only a small proportion of all cases with metastatic growth in the bones develop the typical blood-picture; and though it is commonest when X-rays reveal extensive skeletal metastases, it may occur when the X-ray findings are limited to a single bone or even when they are negative.

Sometimes the blood-picture undergoes very rapid changes; thus the immature red and white cells may entirely disappear and then reappear after an interval. Hence a normal blood-picture can in no sense exclude carcinoma of the bones; on the other hand, the finding of the characteristic blood-picture in an adult makes such a diagnosis extremely probable, owing to the greater rarity of the other possible causes. The next step in the differential diagnosis is to search for evidence of a primary tumour, either a history of its recent removal, or its discovery by means of thorough clinical investigation. If the result is negative one must then look for positive evidence of one of the other causes.

Myelomatosis. Typically *myelomatosis* (or *multiple myeloma*) gives rise to multiple tumours arising from those bones which are the sites of the red marrow: ribs, sternum, skull, vertebrae, and the bones around the shoulder and pelvic girdles. These are associated with pain, bony in character, and may give rise to pathological fractures. Hepatosplenomegaly is unusual. Other features include neurological symptoms, such as paraplegia and root pains due to involvement of the spine, uraemia, a haemorrhagic tendency usually without any detectable abnormality of the platelets or clotting mechanism, and pulmonary infections, particularly recurrent attacks of pneumonia—and one of these may occasionally be the first sign of the disease. The X-ray appearance of the bones is usually typical and sometimes simulates that of carcinomatosis. Not infrequently there may be no radiological changes. In 65 per cent of the cases Bence Jones protein is found in the urine, and in 90 per cent the serum globulins may be grossly raised and may be abnormal; the serum calcium may also be much increased without any diminution in the serum phosphorus. The abnormal globulin is IgG in

67 per cent, IgA in 25 per cent, and IgM in 2 per cent of cases.

The disease often produces a severe anaemia, which may be a typical leuco-erythroblastic anaemia. When anaemia is the only obvious clinical manifestation, the diagnosis may depend entirely upon laboratory findings: hyperglobulin-aemia, Bence Jones protein in the urine, or the presence of the typical myeloma cells in the marrow. These are large cells with bright blue cytoplasm, and nuclei, which are occasionally multiple, with moderately fine chromatin structure. When found in large numbers the diagnosis is obvious, but sometimes only a few are present, and even their complete absence from the marrow-films in about 20 per cent of cases by no means excludes the disease. On occasions these cells are found in the peripheral blood and very rarely they are present in large numbers. A useful finding indicating a very high serum-globulin, and thus suggesting the possibility of this disease, is the coexistence of perfectly smooth blood-films with a sedimentation-rate that is grossly increased even after correction for anaemia (*see under* SEDIMENTATION-RATE, p. 30). In *myelosclerosis* pain, tenderness, and fractures of the bones never occur, while hepatosplenomegaly is commonly present. The symptoms are mainly due to the severe anaemia and the diagnosis is made by marrow biopsy. *Marble-bone disease* is most often seen in children; but, even when the patient is not seen by the physician till adult life, there is usually a history of fractures having occurred in childhood. The spleen is usually enlarged. In both this and the previous disease Bence Jones protein is never found in the urine. Finally, in the differential diagnosis of these four diseases the X-ray changes in the skeleton may be of considerable help. In infancy a blood-picture closely resembling that of leucoerythroblastic anaemia is met with in erythroblastosis foetalis.

Chronic Myeloid Leukaemia is the commonest of the three main types of leukaemia, the other two being *chronic lymphatic leukaemia* and *acute leukaemia*. It is extremely doubtful whether mixed forms of the leukaemias ever occur but chronic myeloid may terminate as acute leukaemia. The age incidences are very different: chronic myeloid leukaemia occurs between the ages of 20 and 50; chronic lymphatic leukaemia occurs in older people and rarely under 40 or 45; acute leukaemia may occur at any age, but most frequently in the first two decades. Typically the leukaemias are characterized by leucocytosis which may be much higher than in any other condition.

Though anaemia does not usually develop in chronic myeloid leukaemia until the disease is well advanced, it is nevertheless the cause of the symptoms for which the patient most frequently first seeks advice—progressive pallor, weakness, tiredness, shortness of breath, etc. Other symptoms that may first attract the patient's attention are referable to the great enlargement of the spleen, which in this condition may reach its largest dimensions and extend across the middle line into the right iliac fossa. Thus there may be dragging sensations or sensations of weight; acute attacks of abdominal pain due to peri-splenitis and infarction; or such symptoms as vomiting, flatulence, constipation, and urinary disturbances due to pressure on the abdominal viscera. There are also a multitude of other manifestations which may appear in the course of the disease, and one or other of which may occasionally give rise to the initial symptom.

Most often the diagnosis is at once obvious from the blood-picture; and since it is very rare for the splenomegaly to be slight or absent, the importance of a blood examination is practically always indicated by the clinical findings. The white cells, apart from treatment, are usually increased to between 100,000 and 500,000 and may occasionally exceed 1 million per c.mm. Even more striking is the appearance of the stained film with its remarkable number of cells (*Fig.* 57). These consist almost entirely of granulocytes, metamyelocytes, and myelocytes with only a few myeloblasts. Though they belong chiefly to the neutrophil series, there will also be numbers of eosinophils and basophils. In an early stage the predominant cell is the mature polymorpho-nuclear, while the numbers of the various other types of cells gradually tail off with diminishing maturity. As the disease develops and approaches its fatal termination, the predominant form shifts gradually in the direction of diminishing maturity. At the same time mature polymorphonuclear cells diminish in number, while myeloblasts, which at first are scarce or absent, appear in increasing numbers.

Although anaemia may be pronounced at a comparatively early stage, there is then usually but little morphological abnormality in the red-cell picture; and this, together with the paucity of reticulocytes, suggests a hypoplastic type of anaemia. In this stage the anaemia tends to improve spontaneously as soon as the white count is lowered by treatment; in later stages, however, nucleated red cells appear in the blood. In this stage the anaemia tends to be progressive and to respond poorly if at all to treatment. The average duration of the disease is about three years, some patients live less than two years, others may survive as long as five or even ten years. On the whole, the older the patient the longer is he likely to live.

In reaching a diagnosis examination of the bone-marrow is essential. This shows extreme replacement by granulocyte precursors, principally myelocytes and metamyelocytes. Chromosome culture is positive for the Philadelphia chromosome in about 90 per cent of cases and in the peripheral blood the neutrophil alkaline phosphatase is usually low (e.g., scores below 20). Late in the course of the disease the marrow may appear hypoplastic or show the changes of acute leukaemia.

Except for early cases treated successfully, when the blood-picture may become completely normal, the diagnosis of chronic myelogenous leukaemia is rarely in doubt. Infections with unusually high white-cell counts approaching 50,000 per c.mm. may resemble the condition superficially.

Chronic Lymphatic Leukaemia is characterized clinically by general enlargement of the lymphatic glands and splenomegaly, which is seldom as great as in chronic myeloid leukaemia and may be comparatively slight. Most often the initial complaint is of the glandular swelling; less often it is of symptoms referable to the enlarged spleen; and occasionally it is of symptoms due to pressure by mediastinal glands or to involvement of the skin. Symptoms due to anaemia are seldom prominent and, if so, usually at a later stage. Pyrexia and a general haemorrhagic tendency are

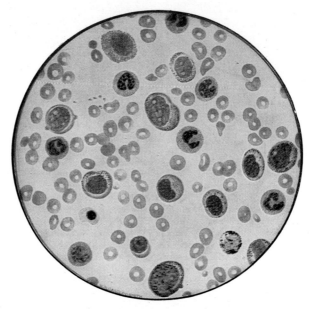

Fig. 57. Part of a blood-film from a case of chronic myelogenous leukaemia, showing a myeloblast, several premyelocytes, myelocytes, metamyelocytes, and polymorphonuclear cells, a basophil and an eosinophil cell, an eosinophil myelocyte, a nucleated red cell, a platelet, and many poikilocytes. (Leishman's stain.)

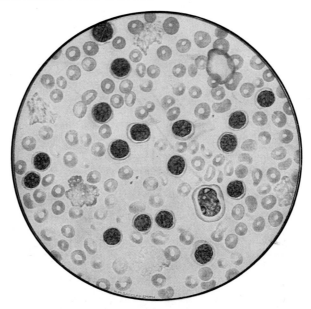

Fig. 58. Part of a blood-film from a case of chronic lymphatic leukaemia, showing a large increase in lymphocytes, one lymphoblast, several 'smudges' or disintegrated lymphocytes, and three platelets. (Leishman's stain.)

also occasional late manifestations. Tenderness over the sternum, though less frequent than in other forms of leukaemia, is sometimes present. The disease, which is often only very slowly progressive, is said to have an average duration of five and a half years; many patients live much longer, and not infrequently die of old age or some other disease, but occasionally when

anaemia or thrombocytopenia are prominent manifestations death may occur much sooner. The diagnosis is usually obvious from the blood, the necessity for the examination of which is suggested by the glandular enlargement and the splenomegaly. The leucocytosis in untreated cases is usually between 50,000 and 200,000 per c.mm.; but sometimes it is scarcely raised above

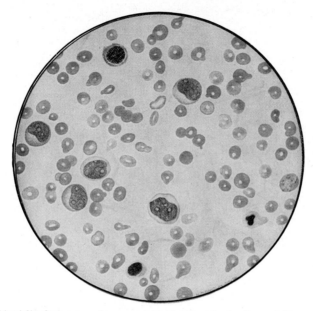

Fig. 59. Part of a blood-film from a case of acute myeloblastic leukaemia, showing myeloblasts, nucleated red cells of different types, and several polychromatic cells. (Leishman's stain.)

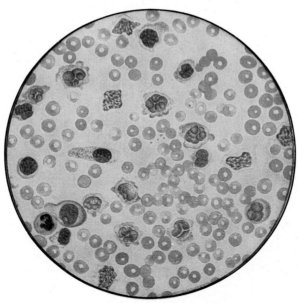

Fig. 60. Blood-film from a case of acute monocytic leukaemia showing monocytes, almost to the exclusion of other white cells, many being primitive.

the upper limit of normal, and rarely it may exceed 1 million per c.mm.

The stained film is striking: its appearance is monotonous; for, with high counts, as many as 95 per cent of the cells may be lymphocytes (*Fig. 58*). Usually these are all normal forms, the majority being small lymphocytes; but occasionally large lymphocytes predominate, and sometimes there is a small proportion of lymphoblasts. The type of cell, however, appears to bear little relation to the stage of the disease or to its rate of progression. In the films there are often large numbers of curious purple smudges, which are partially disintegrated lymphocytes (similar smudges due to disintegrating myeloblasts are often seen in acute leukaemia).

When, as is usual, the white count is above 20,000 per c.mm. the diagnosis is seldom in doubt but should be confirmed by lymph-node biopsy. Most of the high lymphocytoses due to other causes occur in children, whereas chronic lymphatic leukaemia is essentially a disease of older people. Glandular fever will be distinguished by the general signs of an infection, by the presence of numerous *abnormal* lymphocytes, and by a positive Paul-Bunnell test. In a patient with a total white-cell count close to the upper limit of normal, or slightly higher, and a lymphocytosis around 60 per cent, it would be impossible to make a diagnosis of chronic lymphatic leukaemia in the absence of typical clinical findings, such as glandular and splenic enlargement. Fortunately the diagnosis can usually be decided either by gland biopsy or by sternal puncture, for even when the lymphocytes in the blood are only slightly increased the marrow generally shows a marked lymphocytosis. Usually the films show 30 per cent or more lymphocytes scattered among the normal cellular elements, while occasionally the marrow is almost completely replaced by lymphocytes—appearances which are quite different from that of the marrow in aplastic anaemia, when the cells in the films are extremely scarce and the lymphocytosis is only relative. With the glandular enlargement of Hodgkin's disease there is a tendency for a polynuclear leucocytosis, and the absolute number of lymphocytes may even be diminished. With lymphosarcoma there is no characteristic abnormality of the white-cell picture; but at some stage lymphocytes may invade the blood, giving rise to a picture identical to that of lymphatic leukaemia. The disease that is liable to cause confusion is acute leukaemia, owing to the superficial resemblance between the blast cell and the lymphocyte (*see under* ACUTE LEUKAEMIA *below*). One of the many forms of skin involvement—*leukaemic erythrodermia*—merits special mention. It is characterized by a persistent redness of the skin, associated with intolerable itching, which may spread to include the entire body; hence the descriptive term *homme rouge* given to it by the French. In this type of disease glandular and splenic enlargement, though usually present, may be poorly developed, and the lymphocytosis

tends to be moderate and usually between 15,000 and 50,000 per c.mm.

Acute Leukaemia. Three varieties of this disease are described: *lymphoblastic*, *myeloblastic*, and *monocytic*. Acute lymphoblastic leukaemia occurs predominantly in children. The myeloblastic (*Fig. 59*) and monocytic types (*Fig 60*) are classed as acute myeloblastic leukaemia, on the grounds that no definite clinical distinctions can be drawn between them, and further that cases occur in which the type-cell may have any form intermediate between that of an apparently typical monoblast and that of a typical myeloblast. Since clinically they are essentially similar they will be considered here under the title of 'acute myeloblastic leukaemia'. In about half the cases the onset is abrupt. With some this takes the form of high fever, rigors, and prostration, in association with a severe anaemia and often a severe sore throat. In others it is a rapidly developing stomatitis with swelling and purple discoloration of the gums, which may become gangrenous—and this condition may arise spontaneously, or be precipitated by the removal of a tooth. In yet others there is a generalized haemorrhagic tendency; extensive purpura, with oozing from the gums and mucous surfaces, and bleeding from the uterus, bowel, and kidney. In these two latter types also there is severe anaemia and more or less pyrexia. Without treatment a fatal termination is seldom delayed more than two months and may occur within a few days. In about half the cases the only symptoms are those of a severe progressive anaemia. Glandular and splenic enlargement, though generally absent, may be present in a mild degree in all forms. Tenderness over the sternum is common. Rarely there is enlargement of the salivary glands —Mikulicz's syndrome—producing a facial appearance that may be compared to that which would be produced by persistent mumps.

The peripheral blood-count is variable and usually shows a normal or reduced leucocyte count rather than an increased one. Normochromic anaemia is usually present often with thrombocytopenia. The most important diagnostic feature is the presence of 'blast' cells in the blood which may number between 10 and 100 per cent of the total leucocytes.

When there are many blast cells present the diagnosis of acute leukaemia is seldom in doubt. Chronic lymphatic leukaemia is distinguished by the morphological characteristics of the predominant cell, by the absence of intermediate types of granulocytes, by the widespread glandular enlargement and the splenomegaly, by the chronic nature of the disease, and often by the age of the patient. The distinction from glandular fever may be more difficult, owing to the grossly abnormal lymphocytes that may be present, the fever, and the sore throat; but in glandular fever anaemia is absent or slight, while, in the early stages, the patient's serum gives a positive heterophil antibody (Paul-Bunnell) test, which never happens in leukaemia. The terminal, sometimes acute, stage of chronic myelogenous leukaemia can usually be distinguished by the presence of considerable splenomegaly.

In the aleukaemic phase diagnosis may be much more difficult, because only a few myeloblasts may be found during an extensive search. An aleukaemic picture may occur in the most acute form of the disease, in patients suffering from the mouth or throat lesions or from extensive purpura. The picture may be present on admission and persist to the end. Still more difficult are the cases in which the onset is insidious and the chief feature anaemia, which may be severe and associated with neutropenia and thrombocytopenia and normoblasts in the peripheral blood. A picture similar to aplastic anaemia may occur. In children it is necessary to exercise extreme caution before making a diagnosis of acute leukaemia, in order to avoid diagnosing an inevitably and rapidly fatal disease when in actual fact the condition present is comparatively harmless. One cannot emphasize too strongly that the normal lymphocytosis of infancy may persist throughout childhood, and that the blood-picture in a child is peculiarly unstable. Infections that tend to produce a mild lymphocytosis in adults may produce a high lymphocytosis in children, e.g., tuberculosis and syphilis. In whooping-cough the white-cell count may exceed 50,000 per c.mm., and 80 per cent of the cells may be lymphocytes. In addition, infections that produce a polynuclear leucocytosis in adults sometimes produce a lymphocytosis in children. Moreover, whenever there is a lymphocytosis in a child a few lymphoblasts not infrequently make their appearance. It is thus impossible to make a definite diagnosis of acute leukaemia from the blood-picture alone unless perfectly characteristic lymphoblasts or myeloblasts are present in considerable numbers. In doubtful cases perhaps the most useful guide is the condition of the red cells; for it is rare for acute leukaemia to occur in the absence of a rapidly progressive anaemia, while sometimes nucleated red cells of primitive type are present, and platelets are grossly reduced.

F. PANCYTOPENIA

This term describes a deficiency of all the cellular elements of the blood to a greater or lesser degree, so that anaemia, neutropenia, and thrombocytopenia result. Only two causes are usually found for this situation, namely aplastic anaemia (p. 45) and hypersplenism.

T. A. J. Prankerd.

ANGIOMA

The disorders considered under this heading are of two types: (1) Haemangioma or naevus vascularis, in which there is new growth of vascular tissue: (2) Telangiectasis, in which there is dilatation of existing vessels with new vessel formation.

1. Haemangioma or Naevus Vascularis. These may be further divided into cavernous and capillary angiomata.

Cavernous Angioma (Fig. 61). The simplest form is the so-called 'strawberry mark', which is a soft bright red tumour slightly raised above the

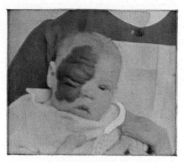

Fig. 61. Cavernous naevus.

level of the skin. It is either present at birth, or appears within the first few weeks, and while it usually grows slowly with the infant, it may occasionally grow with extreme rapidity. There is occasionally a deeper element present also, consisting of vascular tissue, but at times mixed with fatty or fibrous tissue. After a time the tumour ceases to grow and the great majority of cavernous angiomata disappear spontaneously before the child reaches adolescence and usually before the age of 5 years. The main exceptions to this rule are patients in whom the mucous membranes are involved.

The blue rubber-bleb naevus is a rare condition consisting of an angioma of the skin with a rubbery consistency and associated with vascular tumours in the gut, which may be the cause of intestinal bleeding.

Capillary Angiomata, also called 'naevus flammaeus' or 'port-wine stain', may occupy large areas of the body and are not uncommon on the face. In this condition there is closely aggregated capillary hypertrophy and dilatation. As a rule the marking is flush with the skin, but it may be considerably raised and sometimes there are projecting formations. Extensive lesions of this type on the face may be associated with similar lesions on the meninges giving rise to focal epileptiform attacks (Sturge-Weber disease). These lesions are permanent, showing no tendency to spontaneous disappearance except for some examples of the very common nuchal lesion (Unna's naevus). The above forms of haemangiomata are often referred to as 'birth marks'.

The spider naevus (naevus araneus) is an acquired lesion. There is a small central vascular spot from which radiate numerous dilated capillary branches. Spider naevi are often seen in cirrhosis and other affections of the liver. They are also very common in pregnancy. The common distribution is over the base of the neck, front of the chest, the face, and, less often, the hands. Some spider naevi disappear spontaneously and this is especially true of those appearing during the course of pregnancy.

2. Telangiectasis, or vascular dilatation, is usually acquired, but hereditary haemorrhagic telangiectasia (Osler-Rendu-Weber disease, *Fig.* 62) is a familial disease (autosomal dominant)

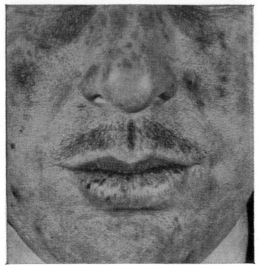

Fig. 62. Multiple telangiectases in a case of hereditary telangiectasia.

in which there occur frequent nose-bleeds in childhood followed by multiple telangiectases in middle life. Some of these appear on the mucosae especially in the mouth. There may be enlargement of the spleen. In *poikilodermia congenitale* there is a familial tendency to telangiectasia in girls. This is followed by pigmentation and atrophy. Acquired telangiectases develop later in life and tend to spread. On the face there may be simple telangiectasis caused by exposure to weather, as in sailors and countrymen or drivers of vehicles without windscreens (brewer's draymen), or they may occur in association with rosacea. They may also occur quite spontaneously. It is unlikely that the excessive consumption of alcohol plays a part in their formation. Telangiectasis is also a well-marked feature of chronic X-ray dermatitis or burn (*see Fig.* 14, p. 19). *Angioma serpiginosum* is a rare disease in which widespread patches of telangiectasis develop on various parts of the body. The origin of the disorder is obscure. In *erythrocyanosis puellarum*, which affects the lower parts of the legs in young women, there may be permanent capillary dilatation. In the tetralogy of Fallot there are sometimes telangiectases on the cheeks. Angiomata developing in later life may be due to capillary dilatation and proliferation. They produce the so-called 'Campbell de Morgan spots' on the trunk with a red colour or small, blue, raised marks on the lips.

P. D. Samman.

ANKLE-CLONUS

Ankle-clonus is best elicited with the patient on his back with the hip slightly abducted, the thigh slightly rotated externally, and the hip and knee slightly flexed. This position is maintained with one hand under the thigh while with the other hand the foot is rapidly dorsiflexed and held in that position by even pressure. A few clonic jerks can occur if the subject is cold and nervous and, indeed, in a nervous person sustained ankle-clonus, if bilaterally symmetrical, can be normal. However, it usually indicates, and always if asymmetrical, damage to the pyramidal tract. Absence of ankle-clonus does not, of course, exclude the presence of such damage.

Ian Mackenzie.

ANTISOCIAL BEHAVIOUR

Whether behaviour can be considered as antisocial or not depends to some extent upon its cultural setting. Homosexuality is a case in point. Homosexual acts between adult males are punishable by law in many countries and were so until fairly recently in the United Kingdom. In contradistinction, homosexual acts among females have never, either in the United Kingdom nor usually elsewhere, been regarded as antisocial enough to have merited legal strictures.

While much antisocial behaviour, even crime, can be regarded as being wholly or in part to mental or personality disorder, crime and mental illness are by no means synonymous. Although the 'professional' criminal cannot be regarded as a *normal* member of society, to regard his abnormal and clearly antisocial acts as the outcome of mental illness would be to stretch the definition of this too wide. There does, however, seem to be a continuum of antisocial behaviour ranging from what can be regarded as 'purely criminal' at one extreme to that which is obviously due to overt mental disorder at the other. The difficulty is to know where to draw the line. Furthermore, the one does not wholly exclude the other.

There are certain groups of psychiatric patients who are prone to delinquency. These include the *mentally subnormal*—who are over-represented among the prison population, especially among *recidivists*—those who are *emotionally* and *physically deprived*, the *emotionally immature*, those of so-called *psychopathic personality*, some *epileptics*, and some with other mental disorders. Qualification is immediately necessary. Most mentally ill persons are as law-abiding as the rest of the population; as are epileptics, some of whose antisocial conduct is a reaction to society's rejecting attitude. The mentally subnormal may be over-represented among criminals, firstly because they are more easily led astray and secondly because they are more easily apprehended. It should also be emphasized that, if properly treated, most mentally ill and mentally subnormal persons are not, as some believe, unduly given to violence.

Juvenile Delinquency. A child's emotional stability and, in consequence, the quality of his behaviour depends largely on how satisfactory are his family relationships. His parents, in particular, serve as a model for identification. Where they are themselves badly behaved, over-protective, over-strict, or above all unduly inconsistent, the child may react with neurotic symptoms, psychosomatic complaints, or delinquent behaviour. Delinquent behaviour is now becoming increasingly common among juveniles and includes such antisocial acts as *truancy, stealing, breaking and entering, vandalism* and *undue cruelty*, all of which can be interpreted as a means of satisfying needs not provided by an environment which is itself unsatisfying. The child who plays truant from school may come from a home in which obedience to authority is too lightly regarded, or may feel an urge for excitement which neither school nor home supplies. Such children often take little or no interest in school-work and for the most part fail to keep up with their school-fellows. Truancy from school is almost invariably associated with stealing. This, however, should not be confused with the *school refusal syndrome* (so-called 'school phobia') which is not associated with delinquent behaviour, but usually occurs in over-anxious depressed children who are fearful of leaving home. *Destructiveness* can to some degree be considered normal among young children, but when purposeful or prolonged may be carried out to obtain revenge on a younger sibling who, it is felt, has usurped the child's place in his mother's affection. Unconcealed *jealousy* is a common reaction of an elder child to the birth of a younger sibling. While it may manifest itself by a direct attack upon the new baby, it does so more often by fits of bad temper, sulking, vague somatic complaints, or a recurrence of *bed-wetting* after bladder control has been gained. Other reactions can occur but all of them have attention-seeking as a common factor and resentment if this need is not immediately met.

Acts of *cruelty* either to animals or undue bullying of other children are evidence of grave maladjustment, particularly when repeated, and call for expert psychiatric help. *Lying* is less serious. It may be a weapon against parental authority or merely a translation of fantasy into words. In the latter instance the child whose real life is dull, unhappy, or emotionally unsatisfying may seek to construct a world of his own and lie to protect it. *Stealing*, likewise, can often be interpreted as an attempt to compensate for an inner feeling of emptiness consequent upon emotional deprivation. However, it may also be the outcome of the bad example of parents or of mixing in a social group which maintains little or no respect for the property of others. In the investigation of all these behaviour disorders it is essential, therefore, to examine the family as a group of which the child is but a part and in which he reacts to or is influenced by the attitudes and behaviour of his parents and siblings.

Adult Delinquency. In adults, delinquency has some of the same but also different roots. Those with antisocial traits, who show a degree of irresponsibility, incorrigibility, and a more or less total disregard for common social obligations, though in the absence of overt mental disorder, may be designated as having *psychopathic* or *sociopathic personalities*. Psychopaths are of several types. Those who are aggressive may be prone to attacks of uncontrolled rage or violence in which much harm may be done to the victim.

Baby-battering is a good case in point. Although it is difficult to construct an exact profile of those prone to inflict violent injuries upon their infant children, it may be observed that the majority belong to the lower socio-economic classes, that they are often markedly immature, and, if married, many married at a younger than average age. These parents are themselves usually socially deprived and may give a history of ill-treatment during childhood, sometimes having themselves been battered. Many are also delinquent in other ways; thus the syndrome of baby-battering is not altogether distinct from violent behaviour as seen in others of psychopathic disposition. Such violent aggressive behaviour is particularly liable to be released by alcohol.

Many psychopaths, on the other hand, are not given to violence but exhibit some form of *inadequacy* as a major personality trait. Such persons seem unable to submit to the ordinary discipline of family or community life, have a poor tolerance of frustration and boredom, and escape their commitments on any pretext. They are also unable to work steadily, to plan, or to make any real progress towards achievement. When short of money they are apt to take to *pilfering* and *petty dishonesty*. They also tend to try to make a living by *gambling, touting,* and *cadging* from various social and charitable agencies. When confronted with their misdeeds they deny them; when denial is no longer possible they admit to everything with a remarkable degree of casualness and *absence of guilt*, which is in itself a most important diagnostic sign. Indeed, the psychopath is adept at putting up a façade of apparent frankness, even amiability, which may at times deceive even a skilled observer. However, the psychopath employs his charm for quite unscrupulous ends.

While *sexual offences* are frequently a symptom of psychopathy, especially such offences as sexual assault and rape, some other kinds of abnormal sexual acts are also committed by those who are not overtly psychopathic and may otherwise appear to be normal. They nevertheless betray a lack of ego strength in their behaviour. While many homosexuals, for example, lead contented and useful social lives, a proportion who engage in overt homosexual practices also show psychopathic traits, particularly those who seduce children (*pederasty*). Psychopathic traits are also evident in those who are not homosexual but make heterosexual assaults on children (*paedophilia*). In either category those who indulge in these kinds of sexual behaviour are so immature as to be incapable of relating adequately to adults of the same or opposite sex.

Other types of sexual anomalies which may be regarded as antisocial are *voyeurism* or *scoptophilia* ('peeping Toms'), *frotteurs* (men who obtain sexual excitement by rubbing against women in crowds—the 'Bakerloo syndrome'), and some perversions having a sadistic tinge, e.g. *clothes-slashing*, *bottom-pinching* and *braid-cutting* which in these days when pigtails are rare is uncommon. Probably the commonest of all deviant sexual behaviour which constitutes a public nuisance is *exhibitionism* ('indecent exposure') in which the offender exposes his genitals to women, usually in some public place such as a park or passage-way or while seated in a motor-car parked close to a pavement. Overt masturbation is a common accompaniment. *Transvestites* may constitute a public nuisance if they parade themselves abroad although on many occasions probably escape detection. Some cases of those who commit *arson* may do so on the basis of disturbed sexuality. Some are young men who are emotionally immature, sexually inhibited, sometimes subnormal, and over-attached to their mothers. *Bestiality* is the name given to sexual intercourse with animals. It is usually only practised by those who are subnormal or grossly emotionally deprived. Nearly all these anomalies are the prerogative of the male sex; if they occur at all among females they are much more likely to escape notice. *Incest* is probably commoner than is generally realized and seems to be of more frequent occurrence in rural areas than in cities, where probably it may come to notice more readily.

Drug dependence, of which alcoholism is still the commonest type, may also, as a rule, be considered a manifestation of a personality disorder or of a neurotic or more rarely a psychotic illness. Chronic alcoholics are on the whole immature, unstable persons to whom drink provides a form of recurrent escape from reality. Dependence on other drugs affects those who are in much the same category—who are in need of a pharmacological crutch, which, by its nature, soon begins to create an intrinsic need for itself. Drug addicts may be led into crime such as 'mugging' for the purpose of obtaining money with which to pay for their drugs, or may break into chemists' shops for the purpose of obtaining drugs. Many addicts are also, at the same time, drug-pushers or pedlars.

Among those who are overtly mentally ill, *depressive illness* may be an important although an uncommon cause of delinquent behaviour. A few depressives may, prior to making a suicidal attempt, murder their relatives in the delusional belief that they might otherwise suffer by being abandoned in a wicked world. Occasionally, and in the face of waning potency, those with depression and diminished libido may commit sexual offences such as exhibitionism as if to try to overcome a lack of confidence brought about by failing sexual prowess. This is rare, but important to recognize, as impotence is more readily treatable when associated with depression. Depressed middle-aged women may also indulge in *shop-lifting*, sometimes under circumstances in which it is difficult not to conclude that they have an almost patent desire to be caught and punished, thereby expiating deep-seated feelings of guilt. The majority of shop-lifters are, however, no more than common-or-garden thieves.

Mania may present problems arising out of over-activity and lack of judgement. Those in a manic or *hypomanic* state may, in the course of a few days, spend wildly beyond their means or run up extravagant bills which they cannot settle later. The *hypereroticism* which sometimes accompanies hypomania may lead to untoward sexual behaviour and in women to unwanted pregnancy.

A proportion of tramps and those charged with *vagrancy* and allied offences may be found on examination to be chronic, deteriorated *schizophrenics*. *Paranoid schizophrenics* are occasionally violent and homicidal, seeking to destroy those who they believe are responsible for persecuting them. This is rare. Rare also are the occasional murderous assaults made by young, often adolescent, schizophrenics upon their parents.

Epileptics, as has been mentioned, also tend to experience psychological difficulties by virtue of the stigma which still attaches itself to being epileptic and by the restrictions placed upon them which prevent them from driving or exclude them from following certain occupations. Apart from this, some epileptics, particularly those with *temporal lobe epilepsy*, have attacks of *automatism*, during which state they may indulge in awkward if not actually criminal behaviour. Temporal lobe epileptics also have a greater tendency to aggressive explosive outbursts than those who suffer only from grand or petit mal seizures.

In later life the onset of *dementia* may sometimes lead to antisocial conduct which arises usually out of lack of judgement and a deterioration in standards. Increased emotionality in the early stages of *cerebral arteriopathy* may lead to outbursts of rage and aggression. Sexual interference with children sometimes occurs in those who are dementing but who hitherto have lived otherwise blameless lives, presumably due to *disinhibition* together with the uncovering of latent, but hitherto well-controlled, tendencies. Some demented patients become unduly secretive, paranoid, and parsimonious, all of which may occasionally give rise to difficulty. They may hoard rubbish, refuse to pay bills or to admit the meter reader, and so on. Those with *frontal lobe* damage with or without overt dementia are particularly prone to conduct disorders. These arise once again out of lack of judgement, disinhibition, tactlessness, reckless-ness, and a lack of appreciation of the feelings of others. Such a state may follow *head injury* or *prefrontal leucotomy*, or be symptomatic of certain degenerative disorders such as *Hunting-ton's chorea*, *general paralysis*, or *Pick's disease* in which the frontal lobes are likely to be involved.

W. H. Trethowan.

ANURIA

Anuria—or suppression of urine—must be distinguished from *retention of urine*, in which urine is secreted from the kidneys but is retained in the bladder from some lesion causing obstruc-tion to the urethra, such as urethral stricture or prostatic enlargement in the male, or pressure or drag upon the urethra by a large pelvic tumour or a retroverted gravid uterus in the female, or without urethral obstruction in various forms of injury or disease of the spinal nervous system affecting the lumbar centres. In acute retention of urine (apart from the neurological variety) there is pain above the pubes, often a constant and urgent desire to pass urine, and the distended bladder forms a tense, oval, dull tumour above the pubes in the middle line. In many cases a pre-vious history of obstruction to the urinary flow will be obtained, while in others the involuntary dribbling of urine from the urethra, from the overdistended bladder of chronic retention, at once distinguishes the case from one of anuria, in which no urine reaches the bladder.

Anuria may be caused by obstruction to the outflow of urine from the kidneys, or to failure of secretion by them. The two causes frequently act in combination.

Anuria may occur and be complete without any other symptom, and it is remarkable that in the obstructive forms, especially with calculus, anuria may be complete for several days without any other symptom—latent uraemia. In the non-obstructive forms anuria may be accompanied from the onset by the various symptoms of uraemia, such as vomiting, drowsiness, convul-sive muscular twitchings, dyspnoea, and headache. In the obstructive form there may be total absence of any urine secreted, or a small quantity may be passed of low specific gravity, containing very little urea or solids. Protein is absent unless there is haematuria, or when there is urinary infection, when pus may be present also. The patient may complain of aching in one or both loin regions but, with the exception that no urine is passed, seems to be in ordinary health. The appetite is good and the mental state clear; but after a variable period, from 7 to 10 days, the patient becomes drowsy, the tongue dry, tem-perature subnormal, appetite deficient, and pupils small. There may be muscular twitching; the

drowsiness gradually becomes deeper, without any true uraemic convulsions, and death may be postponed for as long as twenty days from the onset of the anuria. This sequence is very different from that seen when anuria occurs from non-obstructive causes, when there is frequently marked disturbance of the nervous system; headache and giddiness are followed rapidly by convulsions, delirium, and dyspnoea, with vomiting and small pupils, the patient rapidly becoming comatose and dying within a few days.

Causes of Anuria:

A. OBSTRUCTIVE:

Calculus in kidney or ureter, particularly in a solitary kidney
Vesical carcinoma involving both the ureteric orifices
Ligature of both ureters
Blockage by sulphonamide crystals
Blockage by uric acid crystals
Uterine carcinoma infiltrating and obstructing both ureters
Large pelvic or abdominal tumours obstructing both ureters
Idiopathic or malignant retroperitoneal fibrosis involving the ureters.

B. NON-OBSTRUCTIVE:

In Renal Disease:
Acute and chronic nephritis
Amyloid disease
Systemic lupus erythematosus
Tuberculosis of both kidneys
Polycystic disease of the kidneys
Suppurative and non-suppurative pyelo-nephritis

Other Causes:
Tubular necrosis after operations or trauma, es-pecially after operations on the lower urinary organs, after prostatectomy, or after perineal injury
In severe collapse with low blood-pressure, either from severe injury or in association with severe febrile illnesses, such as dysentery, cholera, yellow fever
After septic abortion
After the rapid emptying of an over-distended bladder in chronic retention
In poisoning from lead, phosphorus, oxalic acid, cantharides, turpentine, or corrosive sublimate
Blackwater fever
After the administration of heavy metals—mercury, gold, arsenic, bismuth
After the administration of pituitary extract
After serum injections
After blood transfusion
In the 'crush syndrome'
From any cause of intravascular haemolysis.
With certain drugs, e.g., amphotericin B.

A. OBSTRUCTIVE ANURIA

Calculous Disease is the most frequent cause of obstructive anuria. It may occur at any age, but is commonest in men of about forty. Suppression of urine may arise from the impaction of a small calculus in the ureter of a kidney which is practically normal, or may be due to the total destruction of the renal secreting substance, which has progressed gradually and without marked symptoms. Between these two extremes there may be many stages, and the two conditions, namely, ureteric impaction and renal destruction, may exist at the same time. Clinically, it is rare for calculous anuria to arise from simultaneous blockage of both ureters by calculi; it is less uncommon to find that one kidney has been partially destroyed by previous disease, the ureter of the remaining organ then becoming obstructed by a stone. Exceptionally, the blockage of one ureter may cause reflex suppression of urine in the other kidney, especially if the function of the latter is impaired already by disease; in these cases the anuria is usually temporary. Calculous anuria may occur suddenly, and in patients who are apparently in good health, for a patient may be in good health though possessing only one kidney, the other being removed, destroyed by slow disease, or congenitally absent; or there may be a history of previous lumbar pain, haematuria, pyuria, or the passage of calculi. At the onset of anuria there is usually pain in the lumbar region and along the course of the ureter of the side most recently affected; it commonly lasts a day or so and then subsides, or it may last throughout the period of anuria. In addition, there is frequently a constant desire to micturate, although no urine is passed, or if the anuria is intermittent, urine of pale colour and low specific gravity, sometimes blood-stained, may be passed. If the anuria remains complete, no other symptoms may occur for several days, a feature which is common to the obstructive forms of anuria, but is in marked contrast to the non-obstructive variety. After a period of anuria lasting from 7 to 10 days, during which time the blood-urea is progressively increasing, the patient becomes drowsy, the tongue is dry, there is disinclination for food, and the general symptoms of uraemia may come on. Thus, it is usual to speak of a *period of tolerance* and a *period of intoxication* in obstructive anuria. The tolerant stage of obstructive anuria may be more prolonged if the functional kidney is already hydronephrotic from previous intermittent obstruction, even to twenty days. The sudden obstruction to the urinary flow in a comparatively normal kidney causes complete suppression, while a partial or intermittent obstruction causes dilatation of the kidney. If such a kidney is the functioning organ, and becomes completely obstructed, the dilatation will increase; a lumbar tumour may be palpable. If there is pain on pressure over the kidney, or along the course of the ureter, the diagnosis is strengthened, or it may be decided to settle the diagnosis by immediate operation. In some cases in which one kidney has been destroyed gradually without pain, and anuria occurs, there may be difficulty in determining which of the two kidneys is the functional organ which has recently become obstructed; in these cases it is a good rule to operate upon the side on which the pain has occurred more recently. A calculus impacted in the vesical end of the ureter may on rare occasions be felt on careful rectal or vaginal examination. If the impaction is close to the bladder, evidence of ureteric calculus may be obtained by the cystoscope, when the ureteric orifice of the obstructed side may be seen to be congested or ecchymosed. A radiograph of the renal and ureteric areas is mandatory; *Fig.* 63 illustrates the way in which the obstruction may be demonstrated and located with the aid of a radio-opaque catheter; large or multiple shadows in one renal area will suggest that the kidney is

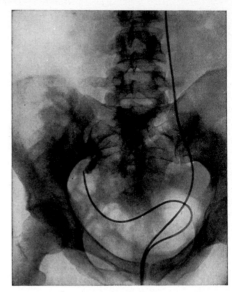

Fig. 63. A radiograph showing the tip of a radio-opaque catheter obstructed by a calculus in the right ureter.

functionally impaired or inactive, whereas a shadow in the line of the opposite ureter will indicate the immediate cause of the anuria. Operation upon the side of the recent pain may be urged strongly, when the offending stone in the ureter can be removed and the patency of the ureter established. If no stone is found on radiography, a pyelostomy or nephrostomy can be performed. In some cases the passage of a ureteric catheter via a cystoscope may dislodge the impacted calculus and may slowly drain the distended renal pelvis. In any case of anuria, with severe elevation of the blood-urea (above 100–150 mg. per cent), renal or peritoneal dialysis may allow more time for the establishment of a complete diagnosis.

Anuria from Vesical Carcinoma implies either that both ureteric orifices are involved in the disease, or that the ureteric orifice of the only functional kidney is implicated. The condition is uncommon as a pure obstructive anuria, for in most cases the kidneys are already the seat of changes due in part to the back-pressure and in part to sepsis, so that when anuria terminates a case of vesical carcinoma it is more often due to renal disease than to ureteric obstruction. If the bladder has remained uninfected the gradually increasing ureteric obstruction may first cause hydro-ureter and hydronephrosis, so that when the obstruction becomes complete the renal distension may increase quickly, and the symptoms of uraemia be delayed. In cases arising from vesical carcinoma it is very rare for the anuria to occur before symptoms of vesical growth are apparent, such as haematuria, pyuria, increased frequency, and pain on micturition; but in the infiltrating type of carcinoma, haematuria and pyuria may be absent for a long time. In all cases, careful vaginal or rectal examination will detect infiltration and thickening of the base of the bladder, and the growth can be seen through the cystoscope (*Fig.* 365, p. 346).

Uterine Carcinoma. Anuria is frequent in the terminal stage of uterine carcinoma when the growth has extended into the cellular tissues of the broad ligament and involved the terminal portions of the ureters, or when the orifices of the latter are implicated in the direct infiltration of the growth into the bladder base. It may supervene on radium treatment in a case where the degree of obstruction has previously been insufficient to produce it. In the majority of cases of death from uterine cancer, the kidneys are hydronephrotic, the ureters and renal pelves dilated, or the renal secreting tissue sclerosed, apart from the frequent infection with septic micro-organisms. In all cases the growth has reached an advanced stage, but it has been recorded that anuria has occurred before the patient has complained of any symptom pointing to the uterine condition. These cases might simulate other forms of obstructive anuria, but the diagnosis is readily established upon vaginal examination.

Pelvic or Abdominal Tumours, such as uterine fibromyomata, ovarian cysts, or carcinomata, or retroperitoneal haematomata following pelvic operations, may cause anuria from direct pressure on the ureters, especially if a part of the tumour is impacted in the pelvic cavity. The cause of the anuria will be apparent on examination of the abdomen and of the pelvic organs.

Ligature of Both Ureters or of that of the only functional kidney is a possible complication of total hysterectomy, abdominoperineal excision of the rectum and other extensive pelvic eviscerative procedures, and will be followed by anuria if the ligation is complete or by a urinary fistula if incomplete.

Sulphonamide Anuria may be due to mechanical blocking of the renal pelves and ureters by crystals, or to tubular damage from toxicity of the drug. In the former case there will be obstruction to a ureteric catheter; when attempts are made to pass such a catheter on cystoscopy masses of sulphonamide crystals and debris will escape into the bladder. In the latter case there will be no obstruction to the catheter but the renal pelvis will contain little or no urine. Sulphapyridine is the drug most likely to cause anuria, but if the urine is kept alkaline and the fluid intake high it is of infrequent occurrence.

Uric Acid Obstruction may cause anuria when radiotherapy or cytotoxic therapy bombards the kidneys with uric acid from broken-down tissues sensitive to such therapy, as, for instance, in chronic leukaemia and lymphosarcoma. Allopurinol may be used prophylactically in such cases.

Idiopathic Retroperitoneal Fibrosis involving the Ureters (Periureteritis plastica). In this condition, of unknown aetiology, a sheath of fibrous tissue envelops the great vessels and extends laterally to surround the ureters. They are gradually compressed with resulting hydronephrosis (*Fig.* 64).

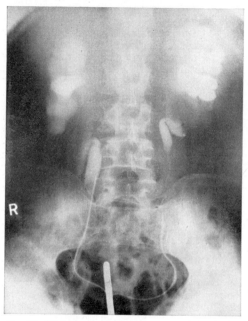

Fig. 64. Bilateral hydronephrosis due to retroperitoneal fibrosis involving the ureters.

There may be no symptoms until the development of malaise, uraemia, and anuria, but sometimes there is oedema of the scrotum or legs and increase in weight, and there may be loin or lumbar back pain and rarely claudication from compression of the iliac arteries. The patients are mostly of middle age and are male more frequently than female. There is often anaemia and the E.S.R. is raised. The urine is usually normal, but there may be transient albuminuria, pyuria, or microscopic haematuria. The diagnosis depends on the finding of a raised blood-urea together with bilateral hydronephrosis and medial displacement of the ureters on retrograde pyelography. There is usually no obstruction to the passage of a ureteric catheter, which results in marked diuresis and relief of symptoms. While the condition is not common several hundred cases have now been reported. Among the suggested aetiological factors are leakage of urine or blood, trauma, infection, lymphatic obstruction secondary to lymphangitis, vitamin-E deficiency, Webber-Christian disease, and polyarteritis nodosa. The condition has been reported following the use of methysergide in prevention of migraine and may regress (although not invariably) when the drug is withdrawn. It has also followed the use of practolol in cardiac practice. It may be part of a more widespread sclerosing fibrosis implicating the mediastinum, bile ducts, and orbital tissues, and may include Dupuytren's contracture, Peyronie's disease of the penis, and Riedel's thyroiditis. It is important to differentiate retroperitoneal diffuse malignant disease, secondary especially to carcinoma of the breast, stomach, prostate, and cervix.

B. NON-OBSTRUCTIVE ANURIA

Marked diminution in the amount of urine, or complete anuria, may occur without obstructive lesions of the urinary apparatus, due in many instances to disease of the renal secreting tissues. In most of these cases the symptoms differ remarkably from those seen in obstructive anuria, in that the anuria is accompanied by symptoms of uraemia in a short time, and not after an interval of days as in the obstructive cases. Anuria may occur under certain toxic conditions, as in acute fevers, or in acute poisoning by mercury, lead, phosphorus, or turpentine; the history and accompanying symptoms of such cases are usually sufficient to point to the nature of the urinary suppression.

Anuria in Renal Disease. In *acute nephritis* anuria may occur early or after the disease is well established, and is usually accompanied by marked disturbance of the nervous system. The sudden onset of the disease in the course of an acute specific fever such as scarlet fever, typhoid, or pneumonia, or in haematogenous renal infections, associated with pallor, puffiness of the face and ankles, and slight pyrexia, together with the small amount of urine passed before the suppression becomes complete, are points all suggesting acute nephritis. If the urine has been tested before the onset of anuria it is often of reddish-brown colour from the presence of blood, and contains abundant albumin, together with epithelial and blood casts. In *chronic nephritis* anuria may occur as a late symptom in the disease, and is often preceded by a period in which polyuria is marked. Anuria in chronic nephritis is accompanied by prominent symptoms of uraemia, such as headache, giddiness, nausea, convulsions, stertor, and coma, and unless the flow of urine is re-established quickly, or renal dialysis instituted, death ensues. The previous history of the case, hypertension, cardiac hypertrophy, retinal changes, raised blood-urea, and signs of back-pressure, with or without ascites and anasarca, will point to the nature of the anuria. In other diseases of the kidney, such as *amyloid disease, suppurative* or *non-suppurative pyelonephritis, bilateral tuberculosis,* or *hydronephrosis,* anuria may be preceded by general failing health, loss of appetite, a dry brown tongue, subnormal temperature, headache, increasing pulse-rate, hiccup, and attacks of dyspnoea; there may be

polyuria before suppression occurs; in these cases the anuria is terminal, the condition of the kidneys having been known previously. With the occurrence of anuria there may be great restlessness, muscular twitching, incontinence of faeces, convulsions, and a slow lapse into coma.

Systemic lupus erythematosus should be considered in any febrile disorder with rashes, joint involvement, and signs of renal disease, for renal failure is a common cause of death in this disorder.

Polycystic disease of the kidneys frequently terminates in anuria and uraemia, but the diagnosis of the disease has probably been arrived at previously. The symptoms in the adult resemble those of chronic nephritis, with the exception that ascites and oedema of the extremities are uncommon. Headache, flatulence, and digestive troubles, sickness, and general lassitude are symptoms of renal inefficiency, while arteriosclerosis, a raised blood-pressure, a bilateral renal tumour, and a low-specific-gravity urine in increased quantity would suggest polycystic disease. There is usually a family history of the condition. Haematuria is the first symptom in not a few of these cases. Clinical examination reveals enlarged nodular kidneys and diagnosis may originally have been made by the discovery of these masses at routine examination.

The infantile type has a more acute course and is associated with death in the neonatal period or in the first two or three years of life.

In all cases of anuria an estimation of the *blood-urea* and electrolytes should be carried out and repeated at regular intervals. The normal blood-urea of 15–40 mg. dl⁻ (2·5–7·5 mmol l⁻) may be enormously increased, even to 350–400 mg. dl⁻ (29–66 mmol l⁻), and an increasing amount in successive estimations forms a valuable guide in prognosis.

Anuria following Operations or Trauma. Anuria may occur in patients who have undergone operation and who are the subjects of renal disease, or may occur occasionally even when no renal disease is present, especially when there has been considerable loss of blood with a marked fall in blood-pressure and diminution in the renal blood-flow. This is particularly seen in elderly patients with rupture of an aortic aneurysm or an exsanguinating haematemesis from a peptic ulcer. Acute tubular necrosis is often present. A patient with renal disease, or in whom the kidneys have been subject to back-pressure, as with prostatic enlargement or uterine myomata, after any operation which involves a good deal of shock, may succumb to anuria unless appropriate measures are undertaken. An apparently trivial operation on the urinary organs, such as mere cystoscopic examination or dilatation of a urethral stricture, even when the kidneys are apparently unaffected by disease, may occasionally cause acute suppression of urine. This must be differentiated carefully from the retention of urine in the bladder often seen after operations such as for haemorrhoids or for hernia. Anuria is particularly liable to occur when a catheter is passed to relieve a long-standing overdistended bladder in a case of prostatic enlargement or urethral stricture, the kidneys being already affected by back-pressure or infected with septic processes, and it is still a golden rule that if a catheter is passed in these cases the urine must be withdrawn very gradually and must not be allowed to re-accumulate. Anuria following operations upon the lower urinary tract is diagnosed by the direct relationship between the operation and the onset of symptoms; by the rigors, pyrexia, increasing blood-urea content, and the profound prostration, rapidly followed by convulsive movements and coma.

Anuria may also occur after a crushing injury or severe wound of a limb, after incompatible blood transfusion, excessive *vomiting, septic abortion,* or in the late stages of *cholera, yellow fever,* and *blackwater fever.* It is likely that the ultimate cause in all these conditions is acute renal ischaemia causing tubular necrosis. When due to drugs, injections of metals or serum, or to blood transfusion, the cause is indicated by the treatment that has been adopted. When due to injury, abortion, or intravascular haemolysis the cause is also apparent.

Drugs. Certain drugs have on occasion been reported to have caused anuria. Amphotericin B, used to treat fungal infections, may cause nephrotoxicity, and total anuria has been reported, as it has with boric acid, used as a dusting powder for napkin rashes in infants or after burns. The indane derivatives, e.g., phenindione, used as an anticoagulant, may very rarely cause oligo- or anuria, as may phenolphthalein, phenylbutazone, mercury salts, oxalic acid, carbon tetrachloride, and a number of other substances.

Harold Ellis.

ANUS, BLOOD PASSED THROUGH

The passage of blood per anum may be: (1) *Obvious to the patient because the blood is still of its recognizable colour;* (2) *Obvious to the doctor, but not the patient, when the blood has become so changed as to be black—Melaena* (p. 523); (3) *Recognizable only when laboratory tests for blood are applied to the faeces—a condition spoken of as 'occult blood in the stools'.*

I. OBVIOUS RED BLOOD PASSED PER ANUM MAY BE DUE TO:

1. Anal Causes:

Piles
Fissure
Fistula
Foreign body
Non-specific inflammation associated with pruritus; sensitivity to certain topically applied drugs, e.g., cinchocaine hydrochloride
Primary syphilis.

2. Rectal Causes:

Neoplasm, e.g., carcinoma or lymphosarcoma
Polypus

Injury, e.g., by sigmoidoscopy or enema nozzle
Invasion of the rectum by carcinoma of the bladder, uterine carcinoma, pelvic sarcoma, pelvic abscess, actinomycosis, schistosomiasis
Infective proctitis including lymphogranuloma venereum and primary syphilis
Tuberculous ulceration
Non-infective proctitis
Solitary simple ulcer.

3. Colonic Causes:

Carcinoma of sigmoid colon, descending colon, splenic flexure, transverse colon, hepatic flexure, ascending colon, and caecum
Polypus of the colon
Tuberculous ulceration of the colon
Intussusception
Dysentery, amoebic or bacillary
Ulcerative colitis
Granulomatous colitis
Actinomycosis of the caecum
Diverticular disease
Colonic vascular occlusion of either artery or vein by thrombosis or embolism
Injury
Acute summer diarrhoea of infants
From irritant drugs; arsenic, phosphorus, calomel, corrosive sublimate
Excessive purgation
Oxyuris vermicularis.

4. Causes in the Ileum:

Intussusception
Typhoid fever
Dysentery
Mesenteric vascular occlusion by thrombosis or embolism
Injury
Meckel's diverticulitis
After delivery, if the stump of the umbilical cord becomes infected
Granulomatous ileitis (Crohn's disease)
Haemangioma
Non-epithelial malignant tumours, e.g., lymphosarcoma, or leiomyosarcoma
Multiple polyps—Peutz-Jeghers syndrome.

5. Causes in the Jejunum:

Peptic ulcer
After gastrojejunostomy.

6. General Infective or Allied Causes:

Cholera
Yellow fever
Sprue
Intermittent fever
Relapsing fever
Scurvy
Septicaemia
Blood diseases: leukaemia, thrombocytopenic purpura, hereditary capillary fragility—von Willebrand's disease, hypoprothrombinaemia
Anticoagulants
Haemophilia and allied disorders
Henoch-Schönlein purpura
Uraemia.

7. Duodenal Causes:

Chronic duodenal ulcer
Duodenal diverticulum
Injury

Carcinoma (rare)
Carcinoma of the ampulla of Vater.

8. Gastric Causes:

Simple ulcer
Drug induced, e.g., aspirin, phenylbutazone, cortisone
Injury—Mallory-Weiss syndrome
Carcinoma
Sarcoma
Hereditary telangiectasia—Osler-Weber-Rendu disease
Grönblad-Strandberg syndrome (pseudoxanthoma elasticum).

9. Oesophageal Lesions:

Oesophageal varices
Hiatus hernia
Carcinoma of the oesophagus.

10. Swallowed Blood, due to:

Epistaxis
Haemoptysis
Ruptured aneurysm
Malingering.

In many of the above conditions blood per anum is but a minor item in the course of some illness whose nature is indicated by other symptoms. When the source of bleeding is high up in the alimentary canal—gastric ulcer, gastric carcinoma, duodenal ulcer, cirrhosis of the liver—or when the blood has been swallowed, from epistaxis, haemoptysis, or a leaking aneurysm, the blood is as a rule so altered by the digestive juices that, by the time it is passed per anum, it is no longer red but black; the differential diagnosis is discussed under MELAENA (p. 523). Occasionally, however, the quantity of blood lost in conditions which usually cause melaena may be so great that when passed it is unchanged and so still recognizable by its red colour.

When blood, recognizable by the patient, is passed per anum and there is no general pyrexial illness—typhoid fever, for example, or infective endocarditis, or some abdominal catastrophe, such as direct injury, or the effects of thrombosis or embolism to account for it, the first point to decide is whether the blood originates from piles or other anal lesion, or from a lesion higher up in the alimentary canal. Examination of the rectum digitally, by sigmoidoscope, and by proctoscope is a vital series of primary procedures necessary to avoid the error of attributing to piles haemorrhage from rectal carcinoma. They should be carried out in every patient presenting in this way.

In the case of *piles*, *fissure*, or *fistula* the blood is passed unmixed with the faeces, and as a rule not associated with much mucus; with lesions of the pelvic colon, or of parts higher up, there may be no mucus. When mucus is passed as well as blood or if the blood is mixed with the faeces rather than passed independently, the lesion is generally more serious than piles, though a rectal carcinoma or a polypus may lead to blood passing in drips or even in gushes quite separate

from faeces. One rule should be regarded therefore as invariable: no case in which blood is passed per anum can be regarded as unimportant until careful examination—visual, digital, and instrumental—has been made to exclude the more serious causes.

In adults, the chief lesions to diagnose or exclude are the following:

1. *Malignant Disease of the Rectum and Colon.*
2. *Polypus*:
   Pedunculated polypus and multiple polypi of the rectum or colon.
3. *Non-malignant Ulceration*:
   Venereal, tuberculous, septic, or stercoral (*Fig.* 69) ulceration of the rectum
   Ulcerative colitis
   Granulomatous colitis (Crohn's disease)
   Dysentery: (*a*) Amoebic (*Fig.* 70), (*b*) Bacillary.

1. Malignant Disease. By a digital examination of the rectum *carcinoma* may be obvious to the finger or a *rectal polypus* may be felt. In the case of carcinoma there is usually an inch or more of normal mucosa above the sphincter before the neoplasm is reached by the finger. Other conditions generally require further investigation for their diagnosis, by means of the proctoscope, the sigmoidoscope, barium-enema X-rays with (Malmo technique) or without air contrast, and microscopical and bacteriological examinations of the stools. The need for these will be indicated by such additional symptoms as spurious diarrhoea (i.e., frequent desire to go to stool but with comparatively little result), pain, constipation, loss of weight, anaemia, or general ill health. *Carcinoma of the sigmoid colon* may be seen with the sigmoidoscope.

Carcinoma of the upper parts of the colon may be suspected by the passage of blood and mucus associated with increasing constipation and discomfort or pain in the left iliac fossa. A tumour may be felt in the left iliac fossa, but the growth may be too high up to be seen through the sigmoidoscope. Barium enema, particularly of the double-contrast type, may serve to demonstrate stenosis of the bowel at the site of growth. Differentiation of chronic diverticulitis from carcinoma may be evident only by laparotomy, and even then doubt is not always dispelled.

2. Polypus. *Single polypi* of the rectum or of the colon may sometimes be difficult to feel with the finger, but they may be detected with the sigmoidoscope (*Fig.* 68). Their pedicle is often an inch or more in length, and no thicker than string; the globular distal end of the polypus is apt to become inflamed and to bleed; there may be no pain and no diarrhoea and the haemorrhage may be attributed to internal piles. So much blood may be lost that Addisonian anaemia or another blood dyscrasia responsible for general bowel haemorrhage may be suspected, when sigmoidoscopy might reveal the polypus, removal of which should terminate the bleeding.

Multiple polypi of the rectum or pelvic colon cause constipation with the passage of bloody mucus rather than profuse haemorrhage, so presenting a close simulation of rectal carcinoma. They may be felt digitally per rectum, or if higher up may need the sigmoidoscope (*Fig.* 68) for their detection. Sometimes they are flat and sessile, occasionally they project like stunted biopsied, but, providing they are not too large and sessile, they may also be removed using a diathermy snare.

3. Non-malignant Ulceration. Non-malignant colitis, with or without ulceration, may be of all degrees from mild, temporary, superficial, to

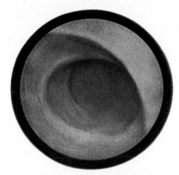

Fig. 65. A normal rectum.

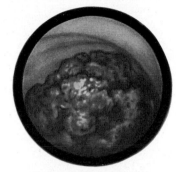

Fig. 66. Carcinoma of the rectum.

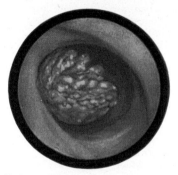

Fig. 67. Large simple papilloma of the rectum; not distinguishable from carcinoma without microscopical examination.

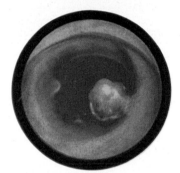

Fig. 68. Polypi of rectum.

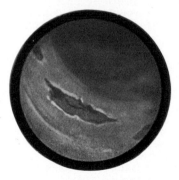

Fig. 69. Simple stercoral ulcer of the rectum.

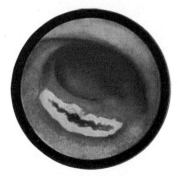

Fig. 70. Amoebic ulcer of the rectum.

Figs. 65–70. SIGMOIDOSCOPIC APPEARANCES IN THE RECTUM.

fingers, and may be sufficiently numerous to produce partial intestinal obstruction. They are liable to develop in the course of *chronic ulcerative colitis* and may become malignant.

Colonoscopy has now become an essential method for the complete examination of the colon. Not only may polyps be located and severe, intractable, persistent, and fatal. Ulcerative colitis, although resembling bacillary dysentery in many respects, is nevertheless a different disease of unknown aetiology.

There are three main types of so-called tropical dysentery: (*a*) Amoebic, (*b*) Bacillary, and (*c*) Malarial.

A. AMOEBIC. The distinction is important in connexion with treatment, amoebic dysentery being curable by intramuscular injections of emetine hydrochloride and then by the administration of other drugs by the mouth. Bacillary dysentery is uninfluenced by emetine, but responds to certain sulphonamides and antibiotics. Malarial dysentery responds to treatment of the primary condition. The amoebic form is likely to be followed by an amoebic abscess of the liver. The onset may be mild—a comparatively trivial diarrhoea, or the illness may start violently with pyrexia, severe abdominal pain, tenesmus, and protracted diarrhoea succeeded by the repeated passage of blood-stained mucus or pure blood. The acute phase may very rarely be rapidly fatal. On the other hand, complete cure may be brought about in a week or two, or temporary improvement may occur followed by a relapse or several relapses to end in gradual recovery. Instead of complete cure, a condition of chronic dysentery with persistent ulceration of the colon may supervene, a state of affairs often met with in patients who have returned, imperfectly treated, from the tropics. The symptoms are then precisely similar to those of ulcerative colitis, that is to say there may be chronic diarrhoea, six or seven motions being passed daily with more or less abdominal griping and tenesmus, the stools being accompanied by mucus and at times blood. On some occasions blood and mucus may be evacuated without faecal matter, or the patient may from time to time pass pure blood without mucus or faecal material. There may be quiescent intervals of weeks or months with stools that may be loose and rather frequent but otherwise not abnormal, such an interval being followed by an exacerbation of the diarrhoea and repetition of the passage of blood and mucus. This state of affairs may persist for years if established ulceration of the colon fails to heal under appropriate treatment by emetine, in combination with other amoebicides such as oxytetracycline, chloroquine, di-iodohydroxyquinoline, metronidazole (Flagyl) and bowel wash-outs. The diagnosis is based partly on the history, especially of residence in the tropics, partly on what is seen through the sigmoidoscope, but mostly upon the results of microscopical and bacteriological examinations of the stools.

Amoebic dysentery (*amoebiasis*) in its chronic form is diagnosed chiefly by three methods, namely: (1) Discovery of the *Entamoeba histolytica* or its encysted forms in the stools; (2) Identifying the characteristic ulcers with the sigmoidoscope (*Fig.* 70); (3) Relief or cure of the condition by the use of emetine, either as emetine hydrochloride given intramuscularly, or as bismuth-emetine-iodide given by the mouth in combination with other drugs.

The *Entamoeba histolytica* is a large motile protoplasmic body with a relatively small nucleus measuring from 30 to 40 μ in diameter. It is seen best when an emulsion of the stools is examined fresh under the medium power of the microscope, a warmed stage being employed. Specialized experience is required to distinguish it from the harmless *Entamoeba coli*. The encysted forms are even more difficult to distinguish at sight than are the motile types. Examination is assisted if a little methylene-blue solution is added to the faecal emulsion, for the stain is at once taken up by pus and epithelial cells and not by the living amoebae which stand out by contrast as light refractile motile bodies.

The sigmoidoscopic appearances of amoebic dysentery differ from those of bacillary dysentery and of ulcerative colitis in that, instead of quite irregular and widespread ulceration with general angry reddening of the mucosa that is not denuded by the ulcerative process, there are usually a number of relatively small, separate, well-defined ulcers with reddened margins and greyish-white and pitted bases (*see Fig.* 70).

The therapeutic test by emetine applies only to amoebic dysentery.

B. BACILLARY DYSENTERY. This is caused by an infection with one of the *Shigella* group of organisms. There are four main groups that are pathogenic to man: *Shigella dysenteriae, S. flexneri, S. boydii, S. sonnei.*

The most severe attacks of dysentery are caused by various types of the first group. *S. shigae* produces a soluble exotoxin which affects the intestine itself and occasionally the nervous system. In the severe types of infection which may occur in tropical regions with this organism, patients have become severely ill with abdominal pain followed by severe diarrhoea with passage of blood, pus, and mucus many times a day. The more common type of infection in England is due to *S. sonnei* which may result in only mild diarrhoea.

C. MALARIAL DYSENTERY. This is usually only seen in acute falciparum malaria and is often associated with vomiting, jaundice, and collapse. The diagnosis depends on the recognition of malaria (q.v.). The condition responds to suitable anti-malarial drugs.

D. CILIATE DYSENTERY. Closely resembles the amoebic variety even to sigmoidoscopic appearances. It may be suspected in those who are in close contact with pigs. The diagnosis is confirmed by finding *Balantidium coli* in the stools (*Fig.* 71).

E. ULCERATIVE COLITIS. The chief points of distinction from bacillary dysentery and amoebic dysentery are the absence of the dysentery bacilli or amoebae from a recently passed stool and of agglutination reactions in blood-serum tests, and with the characteristic picture obtained with a barium enema. The condition may exist as an acute attack which varies from mild to fulminating. In the latter case the patient passes more than six stools per day, haemoglobin is below the lower limit of normal, the temperature is raised, and there is a tachycardia above 120 per minute. Colitis may extend over a period of years with periods of remission, the so-called 'chronic active form'. In this case the patient becomes progressively reduced in health, loses weight, suffers progressive anaemia, and in the long term may develop amyloid disease. Cardinal signs of this condition are diarrhoea associated with the passage of bright red blood per rectum. Abdominal pain may occur and is usually an indication of severe colonic disease particularly when associated with gaseous distension.

The sigmoidoscopic appearances depend upon the degree of activity and vary from a mild granular proctitis to an extensively ulcerated

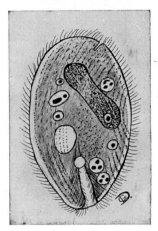

Fig. 71. *Balantidium coli* as seen in faeces in ciliate dysentery.

rectum with blood oozing from the denuded areas. These appearances are readily confused with granulomatous colitis (Crohn's colitis), which, although usually affecting the ileum, may involve colon or rectum. A biopsy of the rectal mucosa may show the characteristic crypt abscesses seen in ulcerative colitis but only too often giant-cell systems are present and there is no clear-cut histological distinction between the two diseases. A barium enema provides the best means of distinguishing ulcerative colitis from other forms of colitis. Although the whole of the colon may not necessarily be affected the disease spreads proximally from the rectum, which is therefore always involved. In granulomatous colitis, on the other hand, there may be 'skip' areas in the colon so that affected parts are interspersed between normal areas. In addition there may be evidence of fistula formation, for example, between the small and the large intestine.

The only certain cure of ulcerative colitis is surgical excision of the entire colon and rectum: panproctocolectomy. This is not always required, however, and certain centres remove the colon but leave the rectum, carrying out an ileorectal anastomosis. Occasionally acute attacks of ulcerative colitis respond to steroids and the chronic form is often controlled by salicylazo-sulphapyridine (Salazopyrin) 1–2 g., four to six times daily with a maintenance dose of 1 g. twice daily.

Ulcerative colitis may be associated with the characteristic lesions of pyoderma gangrenosa, polyarthritis, iritis, portal hepatic cirrhosis, anal fissure and fistula, and later the development of a carcinoma of colon which may be multifocal in origin.

F. URAEMIC COLITIS. This may be quite a severe form of colitis occurring in the late stages of renal failure. It is always possible to distinguish this from other forms of colitis by the presence of a raised blood-urea.

G. SYPHILITIC PROCTITIS. A primary syphilitic ulcer (chancre) of the anus, occasionally extending into the rectum, occurs as a venereal disease in homosexual men. It is becoming more common in large cities and has to be distinguished from fissure-in-ano by bacteriological examination. The tertiary stage of the disease, particularly as it affects the rectum, is very rare; the condition is chronic and may result in the passage of frequent loose stools with blood. The ulceration may simulate carcinoma of the rectum from which it is distinguished by the fact that it starts immediately above the anus. The upper limit of the ulcerated area seldom extends more than 15 cm. from the anal margin; above this the mucosa is perfectly normal.

H. TUBERCULOUS ULCERATION OF THE RECTUM. This also is an uncommon condition. It may simulate carcinoma, venereal ulceration, or ulcerative colitis. It is usually associated with active tuberculous disease in the lungs and tubercle bacilli will generally be found in either swabbings from the lesions or in careful examination of the faeces.

The Passage of Blood per Anum in a Child. When an infant is a few months old, especially about the age of eight or nine months, *acute intussusception* is a condition to be suspected if blood, with or without mucus, is passed per anum. The infant will indicate that it is in pain by screaming and drawing up its legs. After an initial evacuation of the normal contents of the lower bowel no true faeces will be passed, in fact the complete absence of any faecal odour is to be regarded as a crucial feature, the diapers becoming reddened by the bloody mucus that passes in small amounts at intervals. Vomiting is usual. Examination—if need be under an anaesthetic—must be made for a palpable abdominal lump. Although the intussusception generally starts at or near the ileocaecal valve, the right iliac fossa is as a rule the least likely place for the lump to be identified, for as the invagination of the bowel progresses the hardened distal end of the intussusception travels along the colon so that it may be felt under the liver, in the epigastrium, or on the left side of the abdomen; it may even be felt by a finger inserted gently into the rectum. At later ages intussusception is uncommon, and is usually not acute but subacute or chronic, leading to abdominal pains and constipation which may not be absolute, the precise diagnosis being made as a rule only after the abdomen has been opened.

Prolapse of the anal mucosa may cause passage of blood per anum. It is a fairly common condition, associated with constipation and straining at stool, but not necessarily with ill health; it is recognized by inspection, as a globular red swelling that projects from the anus when the child defaecates.

Alarm lest intussusception has occurred may arise when older children pass blood per rectum in association with *acute diarrhoea*, especially common in summer. Many of these cases develop acute enterocolitis with blood oozing from the inflamed and occasionally ulcerated mucosa. Vomiting may be as marked as the diarrhoea, there may be cramp-like attacks of abdominal colic, the motions often present a grass-green colour. Diarrhoea and vomiting may be very serious, often fatal, but the occurrence of blood per anum does not make the prognosis worse. The abdomen will be examined for the possible tumour of an intussusception, but the fact that faecal material is passed, even though only in small quantities after the first few evacuations, will indicate that enterocolitis and not intussusception is the condition.

Henoch's purpura is a striking malady the nature of which may be obscure in the first attack; when, however, the child suffers from recurrences the diagnosis becomes easy, and the trouble generally ceases before adult life is reached. It is seldom fatal. In a typical attack the little patient, previously in good health, is seized with a prostrating illness associated with pyrexia, vomiting, abdominal pains now here, now there, sometimes with diarrhoea, sometimes with constipation. Purpuric spots develop in the skin, recurring in successive crops and perhaps affecting all parts of the limbs and trunk. A severe case might be described as a combination of cyclical vomiting with generalized purpura. The attack may last a week or longer, gradually passing off. After an interval of good health there is a recurrence of precisely similar symptoms; and during the years between 5 and 15 the patient may have from two or three to a dozen or more bouts, ultimately ceasing to be subject to them. Many of the cases exhibit no more than the purpura associated with the gastro-intestinal upsets, but a few present other haemorrhages besides purpura—epistaxis, haematemesis, haemoptysis, haematuria, melaena, anal blood. In some instances there is extensive haemorrhage into the submucosa of the bowel, with violent abdominal pains comparable with those of mesenteric vascular occlusion or of intussusception; indeed, the cessation of peristalsis in a short length of bowel affected by submucosal haemorrhage may on rare occasions cause the active bowel above to drive the haemorrhagic part by invagination into the part below and produce an actual intussusception as a complication of what is primarily Henoch's purpura.

In an obscure occurrence of intestinal haemorrhage in a child, the possibility of ulcer in a *Meckel's diverticulum* should be considered.

There remain for discussion two other groups of causes for the passage of fresh blood per anum, both rare but both important, namely: (1) *Parasites*, especially *Bilharzia haematobia*, *Oxyuris vermicularis*, *Ancylostomum duodenale*; and (2) *Gastro-intestinal irritant drugs* or *chemicals*, especially calomel and arsenic.

Parasites. *Bilharzia haematobia*, known also as *Schistosoma haematobium*, may occur in the rectum, though less frequently here than in the bladder. Its presence gives rise to the passage of mucus and blood per anum. Infection is contracted abroad, especially in Egypt and in parts of South Africa. *S. mansoni* and *S. japonica* may also cause intestinal bleeding. Diagnosis depends on finding the ova of the parasite microscopically in the faeces or in the urine or in the rectal mucosa.

In children the presence of thread-worms (*Oxyuris vermicularis*) in the rectum may lead to the discharge of small amounts of mucus coloured by a trace of blood. The worms will be seen on inspection of the child's motions. They are white, as thick as coarse thread, and 12–16 mm. long.

Infection by *Ancylostomum duodenale*—ancylostomiasis—is characterized by pronounced asthenia and anaemia, though patients may harbour ancylostomes without exhibiting any symptoms at all. Blood occurs in the stools but is seldom obvious, it is generally detected by the tests for occult blood given below. Blood-counts in severe cases exhibit most of the characters of Addisonian anaemia, but with the important difference that EOSINOPHILIA (p. 253) is often conspicuous in ancylostomiasis. Eosinophilia in a case of supposed Addisonian anaemia should always lead to a search for evidence of parasitic infection, especially by tape-worm, ancylostome, or bilharzia. Ancylostomiasis may be suggested by former residence abroad, particularly in Egypt, South Africa, South America, Mexico, India, Assam, or Thailand, though instances occur in European countries in which the infection has been introduced from overseas—for instance, among Cornish lead-miners and in the St. Gotthard tunnel workers.

Gastro-intestinal Irritants of a chemical nature are numerous, but the majority cause blood per anum only when administered in a considerable quantity as for suicidal or homicidal purposes—for instance, sulphuric acid, nitric acid, hydrochloric acid, corrosive sublimate—the diagnosis then depending upon the collateral evidence. Two, however, that may cause haemorrhage per anum even when the dose has been within recognized therapeutic limits are *arsenic* and *calomel*.

Arsenic is well known as liable to cause gastro-intestinal disturbances when employed in pharmacological doses. It is not surprising therefore that when it has been administered with felonious intent in the form of weed-killer, vermin killer, or sheep-dip, the symptoms produced have been attributed to gastric ulcer or to ulcerative colitis.

Calomel is usually a harmless purge, but in particularly susceptible patients or those who are septic or are suffering from renal disease it may lead to severe and even fatal colitis.

II. BLACK BLOOD IN THE STOOLS

(*See* MELAENA, p. 523.)

III. OCCULT BLOOD IN THE STOOLS

The nature of blood passed in the stools depends on the quantity of the bleeding, its position in the gastro-intestinal tract, whether high or low, and the rate of intestinal transit. Thus bleeding in the caecum may appear as bright red blood, melaena, or be in such small quantities as to be undetectable to the naked eye. In this latter case the bleeding is said to be 'occult'. Most of the conditions described above may sometimes lead to the passage in the stools of occult blood that can be identified only by the application of special tests to the motions.

C. Wastell.

ANXIETY

Anxiety, like pain, is a normal biological protective mechanism when occasioned by circumstances which warrant it. Not to feel anxious when confronted by a potentially dangerous situation could be disastrous. In contrast, undue unjustified anxiety may be a crippling neurotic symptom and clearly of morbid origin. Anxiety, indeed, is probably the commonest of all psychiatric symptoms and can occur as part of almost every mental disorder. If it occurs as a primary manifestation, either persistently or in recurrent paroxysms, the diagnostic label: *anxiety state* may be justified.

Anxiety has both mental and physical manifestations with which every normal person is familiar. Whether due to some 'real' anxiety-producing situation or of morbid origin, the experience of anxiety is qualitatively the same although it may differ in its persistence and intensity under varying circumstances.

Mentally, anxiety is characterized by a sense of *expectant dread*, i.e., apprehension of some disaster about to happen. Physically, anxiety gives rise to a large number of autonomic symptoms, both of sympathetic and para-sympathetic origin, which affect nearly every bodily system and tend, in their occurrence, to reinforce mental anxiety. *Palpitations* occur together with *breathlessness* and a sometimes alarming experience of *precordial discomfort*. Respiration may become fast and shallow leading to *paraesthesiae*, *tetany*, and *carpopedal spasm* (*hyperventilation syndrome*). The mouth tends to dry up and there may be an intense desire to *retch*. *Vomiting* may occur. A *sinking feeling* in the abdomen is almost invariable. *Diarrhoea* and *frequency of micturition* are common. *Tremor*, usually of a fairly gross kind, also occurs. In the event of sudden, severe, and acute anxiety there may be a loss of muscle tone leading to a feeling of weakness or loss of control and in states of extreme terror *paralysis*, together with mutism, staring eyes, and widely dilated pupils.

Anxiety may be 'free-floating', i.e., without obvious attachment to any forthcoming event or may be related to some specific circumstance. But as continued free-floating anxiety of any severity soon proves intolerable, ways and means must be found of overcoming it. One of these is *phobia-formation*—the attachment of anxiety to specific objects or situations which may then sometimes be avoided although not usually without considerable inconvenience to the sufferer. Such phobias may be classified in various ways. A currently acceptable classification divides them into phobias of external origin, e.g., agoraphobia (fear of open spaces) or claustrophobia (fear of closed spaces); social phobias (e.g., fear of eating in public); and animal and other highly specific phobias focused on a single object (e.g., phobic fears of cats, dogs, dead birds, etc.). Phobias of internal origin include illness phobias (hypochondriasis) and a variety of symptoms which border on obsessions, e.g., fear of harming others either accidentally or due to some ungovernable impulse. Of all phobic states the so-called agoraphobic syndrome appears to be the most common. Here the sufferer, usually although not invariably a young married woman, becomes increasingly terrified every time she tries to leave home. Within a few yards of her front door she is overcome by panic, fears she may faint, and feels progressively unreal (depersonalization) leading her to flee back home, a state which may soon result in her becoming housebound. This type of phobic condition is much less symptom-specific than are social and animal phobias and is usually associated with other neurotic and depressive symptoms.

Another type of defence against anxiety is by *repression* of the original source of anxiety together with *dissociation*, that is a splitting-off of the repressed anxiety from the mainstream of awareness, and *conversion*, which leads to the production of certain *hysterical symptoms* such as paralyses, anaesthesias, hysterical aphonia, amnesic attacks, and so on. All these have the purpose of divorcing the patient in some way from the source of his or her anxiety. Thus the young girl with intense anxiety concerning sex may develop a hysterical paralysis of her legs which may in turn serve the purpose of preventing her being exposed to certain situations in which anxiety about sex may be aroused. The matter, however, is seldom quite so simple as this. Another form of defence against anxiety which, as has been indicated, is not too far removed from phobia formation, is the production of *obsessions* in which the sufferer finds himself compelled to indulge in all sorts of seemingly senseless rituals (*see* OBSESSIONS, p. 586).

Because of the nature of its physical symptoms, anxiety has a marked tendency to become *somatized*. The triad: *precordial pain, palpitations*, and *breathlessness on exertion*, may be easily misinterpreted by the patient as being due to heart disease when purely the outcome of anxiety; this in turn leads to the production of a *cardiac neurosis* or *effort syndrome* (*Da Costa's syndrome*). This may have to be distinguished from angina which, however, has a different quality and location and is more clearly related to effort. The anxious patient experiences precordial discomfort rather than pain, the location of this being in the region of the apex beat where he believes the mass of his heart to be. Anginal pain by contrast tends to be gripping and located in the region of the sternum. Other combinations of anxiety symptoms may give rise to recognizable though somewhat less well-defined hypochondriacal states. So-called *functional dyspepsia* is an example. In this a patient, often of markedly asthenic physical constitution, complains of more or less continuous vague pain generally in the epigastric region, but without much in the way of localized tenderness. The appetite is poor with a marked aversion to fatty or fried foods. Retching and even vomiting are common, although vomiting when it occurs is rarely of food but of gastric juice. Continuous belching may occur which may be the outcome of air swallowing (*aerophagy*). The pain does not, as in the case of peptic ulcer, bear a fairly well-defined relationship to meals, nor does it tend to wake the patient at night.

Where headaches are prominent migraine may be considered. Migraine headaches are, however, usually severe, throbbing, of hemi-cranial distribution, and often preceded by a characteristic hemi-anopic visual disturbance (*fortification spectrum*). Headaches associated with anxiety, on the other hand, more often consist of sensations of woolliness, pressure as might be caused by a cap, or a sensation as if an iron band is encircling the head. Bitemporal and frontal headaches are commonly described and sometimes an occipital aching sensation which may be the outcome of muscle tension in the neck. If eye symptoms are present these are often complained of as 'spots before the eyes' and almost invariably turn out to be due to *muscae volitantes* to which the attention of the patient is unduly drawn. If giddiness is severe, the possibility of vertigo due to Ménière's disease or some other similar condition may be considered. However, the giddiness of which the anxious patient complains does not have a true rotatory quality as in vertigo; indeed, what the patient usually means in using the term 'giddiness' is more often a vague 'muzzy' feeling as if he is about to faint.

An anxiety state in which psychiatric rather than physical symptoms are more prominent may need to be distinguished from *hyperthyroidism*. Clinically this can sometimes be difficult unless the signs of hyperthyroidism are patently obvious. Anxiety and sweating are features common to both disorders but the patient with an anxiety state is less responsive to climatic conditions. The pulse-rate is also rapid but in anxiety states falls below 80 beats per minute when the patient is asleep. In hyperthyroidism tremor is so fine as sometimes not to be immediately evident, in anxiety states it tends to be coarser and irregular. Studies of thyroid function will usually put the matter beyond doubt.

The diagnosis of a *primary anxiety state* calls for an investigation of its basic nature. It may be of purely neurotic origin having its roots in a difficult upbringing which leads to a persistent sense of insecurity. Anxious children tend to be born of anxious parents or to have undue anxiety engendered in them by parental discord. Inconsistency of parental behaviour towards a child may be an especially potent anxiety-producing factor. Adults with anxiety symptoms have almost invariably had these in one form or another from an early age. They give a history of being shy, timorous children who mix badly with others and cling closely to their mothers' skirts. They tend to be afraid of the dark and are more than ordinarily liable to nightmares. Psychosomatic upsets, principally vague abdominal symptoms which may prevent them going to school (which they attend unwillingly), are common. They are given to respiratory infections and other forms of minor ill health and are often referred to as 'delicate'. Their timidity, shyness, and inability to form social relationships persist into adolescence. At school they are not usually good at sports and prefer solitary pursuits. Day-dreaming is common. They are immature in sexual development and cannot relate adequately to either members of their own or the opposite sex. Although not necessarily unintelligent, they tend to lack drive and to be over-readily discouraged by initial failure.

Secondary anxiety states, i.e., those which are symptomatic of some other psychiatric or physical disorder, are those which tend to arise *de novo* in those who may not have been regarded hitherto of being of neurotic disposition. The most likely cause is *depression*, for indeed anxiety is an integral part of a *depressive illness*. All depressed patients show anxiety; in some it may be overwhelming, leading to intense agitation. In others, although anxiety may be less severe the depressive aspects of the clinical picture may be minimal and obscured to a degree by anxiety symptoms which may lead to an incorrect diagnosis of a neurotic anxiety state being made. Here the key to diagnosis lies in the elucidation of the patient's psychiatric history. But even if anxiety is the outcome of depression, the same kinds of defences as have already been described may be used to keep it at bay. Thus, in some depressive illnesses obsessions may be a prominent feature; in others hysterical symptoms may dominate the clinical picture.

Although in long-standing schizophrenia there is a flattening of emotional response, at the inception of the illness, especially when this is acute, the patient's anxiety level may be considerably heightened. Where, in adolescence, fairly intense anxiety symptoms appear which have not been present before, this possibility should therefore be borne in mind.

Just as anxiety is common in children so does it tend to recur with advancing age, and particularly as degeneration of the central nervous system begins to take place. However, even before then both physical and psychological anxiety-producing factors may start to become operative. In late middle age—the sixties—in many cases some degree of decline of physical health becomes apparent. There may be limitation of movement and activity due to arthritis, chronic bronchitis, heart disease, etc. There may also be some awareness of waning mental powers. Apart from these, there is the notion to be faced that life is possibly nearly over. Retirement, together with the financial insecurity that this may bring in its wake, is another potent source of anxiety. In *cerebral arteriosclerosis* anxiety and depression may be especially prominent. Faced with a social situation or some other task with which he can no longer cope the arteriosclerotic patient is liable to become acutely anxious, agitated, and tearful (*catastrophic reaction*). Anxiety may occur as an early feature of other cerebral disorders, but usually as dementia progresses there is a merciful flattening of emotional responses of all kinds so that with the final onset of 'sans everything' the patient is without anxiety also.

W. H. Trethowan.

AORTA, UNDUE PULSATION OF

Excessive, and easily palpable, pulsation of the abdominal aorta is hardly ever due to an aneurysm. If the pulse is collapsing, due to aortic incompetence or other similar lesion, the abdominal aortic pulse may be palpable; this, of course, is of no great significance. An atheromatous aorta may also be palpable due to the large pulse pressure resulting from the inelastic arterial tree. In thin subjects, especially those with a marked lumbar lordosis, pulsation of a normal aorta may be palpable; this, too, is of no great moment unless the patient has noticed it himself or his attention has been ill-advisedly drawn to it. Such a discovery may lead to various functional symptoms if the patient is temperamentally so predisposed. It is not uncommon in hyperthyroidism.

Excessive aortic pulsation may be transmitted to the overlying liver in the epigastrium and may lead the unwary into making a diagnosis of right ventricular hypertrophy or tricuspid incompetence. A search for a right ventricular impulse in the left parasternal region and for *expansile* pulsation of the liver will clarify the issue.

P. R. Fleming.

APPETITE, ABNORMAL

Appetite may be: (1) *Increased*; (2) *Diminished*; (3) *Perverted*.

Increase of Appetite (hyperorexia, bulimia) is rarely advanced as the primary complaint. Occasionally, in disease of the nervous system, as in the mentally disturbed and with hypothalamic lesions, patients may lose the sense of fullness after meals resulting in excessive consumption of food. Increase of appetite may be a feature of hysteria or may accompany diabetes mellitus, hyperthyroidism, steatorrhoea, gastro-intestinal fistulae, pregnancy, and infestation with intestinal parasites (round worms and tape-worms). In *diabetes mellitus*, especially in its earlier stages, there may be an abnormal craving for food, but, on the whole, this symptom in diabetes is not conspicuous, in contrast with that of thirst.

Diminution of Appetite may be a feature of organic gastric disease, of any chronic disease process, or may be psychological in origin.

Loss of appetite is often an early, occasionally the only, symptom in cases of gastric carcinoma and should lead to an examination for other features of that disease and, if necessary, to a barium-meal examination. However, loss of appetite may occur in many forms of dyspepsia, especially gastric ulcer. Duodenal ulceration accompanied by stenosis may result in loss of appetite and profound weight-loss. Patients with biliary disease often avoid food, sometimes from true hypo- or anorexia, sometimes to avoid attacks of pain (sitophobia). This fear of precipitating unpleasant symptoms of pain and fullness is also seen with peptic ulcers, after partial or complete gastrectomy, in regional enteritis, and with several other conditions.

Any chronic disease process, for example advanced malignant disease, chronic alcoholism, uraemia, severe congestive heart failure, chronic pulmonary disease, and hepatic cirrhosis, may be accompanied by loss of appetite. This is also a feature of any persistent febrile illness.

Patients with emotional upsets, depressive states, and delusions with reference to suspicion of poisoning may have loss of appetite. A special syndrome is *anorexia nervosa*, which affects young women who demonstrate a remarkable loss of appetite and weight and yet remain surprisingly well and active. This syndrome is accompanied by amenorrhoea, subnormal temperature, and a low basal metabolic rate. Obstinate constipation is usually present. There is sometimes a close resemblance to Simmonds's disease.

Perverted Appetite (parorexia) may occur in the course of pregnancy and is then of no special significance. It is met with, too, in nervous children in whom it often takes the form of dirt-eating (pica). Perverted appetite is also a common occurrence in insanity.

Harold Ellis.

ASCITES

Ascites is the term applied to the accumulation of serous fluid in the peritoneal cavity; it may be produced by a large variety of conditions.

Consideration must comprise: (*I*) *its physical signs*; (*II*) *its distinction from other conditions which may simulate it*; (*III*) *a classified list of its causes*; (*IV*) *the chief points which will help in arriving at a correct differential diagnosis in a particular case.*

I. PHYSICAL SIGNS

Inspection. The abdomen is uniformly distended. If the quantity of liquid is large and its accumulation has been rapid, the abdomen is more or less globular, the umbilical region being the most prominent. The skin is tense and shiny. If the quantity of liquid is large but its accumulation has been gradual, bulging of the flanks is more marked, the lower ribs may be pushed outwards and upwards and the epigastric angle widened. If the quantity of liquid is small, only a slight bulging of the flanks may be evident. The appearance of the abdomen depends a good deal on the position of the patient. When lying on one side, the most dependent part is the most prominent owing to the liquid gravitating to that side of the abdomen. If the patient stands or sits upright, the hypogastric and iliac regions will be most distended (*Fig.* 72).

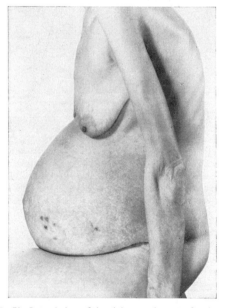

Fig. 72. Lateral view of the abdomen, the seat of ascites of chronic congestive cardiac failure. Puncture marks from repeated paracentesis are visible. In these days of effective diuretics such cardiac cases are extremely rare. (*Dr. C. G. Baker.*)

The umbilicus becomes stretched and may become flush with the surface or even be protruded. In cirrhosis of the liver the veins around the umbilicus may be dilated. The superficial veins all over the abdomen and lower part of the chest may become distended, the blood flowing in an upward direction, this reversal of the stream occurring mainly when the inferior vena cava is obstructed, either by the tension of the ascites or by something related to its cause (*see* VEINS, VARICOSE ABDOMINAL, p. 815). The abdominal respiratory

movements are diminished or may be entirely absent. The cardiac impulse may be displaced upwards and outwards and the legs, thighs, loins, and scrotum or labia may be oedematous.

Palpation. The abdomen demonstrates varying degrees of tenseness. A fluid thrill may be obtained by placing one hand against one flank and gently flicking the opposite flank with the fingers of the other hand. The possibility of an impulse being transmitted in the abdominal wall itself should be eliminated by instructing the patient or an assistant to place the side of his hand on the front of the abdomen in order to stop transmission of a mural current.

The experienced observer will detect a distinct 'heaviness' in the flanks simply by placing each hand beneath either flank with the patient lying on his back and gently lifting the hands upwards; this is due, of course, to the ascitic fluid gravitating into the paracolic compartment on either side.

If the liver or spleen has enlarged, it sinks backwards so that a layer of liquid is present between it and the abdominal wall. If the hand is placed on the abdomen in the right or left hypochondrium, as the case may be, and depressed suddenly, this liquid is displaced and the surface of the enlarged viscus can then be felt. This phenomenon of 'dipping' is almost pathognomonic of ascites.

Percussion. When the patient lies flat on his back the liquid gravitates to the posterior part of the abdomen, and the air-containing viscera float to the anterior part, so that the percussion note is resonant in front and dull in the flanks. As the liquid increases in quantity, the line of dullness creeps forward from the flanks and upwards from the pubes, keeping a concave upper border.

One of the most typical physical signs of ascites is the effect produced on the percussion note by a change in the posture of the patient. If, after examining him lying on the back and finding dullness in the flanks and resonance in the front, he is turned on one side, the uppermost flank becomes resonant and the line of dullness on the other side rises nearer to the midline, owing to the liquid gravitating to the most dependent part (shifting dullness). If only a very small quantity of liquid is present, the abdomen may be resonant all over when the patient lies on his back; on percussion in the knee–elbow position, the umbilical region may be found to be dull.

Tuberculous peritonitis may cause the liquid to be loculated through matting together of the abdominal viscera. The distension may not then be uniform, and a change of posture may not alter the distribution of the dull percussion note. **Auscultation** is sometimes recommended as a diagnostic measure. A tap on one side of the abdomen is said to communicate a characteristic sound to the bell of a stethoscope applied to the opposite side. There is very little to be said for this method of examination and one will never see an experienced clinician using it.

It is always important to examine the abdomen as soon as possible after paracentesis, if this procedure is to be performed. The cause of the ascites may then be discovered through the possibility of palpating tumours or enlargements of organs which were previously obscured by the tenseness of the abdominal wall.

II. DIFFERENTIAL DIAGNOSIS

Ascites has to be distinguished from other conditions which may give rise to general abdominal distension, especially from: (1) tympanites, (2) ovarian cysts, (3) gravid uterus, (4) distended bladder, (5) distension associated with obesity, (6) phantom tumour, (7) large abdominal cysts, (8) dilated stomach, and (9) hydro- or pyonephrosis.

1. Tympanites or gaseous distension of the bowel is distinguished from ascites by the following signs: the outline of distended coils of intestine may be visible, and peristaltic movements may be noticed; there is no fluid thrill if precautions are taken to prevent an impulse being transmitted by the abdominal wall; and the abdomen is resonant both in front and in the flanks. An X-ray of the abdomen will demonstrate the distended coils of bowel.

2. Ovarian Cysts may all but fill the abdomen and may be very difficult to differentiate from ascites. Careful palpation may reveal the uppermost border of the tumour mass. Percussion is useful in that there is usually dullness in front, with resonance in the flanks. A massive ovarian cyst may transmit the aortic pulsations but this phenomenon is not present in ascites. Bimanual examination may confirm that there is a mass arising from the pelvis. Much difficulty in diagnosis occurs when a malignant ovarian cyst and ascites coexist. Rarely a ruptured pseudomucinous cystadenoma of the ovary may be followed by pseudomyxoma peritonei.

3. Gravid Uterus with Hydrops Amnii. In this condition it may be possible to define the outline in its consistency with contractions and relaxations of the uterine muscle. On vaginal examination the cervix is found to be soft. Other signs of pregnancy are present, such as the characteristic condition of the breasts, the presence of foetal heart-sounds, as well as the history of amenorrhoea. There will be dullness in front of the abdomen with a convex upper border and resonance in the flanks.

4. Distended Bladder. This may occur as a globular mass in the midline reaching to the umbilicus or, occasionally, filling most of the abdomen. The mass is dull to percussion, rises up from the pelvis, and is usually accompanied by overflow incontinence of urine. The passage of a catheter should clear up all doubt.

5. General Obesity may cause considerable abdominal distension and it may be almost impossible to determine with certainty the presence of even a considerable amount of ascitic fluid. With obesity the umbilicus remains as a deep pit; with ascites it is pushed forward to become flush with the surface or may even protrude. (*Fig.* 73.)

6. Phantom Tumour. The abdomen may rarely be distended in hysterical women, especially at the time of the climacteric, so that ascites, ovarian tumour, or pregnancy (pseudocyesis) may be simulated. The phantom tumour disappears with the complete relaxation of the abdominal wall which follows administration of a general anaesthetic.

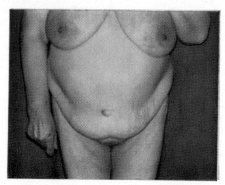

Fig. 73. Grossly obese patient. There is a small umbilical hernia present but even then there is not the protrusion of the navel which so often accompanies a considerable degree of ascites.

7. Large Abdominal Cysts or Cystic Swellings may occasionally simulate ascites, e.g., retroperitoneal cyst, pseudopancreatic cyst, mesenteric cyst, or hydatid cyst. They do not, as a rule, however, cause uniform distension of the abdomen and may have a well-demarcated outline.

8. A Dilated Stomach may occasionally reach an enormous size and be mistaken for ascites. However, a succussion splash can be elicited and visible gastric peristalsis, from left to right, may be seen.

9. Hydro- or Pyonephrosis may again reach an extraordinary size but is distinguished by the way it bulges back into one loin and is bimanually palpable.

III. CAUSES OF ASCITES

Fluid may collect in the peritoneal cavity as a result of transudation or exudation. Rarely, chyle may escape from ruptured lymphatic ducts.

Transudation results from an increase in pressure in the portal or systemic venous systems or lowering of the plasma osmotic pressure. It may, therefore, be a feature of congestive cardiac failure as a result of valvular disease, adherent pericardium, chronic myocardial disease, cardiomyopathy, or cor pulmonale. Portal hypertension alone is only rarely associated with ascites but requires the additional factor of either a lowered plasma protein, as may occur in cirrhosis, or increased hepatic lymphatic pressure which accompanies obstruction of the hepatic veins in the Arnold-Chiari syndrome. Gross depletion of plasma proteins in starvation and the nephrotic syndrome is accompanied by general anasarca.

Exudation occurs either in tuberculous peritonitis or carcinomatosis peritonei.

Chylous Ascites results from escape of chyle from the abdominal lymphatics or the thoracic duct. This may follow trauma, malignant obstruction, or obstruction by *Filaria bancroftii*.

Peritoneal transudate is faint yellow, has a specific gravity of less than 1·015, and contains few or no cells. The peritoneal exudate, in contrast, is deep yellow, is often turbid, and may clot on standing. The specific gravity is above 1·015. The fluid may be blood-stained, especially in malignant disease, and in these circumstances malignant cells may be seen on microscopy. In tuberculous peritonitis, lymphocytes are present.

In chylous ascites the fluid is milky and a cream separates on standing.

IV. DIFFERENTIAL DIAGNOSIS

If ascites is the only liquid accumulation present or if, although there is also oedema of the legs, the ascites is known to have appeared first, or if the ascites is out of proportion to the oedema or fluid collection elsewhere, it is probably due to either some form of cirrhosis or an exudation resulting from peritoneal involvement by tuberculosis or by malignant disease.

If the ascites is associated with general anasarca, that is to say, with oedema of the legs, body, and face, and with other serous effusions, the probable cause is the nephrotic syndrome.

If oedema of the legs is first noted, followed by the ascites, heart failure would be the most probable and commonest cause. It is difficult, however, to ensure reliable information regarding the onset of the oedema or the order in development.

Jaundice accompanying the ascites points to some form of portal obstruction as the cause, e.g., cirrhosis of the liver or hepatic metastases. Enlargement of the liver accompanying the ascites suggests cirrhosis, malignant disease, hydatid disease, or congestive nutmeg change, the result of backward pressure from chronic heart or lung disease. If accompanying multiple abdominal masses can be identified, tuberculous or malignant peritoneal disease, or, in rarer cases, hydatid disease must be considered.

1. Diseases of the Peritoneum

TUBERCULOUS PERITONITIS may occur in children and young adults. The following varieties are distinguished:

a. The acute ascitic form, which may simulate general peritonitis due to perforation of a viscus.

b. The subacute or chronic ascitic form. The peritoneum may be studded with miliary tubercles without any caseous masses. The physical signs are those of ascites without any abdominal tumour, and in adults the condition may be mistaken for cirrhosis of the liver or for malignant ascites. In a child the occurrence of ascites without oedema of the legs suggests tuberculous peritonitis; in an older person tuberculous peritonitis is much less common.

c. The omentum may be contracted and thickened from infiltration from caseous or fibrocaseous material and a hard abdominal 'tumour' may be felt across the upper abdomen. This may mimic an enlarged liver, but may be distinguished by the resonant percussion note between it and the costal margin; moreover, the liver edge may be palpable above and distinct from this omental mass. In cases of this kind ascites is generally less in amount than in the miliary tuberculous form.

d. The intestines may be matted together by adhesions which are thickened and infiltrated with tuberculous deposits, so that the peritoneal cavity may be divided into a number of loculi, the abdominal distension not being uniform.

Pyrexia and abdominal pain and tenderness are in proportion to the acuteness of the tuberculous process. Confirmatory evidence may be supplied by the presence of tuberculous lesions elsewhere; for instance in the spine, kidney, a joint, cervical lymph-nodes, or the chest, although the peritonitis is often the only objective tuberculous lesion. If paracentesis is performed some of the liquid should be injected into the guinea-pig, which may develop general tuberculosis during the succeeding six weeks. A search of the fluid for acid-fast organisms and appropriate culture for the mycobacterium are performed.

Ascites due to SECONDARY DEPOSITS rarely occurs before the age of 40. Fluid in the abdomen may be the first evidence of a growth, and it may be mistaken for that of cirrhosis or tuberculous peritonitis, especially when the abdominal distension is so considerable that no nodules can be felt. In other cases the ascites may develop in a patient with a known preceding tumour, for example, the primary in the stomach or bowel might already have been resected and the ascites is the first evidence of recurrence of the disease, or free fluid is discovered in the abdomen on routine examination in a patient with features of primary malignant disease elsewhere. The ascites usually collects rapidly and is accompanied by progressive emaciation and cachexia. A large quantity of liquid may be present and it is often blood-stained. Other masses may be present in the abdomen, deposits in the liver may be palpable, and a secondary nodule may be felt at the umbilicus. Rectal examination should never be omitted. Intra-abdominal malignant disease is sometimes indicated by enlargement of the left supraclavicular lymph-nodes through secondary deposits (Troisier's sign). Peritoneal spread of gastric carcinoma to the ovaries may be associated with ascites and a pelvic mass due to involvement of both ovaries, the so-called *Krukenberg tumour*.

Microscopic examination of the ascitic fluid by a cytologist may reveal the presence of malignant cells.

HYDATID CYSTS in the peritoneal cavity may be primary, but are more often secondary to hydatid disease of the liver. The malady is rare in this country although comparatively common in Australia and elsewhere. There may be a large globular tumour in the liver giving the 'hydatid thrill' on percussion. Eosinophilia is usual and Casoni's test may be positive. In some cases in which there are hydatid cysts associated with ascites it is possible to make the diagnosis by rectal examination. Globular bodies about the size of grapes may be felt in front of the anterior rectal wall; when these have been pressed upon they have slipped away from under the finger through being pushed up into the ascitic fluid to descend again after an interval into the pouch of Douglas. The ultimate diagnosis depends upon the detection of daughter cysts, hooklets (*Fig.* 74), or scolices (*Figs.* 2 and 3, p. 10), in the liquid

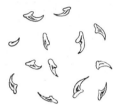

Fig. 74. Echinococcal hooklets. Low power.

obtained by paracentesis. The absence of hooklets does not exclude hydatid disease; the cysts may be sterile, in which case hooklets are not produced.

2. Diseases of the Liver

CIRRHOSIS OF THE LIVER. When ascites is the result of this condition, the diagnosis is usually easy. There may be a history of previous chronic alcoholism or of an episode of severe hepatitis. There may have been previous haematemesis, melaena, or jaundice. Other features in support are the presence of telangiectases on the cheek, spider naevi, a furred and tremulous tongue, nausea, vomiting, loss of appetite, distended veins around the umbilicus, gynaecomastia, loss of hair as well as libido, testicular atrophy, haemorrhoids, enlargement of the liver (the surface of which is hard), enlargement of the spleen, icterus, and the presence of a flapping tremor. Liver-function tests (p. 510) are often of help even in the early stages. In the late stages of the disease, the liver may be shrunken. Since the ascites is largely determined by hypoproteinaemia there is often associated oedema of the legs.

MALIGNANT DISEASE OF THE LIVER is usually due to secondary deposits from carcinoma or malignant melanoma. Primary growths of the liver are rare in this country although hepatoma is particularly likely to occur in the liver already the seat of cirrhosis and is comparatively common in the Far East and East Africa. The liver becomes very hard and greatly enlarged, the edge often extending well below the umbilicus. Besides being very hard, the liver may be tender and umbilicated nodules may be felt on its surface. The ascites associated with this condition may result from a number of causes acting alone or together. The tumour masses themselves may produce portal venous obstruction; extensive destruction of liver tissue may result in a fall in the serum albumin with consequent reduction in serum osmotic pressure; secondary deposits in the liver may be associated with carcinomatosis peritonei so that the free fluid in the peritoneal cavity may result in large part from this cause.

3. Portal Vein Thrombosis. Portal venous obstruction alone will result in portal hypertension, the development of oesophageal varices (with consequent risk of melaena and haematemesis), and splenomegaly. Ascites will not develop in uncomplicated portal vein occlusion unless this is associated with some other factor, usually a fall in plasma protein resulting from haemorrhage.

Portal vein thrombosis may result from umbilical sepsis in the neonatal period, either from infection at the time of division of the cord or as a result of exchange transfusion. It may result from portal pyaemia or operative trauma, particularly an unsuccessful portacaval shunt or consequent upon spreading thrombosis from the divided splenic vein at splenectomy. It may result from pressure of adjacent tumours of the pancreas, stomach, or secondarily involved lymph-nodes and may complicate chronic pancreatitis. It may follow abdominal injuries and finally may occur in association with polycythaemia and other blood diseases.

4. Obstruction of the Hepatic Veins. This condition, the *Budd-Chiari syndrome*, is rare and may be either due to occlusion of the hepatic veins themselves or, more often, due to obstruction of the inferior vena cava at the site of the orifices of the hepatic veins. The most common cause is the extension of a renal carcinoma along the renal vein into the inferior vena cava, but the condition may result from pressure of an enlarged liver, the site of malignant deposits. Thrombosis may complicate polycythaemia or thrombophlebitis migrans. A membranous obliteration of the hepatic segment of the inferior vena cava has been described which may be congenital in origin. The condition is characterized by enlargement of the liver and ascites. If the inferior vena cava is obstructed there will also be gross oedema of the legs and dilatation of the veins of the abdominal wall (*see* VEINS, VARICOSE ABDOMINAL, p. 815).

5. Right-sided Heart Failure. When the right ventricle fails, there is a rise in pressure in the right atrium and hence in the systemic venous system, as demonstrated by engorged neck veins, enlarged and tender liver, oedema, and ascites. Ascites in this condition is nearly always, but not invariably, preceded by oedema of the legs. Signs of the disease causing either the right-heart failure or the left-heart failure which very frequently precedes it may be present. There may be a history of acute rheumatism or of chronic bronchitis or emphysema since many of these patients are examples either of rheumatic valvular disease or of cor pulmonale.

An important group of diseases which may present difficulty in diagnosis are constrictive pericarditis and the cardiomyopathies. *Constrictive pericarditis* (Pick's disease) results from fibrous thickening of the pericardium. This is associated with calcification in about half the cases. Most probably the condition results from healed tuberculous pericarditis, but some examples may follow suppurative bacterial disease. The condition is found in adults of either sex and of any age and is characterized by the triad of a high venous pressure, with engorgement of the jugular veins, a small 'quiet' heart, and ascites. About a quarter of the patients have associated auricular fibrillation. The E.C.G. shows low-voltage QRS complexes as well as pericardial T-wave changes. X-ray screening usually shows a heart of normal size or, if it is enlarged, the enlargement is not proportional to the degree of congestive failure. Movements of the heart are seen to be limited. The initial ascites is followed eventually by generalized oedema together with liver enlargement.

The cardiomyopathies give a similar picture to that of constrictive pericarditis, although the X-rays show no calcification. There are numerous aetiological factors including virus infection, collagen disease, amyloidosis, and alcoholism. In Africa, endomyocardial fibrosis is common among young adults; its origin is unknown.

6. Renal Disease. Ascites may be produced in renal disease under two circumstances. In the nephrotic syndrome there is excessive loss of albumin in the urine leading to a lowered plasma albumin level so that the colloid osmotic pressure is unable to retain the fluid volume within the capillaries. Severe examples of this condition are associated with massive anasarca. In terminal stages of chronic nephritis congestive cardiac failure supervenes with ascites as one of its associated manifestations.

7. Chylous Ascites. This is not in itself a specific malady because there are several conditions in which the ascitic fluid may resemble milk. This may result from obstruction to the main abdominal lymphatics or the thoracic duct by secondary deposits of malignant disease or one of the reticuloses. The best known tropical cause for chylous ascites is *Filaria bancroftii* often with associated elephantiasis. The lymphatic channels may also be damaged by trauma, either at the time of operation or following abdominal injury.

The fluid is yellowish-white in colour and opalescent. Microscopically it contains fine fat globules and generally shows a distinct creamy layer on standing.

Harold Ellis.

ATAXIA

Co-ordination of movement implies the execution of the movement with accuracy and with the most economical expenditure of energy and time. It is disturbed by muscular weakness, spasticity, involuntary movements, sensory loss, and cerebellar disease, but *in clinical practice the term ataxia is restricted to inco-ordination resulting from affections of the sensory and the cerebellar systems*. It may, of course, be aggravated by coexistent spasticity, weakness, or involuntary movements.

Sensory Ataxia refers to the inco-ordination of movement which occurs in a limb or limbs as a result of sensory loss. The motor cortex is dependent on the sensory cortex and on afferent fibres passing to it from the spinal cord and brain-stem for guidance as to the position of the body in space and for 'information' about the movements it controls. In the absence of this sensory evidence, the corticospinal system cannot co-ordinate the activities for which it is responsible any more than an army headquarters can regulate the fighting of forward units the positions of which are unknown. Cutaneous sensory loss causes a comparatively slight degree of ataxia, and that mainly for fine movements. Impairment of sensibility of joints, muscles, and ligaments, on the other hand, gives rise to severe ataxia. Such proprioceptive sensory loss occurs in disease of the peripheral nerves (e.g., polyneuritis), of the posterior roots (e.g., tabes dorsalis), of the posterior columns (e.g., subacute combined degeneration of the cord), and in lesions of the medial lemniscus, thalamus, and sensory cortex. The resulting ataxia is characterized by clumsiness and fumbling in the execution of all movements, and is much aggravated when visual guidance is removed by closing the eyes. Gait is wide-based and uncertain, the feet coming to the ground with undue force; whereas it may be possible to stand still with the eyes open, the body sways when the eyes are closed (Rombergism). Movements of the upper limb are slow and clumsy; fine movements, such as are involved in doing up buttons, are carried out laboriously and may be impossible without visual aid. If the facial and bulbar muscles are affected, dysarthria follows. Diagnosis depends on the demonstration of proprioceptive sensory loss, and on conventional tests, such as the heel–knee and finger–nose tests, which demonstrate the typical aggravation of the ataxia on closing the eyes.

Sensory ataxia is seen in any *polyneuritis* with proprioceptive sensory loss, as in the polyneuritis of *diphtheria, diabetes, visceral carcinoma, polyarteritis nodosa, Hodgkin's disease, alcoholism*, and *arsenical poisoning*; in the infective *polyneuritis of Guillain-Barré*; in the rare *familial hypertrophic polyneuritis*, and the *polyneuritis of acute porphyrinuria*. Ataxia from disease of the posterior roots and subsequent degeneration of the posterior columns is exemplified by *tabes dorsalis*; the legs are usually more severely affected than the arms, but the reverse is seen in the rare 'cervical tabes'. In a minority of tabetics, postural sensibility is either normal or slightly impaired despite the presence of ataxia; this is due to degeneration of Clarke's column and the spinocerebellar tracts which convey afferent impulses from joints and ligaments to the cerebellum; these impulses do not reach the conscious level as a sensation, and such ataxia is 'cerebellar' rather than sensory in its clinical characteristics. *Subacute combined degeneration of the cord*, usually but not exclusively associated with pernicious anaemia, exhibits a sensory ataxia due to degeneration of the posterior columns, but the ataxia is soon overlaid by weakness. Prolonged *starvation*, such as occurred in prisoner-of-war camps in the Far East in 1941–5, can give rise to a syndrome marked by sensory (spinal) ataxia, peripheral neuritis, and visual defect from retrobulbar neuropathy. In some forms of *heredofamilial ataxia*, notably the Friedreich type, proprioceptive sensory loss complicates the degeneration of the spinocerebellar tracts, and the ataxia is of a mixed type. In *disseminated sclerosis* ataxia may be sensory, cerebellar, or mixed, depending on the distribution of the lesions; it usually appears in a cerebellar form. *Gross lesions of the spinal cord*—tumours, transverse myelitis—seldom give rise to obvious ataxia because of the presence of an overriding degree of weakness and spasticity. *Disease of the brain-stem* is more likely to give rise to a cerebellar type of ataxia than the sensory variety because of the concentration of cerebellar afferent and efferent tracts in this region. Injuries and disease of the thalamus, internal capsule, and sensory cortex may cause sensory ataxia of the limbs on the opposite side of the body. In parietal lesions, inability to carry out movements may be due to sensory ataxia, or the disability may on occasion be an expression of apraxia, a condition in which the pattern of voluntary movement is disturbed so that the patient cannot carry out familiar actions although he understands what he is required to do. Thus he may 'forget' how to walk, although there is no ataxia of the legs for other activities or on formal clinical tests.

Cerebellar Ataxia is distinguished from sensory ataxia by the presence of normal postural sensibility. There are important and physiologically interesting differences between the two forms, but the sensory findings provide the diagnostic guide in clinical practice. Each cerebellar hemisphere exerts a controlling influence on the co-ordination of movement of its own side of the body. Afferent impulses from the limbs, trunk, neck, bulbar muscles, eyes, and labyrinth pass to the cerebellum through the cerebellar peduncles. Efferent fibres go to the pontine nuclei and the vestibular nucleus, whence descending tracts convey impulses to the spinal cord. Other efferent fibres cross to the red nucleus and to the thalamus of the opposite side; those to the thalamus are relayed to the premotor cortex. Each hemisphere of the cerebellum is thus linked with the premotor cortex of the opposite side, but since the cerebrospinal and rubrospinal tracts themselves cross the midline on their downward path, the rule of homolateral cerebellar control is maintained.

These connexions explain important clinical observations. They explain why lesions of the frontal lobe sometimes give rise to a cerebellar type of inco-ordination on the opposite side of the body; why diseases affecting the labyrinth and the vestibular nucleus mimic cerebellar symptoms on the same side as the lesion; why destruction of the afferent spinocerebellar tracts in the cord, by denying the cerebellum the information from the periphery which is necessary for its functions, causes homolateral ataxia below the level of the lesion.

The clinical features of cerebellar ataxia depend on loss of the modifying and regulating influence which the cerebellum exerts on muscle movement by augmenting or inhibiting muscular tone in accordance with the needs of the moment. This regulation of tone is exerted on muscles which are directly and indirectly concerned with a given movement.

It controls agonists, antagonists, synergists, and more distant muscles which 'fix' the trunk and limb and so provide the prime movers with a firm basis for action. Impairment of cerebellar function affects all these functions, and the resulting inco-ordination may be analysed by conventional clinical tests. Thus imbalance between agonists and antagonists is seen in jerkiness of movement, as for example when the outstretched finger is brought to the nose (action tremor), and in the tendency for willed movements to be carried out either too forcefully or too weakly, as when the hand, on attempting to grasp an object, either fails to reach it or overshoots it (dysmetria). Loss of normal synergy is most easily demonstrated by asking the patient to make a fist; the synergic dorsiflexion of the wrist, which normally augments the efficiency of the long flexors of the fingers, is absent. Defective postural fixation is seen during rapid pronation–supination movements of the forearm; normally this is carried out smoothly and quickly from the elbows, the upper arm remaining fixed, but in cerebellar disease the whole upper limb takes part in the movement so that there is failure to carry out, regularly and rapidly, alternating movements such as pronation and supination of the forearm or opening and closing the hand (dysdiadochokinesia). In extreme cases this impairment of postural fixation, which depends on the maintenance of postural tone, affects the trunk and legs as well, so that the entire body sways unsteadily when the upper limb is being used. Impairment of postural tone in the extrinsic ocular muscles gives rise to nystagmus, and cerebellar inco-ordination of speech produces dysarthria. In attempting to overcome inco-ordination, complicated movements are broken up into their constituent parts; in performing the heel–knee test, the thigh is flexed, then the knee; the limb is then adducted and the heel is allowed to fall on to the knee (decomposition of movement). This same process is seen in some cases of cerebellar dysarthria; words are broken up into syllables and each is pronounced separately (scanning speech). Cerebellar gait is marked by a tendency to fall towards the affected side; if overcompensation occurs, the patient may then sway to the non-affected side. The feet are put down noisily (dysmetria) and decomposition of leg movements may sometimes be discerned in each forward movement of the affected limb. Because of this imbalance a broad-based gait affords additional stability and is voluntarily adopted by the experienced patient. *These disabilities are not significantly increased by closing the eyes.* The head is sometimes held towards the affected side and the arm fails to swing normally during walking. Tremors of the head and trunk may occur when standing or sitting—an action tremor.

Damage to the midline flocculonodular lobe of the cerebellum or of the vermis causes dysequilibrium in which there is unsteadiness of stance and of gait which may be so severe that the patient is unable to stand or to walk (astasia abasia) but no nystagmus or dysarthria, and no ataxia of the limbs when the patient is sitting or lying down. It is readily mistaken for hysteria because of this seeming contradiction.

Acute cerebellar lesions—cystic degeneration in a glioma, thrombosis, haemorrhage into an angiomatous cyst, penetrating injuries, acute cerebellar abscess—give rise to signs which are not seen in chronic disease. There may be vertigo, vomiting, and forced movements which rotate the patient so that he comes to rest prone, with the side of the face corresponding to the cerebellar lesion in contact with the pillow. Hypotonia and ataxia are general, but soon become limited to the limbs on the affected side. Skew deviation of the eyes may occur. When the pressure below the tentorium is high, as in tumour, attacks of decerebrate rigidity may occur; these are probably due to pressure on the brain-stem.

It has already been noted that cerebellar ataxia may be due to lesions in widely separate sites— the prefrontal area of the cerebral hemispheres, the brain-stem, the cerebellum and its peduncles, the vestibular system, and the spinocerebellar tracts. Of these the brain-stem is the commonest site and then the cerebellum. *Disseminated sclerosis* is a common cause. *Thrombosis of the posterior inferior cerebellar artery* may cause acute unilateral ataxia of abrupt onset.

Gliomata, haemangioblastomata, and *secondary growths* from the lungs and elsewhere are not infrequent. Cerebellar degeneration can occur as a 'toxic' result of a primary carcinoma of the lung, and even more rarely from carcinoma elsewhere in the body. *Cerebellar abscess* (usually otitic in origin) and *tuberculoma* are now infrequent infective lesions, and the rare but transient cerebellar ataxia of the *encephalomyelitis* which follows the exanthemata, particularly measles, must be remembered. Equally uncommon is cerebellar degeneration in *Schilder's disease* and *cerebromacular degeneration. Pelizaeus-Merzbacher disease* is a rare familial disease starting in infancy and characterized by cerebellar ataxia and a wheel nystagmus, to which pyramidal signs are added later on. *Congenital ataxia,* with or without an associated cerebral diplegia, is a rare developmental defect which appears in the first two years of life. Cerebellar ataxia can occur in basilar impression, a condition in which upward displacement of the basi-occiput causes compression of the cerebellar tonsils, which may come to lie below the foramen magnum. It is sometimes

a congenital defect; in other cases it is due to softening of the skull in Paget's disease and in osteomalacia. *Head injuries* which involve severe contusion of the brain-stem, and gunshot wounds of the cerebellum itself, give rise to ataxia; the only diagnostic difficulty likely to arise is confusion with hysterical ataxia following head injuries, but absence of nystagmus, inconsistencies in the physical signs, and the presence of positive psychological manifestations of hysteria will indicate the nature of the malady. Traumatic ataxia is seldom either severe or persistent except in the special variety known as 'punch-drunkenness', or *chronic progressive traumatic encephalopathy* of boxers, i.e., in pugilists who have become punch-drunk as a result of repeated blows to the head during a long and usually undistinguished career in the ring. Dementia and emotional lability develop very slowly. Memory suffers, and both thought and speech slow down. Fatuous cheerfulness, irritability, and uninhibited behaviour are common, and insight is speedily lost so that the victim is quite unaware of his deterioration. A similar encephalopathy occurs in National Hunt jockeys who have had a number of falls on the head. The physical signs are a mixture of cerebellar ataxia and extrapyramidal disorder—an expressionless face, slurred speech, slowness of movement, tremor of the head and hands, unsteady gait, and general clumsiness. The condition may have a superficial resemblance to frontal tumour, general paralysis, or disseminated sclerosis.

Reference has been made to the occurrence of a cerebellar type of ataxia in *frontal lesions.* Caution must be exercised in attributing incoordination to a lesion at this site, because an expanding tumour may displace the brain-stem and cerebellum downwards so that the cerebellar tonsils are forced into the foramen magnum, with a resultant disturbance of cerebellar function; moreover widely infiltrating growths of the cerebral hemisphere may give rise to an apraxia, which may superficially resemble an ataxia of gait and will mislead unless the nature of the disturbance is subject to critical analysis.

Disease affecting the *spinocerebellar tracts,* which convey afferent impulses from muscles and joints to the cerebellum, is not a common cause of ataxia, because the cerebellar component is usually obscured by spasticity and by proprioceptive sensory loss. Nevertheless it is seen in disseminated sclerosis, in some tabetics, in subacute combined degeneration of the cord, and— in a relatively pure form—in the early stages of Friedreich's ataxia.

Ataxia due to Drugs and Chemicals. Acute alcoholism is a familiar example of an intoxication ataxia. Barbiturate poisoning may be followed for days or even weeks by slurring speech, nystagmus, and ataxia of the limbs. Sodium-diphenyl-hydantoinate has a similar effect. Hypoglycaemia, whether due to insulin overdosage or endogenous hyperinsulinism, may be marked by a reeling gait in the early stages of its development. Carbon-monoxide poisoning from incomplete combustion of coal-gas, coke, and petrol may give rise to ataxia amongst other effects.

Hysteria. Ataxia is one of the many somatic symptoms found in hysteria. Diagnosis depends on the demonstration of inconsistencies in the ataxia itself, the absence of organic disease, and above all on the presence of demonstrable psychological disturbance. Difficulties arise when there is an organic nucleus with hysterical exaggeration, and it must be remembered that an entirely 'organic' ataxia may be complicated by a neurosis. A further complication concerns the presence of inconsistencies. In cerebellar disease it may be possible for the patient to carry out the heel–knee test and other formal tests of co-ordination in a normal manner when recumbent but yet be literally unable to stand. This apparent inconsistency is due to the fact that the lateral lobes of the cerebellum are responsible for co-ordination and the middle lobe for balance, each of which may be involved separately in a disease process.

Ian Mackenzie.

AURA

An aura commonly regarded as something heralding an epileptic attack is really the first stage of such an attack. It is recognized in some form in about 30 per cent of patients with epilepsy and usually takes the same form in each individual, although not invariably present. An aura may be motor, sensory, psychical, visceral, or related to some special sense. A *motor* aura may be represented by an involuntary movement of a limb or a part of a limb; or a general movement such as running. A *sensory* aura is common, and is described as a pain, a numbness, or a tingling in some part of the patient's body. Paraesthesiae spreading to one half of the body, or less, may occur in migraine, but in this case they last several minutes whereas in epilepsy they last a few seconds only. A *psychical* aura is often expressed as a vague apprehension, or an indescribable feeling, or a sense of unreality. A *visceral* aura is frequent, usually as an 'epigastric sensation' or queer feeling starting in the region of the stomach and rising to the throat, or less often as a peremptory desire to go to stool. An aura may be *olfactory*, *visual*, *auditory*, or *gustatory*; a pleasant or unpleasant odour or flavour may be perceived by the patient, or some alteration in vision may warn him of the onset of a seizure, or he may hear voices or some particular kind of sound.

The aura of epilepsy is, in relation to diagnosis, important from at least two points of view. In the first place, it often affords a clue to the particular locality in the brain from which the 'fit' or 'storm' originates and spreads. A tumour of the uncinate region of the temporo-sphenoidal lobe, for instance, may be revealed by signs of increased intracranial pressure and the repeated occurrence of an olfactory aura, followed by a vague, dreamy state of consciousness. A lesion of one occipital lobe may be suspected from the occurrence of epileptiform fits immediately preceded by an aura consisting of visual disturbance limited to the opposite field. An aura of pain starting in the left foot, spreading up the left side of the body, and terminating in a generalized convulsion, suggests a lesion of the post-Rolandic region of the right parietal lobe.

In the second place, the importance of recognizing a subjective sensation as an aura, and so recognizing the existence of epilepsy in its simplest and sometimes earliest form, can hardly be over-estimated from the point of view of treatment. When a patient describes himself as being liable to subjective sensations occurring at intervals, and for which he cannot account, careful inquiry should be made as to their nature. The chief characteristics of an aura are: (1) Its spontaneous development without cause, generally during good health; (2) The suddenness of its onset; and (3) Its brevity. An aura may occur alone, or may be followed by momentary loss of consciousness (minor epilepsy), or by loss of consciousness with convulsions (major epilepsy); in some cases an aura may be repeated for many months before a typical epileptic seizure supervenes, and if recognized as such during this stage it is reasonable to expect that treatment will have more chance of success than at a later period when the 'habit' of convulsions has been established firmly. The recurrence of an aura, even without further manifestations of the disease, is evidence that the morbid tendency is not controlled completely, and that discontinuance of treatment will lead to the reappearance of more serious attacks.

Ian Mackenzie.

AXILLA, SWELLING IN

Swelling in the axilla is due in the great majority of cases to enlargement of the lymphatic nodes. If the enlargement is inflammatory, a subsequent abscess, either acute or chronic, is frequent. Any form of tumour other than a nodular one is distinctly rare, but unfortunately it is common to find the node the seat of metastases from carcinoma of the breast.

Acute Abscess may be recognized at once by the well-marked signs of local inflammation and the general febrile disturbance. There is one form of acute abscess that may not be obvious, namely, one situated in the upper part of the axilla and covered by the pectoral muscles. On account of its distance from the surface the local signs of inflammation may not be great, though the general signs are marked. There will be great disinclination to move the arm on account of pain, and there is usually some cause, such as a whitlow on the finger, to account for the trouble. It must be remembered, however, that the abscess may be 'residual'; that is to say, the original source of infection, such as the whitlow, may have healed completely two, three weeks or even longer before the axillary abscess declares itself. Occasionally an empyema points in the axilla; there are generally, but not always, abnormal lung signs to suggest the diagnosis.

Chronic or **Tuberculous Abscess** forms a single fluctuating swelling which, if large, may extend upwards under the pectoralis major. Owing to the fact that few, if any, of the local signs of inflammation may be present, difficulty may arise in distinguishing this form of abscess from a soft lipoma. The duration and the rapidity of growth of the swelling are good guides, for though the duration of a chronic abscess may run into months, it does not exist for years, as does a lipoma. Aspiration will settle the difficulty.

Enlargement of the Lymphatic Nodes. Next, supposing that examination proves that the swelling is not an abscess, attention should be directed to ascertain whether it arises from lymph-nodes, and it is therefore necessary to recall the anatomical position of the nodes. The axillary lymphatic nodes are ten to twelve in number, and are arranged in three sets. One chain surrounds the axillary vessels and receives the lymphatics from the arm; a small chain runs along the border of the pectoralis minor receiving the lymphatics from the front of the chest and the breast; the third chain is placed along the lower margin of the posterior wall, to receive lymphatics from the integuments of the back. If the nodes are affected in any way, all need not necessarily be enlarged, but it would be extremely unusual if only one were picked out, and commonly two or three glands, or one entire group, are affected. Therefore axillary swellings due to nodular enlargement are almost always multiple, and are situated in the part of the axilla where nodes are normally present. This may not be quite accurate when much inflammation has occurred around the glands and they are matted together, as happens with tuberculous infection; but even then the mass may be felt to be made up of many nodes. For the differential diagnosis of nodular swellings, *see* LYMPHATIC NODE ENLARGEMENT (p. 513), axillary nodes in particular being dealt with on p. 516. It is sufficient here to enumerate the principal causes. These are: acute infection, chronic infection with tuberculosis or syphilis; rheumatoid arthritis, lymphatic leukaemia, lymphosarcoma, and Hodgkin's disease; malignant glandular metastases. The first and the last are far the most common in the axilla.

Occasionally a node or group of nodes in the axilla appears malignant and on being removed for histological section is found to be infiltrated with metastatic carcinoma, and yet no source for the primary can be found. The most likely site for such a hidden primary is undoubtedly the breast and, next to this, the lung, so that an energetic search should be instituted by clinical, radiological, and laboratory methods as well as by bronchoscopy to incriminate or exculpate these two organs. Other less common possibilities are the stomach and the ovary, and if all investigations have so far been negative, expert pelvic examination and a complete investigation of the gastro-intestinal tract are called for. If, after careful search in this way, no primary can be detected it must be assumed that this is within the breast. It is probably unwise, however, to perform a 'blind mastectomy', because although cancerous tissue will probably be revealed in the mastectomy specimen, it is very doubtful whether, the breast being left in situ, the next manifestation to obtrude would be in that organ. Indeed, the appearance of supra-clavicular nodes or skeletal metastases are more common and to have removed the breast would have been fruitless. The introduction of mammography has helped to reveal very small breast carcinomas presenting as enlarged axillary glands.

Primary Tumours of the Axilla are distinctly rare, but it is a possible site for an accessory breast, the nipple of which will provide the diagnosis.

LIPOMA is the most common tumour. It may attain a large size and extend up under the pectoral muscles. It should be diagnosed by its long history, slow growth, definite outline, and free mobility. When very soft, the tumour may give the feeling of fluctuation, and so be mistaken for a chronic tuberculous abscess, and as it consists of large lobules of fluid fat, some degree of translucency may be present. The skin wrinkles when one attempts to raise it away from the tumour.

CYSTIC HYGROMA of the axilla is rare. It is usually congenital, but apparently similar cystic swellings may appear in adult life. It forms a soft, fluctuating, quite translucent and painless swelling, which sometimes grows rapidly. It may be mistaken for a lipoma, and the diagnosis may not be certain until excision and microscopical examination are completed.

PRIMARY MALIGNANT TUMOURS may arise, but are of extreme rarity.

ANEURYSM OF THE AXILLARY ARTERY does occur, but is uncommon. It is recognized easily because it is comparatively superficial and it gives an expansile pulsation synchronous with the heart's beat; the veins of the forearm may be distended on account of pressure on the axillary vein, and the radial pulse on the affected side is diminished in size and delayed. There may be a definite history of local injury, or in cases of apparently spontaneous aneurysm there may be signs or symptoms of bacterial endocarditis.

R. G. Beard.

BABINSKI'S SIGN

Babinski's sign is a modification of the plantar reflex. In eliciting the latter the patient should be lying upon his back with the leg straight; the ankle should be grasped firmly while a blunt-pointed instrument firmly strokes from the heel forwards up the outer border of the sole. In healthy adults the toes will adduct and plantar-flex, and the foot may extend and the quadriceps contract—that is to say, there is a lengthening reaction of the limb. When the pyramidal fibres to the leg are interrupted by disease, the response is usually different: there is a shortening reaction. The toes fan out, the big toe is dorsiflexed, the foot is withdrawn, and the hamstrings may con-tract—Babinski's sign of pyramidal disease, otherwise known as an extensor plantar response. It is a sign of interference with the pyramidal system at some point between the motor cortex and the anterior horn cells of the lumbar segment of the cord, but it is also present bilaterally in any organically determined coma—as in an epileptic fit, general anaesthesia, uraemia, concussion, etc. In coma it has no localizing significance. The response will be flexor when a pyramidal lesion is combined with a lower motor neuron paralysis of the physiological flexors of the toes, foot, and knee. An extensor response is associated with loss of the other superficial reflexes on the same side of the body—the abdominals and the cre-masteric reflex—provided that the pyramidal fibres which serve these reflexes are also involved, as is usually the case. It is normal to find an extensor response in infants under the age of twelve months, and it may persist for longer. Moreover, in adults there is ample evidence that the sign may fail to appear in cases of proved trans-section of the pyramidal tracts in the spinal cord.

Ian Mackenzie.

BACK, PAIN IN

Pain in the back is one of the commonest com-plaints in general and specialist practice, and no specialism is immune from it. The differential diagnosis, therefore, covers most of medicine. The first important subdivision is into acute and chronic back pain.

Acute Pain in the Back may occur in any febrile disorder, even after an injection of T.A.B. vac-cine. A good example is dengue or 'break-bone fever'. It may also result from injury: any gar-dener, spring-cleaning housewife, or horse-rider knows how common such minor insults are. Such pains usually rapidly settle either when the cause is removed or as the injured tissues heal. Only when the back aches and pains persist after several days does one look further into the possible causes.

Chronic Backache. In any backache lasting more than 2–3 weeks the conditions listed in the Table (p. 86) should be considered. By far the com-monest are the first four mentioned (1 (*a*)–(*d*)), sometimes associated with depression or anxiety. The list is probably incomplete but covers most of the likely causes. In eliciting the cause, a full history is essential, with particular reference to factors operating at the time of onset and factors known to ease or aggravate the condition. On

examination the way a patient moves, walks, sits, or lies, and how he rises from sitting and lying positions may be highly informative. Spinal range of movement may be measured by various instruments such as Dunham's spondylometer (*Fig.* 75) or Loebl's inclinometer. Another

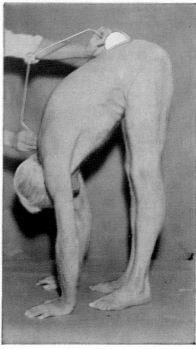

Fig. 75. Ankylosing spondylitis. The patient can touch the floor easily with his hands but measurement with a spondylo-meter shows spinal movement to be restricted to 60 per cent of normal.

method is that of Schober, which depends on stretching of the skin over the lumbar spine in spinal flexion. More sensitive and accurate is Macrae's modification of the same method, which measures stretching of the skin in spinal flexion between a point 10 cm. above the lumbo-sacral junction and a spot 15 cm. below over the sacrum. Ability to touch the toes is a poor measure of spinal movement as it depends greatly on hip flexion; these methods elimi-nate the hip component. They also enable the examiner to give a positive figure for the spinal range of movement, which can be measured repeatedly to assess progression or regression of the spinal disorder. Radiography often helps in diagnosis, but even more often does not. The fact that there are radiological changes does not mean that these are the cause of the symptoms. Radiologically speaking, there is no such thing as a normal spine after middle age is passed.

1. Non-infective Traumatic and Degenerative Dis-orders arising in the bones, joints, and soft tissues of the spine are extremely common. In a structure of such complexity as the human spine, with so many joints, ligaments, and cartilages at risk, it is no wonder that aches and pains are common-place. Too-easy chairs at home, badly placed car seats, and unsatisfactory chairs at work are often the cause of postural strain. Fixed unnatural positions held for hours on end are highly productive of symptoms. Bad posture and fatigue act together to produce one of the most common of backaches. The postural back pain of pregnancy usually goes soon after child-birth but is sometimes replaced by one of lumbo-sacral origin due to the childbirth itself. Obesity is an aggravating factor rather than a sole cause, but chronic backaches may not infrequently be

THE CAUSES OF CHRONIC BACKACHE

1. *Traumatic, Mechanical, or Degenerative*:
(*a*) Low back strain; fatigue; obesity; pregnancy. (*b*) In-juries of bone, joint, or ligament. (*c*) Degenerative dis-ease of the spine (osteo-arthrosis) including ankylosing hyperostosis. (*d*) Intervertebral disk lesions. (*e*) Lumbar instability syndromes, e.g., spondylolisthesis. (*f*) Scoli-osis: primary and secondary.

2. *Metabolic*:
Osteoporosis. Osteomalacia. Hyperparathyroidism. Ochronosis. Fluorosis. Hypophosphataemic rickets.

3. *Unknown Causes*:
Inflammatory arthropathies of the spine, such as anky-losing spondylitis and the spondylitis of Reiter's (Brodie's) disease, psoriasis, ulcerative colitis, Whipple's and Crohn's diseases. Rarely polymyositis and polymyalgia rheumatica. Paget's disease of bone. Epiphysitis (Scheuermann's disease).

4. *Infective Conditions of Bone, Joint, and Theca of Spine*:
Osteomyelitis. Tuberculosis. Undulant fever (abortus and melitensis). Typhoid and paratyphoid fever and other *Salmonella* infections. Syphilis. Yaws. Very rarely Weil's disease (leptospirosis icterohaemorrhagica). Spinal pachymeningitis. Chronic meningitis. Subarachnoid or spinal abscess.

5. *Psychogenic*:
Anxiety. Depression. Hysteria. Compensation neurosis. Malingering.

6. *Neoplastic—Benign or Malignant, Primary or Secon-dary*:
Osteoid osteoma. Eosinophilic granuloma. Metastatic carcinomatosis. Bronchial carcinoma. Oesophageal carcinoma. Sarcoma. Myeloma. Primary and secondary tumours of spinal canal and nerve roots: ependymoma; neurofibroma; glioma; angioma; meningioma; lipoma; rarely cordoma. Reticuloses, e.g., Hodgkin's disease.

7. *Cardiac and Vascular*:
Subarachnoid or spinal haemorrhage. Luetic or dissect-ing aneurysm. Grossly enlarged left atrium in mitral valve disease. Rarely myocardial infarction.

8. *Gynaecological Conditions*:
Tuberculous disease. Rarely prolapse or retroversion of uterus. Dysmenorrhoea. Chronic salpingitis. Pelvic abscess or chronic cervicitis. Tumours.

9. *Gastro-intestinal Conditions*:
Peptic ulcers. Cholelithiasis. Pancreatitis. Rarely appendicitis, or from new growth of intra-abdominal viscus (colon, stomach, pancreas), or from retroperi-toneal structures.

10. *Renal and Genito-urinary Causes*:
Carcinoma of kidney. Calculus. Hydronephrosis. Poly-cystic kidney. Pyelitis and pyelonephritis. Perinephric abscess. Infection or new growth of prostate.

11. *Blood Disorders*:
Sickle-cell crises. Acute haemolytic states.

12. *Drugs*:
Corticosteroids. Methysergide.

13. *Normality*:
(Non-disease).

improved or cured by the loss of 1–3 stones (30–90 kg.) or more in weight.

Degenerative changes of the spine are almost always present after the age of 45 years, but only sometimes are they accompanied by symptoms, and these in turn are often due to some of the factors mentioned above. *Ankylosing hyper-ostosis*, a condition often associated with dia-betes mellitus, is characterized by coarse bridging along the anterior borders of the lower dorsal vertebrae, seen well in lateral radiographs. De-generative changes in the *intervertebral cartilages* may be associated with chronic backache, and such changes may be localized, usually to lower cervical and lumbar areas, or may extend widely throughout the entire spine. More severe symp-toms of compression may occur when a disk herniation protrudes through a tear of the longi-tudinal ligament and presses on root and/or cord causing symptoms and signs of sciatica, femoral neuropathy, or brachialgia, depending on the site of the lesion. Such lesions can cause severe and prostrating pains which may be aggravated by coughing and straining. A sudden strain, such as lifting a heavy weight with the spine flexed, is often the precipitating cause. Par-aesthesia in the distribution of the affected nerve is common and the appropriate reflex may be diminished or absent (*see* Table). In lumbar

NEUROLOGICAL SIGNS OF LUMBAR DISK LESIONS

ROOT	REFLEX CHANGES	SENSORY CHANGES	MOTOR WEAKNESS
L.2	None or re-duced knee reflex	Lateral thigh	Hip flexion
L.3	Reduced knee reflex	Medial thigh	Hip flexion. Knee exten-sion
L.4	Reduced knee reflex	Medial leg	Foot inversion, dorsiflexion
L.5	Nil. Rarely reduced ankle reflex	Lateral leg. Dorsum of foot and hal-lux	Hallux dorsi-flexion. Foot eversion
S.1	Reduced ankle reflex	Lateral leg and sole of foot	Foot plantar flexion. Foot eversion

From 'A Synopsis of Rheumatic Diseases' by D. N. Golding (Bristol: John Wright & Sons Ltd.).

lesions the normal lumbar lordosis may be lost; stooping causes great pain but lateral spinal movement may be painless. The so-called 'scia-tica scoliosis' is a lumbar scoliosis with a limping gait in an attempt by the patient to avoid pain. The back is held stiffly and painfully, the patient feeling the need to press it on to a hard, flat sur-face for support and pain relief. Stiffness and pain are often worst in the morning when rising from the bed and may be agonizing. Straight-leg raising causes pain. A large disk protrusion may not only press directly on nervous tissue but interfere with its blood-supply. Cerebrospinal fluid may show an increase of protein, often with an increase of lymphocytes and perhaps some red blood-cells, and the fluid pressure may be altered. Radiographs of the spine after introduction of a contrast medium may occasionally

low backache and aches extending round into the groins; unilateral or bilateral sciatica is rare, as is a cauda equina lesion. This (cauda equina) lesion, partly due to compression, partly due to traction, the severest of the syndromes associated with spondylolisthesis, is more often seen in adolescent children. Physical signs are often non-existent, but the visible and palpable prominence of the spine of the affected vertebra may become

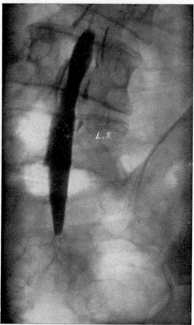

Fig. 76.

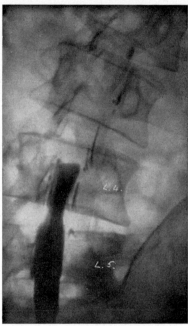

Fig. 77.

Fig. 76. Radiograph (patient supine) after intraspinal injection of lipiodol showing narrowing of the oil column at the level of the interspace between the 4th and 5th lumbar vertebrae and scoliosis due to muscular spasm. A protruded portion of disk was removed with complete relief of pain in the back and sciatica. (*Dr. H. M. Worth.*)

Fig. 77. Radiograph in same case as in *Fig.* 76 with the patient prone.

be necessary to localize the obstruction, as is shown in *Figs.* 76, 77.

Many disk protrusions are posterior rather than posterolateral. In the former case they cause back pain only, rarely cord compression. There may be tenderness over the affected area, in some cases referred to paravertebral muscles or buttocks.

Spondylolisthesis, usually in the lower lumbar spine, occurs as a result of a bilateral lesion in the pars interarticularis, i.e., that bony bridge which unites the superior articular facet and pedicle to the lamina and inferior articular process. A forward or backward (retrospondylolisthesis) displacement may also occur as a result of degeneration of an intervertebral disk ('pseudospondylolisthesis') resulting in instability of the upper vertebra and narrowing of the intervertebral foramina. Well-centred X-rays taken in full flexion and extension will show the lesion. There may be no symptoms in some cases, others have

more obvious as the patient flexes his spine. Cervical spondylolisthesis is much less common than lumbar.

2. Crushed or Wedged Vertebrae due to osteoporosis are seen in radiographs to be part of a diffuse thinning of the texture of the bone without lytic lesions or condensation. There is often wedging of several vertebrae from previous crushes and the back is usually rounded. The patient is in most cases an elderly woman. Blood chemistry (serum alkaline phosphatase, calcium and plasma phosphates) is typically normal, though hypocalcaemia often occurs. In a spine painful from malignant deposits there is actual destruction of bone tissue in the radiographs and porosis is patchy and not generalized; if due to carcinoma of the prostate the bone shadow may be denser and dead-white in the X-ray pictures in the affected areas. The serum alkaline phosphatase is elevated in metastatic malignant disease but normal in multiple myelomatosis. In both cases the sedimentation-rate is raised, usually in carcinomatosis, invariably and to a high figure around 80–100 mm. in 1 hour (Westergren) in myelomatosis; marrow biopsy and electrophoretic studies clinch the diagnosis. The commonest source of spinal malignant deposits today is carcinoma of the breast in the female and of the bronchus in the male, but multiple myeloma should always be kept in mind in any unexplained backache. *Osteomalacia* differs from osteoporosis in that there is often a history of dietetic and/or intestinal insufficiency or of chronic disease and sometimes of a previous gastrectomy. The serum alkaline phosphatase is often elevated, serum calcium and plasma phosphates decreased. Urinary 24-hour calcium output is low. The aches are more diffuse and are not centred on the crushed vertebra, as in osteoporosis; they are nagging and unremitting, are eased by rest, and aggravated by activity. Pain in osteoporosis appears to be due to local fracture of a brittle non-tender vertebral body, in osteomalacia to strain of the tender soft bones of the spine. Radiographs may show stress fractures (pseudo-fractures) and Milkman's lines or Looser zones in pelvis or ribs, rarefied areas consisting of uncalcified osteoid. In *Hyperparathyroidism* (Osteitis fibrosa cystica) there may be generalized osteoporosis in the radiographs. Periarticular bone cysts may occur, but not invariably; resorption of distal ends of clavicles is said to be characteristic. There may be generalized backache and tenderness. Serum calcium is raised, but repeated estimations over a period of time may have to be done to demonstrate this. Plasma phosphorus is low, though it rises with renal failure, and the alkaline phosphatase is usually but not invariably raised; small doses of vitamin D reduce the serum levels of alkaline phosphatase. Serum acid phosphatase, citrate, and magnesium may also be increased. There may be other features of hypercalcaemia, such as nausea and vomiting, muscle weakness or a true myopathy, corneal calcification (band keratitis), and nephrocalcinosis. Peptic ulceration and pancreatitis may occur. The syndrome is usually due to primary hyperparathyroidism, from hyperplasia or adenoma of the parathyroid gland, but it can occur as secondary to renal and other diseases in which case the serum calcium may be normal. The finding of plasma chloride levels consistently less than 100 mEq./l. in the presence of hypercalcaemia virtually excludes the diagnosis of primary hyperparathyroidism.

Paget's disease of bone is often an accidental radiological finding in a patient with no symptoms. It can occasionally, however, cause quite severe backache. Diagnosis is made on X-rays and an elevated serum alkaline phosphatase. The disease may extend throughout the pelvis and spine or involve one or two vertebral bodies only. A small number of the lesions become sarcomatous, and severe pain should arouse suspicions of malignant change.

3. Inflammatory Arthropathies of the Spine. The best example is idiopathic ankylosing spondylitis

(*Fig.* 80). Here the patient is usually a male aged between 16 and 36, and it has been discovered that in the large majority of cases he is of tissue type HLA–B27wz. (*See Figs.* 78–80.) His spine is stiffened and restricted in movement *in all planes*. Neck movements are often restricted and intercostal expansion at nipple level reduced from the normal 5–7·5 to 2·5 cm. or less. This intercostal restriction occurs early in the course of the disease and is not a late complication but an essential and early part of the clinical picture. Diaphragmatic movement is normal. Evidence of active or old iridocyclitis is present in over 20 per cent of the patients, in most cases seen as iritic adhesions or dark spots in the anterior chamber on the posterior surface of the cornea. Tender heels or tender areas over the pelvic brim, ischial tuberosities (*see Fig.* 79), or greater trochanters are not uncommon. Peripheral arthritis occurs in some 25 per cent of cases initially and hydrarthrosis of knees in about 7 per cent of cases. The sedimentation-rate is elevated in almost all cases, but sheep-cell agglutination and Latex tests are negative. Nodules do not occur, nor does lymphadenopathy or splenomegaly. The commonest initial symptom is aching in the buttocks, the patient drawing his hand down the back of the buttocks and thighs as the site of discomfort, but lumbar backache and stiffness soon occur and may be the initial symptoms. Two radiographs help in early diagnosis, a postero-anterior view of the sacro-iliacs and an anteroposterior of the dorsolumbar spine D.8–L.3, but X-ray changes may not be present until symptoms have been present 2–3 years or more. The earliest radiological sacro-iliac changes are blurring of the joint outlines with para-articular ilial sclerosis, erosions, and apparent widening, gradually giving way over the years to narrowing and obliteration of the joint. Small syndesmophytes, resembling bony 'stalagmites and stalactites', are usually seen first along the edges of the intervertebral cartilages between the vertebral bodies of D.10 and L.2; this is where the 'bamboo spine' usually first becomes evident. Lytic lesions with periosteal elevation and 'whiskering' may be seen in the pelvis or in the spine, most commonly in the ischial tuberosities. Ankylosing spondylitis affects the spine primarily (*Fig.* 78), girdle joints (hips and shoulders) secondly (*Fig.* 79), and peripheral joints least often, in contrast to the distribution of joint involvement seen in rheumatoid arthritis, where initial involvement is usually feet, hands, and wrists. The spondylitic pattern of disease may also be seen occasionally in Reiter's (Brodie's) disease, or in association with psoriasis, ulcerative colitis, Crohn's disease, and occasionally Whipple's disease and Behçet's disease and, very rarely, polymyalgia rheumatica. Some male cases of juvenile chronic polyarthritis progress to the spondylitic picture. In the diagnosis of ankylosing spondylitis these variants should always be considered.

4. Infective Conditions of bones and joints are uncommon and the history will often give a lead

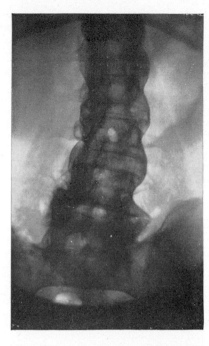

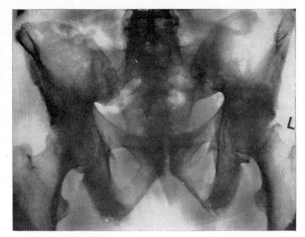

Fig. 79. Radiograph of the pelvis showing obliteration of sacro-iliac joints in ankylosing spondylitis and typical periosteal changes in ischial tuberosities and outer surface of pelvis. The hips are also involved. (*Dr. Cochrane Shanks.*)

Fig. 78. Radiograph of lumbar spine in ankylosing spondylitis (bamboo spine). The coarse bridging at L.5 on the left is due to associated degenerative (disk) changes.

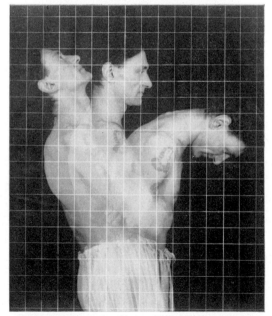

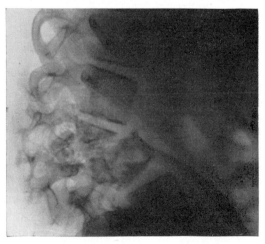

Fig. 81. Radiograph of tuberculous spine showing angulation and vertebral destruction. (*Dr. J. D. Dow.*)

Fig. 80. Triple-exposure photograph showing full extension and spinal flexion in a patient with ankylosing spondylitis.

to the diagnosis. The lesions tend to be lytic and abscesses may form and discharge. The final picture may resemble osteo-arthrosis or even ankylosing spondylitis. *Tuberculosis* of sacro-iliac joint or spine is more painful than these conditions, however, and more incapacitating. The dorsal spine is the most commonly affected

portion of the spine, the vertebral bodies being most commonly involved (*Fig.* 81), though the disease may start in the intervertebral disk. Collapse of vertebral bodies leads to angulation of the spine. Cold-abscess formation and paresis are much less common today than 30 or more years ago. There is pain and weakness in the back and tenderness and muscle spasm in the affected area, the spine being held rigidly. Sacro-iliac disease is usually unilateral in tuberculous disease, bilateral in ankylosing spondylitis.

In *undulant fever* generalized aches, fever, sweats, anorexia, and other features of a febrile infective process may coexist with backache and joint and bone pains; signs of actual joint inflammation are rare. The lesion is essentially an osteomyelitis of the spine or pelvis; both bone and disk may be involved, only occasionally with pus formation. Localization in the spinal column may occur many weeks or months after the original infection, which may have been overlooked and undiagnosed at the time. The same delay of months, or even years, before the advent of spinal symptoms is also seen with typhoid and paratyphoid fevers. *Weil's disease* (leptospirosis icterohaemorrhagica), characterized by fever and high leucocytosis, haemorrhagic manifestations, and jaundice, may give rise at the time to acute backache and later to destructive and degenerative changes in the spine with chronic symptoms.

5. Psychogenic. The essence of hysteria is the theatrical nature of the symptoms it causes. This is true of the hysterical spine, formerly known as the 'soldier's spine', which, though exceedingly rare in British troops in the last war, was by no means uncommon in the 1914–18 War. The spine is held elaborately bent (camptocormia), all attempts at movement being resisted with great drama and much expression of suffering. The back, nevertheless, straightens out readily on bed, couch, or floor. The patient may be able to flex his spine painlessly, but will not straighten it. Palpation or attempts at movement by the examiner may produce much louder groans, grimaces, and excessive reactions than in a patient with a true acute inflammatory spondylitis. It is this 'over-reaction' which is typical of the hysteric. Watched closely, movements previously impossible are later made without discomfort and areas previously acutely tender touched without complaint. *Malingering* may give a similar picture though usually less dramatic. In both cases spinal movements are often more grossly restricted than in severe spinal disease. *Compensation neurosis* tends to improve when the case is settled, whatever the legal decision. The history and features of *anxiety* and *depression* are usually apparent in a well-taken history. Backache may be entirely due to either or both, or features of these disorders may become superimposed on an organic cause. Such a picture is common in the overworked, harassed, anxious housewife.

6. Spinal Tumours may be divided into extradural and intradural, the latter being further subdivided into those outside and those within the cord, i.e., extra- or intramedullary. Endotheliomas and neurofibromas are the commonest extramedullary growths, the latter usually arising from spinal roots, the posterior more often than the anterior. They may be single or multiple and may or may not be part of a generalized neurofibromatosis. Endotheliomata may arise from meninges or spinal roots.

Benign tumours of the spine are uncommon. Bone cysts, giant-cell tumours, osteochondroma, and chondroma may occur but more common are haemangiomata, aneurysmal bone cysts, and

osteoid osteomata. Not all haemangiomata are benign; some lead to extensive destruction of bone. X-rays show vertical striations in the vertebral body which may be partially crushed. Aneurysmal bone cysts form large paraspinal masses, usually posteriorly, with scattered calcific deposits. The osteoid osteoma is a painful lesion in which new bone is formed leading to considerable surrounding bony sclerosis. Tomograms may be necessary to demonstrate the lesion well, a zone of dense bone encircling a small radiolucent centre. The pain is often severe and worse at night.

7. Backache caused by Cardiovascular and Intrathoracic Disorders, of which a good example is the intense, demoralizing, boring pains of an aneurysm invading the dorsal spine. Features of luetic aneurysm of the arch and early descending aorta will probably be present with signs of an aortic reflux, collapsing radial and carotid pulses, and possibly signs of tabes dorsalis also. Lower dissecting atherosclerotic aneurysms of the descending aorta below the arch are less apparent; unequal or delayed pulses in arms and legs should be noted. An arteriosclerotic aneurysm of the abdominal aorta may cause pain in the lower part of the back as well as in the upper abdomen, the groin, and occasionally in the testicles; a pulsating mass may be felt in the abdomen. A carcinoma of the bronchus or oesophagus may cause backache, myocardial infarction only rarely. *Fig.* 82 shows a rare cause, enormous enlargement of the left atrium in mitral disease. The pain in such cases is usually relieved by leaning forwards and to the left.

8. Gynaecological Conditions are, on the whole, a rare cause of backache. Disease of the ovaries and tubes may be responsible in a few cases, prolapse or retroversion of the uterus occasionally, but the cause commonly lies elsewhere and correcting the gynaecological condition leaves the backache in most cases unrelieved. If backache worsens during the menses this may suggest a gynaecological cause, but may also suggest a change in pain threshold at this time. Tuberculous endometritis may cause backache which is relieved by appropriate therapy.

9. Gastro-intestinal Conditions, from which backache may be referred. Chronic pancreatitis and carcinoma of the pancreas may cause a dull, persistent, upper lumbar ache, usually but not always associated with upper abdominal pain and discomfort. Relief of pain may be obtained by leaning forwards. An acute appendicitis when the organ lies behind the caecum or ascending colon may cause pain felt entirely posteriorly in the lumbar region, more to the right side. Muscular rigidity may be present, particularly of the quadratus lumborum, and deep pressure applied at a point halfway between the crest of the ilium and the twelfth rib usually causes definite pain (Baldwin's sign). Enlargement of the liver from any cause may give a dull ache felt to the right of the lower dorsal spine, but aches are usually felt also elsewhere in the abdomen and lower chest. The pain of cholecystitis or cholelithiasis may be experienced posteriorly over the liver, or a little higher, in addition to the upper abdomen.

10. Renal and Genito-urinary Causes are not uncommon. Pyelitis and pyelonephritis may cause lower dorsal and lumbar backaches; the diagnosis is usually evident. It is less obvious with

12. Drugs. Corticosteroids may increase osteoporosis due to other causes and help to precipitate crush fractures. (*Fig.* 83.) Methysergide taken over long periods to prevent migraine may cause backache from retroperitoneal fibrosis.

13. Normality (Non-disease). A chronic backache may be an expression of frustration,

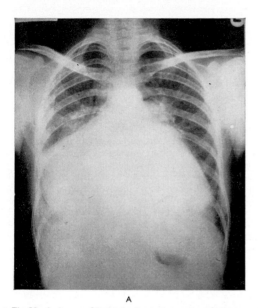 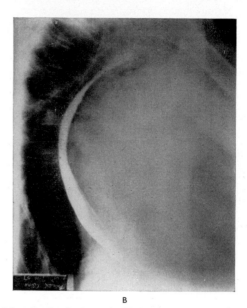

A   B

Fig. 82. **A**, A case of backache due to enormous enlargement of the left atrium in mitral stenosis. The heart shadow to the right of the spine is due to superimposed right and left atrium. **B**, The same case showing scythe-shaped oesophagus from left atrial pressure. (*Dr. A. Schott.*)

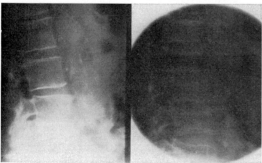

Fig. 83. Rapid advance of spinal osteoporosis over a 1-year period in a rheumatoid patient on prolonged cortical steroid therapy.

renal tumours such as carcinoma, which may remain largely silent since haematuria and the finding of a palpable mass in the flank may only occur late in the course of the disease. Prostatic inflammatory or neoplastic disease may be associated with backache, usually low lumbosacral, but occasionally higher.

11. Blood Disorders. Severe attacks of backache, often with fever, may occur in sickle-cell disease and haemolytic crises in other disorders. Backache may also be a manifestation of acute or chronic leukaemia.

unhappiness, or strain and fatigue. The back is a sounding-board for many persons' dissatisfaction with their lives, and no organic or psychiatric disease need be present.

F. Dudley Hart.

BACTERIURIA

Bacteriuria is a term to indicate that the freshly voided urine contains micro-organisms but little or no pus. *Escherichia coli, Streptococcus faecalis,* and other bowel organisms are the commonest varieties to be encountered. *Bacilluria* is of similar import, but restricted to those cases in which only rod-shaped bacteria are present. The distal segment of the female urethra and the anterior portion of the male urethra are normally inhabited by certain non-pathogenic bacteria (chiefly cocci, such as *Staphylococcus albus*), which are often present in urine and constitute what may be termed 'physiological' bacteriuria. Bacteriuria as a pathological condition due to some lesion of the urinary system posterior to the urethra can be recognized with certainty only by the examination in the laboratory of a mid-stream specimen collected with scrupulous attention to asepsis. A bacterial count is all-important and significance is attached to numbers of 10^5 organisms or more per cubic ml.

Bacteriuria may be persistent and indicate either general or local infection. The commonest variety is *coli bacilluria*, an occasional site of the *Escherichia coli* infection being the pelvis of the right kidney; this occurs with greatest frequency in young female children and pregnant women; it is, however, met with at all ages and in both sexes.

Intermittent bacteriuria, particularly when due to resistant *Pseudomonas aeruginosa* or *Proteus* species, may be associated with urinary calculus—emphasizing the necessity for radiological examination. Haematuria consequent on vesical schistosomiasis may give place to *E. coli* or staphylococcal cystitis; successful treatment depends upon the recognition of the ova of *Schistosoma haematobium* in the urinary deposit or by the result of rectal biopsy. *Staphylococcus albus* bacteriuria sometimes occurs in cases of rheumatoid arthritis; it is not attended by pus or other sign of urinary irritation or infection, and is of no local pathological import.

Slight and transitory simple bacteriuria due to *E. coli* or *Klebsiella aerogenes*, usually subsiding without any treatment, frequently occurs after operation upon the rectum or anus, or the organs of generation. It may follow catheterization or urethral dilatation performed with less than perfect aseptic technique.

In general infections the urine is either normal in appearance, or by admixture with blood may present any tint from 'smoky' to bright red. The reaction is usually acid, often of a degree which if present in an artificial culture medium would inhibit the growth of the infecting micro-organism; protein is present, varying in amount from a trace to a heavy deposit. Microscopically the centrifugalized deposit shows blood-cells, renal tube-casts, and renal epithelium, in addition to the infecting bacterium and a few white cells. The clinical symptoms are those of the general systemic infection together with some degree of increased frequency of micturition as a rule.

In local infection of the genito-urinary tract due to one species of micro-organism only, the urine presents a somewhat similar appearance; blood, however, may be entirely absent, while pus measured by the centrifuge may vary in volume from a trace to 10 or 20 per cent of the total bulk of urine. The presence of pus is an indication of some inflammatory lesion of the urinary tract and the case should no longer be classed as one of bacteriuria. In the early stages of a local infection, however, microscopical examination of the deposit may show the presence of leucocytes only slightly in excess of normal, so that without the microscope the existence of pyuria and the associated bacteriological factor may easily be overlooked. A valuable investigation is the 'one-drop test'. A drop of uncentrifuged urine is placed on a slide, covered with a cover-slip and examined under the one-sixth magnification. More than 5 or 6 pus cells per field is regarded as highly significant.

Occasionally, and particularly in adults, the urine passed during the day is neutral or faintly alkaline—a change in reaction due to physiological causes. In cases where the urine is strongly alkaline the alkalinity is due to ammonia resulting from the decomposition of urea, by urea-splitting organisms such as *B. proteus*, which have gained access to the urine, either after it has been voided or whilst still *intra vesicum*. In the latter instance the contamination may have taken place as a result of careless instrumentation, or (as in the female) by continuity of surface, but its occurrence may also be due to the passage of micro-organisms by lymphatic paths from the lumen of the adjacent large intestine.

The clinical symptoms associated with bacteriuria due to local infection vary widely with different patients (*see* PYURIA, p. 678). Frequency of micturition, scalding, dull aching pains in one or both loins, tenderness on deep pressure over the kidneys or ureters, pains in the perineum and hypogastrium (according to the situation of the primary infection), severe rigors, pyrexia, anorexia, nausea, and vomiting are amongst those commonly observed. Sometimes the abdominal symptoms are so insistent, particularly in children and in the female, as to suggest either appendicitis or peritonitis; in this connexion, too, it is important to remember the relatively common occurrence of bacteriuria with pyuria in children in whom there may be very few symptoms beyond 'delicacy' or gastro-intestinal disturbance, without any special urinary symptoms. The urine generally contains only a trace of albumin and quite frequently no obvious pus; the diagnosis then depends upon routine investigations including the bacteriological investigation of a mid-stream specimen, suggested by the discovery of a decided excess of leucocytes in the centrifugalized deposit from the specimen collected during the first routine examination of the patient. An intravenous pyelogram, which should always be done, may show a congenital lesion of the upper urinary tract. Indeed, a urinary infection in a male child nearly always indicates the presence of an underlying developmental anomaly.

Tubercle Bacilluria. It has been stated that tubercle bacilli can be excreted by a healthy kidney or one not affected by tuberculous disease. Such kidneys may show no lesions to the naked eye, but serial sections always reveal minute cortical foci of tuberculous disease.

Harold Ellis.

BEARING-DOWN PAIN

This form of pain is frequent in women, and is an associate of many pelvic conditions. It is often associated with chronic aching, but it is not every chronic pelvic pain which has the bearing-down character. It usually results from impaction of some pelvic structure, and owes its character to pressure on the rectum, or on the bladder. Displacement of pelvic organs, particularly prolapse, or congestion of them, will produce it. Its source is not always gynaecological, as it may be the result of rectal disease, such as carcinoma, polypi, ulcer, or haemorrhoids; it is thus closely associated with rectal tenesmus. The commonest cause is abnormal uterine descent with backward displacement, and it is most marked in retroversion of the pregnant uterus, especially if impaction of the organ occurs. Impaction of a pelvic tumour may produce it, uterine fibroids, ovarian tumours, and pelvic haematocele being the chief swellings which give rise to it; these produce pain of a different character in addition, due to pressure on nerves; but bearing-down pain referred particularly to the rectum and the perineum may be extreme. A pelvic abscess of peritoneal origin is an unusual impacted swelling giving rise to very severe bearing-down pain—impacted, because it is bound down by peritoneal adhesions, and exercising pressure because of the tension in it; the bearing-down character becomes most marked if the abscess involves the rectal wall, as it frequently does, causing much irritation of the rectum and a flow of mucus from it.

The differential diagnosis of the causes of this type of pain can be made only after a complete pelvic examination by abdominal palpation, and bimanual examination by the vagina and by the rectum. Further, it may be necessary to examine the bladder by the cystoscope, or the rectum by the proctoscope, or sigmoid by the sigmoidoscope. The differential diagnosis of the pelvic disorders mentioned is discussed under PELVIC SWELLING (p. 626).

T. L. T. Lewis.

BLOOD-PRESSURE, ABNORMAL

The apparent ease and accuracy with which the blood-pressure can be measured, using a modern sphygmomanometer, are deceptive. In recent years it has been shown that, apart from errors due to faulty technique, considerable variability is introduced by the habits and preconceptions of the observer. For epidemiological studies, it has been possible to minimize these by using specially designed sphygmomanometers but, in clinical practice, little can be done except to acknowledge their existence. Technical errors, however, can, and should, be eliminated.

Measurement of the Blood-pressure. In 1939 a Joint Committee of the British Cardiac Society and the American Heart Association published recommendations on the technique of sphygmomanometry. Complete international agreement was not achieved and further divergence of opinion was expressed in subsequent American publications in 1951. On most essential points, however, firm recommendations were made on which the following notes are based.

Most modern sphygmomanometers can safely be regarded as accurate but it is wise to calibrate one's instrument from time to time, especially if it is of the aneroid type, against a standard mercurial manometer. The patient should be comfortable and relaxed and should have been allowed to recover from any recent exertion or excitement; for this reason, there is a good case for not recording the blood-pressure until the end of a physical examination. The patient will usually be recumbent; if he is in any other position, the fact should be recorded. The arm should be supported at the patient's side and should be bared to the shoulder to facilitate proper application of the cuff and to avoid constriction by a rolled-up sleeve. The cuff should be fitted closely and evenly round the arm with the centre of the rubber bag over the brachial artery and with its lower edge 3 cm. above the bend of the elbow. For normal adults, the width of the cuff should be 12 cm. but, if the arm is obese—that is, more than 30 cm. in circumference—a 14-cm. cuff should be used. Use of too narrow a cuff, or one which has been applied too loosely, overestimates the blood-pressure; with too wide a cuff the pressure is underestimated. Smaller cuffs should be used for infants and children.

A preliminary estimation of the blood-pressure should be made by palpation of the radial or, better, the brachial artery. The pressure in the cuff should be raised until the pulse is obliterated, but no higher as overdistension of the cuff may cause pain, possibly with arterial spasm, and the blood-pressure may be overestimated. The cuff should then be slowly deflated; the systolic pressure is that at which the pulse is first felt. Further deflation of the cuff causes the pulse to become collapsing in quality and the point at which this abruptly becomes normal is an approximate measure of the diastolic pressure. The cuff pressure should then be raised again to 20–30 mm. above the systolic pressure as estimated by palpation and the stethoscope applied lightly over the brachial artery just below, but not in contact with, the cuff; if the stethoscope is positioned inaccurately the blood-pressure may be underestimated. Deflation of the cuff should be fairly slow, particularly as the systolic and diastolic pressures, as estimated by palpation, are approached. The systolic pressure is that at which the first Korotkow sounds are heard. With further deflation the sounds are replaced by murmurs which themselves become louder and sharper sounds. The point at which these sounds become muffled is regarded, in this country, as the diastolic pressure although the American committee, pointing out that softer sounds may be heard at lower pressures, recommended that the diastolic pressure should be the point at which all sounds cease. The blood-pressure is customarily recorded to the nearest multiple of 5 mm.; greater precision is not possible in view of the variation in the blood-pressure with respiration. In connexion with this practice it has been shown that the pressures recorded by some observers contain a preponderance of figures ending in 0; others tend to record values ending in 5. This 'digit preference' is one of many sources of observer error.

Occasionally, if the blood-pressure is raised, sounds may disappear during deflation of the cuff only to reappear as the pressure is lowered further. This 'auscultatory gap' can cause gross errors if the auscultatory method is used alone. Preliminary measurement of the pressure by palpation will eliminate such errors.

If extrasystoles are present, they and the large amplitude postextrasystolic beats should be ignored in measuring the blood-pressure. In atrial fibrillation the measurement of blood-pressure can be only approximate and the systolic and diastolic pressures should be recorded as the points at which the majority of the sounds appear or become muffled. Pulsus alternans should be noted if present. This is manifest as a sudden doubling of the number of beats heard as the cuff pressure is lowered to the level of the beats of smaller amplitude.

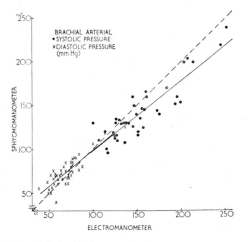

Fig. 84. Relationship between the blood-pressure measured by sphygmomanometry and the pressure recorded via an indwelling needle in the brachial artery. The interrupted line is the line of identity and the two continuous lines are calculated regression lines.

If the radial pulses are unequal, the blood-pressure should be measured in both arms; a small discrepancy is not abnormal, the pressure in the right arm usually exceeding that in the left. If coarctation of the aorta is suspected, the blood-pressure should be taken in the legs. For this purpose, a cuff 15 cm. wide and 30 cm. longer that the arm cuff is used. The patient lies prone and auscultation is carried out over the popliteal artery.

The relationship between the brachial arterial pressure determined by sphygmomanometry and that recorded directly, using an intra-arterial needle and pressure transducer, is of interest. The systolic pressure, measured by sphygmomanometer, is consistently less than that recorded

directly; the opposite is, less consistently, the case with the diastolic pressure (*Fig.* 84). Furthermore, if the artery in which the pressure is being recorded is occluded distally, the direct recording of the blood-pressure shows a rise of 20–30 mm. Hg which is not recorded by the sphygmomanometer. Thus the latter method appears not to record reflected waves and seems to be sensitive only to a pressure wave proceeding distally. The brachial arterial systolic pressure normally exceeds that in the ascending aorta, when both are directly recorded (*Fig.* 85), and

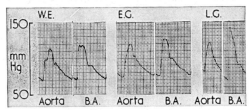

Fig. 85. Simultaneous direct recordings of aortic and brachial arterial pressures of 3 patients.

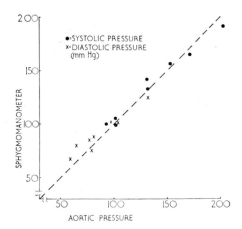

Fig. 86. Relationship between the brachial blood-pressure measured by sphygmomanometry and the pressure recorded via a catheter in the ascending aorta. The interrupted line is the line of identity.

this difference is believed to be due to the superimposition of a reflected wave on the primary aortic pressure pulse. Hence, it has been suggested that the sphygmomanometer records the central aortic pressure more faithfully than the brachial arterial pressure. This suggestion appears to be confirmed by simultaneous measurements (*Fig.* 86).

Normal Blood-pressure. There are some who believe, as a result of large population surveys, that the frequency distribution of blood-pressure is continuous and unimodal and that hypertension represents the upper end of this distribution. Others believe that hypertension is a qualitatively different state from the normal and that the frequency distribution should be regarded as bimodal. Whichever of these views is correct, it is probably true to say that, in an adult, a pressure below 150/90 is normal and values above 160/100 are abnormal; the significance of pressures between these two figures is more debatable. In clinical practice, it is more profitable to discard the concept of a 'normal' blood-pressure and to consider each figure on its merits, having regard to the age and sex of the patient, the circumstances in which the pressure was measured, and other relevant factors. For example, a blood-pressure consistently around 140/95 in a man of 25 would certainly be regarded as abnormal, probably requiring close observation if not treatment, whereas, in a woman of 70, a figure as high as 180/115 might well cause no disquiet.

In children the blood-pressure is much lower than in adults, rising from about 80–90/50–60 in infancy to 90–100/60–70 at about the age of 10. It rises further to reach adult levels in the late teens.

HIGH BLOOD-PRESSURE

The finding of a significantly and consistently raised blood-pressure should stimulate investigation along two distinct, although overlapping, lines. The *severity* is assessed, to a small extent, by the level of blood-pressure itself but, more importantly, by the effects it has produced on the heart, kidneys, eyes, or brain. In addition the *aetiology* should be investigated by a search for clinical or other evidence of renal, endocrine, and other diseases which may cause hypertension. Much more often than not, of course, no such evidence will be found and a diagnosis of essential hypertension will be made.

ESSENTIAL HYPERTENSION. This is a very common disease and causes, together with its direct complications, over 15 per cent of all deaths. The peak age incidence is in the sixth decade and it is uncommon below 40; severe hypertension in young people is commonly renal in origin. Males are more commonly affected below the age of 50 and, although the sex incidence is equal above this age, women are less seriously affected and appear to be able to tolerate hypertension with less disability than men. Various aetiological factors have been postulated; of these, heredity is certainly the most important. The role of vascular disease is difficult to determine as most, if not all, of the changes found in the vessels in established cases are the result rather than the cause of the disease. The renin–angiotensin system and other humoral factors have been extensively investigated and it seems possible that, before very long, a classification of essential hypertension in these terms will become accepted.

Commonly hypertension is found in symptomless subjects at routine examination, for example for life insurance. Occasionally further study of such cases reveals evidence of advanced disease; more often the raised blood-pressure is the only abnormality. Hypertension *per se* causes almost no symptoms except, possibly, headache. Hypertensive headaches are typically worst on waking in the morning and become less severe as the day wears on; the classic localization in the occipital region is not, in fact, very common. This said, it must be admitted that most of the headaches of which hypertensive patients complain are unrelated to the raised blood-pressure.

All the other symptoms of hypertension are those of its complications which, as has been said, may affect the heart, kidneys, eyes, and brain. In hypertensive heart disease left ventricular hypertrophy develops in response to the increased pressure load. The degree of hypertrophy is very variable and is not at all closely related to the level of the blood-pressure. One probable cause of this discrepancy is the failure of occasional sphygmomanometry to reflect the average pressure load imposed on the ventricle. Another important determinant of the degree of left ventricular enlargement is the duration of the hypertension. Little or no cardiac enlargement in a patient with a very high blood-pressure suggests that the hypertension is of recent onset. The most important symptom of hypertensive heart disease is dyspnoea—on exertion and in the form of paroxysmal nocturnal dyspnoea. This implies a raised left ventricular diastolic pressure and, therefore, left ventricular failure. Angina also is common; this may be due to associated coronary artery disease or to the hypertrophied myocardium having 'outgrown' its blood-supply or, not infrequently, to both factors. On examination an important early sign of left ventricular overload is a left atrial gallop rhythm, heard at the displaced apex beat; the loud aortic second sound reflects the level of the blood-pressure only and not the state of the left ventricle. Later, evidence of left ventricular failure, such as a third heart-sound, pulsus alternans, and crepitations at the lung bases, appears. Finally, congestive heart failure, with a raised jugular venous pressure, hepatomegaly, and dependent oedema, may develop. The degree of left ventricular enlargement and the presence of pulmonary venous congestion can be confirmed by X-ray; electrocardiography is even more reliable in the assessment of left ventricular hypertrophy.

Although renal failure is rarely a problem in benign essential hypertension, evidence of a less severe degree of impaired renal function is common. An early feature is failure of urinary concentration, causing nocturnal frequency of micturition. Moderate proteinuria may develop and later, with increasing glomerular damage, the serum-urea may rise; it will, however, rarely exceed 15 mmol/l (90 mg per 100 ml) in the absence of heart failure. The dominant role of renal failure in the natural history of malignant hypertension is discussed below.

The retinal changes of hypertension are well known as an index of the severity of the vascular disease. Grading of the changes is less popular than hitherto as trials have shown considerable observer error in the identification of Grades I and II. An increase in the light reflex, tortuosity of the arteries, and even venous nipping have all been recorded in patients with little or no hypertension; irregularity in arterial calibre and obliteration of arteries ('silver-wiring') are more reliable signs (*Fig.* 87). The later changes (Grade III) include haemorrhages which, as they usually occur in the nerve-fibre layer, are classically linear or 'flame-shaped', and exudates, either small and hard and sometimes disposed around the macula to form the 'macular star' or soft and 'fluffy'; the latter indicate retinal oedema and are usually transient. Grade IV retinopathy is characterized by papilloedema, the clinical hall-mark of malignant hypertension (*Fig.* 88).

The cerebral complications of hypertension are mainly due to associated cerebral vascular

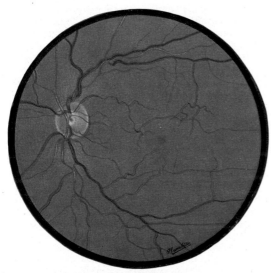

Fig. 87. Optic fundus of a man, aged 40, with a blood-pressure of 230/130. Note the tortuosity of the arteries and the irregularity of their lumen.

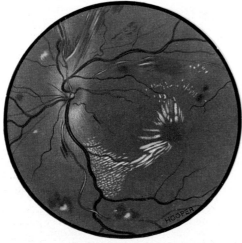

Fig. 88. Optic fundus of a man, aged 47, with malignant hypertension (B.P. 240/140). Note papilloedema, hard exudates forming a 'macular star', softer exudates at the periphery, and haemorrhages, some of which are linear.

disease. The effects of arterial occlusion range from transient mental confusion and motor weakness, paraesthesiae, and other varieties of 'transient ischaemic attack' to complete hemiparesis which may be permanent. Cerebral haemorrhage is more closely related to the level of the blood-pressure itself; it is frequently the terminal event although, with the advent of effective hypotensive therapy, less often than previously. Hypertensive encephalopathy produces many of the clinical manifestations of cerebral haemorrhage but responds dramatically to reduction of the blood-pressure. It is seen in patients whose blood-pressure is very high and is often, although not exclusively, a feature of malignant hypertension.

MALIGNANT HYPERTENSION. In hypertension of almost any aetiology, a very rapid rise of blood-pressure may cause the development of malignant hypertension. This syndrome has been called 'a fast race between renal failure, cardiac failure, and cerebral catastrophe'. The essential pathological feature is arteriolar necrosis which, when it involves the afferent glomerular arterioles, causes proteinuria, haematuria which may be gross, and rapidly advancing renal failure. The clinical diagnosis stands or falls on the presence or absence of papilloedema. Malignant hypertension is commonly seen in patients below the age of 40 but no age-group is exempt. Of all the causes of a raised blood-pressure, only coarctation of the aorta almost never causes malignant hypertension.

RENAL HYPERTENSION. Hypertension in renal disease can be attributed either to ischaemia of part or all of the renal substance or to acute inflammation or fibrosis of the kidney.

Renal artery stenosis is most often due to atherosclerosis; less common causes include fibromuscular hyperplasia, dissecting aneurysm of the aorta, and various forms of arteritis. The renal artery may also be occluded by extrinsic pressure from a neighbouring tumour or cyst, by a fibrous band, or by an aneurysm of the aorta or of the renal artery itself. Renal artery thrombosis may complicate any of these conditions and cause a severe exacerbation of hypertension. Renal embolism may also lead to hypertension which has been attributed to this cause in cases of mitral stenosis, myocardial infarction, and infective endocarditis. Hypertension may, very rarely, result from thrombosis of the renal vein. Congenital anomalies of the renal arteries can cause hypertension, directly or indirectly. Thus, absence of the main renal artery and its replacement by small anomalous vessels may cause significant ischaemia; also aberrant renal arteries may inadvertently be ligated or divided at operation and hypertension may result from the consequent segmental ischaemia.

Clinically, renal artery stenosis may be suspected if a hypertensive patient has evidence of widespread arterial disease or if a bruit is heard over the abdomen or loin. Neither of these features is of great diagnostic value as arterial disease is a common complication of hypertension and an abdominal bruit most often arises from an atherosclerotic aorta. Intravenous pyelography, a routine procedure in the investigation of most hypertensive patients, is a valuable screening test for renal artery stenosis. The affected kidney is smaller than the other and the contrast medium is of greater density in the abnormal kidney although its excretion may be delayed. Further investigation may include study of the function of the two kidneys separately, using ureteric catheterization; suggestive features include a reduced clearance of inulin, creatinine, and PAH together with increased urinary concentrations of these substances on the affected side. Radio-isotopes have also been used to study the function of the two kidneys, without the need for ureteric catheterization, but the reliability of these techniques has not yet been established. The definitive anatomical diagnosis of renal artery stenosis is made by aortography or renal arteriography, but it must be remembered that radiological evidence of arterial narrowing cannot be used alone as evidence of significant renal ischaemia.

In *acute nephritis* hypertension is usually of moderate severity and is almost always reversible, at least in children. More severe hypertension may occur, however, and cause left ventricular failure or hypertensive encephalopathy. The glomerulitis of *Henoch-Schonlein purpura* may also be associated with hypertension; the prognosis is rather worse than that of acute nephritis. Hypertension is also a feature of other causes of glomerular damage such as *systemic lupus erythematosus* and *polyarteritis nodosa*; in the latter condition healing of arteritic lesions of larger vessels is an additional cause of renal ischaemia and hypertension. Lesions of the intrarenal arteries are also seen in *systemic sclerosis* in which progressive renal failure and hypertension may be rapidly fatal in a small proportion of cases.

Hypertension is not a feature of acute pyelonephritis in which inflammation is less widespread than in acute nephritis. In *chronic pyelonephritis*, however, hypertension is common, although less common than in glomerulonephritis. The progress of chronic pyelonephritis is often insidious; there may be no history of overt attacks of urinary infection and patients, often females, commonly present with severe hypertension and advanced irreversible renal damage. Hypertension is also sometimes seen in other forms of chronic interstitial renal inflammation such as *analgesic nephropathy*. The radiological findings in chronic pyelonephritis are small kidneys with focal reductions in the thickness of the renal substance, associated with clubbing of the adjacent calix. *Retention of urine* due to prostatic hypertrophy is sometimes associated with hypertension; the blood-pressure may fall with relief of the obstruction. The mechanism may be renal ischaemia due to the back-pressure but reflex stimuli from the distended bladder may play some part. *Chronic glomerulonephritis* is less common than pyelonephritis, but hypertension is a more constant feature. Diagnosis of this condition and, particularly, of its cause often requires renal biopsy. Other varieties of renal disease in which hypertension is common include *diabetic glomerulosclerosis* (Kimmelstiel-Wilson lesion) and *polycystic*

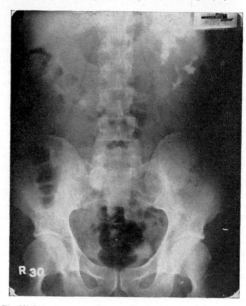

Fig. 89. Intravenous pyelogram showing polycystic kidneys.
(*Film by courtesy of Dr. Basil Strickland.*)

disease of the kidneys (*Fig.* 89); in renal *amyloidosis* hypertension is somewhat unusual and occurs rather late in the course of the disease. Chronic *lead poisoning* also may cause hypertension as a result of renal damage.

The association of hypertension with unilateral renal disease has important therapeutic implications although there is now a good deal less enthusiasm for surgical treatment than hitherto. Renal artery stenosis is commonly, and chronic pyelonephritis occasionally, unilateral. Other, less common, varieties of unilateral renal disease causing hypertension are *radiation fibrosis, perirenal haematoma*, and, very rarely, *renal tuberculosis.*

Hypertension is almost always present in *preeclamptic toxaemia* of pregnancy; the blood-pressure usually falls after delivery but chronic hypertension may develop subsequently. Toxaemia is not the only cause of hypertension during pregnancy and the possibility of pre-existing essential hypertension or chronic pyelonephritis must not be forgotten.

ENDOCRINE CAUSES OF HYPERTENSION. *Phaeochromocytoma*, usually but not always in or near the suprarenal glands, classically causes paroxysms of hypertension associated with headache, palpitations, dyspnoea, nervousness, and, sometimes, profuse sweating. Between the paroxysms, in typical cases, the blood-pressure is normal but, in some cases, the paroxysms may be superimposed on a persistently raised blood-pressure; in a few cases with persistent hypertension no paroxysms occur. Rarely phaeochromocytoma may cause attacks of *hypo*tension; the mechanism is unknown but a reduction in blood-volume may play some part. The diagnosis of phaeochromocytoma is not difficult if a history of paroxysmal hypertension can be elicited; in persistent hypertension without paroxysms phaeochromocytoma may be suspected if the patient has evidence of one of the conditions known to be associated with this lesion; these include neurofibromatosis, Lindau's disease, tuberose sclerosis, and the Sturge-Weber syndrome. On examination of the abdomen it may be possible to feel a suprarenal mass; if palpation causes a paroxysm of hypertension, the diagnosis is almost certain. In some cases no diagnostic clues can be found and phaeochromocytoma should be specifically sought in the investigation of any case of hypertension. The use of histamine to provoke a rise in blood-pressure or of phentolamine to reduce a raised pressure may give useful information, but the results of these tests may be misleading. As a routine investigation, the estimation of the urinary excretion of catecholamines or, more simply, of their metabolite 4-hydroxy-3-methoxymandelic acid (HMMA) is more reliable; HMMA is also known as vanillylmandelic acid (VMA). A phaeochromocytoma, once diagnosed, can be localized radiographically either by noting displacement of a kidney at intravenous pyelography or, better, by retroperitoneal air insufflation or aortography (*Fig.* 90).

Hypertension is a feature of many cases of *Cushing's syndrome*. Other typical features include obesity of the trunk, a plethoric facies, glycosuria, and abnormal glucose tolerance; purple striae on the skin, although typical, are not very common. The diagnosis can be confirmed by estimation of the plasma cortisol.

In *primary aldosteronism* (Conn's syndrome) hypertension is accompanied by hypokalaemia which may cause muscular weakness, polyuria, and polydipsia. In most cases a benign adrenocortical adenoma is the cause of the syndrome. Hypertension may be accompanied by hypokalaemia in a number of other conditions which must be differentiated from Conn's syndrome. In some cases of severe, often malignant, hypertension, most often due to renal disease, aldosterone secretion may be raised and cause hypokalaemia. Such cases of *secondary aldosteronism* differ from Conn's syndrome in that the serum sodium is usually below normal contrasted with the tendency to hypernatraemia in primary aldosteronism. These changes in serum sodium are reciprocally related to changes in plasma renin which is very low in Conn's syndrome and raised in secondary aldosteronism. Primary aldosteronism must also be excluded in those cases of pyelonephritis, causing hypertension, in which potassium loss is directly due to the renal disease.

Liddle's syndrome is a rare familial disorder of renal tubular function causing hypokalaemia and hypertension; it can be distinguished from primary aldosteronism by its failure to respond to spironolactone, an aldosterone antagonist which reverses the electrolyte changes in Conn's syndrome. Liddle's syndrome responds, however, to triamterene.

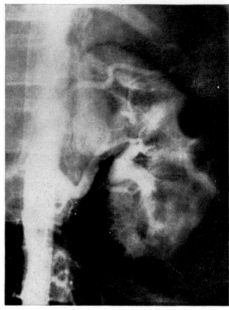

Fig. 90. Aortogram showing phaeochromocytoma of left suprarenal. The highly vascular tumour is visible just above the left renal artery.

Hypertension is not a typical feature of *myxoedema* but it is, nevertheless, statistically more common in this condition although the mechanism is not known.

COARCTATION OF THE AORTA. In this condition the obstruction is usually situated just distal to the origin of the left subclavian artery, at or near the insertion of the ligamentum arteriosum. The so-called 'infantile' type of coarctation, in which the ductus is patent, is irrelevant to the present discussion.

The blood-pressure is raised in the upper half of the body and the most important sign is diminution and delay in the femoral pulses; normally the pulse wave reaches the radial and femoral arteries at the same time and simultaneous palpation of these two vessels allows detection of the characteristic femoral delay. The femoral blood-pressure is, of course, less than that in the brachial artery. Collateral vessels may be visible, and palpable, in the interscapular region; they are more easily seen if the patient bends forward with his arms hanging down. A bruit may be heard over the collateral vessels but a murmur in the interscapular region is more often produced at the coarctation itself and is an important confirmatory sign. A firm diagnosis can often be made from the chest X-ray. The characteristic double aortic knuckle is made up of the dilated left subclavian artery and post-stenotic dilatation of the descending aorta; another, almost pathognomonic, sign is notching of the lower borders of the ribs (*Fig.* 91). These are not to be confused with defects of an erosive nature in the superior

of the vagus and glossopharyngeal nerves, interrupting the afferent pathways from the aortic and carotid baroceptors. The hypertension of *acute intermittent porphyria* is probably related to the neuropathy seen in this disorder.

Familial dysautonomia (the Riley-Day syndrome) is a very rare neurological cause of hypertension.

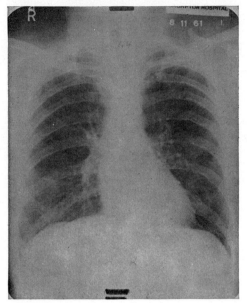

Fig. 91. Postero-anterior chest radiograph of a case of coarctation of the aorta. Note the double aortic knuckle and the widespread rib-notching. (*Film by courtesy of Dr. Basil Strickland.*)

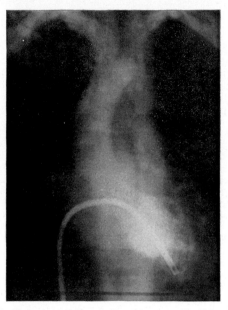

Fig. 92. Angiogram of coarctation of the aorta. The catheter tip is in the right ventricle into which the contrast medium was injected. The film shown was taken several seconds later by which time the contrast medium outlines the left ventricle and the aorta. (*Film by courtesy of Dr. Basil Strickland.*)

margins of the ribs seen (rarely) in poliomyelitis, hyperparathyroidism, rheumatoid arthritis, and scleroderma. The diagnosis can be finally confirmed and the extent of the coarctation delineated by aortography (*Fig.* 92).

HYPERTENSION IN NEUROLOGICAL DISORDERS. The blood-pressure may be raised in a number of conditions involving the brain-stem. The hypertension associated with *raised intracranial pressure* is probably due to brain-stem compression; a similar mechanism may be responsible for the transient elevation of blood-pressure seen in some cases of *head injury*. The association of hypertension with *bulbar poliomyelitis* is well documented. In some cases this may be due to asphyxia but damage to cardiovascular centres in the medulla, causing interruption of homeostatic reflex pathways, is also believed to be an important factor.

Paroxysmal hypertension is sometimes seen with *lesions of the spinal cord* in the cervical or upper thoracic region. These paroxysms are commonly provoked by distension of hollow viscera, such as the bladder or rectum. Hypertension has also been described in patients with *peripheral neuropathy*; this may be due to lesions

WIDE PULSE-PRESSURE

The term 'systolic hypertension' has sometimes been used to describe the situation in conditions such as thyrotoxicosis in which the systolic pressure may be raised without any elevation of the diastolic pressure. The use of this term is to be deprecated as it implies that there is an association between this condition and hypertension, properly so called; this is not so and the expression 'wide pulse-pressure' is suggested as preferable.

In physiological terms there are two factors which may increase the pulse-pressure: the first is an increased left ventricular stroke volume and the other a reduction in the elasticity of the arterial tree. A wide pulse-pressure is, therefore, a feature of aortic incompetence, large persistent ductus arteriosus, arteriovenous fistula, and high output states in general; it is also seen in bradycardia from any cause when the cardiac output can only be maintained by a considerable increase in stroke volume. Finally, it is often seen in elderly arteriosclerotic subjects although in such patients it must be admitted that some elevation of diastolic pressure as well is not uncommon; in that case, of course, the additional diagnosis of hypertension can be made.

LOW BLOOD-PRESSURE

A blood-pressure somewhat below the accepted lower limit of normal may be found, from time to time, in otherwise normal individuals. This is of no importance. Few diseases cause a chronically low blood-pressure; the best known is Addison's disease in which the cause of the hypotension is chronic sodium depletion. The blood-pressure may be low also in the terminal stages of wasting diseases such as carcinomatosis.

An acute fall in blood-pressure is one of the features of 'shock'. This rather unsatisfactory term is used to include a large group of conditions which have in common a fall in cardiac output due either to a reduced venous return or to primary myocardial disease. Thus hypotension is a well-known feature of blood-loss, loss of plasma as in burns, or loss of extracellular fluid as a result of diarrhoea, vomiting, diabetic keto-acidosis, and many other conditions. Cardiac tamponade also prevents adequate cardiac filling and leads to a rapid fall in blood-pressure. Cardiogenic shock is a well-recognized complication of myocardial infarction, and a severe fall in blood-pressure, as a result of a primary fall in cardiac output, may also occur in ectopic tachycardia. In congestive heart failure the blood-pressure is usually little changed until the terminal stages when the cardiac output falls to very low levels.

Postural hypotension and other varieties of vasomotor syncope are discussed in the section on FAINTING (p. 283).

P. R. Fleming.

BONE, SWELLING ON

A simple enumeration of the more important conditions to be considered will indicate the complexity of this subject:

Subperiosteal haematoma (calcified or ossified).
Callus following fracture
Acute osteomyelitis
Chronic osteomyelitis (including Brodie's abscess)
Tuberculous disease of bone
Syphilitic disease of bone
Typhoid (periostitis)
Rickets (*Fig.* 93)
Scurvy
Leontiasis ossea
Acromegaly
Generalized fibrocystic disease (von Reckling-hausen)
Paget's disease
Osteoma
Chondroma
Localized fibrocystic disease
Osteoclastoma ⎫
Aneurysmal bone cyst ⎬ Giant-cell tumours
Non-osteogenic fibroma ⎪
Benign chondroblastoma ⎭
Osteogenic sarcoma
Periosteal fibrosarcoma

Angiomata (innocent and malignant)
Ewing's tumour
Myeloma
Metastatic tumours
Joint conditions such as Charcot's disease and osteo-arthritis give rise to swelling of the ends of the bones involved, but these lesions are more properly considered in the discussion on joints.

This list includes diseases which are prevalent only at certain ages and it can be simplified for diagnostic purposes by sifting the conditions into approximate age-groups:

FROM BIRTH UNTIL THREE YEARS:
Intra-uterine fracture with callus, including those due to osteogenesis imperfecta
Battered baby syndrome
Rickets (*Fig.* 93.)
Scurvy
Congenital syphilitic epiphysitis.

FROM THREE UNTIL FIFTEEN YEARS:
Fracture
Calcified subperiosteal haematomata
Acute osteomyelitis
Tuberculous disease
Congenital syphilitic periostitis
Localized fibrocystic disease
Multiple exostoses usually come under observation at this age
Ewing's tumour
Aneurysmal bone cyst
Non-osteogenic fibroma
Benign chondroblastoma.

FROM FIFTEEN UNTIL TWENTY-FIVE YEARS:
Fracture
Calcified subperiosteal haematomata
Chronic osteomyelitis
Tuberculous rib
Osteoma, osteochondroma, chondroma
Angioma
Osteogenic sarcoma
Ewing's tumour.

FROM TWENTY-FIVE TO FORTY YEARS:
Fracture
Onset of acromegaly
Tuberculous rib
Acquired syphilitic disease of bone
Osteoclastoma
Periosteal fibrosarcoma
Generalized fibrocystic disease (von Reckling-hausen).

FROM FORTY ONWARDS:
Fracture
Acquired syphilitic disease of bone
Paget's disease (in the upper years of age-group)
Acromegaly
Myeloma
Metastatic tumours.

Although these groups are obviously very elastic there are only a certain number of possibilities at any given age and the field is therefore restricted a little. The difficulties of diagnosis lie not only in distinguishing the varieties of bone swelling, but also in deciding whether the condition is arising from the bone or not, which may be particularly difficult in the case of inflammatory lesions where there is surrounding oedema of soft parts and very little enlargement of the bone itself. If careful palpation fails to reveal alteration in the normal bony contour in a patient where a bone lesion is suspected, the character of any overlying soft-tissue swelling that may be present will sometimes act as a guide. If present it involves all layers, arising from the deep tissues and radiating more or less symmetrically outwards. A central bone lesion

Awareness of the *Battered baby syndrome* in infants with multiple fractures may save more injuries being inflicted by parents or guardians. RICKETS is rarely recognized before the age of 6 months and more usually at a year to 18 months. General backwardness often calls attention to the disease, the child being late in sitting up and in dentition, and making little attempt to walk. Restlessness, fretfulness, sweating of the head,

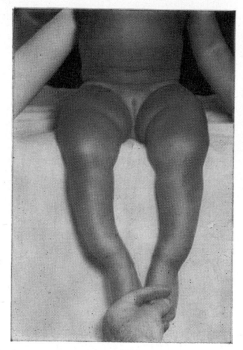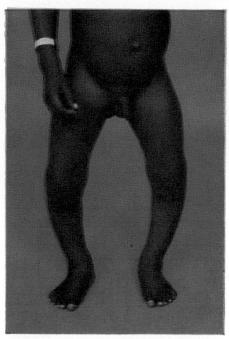

Fig. 93. Rickets: Note bow legs and swelling in the region of the epiphyses at the knee. (*Courtesy of the Gordon Museum, Guy's Hospital.*)

will result in swelling of the whole contour of the limb in the area at fault. Pain originating in bone is deep and boring in character and often very intense. In all cases a radiograph is essential and the differential diagnosis of many of these conditions often resolves itself into a question of interpreting the radiograph.

Bony Swellings prevalent in Infancy. These are often first made apparent by a disinclination on the part of the infant to use the limb or limbs affected; occasionally swelling or deformity are the first signs. In osteogenesis imperfecta, rickets, scurvy, and syphilis the bone lesions are multiple, and in scurvy and rickets symmetrical.

INTRA-UTERINE FRACTURE is the only likely cause of swelling or deformity at birth. There may be an isolated fracture of one bone or the condition known as osteogenesis imperfecta may be present, resulting in multiple fractures, some united and some recent, often with gross deformity. There may also be deficient ossification of the skull. The disease may be familial and is typically accompanied by the presence of blue sclerotics.

and abdominal distension are other features. The bone swellings occur in the region of the epiphyses and are often most marked in the lower end of the radius. The ribs are another situation where the deformity occurs, with resulting 'rickety rosary'. Bossing of the frontal and parietal bones leads to the 'hot-cross bun' head. Bow legs, sinking in of the ribs at the costochondral junctions, and other bending deformities are due to softening of the bones. The history may reveal that the diet has been inadequate and that there has been a lack of fresh air and sunlight. Radiographic examination shows general osteoporosis with considerable broadening and cupping of the metaphyses, which have a hazy irregular margin as if the bone had melted away. The lower end of the radius is usually the best area to choose to obtain a good radiograph. The diagnosis is not difficult except in the mildest cases (*Fig.* 94).

SCURVY is commonly manifest about the age of 12 months or later. The child is restless and irritable and develops extreme tenderness of the affected bones. These are usually the lower end of the femur and upper end of the tibia, and to touch them or even to approach the infant results in paroxysms of screaming. The bone lesion is one of subperiosteal haemorrhage, to which the swelling is due. The overlying skin may become glossy although signs of inflammation are absent. The gums may become swollen and dusky, and haematuria is an occasional feature. In the radiograph the bones show loss of cancellous structure

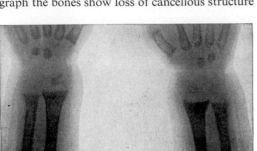

Fig. 94. Rickets. Typical thickening and lengthening of the epiphysis of the lower end of the radius and ulna. (*Dr. T. H. Hills.*)

and extreme thinning of the cortex. Lime salts are deposited in the haematoma, beginning on the deep surface of the periosteum; as soon as this has occurred the haemorrhages can be delineated on the radiograph. Here as in rickets a history of inadequate nutrition may be obtained.

CONGENITAL SYPHILITIC EPIPHYSITIS appears earlier than rickets or scurvy and can sometimes be demonstrated radiographically as early as the second month. The bones of the knee- and wrist-joints are the commonest to show the characteristic changes, and the pain of the lesion is such that the affected limb is often held quite still (syphilitic pseudo-paralysis). The pseudo-paresis which accompanies syphilitic epiphysitis can be distinguished from that occurring in rickets or scurvy by the younger age of onset in the syphilitic form and by other stigmata of congenital syphilis (*see below*). The radiograph shows broadening and irregularity of the metaphysis which is quite different from rickets in that the outline, although irregular, is dense and sclerosis is predominant, whereas in rickets the outline is hazy and ill defined and osteoporosis is marked. Typically the layer of dense irregular bone capping the metaphysis is bounded on the shaft side by a thin layer appearing translucent in the radiograph, while the cortical region of this part of the bone shows punched-out areas of subperiosteal erosion (*Fig.* 95). Other bone manifestations present in syphilis of infancy include areas of periosteal new-bone formation, syphilitic dactylitis, and also Parrot's nodes. These last are bosses on the bones of the vertex of the skull which result in a 'hot-cross bun' head often of more exaggerated shape than in rickets. Syphilitic dactylitis is discussed with tuberculous dactylitis

in the next section. Other signs of syphilis will of course aid the diagnosis. Pemphigus and other skin eruptions, snuffles, condylomata, mucous patches and fissures at the corners of the mouth are all stigmata to be looked for, while in any suspicious case the Wassermann reaction will be tested both of the infant and the parents.

Bone Swellings prevalent in Childhood and Early Adolescence. Fractures and subperiosteal haematomata are considered in the next age-group.

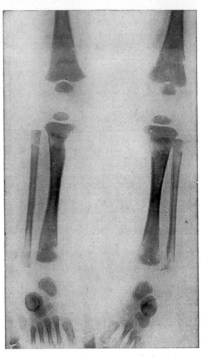

Fig. 95. Radiograph of the lower limbs in a case of congenital syphilitic epiphysitis, showing alternating layers of dense and translucent bone and punched-out areas of subperiosteal erosion. (*Dr. D. N. Nabarro.*)

ACUTE OSTEOMYELITIS occurs in this period in the great majority of cases. The diagnosis does not present itself as a bony swelling of doubtful nature, but as an acute inflammatory condition whose anatomical origin is the matter for decision. A history of chronic sepsis such as boils or impetigo is frequently obtained. The lesion is usually found at one end of a long bone and the severe pain with which it is accompanied causes the child to cry when the limb is touched or moved. There is hot tender brawny oedema of the part, with subsequent reddening and glossiness of the skin; the temperature and the leucocyte count are high and the patient is very toxic. The differential diagnosis is from cellulitis of soft parts and from an acute joint lesion. Cellulitis does not usually result in such severe toxaemia as does osteomyelitis and there may be a skin lesion such as a septic abrasion over the area of cellulitis to indicate its origin, in which case the diagnosis will be rendered much easier. The swelling of a cellulitis tends to be localized at least in the early stages to one aspect of the limb and its limits can be approximately gauged, whereas the swelling over an osteomyelitis is more generalized and less defined. Furthermore, cellulitis is usually accompanied by lymphangitis and lymphadenitis, whereas osteomyelitis, unless it has extended through the periosteum and invaded the soft tissues around, is not commonly associated with these complications. The diagnosis from a joint lesion such as an acute infective arthritis is made more difficult by the frequent presence of a sympathetic effusion into the joint in cases of osteomyelitis. The maximum swelling in the bone lesion, however, is not over the joint but over the end of the bone, and gentle passive movements of the joint are just possible; in the primary arthritic condition movement is exquisitely painful and the maximum swelling is confined to the joint. Rheumatic fever is differentiated by the unusually rapid pulse-rate as compared with the rise in temperature, by the 'flitting' nature of the pains, and by the response to salicylate therapy. Osteomyelitis is unaffected by salicylates, but may respond to penicillin. In case of doubt the therapeutic agent considered most likely to be effective may be prescribed first, followed by the other if no response is obtained.

CHRONIC OSTEOMYELITIS may follow acute osteomyelitis, the infection persisting and chronic discharging sinuses developing as a result of sequestra still present. A subacute or chronic abscess may also form as a metastasis in another bone or may arise as a chronic infection from the beginning. A Brodie's abscess, as it is called, is usually found near the end of a long bone and is evidenced by palpable thickening of the bone. Radiographs show a central area of rarefaction with more or less surrounding sclerosis, with a deposition of subperiosteal new bone and sometimes with a sequestrum in the cavity (Fig. 96). The diagnosis is chiefly from a tuberculous lesion. This may be impossible without exploration, although sclerosis and subperiosteal new bone are in favour of pyogenic infection. On opening a Brodie's abscess pus and granulation tissue, usually not exuberant, are found. A tuberculous abscess contains caseous material and the granulations are thick and juicy. If microscopy does not reveal tubercle bacilli in a suspicious case guinea-pig inoculation is essential. It may not be possible to distinguish radiologically a Brodie's abscess in an older patient from a central gumma. Other signs of syphilis and the serological reactions will give help in this direction.

There are two likely situations for *tuberculosis* to present itself as a bony swelling of doubtful origin. One is the digits, when one or more of the phalanges, metacarpals, or metatarsals may be the subject of tuberculous dactylitis; and the other is the ends of the long bones where a focus may remain localized for some time before spreading, as eventually it frequently does, into the joint. Tuberculous dactylitis begins early in

life, usually before the age of 5, and results in a spindle-shaped swelling of the affected segment of the digit. Radiography shows central erosion with deposition of subperiosteal new bone with consequent expansion (*Fig.* 97). The erosion may spread outwards, destroying the new bone laid down, and finally breaking through the skin already red and shiny. At the stage when the original cortex has been destroyed and there is just a shell of the new bone left the appearance in the radiograph is of the shaft distended as if

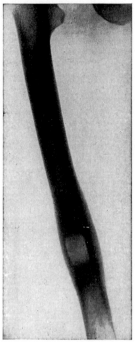

Fig. 96. Radiograph of femur showing Brodie's abscess. (*Mr. C. A. Joll, Royal Cancer Hospital.*)

by gas bubbles, to which the term 'spina ventosa' has been applied. Pain is not a marked feature of the disease. The diagnosis is from syphilitic dactylitis. This latter condition occurs at an even earlier age than tuberculosis, usually before 12 months. Other signs of syphilis (skin rashes, snuffles, thick mop of coarse hair, oral fissures, etc.) and positive serological tests of infant and parents will in most cases aid the diagnosis. Locally the distinction is difficult; there is not the same tendency in syphilis to erosion of the bone or the formation of sinuses, and the new bone is usually thicker and denser, but these slight differences are unreliable. Enchondromata should not enter into the differential diagnosis as they occur in adult life, rarely in childhood, never in infancy; and the radiograph shows clear-cut central rarefaction without erosion, and expansion without new bone formation. The only other site of bone tuberculosis where periosteal new bone formation is common is in the ribs. This is a disease of adult life and is not usually presented as a bony swelling but as a cystic swelling, the result of abscess formation. Tuberculosis of the ends of long bones results in an ill-defined swelling with slight pain and some evidence of loss of function, for example a persistent slight limp if the lower limb is involved. Clinically some thickening can be detected, but the diagnosis really rests on the radiograph, which shows an area of rarefaction sometimes containing an ill-defined sequestrum and with little or no new bone formation. The

BONE CYST commonly occurs between the ages of 10 and 15 and usually arises in the upper ends of the humerus, femur, or tibia, the patient most often coming under observation for a pathological fracture. The fracture is notably caused by comparatively slight violence, and the radiograph shows the well-defined outline of a cyst with cortical thinning but no erosion. There are usually trabeculae running across the cyst cavity which may lead to confusion with a giant-cell

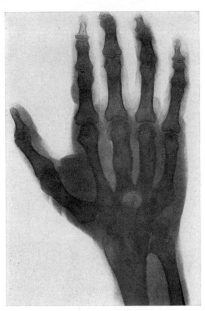

Fig. 97.   Old tuberculosis of the carpus and metacarpus. (*Dr. T. H. Hills.*)

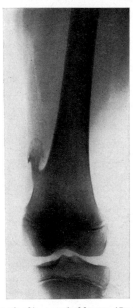

Fig. 98.   Exostosis of lower end of femur.   (*Dr. T. H. Hills.*)

differential diagnosis is from a lesion due to non-specific pyogenic organisms and is discussed under *Chronic Osteomyelitis*, above. Tuberculosis of bone is a condition insidious in onset and chronic in progress: there may be slight pyrexia, there is no increase in polymorph leucocytes, but usually a slight lymphocytosis. Abscess formation is common in the late stages; the abscess is of the cold variety and tends to break down through an indolent undermined opening on to the skin. Wasting, reflex guarding, and starting pains are marked only when the adjacent joint is invaded.
SYPHILITIC PERIOSTITIS. At about the age of 9 or 10 congenital syphilitics are liable to develop local or diffuse deposition of dense periosteal bone. This typically occurs in the tibiae, which also undergo some elongation resulting in the well-known sabre shape. Other signs of congenital syphilis appear at this age, including Clutton's joints, interstitial keratitis, and Hutchinson's teeth (affecting the permanent incisors), and these, together with signs present since infancy (rhagades, saddle-shaped nose, etc.), and the positive serology will give the diagnosis.
LOCALIZED FIBROCYSTIC DISEASE or SOLITARY

tumour, but the simple cyst occurs at a younger age, does not invade the epiphysis, and does not expand to the same extent as an osteoclastoma and therefore does not perforate the cortex. The clear-cut margins and the absence of erosion or melting away of the bone differentiate the condition from a sarcoma. Following a fracture healing may occur. Any extension should encourage the surgeon to explore the lesion and have the tissues microscoped, although this is not necessary for diagnosis in most cases.
MULTIPLE EXOSTOSES. A hereditary disease where the multiple bony outgrowths are accompanied in many instances by dwarfing and crooked limbs. The deformities are usually quite obvious and the radiographs typical (*Fig. 98*).
EWING'S TUMOUR. This is a condition closely resembling osteomyelitis. There is often a history of trauma, pain is a marked feature, there is swelling either localized to one end of the bone or diffuse throughout its length, with pyrexia and usually leucocytosis. The symptoms are occasionally intermittent. The common sites are the humerus, femur, and tibia, usually starting in the middle of the shaft. Radiographs show

the systemic vascular resistance, increases the shunt and reduces the intensity of the murmur; also, in cyanotic attacks associated with infundibular 'shut-down', the murmur may disappear completely.

Apart from obstructive lesions of the ventricular outflow tracts, ejection systolic murmurs are frequently due to a rapid flow rate through a normal semilunar valve orifice. Thus, in *high-output states*, a pulmonary or aortic systolic murmur is commonly heard. This is the case also in

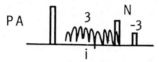

Fig. 128. Diagram of typical auscultatory findings in pulmonary stenosis. At the pulmonary area a grade 3 (loud) systolic murmur, louder during inspiration, encroaches on the aortic second sound, but ends before the markedly attenuated pulmonary second sound. The behaviour of the second sound with respiration is normal.

bradycardia, especially the very slow rate of complete heart-block; the cardiac output can be maintained at such a rate only by a large increase in stroke volume. With an *atrial septal defect* a pulmonary mid-systolic murmur is an almost invariable finding; this is due to the large pulmonary blood-flow. Probably the commonest mid-systolic murmur of all is the *innocent murmur* of childhood and adolescence. It is clearly most important to differentiate this murmur from those due to organic disease to avoid unnecessary invalidism. Innocent murmurs are short and soft and often vary considerably with changes in posture. No other auscultatory abnormalities are present; in particular the behaviour of the second heart-sound with respiration is quite normal. Such murmurs are usually best, or only, heard at the base of the heart but an innocent aortic systolic murmur may be maximal at the apex. In that case it must be clearly identified as mid-systolic, as pansystolic murmurs can never be regarded as innocent. Electrocardiography and radiography will help to confirm the normality of the cardiovascular system; rarely cardiac catheterization may be needed to prove, beyond reasonable doubt, that a murmur is innocent.

Coarctation of the aorta causes a rather late systolic murmur, heard best in the midline of the back of the chest. The murmur may run on a little into diastole if the obstruction is severe.

II. DIASTOLIC MURMURS

The two commonest causes of a diastolic murmur are turbulent atrioventricular flow and semilunar valve regurgitation. The two types of murmur differ in several respects but most significantly in their timing. Atrioventricular flow cannot begin until the pressure in the ventricle has fallen to atrial level. The onset of the murmur is thus delayed until the end of ventricular isovolumic relaxation, that is about 0·08 second after the second heart-sound. Conventionally

this murmur is described as 'mid-diastolic' although latterly there has been a tendency to designate it 'delayed diastolic'. The greater precision of the latter term cannot be denied but there can rarely have been any misunderstanding as a result of the use of the term 'mid-diastolic'. In sinus rhythm, atrioventricular filling is accelerated by atrial systole so that a presystolic, or atrial systolic, murmur is often present in association with a delayed diastolic murmur. Regurgitation through a semilunar valve orifice begins immediately the pressure in a ventricle falls below that in the corresponding great artery. The murmur, therefore, starts at the second heart-sound and is known as an 'early', or 'immediate', diastolic murmur. The terms 'immediate' and 'delayed', which appear to be gradually gaining favour, will be used in this section.

The delayed diastolic murmur of *mitral stenosis* is heard in a rather restricted area at, and just medial to, the apex beat (*Fig.* 129). It is low-pitched and rumbling in character—like the rumble of distant thunder—and is, therefore,

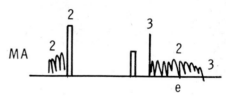

Fig. 129. Diagram of typical auscultatory findings in mitral stenosis. At the mitral area a grade 2 (moderately loud) presystolic murmur precedes a moderately accentuated first sound. A grade 3 (loud) opening snap follows the second sound fairly closely and precedes a long grade 2 (moderately loud) delayed diastolic murmur which is louder during expiration.

better heard with the bell of the stethoscope, lightly applied. It is louder when the patient is lying on his left side, a position which he should be asked to adopt whenever there is doubt about the presence of this murmur. Loud mitral diastolic murmurs are harsh and may be accompanied by thrills. The intensity of the murmur is of no great significance but its length is a useful indication of the severity of the lesion; a long murmur implies that the atrioventricular pressure gradient persists throughout diastole and that the stenosis is severe. The murmur is often immediate'y preceded by an opening snap.

In sinus rhythm mitral stenosis is also characterized by a presystolic murmur (*Fig.* 129). The terms 'atrial systolic' or 'atriosystolic' are also applied to this murmur; clinicians will each decide for themselves between the competing claims of tradition and semantic precision. Terminating, as it often does, at a loud first sound, this murmur gives the impression of having a crescendo quality; this is not borne out by phonocardiography. A common error is to confuse the murmur with a split first sound, an atrial gallop, or an ejection sound. Auscultation with the patient lying on his left side after light exercise will usually clarify the issue.

The *Austin Flint murmur*, heard at the apex in a few cases of free aortic regurgitation, has all the characteristics of the diastolic murmur of mitral stenosis, including accentuation at the time of left atrial systole. If the aortic incompetence is rheumatic, such a murmur must be presumed to indicate mitral stenosis but, if the cause of the aortic valve lesion is syphilis, ankylosing spondylitis, Reiter's syndrome, or other condition in which the mitral valve is not involved, it may be justifiable to diagnose an Austin Flint murmur. The mechanism is probably the impingement of the regurgitant jet on the anterior cusp of the normal mitral valve, tending to close it in the path of the blood flowing from the left atrium. A short delayed diastolic murmur may be heard at the apex in *congenital aortic stenosis* and in *coarctation of the aorta*; there is no pre-systolic accentuation and the mechanism is not clear. The *Carey Coombs murmur* also has the same timing as the murmur of mitral stenosis but is very short and often soft. It appears in the course of acute rheumatic fever and is regarded as evidence of inflammation of the mitral valve. As rheumatic activity subsides the murmur disappears; in some, but not all, cases, evidence of mitral stenosis appears subsequently.

The third group of conditions in which a delayed diastolic murmur may be present at the apex is that in which atrioventricular flow is rapid on account of its large volume. In severe *mitral incompetence* left atrial systolic filling is augmented by the large volume of blood regurgitated from the left ventricle so that, when the atrium empties, a short delayed diastolic murmur is often heard (*Fig. 126, p. 120*); in this context, such a murmur cannot be regarded as evidence of associated mitral stenosis. The large volume of blood returning to the left atrium and flowing through the mitral orifice in *ventricular septal defect* and *persistent ductus arteriosus* also produces a delayed diastolic murmur. Such a murmur implies that the shunt is large; if severe pulmonary hypertension develops the consequent reduction in the pulmonary blood-flow may cause the murmur to disappear. Finally, in *high output states*, a similar murmur may be heard.

Tricuspid stenosis produces a delayed diastolic murmur, with presystolic accentuation in sinus rhythm, in the tricuspid area; the murmurs are increased in intensity during inspiration. Similar diastolic murmurs, without presystolic accentuation, may be heard in organic *tricuspid incompetence* and *atrial septal defect*. The mechanism is a large flow volume analogous to that producing a mitral diastolic murmur in mitral incompetence and ventricular septal defect. In *Ebstein's malformation* of the tricuspid valve a delayed tricuspid diastolic murmur is heard widely over the dilated right atrium and has a curious superficial 'scratchy' quality.

The commonest cause of an immediate diastolic murmur is *aortic incompetence*. This murmur is heard in the aortic area and radiates to the third and fourth left interspaces and to the apex; it is often most easily heard at the left sternal border. It begins at the second heart-sound and diminishes in intensity throughout diastole (*Fig. 130*). Being high-pitched and 'blowing' in character, it is better heard with the diaphragm of the stethoscope. Very soft aortic diastolic murmurs may only be audible when listening at the left sternal border with the patient leaning forward slightly and holding his breath in full expiration. When it is well heard at the apex, it has to be distinguished from a mitral diastolic murmur; its timing and pitch are the most important features in this distinction. Occasionally both mitral and aortic diastolic murmurs may be audible at the apex and, in such cases, it may be helpful to apply the bell with varying amounts of pressure. The delayed diastolic murmur of mitral stenosis is heard best with light pressure and is attenuated by firmer

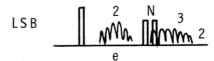

Fig. 130. Diagram of typical auscultatory findings in aortic incompetence. At the left sternal border a grade 2 (moderately loud) mid-systolic murmur is heard best during expiration; this is due to the large left ventricular stroke volume and does not necessarily imply associated aortic stenosis. Splitting of the second sound is normal and a grade 3 (loud) immediate diastolic murmur of moderate length is present.

pressure which selectively increases the intensity of the aortic murmur. If aortic regurgitation is so severe that the left ventricular and aortic pressures become equal early in diastole, the diastolic murmur is very short and may, rarely, be absent.

An immediate diastolic murmur is also heard in *pulmonary incompetence*—along the left sternal border. Rheumatic disease of the pulmonary valve is very rare and the commonest cause is pulmonary hypertension causing the so-called *Graham Steell murmur*. This is most often heard in pulmonary hypertension secondary to mitral stenosis but may be present in association with any other cause of raised pulmonary artery pressure. It may be difficult to distinguish from the murmur of aortic incompetence as it has the same 'blowing' quality and begins at the accentuated pulmonary second sound. However, it is rarely audible to the right of the sternum or at the apex and an immediate diastolic murmur in these areas is almost certainly aortic in origin. Relief of the pulmonary hypertension, as by a successful mitral valvotomy, may cause the Graham Steell murmur to disappear. The pulmonary diastolic murmur which may be heard after valvotomy for pulmonary stenosis differs somewhat from the Graham Steell murmur. The very much lower pulmonary arterial pressure and the prolongation of right ventricular ejection which may persist for a time after valvotomy cause the pulmonary second sound to be soft and considerably delayed. Hence the diastolic murmur, beginning at the pulmonary second sound, seems to be delayed in relation to the much more easily audible aortic second sound and may be confused with a tricuspid diastolic murmur.

III. CONTINUOUS MURMURS

A murmur which is heard, without interruption, both in systole and diastole is most commonly due to flow from the aorta into a relatively low-pressure region. The continuity of the murmur must be emphasized and it must be distinguished from the to-and-fro cadence of combined aortic stenosis and incompetence. This should present little difficulty but the rarer combination of loud murmurs of mitral and aortic incompetence simulates a continuous murmur more closely.

The best-known cause of a continuous murmur is *persistent ductus arteriosus*; this murmur is also known as a 'machinery' murmur or, less often, a Gibson murmur. It is best heard in the pulmonary area and is at its loudest around the time of the second heart-sound (*Fig*. 131). If pulmonary hypertension develops, a systolic murmur

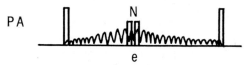

Fig. 131. Diagram of typical auscultatory findings in persistent ductus arteriosus. In the pulmonary area a continuous murmur is present reaching its maximum intensity at the time of the normally split second sound; the murmur is louder during expiration.

only may be heard. An exactly similar murmur is heard over the site of a *subclavian-pulmonary anastomosis*, performed for cyanotic congenital heart disease, and in *aortopulmonary septal defect* in which there is a communication between the great vessels just above the semilunar valves. The sudden development of a continuous murmur over the base of the heart is a feature of *rupture of an aneurysm of a sinus of Valsalva* into a right heart-chamber or into the pulmonary artery. Arteriovenous fistulae in general produce continuous murmurs but these can rarely be designated 'cardiac' murmurs except in the case of a *coronary arteriovenous fistula*. In *pulmonary atresia*, or severe Fallot's tetralogy, anastomoses between the bronchial and pulmonary arteries enlarge enormously and continuous murmurs may be heard over the lungs. A similar murmur localized to one region of the chest wall would suggest a *pulmonary arteriovenous fistula*, sometimes found in association with hereditary haemorrhagic telangiectasia.

Apart from arteriovenous shunts, a few other conditions cause continuous murmurs. Perhaps the commonest of these is the *venous hum*. This is most often heard over the jugular veins but may be audible at the base of the heart. It is much louder in the sitting posture than when the patient is recumbent, is accentuated by inspiration, and can be abolished by digital occlusion of the jugular vein. The murmur produced by *stenosis of a branch of the pulmonary artery* is

usually systolic in timing but, if the proximal pulmonary arterial pressure is significantly raised, it may be continuous. Finally, and very rarely, if an *atrial septal defect* is small and the left atrial pressure is significantly higher than that in the right, a soft continuous murmur may be heard at the right and left sternal borders. Usually, of course, no murmur is produced by flow through an atrial septal defect.

IV. EXOCARDIAC SOUNDS

Various sounds may be heard, over and near the precordium, which are temporally related to the action of the heart and must be distinguished from cardiac murmurs. An important example of these is the *pericardial friction rub*, described in detail on page 137. *Cardiorespiratory murmurs* are also common; they are systolic in timing and are heard in one phase of respiration only as a series of short 'puffs'. They are louder in the erect than in the recumbent position and are most commonly heard at and just lateral to the apex beat. Precordial clicks may occasionally be heard in the presence of a *spontaneous pneumothorax*, and *mediastinal emphysema* produces a loud 'crunching' sound which the patient himself may notice; this is sometimes known as Hamman's sign.

P. R. Fleming.

CEREBROSPINAL FLUID, EXAMINATION OF

A. PRESSURES

Measurement of the cerebrospinal fluid pressure with the subject upright shows the following results: it is slightly lower than atmospheric pressure in the lateral ventricles, and equal to atmospheric pressure in the cisterna magna, while in the lower lumbar sac it equals a column of water as high as the distance between the needle and the foramen magnum. The fluid therefore spurts out through a lumbar puncture needle in the lumbar sac but has to be withdrawn by syringe-suction from the ventricles and the cisterna magna. For most diagnostic purposes the fluid is conveniently obtained by lumbar puncture, the patient lying on his side with the spine horizontal and flexed, and the back vertical. In this position the pressure varies between about 60 mm. and 180 mm. of fluid in normal subjects, and it exhibits small oscillations due to the pulse and respiration.

Pressures between 60 mm. and 30 mm. are suspicious, and those below 30 mm. are abnormal. *Low pressures* may be seen in the following conditions: (1) in the presence of spinal block by tumour, etc.; (2) when lumbar puncture is repeated a day or two after a previous tap; (3) occasionally after head injuries without subdural haematoma and also, as an intermittent phenomenon, in some subdural haematomas; (4) in otherwise normal persons suffering from paroxysmal headaches, a syndrome which awaits elucidation; (5) in intracranial space-occupying lesions where displacement of normal structures has produced coning at the foramen magnum or tentorial opening. Lumbar puncture is dangerous in the last and *should never be performed when there is high pressure as manifested by papill-oedema* or *reason to suspect a space-occupying lesion.*

Pressures above 180 mm. are probably abnormal, and those in excess of 250 mm. are certainly so, *provided that the patient is relaxed* at the time of reading. Obese and tense individuals often give figures between 180 mm. and 250 mm. in the absence of disease, especially if

manometer attached to the needle in the lumbar sac—it means that there is a block in the subarachnoid space somewhere between the site of the needle and the foramen magnum. This is seen in a variety of neoplastic and inflammatory conditions, as also in fracture-dislocations, soft-disk protrusions, and advanced syringomyelia. A second but less reliable application of Queckenstedt's test is its use in looking for evidence of sinus thrombosis in mastoiditis and allied conditions. If the sigmoid sinus is thrombosed, there will be no rise of intracranial pressure when the jugular vein on that side is compressed, whereas there will be a normal response on the other, normal, side.

Table I. NORMAL VALUES FOR CONSTITUENTS OF CEREBROSPINAL FLUID AND PLASMA

SUBSTANCE	CEREBROSPINAL FLUID			PLASMA
	Lateral Ventricle	Cistern	Lumbar Sac	
Protein	5–15 mg.	15–25 mg.	15–40 mg.	5–7 g.
Cells	0	1	1–5	
Glucose	50–80 mg.	50–80 mg.	50–80 mg.	50–100 mg.
Urea	5–25 mg.	5–25 mg.	5–25 mg.	5–25 mg.
Cholesterol ..	trace	trace	trace	150 mg.
Uric acid	trace	trace	trace	2–4 mg.
Inorg. phosphorus	1–2 mg.	1–2 mg.	1–2 mg.	2–4 mg.
Calcium	4–7 mg.	4–7 mg.	4–7 mg.	8–10 mg.
Sodium	325 mg.	325 mg.	325 mg.	325 mg.
Potassium ..	12–17 mg.	12–17 mg.	12–17 mg.	18–20 mg.
Chlorides	720–750 mg.	720–750 mg.	720–750 mg.	

the knees are drawn up too high in an effort to flex the spine. *Raised pressure* may occur in the following conditions: (1) intracranial tumour; (2) suppurative encephalitis and cerebral abscess; (3) hydatid cysts; (4) extradural, subdural, subarachnoid, and intracerebral haemorrhage; (5) meningism and meningitis; (6) acute encephalitis and encephalopathy; (7) hydrocephalus from any cause; (8) craniostenosis; (9) cerebral oedema following head injury and cerebral infarction; (10) acute nephritis; (11) hypertensive encephalopathy and eclampsia; (12) otitic hydrocephalus, the name given by Symonds to intracranial hypertension due to dural sinus thrombosis arising as a result of otitis. It is a misnomer because there is no ventricular dilatation and sinus thrombosis, likewise causing intracranial hypertension, can arise from other causes, such as trauma, in pregnancy and the puerperium, and with the use of some drugs, such as the tetracyclines and nalidixic acid (Negram). However, the clinical picture in the otitic cases differs from that of sinus thrombosis from most other causes. It is generally the story of a child who has recently had otitis, develops a squint due to an external rectus palsy, and may complain of headache. Examination of the fundi shows papilloedema. In spite of this the patient is alert and active. The cerebrospinal fluid, although under increased pressure, is usually normal in composition.

QUECKENSTEDT'S TEST: Compression of the jugular veins causes a rise of intracranial pressure which is transmitted along the spinal subarachnoid space. If there is no rise—as judged by a

B. CONTENTS

Normal cerebrospinal fluid is clear, colourless, faintly alkaline; it has a specific gravity of from 1006 to 1008. Its protein and cell contents vary with the site from which the sample is drawn, whereas the quantities of glucose, urea, electrolytes, etc., are constant throughout. A scrutiny of normal values, listed in *Table I*, reveals that the concentration of some substances is identical in the plasma and cerebrospinal fluid, but that in other cases the cerebrospinal fluid concentration is either higher or lower than the plasma level. Further, many substances do not normally reach the spinal fluid, e.g., lipoids, bile-pigments, penicillin, streptomycin, but they may do so when the permeability of the choroid plexuses and other capillaries is increased by disease.

Turbidity is usually due to the presence of excess cells—erythrocytes, white cells, or micro-organisms. Spontaneous *clotting* indicates the presence of fibrinogen and fibrin ferment; a fine spider-web clot occurs in tuberculous meningitis, and less often in meningitis due to other organisms. Massive coagulation may be seen in polyneuritis and spinal block. *Blood staining* may be caused by accidental puncture of an intrathecal vein by the needle, in which case the contamination is greater in the first few ml. than in what is withdrawn later; when the red cells settle the supernatant fluid is colourless. If, however, the blood was present before the puncture, staining will be uniform and the supernatant fluid slightly yellow. This colour bleaches in sunlight, so that it is desirable to avoid such exposure. Yellow coloration is also seen in the absence of sub-arachnoid haemorrhage, as, for instance, when pus is present, and also in fluids with a high protein content such as occur in spinal block and some cases of polyneuritis. The cerebrospinal fluid usually remains colourless in jaundice; exceptionally, it may be yellow. Subarachnoid haemorrhage, however, is by far the commonest cause of xanthochromia; it may arise from rupture of an aneurysm, leakage of blood from an angioma, or from a haemorrhagic infarct, haemorrhagic encephalitis, anthrax meningitis, head injury, intracerebral haemorrhage with rupture into the ventricles or basal cisterns, and cerebral tumour.

Cytology. Normal cerebrospinal fluid obtained from the lumbar sac contains not more than 5 lymphocytes per c.mm. They are usually small, but occasional large hyaline cells are seen. Cells of the polymorph series, plasma cells, and compound granular corpuscles are always due to disease. Polymorphs predominate in coccal meningitis, and may also appear, along with lymphocytes, in tuberculous meningitis, cerebral abscess, and the early stages of poliomyelitis. Eosinophils in small numbers are sometimes seen in neurosyphilis and acute meningitis, but are often absent in parasitic infections of the nervous system even in the presence of eosinophilia in the blood. A lymphocytosis occurs in many virus infections, active neurosyphilis, tuberculous meningitis, encephalitis, and a large number of other infections and intoxications listed in *Table II*.

Table II. CEREBROSPINAL FLUID CHANGES IN DISEASE

DISEASE	CHARACTERISTIC CEREBROSPINAL FLUID CHANGES
Abscess:	
Cerebral	Pressure raised in acute cases. Pleocytosis, mainly lymphocytes, few poly-morphonuclears. Cells occasionally normal. Moderate rise of protein. Fall of glucose and chlorides if meningitis present. Bacteria rare
Epidural	Spinal block common. Cell count raised, polymorphonuclears predominating. Protein raised. Changes very slight in early stages
Arteriosclerosis, cerebral	Usually normal. Moderate increase of protein—rare
Chorea (Sydenham's)..	Usually normal. Slight lymphocytosis occasionally in early stages
Congenital and heredofamilial conditions	Normal
Craniostenoses (e.g., oxycephaly) ..	Pressure raised, contents normal
Cysticercosis	Pressure normal. In chronic cases may be increase of protein and cells. 'Paretic' Lange may occur
Disseminated sclerosis	Usually normal, but may contain slight excess of lymphocytes, protein, globulin. 'Paretic' Lange may occur, with negative Wassermann reaction
Encephalitis:	
Equine encephalomyelitis	Increase of polymorphonuclears and lymphocytes, protein slightly raised, glucose normal
Encephalitis lethargica	Normal, or slight lymphocytosis only
Japanese B encephalitis	Lymphocytosis. Protein rises as cells fall
Louping-ill	Moderate lymphocytosis. Otherwise normal
St. Louis encephalitis	Moderate lymphocytosis and slight increase of protein
Subacute inclusion encephalitis ..	Normal apart from a 'paretic' Lange curve in some cases
Encephalomyelitis:	
Acute disseminated form ..	Normal, or slight lymphocytosis
After exanthemata, vaccination, and inoculation against rabies ..	Normal, or slight lymphocytosis
Encephalopathy:	
Arsenical	Pressure normal or raised. Moderate lymphocytosis
Hypertensive	Pressure normal or raised. Occasional increase of protein after repeated convulsions
Lead	Pressure raised. Moderate rise of lymphocytes and protein. Contents sometimes normal
Wernicke's	Pressure and contents usually normal. Exceptionally, a rise of protein
Hepatitis, infective	Lymphocytes and protein increased in meningitic cases. Fluid rarely icteric
Herpes zoster	Often normal. May be slight lymphocytosis
Hydatid cyst, cerebral and spinal ..	As for cerebral and spinal tumour. Eosinophil cells exceptional
Lathyrism	Normal
Malaria, cerebral	Pressure normal or raised. Contents often normal, but increase of lymphocytes and protein may occur

Table II. CEREBROSPINAL FLUID CHANGES IN DISEASE—*continued*

DISEASE	CHARACTERISTIC CEREBROSPINAL FLUID CHANGES
Meningism	Pressure often raised, but contents normal
Meningitis (*see* HEAD, RETRACTION OF, p. 358): Anthrax	A moderate rise of pressure is usual in all acute forms of meningitis Red cells present. Abundance of polymorphonuclears. Protein raised, glucose reduced. Bacilli present
Brucellosis	Moderate lymphocytosis. Protein increased. Glucose and chlorides reduced
H. influenzae	Polymorphonuclear response; glucose and chlorides reduced
Meningitis (*contd.*): Glandular fever	Lymphocytosis and slight rise of protein. Glucose and chlorides normal
Leptospiral meningitis	Considerable lymphocytosis, few polymorphonuclears; protein raised; glucose and chlorides normal
Lymphocytic choriomeningitis ..	Lymphocytosis; fibrin clot may form; otherwise normal
Meningococcal meningitis ..	Fluid at first clear, then turbid, finally purulent. Large numbers of poly-morphonuclears, some of which contain diplococci. Protein increased, glucose and chloride diminished. Smears and cultures positive
Mumps meningo-encephalitis ..	Lymphocytosis and a few polymorphonuclears. Protein raised, glucose and chlorides normal. Sterile
Plague	Purulent fluid with polymorph excess. Bacilli present
Pneumococcal	Similar to meningococcal apart from bacteriology
Post-basic	Slight increase of cells and protein; usually sterile
Relapsing fever	Considerable pleocytosis, protein raised, glucose and chlorides slightly reduced; *B. recurrentis* is present in fluid
Staphylo- and streptococcal ..	Similar to meningococcal apart from bacteriology
Torulosis	Clear or turbid, with mucoid deposit in later stages. May be xanthochromic. Excess of lymphocytes and protein. Cryptococcus present; may be mistaken for lymphocytes
Motor neuron disease	Normal
Myelitis: Acute transverse myelitis	Occasionally normal; often partial block, with rise of lymphocytes and protein, in early stages only. Wassermann reaction positive in syphilitic cases
Subacute necrotic myelitis ..	Considerable increase of protein; lymphocytes may be slightly increased, or normal
Neuromyelitis optica (Devic) ..	Often normal, but may contain moderate excess of lymphocytes and protein
Nutritional neuropathies—beriberi, pellagra, 'captivity' syndrome ..	Normal
Paralysis agitans	Normal
Poliomyelitis, acute anterior ..	Pressure normal. Clear fluid, rarely containing fibrin clot. Lymphocytosis, 10–300, polymorphonuclears present in early stages. Rarely, cells normal. Protein at first normal, but rises as cells fall and may remain as high as 150 mg. for several weeks. Virus present but cultured with difficulty
Polyneuritis: Acute febrile polyneuritis	Cells normal or slight lymphocytosis. Protein may be grossly increased, with xanthochromia, but is sometimes normal
Alcoholic	Usually normal
Diphtheritic	Normal, or slight lymphocytosis and protein increase
Lead	Normal
Other forms..	Usually normal; protein raised in severe cases, irrespective of the cause
Presenile dementia (Pick and Alzheimer)	Normal
Prolapsed intervertebral disk ..	Often normal, or moderate increase of protein. Large herniations can cause spinal block and Froin syndrome
Sarcoidosis	Often normal. May be lymphocytosis and considerable increase of protein
Schilder's disease	Pressure and contents normal except in acute cases, in which pressure, lymphocytes, and protein may be raised (rare)
Schistosomiasis—cerebral and spinal	As in cerebral tumour and spinal compression respectively. Eosinophil cells absent, though present in blood
Spinal compression—tumour, para-sites, Pott's disease, syringomyelia, etc.	Partial or complete block on Queckenstedt's test. Protein increased (60–1000 mg.). May be slight lymphocytosis. Tumour cells rarely found. Xanthochromia common but not constant
Subacute combined degeneration of the cord	Normal

Table II. CEREBROSPINAL FLUID CHANGES IN DISEASE—continued

DISEASE	CHARACTERISTIC CEREBROSPINAL FLUID CHANGES
Subdural haematoma in adults ..	Pressure high, subnormal, or variable at successive punctures. Contents usually normal but may be excess of lymphocytes
Syphilis of Nervous System: Asymptomatic neurosyphilis ..	Increase of lymphocytes; albumin slightly raised, excess globulin. Wassermann reaction positive
Cerebral thrombosis	Fluid may be normal, but blood Wassermann reaction positive. Usually evidence of meningitic inflammation as above
Syphilis of Nervous System (contd.): Congenital neurosyphilis	As for acquired forms
General paralysis	Moderate increase of lymphocytes. Plasma cells may appear. Albumin and globulin increased. Lange curve usually 'paretic'—see text. Wassermann reaction always positive in fluid
Meningovascular type	Pressure usually normal but may be high in acute syphilitic meningitis and chronic basal form with hydrocephalus. Features of spinal block may appear with transverse myelitis, gumma of cord, and hypertrophic pacchymeningitis. Variable degree of lymphocytosis. Protein raised, especially globulin. Lange variable. Wassermann reaction positive in 90 per cent
Tabes dorsalis	Normal in at least 20 per cent of untreated cases. Usually slight excess of lymphocytes, albumin, and globulin. Lange variable, usually a mid-zone curve. Wassermann reaction negative in more than 20 per cent
Syringomyelia	Fluid normal until expansion of syrinx blocks subarachnoid space and produces compression syndrome
Toxoplasmosis	May be normal. Protein may be increased, sometimes with xanthochromia. Protozoon present in fluid
Trichiniasis	Normal in published cases
Trypanosomiasis	Changes may precede neurological symptoms. Pressure normal. Lymphocytosis; plasma cells and morular cells in severe cases. Protein raised, globulin prominent. Trypanosomes sometimes present
Tumour: Cerebral	Pressure normal in early stages, ultimately raised. Cells normal or slight lymphocytosis; tumour cells rarely found. Protein increased if tumour involves ventricles, surface of brain, or subarachnoid space; may be very high in acoustic neurinoma. Chlorides and glucose normal
Spinal	See Spinal compression, above
Vascular Accidents: Cerebral haemorrhage	Pressure usually raised. Contents normal until blood reaches the subarachnoid space
Embolism	Normal except in haemorrhagic infarction (rare)
Subarachnoid haemorrhage ..	Pressure usually raised. Fluid uniformly blood-stained, and xanthochromic after centrifuging. Proteins raised. Cell-count appropriate to degree of haemorrhage; lymphocytosis during period of absorption
Thrombosis and softening ..	Pressure normal. Fluid usually normal, but may be xanthochromic, with raised protein and lymphocytes if haemorrhagic softening reaches ventricles or surface of brain
Weil's disease: see Leptospiral meningitis	

Protein. A rise of protein content may involve the albumin fraction, the globulins, or both. In most diseases the albumin increases more than the globulin, but in neurosyphilis the latter is prominent. Excess of globulin, as judged by the Pandy test, is always pathological. The latter is so sensitive that it sometimes gives a faint reaction in normal fluids, whereas the former is positive in disease only. Taking the protein as a whole, the upper limit of normal is probably about 40 mg. per cent, but figures up to 60 mg. are not uncommon in otherwise normal persons. Spontaneous coagulation occurs when fibrinogen and fibrin ferment are present; in their absence it does not occur even in highly albuminous fluids. The protein may be raised in subarachnoid haemorrhage, in most infections of the brain and cord, in certain intoxications, and in spinal block. In the last it may reach 1000 mg. or more, and the fluid is often xanthochromic. These changes constitute the Froin syndrome, which may also be found in some cases of acute polyneuritis and chronic syphilitic meningomyelitis. A lymphocytic pleocytosis, originally mentioned by Froin as part of the syndrome, is nowadays regarded as an inessential but allowable ingredient.

Glucose. This varies between 50 mg. and 85 mg. per cent. It follows the fluctuations of the blood-glucose, albeit more slowly. Thus, after a large meal it may reach 105 mg. It is raised in uncontrolled diabetes and is often high in uraemia. It is diminished and may disappear in coccal meningitis, but is usually normal in tuberculous meningitis and virus infections.

Chlorides. A reduction of chlorides from the normal, 720–750 mg. per cent, occurs in most forms of acute meningitis, but the fall is most marked in the tuberculous form, in which readings of 500–600 mg. are not uncommon when the disease is well established. A rise may occur in uraemia, and this can be of diagnostic value in cases with cerebral symptoms but with few other features of the condition.

Urea. The urea level follows that of the plasma so closely that separate assessment is not necessary.

Calcium. The normal figure, 5·7 6·8 mg., may be exceeded in the Froin syndromeand may fal l in tetany.

Colloidal Reactions. The addition of albuminous cerebrospinal fluid to colloidal suspensions of various substances causes a precipitate of those substances. Lange's colloidal gold curve is the most satisfactory of these tests: he found that the curve obtained by adding 5 ml. of colloidal gold to 1 ml. of progressive dilutions of cerebrospinal fluid from 1 in 10 to 1 in 10,000 differed according to whether the fluid came from a case of meningovascular syphilis, tabes, or general paralysis. In practice this test is of little value in neurosyphilis but is useful in the diagnosis of disseminated sclerosis and subacute inclusion encephalitis since a 'paretic' curve (e.g., 5 5 5 4 4 4 3 3 2 2 1) is sometimes present, the Wassermann reaction being negative in both blood and fluid.

Ian Mackenzie.

CHEST, BLOODY EFFUSION IN

When on needling a chest a blood-stained serous effusion is found, the first question to be decided is whether the presence of the blood is due to the trauma of the needling. This can generally be decided immediately, since if the effusion is of any considerable size and the blood-staining is due to the diagnostic procedure itself, it will generally be found that though the first specimen removed is blood-stained, subsequent specimens are progressively less so, and ultimately unstained serous fluid is obtained. This test is impossible when the effusion is so small that a free flow of fluid cannot be obtained. Discoloration of the supernatant after centrifugation, due to haemoglobin, suggests that a pleural fluid is intrinsically blood-stained. The finding of blood in an effusion at a second tapping when it was not present at the first is of little significance, since the most probable cause of the bleeding is the previous paracentesis.

If it is decided that the effusion is intrinsically blood-stained, the possible causes of the effusion are exactly the same as those for any other serous effusion in the chest (*see* CHEST, SEROUS EFFUSION IN, p. 146); but the probabilities are slightly altered by the finding of a blood-stained effusion. The finding of a blood-stained effusion, especially in a middle-aged man, will arouse suspicion of the presence of malignant disease, since the proportion of cases of serous effusion which are blood-stained is higher among those due to malignant disease of the lung and pleura than among those due to the other common causes. Post-pneumonic effusions and those secondary to pulmonary infarction may also be blood-stained, though less frequently than those associated with malignant disease. The finding of a blood-stained effusion which re-accumulates rapidly and remains blood-stained or becomes more and more blood-stained is highly suggestive of malignant disease involving the pleura. This is most frequently due to invasion of the pleura by bronchial carcinoma, but may also be due to metastases in the lung or mediastinal lymph-nodes from tumours in other sites, either carcinomata or sarcomata. Mesothelioma of the pleura should be considered in patients who present with a pleural effusion of malignant type without evidence of a primary tumour in the lung or elsewhere, especially if there is a past history of exposure to asbestos. Apart from these rapidly reaccumulating heavily blood-stained effusions, the differential diagnosis of cases of blood-stained serous effusion follows the general lines indicated in the article on Serous Effusion in the Chest.

There are certain rare cases of *spontaneous haemothorax* in which, in the absence of trauma, paracentesis produces pure blood from the pleura. In the majority of these the cause of the haemothorax is difficult to determine, though it seems most likely that the condition is related to spontaneous pneumothorax, and that the bleeding is due to rupture of a vascular pleural adhesion or to a small tear in the lung. The symptoms consist of sudden pain in the chest followed by progressive dyspnoea, as in spontaneous pneumothorax; but in addition to these symptoms the patient quite rapidly develops a shock-like state with pallor, sweating, and rapid feeble pulse, indicative of internal bleeding. This condition demands energetic treatment by aspiration of the haemothorax and blood transfusion, and sometimes operative intervention. A rarer cause of spontaneous haemothorax is rupture of an aneurysm of the thoracic aorta, either dissecting or syphilitic. Diagnosis may be difficult, and depends upon the recognition both of the symptoms and signs of spontaneous haemothorax and of the presence of an aneurysm, either from the history or from physical and radiological signs. In some instances the patient dies so rapidly that nothing can be done: if he survives long enough for the diagnosis to be made, surgical treatment provides his only chance of survival.

An old-standing traumatic haemothorax steadily diminishes in haemoglobin content as the pleura, irritated by the blood, produces secondary serous exudate; and hence if the first aspiration is performed at an interval after the injury, serous fluid heavily stained with old blood may be obtained. It sometimes happens that a patient who has made light of a non-penetrating injury of the chest first comes under observation several weeks later with a small blood-stained pleural effusion, and direct questioning may be needed to elicit the history of injury; radiological evidence of fractures of ribs may be helpful in such cases, but sometimes traumatic haemothorax may follow non-penetrating injury without rib-fracture.

J. G. Scadding.

CHEST, DEFORMITY OF

The normal configuration of the chest is variable both with age and according to the physical build of subjects within the same age group. In infants the cross-section of the chest is normally almost circular, and the chest is as deep as it is wide. In the normal course of development, the chest

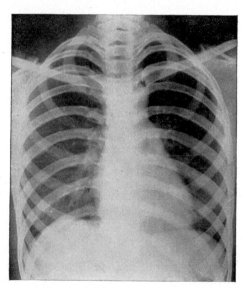

Fig. 132. Radiograph of normal chest. Patient of stocky build with transversely disposed heart.

becomes flattened anteroposteriorly, so that in older children and in adults it is wider transversely than it is deep. However, there are considerable variations within the normal. In persons of stocky build the chest tends to be relatively deep anteroposteriorly and short from above downwards, and the heart tends to lie horizontally (*Fig.* 132). In persons of tall spare build, the chest is long from above downwards and shallow anteroposteriorly, and the heart tends to lie vertically (*Fig.* 133). There is no evidence that any of these varieties of normal configuration of the chest can be correlated with liability to any particular disease.

5

Congenital Deformities of the Chest. Congenital abnormalities of the chest evident clinically are comparatively rare. Occasionally an infant is born with *incomplete fusion of the sternum*, producing the appearance of a split sternum. If this is of moderate or severe degree there is apt to be indrawing of the soft tissues over the central fissure during inspiration, with bulging in expiration. This paradoxical respiratory movement is much increased in the presence of respiratory obstruction such as may be produced by an attack of bronchitis, and then constitutes a severe embarrassment to respiration. There should be no difficulty in recognizing this condition if the possibility of its occurrence is borne in mind.

Another rare congenital anomaly is partial or complete *absence of pectoral muscles*. This is usually unilateral, and generally affects the lower part of the pectoralis major, though more severe defects may occur. The condition produces no symptoms, but if it is of severe degree a deformity

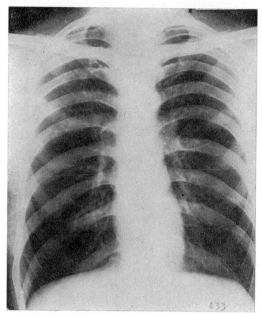

Fig. 133. Radiograph of normal chest. Patient of tall thin build with vertically disposed heart.

of the bony chest results, the anterior chest wall on the affected side being sunken in, since it is not subjected to the lateral pull of the pectoral muscle. In radiographs of the chest, absence of the pectoral muscles gives rise to abnormal transradiancy of the affected side, which may give rise to an erroneous impression of pulmonary disease (*Fig.* 134).

Funnel chest, or pectus excavatum, is generally thought to be initially of congenital origin, though the deformity may be increased by subsequent respiratory infections. This deformity consists of a depression of the lower end of the sternum into a rounded hollow, which in the most extreme cases may be so deep that the sternum almost touches the vertebral column. In such severe cases the heart is of necessity displaced into the left side of the chest. The condition can hardly be missed clinically. It is not related to rickets, but is due to a congenital anomaly of the diaphragm, probably deficient development of muscle in the anterior part. *Congenital sternal prominence*, which constitutes one of the varieties of 'pigeon-breast' deformity (*see below*), is also

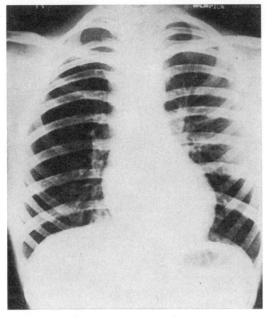

Fig. 134. Radiograph of chest of a patient with congenital absence of the right pectoral muscles. Note the greater transradiancy of the right side.

thought to be due to a congenital anomaly of the diaphragm.

General Changes in the Conformation of the Chest resulting from Disease. *Rickets* produces important changes in the shape of the chest. The active phase of rickets in infants and young children produces the so-called 'rickety rosary', composed of the swollen costochondral junctions. When the ribs are soft and plastic in active rickets, they tend to become indrawn on inspiration, especially during intercurrent respiratory infections with bronchitis causing slight respiratory obstruction. The chest wall is supported at the costal margin by the abdominal viscera, and hence a depression just above the costal margin, usually of the 5th to 8th ribs, with flaring outwards of the costal margin itself, is produced. This deformity remains after the rickets is healed, and is known as *Harrison's sulcus*. By a similar mechanism the chest wall in the region of the costochondral junctions may become indrawn and produce a longitudinal depression parallel to the sternum, which is usually deeper on the right side since the heart gives some support to the left side. This is a factor in the production

of pigeon-breast deformities (*see below*). Rachitic deformities of the chest are often asymmetrical, and may be accompanied by deformities of other bones.

Pigeon-breast, or pectus carinatum, is a not uncommon deformity in which the sternum bulges forwards and the ribs incline forwards to it, causing a greatly increased anteroposterior depth of the chest. It may be acquired as a result of rickets and chronic bronchopulmonary infections in childhood, but, as noted above, a similar deformity can arise congenitally.

Barrel chest is the name given to the deep chest, in which the anteroposterior diameter is increased, often to equal the transverse diameter, the subcostal angle is abnormally wide, and in a radiograph the ribs appear more horizontally disposed than normal. This conformation of the chest has in the past been regarded as related to the presence of pulmonary emphysema; but it is more constantly related to over-inflation of the lungs than to irreversible structural emphysema. It may be observed in acute attacks of asthma, and in patients with chronic obstructive bronchitis with relatively little emphysema. Many patients with 'primary' emphysema, e.g., those with α-1-antitrypsin deficiency, have a long thorax with increased anteroposterior diameter, giving a more or less circular cross-section; radiologically the heart is vertically disposed and narrow, and the diaphragm very low in position and flat in outline. Additional signs, such as lack of respiratory expansion, action of the accessory muscles of respiration, feeble or impalpable apex beat of the heart, distant heart-sounds, hyper-resonant percussion note over the lungs with diminution in the areas of cardiac and hepatic dullness, and weak breath-sounds must be present before a clinical diagnosis of emphysema can be suggested.

Changes in the Chest Wall resulting from Scoliosis. It is important to recognize the changes in the chest wall which are produced by a *scoliosis*. In an 'idiopathic' (congenital, juvenile, or adolescent) scoliosis, the vertebrae at the most prominent part of the curve of a postural scoliosis rotate in such a way that the degree of curvature indicated to external inspection by the line of the spinous processes is less than the degree of curvature shown by the vertebral bodies; and this rotation causes corresponding displacement of the ribs. Hence with a thoracic scoliosis the ribs at the back tend to be prominent on the side of the convexity and flattened on the side of the concavity; and conversely in front there is prominence on the side of the concavity and flattening on the side of the convexity. These considerations apply without modification only to cases where there is a wide curve throughout the thoracic spine. If there is a double curve of the thoracic spine, the resulting deformity of the chest wall is naturally more complex.

In *paralytic scoliosis*, e.g., that due to poliomyelitis or syringomyelia, the changes in the chest wall are of generally similar type, but may be modified by the effects of weakness of the shoulder-girdle muscles. Similarly in *scoliosis or kyphosis due to disease of the spine* the chest wall changes are dependent upon the site and extent of the vertebral changes; e.g., in *tuberculosis of the spine*, destruction of vertebral bodies causes a sharp kyphosis with a variable amount of scoliosis. Other spinal diseases causing kyphosis or scoliosis include *osteoporosis* and *congenital anomalies of the vertebrae*.

Local Changes in the Chest Wall resulting from Disease

1. UNILATERAL CHANGES. *General expansion* of one side of the chest may be produced by a large *spontaneous pneumothorax* or a large rapidly accumulating *pleural effusion*. The prominent side will be less mobile, and this distinguishes the condition on inspection from those in which the opposite side of the chest is abnormally con-tracted. This abnormal prominence of the chest wall produced by a large amount of air or liquid in the pleura is to be expected only in children and young adults; in older persons the chest wall is generally too rigid to be over-inflated in this way. With large pleural effusions, even if they are not absorbed or removed by aspiration, the phase of over-distension is generally fairly short-lived. Distinction between pneumothorax and pleural effusion can easily be made by physical examination, since the percussion note over the affected side of the chest is resonant in pneumo-thorax but dull with effusion. There may, of course, be both gas and liquid in the chest; in this case there is dullness at the base separated from resonance above by a horizontal line which shifts with movement of the patient, but remains hori-zontal. A very rare cause of general expansion of one side of the chest is a very large *intrathoracic tumour*, such as a dermoid or a neurofibroma. Other very rare causes are *unilateral obstructive emphysema*, which is an occasional effect of a foreign body in a main bronchus, and over-disten-sion of giant air-containing cysts in the lung; both of these events are more frequent as causes of expansion of one side of the chest in young children and infants than in adults.

General contraction of one side of the chest may be produced by a variety of causes, some of them complex; among these, the most frequent common factor is pleural thickening. This may be caused by primarily pleural processes such as *chronic empyema* (*Fig.* 135) or *tuberculous pleural effusion*. Although most tuberculous pleural effusions absorb leaving no clinically detectable pleural thickening, a few show delayed absorp-tion and progressive pleural thickening, with considerable contraction of the affected hemi-thorax. Pulmonary fibrosis due to inflammatory processes, such as *chronic pulmonary tuberculosis*, *chronic lung abscess*, or the slow resolution of some forms of *pneumonia*, causes contraction of one side of the chest, and in the most extreme examples is found to be associated with gross pleural thickening. *Atelectasis* of the lung will also produce unilateral contraction of the chest

wall; it may be due to organic obstruction such as a new growth of the bronchus or a foreign body, or to past obstruction by excessive secre-tions, as in postoperative atelectasis. The con-tracted fibrotic lung due to chronic pulmonary suppuration, to organization of unresolved pneu-monia, or to unrelieved atelectasis is frequently

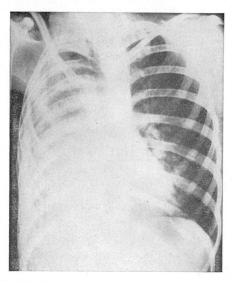

Fig. 135. Radiograph of chest showing contraction of the right side with gross pleural thickening due to a chronic empyema. Note the scoliosis and the periosteal thickening of the ribs on the affected side.

the site of *bronchiectasis* (*Figs.* 136, 137), which gives rise to characteristic symptoms and signs. The contraction of the chest wall due to these intrathoracic changes is equally evident in front and at the back of the same side of the chest, and if there is also a scoliosis secondary to the intra-thoracic disease the concavity of the curve will be towards the contracted side. The deformity should thus be distinguished quite easily from that due to a postural scoliosis. When uni-lateral contraction of the chest with gross pleural thickening arises from any cause during childhood or adolescence, the resulting scoliosis may become extreme as growth proceeds over the years.

2. LOCALIZED CHANGES IN THE CHEST WALL IN DISEASE. *Localized swellings of the chest wall* may be due to lesions of the chest wall itself or to intrathoracic disease.

The chief lesions of the chest wall producing swellings are tuberculosis, simple inflammations, and tumours, especially of the ribs. *Tubercu-losis* of the chest wall usually originates in a lymph-node in an intercostal space; the tubercu-lous process in this node progresses to caseation and finally formation of a cold abscess, which tracks through the intercostal space in collar-stud fashion to cause a cold abscess in the chest wall. Tuberculosis of the sternum may cause a cold abscess over the anterior chest wall. Rarely a cold abscess associated with Pott's disease of the thoracic spine may point over the lower ribs at the back. *Simple inflammations* of the skin and subcutaneous tissues may occur on the chest wall as elsewhere; occasionally *osteomyelitis of the ribs or sternum*, which may be chronic, gives rise to chest-wall swellings. A rare though important type of chronic osteochondritis of the ribs, usually localized to the costochondral junctions, is that

When it is not the result of a gross injury it occurs through an intercostal space, especially a congenitally wide one. More rarely still, herniation of the lung into the neck, through a weak part of Sibson's fascia, has been reported. These herniations of the lung will be recognized by the fact that they inflate during expiration, especially a forced expiration against the closed glottis, and collapse during inspiration; and by the fact that

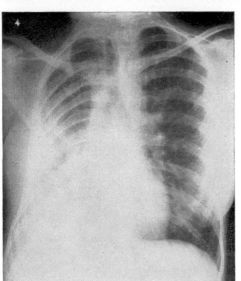

Fig. 136. Radiograph of chest showing contraction of the right side due to fibrosis of the lung, pleural thickening, and bronchiectasis.

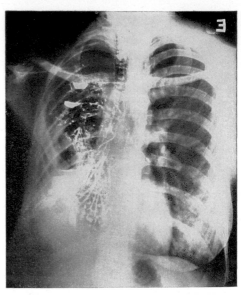

Fig. 137. Bronchogram in the same case as *Fig*. 126.

due to the typhoid bacillus; it may first become evident during convalescence, or even months after recovery, from typhoid fever. In tertiary syphilis *gummata* may appear in association with the ribs or the sternum, though they are now rarely seen. The commonest *tumours* of the ribs are chondromata, osteochondromata, and chondrosarcomata. Isolated myelomas may occur, and the ribs may be involved in multiple myelomatosis. Metastases of malignant disease may appear in the ribs; they may be associated with primary growths anywhere, but especially in the lung. The innocent tumours and some of those of low malignancy present as hard, often lobulated, usually painless swellings; the malignant ones often cause pain and localized tenderness, sometimes with pathological fractures.

Occasionally, in association with a bronchitis or other acute or chronic respiratory infection, small painful swellings appear at the costochondral junctions, especially the second. They generally subside after the subsidence of the associated respiratory infection; the name *Tietze's disease* has been given to this syndrome.

Very rarely *herniation of the lung* occurs by protrusion of the lung into a bulge of parietal pleura through a weak part of the chest wall.

transillumination in the inflated state shows them to be translucent.

The commonest localized swelling of the chest wall due to intrathoracic disease is that caused by the pointing of a neglected empyema externally. This produces a swelling which may be anywhere on the costal part of the chest wall; at first diffuse and brawny, it later softens in the middle and sometimes gives an impulse on coughing, and may be partially reducible by pressure into the chest. This condition is called *empyema necessitatis*. Any type of empyema may point in this way.

Intrathoracic *actinomycosis* tends to cause diffuse indurated swelling of the chest wall, especially over its lower part; if the condition is undiagnosed and untreated it progresses to the formation of the characteristic multiple sinuses discharging 'sulphur-granule' pus.

Intrathoracic tumours of all sorts may invade the chest wall and cause local swellings; rarely *carcinoma of the lung* invades the chest wall directly from the lung, and various mediastinal tumours, for example *Hodgkin's disease* of mediastinal lymph-nodes, may directly invade the chest wall and cause local swelling. *Aortic aneurysms* involving the ascending part of the aorta may cause pulsating swellings over the upper part of the chest anteriorly; they should be easily recognizable by the characteristic expansile pulsation and by the other signs and symptoms of aneurysm; the commonest situation for such a swelling is to the right of the sternum in the 1st, 2nd, and 3rd intercostal spaces. The *precordium* may become prominent as the result of the presence of a grossly enlarged heart; this is most frequently seen in children suffering from severe rheumatic or congenital heart disease. It may also become prominent in children with large pericardial effusions.

Localized contraction of the chest wall may be caused by any of the intrathoracic conditions which are mentioned above as possibly causing general contraction of the chest wall, if they are confined to a lobe or part of a lobe of the lung. Thus chronic pulmonary tuberculosis affecting the apex of the lung, or atelectasis of a lower lobe, will cause contraction and restricted movement of the corresponding part of the chest wall. An important group of changes in the chest wall and the neighbouring muscles is associated with *chronic apical fibrotic lesions*, of which the great majority are tuberculous. These consist of contraction and limitation of movement together with wasting of the trapezius, sternomastoid, and pectoral muscles.

J. G. Scadding.

CHEST, PAIN IN

Pain in the chest is one of the commonest of all complaints. However slight it may be, it only too often conjures up in the mind of the sufferer a vision of serious organic disease of the lungs or, more often, of the heart. Accurate diagnosis depends, to a considerable extent, on physical examination and special investigations but, most of all, on a detailed and precise history of the site and radiation of the pain, of its character and duration, and of factors by which it is aggravated or relieved. To emphasize this point, chest pain will be considered according to whether it is felt mainly in the centre of the chest or in its lateral aspects. Pain in the precordium will be included in the discussion of central chest pain. The adjectives 'central' and 'precordial' are not, of course, synonymous—the precordium being that area of the anterior chest wall circumscribed by the surface markings of the heart—but the two sites are naturally associated in the diagnosis of pain which arises, or is thought to arise, from the heart. Before proceeding to the main discussion, a brief account will be given, for the sake of completeness, of several causes of chest pain which are immediately obvious on superficial examination.

1. Pain due to Superficial Lesions. Pain due to *inflammation of the superficial tissues* of the chest wall poses no great diagnostic problem. It is important to remember, however, that the inflammation may have spread from a deeper lesion such as an empyema. *Herpes zoster*, which involves thoracic nerve roots in at least 50 per cent

of cases, is also obvious once the eruption has appeared but pain and paraesthesiae may be present for a few days before this and cause temporary diagnostic confusion. The vesicles are implanted on an erythematous base and may be discrete or confluent; they are strictly unilateral and occupy the area of one or more dermatomes (*Fig.* 138). Fever and malaise occur in a few patients and the axillary lymph-nodes

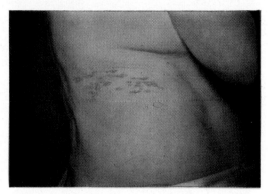

Fig. 138. Intercostal herpes zoster.

may be enlarged. Scabs form and the lesions heal in a week or two, without scarring unless they have become secondarily infected. Postherpetic neuralgia may, occasionally, cause severe pain for a long period after the eruption has disappeared, especially in the elderly. Very rarely *Mondor's disease*, which is phlebitis of the subcutaneous anterior thoracic veins, produces pain, either pleuritic in type or provoked by raising the arms. The inflamed vein may be palpable as a tender cord. Resolution occurs in a few weeks or a month or two.

2. Central Chest Pain. Much the most important cause of central chest pain is myocardial ischaemia. Three separate clinical syndromes are recognized—angina of effort, acute coronary insufficiency, and myocardial infarction—although there is some overlap, at least between the first two.

The diagnosis of *angina* turns, in the great majority of cases, on an accurate history. The pain is typically symmetrical in the chest, or nearly so, being felt in the region of the sternum, or slightly to the left, and radiating laterally towards the axillae and down the inner sides of the arms; the left is involved a little more often than the right but this is of no diagnostic importance as bilateral radiation is the rule. Radiation to the epigastrium, the side of the neck, jaw, and tongue also occurs. Very occasionally the pain is felt in the midline of the back or in one or other scapular region. The pain is described as 'tight', 'gripping', or 'like indigestion', or the patient may deny actual pain and describe only a feeling of pressure or of tightness. A particularly revealing gesture is the clenched fist placed on the sternum to indicate both the site and, presumably, the character of the sensation. A pain described as 'stabbing' is probably not angina, but patients do not always choose their words with care and each statement must be carefully analysed to ascertain the patient's meaning exactly. Certainly a pain which comes in sharp jabs, lasting a second only, is not angina and adjectives such as 'shooting' and 'stabbing' are suspect on this account. The typical duration of an attack is a few minutes only and a pain lasting for a much longer or shorter time than this is unlikely to be angina; there are exceptions, however, which will be discussed. Perhaps the most important aspect is the relationship to exertion. A pain in the anterior part of the chest which is consistently provoked by effort and relieved by rest must be presumed to be angina unless there is overwhelming evidence to the contrary. The pain may be provoked more easily after meals or in cold weather, but it is the relationship to effort which is of paramount importance provided that the pain develops *during* the exercise; a pain starting *after* exercise is not angina. The effect of sublingual trinitrin may be of diagnostic importance but, again, the time relationship is important. If the pain is relieved within a minute by trinitrin, angina is probable; patients are, however, unfamiliar with such a rapid effect from oral medication and may claim that trinitrin relieves their pain, omitting the essential fact that the pain does not cease until, perhaps, half an hour after the tablet was taken. Occasionally variants of angina are seen such as pain felt only in one of the distal sites of radiation; even 'tennis-elbow' and 'toothache' may prove to be angina if the constant relationship to exertion can be elicited.

Apart from exercise, angina may be precipitated by sympathetic overactivity. This is the mechanism of angina provoked by emotion as in the case of John Hunter who said, some time before he died after an acrimonious Board Meeting, 'My life is in the hands of any rascal who chooses to annoy and tease me.' Nocturnal angina is also related to sympathetic overactivity as it has been shown to occur after a period of REM (rapid eye movements) sleep which is associated with dreaming. Angina decubitus, provoked by lying down, is probably due to the increase in cardiac output in this posture; it is rather characteristic of syphilitic aortic valve disease. In general, angina which is easily provoked or occurs, apparently spontaneously, at rest is associated with severe disease involving all three coronary arteries (right, left circumflex, and anterior descending).

In the majority of cases of angina no abnormal physical signs are found but two important signs should be specifically sought. A left atrial impulse may be palpable at the apex and an atrial gallop rhythm heard particularly during an actual attack of pain. Paradoxical splitting of the second heart-sound is less common and is difficult to elicit but, if present, implies prolongation of left ventricular systole and a serious

disturbance of left ventricular function. The electrocardiogram is usually normal at rest but the typical depression of the RS-T segment may be present to confirm the diagnosis of ischaemia (*Fig.* 139); evidence of previous infarction may also be present or non-specific changes such as bundle branch block. Diagnostic changes may sometimes be produced in the electrocardiogram by exercise (*Fig.* 140), but this test requires very careful interpretation. The diagnosis can also be confirmed and the severity quantified by using an artificial pacemaker to drive the heart at increasing rates until pain is produced. The results of

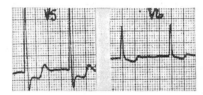

Fig. 139. RS-T segment depression. The record on the left (V5) is from a patient with severe ischaemic heart disease, causing angina on the slightest exertion. Depression of the whole of the RS-T segment, which remains horizontal, should be compared with the downward sloping RS-T segment due to digitalis seen in the record, from another patient, on the right (V6).

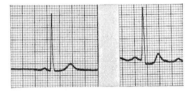

Fig. 140. Positive exercise test. The complex on the left was recorded at rest from a patient with chest pain suspicious of angina. The complex on the right from the same lead, recorded after exercise, shows depression of the whole RS-T segment which remains horizontal. The diagnosis of myocardial ischaemia is confirmed.

this test are very reproducible and are uninfluenced by the subjective effects of the exercise test.

In practically all cases of angina the underlying lesion is coronary atherosclerosis. It must not be forgotten, however, that other forms of arterial disease can, occasionally, cause myocardial ischaemia. Angina is a well-recognized, though rare, symptom of polyarteritis nodosa and giant-cell arteritis; smaller vessels may be involved in rheumatoid arteritis and in association with livedo reticularis. Disease of small coronary vessels is rare as a cause of angina but its presence may be inferred if a normal coronary arteriogram is found in a patient with an unequivocal diagnosis of angina. It is for this reason that coronary arteriography, which delineates the larger vessels only, cannot be used to exclude myocardial ischaemia as a cause of obscure chest pain. Another important inflammatory cause of angina is involvement of the coronary ostia in syphilitic aortitis; the attacks of pain tend to last longer and occur rather characteristically at night although the relationship to effort is as in other varieties of angina.

Ischaemic pain is aggravated by left ventricular hypertrophy due to hypertension and, particularly, aortic valve disease. In these conditions, and in hypertrophic obstructive cardiomyopathy, the disease of the coronary arteries themselves may be trivial and the pain due to relative ischaemia of the hypertrophied muscle. Severe anaemia, for example pernicious anaemia or following gastro-intestinal haemorrhage, thyrotoxicosis, and rapid ectopic tachycardia can also cause angina in patients with minor coronary disease only. All these factors must be borne in mind particularly when dealing with a case of angina in a premenopausal woman. Coronary atherosclerosis is rare in such patients and angina is likely to be due to one of the precipitating factors mentioned or to premature atherosclerosis resulting from hyperlipidaemia, as in diabetes, myxoedema, or hereditary hypercholesterolaemic xanthomatosis (Type II hyperlipidaemia in Fredrickson's classification) (*Fig.* 141).

Acute coronary insufficiency is the least common clinical variety of ischaemic heart disease. This is one of a number of terms used to describe cases in which prolonged cardiac pain occurs at rest without evidence of myocardial necrosis. Other terms used include 'pre-infarction angina' and 'crescendo angina' which carry the, often correct, implication that myocardial infarction is imminent; the non-committal term 'intermediate coronary syndrome' has also been used. A variant of this condition is the so-called 'angina inversa', described by Prinzmetal, in which RS-T *elevation* occurs briefly in association with ischaemic pain at rest; this is believed to be due to severe ischaemia of a rather localized area of myocardium (*Fig.* 142).

Myocardial infarction is nearly always due to occlusion of a coronary artery by atherosclerosis, with or without superadded thrombosis; a much rarer cause is coronary embolus in association with, for example, atrial fibrillation or infective endocarditis. The pain of myocardial infarction has exactly the same character and areas of radiation as angina. It is not, however, related to exercise and typically lasts for several hours, if untreated, rather than the few minutes of an anginal attack. Myocardial infarction can, rarely, be painless, especially in the elderly in whom it may manifest itself as syncope or a dysrhythmia or as otherwise unexplained left ventricular failure. In contrast to the paucity of physical signs in angina, it is unusual to find no abnormal physical signs in a case of myocardial infarction provided that frequent examination is carried out as many of the signs may be very transient. Some fall in blood-pressure is common but may not be detected if the previous level is unknown. Slight elevation of the jugular venous pressure is seen in many cases and an audible or palpable atrial gallop is found even more frequently. Paradoxical splitting of the second sound may occasionally be detected and, after a day or two, a pericardial rub may be heard.

The three most common complications are dysrhythmias, cardiac failure, and shock, in that order. Continuous monitoring has demonstrated that over 90 per cent of cases of myocardial infarction have some form of dysrhythmia, of which ventricular extrasystoles are the most common and may presage ventricular tachycardia and fibrillation. Supraventricular dysrhythmias also occur, often in association with cardiac failure. Atrioventricular block is an ominous complication, especially if it develops in a case of anterior infarction. Congestive heart failure or frank pulmonary oedema occur from time to time but lesser degrees of left ventricular failure are common. As a result of the consequent pulmonary venous congestion, with the probable addition of multiple alveolar collapse, mild arterial hypoxaemia is seen very frequently, the arterial Po_2 being around 9 kPa (65 mmHg); this often causes sufficient hyperventilation to reduce the arterial Pco_2 to about 5 kPa (37 mmHg). The term 'cardiogenic shock' should be reserved for cases with severe hypotension, cold, clammy skin, oliguria, and clouding of consciousness.

Less common complications include rupture of the infarct which will usually cause rapidly fatal haemopericardium or, if a papillary muscle is involved, acute mitral regurgitation with pulmonary oedema; rupture of the interventricular septum causes acute right ventricular failure. Systemic embolism from a mural thrombus is not uncommon; pulmonary embolism arises most often from phlebothrombosis of the calf veins secondary to the enforced recumbency. Later sequelae are ventricular aneurysm, which may rarely calcify (*Fig.* 143), Dressler's syndrome of recurrent pericarditis and pleurisy (*see* POST-PERI-CARDIOTOMY SYNDROME, p. 655) and the shoulder–hand syndrome, which consists of 'frozen shoulder' and Raynaud's phenomenon, usually on the left.

Electrocardiography remains the most commonly used method of confirming a diagnosis of myocardial infarction but estimation of various serum enzymes is also valuable particularly in the, not infrequent, cases in which the electrocardiographic signs are equivocal. There are three cardinal electrocardiographic signs of myocardial infarction: a pathological Q wave, at least a third the amplitude of the R wave in the same lead and at least 0·04 second in duration; RS-T segment elevation with an upward convexity; and T wave inversion which may not be seen until the RS-T segment is returning to the iso-electric line as it does during the first few weeks after the episode. The T wave may also return to, or towards, normal after some months, but the Q wave, the sign of irreversible muscle necrosis, virtually always remains indefinitely. These changes are seen in leads whose positive terminals face the infarcted area of myocardium; in leads 'facing' the diametrically opposite part of the heart reciprocal changes are seen which may, occasionally, be of diagnostic significance. For descriptive purposes, infarcts are subdivided into anterior, inferior (or diaphragmatic), and 'true' posterior. Until quite recently the term 'posterior' was applied to the diaphragmatic surface of the heart but, now that it is possible to diagnose infarction of the small part of the left ventricle which lies posteriorly, the anatomically more correct term 'inferior' is preferred. To avoid confusion with the older nomenclature, infarcts at the back of the left ventricle are designated *true* posterior (*Figs*. 144–147).

Many intracellular enzymes are released into the circulation from the infarcted myocardium and the rise and fall of their serum levels can be of great diagnostic value. Those most commonly estimated clinically are aspartate aminotransferase (previously known as 'glutamic-oxalacetic transaminase'), creatine phosphokinase, and lactate dehydrogenase. The first two remain elevated for three or four days only but elevation of the serum lactate dehydrogenase persists for up to two weeks. Greater specificity for myocardial damage can be achieved by estimating the isoenzymes of lactate dehydrogenase separately; the

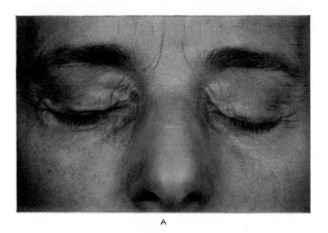

A

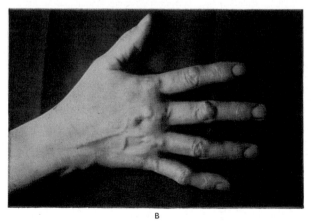

B

Fig. 141. Xanthelasma palpebrarum and xanthomata on the hand of a female aged 52 with angina of effort. The serum cholesterol was 15·5 mmol/l (600 mg per 100 ml).

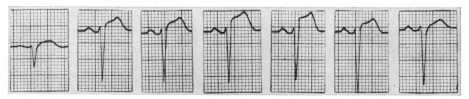

Fig. 142. 'Angina inversa'. Male, aged 50, with angina at rest. RS-T elevation appeared and disappeared over a period of about 2 minutes. Recorded via a monitoring chest electrode.

iso-enzyme released in largest amounts from myocardium also acts upon hydroxybutyrate and can be conveniently estimated as hydroxybutyrate dehydrogenase. Apart from the changes in the serum enzymes, non-specific evidence of tissue necrosis is also present following myocardial infarction; such evidence includes pyrexia, leucocytosis, and raised sedimentation rate. Such

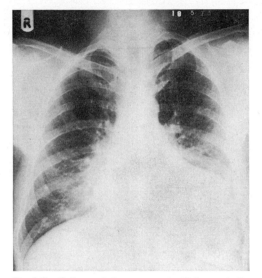

Fig. 143. Left ventricular aneurysm. Male, aged 48, who had had an anterior myocardial infarction 6 months previously.

changes, although characteristic, are of little or no diagnostic value.

The pain of *pericarditis* is, in some respects, similar to that of myocardial infarction and, as localized pericarditis is common in the latter, the differentiation may present some difficulty. Pericardial pain is felt in the sternal region and towards the left and may radiate to the epigastrium, neck, back, shoulders, and, occasionally, to the arms. The severity varies markedly, from a mild discomfort to extreme agony and the pain is described either as 'stabbing' or 'like a knife' or in terms very reminiscent of those used to describe the pain of myocardial ischaemia. It is aggravated by deep breathing, coughing, and by twisting movements involving the muscles of the chest wall. There is therefore some relationship with exertion, on account of the associated hyperventilation, but the aggravation by specific movements such as turning over in bed serves to distinguish it from angina. The pain is also worse in the recumbent position and is relieved by sitting up; it may also be aggravated by swallowing. The characteristic physical sign is the friction rub, heard over all or part of the precordium. It may be markedly influenced by respiration, becoming inaudible in full inspiration. The rub is usually easily distinguishable from murmurs by its characteristic quality and to-and-fro cadence but occasionally, especially as it is fading, it may resemble a murmur or a systolic click. The third cardinal feature of pericarditis is the electrocardiogram. RS-T elevation is seen in all epicardial leads, that is in all the leads of a conventional 12-lead record except aVR (*Fig.* 148).

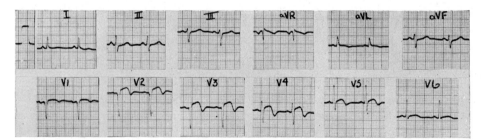

Fig. 144. Anteroseptal myocardial infarction. Pathological Q waves are present in V1 and 2 and RV3 is diminutive. RS-T elevation is seen in V1–6 and aVL. The T wave is inverted in V1–5 and in aVL.

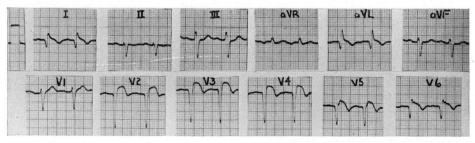

Fig. 145. Anterolateral myocardial infarction. Pathological Q waves are present in I, aVL and V2–6 with RS-T segment elevation and T inversion.

The RS-T elevation is concave upwards unlike that of myocardial infarction; pathological Q waves are, of course, absent. Later in the course of the disease, T-wave inversion appears and, at this stage, the differentiation from myocardial ischaemia may be difficult. The diagnosis of pericarditis is incomplete unless the aetiology is determined. Common causes include virus infection (often Coxsackie B), connective-tissue disorders such as systemic lupus erythematosus, rheumatic fever, rheumatoid arthritis, bacterial infections, and Dressler's and other similar syndromes. Uraemia is a well-known cause but the commonest cause of all is myocardial infarction; in that condition the pericarditis probably contributes little to the pain.

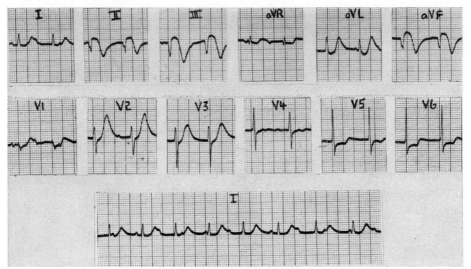

Fig. 146. Inferior myocardial infarction. Pathological Q waves, RS-T elevation, and T wave inversion are present in II and III and aVF. The tall T waves in V2 and V3 and the RS-T depression in V5 and V6 are probably reciprocal to the primary inferior changes. Atrioventricular dissociation is also present.

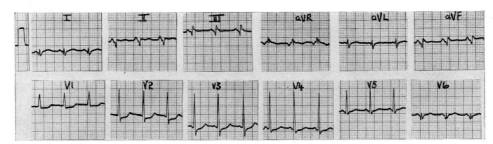

Fig. 147. Postero-inferior myocardial infarction. The pathological Q waves in II, III, and aVF are evidence of infarction of the inferior (diaphragmatic) surface of the left ventricle. The dominant R wave and RS-T depression in V1–3, were known to have been absent before the episode of pain. This pattern is reciprocal to a, presumed, pathological Q wave and RS-T elevation which would have been recorded from an electrode diametrically opposite to V1–3. These changes, in this context, are those of true posterior infarction but the pattern of V1–3, taken alone, is also compatible with right ventricular hypertrophy.

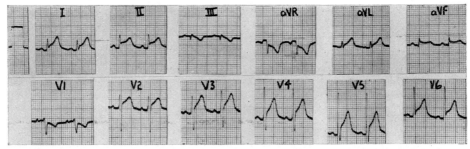

Fig. 148. Acute pericarditis. RS-T elevation, concave upwards, is present in I, II, aVL, aVF, and V2–6. There are no pathological Q waves and the T waves are upright in most leads. These features, together with the *widespread* RS-T elevation, confirm the diagnosis of pericarditis.

Pericardial fat necrosis is a rare cause of pain simulating that of pericarditis. No friction rub can be heard and the electrocardiogram is normal. A paracardiac mass may be visible in the chest X-ray.

the pain may begin in the back. The resemblance to myocardial infarction is close and, indeed, if the dissection involves a coronary artery, infarction may, in fact, occur and confuse the diagnostic

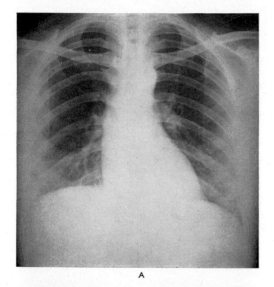

A

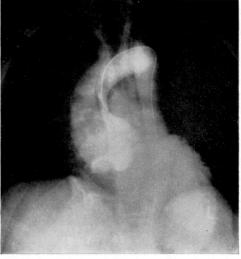

B

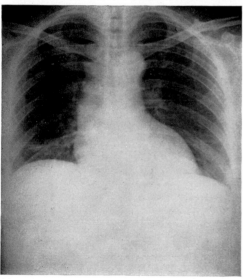

C

Fig. 149. Dissecting aneurysm of the aorta. Male, aged 39, admitted with severe central chest pain. **A,** As late as 6 weeks after admission a chest X-ray showed very little cardiac enlargement or widening of the mediastinum. **B,** Aortography, however, showed dissection of the ascending aorta and gross aortic incompetence. **C,** A month later the mediastinal shadow was a good deal wider and the heart was considerably enlarged. The patient was in left ventricular failure and died following surgical repair.

Dissecting aneurysm causes very severe anterior chest pain radiating to the neck, back, and, later, to the abdomen; it rarely spreads to the arms. With dissection of the descending thoracic aorta

issue further. Important differentiating features include the absence of one or more peripheral pulses, particularly if a pulse disappears while the patient is under observation, or other evidence of arterial occlusion such as hemiparesis, blindness in one eye, or haematuria. The development of aortic incompetence, due to involvement of the aortic valve ring by the dissection, is a valuable diagnostic feature. Also the blood-pressure is little changed compared with the fall commonly seen in myocardial infarction. The severity of the pain is of some diagnostic significance; chest pain which is hardly influenced by morphine or diamorphine may well be due to a dissecting aneurysm. The electrocardiogram is normal unless a coronary artery is involved or pre-existing hypertensive changes are present. Much reliance is placed on radiography in diagnosis: gross dilatation of the thoracic aorta may be seen but this is not always easy to distinguish from unfolding unless a previous film is available. Also the dilatation may not be very marked in the early stages. In practice, a firm diagnosis is rarely possible from the plain X-ray; the definitive diagnosis can only be made by aortography and even this can be misleading at times (*Fig.* 149).

Another important cause of sudden anterior chest pain is massive *pulmonary embolism.* Smaller pulmonary emboli cause pulmonary infarction which is discussed below among the causes of lateral, pleuritic chest pain. Pulmonary embolism occurs commonly in the post-operative period or during a period of enforced recumbency associated with a low cardiac output, as after myocardial infarction or in cardiac failure; in young women oral contraceptive agents have been incriminated as the cause of the initiating venous thrombosis. The same complication may, of course, occur in pregnancy. The source of the embolism is commonly thrombosis in veins of the leg or pelvis but this may not have been clinically manifest except, perhaps, as a small 'spike' of temperature. The patient rapidly becomes severely ill with central chest pain, nearly identical to that of myocardial infarction, breathlessness, and, often, faintness or even loss of consciousness. Peripheral cyanosis is present, the pulse is rapid, and the blood-pressure very low. Elevation of the jugular venous pressure is nearly always present; it is usually a good deal higher than in myocardial infarction causing a comparable degree of hypotension. Gallop rhythm may be heard over the right ventricle. The chest X-ray may show dilatation of one or both main branches of the pulmonary artery, and one lung, or part thereof, may appear unusually translucent. Pulmonary angiography, which is less hazardous than might have been expected in this situation, may show the occlusion of the pulmonary artery clearly (*Fig.* 150). In the electrocardiogram the appearances may simulate those of antero-inferior infarction with a Q wave and inverted T in Lead III and T inversion in Leads VI–4; right axis deviation, with a prominent S wave in Lead II, and clockwise rotation, causing an RS pattern from V1 to V5, are other common features.

Chronic *pulmonary hypertension*, as in mitral stenosis or the Eisenmenger syndrome, can produce a pain indistinguishable from angina. The cause, indeed, is almost certainly myocardial ischaemia as a result of the severely limited cardiac output. Severe *pulmonary stenosis* can cause a similar pain.

The anterior chest pain associated with *prolapse of a mitral valve cusp* is not ischaemic in origin. This lesion, which is not very rare, is often associated with a mid-systolic click and late systolic murmur. The diagnosis can be confirmed by echocardiography or angiocardiography. The pain is very variable in site, duration, and severity and has no clear-cut diagnostic features.

Pain arising from the oesophagus is felt in the midline of the chest with radiation to the jaw, back, shoulders, and, to a small extent, down the inner sides of the arms. The resemblance to angina is close and oesophageal pain may even have some relationship to exertion although this is never constant. The pain may be due to *oesophageal spasm* without any other lesion, it may occur early in the evolution of *achalasia of the cardia* or it may be due to *hiatus hernia* with oesophageal reflux and oesophagitis. Heartburn, with radiation of sternal pain upwards from the xiphoid, is very characteristic of the last. Helpful diagnostic features include the association of the pain with taking food and relief from belching; the pain of oesophageal reflux is commonly worse in the recumbent position or in other postures favouring regurgitation, such as bending forward or the cramped position of the driver of a small car, especially if wearing a tight safety belt. If the pain can be reproduced by the instillation of 0·1 N hydrochloric acid into the lower oesophagus, this is good evidence that it is due to reflux. The demonstration of a hiatus hernia by a barium swallow is only too easy. Most hiatus hernias produce no symptoms at all and chest pain in a patient in whom such a lesion has been demonstrated is as likely to be due to myocardial ischaemia or other conditions as to the

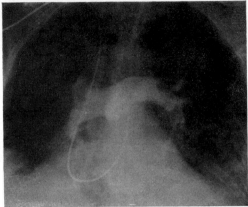

Fig. 150. Pulmonary angiogram showing occlusion of all the branches of the right pulmonary artery by emboli. Emboli are also visible lying free in the left pulmonary artery. (*Film by courtesy of Dr. Basil Strickland.*)

hernia. There is no substitute for a detailed analysis of the symptoms.

Other upper abdominal lesions can cause pain felt in the midline of the front of the chest. The frequency with which angina is regarded as 'indigestion' even by experienced physicians suffering from this condition bears witness to this. Catastrophes such as perforated peptic ulcer and acute pancreatitis must be remembered in the differential diagnosis of myocardial infarction. Gastric distension due to aerophagy or other causes can cause substernal discomfort, but peptic ulcer and chronic relapsing pancreatitis are less common causes of confusion; in the former, the relationship of the pain to meals is obviously important. Finally, there is the, almost mystical, association of gall-bladder disease with ischaemic heart disease. Both conditions are common and can certainly coexist. Much debate has centred around whether this coexistence occurs more commonly than would have been expected by chance; many experienced clinicians have a strong impression that this is so but none of the theories to account for it is very convincing. Suffice it to say that gall-bladder pain can certainly radiate into the front of the chest and simulate angina; also, central chest pain with a constant relationship to exertion must be regarded as angina even if gall-bladder disease is present in addition.

There are numerous musculo-skeletal causes of anterior chest pain. Local *trauma* is usually obvious but recurrent mild trauma, for example in some particular occupation, may not be mentioned by the patient as a possible cause for his pain. The pain may be a dull ache on one or other side of the chest, rarely exactly in the midline, or it may be possible to relate it to particular movements if anterior thoracic muscles are the site of origin. Pain from *spondylosis* or spondylitis of the thoracic, or even the cervical, spine can be referred to the front of the chest. The distribution can occasionally simulate that of angina and radiological proof of the spondylosis is of little diagnostic significance. Relief of the pain from wearing a cervical collar is, however, good evidence of a skeletal origin. Less obvious spinal disease may also be a cause of pain felt diffusely over the precordium or in the corresponding area on the right. Experimentally, the injection of hypertonic saline into an interspinous ligament produces pain referred to the anterior part of the corresponding dermatome with some radiation upwards and downwards. It is difficult to prove this aetiology in any particular patient but it has been suggested that chronic mild trauma to interspinous ligaments, for example due to scoliosis, may be a cause of otherwise unexplained precordial pain.

Less common musculo-skeletal lesions include *Tietze's disease*. This causes pain of sudden or gradual onset in one or more upper costal cartilages. The pain is worse on coughing or deep breathing and the affected cartilage is swollen and tender. *Xiphoidalgia* is a similar condition involving the xiphisternum which is possibly a variant of Tietze's disease or, more likely, due to recurrent mild trauma (*see* Xiphoid syndrome, p. 469). Ankylosing spondylitis can cause a diffuse pain in the anterior chest wall often associated with local tenderness over the sternum and costal cartilages. Pain arising in the sternum itself may be due to *myelomatosis, metastases, ankylosing spondylitis, osteomyelitis*, or *fracture*; it is of interest to note that too-vigorous aspiration of the sternal marrow during diagnostic puncture can produce a poorly localized pain felt widely across the anterior part of the chest. The sudden, sharp pain at, or near, the cardiac apex, known as *precordial catch*, is probably quite common although rare as a spontaneous complaint. There is rarely any diagnostic confusion with other causes of chest pain as the history is quite characteristic. The pain occurs most often when the subject is seated and lasts for a few minutes only. It can be relieved by a single, painful, deep inspiration.

Respiratory disease most often causes pain, if at all, in one or other side of the chest, but *tracheitis* should be mentioned as a cause of upper sternal pain. It is aggravated by the hyperventilation of exercise and may thus, very occasionally, have to be distinguished from angina. *Mycoplasma pneumonia*, unlike other varieties of pneumonia, is never associated with pleurisy but may cause a substernal pain aggravated by coughing. *Dyspnoea* itself, especially if it is associated with obstruction of airways, may be

described as 'tightness in the chest' and an injudicious series of leading questions may persuade the patient that he has a 'tight pain' across his chest and lead to an erroneous diagnosis of angina.

Two psychological conditions are important in the differential diagnosis of anterior chest pain. The terrifying panic of an attack of *acute anxiety* can be confused with a myocardial infarction or other intrathoracic vascular catastrophe. The patient, very often a woman, complains of dizziness, palpitations, dyspnoea, and precordial oppression or pain. Angor animi—the fear of impending death—is a prominent feature, much more so than in genuine myocardial ischaemia, and further exacerbates the anxiety. The circumstances in which the attack occurs and the complete absence of objective evidence of organic disease are important distinguishing features, and doubt about the nature of the condition should rarely persist for long. Chronic anxiety is the commonest underlying disorder in *Da Costa's syndrome*; the non-committal eponymous title is preferred to the numerous other terms, such as 'effort syndrome', 'cardiac neurosis', and 'disordered action of the heart', which have been used—with no great semantic accuracy—to describe this condition. Apart from the pain, the features of the syndrome are dyspnoea, palpitations, fatigue, and dizziness. The pain is most commonly felt in the left submammary region although it may be nearer the midline or, indeed, anywhere on the left side of the chest, even radiating into the left arm. In character it is sharp and stabbing, with occasional momentary twinges superimposed on a dull ache which persists for many hours at a time. It often occurs *after*, rarely during, exertion; this important point may be elicited only after careful questioning. In summary, it differs from angina in almost all respects except in the rare, difficult case in which it has a more constricting quality and is felt near the left border of the sternum. The mechanism of the pain is unknown but it seems likely that, in some cases at least, the original cause was a minor musculo-skeletal abnormality. The pain convinces the patient that his heart is diseased and is perpetuated by the anxiety engendered by this conviction.

Lateral Chest Pain. Almost all the tissues of the lateral chest wall, the pleura, muscles, ribs, and intercostal nerves, can be the site of painful lesions. Frequently the pain is closely related to respiration as exemplified most clearly in *pleurisy*. The visceral pleura is insensitive but the parietal pleura is plentifully supplied with pain fibres from the intercostal nerves. The pain is felt, therefore, in the cutaneous areas supplied by these nerves which, it is important to remember, include a large area of the anterior abdominal wall. Apart from inflammation of the pleura itself, there is some evidence that spasm of the intercostal muscles may be a factor in producing the pain. The pain is characteristically sharp, superficial, of any degree of severity, and is aggravated by deep breathing and by coughing. Inspiration is abruptly halted by the pain so that respiration is often very shallow. Holding the breath in expiration will usually relieve the pain completely and a change in the patient's posture in bed can produce considerable relief or exacerbation. The only physical sign of pleurisy, in the absence of effusion, is the pleural friction rub, a characteristic creaking sound present during inspiration and expiration. The sound is difficult

diagnosis would be supported by finding periorbital or generalized oedema and by eosinophilia in the peripheral blood. Pain arising from the capsule of the spleen is also related to respiration; it is commonly due to *splenic infarction* and may be accompanied by a friction rub so that the resemblance to pleurisy is very close. Splenic pain is not uncommon in Hodgkin's disease and in other reticuloses.

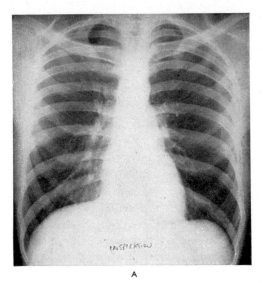

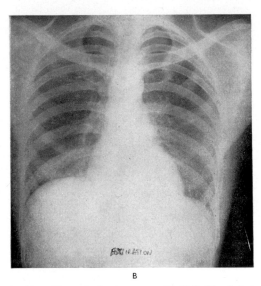

A   B

Fig. 151. Spontaneous pneumothorax. Male, aged 27, admitted with sudden pain in the upper part of left side of chest. A, In a film taken in inspiration the edge of the left lung is only just visible between the posterior parts of the fourth and fifth ribs. B, It is more clearly visible in an expiratory film, just below the posterior part of the fifth rib.

to describe but easy to recognize with a little experience although a coarse rhonchus may sometimes be mistaken for a rub. The pain is not at all closely related to the rub as one may be present without the other; neither alone is essential for the diagnosis of pleurisy. The pain of diaphragmatic pleurisy is typically referred to the shoulder; this is a common feature of pleurisy due to subdiaphragmatic lesions such as liver abscess or subphrenic abscess.

Pleurisy may be due to pulmonary infections such as lobar pneumonia or tuberculosis, to vascular lesions such as pulmonary infarction, or to connective-tissue disorders such as systemic lupus erythematosus. In many of these conditions, the clinical picture is modified by the development of an effusion which usually results in the disappearance of the pain and the rub.

A pain identical to that of pleurisy is felt in epidemic pleurodynia or *Bornholm disease*, due to Group B Coxsackie viruses. The pain is the presenting symptom and may be extremely severe; fever quickly develops and headache and malaise are common. Recovery is usually rapid but relapses are frequent and may continue for several weeks. *Trichinosis*, involving the intercostal muscles, can also produce pleuritic pain; the

The pain of *spontaneous pneumothorax* is usually abrupt in onset and pleuritic in type. Some patients, however, complain only of a dull ache or a sense of tightness and a few have no pain at all. The typical physical signs are a diminution in movement and in breath-sounds on the affected side, often with a hyper-resonant percussion note and, especially if the pneumothorax is under tension, deviation of the trachea towards the normal side. Dissection of the air into the mediastinum may cause central chest pain and the patient may notice a 'crunching' sound over the heart which is also audible on auscultation. The diagnosis of spontaneous pneumothorax can be confirmed by radiography but careful study may be needed if the pneumothorax is shallow; a film taken in expiration will show the lesion more clearly (*Fig.* 151).

Involvement of the intercostal nerves in many pathological processes can cause pain in the corresponding areas of the chest wall. *Spinal disease* has already been mentioned as a cause of referred pain in the anterolateral regions of the chest. Direct pressure on nerves may occur in fracture of the thoracic spine, from malignant metastases in that region, or in tuberculosis of the spine. Spondylosis with disk protrusion is not common as a cause of nerve-root compression in the thoracic spine. Neurofibromatosis may affect the thoracic nerve roots but does not often cause pain.

Aortic aneurysm is not a common lesion although, in former years, it was an important cause of chest pain. Aneurysm of the ascending aorta may cause chest pain by eroding the sternum but much more often causes no symptoms

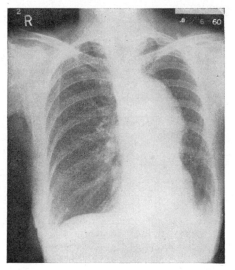

Fig. 152. Aortic aneurysm. Female, aged 67, complaining of pain in the left side of the chest. Autopsy confirmed a huge aneurysm involving the arch and most of the descending aorta. (*Film by courtesy of Dr. Basil Strickland.*)

at all. Aneurysm of the arch and descending thoracic aorta can cause very severe radiating pain by vertebral erosion and pressure on nerve-roots (*Fig.* 152). Other symptoms and signs result from pressure on mediastinal structures. Thus, pressure on the left recurrent laryngeal nerve will cause paralysis of the left vocal cord, cough and stridor may follow pressure on the trachea, and dysphagia results from pressure on the oesophagus. Pressure on the left main bronchus may cause collapse of the left lung with subsequent infection; a tracheal tug is a well-known physical sign of aneurysm depressing the left main bronchus.

Primary or secondary intrathoracic *malignant disease* may cause pain in various ways. Direct invasion of the pleura by a bronchial carcinoma can cause pleurisy, often with effusion; more often pleural pain occurs as a result of infection in the lung distal to a blocked bronchus. Primary tumours of the pleura, such as mesothelioma, cause pleuritic pain directly. Apart from the pleura, the ribs and intercostal nerves may be involved by tumour with the production of severe pain. Metastases in the thoracic spine have been mentioned as a cause of intercostal pain; secondary deposits in the ribs can also be extremely painful. Rarely, tumours in the mediastinum can apparently cause a poorly localized

central chest pain without other pressure symptoms; the mechanism is not known.

P. R. Fleming.

CHEST, PUS IN

When paracentesis of the chest produces pus, the most probable cause is pleural empyema. Other causes are possible, however, and even when the diagnosis of pleural empyema has been established, its cause should be sought. The problem is best considered in two sections: the diagnosis of the presence of a pleural empyema, and the diagnosis of its cause. The latter will be discussed first.

Empyema of the Pleura is invariably secondary to some antecedent inflammatory lesion in the organs and tissues adjacent to the pleura; but it may happen that the antecedent condition has so far progressed towards healing as to be insignificant by the time the empyema is diagnosed. The most frequent antecedents of pleural empyema are:

1. BACTERIAL PNEUMONIAS. Of these the most frequent is the pneumococcal, but pneumonias due to staphylococci, haemolytic streptococci, Friedländer's bacilli, and mixed organisms are also often followed by empyemata. In the absence of bacterial superinfection, pneumonias due to *Mycoplasma pneumoniae* (Eaton's agent), organisms of the psittacosis-ornithosis group, and viruses are not followed by empyema. The pneumonias associated with influenza, however, are usually of mixed virus and bacterial origin, and the bacterial element in the infection is as liable to give rise to empyema in these cases as in pure bacterial pneumonias. If the patient has been under treatment from the beginning of his pneumonia, the points which suggest the development of empyema are failure to respond to adequate treatment by antibacterial drugs to which the infecting organism is known to be sensitive, or a secondary rise of temperature after a satisfactory response to such treatment; a high leucocyte count; the persistence of physical signs, and especially the development of a more or less extensive area of stony dullness, usually over the base of the affected lung; and apparently delayed resolution. In cases showing any of these features, careful examination of the chest to ascertain the area of maximal dullness, followed by paracentesis in this region, is required. Radiography should be carried out in the lateral as well as postero-anterior views to help in the localization of the empyema. Careful physical examination may be as useful as radiography in localization, especially if persistent consolidation is still present in the underlying lung to obscure the radiographic picture. A point in physical examination which is of especial importance is that if the underlying lung is still consolidated or if the empyema is so large that the lung is firmly collapsed under it, bronchial breath-sounds may be heard over the

empyema. This is of especial importance in children. A common error in paracentesis is to choose a site too low on the chest wall. A site just below the upper limit of the area of stony dullness should be chosen, since in empyema the diaphragm is often raised, and the insertion of a needle into the costophrenic angle is apt to give rise to difficulties, both from the shallowness of the pleural space in this region and from the fact that fibrinous debris tends to collect in this lowest part of the pleural space and may lead to a misleading dry tap from blockage of the needle.

2. PULMONARY SUPPURATION. This can be considered as an extension of (1), since the various forms of lung abscess can be regarded as suppurative pneumonias of various grades of severity. The organisms causing these suppurative pneumonias are generally mixed and often include anaerobes. Hence the empyemata associated with them usually contain a mixture of organisms, some of which may be anaerobic. If the presence of a lung abscess or infected bronchiectasis has been already recognized, the diagnosis of a complicating empyema should not be difficult, and is based upon the same principles as those underlying the diagnosis of post-pneumonic empyema. The possibility that underlying bronchopulmonary suppuration may be related to an unsuspected bronchial foreign body should not be forgotten. If, without a previous history of pulmonary suppuration, malodorous pus is found in the pleura, it is probable that the condition is secondary to a previously undiagnosed lung abscess, even though this may have been very small and have resolved by the time treatment of the empyema is completed. Malodorous pus which is sterile on aerobic culture is almost diagnostic of empyema secondary to pulmonary suppuration; even with appropriate cultural methods the anaerobic organisms may be difficult to grow. Empyema secondary to lung abscess may be complicated from the beginning by a pleurobronchial fistula, the abscess cavity in the lung being in communication with the pleural empyema. In such cases a pyopneumothorax results, the patient coughs up pus both from the abscess and from the empyema, expectoration is postural, on physical examination the area of dullness has a horizontal upper border which moves on changes of the patient's posture, and radiography will show a fluid level.

3. TUBERCULOUS EMPYEMA can be considered as a special variety of bacterial empyema. It is nearly always secondary to active pulmonary tuberculosis. It used to be a frequent complication of artificial pneumothorax treatment. The most frequent cause of tuberculous empyema is now spontaneous pneumothorax occurring in the course of active pulmonary tuberculosis. Very rarely an apparently primary tuberculous serous pleural effusion progresses gradually to become an empyema. Tuberculous empyema should be suspected when odourless pus which is sterile on ordinary bacterial culture is found in the chest.

In these circumstances evidence of tuberculous infection should be sought both by a search for tubercle bacilli in the pus by direct examination and by culture on special media or guinea-pig inoculation, and by investigation of the lungs for evidence of tuberculosis both radiologically and by examination of sputum or gastric contents for tubercle bacilli. The diagnosis of tuberculous empyema is of special importance, not only because it leads to specific antimycobacterial chemotherapy, but because surgical drainage is contra-indicated in the absence of secondary pyogenic bacterial infection.

4. SECONDARY TO NEW GROWTHS, ESPECIALLY BRONCHIAL CARCINOMA. Bronchial carcinoma often causes its first symptoms by giving rise to inflammatory changes in the lung beyond an obstructed bronchus. The pneumonia so caused may be due to various types of bacteria, and like other pneumonias is liable to be complicated by empyemata. Hence in empyemata of obscure origin, especially in men of middle age or older, and in those who are heavy smokers, the possibility of an underlying bronchial carcinoma should be considered. The empyema may be of any type bacteriologically. The diagnosis in such cases depends upon careful consideration of the history, the radiographic findings, and above all upon bronchoscopy, which is required in any case in which there is serious suspicion of an underlying carcinoma. In younger persons it occasionally happens that a bronchial adenoma similarly underlies an empyema.

5. INFECTED HAEMOTHORAX. Traumatic haemothorax may be due to either penetrating or non-penetrating injuries of the chest. Depending upon the type of injury, a variable number of such cases becomes infected and develops into empyemata.

6. 'MISSED EMPYEMA.' In this small but important group of empyemata, the empyema is not diagnosed in the acute stage, either because the patient fails to seek advice, or because the condition is treated as a pneumonia, and the presence of a small empyema is not diagnosed. In such cases a pleurobronchial fistula usually develops, and the patient coughs up the pus. This gives rise to symptoms suggestive of bronchiectasis, especially as expectoration will tend to be postural, and the pus may be offensive. Diagnosis of these cases depends upon radiography, which will usually show in the erect plane a fluid level (*Figs.* 153, 154). Sometimes, however, there is no fluid level, and all that is found is an area of apparent pleural thickening. In such cases, if the history suggests the possibility of a missed empyema, paracentesis over the area of pleural thickening after careful radiographic localization is required. If a fluid level is found it is best to direct the exploring needle at the fluid level; this should ensure the obtaining of a sample of pus, which is the object of the procedure rather than complete aspiration.

In other instances in which the diagnosis of empyema is delayed, the pus may point through the chest wall, giving rise to fluctuating inflammatory swelling, which is sometimes reducible into the chest. This is called an *empyema necessitatis*.

7. SECONDARY TO SEPTIC INFARCTION OF THE LUNGS. Rarely the lungs are the site of septic emboli from such lesions as suppurative thrombophlebitis of cerebral venous sinuses (as may occur

involvement of intrathoracic organs or of the liver may be obtained; the organism is found in the pus either by examination of direct smears or by appropriate cultural methods; and the chest wall may become involved in a characteristic brawny induration, in which multiple sinuses discharging typical sulphur-granule pus sometimes develop.

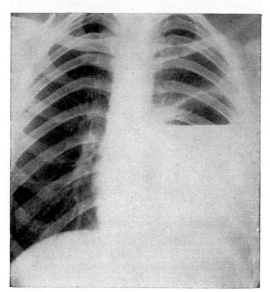

Fig. 153. Radiograph of chest of a patient with a pleural empyema with pleurobronchial fistula. Note the horizontal fluid level.

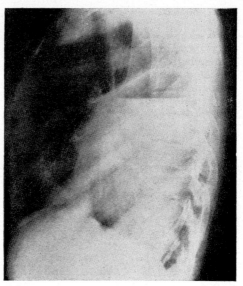

Fig. 154. The same, left lateral view.

in acute mastoiditis or cavernous sinus thrombosis) or from pelvic veins (for instance, in puerperal infections), or from staphylococcal and other pyaemias. In such cases empyema, which may be bilateral, may develop.

8. SECONDARY TO SUBPHRENIC INFLAMMATORY CONDITIONS. The commonest of these is subphrenic abscess. The most frequent pleural complication of subphrenic suppuration is a serous effusion, but sometimes this progresses to empyema. In any patient who has recently had an operation for an acute abdominal emergency and in whom an empyema develops, especially at the right base, the possibility of its being secondary to subphrenic abscess should be considered. Other rarer subphrenic causes of empyema are hepatic abscess, either pyogenic and secondary to an abdominal focus of suppuration, usually appendicular, or more rarely secondarily infected amoebic abscess or hydatid cyst.

9. SECONDARY TO INFECTIONS OF THE CHEST WALL. This is a very rare cause which must be distinguished from empyema necessitatis, in which a neglected empyema points through the chest wall.

10. ACTINOMYCOTIC. Pulmonary, mediastinal, or hepatic actinomycosis sometimes first declares itself in the form of an empyema. Evidence of

The chief conditions with which pleural empyema may be confused are:

1. LUNG ABSCESS (*Fig.* 155). In most instances this should give rise to no difficulty in diagnosis since the history and clinical and radiographic findings should be unmistakable; and it is important to arrive at the diagnosis before attempting paracentesis, since attempts at needling lung abscesses are apt to be followed by contamination of the pleura and the development of empyema. As noted above, lung abscess may be complicated by pleural empyema, and the possibility of the coincidence of the two conditions should be borne in mind.

A 'missed empyema' (p. 144) may simulate a lung abscess, both symptomatically and on physical examination; but careful radiography should serve to reveal that the pus is located in the pleura.

2. INFECTED LUNG CYST. An infected lung cyst may simulate empyema. This is especially important in the case of the large solitary cysts which sometimes become infected and distended with pus and simulate pleural empyema so closely that the diagnosis is only made when on rib resection and drainage the space is found to be within the lung and not in the pleura.

More rarely a large infected hydatid cyst of the lung may simulate a pleural empyema, but there may be a history of coughing up the watery contents of the hydatid, together with anaphylactic symptoms at the same time, and the Casoni or complement-fixation tests may be helpful.

3. SUBPHRENIC ABSCESS. This may be misdiagnosed as pleural empyema, since the diaphragm is usually raised on the affected side and there is often a small effusion in the pleura. The physical

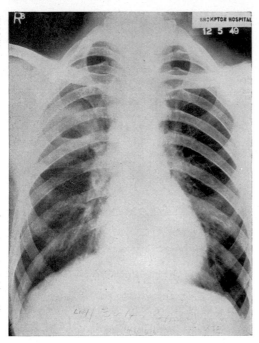

Fig. 155. Radiograph of chest, showing an abscess cavity with small fluid level in the right upper lobe. Lateral radiography showed the abscess to be lying in the posterior segment of the lobe.

signs may be entirely compatible with the presence of an empyema, and needling, especially if it is carried out rather low, may produce pus. Consideration of the history and a careful examination of the abdomen should lead to a correct diagnosis in such cases.

Other conditions characterized by pus within the thorax, but unlikely to be confused with pleural empyema, include *paravertebral abscess*, most commonly tuberculous or staphylococcal, arising from upper or middle thoracic vertebrae; *suppurative pericarditis*; and *mediastinal abscess*, in many instances secondary to instrumental perforation of the oesophagus.

J. G. Scadding.

CHEST, SEROUS EFFUSION IN

The diagnosis of a serous effusion in the chest may be divided into two parts: first, the diagnosis of the presence of a serous effusion in the chest; and, secondly, the diagnosis of the cause of the effusion.

Pleural effusions in general may be confused with *pneumonias* of various sorts, with *lobar atelectasis*, with conditions giving rise to *elevation of the diaphragm*, with *diaphragmatic hernia*, and with large *intrathoracic tumours*.

The symptoms of *pneumonias* may in some instances simulate those of a pleural effusion, but expectoration does not occur in pleural effusion unless there is a complicating broncho-pulmonary infection, and physical examination should serve to differentiate intrapulmonary processes from pleural effusion. However, some pneumonias, notably some of those associated with influenza, are associated with extreme dullness and weakness or absence of breath-sounds rather than the usual tubular or bronchial breath-sounds, and these signs may sometimes erroneously suggest pleural effusion. In such cases consideration of the shape of the area of dullness will usually lead to a correct diagnosis; in pneumonia the dullness generally corresponds with the surface marking of a lobe or lobes, whereas pleural effusions in a free pleura give rise to an area of dullness at the base with a characteristic curved upper border having its highest point in the axilla and a smaller rise at the back towards the spine. Conversely pleural effusions may occasionally be erroneously diagnosed as pneumonias, since, especially in children, bronchial breath-sounds instead of the usual absent breath-sounds may be found over a large pleural effusion which has caused complete collapse of the lung; in such cases the stony dullness and the displacement of the heart towards the opposite side should lead to a correct diagnosis. *Atelectasis of the lung* should be distinguished from pleural effusion by the characteristic displacement of the apex beat towards the affected side, as well as by the history and the symptoms. Occasionally a very *full stomach* without an associated gas bubble may so elevate the left dome of the diaphragm as to give rise to signs erroneously interpreted as pleural effusion on the left side; in left-sided pleural effusion percussion below the level of the effusion in front will generally reveal the normal gastric resonance. Occasionally abdominal distension due to other causes, such as extreme ascites or large abdominal tumours, may give rise to physical signs erroneously interpreted as those of pleural effusion at one or both bases, but knowledge of the possibility of this error will generally lead to its avoidance. *Solid intrathoracic tumours* may rarely occupy the entire cross-section of the thorax, and thus give rise to physical signs suggestive of pleural effusion (*Fig.* 156). Large liquid-containing cysts, notably *hydatids*, in the lung may produce similar signs. The history will generally cast doubt upon a diagnosis of pleurisy with effusion, and usually radiography will lead to a correct diagnosis. Large *diaphragmatic hernias* containing solid viscera or hollow viscera which at the time of examination are filled with liquid contents may similarly give rise to diagnostic difficulty. Radiography (*Fig.* 157) generally provides useful evidence. If it excludes conditions which contra-indicate needling, and there is still doubt about the diagnosis, a paracentesis, best performed over the dullest area, is the best diagnostic procedure.

The presence of an effusion having been established, the next question to be considered is its

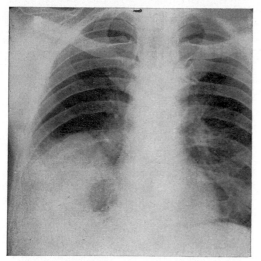

Fig. 156. Radiograph of chest showing a large solid tumour at the right base. This was due to a carcinoma of the bronchus. The physical signs to which it gave rise could well be confused with those of a small right pleural effusion.

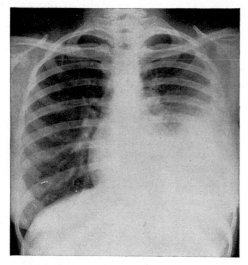

Fig. 157. Radiograph of the chest showing a moderate-sized left pleural effusion. Note the shape of the upper border of the shadow of the effusion, extending up towards the apex of the lung along the lateral wall of the thorax.

aetiology. Pleural effusions are customarily divided into *transudates* and *exudates*. Transudates are those effusions which are caused not by inflammatory changes in the pleura, but by cardiac or renal disease or other conditions such as deficiency diseases in which there is general anasarca. Exudates are due to inflammatory

changes in the pleura itself. The differentiation is usually not difficult since with pleural transudates there is usually obvious evidence of the primary disease and the transudate often appears as part of a generalized oedema. However, in certain cases of cardiac disease a pleural transudate or hydrothorax may occur in the absence of gross evidence of oedema elsewhere. In these instances examination of the pleural fluid is helpful. Exudates from active inflammatory or neoplastic processes clot on standing, and have a specific gravity usually above 1·018 and a protein content higher than 3 per cent and often up to 5 per cent; whereas transudates do not clot on standing, and have a specific gravity below 1·015 and a protein content varying from 0·5 per cent to 1·5 per cent. Sometimes the picture of a pleural transudate is complicated by secondary inflammatory changes, as in heart disease where there has been pulmonary infarction, and hence intermediate figures for specific gravity and protein content may be found.

Pleural transudates occur in:

1. *Heart disease*, especially with congestive failure.

2. *Renal disease* with oedema; sometimes in an acute glomerulonephritis, more commonly in the nephrotic syndrome.

3. *Malnutrition*, including hunger oedema, beri-beri (vitamin-B_1 deficiency), the cachexia of the terminal stages of wasting diseases.

4. *Severe anaemia* from any cause.

Pleural exudates may be due to a great variety of causes:

1. TUBERCULOSIS. Although tuberculosis is a much less frequent cause of pleural effusion in Great Britain than formerly, it remains the most frequent cause in countries with an uncontrolled tuberculosis problem, and should be regarded as a possible cause in all apparently primary pleural effusions wherever they occur. A tuberculous origin for such an effusion is suggested by the absence of symptoms suggestive of an antecedent acute respiratory infection, by a history of recent close contact with open tuberculosis, and by the absence of clinical or radiological signs of a pneumonia or other gross lesion in the lungs. Characteristically the effusion is persistently lymphocytic; but in the earliest stages a tuberculous effusion may show 20 per cent or 30 per cent of polymorphs, and conversely a postpneumonic effusion or one secondary to a neoplasm of the lung will quite often be found on a single or even on several examinations to contain a preponderance of lymphocytes. Proof of the tuberculous nature of an effusion may be obtained by the finding of tubercle bacilli in the effusion; as a general rule the more carefully the examination for bacilli is made the more often will they be found, and culture or guinea-pig inoculation is usually necessary. Failure to find tubercle bacilli should not be taken to contradict a diagnosis of tuberculous pleural effusion which seems to be well established on general clinical grounds. Although the Mantoux test is generally positive, in

a few cases subsequently proved to be tuberculous it has been negative during the early acute stage, becoming positive later. Typical histological changes may be found in the fragment of pleura obtained with one of the special pleural biopsy needles, but the absence of such changes does not exclude the diagnosis of tuberculosis. Formal surgical biopsy of the pleura is justified in cases where no satisfactory evidence has been obtained by other means, and sometimes establishes the diagnosis of tuberculosis when needle-biopsy has failed. Only occasionally will radiological evidence of active tuberculosis in the lungs be found in association with a tuberculous pleural effusion. It is important to remember that a high proportion of cases of pleural effusion, perhaps as many as half, have a relatively insidious onset, and the patient may be still ambulant at the time of diagnosis.

2. SECONDARY TO PNEUMONIAS. Pneumonias due to any cause may be complicated by pleural effusions, but the virus pneumonias are less liable to this complication than bacterial pneumonias. This gives rise to a double diagnostic difficulty; on the one hand a tendency for any febrile illness accompanied by abnormal signs in the chest to be diagnosed and treated as a pneumonia has led to cases of primary tuberculous pleural effusion being misdiagnosed as postpneumonic, while on the other hand the development of serous pleural effusion after a pneumonia tends to give rise to suspicion of underlying tuberculosis. Postpneumonic effusions may occur at any age. The history of the preceding pneumonia may be obvious, and residual signs of it either on physical examination or on radiography can usually be found. The cytology of the effusion may be of very little help on a single examination, since it may show a preponderance of lymphocytes. However, if the effusion persists, a mounting proportion of polymorphonuclear neutrophils suggests a postpneumonic origin; in addition it may occasionally be possible to culture the causative organism of the pneumonia from the effusion, even if this is not purulent. Cultures for tubercle bacilli should of course be done, but the results of these will not be available for several weeks. Postpneumonic serous effusions are usually small and rarely exceed a moderate size.

3. MALIGNANT OR ASSOCIATED WITH MALIGNANT DISEASE (*Fig.* 158). Intrathoracic malignant disease may cause pleural effusions in two chief ways. The pleura may be directly invaded, usually by bronchial carcinoma, causing a true malignant pleurisy; or a bronchial carcinoma may cause bronchial obstruction with secondary pneumonic changes, which then give rise to a pleurisy of the sort described under (2). In this latter group, both the secondary pneumonia and the accompanying pleurisy may resolve with appropriate antibiotic and other treatment, and the effusion behaves generally in a similar manner to the ordinary postpneumonic effusion; it does not necessarily contra-indicate attempts at radical surgical treatment of the underlying carcinoma. The true

neoplastic effusions usually either are, or soon become, blood-stained; they are persistent and reaccumulate after aspiration. They may be due to primary bronchial carcinoma or to metastasis from tumours in other parts of the body. The differential diagnosis from tuberculous and postpneumonic effusions may be difficult. Although the occurrence of a pleural effusion in a middle-aged man inevitably gives rise to suspicion of

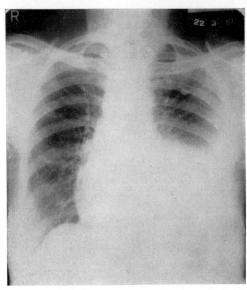

Fig. 158. Radiograph showing malignant pleural effusion shown by biopsy to be due to infiltration of the pleura with an adenocarcinoma. At necropsy, the primary was found to be a small non-obstructive tumour at the ampulla of Vater. Note that the radiographic appearances are indistinguishable from those of the effusion shown in *Fig.* 157, which was due to tuberculosis.

bronchial carcinoma, effusions both of the postpneumonic and of the tuberculous groups also occur at this age. Bronchoscopy may show a carcinoma in an accessible bronchus. If the pleura is directly invaded, malignant cells may be found in the effusion. Biopsy of the parietal pleura by one of the special needles may show infiltration by tumour cells. Thoracoscopy after air replacement of the effusion may show deposits of tumour in the visceral pleura, from which tissue may be removed for biopsy. A history of previous treatment for malignant tumour elsewhere will necessarily give rise to suspicion that a pleural effusion is due to intrathoracic metastasis.

4. PULMONARY INFARCTION. Pulmonary infarction occurs as the result of embolism in peripheral pulmonary arteries either in association with heart disease, or secondary to thrombophlebitis, generally of the veins of the leg or pelvis, often either postoperatively or during an illness leading to a prolonged stay in bed. The diagnosis is simple if there have been obvious symptoms of pulmonary infarction, such as a sudden pleuritic pain in the chest, haemoptysis, and slight fever,

and if there is evidence of the site from which the causative embolism has arisen; the chief possibilities to be considered are either a diseased heart, usually with atrial fibrillation, or a peripheral thrombophlebitis. Sometimes, however, pulmonary infarction may occur without acute symptoms and an effusion which may be blood-stained is the first evidence of it; and in cases secondary to thrombophlebitis, the original thrombophlebitis may have given rise to no special symptoms, and the diagnosis may be difficult.

In some cases, pain in the calf and oedema of the lower leg, as a result of peripheral venous thrombosis, become evident some days after symptoms and signs of pulmonary infarction, providing retrospective confirmation of the diagnosis.

5. SECONDARY TO SUBDIAPHRAGMATIC CONDITIONS. Inflammatory lesions under the diaphragm may give rise to pleural effusions which are generally small and rarely exceed a moderate size. The conditions most frequently causing such effusions are subdiaphragmatic abscess, which is usually secondary to appendicitis, to perforation of a peptic ulcer, to suppurative cholecystitis, or to any other cause of acute peritonitis; and hepatic abscess, which is most frequently amoebic in origin. Since all these conditions occur most frequently on the right side, the pleural changes associated with them are nearly always on the right side. A subdiaphragmatic condition more rarely causing pleural effusion is perinephric abscess. The diagnosis of these conditions depends upon careful consideration of the history and physical signs. An abdominal condition which may give rise to pleural effusion and which, though rare, is of some importance, is Meigs's syndrome, in which certain apparently non-malignant tumours of the ovary are associated with pleural effusions which recur after aspiration, but clear up after surgical removal of the ovarian tumour.

6. EOSINOPHILIC EFFUSIONS. Serous effusions complicating pneumonia, pulmonary infarction, and more rarely tuberculous effusions may as a transient phenomenon show a considerable proportion of eosinophil polymorphs. Persistently eosinophil-containing effusions may occur in association with eosinophilic infiltrations of the lungs, and in association with polyarteritis nodosa.

7. RHEUMATIC. Very occasionally acute rheumatism causes pleural effusion. This occurs only in very severe cases of acute rheumatism in which there either is or has been a recent acute arthritis, and the heart and usually the pericardium are severely involved. Only in such cases should the diagnosis of rheumatic pleurisy be considered.

8. RHEUMATOID ARTHRITIS. Serous effusions into the pleura occasionally appear during the acute phases of rheumatoid arthritis. In a few cases, changes in the pleura resembling histologically those of a rheumatoid nodule have been described. The effusion has been reported to contain a very low glucose content.

9. SYSTEMIC LUPUS ERYTHEMATOSUS. Pleural effusions may be one of the usually multiple clinical manifestations of systemic lupus erythematosus. Other serous effusions, notably pericardial, may coexist. Diagnosis is based upon consideration of the complex total clinical picture and upon such findings as leucopenia, L.E. cells, and positive tests for antinuclear factor.

10. Pleural effusion, usually on the left side, may complicate *acute pancreatitis*; characteristically it contains a very high level of amylase.

11. Pleural effusion is a possible feature of the *post-myocardial-infarction syndrome*, in which fever, pericarditis, and pleuropulmonary changes appear in the weeks following myocardial infarction. Diagnosis, especially from pulmonary infarction, may be difficult; response to corticosteroid treatment is usual.

12. There is a rare syndrome of *yellow nails, lymphoedema, and chronic or recurrent pleural effusion* (p. 560); this seems to be associated with a widespread abnormality of the lymphatic system.

13. POLYSEROSITIS is the name given to a group of cases in which several serous sacs—pleura, pericardium, peritoneum—are involved in an inflammatory process. Some of these are of tuberculous origin. Effusions into the peritoneum and into one or both pleurae may be seen in *constrictive pericarditis* and in *cirrhosis of the liver*.

J. G. Scadding.

CHEST, TENDERNESS IN

Pain that is felt when some part of the chest wall is pressed or even only touched will in some instances be a direct pain due to stimulation of sensory nerves actually in the diseased area; in others the pain is a referred pain (p. 151), due to a visceral lesion remote from the tender area. The causes of tenderness in the chest may be classified according to the situation or character of the responsible lesion.

1. LESIONS OF THE CHEST WALL:

Inflammation of the skin and underlying tissue including the breasts
Intercostal myositis
Myalgia
Affections of the ribs and sternum
Blood diseases
Intercostal neuritis and neuralgia
Injury of the intercostal nerves
Ankylosing spondylitis
Herpes zoster
Tietze's syndrome.

2. LESIONS OF THORACIC AND ABDOMINAL VISCERA:

Lungs
Heart and aorta
Diaphragm
Stomach and oesophagus
Liver.

1. Lesions of the Chest Wall. Tenderness is always present in *superficial inflammatory lesions* of the chest wall, such as bruises, burns, cuts, mastitis, and superficial infections the diagnosis of which will usually be evident on examination.

Pain will be the chief complaint in the so-called *intercostal myositis* that occurs after chill or strain of an intercostal muscle; the affected muscle will also be tender on pressure, the tenderness being in the deeper structures. The condition is also known as *intercostal myalgia* or *pleurodynia*.

previously established. Tenderness of the ribs and sternum occurs in certain *blood diseases* such as leukaemia. The tenderness is due to irritation of the sensory nerves of the periosteum or bone, although the pain felt on pressure is a direct pain. Diagnosis depends on examination of the blood. Tenderness over sternum and ribs also occurs as part of the clinical picture of ankylosing spondylitis.

In this disease the sternomanubrial and sternoclavicular joints may become acutely

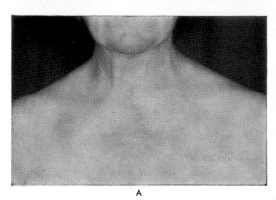 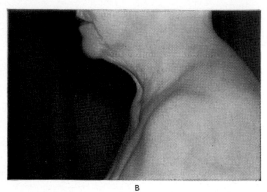

A   B

Fig. 159. Prominent and tender sternoclavicular joints in ankylosing spondylitis. The sternomanubrial joint (angle of Louis) may also be affected in this disease.

It is distinguished from pleurisy by the absence of friction-sounds on auscultation. Similar but more transient pain with a variable degree of tenderness is met with in the *stitch* to which some athletes are prone.

The acute pain of Bornholm disease, due to Coxsackie virus B infection, may be accompanied by hyperaesthesia of skin but less often by muscle tenderness. The myalgia of Phlebotomus (Sandfly) fever and dengue may also be accompanied by tenderness, often mild.

Tenderness of the *breasts* in the absence of mastitis is a common occurrence at the menstrual periods, and with high-dosage oestrogen therapy. Gynaecomastia in males (*see* p. 325), whatever the cause, is accompanied by tenderness of the breasts.

Tenderness in the chest may result from *disease* or *injury of a rib* or *the sternum* when it will be localized to the injured spot; fracture, inflammation, tuberculosis, or new growth may be the immediate cause. If *fracture* is present, X-rays may show the lesion or crepitus between the fragments on movement may be obtainable. *Sternal* or *costal osteitis* or *periostitis* may follow injury and may also occur in such diseases as enteric, tuberculosis, pyaemia. The local signs of inflammation (pain, redness, heat, swelling) will usually but not invariably be present. Tenderness in the chest due to *new growth* in a rib or in the sternum—such as multiple myelomatosis, sarcoma, secondary deposit from carcinoma— is generally a late occurrence, the existence of malignant disease elsewhere having usually been

swollen and tender, causing considerable discomfort (*Fig.* 159).

The particularly tender spots in the course of an *intercostal nerve* are three in number, corresponding to the points at which the posterior primary, the lateral cutaneous, and the anterior cutaneous branches are given off, that is to say near the spinal column, in the mid-axillary line, and at the sternal margin respectively. Such tenderness may be marked in so-called *intercostal neuritis*, which may be diagnosed when some more serious intrathoracic disorder such as pneumonia or pleurisy is present and in cases of pressure on an intercostal nerve, as for example by *abscess* about the spinal column, *aneurysm* of the descending aorta, or *new growth* invading the spinal canal. Local tenderness may more commonly result from external pressure by such a thing, for instance, as a fountain-pen carried in the waistcoat, the buckle of the braces, or some tool used at work, a simple detail but one not infrequently overlooked.

Pain and tenderness along an intercostal nerve are common in *herpes zoster* and may be present before, during, and after the appearance of the characteristic rash. Tenderness can often be elicited at the three spots mentioned above; it is particularly when it occurs in the second half of life that herpes may be followed by a long period of pain and tenderness along the course of the affected nerve. The rash, once seen, can hardly be mistaken; to expect its subsequent appearance on the ground of pain is a diagnostic *tour de force*.

Tietze's syndrome is an unexplained disorder where pain and swelling are found in the upper costochondral junctions of the anterior chest wall. Biopsies of costal cartilages show nothing characteristically abnormal. One or several costal cartilages may be affected. Spontaneous remission occurs in weeks, months, or, occasionally, years.

2. Lesions of the Underlying Viscera. Tenderness in the chest may sometimes be a symptom of disease in the thoracic or abdominal viscera. The tenderness is as a rule superficial, confined to the skin and subjacent areolar and fatty tissues. Tactile hyperaesthesia or the production of unpleasant sensations or pain by the lightest touch may occur in neuralgia and in neuroses or in cases of referred pain. A similar hyperaesthesia for cold or less often for heat sometimes occurs in the chest of tabetic patients. Hyperaesthesia for pain, or hyperalgesia, in which a normally painless stimulus or impression becomes transformed into an acutely painful sensation, is to be regarded as a form of 'tenderness' in the chest. This occurs in patients suffering from anxiety states, often with added depression. Further, perversions of sensation sometimes occur in organic nervous diseases, such as syringomyelia or tabes.

Tenderness of the chest may occur in *pleurisy.* The tenderness is as a rule deeply seated and not in the skin and loose subcutaneous tissues.

The sternum may be tender as the result of *mediastinal inflammation, tumour,* or *aneurysm.* The diagnosis in these cases is made by physical and X-ray examination.

Tenderness with pain over the precordia may occur in *pericarditis,* diagnosed by the pericarditic rub. It may be so severe as to preclude percussion or even the application of a stethoscope. Similar pain and tenderness have also been found at the epigastrium and the upper costal angles.

Chest tenderness is sometimes found in cases of *acute* or *chronic disease of the lungs,* particularly *tuberculosis.* The tenderness may be either superficial or deep. It is generally felt most about the region of the apices of the lungs, the curve of the shoulder, or the scapula. Similar tenderness is met with occasionally in *acute bronchitis,* or in *chronic bronchitis and emphysema.* Tenderness along the lower chest wall is a relatively common symptom in any sufferer from recurrent or excessive *cough* from any cause. Tenderness and pain may also occur between the ribs in the chest wall anteriorly after vigorous coughing, probably from trauma in the soft tissues, the muscles particularly. A rib may be fractured by vigorous coughing.

Direct tenderness about the precordia is rarely prominent in *heart disease.* It is more generally associated with cardiac neuroses than with organic heart disease. Tenderness at the area of the apex beat is common in the Da Costa syndrome ('soldier's heart' or neurocirculatory asthenia), a nervous condition in which there is no cardiac abnormality. The tenderness, which may be extreme, felt by some patients with heart disease such as mitral stenosis at the cardiac apex is of functional (anxiety) type rather than any organic lesion present.

Tenderness in the chest may result from diaphragmatic or basal pleurisy. The central portion of the diaphragm is innervated by the phrenic nerves, and so is connected with the third, fourth, and fifth cervical nerve-roots; accordingly, referred diaphragmatic pain and tenderness may also be felt at the top of the shoulder, an area innervated by the fourth cervical nerve.

Tenderness in the right side of the chest near the costal margin is not rare in *diseases of the liver* and *gall-bladder* corresponding to the cutaneous distribution of the seventh, eighth, and ninth dorsal nerves; for the most part, however, the pain and tenderness are in the epigastrium and the right hypochondrium. The right phrenic nerve (third to fifth cervical) sends twigs to the liver and gall-bladder, so that tenderness and pain may also be felt in the right shoulder as in the case of disorders of the diaphragm. It is particularly in cases of gall-stone or biliary colic that these areas of tenderness are likely to be found. In patients with hepatic abscess the spread of inflammation to the chest wall may give rise to direct pain and tenderness. In this condition the diagnosis will have to be made from the axillary abscess, empyema extending through the chest wall, and abscess arising in the chest wall itself. On the whole, with the exception of obviously superficial lesions of the chest wall, a complaint of tenderness is rarely advanced without that of pain, the causation of which must be the prime consideration. (*See* CHEST, PAIN IN, p. 133.)

F. Dudley Hart.

CHEST X-RAY ABNORMALITY IN 'SYMPTOMLESS' SUBJECTS

The use of chest radiography as a screening procedure, either in personal health examinations or in surveys of groups, leads to the discovery of abnormalities in some individuals who regard themselves as healthy. Some of these deny all symptoms on inquiry, others admit to minor symptoms which they have regarded as unimportant or even 'normal'. For brevity, both these groups will be described as 'symptomless'. Thus an abnormal chest X-ray may be the event that first leads a patient to seek medical advice. The following discussion concerns the problems of diagnosis that arise in this way, rather than those of patients who present with symptoms in the investigation of which abnormalities are found in chest radiographs. Radiographic abnormalities that may present with no or trivial symptoms can be considered in three groups: localized shadows in the lung-fields, generalized abnormal patterns, and central (mediastinal and paramediastinal) shadows.

Localized Shadows. Shadows arising from normal or abnormal structures in or on the chest-wall and in the pleura may appear in the lung fields in a radiograph, as well as those due to abnormalities in the lungs. Localization, both in relation to the chest-wall, the pleura, and the lung and within the lung, requires at least the relevant lateral as well as the postero-anterior (PA) radiograph.

The shadows of one or both *nipples* may be seen in a normal PA radiograph. If both are visible symmetrically in appropriate positions the interpretation is usually obvious, but often only one is visible. They are more often seen in radiographs of women, but may be present in

in a 'symptomless' patient, but those produced by *pleural thickening* consequent upon inflammatory pleurisy are frequently found at routine examinations. There is usually little difficulty in recognizing such a shadow. If it is situated over the lower parts of the lungs, there will be obliteration of the costophrenic angle by adhesions at this site, with a linear opacity, produced by the thickened pleura, extending upwards from it

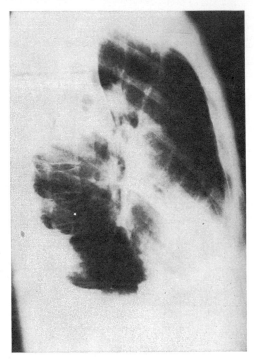

Fig. 160. PA and lateral X-rays of the chest of a symptomless man aged 50. Five years previously he had had a feverish 'chest cold', treated with tetracycline. Thoracotomy showed thickened pleura with a small encysted effusion; the shadow seen posteriorly in the lateral view was due to infolding of the thick pleura.

those of men. *Soft-tissue tumours in the chest wall*, especially those arising in the skin or subcutaneous tissue, such as neurofibromas in von Recklinghausen's disease or lipomas, may produce well-defined rounded shadows. The finding of tumours in an appropriate position on inspection is the essential clue to interpretation. All shadows cast by structures in the chest wall are moved in relation to the vascular pattern of the lungs by small changes in positioning, and radiography, after the soft tissue structure has been encircled with a metallic wire marker, will remove all doubt.

Tumours arising from ribs usually cause radiologically evident changes in the affected ribs, and are thus unlikely to be confused with other abnormalities projecting shadows in the lung-fields. If there is any doubt, further radiographic studies, including tomography, will resolve it.

The shadows produced by pleural effusions, either serous (p. 146) or purulent (p. 143), are usually distinctive and are unlikely to be found

between the lung and the ribs. Occasionally, a pleural effusion becomes loculated as it absorbs; if this occurs laterally, the usual postero-anterior (PA) radiograph will show it in profile and no difficulty in interpretation arises. But if such loculation occurs posteriorly, it will appear in the PA view as a localized shadow usually with ill-defined margins; and in rare instances, such loculated effusions may become better defined in very localized pockets of thick pleura (*Fig.* 160). In such cases, confusion with intrapulmonary conditions may arise: radiography with the patient positioned so that the rays are tangential to the pleura at the site of the loculated effusion will show it in profile. A past history of pleurisy or of trauma that might have given rise to haemothorax will of course support the interpretation of the shadow as pleural in origin.

Localized *pleural thickening* may be a consequence of various inflammatory processes, both tuberculous and non-tuberculous, and is sometimes situated elsewhere than at the bases of the lungs. Tuberculosis especially may cause apical pleural thickening, easily recognized as a cap of uniform density over the apex of the lung. An important cause of localized plaques of pleural thickening is exposure to asbestos. These may be indistinguishable from those consequent upon inflammatory pleurisy, but certain features are more frequently seen in them. They are usually bilateral, sparing the apices and costophrenic angles, and tend to be irregular in shape and sharply defined. They often show irregular calcification. Only a minority of patients in whom they are found have radiological evidence of asbestosis, and many of them are symptom-free. Exposure to asbestos may have been slight.

Diaphragmatic hernias (p. 211), congenital and traumatic, and especially the common oesophageal and para-oesophageal hiatus hernias, not infrequently first come to light as a result of routine examination of 'symptomless' subjects.

When it has been shown that the abnormal shadow is due to something located in the lung, its size, shape, density, and definition and its location within the lung must be considered in assessing its probable nature, as must the age of the patient and the diseases prevalent in the population from which he comes. But in most instances further investigation is required to establish a diagnosis.

Rounded or oval more or less well-defined shadows in otherwise normal-looking lung fields, so-called *coin lesions*, constitute one of the more frequent abnormalities found in 'symptomless' individuals. The first suspicion in a person of middle age or over, especially if he is a cigarette-smoker, must be *bronchial carcinoma*, and in a younger individual *tuberculosis*, especially in populations where this disease is prevalent. But there are many other causes of such shadows, which will be considered as they arise in consideration of differential diagnosis, rather than in any approximation to order of frequency.

If there has been a previous chest X-ray examination, at least a report on it and preferably the film itself, for direct comparison with the current one, should be obtained. This may set limits to the duration of the abnormal shadow; and occasionally it will be found to have been present, possibly smaller in the earlier film, but missed or regarded as unimportant. Information of this sort evidently alters the probabilities about the cause of the shadow.

Careful inquiry into symptoms, which may in fact have been present but disregarded by the patient, and into previous illnesses should be made. Symptoms referable to all systems may be relevant, especially in relation to malignant disease, since primary carcinoma of the lung may produce its first symptoms by distant effects, metastatic and non-metastatic, and metastases may be found in the lung before a primary tumour elsewhere has become evident. A history of treatment for a malignant tumour at any site in the past will raise the possibility of a *solitary metastasis* in the lung, which may appear a long

time after apparently successful treatment of the primary tumour.

Physical examination, though frequently non-contributory, is important. Special attention should be paid to superficial lymph-nodes, and to those organs that are common sites of primary carcinoma and which are accessible to clinical examination.

Details of radiographic appearances, usefully supplemented by tomography, should be considered. A sharply defined edge to a round or oval shadow suggests a *benign tumour* (adenoma or hamartoma), an old, inactive, well-encapsulated *caseous focus of tuberculosis*, or a *hydatid cyst* (*Fig.* 161). The presence of calcification,

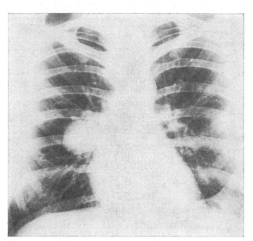

Fig. 161. This round shadow in the chest X-ray of a symptomless sheep-farmer aged 25 was due to a hydatid cyst.

possibly evident only on tomography, suggests either an old tuberculous focus or a hamartoma. The finding of small well-defined transradiant areas, indicative of cavitation in the structure causing the shadow, suggests a *tuberculous focus*, especially in a small shadow. In a larger shadow, such a finding is compatible with *squamous-cell carcinoma* (*Fig.* 162), which can present as a tumour-mass with central ischaemic necrosis. A *ruptured hydatid cyst* will show a clear zone due to air between the ectocyst and the endocyst, possibly with a fluid level, but the patient is likely to have had symptoms. A carcinoma or a still active, not completely encapsulated tuberculous focus usually has an incompletely defined edge, often with irregular projections. A tuberculous focus may show smaller 'satellite' foci on tomography. Enlargement of related lymph-nodes at the hilum of the lung may be seen with carcinoma or tuberculosis; the presence of well-defined calcification in these nodes favours a diagnosis of tuberculosis (or in patients from relevant areas, other infectious granulomatoses, such as *histoplasmosis* or *coccidioidomycosis*). *Cryptococcal granuloma* (toruloma) may present as a localized opacity in a routine chest X-ray;

it is rare and occurs principally in men coming from agricultural areas.

Localized opacities of uniform density and less well-defined borders, except where they abut on interlobar septa, may be caused by pneumonic consolidation, infarcts, or infiltrating tumours. *Pneumonia* may be seen in a patient now claiming to be symptom-free, but having recently had a febrile respiratory illness. Radiologically, the

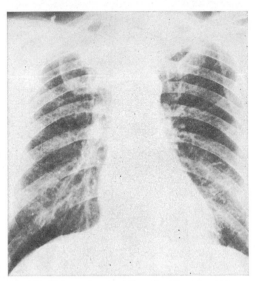

Fig. 162. This round cavity with walls of irregular thickness was found in a symptomless man aged 58. It was due to a cavitated squamous-cell carcinoma.

shadow is likely to correspond in situation and shape to an element or elements in the segmental or lobar anatomy of the lung. It is important to bear in mind that the lung beyond an obstruction in a bronchus may develop inflammatory consolidation; the diagnosis of 'unresolved pneumonia' needs confirmation by either the demonstration at bronchoscopy of a normal bronchial anatomy at the relevant site, or subsequent complete resolution, or both these favourable observations. Patients with long-standing asthma occasionally develop localized consolidations associated with aspergillus hypersensitivity—*allergic aspergillosis*—without noticing symptoms other than those of their accustomed asthma, so that the first evidence is an abnormal routine chest X-ray; the history of asthma and the finding of eosinophilia in blood and sputum should lead to appropriate immunological investigations which will establish the diagnosis. Although *pulmonary infarction* (p. 145) nearly always produces symptoms, occasionally the first evidence is the finding of a shadow suggesting localized consolidation in a routine chest X-ray. A previous history of several episodes of unexplained pleural pain, or of slight haemoptysis, or of the use of an oestrogen-containing contraceptive pill, or the finding of clinical evidence of peripheral venous thrombosis would increase

the likelihood of this diagnosis, as would the presence in the X-ray of one or more horizontal line-shadows in the lower zones of the lungs suggest the scars left by previous infarcts. Infiltrating tumours that may cause localized shadows suggesting consolidation include not only some cases of *bronchial carcinoma*, but *bronchiolo-alveolar cell carcinoma* and *lymphoma of the lung*.

In patients with rheumatoid arthritis, *necrobiotic nodules* sometimes appear in the lungs without respiratory symptoms. Although they usually become multiple, they may at first appear singly as well-defined, rounded, solitary shadows. Sometimes they undergo central necrosis, leading to small cavities, which may be thin-walled. In rare cases, such necrobiotic nodules appear before clinical symptoms or signs of arthritis, and thus in symptomless individuals.

Arteriovenous aneurysm of the lung may be found in a routine X-ray before it causes symptoms. The radiographic appearances (p. 198) especially after tomography are usually pathognomonic.

Although the foregoing points should be considered carefully whenever a patient presents with a symptomless localized shadow in a routine chest X-ray, this will rarely lead to a definitive diagnosis, and the important decision initially is how far investigation should be taken. Examination of sputum, if any, cytologically for malignant cells and by microscopy and culture for tubercle bacilli, and if sputum is not produced, of fasting gastric contents for tubercle bacilli, should be carried out in any case in which there is suspicion of cancer or tuberculosis, but with the sort of X-ray shadow under consideration it is unlikely to give a positive result. In cases in which the X-ray appearances are characteristic of inactive residues of old disease—e.g., calcifying well-encapsulated tuberculous foci or localized pleural thickening, especially where there is indubitable evidence from previous X-rays of the non-progressive nature of the condition—no further action may be necessary. In other cases, bronchoscopy should be performed, although the chance that it will be directly diagnostic in the case of 'coin lesions' is small; it may be possible to carry out needle biopsy through the bronchoscope, preferably under fluoroscopic control, to provide histological evidence, and in all cases material may be obtained by aspiration of secretions or by bronchial lavage for cytology and bacteriology. Other procedures for obtaining material for histology or cytology, such as brush biopsy, are available. Percutaneous needle biopsy under fluoroscopic control is often successful in providing histological diagnosis of tumours, primary or metastatic; it may be considered inadvisable in patients in whom there is no contra-indication to thoracotomy for effective surgical treatment of a probable primary lung tumour, in view of the possibility of implanting tumour cells in the needle track, particularly in the pleura. Mediastinoscopy provides a means of obtaining lymph-nodes from the tracheal and right bronchial groups. If these show metastatic carcinoma, it is almost certain that the lung shadow is that of the primary tumour, and an unnecessary thoracotomy is avoided. Similarly, the finding of caseating tuberculosis in the lymph-node would strongly favour the view that the lung shadow is due to the same disease. It is important that all lymph-nodes removed for diagnosis should be examined by culture for tubercle bacilli. In many instances it will be appropriate to proceed to thoracotomy without delay after a limited number of preliminary investigations; in a patient in good general condition with no contra-indications this often provides not only immediate solution of the diagnostic problem, especially with the aid of histology of a frozen section, but also the possibility of definitive surgical treatment.

Generalized Abnormalities in the Lung Fields. If an abnormal pattern involving the whole or large parts of both lungs is found in a routine chest X-ray, the fact that it has been found in a 'symptomless' individual greatly affects the diagnostic possibilities. Those that should be considered first include sarcoidosis, pneumoconiosis, histiocytosis X, and blood-borne metastases of malignant tumours.

Sarcoidosis may cause remarkably dense mottled shadowing in the chest X-ray in a patient who denies symptoms (*Fig.* 163). In

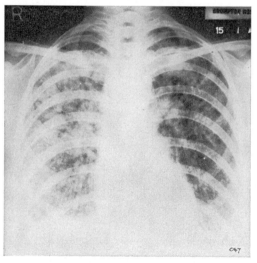

Fig. 163. Widespread mottling rather irregularly distributed through both lungs, found by mass radiography in a symptomless woman aged 22. The diagnosis of sarcoidosis was established by the finding of non-caseating epithelioid granulomas in scalene node and liver biopsies and a negative tuberculin text. The condition resolved spontaneously within two years.

such cases the disease is likely to be at a pre-fibrotic granulomatous stage. Hilar lymph-nodes may be symmetrically enlarged, but this is not invariable, and the absence of hilar node enlargement does not militate against the diagnosis of

sarcoidosis. At this stage of the disease, the abnormal pattern, consisting in multiple rounded opacities of variable size ranging from 1 to 5 mm. in diameter, with ill-defined margins, scattered fairly uniformly through the lungs, but tending if anything to be denser in the middle zones, is accompanied by no distortion of the vascular shadows. A history of erythema nodosum, a self-limiting febrile arthropathy, or an unexplained episode of iritis, or of the finding of bilateral hilar lymph-node enlargement in a previous X-ray would favour a diagnosis of sarcoidosis. Enlargement of superficial lymph-nodes, minor changes in the skin that might be sarcoid infiltrations, especially in old scars, and evidence of uveitis should be carefully sought. Palpable lymph-nodes, especially above the clavicles, and skin infiltrations provide safe and convenient sites for biopsy. The significance of a Kveim test can be deduced from knowledge that the proportion of cases of otherwise confirmed sarcoidosis that present with pulmonary infiltration giving a granulomatous response to a validated test suspension ranges from 30 to 50 per cent; an unequivocally granulomatous response thus greatly increases the likelihood of sarcoidosis, but a negative or non-specific inflammatory response is of no significance in excluding it. Low or absent tuberculin sensitivity, especially if an earlier tuberculin test is known to have been positive, or the patient has received B.C.G., is a point in favour of the diagnosis of sarcoidosis but in a minority of cases tuberculin sensitivity is retained.

The principal clue to the diagnosis of *pneumoconiosis* is, of course, the history of exposure to mineral dust. A complete occupational history, including all employments throughout life, should be taken, since symptomless mottling in the chest X-ray may be the consequence of mineral dust exposure in an occupation which the individual left many years previously. Moreover, it may be necessary to inquire into the exact nature and conditions of occupations with the details of which the physician is not familiar. Of the mineral dusts causing pneumoconiosis, that of coal is most commonly associated with symptomless X-ray shadows, the simple *pneumoconiosis of coal-workers*, uncomplicated by progressive massive fibrosis, producing few symptoms. A smaller proportion of patients with simple *silicosis*, which occurs principally in miners and quarrymen working in siliceous rocks, stone masons, foundry workers and potters, have no symptoms; and exposure to heavy concentrations of talc and kaolin produces a pneumoconiosis which at least initially may produce no symptoms. Certain dusts of high atomic weight are relatively non-fibrogenic and may be retained in the lungs of workers exposed to them and produce widespread mottling, without symptoms; these include iron oxide inhaled in the fume from iron-welding, causing siderosis, and the dust encountered in mining barium (barytosis). Tin oxide to which workers may be exposed in the smelting produces a pneumoconiosis with dense radiographic shadows but little functional defect (stannosis). On the other hand, asbestos is highly fibrogenic in susceptible individuals, and a radiologically evident *asbestosis* is unlikely to be found in a symptomless individual. Similar considerations apply to beryllium, which may cause a granulomatous fibrosing reaction in the lungs of sensitized individuals (*chronic beryllium disease*).

Histiocytosis X, or *eosinophilic granuloma*, occasionally presents as a symptomless abnormality in a routine chest X-ray. The lung changes start as a widespread infiltration producing irregular mottling in the X-ray; later there is a strong tendency to the formation of small air-containing spaces, giving rise to a 'honeycomb' appearance. The commonest localization of this granulomatosis outside the lungs is the bones, especially the long bones and the flat bones of the skull. Radiological changes in these are therefore helpful in diagnosis, and if present may indicate a convenient site for biopsy.

Blood-borne metastases in the lungs from malignant tumours elsewhere may be found by routine radiography before they cause symptoms. If there is a history of previous treatment for malignant disease, and especially if the X-ray abnormality consists in well-defined opacities scattered discretely, and possibly irregularly, through the lungs, the presumptive diagnosis is evident, though it should not be assumed without exclusion of other possibilities. But lung metastases may arise from as yet inapparent primary carcinomas, especially in the alimentary tract, the pancreas, the breast, the ovaries, the uterus, the testes, and the thyroid gland; and they may be in the form of widely scattered small nodules, producing a mottled appearance in the chest X-ray similar to that produced by granulomatous infiltrations or pneumoconioses. *Adenocarcinomas*, sometimes mucus-secreting, are especially liable to be associated with this rare and diagnostically difficult presentation; the primary tumour may never produce symptoms and remain unlocated except at necropsy. Special attention should be directed to those organs, such as the breast, the uterus, and the thyroid, from which a tumour susceptible to effective control by hormones, cytotoxic drugs or radioisotopes may arise. For instance, it is very unusual for a choriocarcinoma to present in this way; but the possibility of effective treatment makes it essential that in a 'symptomless' woman a history of a recent miscarriage, menstrual irregularity, or complicated pregnancy should lead to estimation of urinary gonadotrophins. Radiographically apparent blood-borne pulmonary metastases may be associated, at least initially, with no symptoms. By contrast, *lymphangitis carcinomatosa*, the diffuse spread of secondary carcinoma through the lung by permeation of lymphatics, causes dyspnoea early in its course, largely by making the lungs stiff, and is very unlikely to be found in a symptomless person; the X-ray abnormality is likely to include fine linear shadows indicative of lymphatic permeation or distension.

Very rarely, *chronic miliary tuberculosis* of the lungs presents as a symptomless fine, more or less uniform mottling in a chest X-ray. Diagnosis depends upon the demonstration of *Mycobacterium tuberculosis*; possibly from gastric contents, or in bronchial washings at bronchoscopy, but in some cases only by culture from lung samples obtained for biopsy (*see below*). Differential diagnosis from sarcoidosis depends also upon failure to find extrathoracic manifestations of sarcoidosis.

Scattered, small, well-defined, very dense opacities, indicative of multiple foci of calcification in otherwise normal lungs, suggest healed foci of *tuberculosis* or, in persons who have lived in endemic areas of these diseases, *histoplasmosis* or *coccioidomycosis*. They are a possible consequence of severe *chicken-pox* in an adult, becoming evident in the chest X-ray several years after the acute illness.

A very rare cause of initially symptomless diffuse X-ray changes is *pulmonary alveolar microlithiasis*, a familial disease in which the alveoli become occupied progressively by densely calcified material. The accumulation of extremely dense punctate opacities, tending to confluence in the middle zones of the lung, and in places obscuring all vascular shadows, in a patient with few or no symptoms is virtually diagnostic.

Extrinsic allergic alveolitis (farmer's lung, bird-fancier's lung, and pathogenetically similar diseases) is very unlikely to present in a truly symptomless patient. A patient recovering from an episode may still show some abnormal shadowing, consisting in probably not very dense mottling maximal in the lower parts of the lungs; the history of recent illness and of contact with organic dust should suggest the diagnosis, and lead to appropriate immunological studies.

Cryptogenic fibrosing alveolitis (diffuse interstitial fibrosis of the lungs) is characteristically a symptomatic disease, with dyspnoea as the principal symptom. In some cases, especially in older patients, the course is only very slowly progressive, so that patients may accept the increasing dyspnoea as a consequence of ageing. In such instances, the X-ray changes are likely to consist in a finely honeycombed appearance, most prominent, and possibly evident only, at the bases of the lungs. Persistent crepitations are likely to be found over the principally affected parts, and there may be clubbing of the fingers.

Idiopathic pulmonary haemosiderosis is characterized by recurrent episodes of haemoptysis, during which haemosiderin is deposited in the lung, causing widespread fine mottling, and anaemia. The mottled shadowing diminishes in density between the episodes, and at first may entirely disappear, but eventually it becomes persistent. The prominence of the haemoptysis varies from case to case, and in a few the episodic alveolar bleeding causing the haemosiderosis may be too gradual to cause haemoptysis. Thus this disease very occasionally presents as an X-ray abnormality in a 'symptomless' patient. The haemosiderosis which develops in the lungs of some patients with mitral stenosis presents similar X-ray appearances in the lungs; but with clinical and other evidence of mitral stenosis the characteristic pattern of well-defined punctate opacities scattered over the lungs is unlikely to be due to anything but *secondary haemosiderosis*.

The pattern of functional defect associated with most of the diagnostic possibilities is that common to diseases affecting the peripheral gas-exchanging part of the lungs. It consists in the combination of a restrictive ventilatory defect with a defect in gas transfer. The ventilatory defect can be demonstrated most simply by spirometry, which shows a reduced vital capacity of which a normal or even higher than normal proportion is expelled in the first second of a forced expiration. The defective gas transfer may be demonstrated by measurement of arterial blood gases at rest and after exercise; the oxygen pressure at rest in a patient who denies symptoms is likely to be within the normal range, though it may be below it, but will fall on exercise, while the carbon dioxide pressure is likely to be at or below the lower limit of normal. Estimation of the transfer factor for carbon monoxide is a convenient way of quantifying in one variable the complex set of factors concerned in the transfer of gases between the air-spaces and pulmonary capillary blood throughout the lungs; it will be likely to give a result below the predicted figure. The only difference between the possible diagnostic categories that may assist in discriminating between them is the differing relation between radiographic and functional changes. A dense radiographic pattern with little functional defect, especially if gas transfer is well maintained, favours sarcoidosis; whereas a not very striking radiographic abnormality with an evident functional defect, especially in gas transfer, favours fibrosing alveolitis. In the pre-fibrotic stages of histiocytosis X, as in sarcoidosis, the radiographic changes tend to be more striking than the functional defect. In extrinsic allergic alveolitis, there may be an additional factor of increased air-flow resistance. A further complication is that any individual who is a cigarette smoker may have high air-flow resistance due to this, and unrelated to whatever is causing the radiographic abnormality. Thus, pulmonary function tests are of little differential diagnostic value in this context.

Investigation of a 'symptomless' patient presenting with widespread X-ray changes must start with careful inquiry into previous health and occupation, and physical examination with special attention to the possible clues in other systems mentioned in the foregoing discussion. Any such clue should, of course, be followed up appropriately. But in many cases the abnormal X-ray appearance remains the only evidence obtainable by non-invasive procedures, and decision must be made about biopsy. In the few cases in which enlarged superficial lymph-nodes, or a possibly relevant abnormality in the skin or in bone are discovered, the indirect evidence that may be found by biopsy of these, a simple and safe procedure, is worth obtaining. But 'blind' biopsies of lymph-nodes obtained by exploration of the pre-scalene space or by mediastinoscopy are in general not worth while in this context, and the need for biopsy of the lung itself must be considered. The decision about this can be made only in relation to the circumstances of the individual case, after assessment of the *a priori* probabilities and the possible benefits to the patient of carrying investigations further. Especially in older patients with X-ray changes that suggest a non-progressive condition or one in which no treatment is likely to be effective, an expectant policy may be best; but, of course, when important decisions about management depend upon exact diagnosis, as is usually the case in younger patients, lung biopsy is indicated if diagnosis cannot be established otherwise.

Of the available methods, surgical biopsy through a small thoracotomy has the advantages of providing the occasion for inspection of the lung and the choice of biopsy site, if appropriate the taking of samples from areas of differing naked-eye appearance, and the obtaining of samples large enough to be submitted to all of the several sorts of study—histological, bacteriological, immunological, and in some instances mineralogical and chemical—that may be desirable. It should be undertaken only by experienced surgeons, in whose hands its hazards are probably less than those of either transbronchial or percutaneous biopsy procedures. These seem less formidable to the patient, but carry small risks of haemoptysis or bleeding into the pleura, and of pneumothorax which may need tube drainage; they produce much smaller specimens, usually sufficient only for histology and often with a distorted pattern. Choice between these procedures will depend to some extent upon availability. In general, if diagnosis seems likely to be difficult and to depend upon refinements of histological interpretation and also upon the results of other laboratory studies, open biopsy is to be preferred. If the problem is a decision between two contrasting possibilities—e.g., granulomatous or malignant? or pneumoconiosis or not?—transbronchial needle or percutaneous needle or drill biopsy may be sufficient.

Central (mediastinal and para-mediastinal) shadows. When an abnormality of the central shadow is found, a lateral view is required to localize it in relation to mediastinal structures. A shadow which appears parahilar in the PA view may be shown in this way to be located in the lung, in the apical segment of a lower lobe, the anterior segment of an upper lobe, the middle lobe or the lingula; the differential diagnosis is then that of a localized shadow arising from the lung. The shadows of bronchial adenomas and hamartomas often appear close to the hilum in this way in PA films. Mediastinal shadows can be considered according to their location: in hilar (bronchopulmonary) and paratracheal lymph-nodes and in the mediastinum anteriorly, centrally, and posteriorly.

Bilateral hilar lymph-node enlargement (BHL), with or without right paratracheal node enlargement, is one of the commoner findings in symptomless individuals at routine chest X-ray examinations. If the shadows of the enlarged nodes are well defined, with a polycyclic outline, often with a clear transradiant band between the lower pole of the shadow and the heart-shadow, and the patient is symptom-free and shows no abnormality on physical examination, the diagnosis of *sarcoidosis* is virtually certain (*Fig.* 164). A history of erythema nodosum or

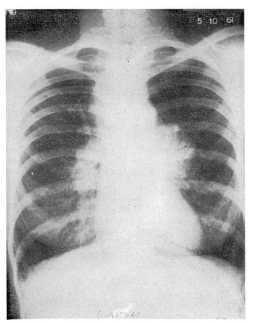

Fig. 164. Bilateral hilar and right paratracheal lymph node enlargement in a symptomless woman aged 30. Spontaneous resolution confirmed that it was due to sarcoidosis.

febrile arthropathy in the recent past puts it beyond reasonable doubt.

If the lymph-node enlargement is not bilaterally symmetrical, or if the outline of the shadow produced by it is a smooth curve suggesting that the nodes are confluent, or the patient admits to constitutional or local symptoms, additional possibilities must be considered. These include *Hodgkin's disease* and other *lymphomas*, *tuberculosis*, and metastatic *malignant disease*. Tuberculin test, examination of sputum, if any, for tubercle bacilli and cytologically, and bronchoscopy may be helpful, but diagnosis in most cases depends upon biopsy.

A careful search for enlarged superficial lymph-nodes, especially in the neck, may lead to the discovery of one that can conveniently be removed. If none can be found, mediastinoscopy is the most favourable procedure by which a node likely to be involved in the disease-process can be obtained. Alternatively, but with less chance of contributory findings, scalene node biopsy may be performed. Nodes removed for biopsy should be submitted to bacteriological examination, especially for tubercle bacilli, as well as histology. A Kveim test is of limited value in this context. A granulomatous response to a well-validated suspension virtually excludes Hodgkin's disease, and makes a diagnosis of other forms of lymphoma or metastatic cancer unlikely; it strongly supports a diagnosis of sarcoidosis, but may also occur in the presence of a hilar lymphadenopathy proved bacteriologically to be due to *M. tuberculosis*.

Similar considerations apply to unilateral hilar node enlargement, with the additional point that *tuberculosis* must be especially considered, especially in persons from communities in which this is a common disease and in the young. A small shadow may be present in the part of the lung which drains into the enlarged nodes if, as is often the case, these are part of the complex of primary tuberculous infection; and the tuberculin test can be expected to be positive. In the presence of these findings, a determined search should be made for tubercle bacilli in sputum or gastric contents.

Abnormalities of the central mediastinal shadow may be produced by tumours, by foregut cysts, by anomalies of the oesophagus, and by abnormalities of the great vessels. Among tumours, *intrathoracic goitre* is located high in the anterior part of the superior mediastinum: it may extend laterally from either or both sides of the normal central shadow, it may or may not be continuous with a goitre in the neck, and may itself become palpable in the suprasternal notch when the patient swallows. *Thymic tumours* are also located anteriorly, and may project to either or both sides of the central shadow; the upper pole is often visible in the PA film, and in the lateral view the tumour abuts on the posterior surface of the sternum (*Fig.* 165). *Teratomas* and *dermoid cysts* appear as round or oval well-circumscribed shadows in the anterior mediastinum, best seen in the lateral view, but extending into the lung fields on either side in the PA view; calcification may occur in their walls, and occasionally tomography detects teeth within them.

Neurogenic tumours present as round or oval sharply defined shadows in the posterior half of the chest and usually in its upper half (*Fig.* 166). They often lie in the costovertebral sulcus, and are liable to cause local thinning of adjacent ribs by pressure, and sometimes enlargement of intervertebral foramina. The rare tumours of the vagus are situated less posteriorly. Neurofibromas may be associated with neurofibromatosis (von Recklinghausen's disease), evident from its cutaneous manifestations. Occasionally, a neurofibroma is associated with a secondary meningocele protruding through an enlarged intervertebral foramen. Very rarely, an intrathoracic meningocele develops through a presumably congenital defect in a vertebra, usually on the right side.

Bronchogenic foregut cysts are not infrequently present as symptomless radiographic findings; they usually appear near the tracheal bifurcation, and may be attached to the trachea, the main bronchi, or the oesophagus; they

produce round or oval opacities overlapping or just anterior to the vertebral bodies in the lateral view (*Fig.* 167).

The gross dilatation of the oesophagus due to *achalasia of the cardia* (p. 235) is, surprisingly, sometimes seen for the first time in a routine chest radiograph in a patient who has not sought advice about dysphagia; it produces a continuous central band of opacity with broadly sinuous borders, which project on either side into the

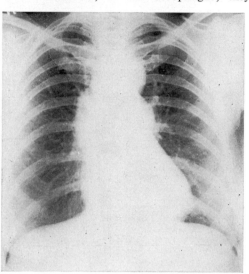

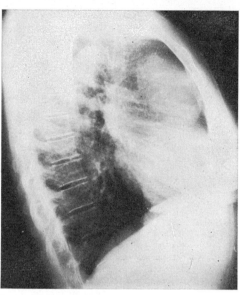

Fig. 165. PA and lateral X-rays showing a well-defined oval shadow anteriorly in the mediastinum of a woman aged 48. At thoracotomy a well-encapsulated thymic tumour was found.

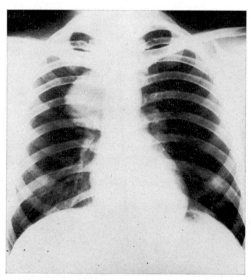

Fig. 166. This well-defined oval opacity to the right of the upper mediastinum was found by mass radiography in a man aged 20. In the lateral view, it lay posteriorly. At thoracotomy a neurilemmoma arising from the sympathetic chain was found.

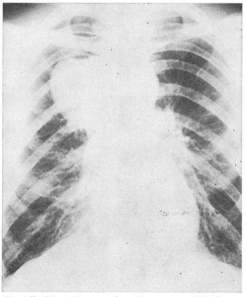

Fig. 167. This shadow was found in a man aged 48. In the lateral view, it lay in the line of the trachea. At thoracotomy a bronchogenic cyst was found.

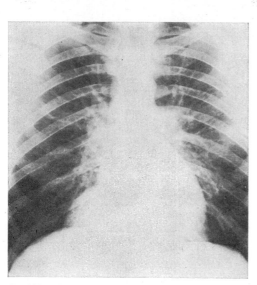 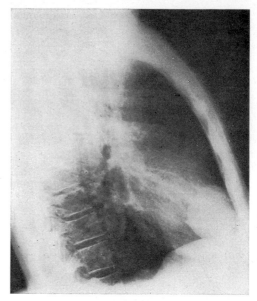

Fig. 168. This well-defined shadow adjacent to the heart, anteriorly in the cardiophrenic angle, was found by mass radiography in a man aged 30. At thoracotomy a parapericardial cyst containing clear fluid was found.

lung-fields, and may be visible through the heart-shadow. Similarly, an *oesophageal diverticulum* at the level of the bifurcation of the trachea is occasionally seen as a rounded shadow at this level in a routine chest X-ray. In either of these situations, radiography after barium swallow resolves the diagnostic problem.

Aneurysm of the aorta may be found in a symptomless subject. If it affects the ascending part of the arch, physical signs, such as those of aortic valve disease, inequalities of the pulses in the arms, or of the pupils, may be found. Usually careful radiological studies, including tomography, showing continuity of the abnormal shadow with that of the aorta make the diagnosis evident, but angiography may be needed.

Pleuropericardial cysts are situated alongside the pericardium, in the cardiophrenic angle anteriorly, on either side but more frequently on the right (*Fig.* 168). They rarely produce symptoms, and thus usually become apparent in routine X-ray examinations as well-defined extensions of the cardiac shadow in the appropriate position.

J. G. Scadding.

CHEYNE-STOKES RESPIRATION

This well-known abnormality of respiration, described independently by John Cheyne in 1818 and William Stokes in 1846, is probably referred to in the Hippocratic writings in an account of a patient whose breathing was 'like that of a man recollecting himself, and rare and large'.

Cheyne-Stokes respiration, the commonest form of periodic breathing, consists of a series of breaths, beginning with hardly perceptible movements, gradually increasing until the tidal volume is much above normal, and then dying away to end in apnoea (*Fig.* 169). The apnoeic period lasts for 10–30 seconds or more and the hyperpnoeic phase comprises thirty or more breaths and usually lasts between 1 and 3 minutes. The condition is obvious to the experienced observer but untrained persons will often describe the hyperpnoeic phase as 'breathlessness'. The patient himself is frequently unaware of the abnormality in his breathing. It is particularly prominent at night and the hyperpnoea may wake the patient repeatedly so that symptomatic treatment of the respiratory disorder may be well worth while.

The mechanism is complex, but there appear to be two prerequisites for the appearance of Cheyne-Stokes breathing: a reduced sensitivity of the respiratory centre and a reduction in the arterial P_{CO_2}. Thus, in a normal subject, voluntary hyperventilation in room air will lead to a short period of apnoea followed by a few cycles of Cheyne-Stokes breathing; this does not occur after hyperventilation with 5 per cent CO_2. It is, therefore, possible to reduce the arterial P_{CO_2} to such a level that even a normal respiratory centre fails to discharge normally. The slow decline in arterial oxygen saturation and rise in carbon dioxide during the apnoea begin to stimulate the respiratory centre and respiration is resumed leading to a second fall in P_{CO_2} with repetition of the cycle. The changes in the blood gases during the cycle are shown in *Fig.* 170. It will be

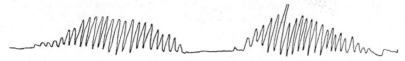

Fig. 169. Spirogram from a patient with severe cerebral vascular disease. Two cycles of Cheyne-Stokes breathing are shown, over a period of 143 seconds.

noted that they are not exactly as might have been expected from the account which has been given and are out of phase with the respiratory movements. This may be due to a relatively long lung–brain circulation time which some believe is a third factor needed for the development of Cheyne-Stokes respiration in disease.

Cheyne-Stokes respiration occurs in normal subjects not only after hyperventilation but also at high altitudes where the hypoxic stimulus to respiration reduces the arterial P_{CO_2}. It may also

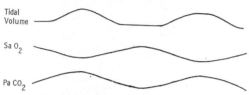

Fig. 170. Diagram of changes in tidal volume, arterial oxygen saturation (Sa_{O_2}), and partial pressure of carbon dioxide in arterial blood (Pa_{CO_2}) over two cycles of Cheyne-Stokes breathing.

be seen in apparently healthy elderly subjects during sleep; it is difficult, however, to exclude minor degrees of cerebral vascular disease causing depression of the respiratory centre in such cases. In clinical practice the commonest cause is left ventricular failure, especially in patients with degenerative arterial disease in whom the blood-supply to the brain-stem may be reduced as a result both of the low cardiac output and local arterial disease. Cheyne-Stokes respiration is commonly regarded as indicating a poor prognosis in left ventricular failure, but it may disappear with treatment of the failure and, rarely, may persist for many months in patients in whom the other symptoms and signs of failure are unobtrusive.

Bronchopneumonia or other respiratory infections may also precipitate Cheyne-Stokes breathing in the elderly; hyperventilation is the mechanism, as in left ventricular failure. However, it must be realized that, in chronic respiratory failure in which a raised rather than a lowered arterial P_{CO_2} is the rule, Cheyne-Stokes respiration does not occur. Occasionally there may be a few cycles in the recovery period following a Stokes-Adams attack. Respiration continues during the period of circulatory arrest and the first blood to enter the cerebral circulation after cardiac action is resumed contains very little carbon dioxide. The sensitivity of the respiratory centre is reduced by hypoxia during the circulatory arrest and this combines with the hypocapnia to cause Cheyne-Stokes breathing. Rarely Cheyne-Stokes breathing is complicated by cardiac dysrhythmias,

including junctional rhythm and atrioventricular block, which occur intermittently in phase with the respiratory dysrhythmia; the mechanism is unknown.

Primary depression of the sensitivity of the respiratory centre in the absence of much change in the arterial P_{CO_2} can also cause Cheyne-Stokes respiration. Thus it occurs in many diseases of the central nervous system. These include cerebral vascular disease with or without haemorrhage or thrombosis, cerebral tumours especially those involving the brain-stem, and severe head injuries. Cheyne-Stokes respiration is always more prominent during sleep and can be precipitated by the administration of narcotic or hypnotic drugs such as morphine or barbiturates. It is also seen quite often in uraemia but is probably not due to the renal failure *per se*. Hyperventilation in renal failure is caused by acidosis, the effect of which persists despite the fall in arterial P_{CO_2}. Probably it is the left ventricular failure resulting from renal hypertension which is mainly responsible for Cheyne-Stokes breathing in this situation although it may occur in patients whose blood-pressure is normal.

Cheyne-Stokes respiration must not be confused with Biot's breathing which is much rarer. This may occur in primary lesions of the brain-stem or if the intracranial pressure is raised from any cause. The respiratory pattern is only superficially similar as, in Biot's breathing, the hyperpnoeic phase consists of four or five breaths only, all of which are of the same amplitude, so that the beginning and end of the phases are abrupt.

P. R. Fleming.

CHORDEE

Chordee is the name given to a condition in which, during erection, the penis is curved to one side and severe pain is present. It used to occur during the early stages of an acute urethritis—usually gonorrhoeal—but is today, when effective early treatment is usually the rule, extremely rare. It is caused by inflammation in the corpus spongiosum or corpora cavernosa. The condition must not be confused with the curved erection which follows chronic indurative cavernositis (Peyronie's disease), in which a firm induration can be felt in either one or both corpora cavernosa and which prevents true erection in the part of the penis distal to the fibrous thickening. If the condition is bilateral, the distal penis may be entirely flaccid during erection. This condition may follow trauma, or may be a fibrosis allied to, and associated with, Dupuytren's contracture. The cause is unknown.

In hypospadias the urethra opens proximal to its usual position and there is usually an associated ventral contraction of the penis caused by a fibrous band along the usual course of the corpus spongiosum. This also causes changes which have been termed chordee, but acute pain is here absent.

F. Dudley Hart.

CHYLURIA

The passage of urine which is milky in appearance is due to the presence of emulsified fat. The fat usually originates from the intestinal lymphatics, but the term *lipuria* has been used to indicate the presence of fat from other sources. The condition must be distinguished from phosphaturia, in which the turbidity is removed by acidification of the urine with acetic acid, from a deposit of urates which is dissolved by warming, from extraneous fat introduced as a lubricant, from rectal contamination with oily purgatives, and from the deliberate addition of milk. In true chyluria the fat is usually finely emulsified so that fat droplets are visible with the $\frac{1}{12}$-in. but not with the $\frac{1}{6}$-in. objective; protein and a few red cells are also present and fibrin clots may be seen. The turbidity may not be completely removed by simple ether extraction, but will be intensified by feeding the patient with 0·1 g. of Sudan III in 10 g. of butter, after which the ether extract of the urine will be red.

True chyluria implies a connexion between the intestinal lymphatics and the urinary tract. This is usually in the neighbourhood of the bladder or renal pelvis and is the result of lymphatic blockage. Causes include tuberculosis, neoplasm, peritonitis with abscess formation, and filariasis. Chyluria (or lipuria) has also been described in chronic nephritis, phosphorus poisoning, eclampsia, and after fractures of the long bones or trauma to subcutaneous fat. In the case of filariasis there may or may not be elephantiasis; this diagnosis will be supported by the presence of eosinophilia and the presence of microfilariae in the blood at a suitable time of day. In the other examples chyluria is usually an incidental symptom in a condition which has already been diagnosed by other means.

Joan F. Zilva.

CLAW-FOOT (PIED-EN-GRIFFE)

Claw-foot (*Fig.* 171) is less common than claw-hand, but it may arise from similar causes. The tibial nerve, which supplies the interossei and lumbricals of the foot through its lateral plantar branch, is homologous to the ulnar nerve in the upper extremity. Its buried course

in the leg does not, however, expose it to the same chances of injury as is the case with the more superficial ulnar nerve, and consequently claw-foot is not often the result of injury. Disease or injury of the first and second sacral segments of the spinal cord or of the corresponding spinal nerve-roots may produce the characteristic deformity of the toes, in which case there may be disturbances of sensibility in the corresponding cutaneous areas. In acute poliomyelitis affecting

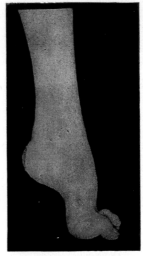

Fig. 171. Claw-foot.

those segments the diagnosis depends on the history of onset, as in the case of claw-hand of similar origin.

In *peroneal atrophy* (Tooth's paralysis) the diagnosis depends on the symmetry of the affection, the insidious way it starts, the affection of other members of the family, and the preceding or concomitant atrophy of the leg muscles, generally beginning in those supplied by the peroneal nerve.

Ian Mackenzie.

CLAW-HAND (MAIN-EN-GRIFFE)

Claw-hand is the name used to describe a hand characterized by a claw-like position of the fingers (*Fig.* 172). The fingers are extended at the metacarpophalangeal joints and flexed at both interphalangeal joints. This position is the result of over-action of the extensor communis digitorum and flexores digitorum when unopposed by the normal antagonism of the interossei and lumbricals. It is not symptomatic of any particular disease, but results from any morbid condition which produces atrophic paralysis of the intrinsic hand muscles, so long as the long extensors of the fingers remain intact. *Progressive muscular atrophy* and *amyotrophic lateral sclerosis, ulnar paralysis, syringomyelia, cervical pachymeningitis, acute poliomyelitis, supernumerary rib*, and *spondylosis* are among the conditions which may give rise to claw-hand to a lesser or greater degree. In any particular case the diagnosis of the underlying condition depends on the results of further investigation.

In *progressive muscular atrophy* (*Fig.* 173) wasting of the intrinsic hand muscles is often an early symptom, and a claw-hand may develop before the long extensor muscles of the fingers have become involved in the disease. All four fingers are usually affected to an approximately

the deep palmar branch of the ulnar nerve is compressed there is no sensory loss.

The claw-hand of *syringomyelia* (*Fig.* 172) resembles that of progressive muscular atrophy in general appearance, and may show the modifications to which the terms 'ape's hand' and 'preacher's hand' have been applied. The muscular atrophy is not limited to the distribution of a single nerve, but involves the musculature innervated by the 8th cervical and 1st dorsal spinal segments—segments in which the cavitation frequently begins. The diagnosis depends on the

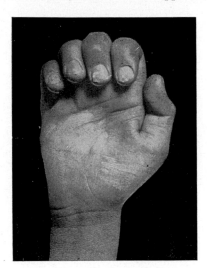

Fig. 172. Syringomyelic claw-hand.

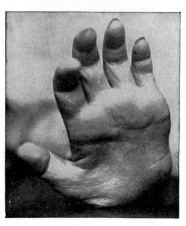

Fig. 173. Ape's hand due to progressive muscular atrophy; note the wasting of the thenar and hypothenar muscles, and the early stage of claw-hand. (*Sir Charles Symonds.*)

equal extent, and there is often marked wasting of the thenar and hypothenar eminences. When the abductor pollicis is also involved the thumb tends to fall into line with the fingers and gives an 'ape's hand' appearance (*Fig.* 173). The flexors of the wrist often become involved before the extensors, with the result that the wrist is hyperextended, and a 'preacher's hand' results. The absence of pain and of all sensory disturbance, the gradual onset, and the general exaggeration of the deep reflexes, serve to distinguish this condition from some of the other causes of claw-hand.

In *ulnar paralysis* the claw position is more marked in the ring and little fingers than in the middle and first fingers, owing to the fact that the two outer lumbricals are supplied by the median nerve. The adductor pollicis is the only thenar muscle to suffer, but the hypothenar eminence is wasted. If the injury to the nerve is above the point where it gives off the branch to the flexor carpi ulnaris this will also be paralysed, and flexion of the wrist will be carried out with a deviation towards the radial side. In ulnar paralysis the palsy is limited to the muscles supplied by the ulnar nerve, and there is usually some sensory loss in the area of skin innervated by this nerve if the lesion is above the wrist. If

presence of areflexia in the arms and dissociated anaesthesia, which means that with regard to cutaneous sensation pain and temperature sense are lost and touch is preserved. Scoliosis and a spastic paraparesis may also be present, as may trophic and vasomotor disturbances such as whitlows, glossy skin (*peau lisse*), and *main succulente*. Horner's syndrome, nystagmus, and variable loss of pain and temperature over the face would suggest associated syringobulbia.

Cervical pachymeningitis only leads to a claw-hand when it interferes with the function of the 8th cervical and 1st dorsal anterior roots and leaves uninjured the 6th and 7th cervical roots. The condition is generally bilateral, with some asymmetry, and it is usually associated with pain and ill-defined disturbances of sensibility in the arms.

Acute poliomyelitis (*Fig.* 174) affecting the 8th cervical and 1st dorsal segments, and leaving intact the 6th and 7th cervical segments, is uncommon. The history of acute onset, with constitutional symptoms such as headache, fever, and vomiting, affords a clue to the diagnosis. The absence of sensory loss, and the possible presence of atrophic palsies in other parts of the body, form additional data in these cases.

Supernumerary cervical rib may produce a claw-hand when it causes neuritic changes in the trunk formed by the 8th cervical and 1st dorsal contributions to the brachial plexus. The muscular atrophy is preceded by pain in the arm and neck, and sometimes by vasomotor changes and diminution of the radial pulse. Analgesia in the

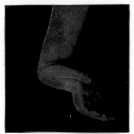

Fig. 174. Claw-hand caused by acute anterior poliomyelitis affecting the forearm.

distribution of the 8th cervical and 1st dorsal root areas may also be detected, but the diagnosis may depend mainly on the radiographic discovery of the rudimentary rib.

Ian Mackenzie.

CLUB-FOOT OR TALIPES

Any deformity of the foot not limited to the toes commonly goes under the name of club-foot, or talipes. The chief varieties are as follows:

1. Talipes Equinus. In this condition the forepart of the foot cannot be raised to the normal degree. A healthy adult, with the knee straight, can dorsiflex the ankle to such an extent that the ball of the great toe is two or three inches higher than the prominence of the heel. The degree of dorsiflexion is even greater in infants. With advancing years the movement becomes limited, especially in women who use high heels; old people may be unable to dorsiflex the foot beyond the right angle.

2. Talipes Calcaneus. In this condition the heel is depressed and the forepart of the foot elevated. Extension of the ankle is limited, so that the forepart of the foot cannot touch the ground in walking.

3. Talipes Valgus. The foot is everted and abducted at the ankle-joint, so that the inner malleolus is too prominent and too near the ground.

4. Talipes Varus. The foot is inverted and adducted at the ankle-joint, so that the outer malleolus is too prominent and too near the ground; in this condition there is in addition serious deformity at the medio-tarsal joint, at which the forepart of the foot is abnormally adducted and inverted.

5. Talipes Cavus. The arch of the foot is too high or hollow. This may be due to depression of the forepart of the foot, of the heel, or of both.

Combinations of these deformities, especially talipes equinovarus, talipes calcaneocavus, and talipes calcaneovalgus, are frequently encountered.

Club-foot cases may be divided into: (I) Congenital; (II) Acquired.

I. CONGENITAL TALIPES

1. A primary deformity present at birth. The terms 'club-foot' and 'congenital talipes' are often limited to a condition in which one or both feet are in the position of extreme equinovarus at birth. Rarely the deformity is one of calcaneovalgus. Congenital club-foot is more common in boys, and in the majority of cases is bilateral. The abnormal position of the foot is probably caused by compression during intra-uterine development, due to abnormal position of the foetal legs in utero, deficient liquor amnii, or pathological changes in the uterine wall; that developmental factors are sometimes responsible is indicated by the occasional coexistence of other malformations, and the appearance of the deformity in several generations. The foot, besides being inverted and adducted, is shorter and broader than normal (*Fig.* 175). The heel is small, raised, turned inwards, and marked off by deep furrows above and to the inner side; another furrow lies on the inner side of the foot opposite the midtarsal joint. There is flattening on the inner side of the foot just in front of the external malleolus, where the skin is dimpled and loose. The varus is worse than the equinus, whereas in paralytic cases the equinus is usually worse than the varus. The limb is pink and warm, and shortening or muscular wasting is slight or absent.

2. Due to absence or faulty development of bones in the leg or foot. Talipes equinovalgus associated with congenital absence of the fibula is the commonest deformity of this class.

3. Due to spina bifida. A spinal defect in the usual situation (lower lumbar region) gives rise to a lower motor neuron lesion involving the lower limbs, often associated with paralysis of the bladder and rectum. The commonest deformity of the foot is talipes calcaneovalgus, but an equinus position associated with varus or valgus may be seen. Both feet are usually affected, but unilateral cases have been reported.

II. ACQUIRED TALIPES

1. The Paralytic. Theoretically it is possible for any paralytic condition, whether of neurological origin or due to rare muscular dystrophies, to produce deformities of the feet. In practice some of these conditions carry a much greater liability to talipes than others; they may be placed in four groups: (*a*) The spastic paralyses due to upper motor neuron lesions; (*b*) The flaccid paralyses due to lower motor neuron lesions; (*c*) The cerebellar ataxias; (*d*) The muscular dystrophies. *a.* DUE TO LESIONS OF THE UPPER MOTOR NEURON. *In the Brain.*

Congenital: Cerebral defects; birth injuries. Although the nerve lesion is present at birth, the talipes appears later, and is therefore grouped with the acquired deformities. This is the commonest of the upper motor lesions to cause talipes.

Acquired: Meningeal haemorrhage, thrombosis, or embolism, from injury, fevers, or wasting conditions; chronic meningitis, hydrocephalus.

In the Cord. Injury; haemorrhage; thrombosis; tumour; and nervous diseases whose pathology includes an upper motor neuron element, such as subacute combined sclerosis of the cord. Talipes is not a prominent symptom in any and

delivery by forceps, indicating injury to the cerebral cortex or meningeal haemorrhage. There may have been difficulty in getting the child to breathe, and later in feeding him. The deformity is rarely obvious for a year or two after birth, and is usually noticed when the child begins to walk abnormally late. In other cases *thrombosis of the cerebral veins* may follow measles or influenza, or rupture of the cortical veins may occur during whooping-cough or fits of passion. The paralysis

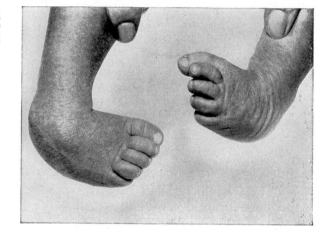

Fig. 175. Talipes deformity from meningocele. The left-hand picture shows a typical talipes equinovarus. The right-hand picture shows the deformity more advanced, and the foot has been drawn up into the position of talipes equinocalcaneus. (*J. B. Blaikley.*)

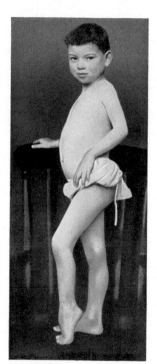

Fig. 176. Infantile hemiplegia causing extreme talipes equinus of the left foot.

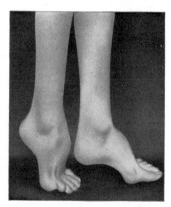

Fig. 177. Bilateral talipes equinus from congenital spastic paraplegia.

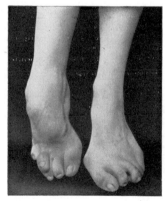

Fig. 178. Talipes equinovarus and equinovalgus, due to spina bifida.

is usually overshadowed by other major disturbances.

In lesions of the upper neuron the tendon reflexes are exaggerated and the plantar reflex is extensor. The electrical reactions of the muscles are normal. Coldness and blueness of the feet and trophic sores are usually absent, but may occur when the lesion involves Clarke's column in the cord. The deformity is characteristically one of equinus, often with slight varus. The history and distribution of the paralysis may help in distinguishing various destructive lesions of the upper motor neuron. In *cerebral paralysis* there may be a history of difficult labour, with

may involve half the body—*cerebral hemiplegia* (*Fig.* 176); it may be limited to the lower extremities—*cerebral paraplegia* (*Fig.* 177); or it may involve both the upper and lower extremities—*cerebral diplegia.* In rare instances one extremity only is affected—*cerebral monoplegia.* There is usually some mental impairment, especially in cases of cerebral defect or birth injury.

b. DUE TO LESIONS OF THE LOWER MOTOR NEURON.

In the Cord. Spina bifida occulta; infantile paralysis; progressive muscular atrophy; peroneal muscular atrophy; amyotrophic lateral sclerosis.

In the Peripheral Nerves. Compression or injury

of nerve-trunks in the cauda equina or the lumbar or sacral plexus, or of peripheral nerves in the limb; tumours (neuroma) of nerves; peripheral neuritis; Tooth's neuromuscular paralysis.

In lesions of the lower neuron the tendon reflexes are diminished or lost. The reaction of degeneration may be found in the muscles, and wasting is always marked. The feet are often cold and blue, and trophic sores may appear. The limb is short when the lesion has appeared during the growth period.

It is important to examine for *spina bifida occulta*, which is usually indicated by a fatty pad or a tuft of hair over the sacrum. A radiograph will usually demonstrate deficiency in the lower vertebral arches. The talipes, while usually bilateral and symmetrical, is not necessarily so (*Fig.* 178). *Infantile paralysis* results from acute anterior poliomyelitis, and is distinguished by its irregular distribution, reaction of degeneration, the shortening, and the vasomotor changes. It is usually possible to show that the patient is unable to use certain muscles or groups of muscles, especially the anterior tibial and peroneal group. It is unusual for the paralysis to be limited to one leg: the thigh muscles, especially the quadriceps and gluteal group, are usually affected to some extent, and often the opposite leg or the trunk or arm muscles. *Progressive muscular atrophy* appears after the age of 30, and shows a steady advance; in the lower limbs it produces a deformity of equinus or equinovarus type. *Peroneal muscular atrophy* usually commences before 25, and also gives rise to talipes equinus and equinovarus. The disease is familial. *Amyotrophic lateral sclerosis*, which involves both the anterior-horn cells and the pyramidal fibres of the cord, gives rise to a paralysis of mixed upper and lower neuron type, the former predominating in the lower, the latter in the upper limbs.

The nerves of the cauda equina or the lumbar and sacral plexuses may be compressed by tumours of the meninges, vertebrae, or sacrum, by carcinoma of the rectum, or by secondary deposits from growth elsewhere. The sciatic nerve, especially the external popliteal branch, may be injured by wounds, the pressure of tight splints in the treatment of fracture, or the forcible extension of a contracted knee. *Peripheral neuritis* due to diphtheria, lead poisoning, or alcoholism may cause foot-drop; in each case there is other evidence of the disease. *Tooth's neuromuscular paralysis* causes paresis of the anterior tibial and peroneal muscles, with talipes equinus and marked cavus, and deformity of the toes. It may be distinguished from infantile paralysis by the symmetrical affection of both feet and the history of similar deformity in others in the family (*see* CONTRACTURES *and* MUSCULAR ATROPHY) and from the primary muscular dystrophies by the occurrence of the reaction of degeneration.

c. DUE TO LESIONS OF THE CEREBELLUM AND ITS AFFERENT TRACTS. *Friedreich's hereditary ataxia.* This can be recognized by the family history, the age of onset, which is usually about 6 to 9 years, the incoordination, nystagmus, slurring speech, absent knee-jerks, and hallux erectus.

d. DUE TO PRIMARY MUSCULAR DISEASE. *Pseudohypertrophic muscular paralysis.* The family history, the enlargement of the calves (*Fig.* 646, p. 626), and the characteristic way in which the patient raises himself from the supine position by rolling into the prone position, and then lifting himself on his toes and hands and working his hands up the front of his thighs, all assist the diagnosis. The usual deformity is one of equinus or equinovarus. *Amyotonia congenita* is a similar condition occurring in infants and without the false hypertrophy.

2. Postural or Static. Talipes valgus may be due to faulty posture, often combined with a deficiency in postural tone of the tibial muscles, either absolute or relative to the weight of the patient. The deformity is commonly seen in older children and adolescents who are growing rapidly and are in poor general health; it is often accompanied by knock-knee. Talipes cavus and equinocavus are often caused by wearing boots which are too short, or whose heels are too high. This condition must not be confounded with a similar one due to paralysis of the small muscles of the foot, especially the interossei and lumbricales, such as may result from infantile paralysis or peripheral neuritis. Talipes equinus may be caused by the weight of the bedclothes in long illnesses.

3. Compensatory. The attitude of talipes equinus is often assumed to compensate for shortness of the limb, such as that due to old hip disease.

4. Due to Fractures and Dislocations. After fracture, dislocations of the ankle-joint, such as Pott's and Dupuytren's fractures, an extreme talipes equinovalgus may develop unless care is taken to correct the deformity whilst the fractures are healing.

5. Due to Bone Disease. Injury or inflammation near the epiphysial line of the tibia may lead to arrest or overgrowth, with the production of a varus or valgus deformity. This is a fairly common cause of talipes, which can be recognized if care is taken to make comparative measurements and radiographic examinations of the bones.

6. Due to Disease of Joints and Ligaments. Talipes equinus may arise as a result of faulty treatment of arthritis of the ankle, unless care is taken to keep the foot at right angles to the leg during treatment. The deformity is a common sequel of Still's disease in children and rheumatoid arthritis in adults.

Acute flat-foot may be due to inflammatory softening of the plantar ligaments in gonorrhoea. Spasmodic flat-foot is often caused by a toxic arthritis of the tarsal joints.

7. Due to Fibrosis of Muscle. Very rarely the calf muscles may contract as the result of an ischaemia analogous to that occurring in the forearm (*see* Volkmann's contracture, *Fig.* 189, p. 179). The same condition may develop as a result of cellulitis of the calf muscles associated with compound fractures of the leg with gross backward displacement of the lower fragment in fractures of the lower end of the shaft of the femur, or with acute necrosis of the tibia. In all these conditions it is important to prevent the development of talipes equinus. Fibrosis of the short muscles of the sole is one cause of talipes cavus.

8. Due to Contracting Scars. Occasionally talipes equinus follows severe burns or lacerations of the skin of the leg or foot. The diagnosis is usually obvious from the scars.

9. Hysterical. Hysterical club-foot may be suspected from the associated symptoms, and confirmed by the absence of any wasting or change in the electrical reactions of the muscles, by the variation of the deformity on different occasions, and by the disproportionate amount of spasm, which passes off during sleep or under an anaesthetic.

DIFFERENTIAL DIAGNOSIS OF THE COMMON VARIETIES OF TALIPES

Equinovarus

CONGENITAL. Bilateral, but often not detected till the baby starts to try to stand or walk.
ACQUIRED. Due to: Poliomyelitis; Injury of the external popliteal nerve. Equinus with a moderate degree of varus is seen in spastic paralysis due to lesions of the brain and cord, spina bifida, peripheral neuritis, and muscular dystrophy.

The main points in the differentiation between congenital talipes equinovarus and that due to poliomyelitis are:

Congenital
  Often bilateral
  Chiefly in boys
  Circulation good
  Wasting moderate
  Tendon reflexes normal
  Shortening moderate
  Radiographs show small os calcis and neck of astragalus inclined inwards. Structure of bones normal.

Acquired
  Usually unilateral
  Sex incidence equal
  Foot blue and cold
  Wasting marked and uneven
  Tendon reflexes diminished or absent
  Shortening marked
  Radiographs show atrophy of bone.

Equinus. Nearly always acquired. May be due to: Poliomyelitis involving the extensors of the ankle; Spastic paralysis, from lesions of the brain or spinal cord; Peripheral neuritis—lead, alcohol, diphtheria; Posture during illness; Compensation for a short limb; Old disease of the ankle-joint; Fibrosis of calf muscles.

Calcaneus

CONGENITAL. Usually pure calcaneus.
ACQUIRED. Due to: Poliomyelitis, usually combined with cavus; Following tenotomy of tendo Achillis.

Varus

CONGENITAL. Due to: Absence of tibia.
ACQUIRED. Due to: Injury of external popliteal nerve; Injury of epiphysial line of tibia.

Valgus

CONGENITAL. Due to: Absence of fibula, spina bifida.
ACQUIRED. Due to: Paralysis of tibial group of muscles in poliomyelitis, injury of internal popliteal nerve; Faulty posture; Pott's or Dupuytren's fracture; Infections of the tarsal joints or plantar ligaments.

Cavus

CONGENITAL. A familial deformity.
ACQUIRED. Due to: Posture; Peripheral neuritis; Poliomyelitis. Combined with calcaneus in poliomyelitis. Combined with equinus in spastic paralysis.

R. G. Beard.

COMA

Coma is a state of deep unconsciousness from which the patient cannot be roused by speech, shaking, or other ordinary form of stimulus such as might prove effective in conditions of stupor. It may be due to many different causes, classified into two main groups, namely: (*A*) Cases in which coma is a late development of a disease, the nature of which has been suggested by other symptoms; (*B*) Cases in which coma comes on early and is the most prominent feature of the case. This broad distinction, although useful practically, has obvious deficiencies, for it is clear that in conditions such as diabetes, cerebral tumour, head injuries, etc., coma may occur either early or late. But generally speaking, the diagnostic difficulties which invest this subject arise in the second group, and it is with these that the present section is mainly concerned.

Group A includes:

1. Severe Infections:

Typhoid fever	Malaria, etc.
Septicaemia	

2. Infections of the Nervous System:

All forms of meningitis	Cerebral abscess
Encephalomyelitis	Encephalitis
Trypanosomiasis	

3. Cerebral Tumours, primary or secondary.

4. Endogenous Intoxications and metabolic diseases:

Uraemia	Diabetes
Cholaemia	

5. Exogenous Poisons:

Arsenic	Lead, etc.

6. Cerebral Anaemia:

Terminal congestive heart failure	Severe anaemia Leukaemia

Group B. Coma occurring as the presenting sign in a previously healthy subject, or in one about whom no medical data are known:

1. Cerebral Vascular Accidents:

Cerebral thrombosis	Cerebral embolism
Cerebral haemorrhage	Subarachnoid haemorrhage

2. Head Injuries:

Cerebral concussion	Subdural haematoma
Cerebral contusion	Late traumatic apoplexy,
Middle meningeal haemorrhage	or delayed cerebral haemorrhage

3. The Acute Effects of Drugs and Poisons:

Alcohol	Insulin
Sedatives and hypnotics	Carbon monoxide, etc.

4. Endogenous Poisons:

Diabetic coma	Hyperinsulinism
Uraemia	Cholaemia
	Hypopituitarism

5. Cerebral Infections:

Fulminating meningococcal meningitis
Cerebral malaria
Rupture of cerebral abscess into the ventricles

6. Cerebral Tumours:

Cystic degeneration of a glioma	Haemorrhage into a tumour, primary or secondary

7. Postepileptic Coma.

8. Cerebral Ischaemia:

Hypertensive encephalopathy
Stokes-Adams syndrome
Cerebral anaemia from haemorrhage

9. The Effect of Physical Agents:

Heat-stroke	Extreme cold
Caisson disease	

10. 'Coma' in Psychological Illness.

When confronted with a case of coma, much help may be got from an interrogation of relatives or witnesses if these are available. Points of importance are the previous health of the patient, with particular reference to cardio-vascular symptoms, hypertension, recent head injury, factors indicating suicidal intentions, diabetes, renal disease, epileptic fits, exposure to malaria, and any abnormal conduct which might indicate either organic cerebral disease or a psychiatric illness. The circumstances under which the patient was discovered may be either relevant or misleading: a man found unconscious in the street, with head injuries, may have been knocked down or he may have fallen down as a result of a stroke; a smell of alcohol in the breath does not necessarily mean that the coma is due to alcohol. A woman found unconscious in her locked bedroom, with a half-empty bottle of aspirin tablets by her bedside, was found to be

suffering from fulminating meningococcal meningitis. Circumstantial evidence, however strong, must always be scrutinized with care, and the conclusions drawn therefrom must be checked by a meticulous physical examination. A stoker found unconscious in the tropics may have heat-stroke, but on the other hand he may be suffering from cerebral malaria; this circumstantial evidence will be put into correct perspective by physical examination, because if it is heat-stroke the skin will be dry whereas if it is cerebral malaria sweating will be normal or excessive. It is necessary, therefore, to conduct a careful and complete examination in every case of coma.

Vascular Accidents. *Cerebral thrombosis,* a common cause of coma, occurs in arteriosclerotics and syphilitics. There is usually some indication of a local unilateral lesion, such as facial asymmetry, conjugate deviation of the eyes, or undue flaccidity of the arm and leg on one side. The tendon reflexes are uniformly depressed in the early stages, but those on the affected side may ultimately become unduly brisk. Bilateral extensor plantar responses are the rule in deep coma from any cause, central or toxic, but if the coma lightens a unilateral extensor response may be obtained.

Cerebral haemorrhage is usually fatal, coma rapidly deepening to a fatal issue; there is usually a raised blood-pressure and a slow pulse; the left ventricle is enlarged, and hypertensive retinopathy may be present. If blood has escaped into the ventricles, the temperature may be raised, and if it has spread to the cervical subarachnoid space the neck may be stiff. Localizing signs, as described above, may or may not be present. Pontine haemorrhage produces hyperpyrexia and pin-point pupils (*Fig.* 179).

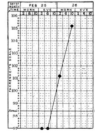

Fig. 179. Temperature chart showing typical pyrexia due to pontine haemorrhage of rapidly fatal type.

The diagnosis of *cerebral embolism* depends on the combination of a sudden cerebral catastrophe with a cardiac or pulmonary lesion capable of giving rise to an embolus—endocarditis, coronary thrombosis, auricular fibrillation or flutter, pulmonary infarct, bronchiectasis, lung abscess, etc. Detachment of a clot from an atheromatous plaque in the arch of the aorta or one of the common carotid arteries may cause cerebral embolism in the absence of any cardiac or pulmonary disease. *Subarachnoid haemorrhage* occurs in young adults from a rupture of a congenital aneurysm and in elderly arteriopaths from bursting of an atheromatous vessel. The onset is abrupt, and there is usually some stiffness of the neck. The temperature may be slightly raised, and glycosuria and albuminuria may be present. Oculomotor palsies (manifested as strabismus, sometimes by inequality of the pupils and drooping of the lid) are not uncommon. The spinal fluid is heavily blood-stained, and if the haemorrhage has been present for some hours, the supernatant fluid obtained by centrifuging a specimen will show xanthochromia.

comparatively mild head injury in adults, but it may occur in infants as a result of excessive moulding of the head in difficult labour. In adults it gives rise to a relapsing impairment of consciousness which varies from drowsiness to coma, with remarkable intermissions. Headache is often severe. Localizing symptoms are either absent or slight; evidence of pyramidal interference may be present on one side of the body, but it varies in degree from time to time and is sometimes found on the 'wrong' side of the body—a false localizing sign. A large subdural collection over the vertex may push the

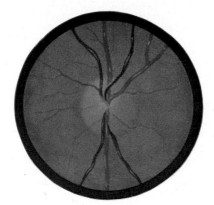 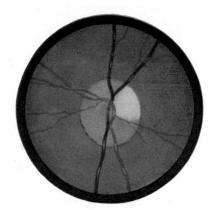

| Right optic disk | Left optic disk |

Fig. 180. Optic neuritis in the right eye, and segmental optic atrophy in the left eye, in the same patient, a case of chronic plumbism. The white segment of atrophy in the left optic disk results from degeneration of those fibres which come from the macular region, the remaining optic fibres not being atrophic.

Head Injuries may or may not be obvious. Inspection and palpation may reveal bruises and depression of the skull. Leakage of spinal fluid from the nose or ear is significant. Subconjunctival haemorrhage spreading forwards from the back of the eye indicates a fracture of the anterior or middle fossa. Localizing signs are rare in concussion, but may be found in cases with severe contusion of the motor cortex. Haemorrhage from the middle meningeal artery may complicate fractures of the squamous portion of the temporal bone; the 'classic' history of concussion, followed by recovery of consciousness and subsequent relapse into deepening coma with signs of increasing intracranial pressure, is not always present, for if the initial concussion has been severe there may be no lucid interval, the picture being one of steadily deepening coma. Radiological evidence of fracture at the appropriate site strengthens the case for immediate exploration when this condition is suspected. *Delayed traumatic apoplexy* — intracerebral haemorrhage occurring hours or days after a closed head injury—is a rare condition characterized by abrupt aggravation of symptoms, with the appearance of focal or localizing signs. Immediate craniotomy with aspiration of the blood-clot affords the only chance of survival. *Chronic subdural haematoma* is usually the result of a

brain downwards, with herniation of the inner margin of the temporal lobes into the posterior fossa; this compresses the brain-stem and may give rise to nuclear and supranuclear ocular palsies, which show the same fluctuations in severity as the coma. The pressure of the spinal fluid may be raised, or very low, or it may fluctuate from high to low on successive examinations. The contents are usually normal. Papilloedema is rare. Recurrent and fluctuating coma should always suggest the possibility of subdural haematoma, but it occurs in both primary and secondary cerebral tumours. The intermittent 'sleepiness' of trypanosomiasis is unlikely to cause confusion.

Coma due to Poisoning is a common event. *Carbon monoxide*, which is present in coal-gas, in the exhaust gases of petrol engines, and in the fumes given off by any fire or explosion if the supply of oxygen is defective, unites with the haemoglobin of the blood to form carboxyhaemoglobin, which is cherry-red in colour and imparts this hue to the complexion of the patient; the colour is not always obvious, and spectroscopic examination of the blood may then become necessary, but in most cases the circumstances under which the comatose patient was found will indicate the precise nature of the condition.

Acute alcoholic coma is marked by pallor,

sweating, collapse, and stertorous breathing. The pupils are first dilated, and later contracted: the reflexes are reduced and the plantar responses may be extensor or flexor. The smell of alcohol in the breath, or its presence in the stomach contents, does not necessarily mean that the coma is due to alcohol. Moreover, alcohol can precipitate other comas, notably epileptic and diabetic coma. Examination of the blood will show an alcohol content in excess of 300 mg. per 100 ml. in true alcoholic coma.

Opium and its derivatives, and morphine, are to be suspected when coma is accompanied by pin-point pupils and a normal or subnormal temperature. Coma with pin-point pupils also occurs in pontine haemorrhage, but in this condition the temperature is usually high.

Barbiturate poisoning has become increasingly frequent in recent years as a means of committing suicide. The general appearance is that of severe depression of the central nervous system, with slow respiration and generalized flaccidity. Coma due to *bromide* poisoning is associated with a blood-bromide level in the region of 250 mg. per cent; a bromide rash may be present in cases of chronic bromism, but is often absent. Poisoning with *acetylsalicylic acid* (aspirin) is marked by hyperpnoea (due to acidaemia) and by muscular twitches; the urine and the cerebrospinal fluid give a violet colour reaction with ferric perchloride.

Lead poisoning occasionally gives rise to lead encephalopathy, particularly in young children, with convulsive fits and coma. The blood-pressure and cerebrospinal pressure are raised, and there may be papilloedema (*Fig.* 180). Other features of plumbism—the 'lead line' in the gums, punctate basophilia, and the presence in abnormal amounts of lead in the urine—are occasionally present. *Arsenic* and *gold* may cause coma, with or without convulsions; in the past this was usually seen as a result of overdosage with intravenous preparations of these substances; today they are practically never given by this route.

Petrol fumes may cause sudden unconsciousness in men engaged in cleaning out petrol storage tanks under conditions of defective ventilation.

Insulin coma, whether the result of overdosage or of hypersecretion by a tumour of the islets of Langerhans, is marked by collapse, low blood-pressure, sweating, and low blood-sugar. Convulsions frequently occur in the early stages of the condition. Careful search of the skin for signs of hypodermic injections is essential in this as in all cases of coma. *Carbolic acid,* present in certain disinfectants, is usually taken by mouth with suicidal intent. The mucous membrane of the mouth may be whitened, and the characteristic smell will be conspicuous.

Poisoning with *Cannabis indica* gives rise to a condition akin to drunkenness, followed by delirium and coma.

Hypercalcaemia arising from an excessive intake of milk and alkalis in the treatment of peptic ulcer over a long period may cause confusion, irritability, aggression, nausea, generalized pruritus, and—rarely—coma. Renal damage is present, with albuminuria, a raised blood-urea, and polyuria. This so-called 'milk-alkali syndrome' is both avoidable and reversible.

Endogenous Poisons. In diabetic coma the patient is dehydrated and collapsed; acetone will be smelt in the breath and the urine will contain sugar and ketones. An examination of the urine for these abnormal constituents should be carried out as a routine in every case of coma, whether diabetes appears probable or not.

Uraemia is marked by dehydration, dyspnoea, high blood-pressure, hypertensive retinopathy, and the presence of albumin in the urine, the specific gravity of which will usually be in the region of 1010. The blood-urea will be much elevated, and the alkali reserve diminished. Hepatic coma usually terminates a period of prolonged illness, a circumstance which usually brings the patient under medical observation before coma supervenes but this may not be the case when the failure of liver function is due to acute hepatic necrosis.

In more chronic liver disease and before coma supervenes there may be the picture of an organic psychosis which may be accompanied by a 'flapping' tremor. This tremor is coarse, irregular, and bilateral and is characterized by flexion–extension movements at the wrists. This tremor may also precede or follow the period of mental confusion. These features are not specific for hepatic pre-coma, occurring also in uraemia and respiratory failure, so the diagnosis rests on other features of liver disease such as foetor hepaticus, jaundice, or ascites.

Coma occurs in and is a frequent terminal complication of hypopituitarism and is especially liable to follow infections. It is probably due to a complex interaction of several factors which include hypoglycaemia, hypothermia, water intoxication, and adrenal insufficiency.

A patient with myxoedema may gradually become comatose and this coma is associated with hypothermia, developing usually when the weather is cold. This coma is clinically indistinguishable from that due to hypopituitarism.

Cerebral Infections. *Fulminating meningococcal meningitis* may cause coma and death within 24 hours. The temperature is usually elevated, but may be subnormal; stiffness of the neck may or may not be present; a fine purpuric rash is common. Diagnosis is by lumbar puncture, which will reveal a cloudy fluid containing the organisms and polymorph leucocytes. *Lumbar puncture should be carried out at an early stage in any case of coma in which the diagnosis is not obvious. Cerebral malaria* is an important cause of sudden coma in subjects who have been exposed to the infection. Whereas this possibility is in the mind of all who work in malarial regions, it is often forgotten by clinicians in temperate zones, and an inquiry as to the recent movements of the patient is therefore an important matter in any case of coma. The temperature may be normal or high; the spleen may or may not be enlarged. Diagnosis, a matter of great urgency if life is to be saved, depends on a careful and prolonged search for *P. falciparum* in blood-smears stained by Leishman's or Giemsa's stain. *Cerebral abscess* usually brings the patient under medical supervision before the onset of coma, but occasionally the early symptoms are mild and there is a sudden lapse into coma when the abscess bursts into the ventricles or into the subarachnoid space. High temperature, rigidity of the neck, and the presence of pus in the spinal fluid will indicate the nature of the disease. But this is a very rare cause of coma of sudden onset.

Cerebral Tumour. Coma is usually late or terminal in cerebral neoplasms, whether primary or secondary, but there are rare cases in which haemorrhage into a small tumour causes sudden unconsciousness in a subject who has not been aware of any disability: cystic degeneration of a glioma may also cause a rapid aggravation of symptoms, ending in coma. The presence of papilloedema and a raised cerebrospinal pressure are suggestive, but the presence of coma precludes the identification of localizing signs with the exception of those indicating interruption of the pyramidal tracts. Jacksonian attacks during the period of coma may provide confirmation, but the final diagnosis depends on the demonstration of a mass by gamma or EMI-scan; in some cases of haemorrhage into a tumour, a diagnosis of cerebral haemorrhage is made during life and the cause of the haemorrhage, the tumour, is discovered post mortem.

Epilepsy. Coma may last for a few minutes after a single epileptic attack, or it may persist for hours between the repeated attacks of status epilepticus. This statement holds for both idiopathic and symptomatic forms of epileptic attack. The brief coma which follows a single attack is no problem, for recovery ensues and allows a history to be taken from the patient. The coma of status epilepticus is not in itself a problem, although the cause of the fits—whether idiopathic or due to organic disease of the brain—may require detailed investigation. In all cases of coma, an examination of the lips, cheeks, and tongue should be made in search of the recent cuts or old scars which may mean that there have been previous fits.

Coma in Cerebral Ischaemia. Coma results from cerebral ischaemia in severe acute haemorrhage; the blanched aspect, air hunger, and indication of external or internal haemorrhage will be obvious on clinical examination. The sudden rises of blood-pressure which are encountered in severe essential hypertension, in malignant hypertension, eclampsia, chronic nephritis, and lead poisoning with hypertension, give rise to *hypertensive encephalopathy*, which is characterized either by transient focal symptoms such as aphasia, monoplegia, hemianopia, etc., or by epileptiform fits with coma between the attacks. The association of coma with fits and a very high blood-pressure will suggest either a cerebral haemorrhage or hypertensive encephalopathy; removal of 20–30 oz. of blood by venesection is a safe and helpful procedure which has diagnostic value inasmuch as it usually arrests an encephalopathic attack but has little influence on cerebral haemorrhage. *Stokes-Adams attacks* (p. 111)—syncopal or epileptiform fits resulting from sudden slowing of the pulse by heart-block—are usually transient incidents except in elderly arteriopaths, in whom the sudden slowing of the circulation may favour the occurrence of cerebral thrombosis which perpetuates the coma and produces appropriate clinical signs of a focal cerebral lesion.

Physical Agents. *Heat-stroke*, with its hyperpyrexia and absence of sweating, is easily diagnosed by the circumstances of its occurrence in tropical conditions or in stokeholds. Reference has already been made to the danger of ascribing every case of coma arising in such conditions to the effects of heat; stokers and residents in the tropics are equally subject to cerebral malaria, cerebral vascular accidents, diabetic coma, and so on. The coma which ends life under conditions of *extreme cold* presents no difficulties. *Caisson disease* is the name given to the symptoms which result when a man returns too quickly to normal atmospheric pressure after being exposed to a pressure which exceeds the normal by 18 lb. to the square inch or more. Under such conditions the tissues—in particular the fat and relatively avascular structures—are saturated with nitrogen, which is released in the form of bubbles when the pressure is reduced. These bubbles exert a mechanical effect on the affected tissues, with the production of pain in the joints ('the bends'), epigastric pain and abdominal distension, paraplegia, hemiplegia, and coma. The diagnosis is made obvious by the circumstances of its occurrence. Similar symptoms occur as a result of rapid climbs in aircraft, the danger being particularly marked at altitudes over 30,000 ft.

'Coma' in Psychological Illness. Conditions of impaired consciousness are not uncommon in certain psychological illnesses, but the term coma, with its conventional organic meaning, is hardly applicable to them and the only reason for their inclusion here is that they may be mistaken for other conditions. Stupor occurs in schizophrenia and severe melancholia, and trance states are not uncommon in hysterical subjects. Diagnosis rests upon the absence of physical signs of organic disease, the presence of psychiatric features in the history, and on an impression difficult to describe but very real, that the subject is aware of what is going on around him.

Ian Mackenzie.

CONFABULATION

Confabulation may occur in patients who suffer from a disorder of registration or of retentive memory who, without insight into their defect, tend to fill the gaps so caused, with irrelevant or seemingly invented material. Thus a patient who has been continuously in hospital over a period of time may, for example, insist, on questioning, that he has been out all the morning travelling by train, and will describe places he has seen and people he has met. Such tales are not deliberate lies but falsifications which arise from an incapacity to remember what really has been happening, together with an inability to distinguish fantasy from fact.

Confabulation is a common feature of *Korsakow's syndrome* (and of *Wernicke's encephalopathy* with which it may be associated). Although most patients with Korsakow's syndrome, being highly suggestible, can usually be induced to confabulate, confabulation is not evident in every case, despite the fact that the characteristic disorder of *retentive memory* and, consequent upon this, *disorientation* of time and place are invariably present. The causal lesion of the mental manifestations of Korsakow's syndrome lies in the mamillary bodies or in the mamillothalamic tracts. The usual overall cause is alcoholism, giving rise to thiamine deficiency. *Peripheral neuropathy* is commonly present and, in the case of Wernicke's encephalopathy, *ophthalmoplegia* and other more central symptoms also.

A similar psychosis known as the *dysmnesic-confabulatory syndrome*, having a number of other somewhat rarer causes, may be encountered. These include *gastric carcinoma*, *anoxia*—due perhaps to strangulation or anaesthetic accidents —*head injury*, etc. In *senile psychoses* and in *Alzheimer's disease*, confabulation may occur in a setting of overall dementia in patients who at first sight may seem to be relatively well preserved. Indeed their tendency to confabulate may actually mask the degree of dementia which closer and more detailed examination will reveal, so much so that in an ordinary social setting they will discuss a variety of topics in an apparently sensible though superficial manner. This state, when marked, is known as *presbyophrenia*.

Confabulation must be distinguished from the conscious lying of the malingerer and that of certain psychopaths; also from *pseudologia phantastica*, which is the name given to fantastic tale-telling by those of markedly hysterical disposition who prefer fantasy to fact and have a neurotic need for aggrandizement ('Walter Mitty' syndrome). The confabulation of patients with Korsakow's syndrome is never of this order but merely mundane and concerned largely with trivia. Some paranoid schizophrenics will tell tales based upon a delusional system often of a grandiose kind and thus claim to be of royal blood, etc. But as their memory for everyday events is simultaneously preserved this, too, is not true confabulation but an outcome of what is known as *double orientation*.

Finally, some other patients showing *hysterical pseudodementia* or the *Ganser syndrome* may give remarkable and, at first sight, confabulatory answers to direct questions. Those answers are characterized by a 'near-miss' quality (*approximate answers*) and are given so consistently that it soon becomes obvious to the listener that the subject must be aware of the correct answer in order to give incorrect replies in so consistent a manner. This, again, is not true confabulation but a near-conscious phenomenon which in some cases is not far short of malingering.

W. H. Trethowan.

CONJUNCTIVA, NON-INFLAMMATORY AFFECTIONS OF

Pinguecula is a yellowish thickening of the conjunctiva, to either side of the cornea. It is usually found in elderly people, especially those exposed to dust and wind, and is due to a hyaline degeneration. It is harmless and needs no treatment.

Pterygium is a wing-shaped encroachment of the conjunctiva on the cornea, which may grow across the pupillary area if left long enough and then demands surgical removal (*Fig.* 181). It is more commonly found in coloured people. It is to be distinguished from *pseudo-pterygium*, which

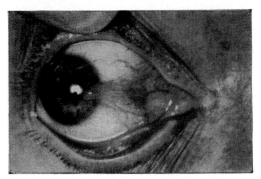

Fig. 181. Pterygium. (*Institute of Ophthalmology.*)

is due to adhesion of a fold of chemotic conjunctiva to a corneal ulcer, and is not attached except at its tip.

Cysts of the conjunctiva may be *retention cysts*, which are usually single and relatively large, or *lymphangiectatic*, which are commonly multiple. In both cases they usually disappear when the outer layer has been snipped off (after inserting a drop of local anaesthetic). Occasionally single multilocular lymphangiomata occur. Sometimes an *implantation cyst* follows an injury or operation.

Papilloma of the conjunctiva is commonest at the inner canthus or at the lid-margin. The growth is often exuberant and tends to bleed readily; it is usually moulded in shape by the lids, and consequently may be polypoid. They occasionally become malignant, and should be removed.

A *granuloma* may derive from a chalazion, sometimes after incision and curettage, and has a characteristic flattened appearance. Granulomas may also develop in a socket after excision of the globe. *Naevi* or congenital moles may be pale or pigmented. They may occur in connexion with a similar growth of the skin at the lid margin, or separately at the limbus or on the plica semilunaris. The favourite site for a *dermolipoma of the conjunctiva* is at the limbus; it is a white or yellow lenticular tumour and occasionally bears hairs. *Dermolipomas*, often of considerable size, may be found at the outer canthus, often in continuity with the normal orbital fat. Any *hyperplasia at the limbus* should be removed for biopsy, lest it prove malignant.

P. Trevor-Roper.

CONSCIOUSNESS, DISORDERS OF

Consciousness, although not wholly definable, is clearly a function of the activity of the nervous system. Impairment of this by injury, disease, or intoxication may produce changes in behaviour which may be the outcome of alterations in the level of awareness.

Levels of impairment are well illustrated by the stages of recovery from *head injury*. After a head injury of moderate severity, the patient may be completely unconscious, with flaccid paralysis and absent tendon reflexes. During recovery, this state of *coma* is followed by *stupor*, a condition in which the tendon reflexes can be elicited and apparently purposive movements of a protective kind may occur. He may even, at this stage, open his eyes and turn his head from side to side as if examining his environment (*coma vigil*). However, this appearance is probably deceptive; for it is more likely that he is actually inaccessible and completely unaware of his surroundings. The first evidence of returning consciousness is a positive response to a simple command. A phase of *restless confusion* succeeds stupor during which the patient may be resistive and violent, a state of *delirium* which tends to be worse at night. Later, he becomes quieter and is capable of conversation, but his thoughts are not fully coherent. Because he may misinterpret his environment he may give way to impulsive actions. Alternatively, a state of automatism may occur in which there is adequate response to inner needs and external stimuli, so that general behaviour does not differ greatly from normal. Mental examination will, however, reveal lack of insight and judgement together with a gross defect of memory for recent events, and more or less complete *disorientation* for time and place. A *tendency to confabulate* may be evident. This phase is not invariable, and is often brief. The fact that subsequently there is *amnesia* for events during this phase demonstrates that consciousness has not fully returned. The final stage of *recovery* is marked by return of the capacity to recall current events, with correct orientation and insight. The duration of these phases of recovery may be an hour or two, several days, or sometimes weeks. Their sequence is, however, more or less regular. There is loss of memory for the injury, often for the period immediately before it, and for all the phases of recovery, including the phase of automatism.

States of altered consciousness resembling one or other of these phases may be, for example, due to intoxication with barbiturates or alcohol (*alcoholic 'blackouts'* in which inability to remember the 'night before' is the main feature). The same may occur in other *delirious* conditions (*see* DELIRIUM, p. 205) and in epilepsy. Periods of confusion with clouding of consciousness sometimes occur in association with *cerebral arteriosclerosis* and may be accompanied by signs of a focal cerebral lesion. Sudden interruption of consciousness may also occur as a result of spinal fluid blockage due to the ball-valve action of *paraphyseal (colloid) cysts* of the third ventricle. Such attacks are more liable to occur when the patient is in the supine position.

Repeated attacks, of which altered consciousness is a feature, may be symptomatic of epilepsy. Sudden and transient 'absences' are one form of *petit mal*. During a temporal lobe seizure— so-called *psychomotor epilepsy*—there may be periods of clouded consciousness accompanied by *automatism*. During this the patient may be hallucinated but later have no recollection of or insight into his experience. Some patients, on the other hand, remain partially in touch with the environment but although aware of what is going on around them are unable to respond. Such states may persist only for a few minutes, for days, or even a week or two (*twilight states*). An E.E.G. will usually show epileptic activity during these episodes.

States of confusion, with irrational or violent actions, may also accompany *hypoglycaemia*; tremor, giddiness, tachycardia, and apprehension may occur, and the condition can resemble a hysterical seizure, a bout of drunkenness (which may have disastrous results if a patient is incarcerated in a police cell on this mistaken account), or an anxiety attack. In hypoglycaemia the blood-sugar is invariably low. *Hyperventilation* attacks can produce a similar clinical picture though, in this instance, the blood-sugar level will be normal.

Hysterical and severely depressed patients may also occasionally be subject to spells of intense emotional disturbance in which consciousness seems to be altered. The content of their experiences may often be shown to have a comprehensible and understandable meaning when the patient's life situation is known. Episodes of wandering (*fugues*), in which the patient breaks away from his ordinary life and claims that he has lost his identity, can occur in depression and in hysterical and some *psychopathic* subjects. As the immediate precipitant is usually an unpleasant situation, the fugue represents an attempt to escape from it. In such circumstances *simulation* may sometimes be suspected depending on the type and extent of the motivation underlying the patient's condition.

W. H. Trethowan.

CONSTIPATION

I. ACUTE

Acute constipation may be: (A) due to acute intestinal obstruction; (B) a symptom of some general disease or of some other acute abdominal disease; or (C) to a sudden alteration in daily habits, e.g., admission to hospital.

A. ACUTE INTESTINAL OBSTRUCTION

The following points help in the distinction between acute intestinal obstruction and severe cases of acute constipation of other origin:

1. In other conditions the constipation is incomplete, in that flatus, and even a small quantity of faeces, may be passed spontaneously. A rectal examination should always be made. In organic intestinal obstruction the rectum is usually empty. If it contains faeces these may be present below an obstruction or, if impacted, may themselves be responsible for the occlusion, but it is exceedingly rare for faecal impaction to produce symptoms quite comparable in severity with those due to acute obstruction. In doubtful cases, it used to be the custom to carry out the two-enema test; the first enema generally brought away a certain amount of faeces even if obstruction was complete; the second, given at an interval of half to one hour, resulted in the passage of faeces or flatus if obstruction was incomplete, whereas, in complete obstruction, the second enema was either retained or expelled unaltered. This test should never be employed; it is exhausting to the patient, time wasting, and the information obtained is often equivocal. Diagnosis can usually be made on clinical grounds supplemented by abdominal X-rays.

2. Vomiting is rarely a feature of constipation, whereas it is frequently present in small-bowel obstruction, and in late cases becomes faeculent.

3. Visible peristalsis, accompanied by noisy borborygmi, is never present except in obstruction.

4. Obstruction is accompanied by progressive distension of the abdomen.

5. Pain is usually the first symptom of intestinal obstruction and is colicky in nature; its severity is out of all proportion to the mild abdominal discomfort that may accompany simple constipation.

Plain X-rays of the abdomen are essential in the diagnosis of intestinal obstruction and in attempting to localize its site. A loop or loops of distended bowel are usually seen, together with multiple fluid levels. Small bowel is suggested by a ladder pattern of distended loops, by their central position, and by striations which pass completely across the width of the distended loop and which are produced by its circular mucosal folds (*Fig.* 182). Distended large bowel tends to lie peripherally and to show the corrugations produced by the taenia coli (*Fig.* 183). A small percentage, perhaps 5 per cent of intestinal obstructions, shows no abnormality on plain X-rays. This is due to the bowel being completely distended with fluid in a closed loop and thus without the fluid levels which are produced by coexistent gas.

Aetiology of Acute Intestinal Obstructions. The causes of intestinal obstruction may be classified as:

1. In the lumen—faecal impaction, gall-stone ileus, pedunculated tumour, and meconium ileus.

2. In the wall—congenital atresia, Crohn's disease, tumours, diverticular disease of the colon, and tuberculous stricture.

3. Outside the wall—strangulated hernia (external or internal), volvulus, intussusception, adhesions, and bands.

Before considering any other possibility, all the hernial apertures should be examined, even in the absence of local pain, as a small strangulated femoral hernia in an obese woman, for example, may easily be overlooked.

The following points should be considered in determining the cause of the acute intestinal obstruction.

1. AGE. Intestinal obstruction in the newborn should always be suspected in the presence of bile-vomiting; the rectum should be examined first for the presence of an imperforate anus; other possibilities are congenital atresia or stenosis of the intestine, volvulus neonatorum, meconium ileus, and Hirschsprung's disease. In infants the commonest cause of intestinal obstruction is intussusception, but Hirschsprung's disease, strangulated inguinal hernia, and obstruction due to a band from the tip of a Meckel's diverticulum should be considered. In young adults and patients of middle age, adhesions and bands from previous surgery or intraperitoneal inflammation are common, but strangulated hernia and Crohn's disease are also encountered. In older patients strangulated herniae, carcinoma of the bowel, and diverticular disease, as well as postoperative adhesions, are all common conditions.

2. HISTORY. The history of a previous abdominal operation, or of inflammatory pelvic disease in females, suggest the possibility of bands or adhesions. A history of biliary colic or of the symptoms which may result from cholecystitis may suggest that obstruction might be due to impaction of a gall-stone in the ileum. Obstruction following a period of increasing constipation, perhaps with blood or slime in the stools or spurious diarrhoea, in a middle-aged or elderly patient, suggests cancer or diverticular disease of the colon. The history in an infant or child that blood and mucus have been passed per rectum is suggestive of an intussusception.

3. ABDOMINAL EXAMINATION. We have already mentioned the importance of searching specifically for a strangulated hernia. The presence of a recent or old laparotomy scar always raises the possibility of postoperative adhesions. Gross distension generally means that the obstruction is in the colon; if occurring very soon after the onset of symptoms it suggests volvulus of the sigmoid or, less commonly, the caecum. If distension has been present to a less extent for some time before the onset of acute symptoms, a growth is likely.

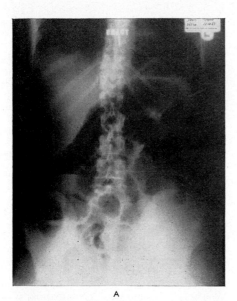

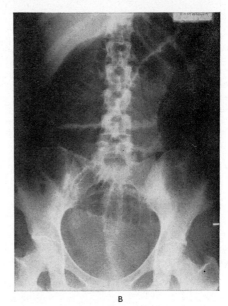

Fig. 182. Small bowel obstruction due to a band. A, Erect, showing fluid levels. B, Supine, showing ladder pattern of distended small bowel loops; the valvulae conniventes make complete bands across the width of the gut.

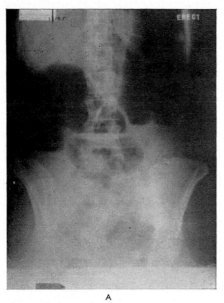

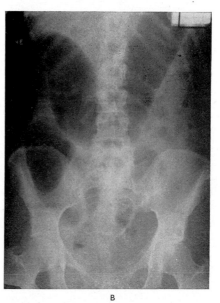

Fig. 183. Large bowel obstruction due to carcinoma of sigmoid colon. A, Erect, showing fluid levels. B, Supine: gas distends the colon and caecum; the haustrae make incomplete bands across the width of the gut.

In infants and small children great distension suggests Hirschsprung's disease. Slight distension occurs when the obstruction is in the duodenum or high in the jejunum.

The diagnosis of intussusception can be made with certainty only when the characteristic sausage-shaped tumour situated somewhere in the course of the colon is felt. In acute obstruction due to cancer the tumour is often not palpable as it may be disguised by the dilated intestine; however, large masses are sometimes felt, especially when present in the right or left iliac fossa. On the right side, they are generally due to cancer of the caecum, on the left to cancer of the sigmoid colon or diverticular disease.

4. RECTAL EXAMINATION. A growth of the rectum should be recognized easily, although this is rather unusual as a cause of obstruction.

Sometimes a growth of the pelvic colon can be felt through the front wall of the rectum. In infants, the tip of an intussusception may be felt in the lumen of the rectum and the typical red-currant-jelly stool (a mixture of blood and mucus) will be seen on the examining finger. Occasionally the mother will report that a sausage-like structure actually prolapses from the child's anal verge during the attacks of colic accompanying the intussusception. I have only seen this on one occasion.* A much-ballooned rectum suggests obstruction in the colon; this is an undoubted fact but its cause is obscure.

5. VOMITING. The more frequent the vomiting and the earlier the onset of faeculent vomiting the higher in the intestine is the obstruction likely to be. Its onset is later and its occurrence less frequent in cases of colonic obstruction.

B. SYMPTOMATIC

1. IN ACUTE GENERAL DISEASES. Constipation beginning acutely is a frequent symptom of a large variety of acute infective and other diseases. It is never so severe as to become a presenting symptom and the other features in the majority of cases are so much more striking that the presence of constipation has little influence on making a diagnosis.

2. IN ACUTE ABDOMINAL CONDITIONS. Constipation is a conpicuous symptom in most acute abdominal conditions. However, once again, other symptoms are often so well marked that the question of intestinal obstruction hardly arises. Thus it frequently accompanies acute appendicitis, salpingitis, perforation of a peptic ulcer, and biliary and renal colic. In lead colic the constipation is not absolute and the occupation of the patient, the blue line on the gums, and the presence of punctate basophilia point to the diagnosis.

3. CHANGES OF DAILY ROUTINE may precipitate constipation as in patients admitted to hospital, children going to boarding school, or patients suddenly being confined to bed from illness.

II. CHRONIC

Constipation can be defined as delay in the passage of faeces through the large bowel and is frequently associated with difficulty in defaecation. Most people empty the bowel once in every 24 hours, but there is a considerable range of variation in perfectly normal individuals; in one recent study this varied from three bowel actions daily to one act every three days.

The abnormal action of the bowel in constipation may manifest itself in three different ways:

1. Defaecation may occur with insufficient frequency.

---

* The editor (F. D. H.) has seen it in an adult woman suffering from systemic lupus erythematosus treated on high dosage of corticosteroids. She finally passed 18 cm. of her large intestine, felt much improved, and lived a year thereafter before dying of vascular complications of her disease.

2. The stools may be insufficient in quantity and a certain amount of faeces is retained although the bowels may be opened once daily or more often (cumulative constipation).

3. The bowels may be open daily yet the faeces are hard and dry owing to prolonged retention in the bowel, dehydration, or insufficient residue in the food consumed.

The commoner causes of constipation are as follows:

1. Organic obstructions, for example carcinoma of the colon or diverticular disease.

2. Painful anal conditions, e.g., fissure in ano or prolapsed piles.

3. Adynamic bowel as may occur in Hirschsprung's disease, senility, spinal cord injuries and diseases, and myxoedema.

4. Drugs which decrease peristaltic activity of the bowel—including codeine, probanthine and other ganglion-blocking agents, and morphine.

5. Habit and diet, for example dehydration, starvation, lack of suitable bulk in the diet, and dyschezia.

It is comparatively rare for a patient to consult a doctor on account of constipation without having already attempted to cure himself with aperients. The symptoms generally ascribed to 'auto-intoxication' caused by intestinal stasis are usually really caused by the purgatives themselves, which may produce depletion of sodium and potassium in the resultant watery stools, or from the abdominal colic and flatulence produced by powerful aperients.

In spite of his probable protests, the patient is instructed to see what happens if no drugs are taken for a few days, an attempt being made to open the bowels each morning on a normal diet containing plenty of fruit and vegetables. In most cases he loses his abdominal pains and so-called 'toxic' symptoms. During this test the bowels are often opened daily, in which case a diagnosis of functional pseudoconstipation can be made, the patient having suggested to himself, as a result of faulty education combined with advice of his friends and with the reading of pernicious advertisements, that he was constipated and required aperients to keep himself well; whereas a little psychotherapy in the form of explanation of the physiology of his bowels and the origin of his symptoms, and persuasion to try to open his bowels each morning without artificial help results in a cure.

The investigation of constipation entails a careful and accurate history, full examination including, of course, examination of the rectum and sigmoidoscopy, followed, in some cases, by special laboratory tests and a barium-enema X-ray examination.

Organic Obstructions. The two common causes of narrowing of the lumen of the large bowel are diverticular disease and carcinoma of the colon. Other non-malignant strictures are rare but include Crohn's disease of the large bowel, stricture complicating ulcerative colitis, and tuberculous stricture.

Organic stricture of the colon is most commonly due to carcinoma. The possibility of cancer should always be considered when an individual above the age of 40, whose bowels have been regular previously, without change of diet or habit develops constipation of increasing severity, or when a patient who is habitually constipated becomes more so without obvious reason. The constipation is at first intermittent and may alternate with diarrhoea, or rather with a frequent desire to go to stool without effective evacuation. Aperients become steadily less helpful. There may be colicky pain and episodes of distension and the patient may notice blood, pus, and mucus in the faeces. Examination of the abdomen may reveal a palpable mass due to the presence of the tumour itself or to inspissated faeces which have become impacted above a cancerous stricture which is itself impalpable. Progressive loss of weight and strength, anorexia, and anaemia are rather late features of the disease. A rectal examination reveals a usually empty rectum but not infrequently a carcinoma in the sigmoid colon can be felt through the rectal wall as the mass in this loop of bowel prolapses into the pelvis. An occult blood-test on any faecal material is often positive. Sigmoidoscopy may visualize the tumour and its nature can be confirmed by biopsy and histological examination. A barium-enema examination is invaluable (*Fig.* 184).

DIVERTICULAR DISEASE of the sigmoid colon can mimic carcinoma exactly and indeed the surgeon, even at laparotomy, may not be able to differentiate between the two conditions. The barium-enema examination (*Fig.* 185) is often helpful, but the radiologist may have difficulty himself in distinguishing a stricture due to one or other cause; indeed not infrequently these two common diseases may coexist.

Occasionally extracolonic masses may press upon the rectum or sigmoid colon with resultant constipation; for example, the pregnant uterus, a mass of fibroids, a large ovarian cyst, or other pelvic tumours.

Painful Anal Conditions. When defaecation is painful, reflex spasm of the anal sphincter may be produced with resultant acute constipation. A local cause of the pain such as a fissure in ano, strangulated haemorrhoids, or a perianal abscess is obvious on careful local examination.

Adynamic Bowel. In Hirschsprung's disease there is always a history of constipation dating from the first few months of life. The abdomen becomes greatly enlarged soon after birth and the outline of distended colon can be seen, often with visible peristalsis. The abdomen finally becomes enormous and it is then tense and tympanitic. There may be eversion of the umbilicus and marked widening of the subcostal angle. The condition is due to the absence of ganglion cells in the wall of the rectosigmoid region of the large bowel, although in some cases a more extensive part of the colon may be involved. Males are affected more often than females.

A barium-enema examination reveals gross dilatation of the colon leading down to a narrow funnel in the aganglionic rectum (*Fig.* 186).

Deficient motor activity of the bowel may be due to senile changes in the elderly and may be a

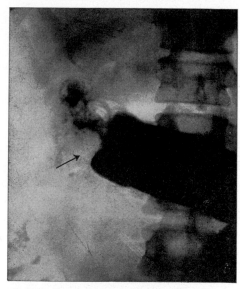

Fig. 184. Radiograph from a case of carcinoma near the end of the pelvic colon which obstructed a barium enema at the site marked by the arrow.

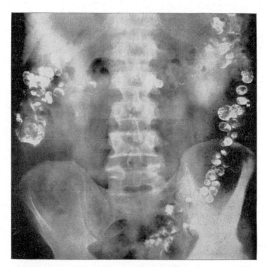

Fig. 185. Extensive diverticulosis in a patient showing a large duodenal diverticulum. (*Dr. Cochrane Shanks.*)

prominent feature of myxoedemic patients. Constipation may occur in the course of organic nervous diseases, including tabes dorsalis, spinal compression from tumour, transverse myelitis, and disseminated sclerosis, as well as cord transection in trauma. This is due to disturbance of the motor and sensory pathways responsible for defaecation.

Drugs. Many commonly employed drugs have a constipating effect on the bowel; these include codeine, morphine, and the ganglion-blocking agents. Constipation accompanied by abdominal pain may be a feature of lead-poisoning.

Habit and Diet. By far the greatest number of patients complaining of constipation fall into this group. When the faeces are abnormally hard as a result of dehydration, inadequate liquid intake, or

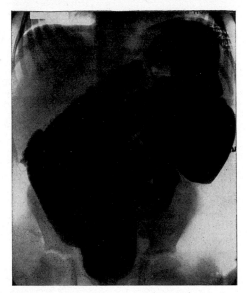

Fig. 186. Barium enema in a case of Hirschsprung's disease showing enormous dilatation of the pelvic colon. (*Dr. T. H. Hills.*)

inadequate cellulose material in the diet, rectal examination will reveal impacted faeces of rock-like consistency. This may occur as an acute phenomenon following barium-meal examination when masses of inspissated barium may lodge in the rectum.

Dyschezia is the term applied to difficulty in defaecation due to faulty bowel habit. The patient ignores the normal call to stool, the rectum distends with faeces with eventual loss of the defaecation reflex. The very same patient who gets into this habit is probably one who lives on the modern synthetic diet grossly deficient in roughage. As we have mentioned above, the so-called symptoms of constipation usually result from the purgatives that the patient ingests when he becomes anxious about the scarcity of his bowel actions. Rectal examination in such individuals often reveals large amounts of faeces in the rectum and more scybala may be palpated in the sigmoid colon. Dyschezia is, of course, present in those patients who have to remove faeces from the rectum digitally.

Harold Ellis.

CONTRACTURES

Contractures occur in five main groups of conditions—in spastic states, in lesions of the lower motor neuron, in hysteria, in diseases of joints, and as a result of disease or injury affecting the muscles themselves. In all cases, however, they can be either prevented or minimized if appropriate physiotherapy is applied in the early stages; severe contracture may therefore be regarded as evidence of neglect in most instances. In the section on spastic states it is pointed out that contractures may result when rigidity of posture has been long-standing and unopposed by any preventive measures. The outstanding example of contractures from disease of the lower motor neuron is *acute anterior poliomyelitis*, which begins suddenly with malaise, pains, and an acute febrile attack; flaccid paralysis appears early, and contractures begin to show themselves within a few months. The limbs are the parts most involved, isolated muscles or groups of muscles being paralysed; and it should be noted that the paralysis is distributed in accordance with the segmental grouping of the muscles in the anterior cornual region of the cord (*Fig.* 187). Sensibility is not affected, and

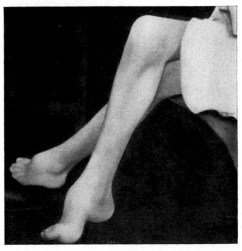

Fig. 187. Bilateral talipes equinovarus in a case of infantile paralysis. (*Dr. P. W. Saunders.*)

there is usually no disturbance of sphincter control. If many muscles in a limb are paralysed, its growth is much impaired. Contractures are less common in *motor neuron disease*; the hands and feet are mainly involved, with the production of various forms of club-foot (p. 162) and claw-hand (p. 162); fibrillation can be seen in the degenerating muscles, provided that they are not covered too thickly with subcutaneous tissue. The onset is insidious, and the disease occurs most often in middle age; the commonest type is that in which the hands are first and most involved, but in other cases the legs, and in others the upper arm and shoulder, first give evidence of the disease. Contractures are common in *neglected alcoholic neuritis* of the motor type, and also in *arsenical neuritis*, talipes equinovarus (*Fig.* 188) or flexor contracture of the wrist being noted; such deformities are rare in other forms of neuritis, such as those due to lead, diabetes, or diphtheria. Secondary contracture of the muscles on the affected side in *Bell's facial paralysis* may occur, and give rise to the impression

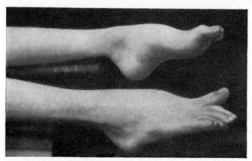

Fig. 188. Bilateral foot-drop (talipes equinus) in a case of peripheral neuritis. (*Dr. P. W. Saunders.*)

that the sound side of the face is paralysed while the face is at rest, for the face as a whole is pulled over to the affected side: on voluntary movement, however, the healthy side will be found to move normally, while the paralysed side remains comparatively still. Contractures are apt to follow severe *injury of nerves* unless appropriate measures are taken to prevent them.

Contractures from disuse may occur in otherwise healthy subjects who for any reason may have been kept too long in one position. Patients who have lain on their backs in bed for long periods may have a temporary talipes equinus when they get up—a contracture due to the weight of the bedclothes resting on the toes and keeping the feet extended. Fractured or injured limbs that have been splinted and kept too long in one position often exhibit contractures when the splints are removed (*Fig.* 189). In some cases, the contracture is due to fixation of the muscles, tendons, or muscle-sheaths by inflammatory products or haemorrhagic extravasations that have become organized, in others to adhesions or bony deposits that have formed in or about the joints, while in others mere disuse, without inflammatory changes, may underlie the contractures, which can be minimized by timely massage and movement.

'Paralyses' occur in many patients with *hysteria*. They may be spastic or flaccid. In hysterical contracture the affected muscles are not wasted except in severe cases of long duration; the deep reflexes are increased; a spurious ankle-clonus may be present; but Babinski's sign is not observed. The limbs are most affected (hemi-, mono-, or paraplegia), less often the muscles of the face. Certain attitudes are characteristic of hysterical paralyses; the elbows, wrists,

and fingers are kept flexed, the arms adducted; the hip and knee are extended, and the foot is held in a position of talipes equinovarus; ptosis may be simulated by spasm of the orbicularis palpebrarum; torticollis by contracture of the sternomastoid. In the less severe cases the stiffness and paresis are neither complete nor marked enough for the condition to be referred to as a contracture. The deformity produced is the result of active muscular spasm, and in severe

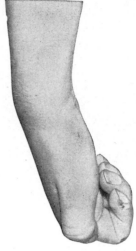

Fig. 189. Volkmann's ischaemic paralysis following the use of an anterior splint for fracture of the bones of the forearm. Note clenched fingers and the trophic sore on the forefinger.

and long-standing cases a true contracture results and the limb cannot be straightened by ordinary mechanical means, on account of adhesions around the joints and shortening of the muscles. Highly characteristic of hysterical contracture is the patient's use of antagonistic muscles to prevent passive or active correction of the deformity exhibited. If, for example, the arm is semiflexed by contracture of the biceps, the triceps can be felt to contract and resist the movement when the attempt is made to flex the arm farther. A similar contraction of the triceps can be felt or seen if the patient is asked to bend the joint herself; with the result that the joint remains unmoved, although all signs of great effort to bend the arm may be displayed. Pain and tenderness in the contracted muscles are usual; and other features such as hemi-anaesthesia, paraesthesia, clavus, globus hystericus, and the hysterical temperament, may be present. Special forms of hysterical contracture may give rise to great trouble in diagnosis by imitating other conditions or diseases. Thus a hysterical contraction of the rectus abdominis may simulate an abdominal tumour, and the maintenance of slight flexion of the hip, plus the aching pain to which such muscular spasm gives rise, may mimic a tuberculous hip-joint.

Other contractures are due to affections of the bones, joints, or soft tissues that mechanically obstruct correction of the deformities they produce. The contracted limbs can be straightened only by surgical measures, or by manipulations severe enough to rupture the obstructions.

Dupuytren's contracture of the palmar fascia, leading to deformity of the little and ring fingers, can seldom be mistaken (*Figs.* 190–192). It is

the movements of these structures. Injury to the sternomastoid at birth, leading either to a haematoma within the sheath of the muscle or to rupture of muscle-fibres, produces one form of 'congenital' torticollis. Large superficial *scars* due to extensive burns or losses of skin and the superficial tissues, being composed mainly of fibrous tissue, may contract, and so bring about marked contractures (*Fig.* 193).

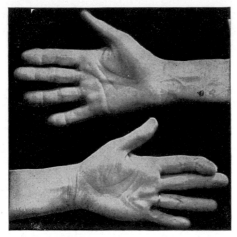

Fig. 190. Dupuytren's contracture of the palmar fascia in an early phase.

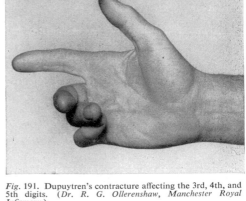

Fig. 191. Dupuytren's contracture affecting the 3rd, 4th, and 5th digits. (*Dr. R. G. Ollerenshaw, Manchester Royal Infirmary.*)

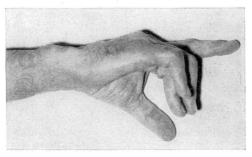

Fig. 192. Severe form of Dupuytren's contracture showing involvement of the middle as well as the little and ring fingers.

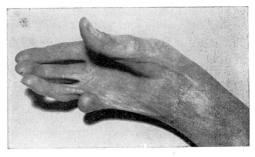

Fig. 193. Cicatricial contracture after a burn. (*Mr. Nils Eckhoff.*)

prone to occur in subjects whose work entails repeated strain on the palms of their hands, as in the case of those who use spades, etc.

In diseases of the *joints*, such as rheumatoid and other types of arthritis, ankylosing spondylitis, tuberculosis, osteoarthrosis, etc., the patient may lie in bed or go about for weeks or months in some bent or contorted position that involves the minimum of discomfort: ankylosis of the affected joints can result.

Corresponding shortening will take place in the muscles that are relaxed, and a passive contracture results. The growth of a tumour in or about a joint may produce identical results. Traumatic or inflammatory lesions about the *muscles* or their *tendons* may establish inflammatory products locally that permanently limit

In *scleroderma* (progressive systemic sclerosis) contraction of the fingers occurs commonly; less commonly knees and ankles are affected.

Dermatomyositis is characterized by progressive inflammatory fibrosis of the affected muscles, which become wooden in consistency; the subcutaneous tissue disappears and the skin becomes thin and pigmented. A somewhat similar condition, but localized to the ankle and foot, occurs as a result of long-standing *varicose ulceration of the leg*, and extreme deformity may also arise from *myositis ossificans*, a rare but easily diagnosed affection in which the muscles all over the body gradually become rigid from calcification; the patient has generally been normal up to adult life, and then becomes the subject of acute attacks of pain in various muscles, accompanied by local myositic swelling and some pyrexia; after the local inflammation subsides, calcium salts are deposited in the site that has been inflamed and the affected muscle becomes stiff and hard. Weeks or months may elapse between successive attacks of this kind, but the number of calcified muscles slowly mounts up, until in extreme instances the patient is rigid almost from head to foot—the 'ossified man'.

Ian Mackenzie.

CONVULSIONS AND FITS

The terms 'convulsion' and 'fit' are used interchangeably to describe attacks of involuntary tonic or clonic movements of the limbs, trunk, and face, with or without loss of consciousness. Thus defined, they embrace epilepsy, tetanus, tetany, rigors, and strychnine poisoning, but the present section will deal more particularly with epileptiform convulsions of cerebral origin, leaving aside the question of rigors, tetanus, tetany, and strychnine poisoning, which are discussed elsewhere.

The motor discharge which causes a convulsion may be due to the action on the brain of some local disease (symptomatic epilepsy) or—as in the majority of cases—it may be due to an inherent instability of the brain (idiopathic epilepsy). This division will serve as the basis for classifying convulsions, but there is one important group which it is difficult to place with certainty, viz., the convulsions of infancy. Some of these are obviously idiopathic in that they occur in otherwise healthy infants and continue to plague the patient at intervals for many years. Others are equally obviously a complication of some well-defined cerebral lesion, such as a cerebral diplegia, hydrocephalus, or birth injury. But between these clearly appreciated extremes there are many cases in which convulsions appear to be the result of general infections, gastro-intestinal disturbances, teething, worm infestations, rickets, otitis media, and so on. There is no doubt at all that infants are prone to have a convulsion in place of a rigor at the onset of acute infections such as pyelitis or pneumonia. It seems that the infantile brain is susceptible to these conditions, and the case-histories of innumerable adults show that convulsions in infancy do not necessarily mean that epileptic fits will occur later in life. For the moment, these infantile convulsions occupy a position somewhere between idiopathic epilepsy and the symptomatic variety:

A. Idiopathic Epilepsy.

B. Symptomatic Convulsions:

1. CONGENITAL CEREBRAL DEFECTS:

Congenital diplegia	Epiloia
Congenital hemiplegia	Congenital idiocy
Congenital microcephaly	Cerebral angioma
Hydrocephalus	

2. HEAD INJURIES:

Birth injuries	Closed head injuries
Open head injuries	

3. INTRACRANIAL INFECTIONS:

Meningitis	Encephalomyelitis
Cerebral abscess	Encephalitis
Syphilis	Cysticercosis
Tuberculoma	Hydatid cyst
Sinus thrombosis	Cerebral malaria
Cortical thrombo-phlebitis	Rabies
Polio-encephalitis	Tetanus

4. GENERAL INFECTIONS (*in infants*):

Gastro-enteritis	Specific fevers
Pneumonia	Osteomyelitis
Pyelitis	Pertussis
Otitis media	

5. PYRIDOXINE DEFICIENCY (*in children*).

6. INTOXICATIONS:

Uraemia	Ether convulsions
Cholaemia	Poisonous insects and snakes
Camphor derivatives	Strychnine
Arsenic, lead, alcohol	Picrotoxin

7. CEREBRAL TUMOURS:

Primary tumour	Secondary metastases

8. CARDIOVASCULAR DISORDERS:

Cerebral thrombosis	Stokes-Adams syndrome
Cerebral haemorrhage	Syncope (postural)
Subarachnoid haemorrhage	Paroxysmal tachycardia
Embolism	Paroxysmal fibrillation
	The cough syndrome

Hypertensive encephalopathy (in essential hypertension, nephritis, eclampsia, and lead poisoning)

9. CAROTID SINUS EPILEPSY.

10. HYPOGLYCAEMIA:

Insulin overdosage	Phenylketonuria
Pancreatic tumours	Metabolic disturbances
Hypoparathyroidism	Von Gierke's disease

11. CEREBRAL DEGENERATION:

Cerebromacular degeneration	Kernicterus
Schilder's disease	Presenile dementia
Arteriosclerosis	Disseminated sclerosis

12. HYPERPYREXIA. (Acute infection, heat stroke.)

13. HYSTERIA.

When confronted with a history of convulsions or fits, it is necessary to make sure that the seizures are epileptiform and not due to tetany, tetanus, or a rigor. The former are characterized by a premonitory aura, loss or disturbance of consciousness, tonic and/or clonic movements of the extremities, trunk, and face, and in many instances incontinence of urine. Consciousness slowly returns, and headache and a sense of fatigue are usually complained of. Respiration is stopped in the tonic phase, with consequent cyanosis, and the tongue may be bitten by clonic movements of the jaws. These symptoms occur in varying combination from case to case, but common to them all is an episodic disturbance of consciousness, which varies from complete un-consciousness to a 'far away' feeling in which the patient is dimly aware of his surroundings but is unable to answer questions.

Having decided that the case is one of true epileptiform convulsions, the next step is to decide whether it is due to idiopathic epilepsy or falls into the symptomatic group. Points in favour of the former are: a family history of epilepsy, alcoholism, or mental disease; the ocur-rence of major or minor fits in the patient's past history; the presence of psychological abnor-mality in the shape of moodiness, egocentricity, and boastfulness; absence of any sign of organic disease, within or without the nervous system; diffuse cortical dysrhythmia on the electro-encephalogram—but this is often absent in major epilepsy. None of these features has an absolute value. Convulsions starting for the first time after the age of thirty are more likely to be symptomatic of organic disease. Jacksonian epilepsy may be either idiopathic, or symptomatic of a focal cerebral lesion. A unilateral fit may be followed by transient paralysis of the limbs on that side (Todd's paralysis), and this is more likely to occur in symptomatic epilepsy than in the idio-pathic variety. 'Adversive epilepsy', in which the head and eyes are tonically deviated to one side, sometimes means a premotor lesion, but it is also seen in idiopathic cases.

The investigation of convulsions should include a careful case-history, attention being paid to each system of the body in turn, followed by a meticulous physical examination. Special investi-gations include lumbar puncture, X-ray examina-tion of the skull and, when relevant, of the chest (for primary carcinoma or bronchiectasis), of the gastro-intestinal tract, and of the limbs (for evidence of cysticercosis). Electro-encephalo-graphy is used to search for focal disturbances around organic lesions. If there is reason to suspect an intracranial lesion, gamma or E.M.I.-scanning and possibly arteriography are neces-sary. Electrocardiography may reveal heart-block. If hypertension is present, renal function must be investigated to determine whether the convulsions are related to the blood-pressure itself (hypertensive encephalopathy) or to renal failure. Thus, nephritis can be ushered in by one or more fits.

Convulsions due to the cerebral lesions under-lying congenital spastic paralysis, congenital hydrocephalus, microcephaly, and idiocy present no problem. They are present from an early age and the underlying lesion is unmistakable. *Epiloia* (syn. tuberose sclerosis, Bournville's disease, Pringle's disease) is characterized by the combination of epilepsy, mental defect with or without spastic paralyses or other focal signs, and the pathognomonic adenoma sebaceum over the cheeks, to which may be added a variety of cutaneous and skeletal abnormalities. *Head injuries* at birth or in later life are a fruitful source of convulsions. In adults, the fits are apt to appear after a delay of several months following the injury. *Cerebral tumours* are an important cause of epileptiform attacks at all ages. Primary neoplasms of slow growth, such as an oligo-dendroglioma or a meningioma, may cause fits for months or even years before providing other evidence of their presence. Rapidly growing gliomata and secondary metastases from growths elsewhere in the body (notably the lung) usually give rise to focal symptoms and signs at an early stage of their development. Congenital cerebral capillary angiomata associated with cutaneous naevi on the face on the affected side (Sturge-Weber disease) are not uncommon, and may cause either general or Jacksonian convulsions, with or without focal neurological signs between the attacks. It is important to remember that epileptiform convulsions are often the only sign of a cerebral neoplasm, and that early diag-nosis may afford the only chance of successful surgical intervention.

Intracranial infections are more likely to pro-duce convulsions in children than in adults. Any form of *meningitis* can do it, and there is no excuse whatever for failing to examine the spinal fluid (p. 124) of any case exhibiting a raised temperature and convulsions; diagnosis depends essentially on the demonstration of a pleocytosis and the causal organisms in the fluid. *Cerebral abscess*, usually due to spread into the temporal lobe from the middle ear or into the frontal lobe from sinusitis, but sometimes metastatic (e.g., from bronchiectasis or other pulmonary suppura-tion) is usually rapid in onset, but sporadic fits over a period of months may be the only sign of a chronic encapsulated abscess. Diagnosis may be very difficult or very easy, depending on whether the source of infection is obvious or not. Increase of cells and protein in the spinal fluid—the pressure of which may be normal or raised—is helpful when present. Pyrexia is often absent, and the blood-count may be normal. When localizing signs are absent, the electro-encephalo-graph may reveal the situation of the abscess; ventriculography may have to be carried out. Infection and thrombosis of the *dural sinuses* and *cortical veins* may cause fits, either general or Jacksonian. The pressure of the spinal fluid is raised, and there may be a moderate pleocytosis in the fluid. The condition usually arises in the course of an infected head wound, but occasion-ally it occurs in the course of some general infec-tion.

Syphilis can cause fits in several ways. They occur in congenital syphilis of infancy, in acquired meningovascular syphilis, in thrombosis of cere-bral arteries, and in general paralysis of the insane. Diagnosis depends on examination of the Wassermann reaction in the blood and spinal fluid, but it is scarcely necessary to add that in communities with a high incidence of the disease a positive Wassermann does not prove that the symptoms are due to syphilis and every care must be taken to exclude other possibilities. The cura-tive effect of modern therapy may prove the decisive diagnostic factor. *Tuberculomata* are rarely a cause of convulsions, largely because they are more often situated in the posterior fossa than in the cerebral hemisphere. When in the latter, the features and diagnostic problems are similar to those described in the case of chronic encapsulated abscesses.

Virus diseases are not an important source of convulsions. They occasionally occur during the acute phase of encephalitis lethargica, polio-encephalitis, and the encephalomyelitis which follows the specific fevers of childhood and vaccination, but in such cases the fits are but one feature of a more complex symptomatology. *Disseminated sclerosis* may not belong to this aetiological group, but it is conveniently considered here. As in the virus diseases, fits are uncommon and when they occur in this disease the question of a coincidental idiopathic epilepsy or symptomatic epilepsy due to another cause must always be considered. Diagnosis is based, not on fits, but on the evidence, from the history, and from the physical examination, of multiple lesions and remissions.

Cerebral malaria can cause coma, convulsions, and fever. Diagnosis depends on a history of exposure to the disease and on the presence of parasites in the blood-film.

Cysticercosis is important. The fits are due to the presence in the brain of the *Cysticercus cellulosae*, derived from the tape-worm, *Taenia solium*. Infestation rarely occurs in the United Kingdom, Western Europe, or other areas where hygiene is highly developed, but is common in India, Egypt, and other Eastern countries. Convulsions of epileptiform type occur months or years after cerebral invasion, and although focal signs do not usually appear multifocal epilepsy is very suggestive. Radiographs may show calcified cysts in the brain or in muscles, but absence of this sign does not exclude the possibility of the disease in the years immediately following infestation, since it takes several years for calcification to occur. In rare cases the period of invasion is marked by fits, raised intracranial pressure, psychotic symptoms, or transient focal disturbances such as hemiparesis, and such cases may show a pleocytosis in the spinal fluid during the acute phase.

Hydatid cysts are the larval form of *Taenia echinococcus*, which normally inhabits the intestinal tract of the dog. For this reason it is common in sheep-rearing countries where contact between dog and man is continuous. Symptoms are more common in children than adults, and take the form of a space-occupying lesion, with headache, papilloedema, convulsions, and focal signs which depend on the situation of the growing cyst. The Casoni test may be positive, but it is an unreliable guide, and the diagnosis is usually established at operation only.

Convulsions due to cardiovascular disease are infrequent, but loss of consciousness without jactitation is fairly common. Either form of seizure may occur at the time of a cerebral vascular accident—haemorrhage, thrombosis,

embolism, or subarachnoid haemorrhage—and they may recur in cases which survive the initial disaster. They also occur in response to a sudden fall of blood-pressure, e.g., coronary thrombosis, paroxysmal tachycardia, intermittent heartblock, and severe fits of coughing in obese emphysematous subjects. Hypertensive encephalopathy is seen in essential hypertension, malignant hypertension, and in hypertension due to nephritis, eclampsia, and lead poisoning. There is a sudden rise of an already elevated blood-pressure followed by unconsciousness with or without convulsions. Hypertensive retinopathy may be present, and papilloedema may occur in cases with cerebral oedema. The blood-urea is not necessarily raised, and the attacks are not due to uraemia.

Hypoglycaemic convulsions are seen as the result of overdosage with insulin. They may also occur in a variety of other conditions, including tumour or diffuse hypertrophy of the islets of Langerhans, disease of the liver, von Gierke's disease, hypopituitarism, Addison's disease, hypothyroidism, hypothalamic lesions, following gastrectomy and other causes of the mal-absorption syndrome, and occasionally without any obvious cause. The attacks may be convulsive, but more often take the form of a feeling of weakness with tachycardia, sweating, and light-headedness or vertigo. They are apt to occur in the early part of the day, or when a meal has been missed, and are frequently precipitated by unwonted physical exertion. The blood-sugar level varies, and is usually in the neighbourhood of 50 mg. per cent, but symptoms may occur when the level is as high as 100 mg. per cent in diabetics who are accustomed to a high blood-sugar.

Intoxications may cause fits—some cases of *uraemia*, *cholaemia* in advanced atrophy of the liver, *heavy metals* such as arsenic and gold when given in excessive doses intravenously, *acute alcoholic* and *absinthe* and *camphor poisoning*, and the bite of the wood tick (*see Fig. 548, p. 557*), etc. Many drugs may cause fits if given in high dosage, e.g., picrotoxin, strychnine, atropine. Conversely, withdrawal of hypnotics or large amounts of alcohol may precipitate convulsions. *Ether convulsions* are not due to the toxic action of ether, but to alkalosis induced by hyperventilation during operation under ether anaesthesia.

A rare form of fit occurs in persons possessing a carotid sinus which is unduly sensitive to mechanical stimuli. Unconsciousness, with or without a convulsion, can be produced by digital compression of the sinus, or by certain movements of the head on the neck. Such cases must be distinguished from (*a*) those in whom compression of one carotid artery induces cerebral anaemia because the opposite carotid is stenosed by thrombosis or atheroma; (*b*) those in whom carotid compression slows the heart; (*c*) those in whom stimulation of the carotid sinus causes a marked fall of blood-pressure without significant bradycardia. In carotid sinus epilepsy there is no fall of pressure, and no slowing of the pulse, but pressure on the sinus induces epileptic discharges in the electro-encephalogram. Denervation of the sinus can abolish these attacks. In another type of case, either Stokes-Adams attacks or epilepsy can be triggered-off by paroxysms of glossopharyngeal neuralgia, and these respond to section of the glossopharyngeal nerve and the upper filaments of the vagus. Still less common are the cases in which the act of swallowing will, on occasion, cause unconsciousness or a feeling of vertigo or light-headedness, and here, too, a neural rather than a circulatory mechanism seems to be involved.

Cerebromacular degeneration (syn. amaurotic idiocy of Tay-Sachs) is a degenerative disease of the brain and ganglion cells of the retina, coming on after the first few months of life and progressing to a fatal termination before the fourth year. It is almost entirely confined to Jews and is familial rather than hereditary in incidence. Progressive idiocy, blindness, and helplessness are the main features. The macula stands out as a cherry-red spot in the pale retina. Convulsions are common. *Schilder's disease* is predominantly a disease of children. It is characterized pathologically by areas of demyelination of the sub-cortical white matter, and clinically by progressive focal signs—hemianopia, hemiparesis, paraplegia, aphasia, dementia, etc., with death within a year or two of the onset. Convulsions are a prominent feature of some cases. When the disease advances rapidly, intracranial pressure is raised and the presence of headache, vomiting, and papilloedema in conjunction with signs of a local lesion in the brain may lead to a mistaken diagnosis of cerebral tumour. *Kernicterus* is an interesting complication of icterus gravis neonatorum, itself the result of rhesus incompatibility in the parents. The jaundice leaves an intense pigmentation of the lenticular, caudate, and some of the hypothalamic and brain-stem nuclei, the cells of which are severely injured. Convulsions, jaundice, and a severe anaemia are present within a day or two of birth. If the child survives the acute phase there is a grave risk of subsequent mental defect, athetosis, rigidity, and epilepsy.

Heat-stroke is characterized by a rising body temperature, dryness of the skin, and either coma or epileptiform convulsions. Diagnosis will be plain owing to the circumstances of its occurrence, but it will be remembered that there are other causes of convulsions which are just as common in the tropics or in stokeholds of ships as elsewhere.

Hysterical convulsions occur in hysterical subjects in the presence of an audience, and for some specific reason. They are usually exaggerated and unconvincing; the tongue is not bitten nor urine voided, and the plantar response—if it can be got at all—is flexor, in contrast to the extensor reflex of any true convulsions. A confusing circumstance arises when true tetany occurs as a result of hysterical overbreathing.

Ian Mackenzie.

CORNEAL AFFECTIONS

Most affections of the cornea cause a loss of its transparency, which may persist, with consequent impairment of vision. Such an opacity, the immediate evidence of some corneal affection may be faint and easily overlooked (as in the case of small corneal ulcers, a frequent cause of a painful red eye). Damage to the corneal epithelium is readily disclosed by inserting a vital stain, such as fluorescein.

The cornea may be affected symptomatically. For example, a diffuse haze is present in *acute glaucoma*, due to corneal oedema; deep *striate opacities* often follow a lowering of tension (as after operation), though they may develop in simple inflammatory conditions. Punctate deposits on the back of the cornea (*keratic precipitates*) are the pathognomonic sequels to an iridocyclitis, though usually visible only under magnification.

The commonest *degenerative condition* of the cornea is the *arcus senilis*—concentric grey crescents, separated by a rim of clear cornea from the extreme periphery, which in time completely encircles the cornea (*Fig*. 194). It very occasionally

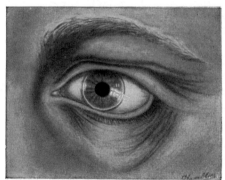

Fig. 194. Arcus senilis.

develops at an early age, and has no clinical importance. *Band-shaped opacity*, extending over the area of cornea normally exposed between the eyelids, is rarely found in otherwise healthy eyes, but occurs fairly frequently in blind, shrunken eyes, and following prolonged uveitis.

An *anterior staphyloma*, a protuberant cicatrix lined by iris and involving part or all of the cornea, usually occurs after perforation of an ulcer; a localized bulge of the cornea (*keratectasia*) may follow thinning of the cornea from ulcerations, under the influence of the intra-ocular tension. *Keratoconus*, or conical cornea, is probably due to a genetic weakness, though it usually does not manifest itself until after puberty.

Inflammation of the cornea—*keratitis*—may be: (1) *Exogenous*, deriving from exogenous infectors, usually promoted by trauma, and thus presenting as a *corneal ulcer*, or (2) (less commonly)

Endogenous, from systemic causes, and presenting as a deep corneal infiltrate, which (if the keratitis is severe) will become vascularized; the commonest of these endogenous keratites is *Interstitial keratitis*, a late manifestation of congenital syphilis, discussed on p. 275 (*Fig.* 291).

Superficial Keratitis may involve (*a*) the corneal *eriphery*, the commonest form of this being catarrhal ulcers, or (*b*) the *axial* (central) region, when they are usually secondary to viral infection

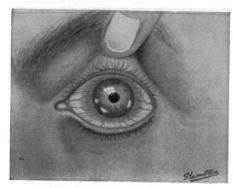

Fig. 195. Catarrhal ulcers.

(especially herpes simplex—the 'dendritic ulcer'), bacterial infection, or devitalization from exposure, vitamin lack, etc.

Catarrhal ulcers are due to the spread of infection from an indolent conjunctivitis of moderate severity, hence their site around the margin of the cornea; for the same reason they are frequently multiple, and (being close to the limbal capillary loops) they tend to remain superficial and simple (*Fig.* 195). They are usually due to *Staphylococcus aureus* (the commonest of conjunctival pathogens) and they are particularly liable to occur where the infection is persistent, as in the presence of a coincidental staphylococcal blepharitis, or with pathogens which are by nature indolent, such as Morax-Axenfeld bacillus. Such ulcers are generally benign, and rarely do they cause enough infiltration to encroach on the axial region of the cornea and interfere with vision.

Dendritic ulcers start as a catarrhal conjunctivitis, which is followed after about four days by a crop of minute punctate opacities on either side of Bowman's membrane; these vesicate, and then rupture almost immediately, so that when the cornea is stained with fluorescein they form a classic jagged pattern on the cornea (*Fig.* 196). Relapses are usual, with fresh branches arising every few days or new foci appearing isolated from the main 'tree'; around these linear erosions is a greyish halo of oedematous corneal epithelium, and this readily becomes destroyed when secondary infection sets in. The ulcer may continue for weeks or even months with repeated relapses in spite of all treatment, but gradually it fades away, leaving a superficial scar that may be

a visual impediment, especially if the damage has been augmented by secondary infection.

Dendritic ulcers may leave the cornea with its epithelial sensitivity impaired (which can easily be tested by touching it with a wisp of cotton-wool, and contrasting the blink reflex with that on the other side); this renders the cornea less resistant

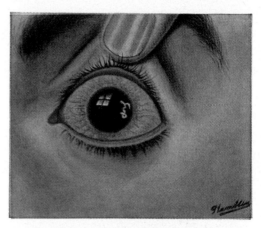

Fig. 196. Dendritic ulcer stained with fluorescein.

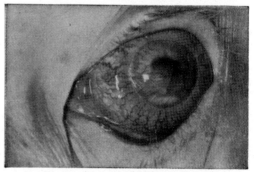

Fig. 197. Hypopyon ulcer (*see* p. 265). (*Institute of Ophthalmology.*)

to subsequent ulceration, and a *keratitis metaherpetica* may be the indolent sequel.

The *pyogenic ulcer* (the 'pneumococcal ulcer') was formerly the commonest form of central corneal ulcer. It arises normally from the coincidence of trauma and the presence of virulent organisms which can then lodge in the exposed corneal stroma; the pneumococcus is usually responsible, being the most common of the more virulent conjunctival pathogens, and generally coming from a focus in the lacrimal sac, but *Pseudomonas pyocyanea* (*aeruginosa*), β-haemolytic *Streptococcus*, and *Klebsiella pneumoniae* (Friedländer's bacillus) are occasionally found.

Clinically the pyogenic ulcer appears as a yellowish, irregular ulcer associated with much necrosis, and tending to spread rapidly along and through the corneal parenchyma so that the margin is often undermined. It is usually associated with an exudative iritis, with the result that the pyogenic ulcer is also known as 'hypopyon ulcer' since a hypopyon is so characteristic a sequel. The symptoms are more severe than those of a catarrhal ulcer, yet in the majority that escape a secondary glaucoma the pain often seems slight for so corrosive a lesion. The ulcer may heal without perforation, but the resulting scar is both large and centrally placed so that ultimate vision is often much impaired; otherwise perforation may be followed by a panophthalmitis or, if the inflammation subsides, a dense corneal scar, to which the underlying iris is adherent, an 'adherent leucoma', which may distend to form an anterior staphyloma (p. 184).

Neurotrophic keratitis, due to loss of sensation in the ophthalmic division of the trigeminal nerve, is the common sequel to herpes zoster ophthalmicus. The mechanism of the degenerative changes that follow damage to a sensory nerve remains obscure, although not through any lack of hypotheses; probably the absence of the axon reflexes that regulate the disposal of toxins and metabolites is largely responsible. The affected tissues tend to become congested and oedematous, and in the cornea this may lead to an epithelial exfoliation and ulceration. As a consequence, such ulcers show little tendency to heal with the usual ulcer therapy, but when protected by a tarsorrhaphy the recovery is often striking.

Nutritional ulcers include *atheromatous ulcers* which arise in long-standing corneal scars, usually the seat of fatty or calcareous degeneration, where nutrition of the overlying epithelium can no longer be maintained; epithelial necrosis is usually precipitated by some incidental trauma or foreign body, but may arise more dramatically when calcified plaques break away from the surface. Such ulcers most commonly form in the lower axial region, since this is the centre of the exposed area and at the same time farthest from the limbal supply of nourishment. They demand protective treatment with lubricants, tarsorrhaphy, and antibiotics should infection supervene.

Keratomalacia due to vitamin-A deficiency is characterized by a desiccation and subsequent necrosis of the cornea and conjunctiva. It affects undernourished infants and is of extreme rarity in England. At first the conjunctiva becomes dry ('xerophthalmia') and patches of frothy Meibomian secretion ('Bitot's spots') may then adhere to the exposed area of conjunctiva on either side of the cornea. At the same time the cornea becomes dry and insensitive, and may ultimately melt away, often with alarming speed since there is a negligible inflammatory reaction and the apathetic child makes little effort to close and protect his eyes; if the child survives, dense corneal scars will remain. The night-blindness, by which lack of vitamin A may be manifested in adults, is occasionally observed by older children before the corneal and conjunctival changes appear. Urgent administration of vitamin A is needed, along with the routine ulcer therapy.

P. Trevor-Roper.

COUGH

Cough is one of the physiological mechanisms for the protection of the lower respiratory tract against infection and invasion by foreign bodies. In disease it also has the function of expelling excessive secretions and exudates from the bronchi and lungs. It is important to remember that there are other mechanisms by which secretions may be removed from the bronchi. The chief of these is provided by ciliary action; this keeps a thin sheet of mucus constantly moving up the tracheobronchial tree towards the larynx. On reaching the pharynx the secretions raised in this way are disposed of into the alimentary tract by unconscious acts of swallowing. In this way even pathological secretions may be removed from the respiratory tract, and in this way it happens that in pulmonary tuberculosis there may be insufficient excess of secretions in the bronchopulmonary tree to excite cough, and yet tubercle bacilli may be found in gastric contents; it is not only in patients who deliberately swallow their sputum that examination of gastric contents may give useful information.

There are three chief phases of the cough mechanism. The first is a preliminary inspiration; the second is closure of the glottis accompanied by contraction of the muscles of expiration, including in the most forceful coughs the accessory muscles; and the third is the opening of the glottis, leading to a sudden blast of air up the respiratory passages, propelling any foreign substance or excessive secretions contained in them upwards. Cough is a reflex mechanism, but is also under voluntary control. This voluntary control is more complete than that which exists with certain comparable reflex mechanisms, for instance that of sneezing. Cough can be produced entirely voluntarily, and to a less extent can be suppressed voluntarily. These facts are well illustrated by the outbreak of coughing which occurs at public gatherings in the course of a boring speech, whereas while the audience's attention is held by the proceedings there may be complete silence. The sensory stimulus is normally derived from nerve-endings in the laryngeal, tracheal, or bronchial mucosa, all of which are supplied by branches of the vagus nerve; in rare instances stimulation of some other branch of the vagus may cause cough. On the motor side, coughing is a co-ordinated act involving the muscles of the larynx and of respiration; hence the motor nerves involved are those of the larynx, that is the inferior laryngeals, and the nerves supplying respiratory muscles. An effective sensory stimulus for cough can be applied to the mucosa of the bronchial tree certainly as far as can be reached by the bronchoscope. It is doubtful whether stimulation of branches of the vagus distributed outside the respiratory tract is effective in producing cough, with one important exception: that is Arnold's nerve, which supplies part of the external meatus of the ear and the adjacent part of the lobule. Stimulation of the part of the meatus supplied by this branch causes an irrepressible desire to cough. This is important clinically since the presence of wax in the ears, foreign bodies in the external meatus in children, or even sometimes inflammatory conditions of the meatus, may cause a constant, dry irritating cough.

The causes of cough are so numerous that they are difficult to classify. The general categories under which they can be considered include exposure to irritants, either gaseous, liquid, or solid; increased irritability of the mucosa to the minor stimuli encountered in normal respiration, as may occur in the early stage of inflammation of the larynx, trachea, and bronchi; excessive secretion in the trachea or bronchi; abnormal exudates from pulmonary disease; pressure on sensitive parts of the respiratory tract from without; and voluntary action. The cough reflex may be depressed by atrophic destructive changes in the sensitive mucosa of the respiratory tract; by medullary depressant drugs, especially morphine and its analogues; and during sleep.

In an Acute Illness cough as a leading symptom suggests either an infection of the respiratory tract—*laryngitis, tracheobronchitis, pneumonia, lung abscess,* or certain acute specific fevers. *Acute laryngitis* is generally preceded by an upper respiratory infection, and accompanied by hoarseness of the voice. *Acute tracheobronchitis* also generally follows an upper respiratory tract infection; the cough is characteristically unproductive and painful at first, with retrosternal pain, and only ater with expectoration at first scanty and mucoid, later more profuse and purulent. The severity of cough in the early stage of pneumonia will depend upon whether or no there has been a preceding descending infection of the respiratory tract. In the *pneumococcal pneumonia* of previously healthy adults, cough may not be apparent at the beginning, and when it first appears is short, painful, and only slightly productive; characteristically the sputa when produced are stained with altered blood, and are usually described as rusty. In *virus pneumonias* cough may not appear until the patient has been febrile, with constitutional symptoms, for several days. In secondary *bronchopneumonias* (aspiration pneumonias) there is either a preceding severe illness or operation or an upper respiratory tract infection, and cough is present from the beginning; there may be nothing distinctive about the sputum.

In *lung abscess* the sputum is characteristically purulent, and may be offensive; it may be blood-stained; and expectoration is often greatly affected by posture. Gangrene of the lung may be considered as the most acute form of lung abscess, with massive necrosis of the centre of the affected part of the lung. In such cases there is extreme foetor, the patient is prostrated, with high fever, and the expectoration is purulent, usually blood-stained, and has a disgustingly offensive odour. Pulmonary suppuration of all types is nearly always due to aspiration of infected material into

the bronchial tree of the affected segment—a process which has been aptly termed 'bronchial embolism'. The material so aspirated may be endogenous secretions, commonly from the upper respiratory tract and often carrying organisms from septic teeth or gums or from nasal sinus infection. Factors favouring the aspiration of such secretions are operations under general anaesthesia, acute upper respiratory infections, and unconsciousness from any cause, including deep sleep. Local disease of the larynx or interference with its motor or sensory nerve-supply, aspiration of gastric contents during vomiting under anaesthesia or in coma, and exogenous *foreign bodies in the bronchi* are important though rarer causes. Pulmonary suppuration of all sorts may be secondary to obstruction of the bronchi by growths, usually carcinomata, more rarely innocent. Some of the less frequent types of bacterial pneumonia, notably those due to *Staphylococcus aureus* and to Friedländer's bacillus, may enter a suppurative phase and break down into lung abscesses. Lung abscesses due to pulmonary arterial embolism are not common and are usually multiple; they may occur in the course of such conditions as staphylococcal pyaemia, often associated with focal staphylococcal lesions elsewhere, such as osteomyelitis.

Of the acute specific fevers characterized by early cough, *measles* is the most frequent. The early bronchitis of *typhoid* and *paratyphoid* fevers is important to bear in mind since in the early days no localizing symptoms or signs are likely to be found. The characteristic cough of *pertussis* may be considered here, though the affected child is often not acutely ill. The differential diagnosis between pertussis and simple bronchitis in children is usually not difficult. A history of contact or the knowledge that pertussis is epidemic is helpful. At the onset the cough of pertussis is usually lacking in the characteristic features which appear later. In its most characteristic form the cough is paroxysmal in bouts which may last for a minute or two and culminate in vomiting, in addition to the characteristic terminal whoop. In severe paroxysms the child may become cyanosed. On examination the most striking finding in the chest is a negative one, the rhonchi characteristic of ordinary acute bronchitis being generally absent. A sublingual ulcer on the fraenum linguae due to the friction of the protruding tongue on the lower front teeth during long paroxysms of cough is a helpful finding.

There is no evidence that dry *pleurisy* itself gives rise to cough, but it is often due to causes which also involve the bronchi and lungs and may thus be associated with cough. In *pleurisy with effusion* of tuberculous origin, cough is usually not a prominent symptom unless the effusion becomes very large. A very large pleural effusion gives rise to troublesome bouts of short ineffective cough, probably due to incipient or actual oedema of the congested opposite lung; this symptom is an indication for aspiration which will relieve it. Similarly empyemata do not of themselves cause cough, though they are usually associated with bronchopulmonary infections which do; in cases of *empyema with pleuro-bronchial fistula*, expectoration of large amounts of pus, usually much affected by changes of posture, is characteristic.

In a Chronic Illness the investigation of the cause of cough is generally a more complex matter. The points to be noted especially in the history are:

1. *The duration of the cough*: A cough which the adult patient has had intermittently since

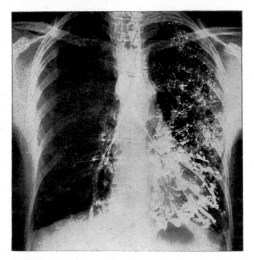

Fig. 198. Bronchogram showing saccular bronchiectasis in the left lower lobe.

childhood is more likely to be associated with bronchiectasis than one the onset of which can be dated more recently. Correlated with this, inquiries should be made whether the cough is seasonal. In simple *chronic bronchitis* the cough is usually worse in the winter.

In children with persistent or recurrent cough, the possibility of *cystic fibrosis* must be borne in mind; the presence of associated bowel symptoms should lead to an estimate of sweat sodium level.

2. *In coughs of which the onset can be dated*, did it come on after an acute upper respiratory infection of the common cold type? Although this is useful information, it must be interpreted with caution, since in many chronic pulmonary diseases, especially pulmonary tuberculosis and bronchial carcinoma, the cough frequently first becomes manifest after an intercurrent simple upper respiratory tract infection. The symptoms of most chronic diseases of the bronchi and lungs are temporarily exacerbated by such infections. For this reason a cough appearing for the first time in a young adult must give rise to suspicion of *pulmonary tuberculosis*, and calls for complete investigation including radiography and sputum examination to exclude this disease. Similarly a cough appearing for the first time in middle age,

especially in men, must raise suspicion of *bronchial carcinoma* which should only be dismissed after complete investigation.

3. *The time of maximal incidence* of the cough is important. The characteristic morning cough of the *cigarette-smoker* is due to a chronic pharyngo-tracheobronchitis. It is so frequent that many cigarette-smokers regard it as a normal part of their lives and refer to it as 'clearing the throat'; such people may say that they do not cough though they raise phlegm. This morning cough and expectoration is the early symptom of *chronic bronchitis*. Chronic nasal sinusitis may produce or contribute to this symptom, secretions which have trickled down into the trachea during sleep being expelled when the patient wakes. A cough which appears on first lying down at night or on some other change of posture is suggestive of localized *bronchiectasis* or chronic pulmonary suppuration. *Asthmatic* patients sometimes complain of cough as a prominent feature of their attacks, although there will always be associated wheezing dyspnoea, and in the typical attacks cough appears towards the end of the attack; asthmatic attacks of any type may appear at any time of the day or night, but frequently occur at night, either when the patient first goes to bed or waking him from sleep. A cough with dyspnoea or orthopnoea waking the patient from sleep is suggestive of left ventricular failure in *hypertension, aortic valvular disease*, or *cardio-renal disease*; the nocturnal attacks of paroxysmal dyspnoea in these conditions may or may not be accompanied by wheezing. If the patient is seen in the attack physical examination will usually enable a decision to be made whether the patient is suffering from bronchial asthma or paroxysmal cardiac dyspnoea. In asthma, the characteristic physical sign of an acutely overdistended chest, with universal wheezy rhonchi higher pitched during a prolonged expiratory phase, will be found. Paroxysmal cardiac dyspnoea is due to pulmonary oedema, and the characteristic physical signs are râles, which in a mild attack or at the beginning of a severe attack are basal, and gradually extend upwards until in a severe case they can be heard all over the thorax. Difficulty is sometimes encountered in cases of paroxysmal cardiac dyspnoea, since secondary bronchial spasm giving rise to rhonchi may occur; but the characteristic râles are always present. Some patients with *cryptogenic fibrosing alveolitis* (diffuse interstitial fibrosis of the lungs) are much troubled by paroxysmal cough tending to occur during the night or on exertion.

4. *The presence or absence of expectoration* and the quality of expectoration should be the next inquiry. *A dry cough* suggests a condition which is not associated with the presence of excessive secretions in the respiratory tract. It should be remembered, however, that many patients find it difficult to expectorate and habitually expel small amounts of secretion through the larynx by cough and swallow it. This is the rule in children. A dry cough, or one producing only scanty

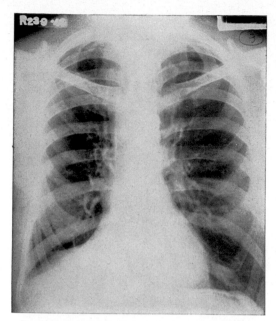

Fig. 199. Radiograph of chest showing atelectasis of the right lower lobe, due to carcinoma of the bronchus. Note the roughly triangular shadow filling the right cardiophrenic angle, with slight displacement of the heart to the right.

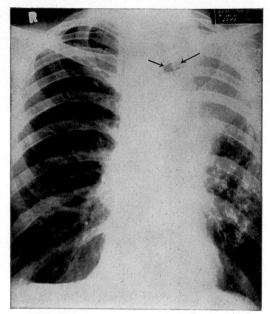

Fig. 200. Radiograph of chest showing atelectasis of left upper lobe due to carcinoma. Note the uniform shadow at the upper part of the left lung with gross displacement to the left of the trachea (indicated by an arrow). The shadows in the lower part of the left lung are due to residual iodized oil.

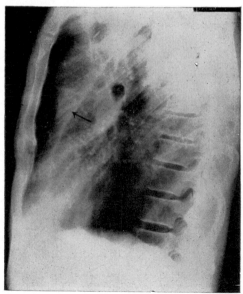

Fig. 201. The same as Fig. 200, in left lateral view. Note the displacement forwards and upwards of the interlobar fissure delimiting the contracted upper lobe.

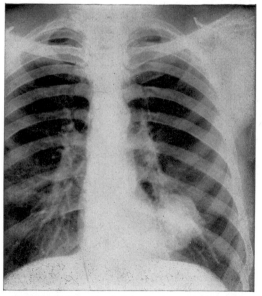

Fig. 202. Radiograph of chest showing an isolated well-defined shadow in the lower part of the left lung. This was due to carcinoma of the bronchus giving rise to a well-defined tumour without obstruction of a major bronchus.

mucoid sputum, may be due to a *chronic laryngitis*; to pressure on the trachea or bronchi from without, as by enlarged mediastinal lymph-nodes, especially *tuberculous mediastinal lymph-nodes* in children, by *aortic aneurysm*, or by *mediastinal tumours* of various sorts both malignant and innocent; to a *new growth of the bronchus*; to the various causes noted above of *irritation of the external auditory meatus*; to a *foreign body* in a bronchus in the earliest stage before infection has occurred; to *carcinoma of the larynx*, when it will be accompanied by changes

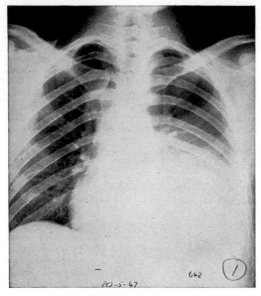

Fig. 203. Radiograph of chest showing consolidation of left lower lobe.

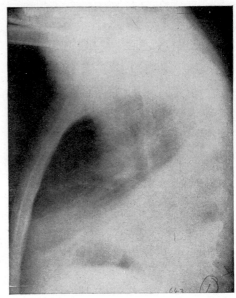

Fig. 204. The same, left lateral view.

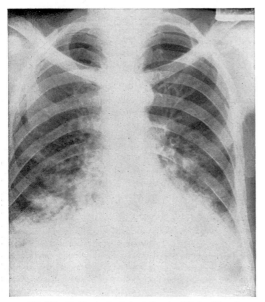

Fig. 205. Radiograph of chest showing bilateral basal bronchopneumonia (postoperative).

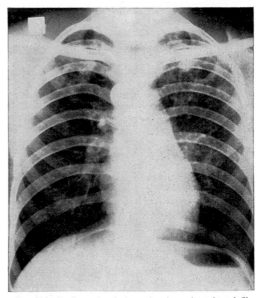

Fig. 206. Radiograph of chest showing tuberculous infiltration of the upper parts of both lungs, with a moderate-sized cavity on the left.

in the voice; occasionally it may be due to *psychological causes*, being little more than a tic.

If the *cough is productive* the quality and mode of production of the sputum should be noted. Frankly purulent sputum suggests either *bronchiectasis, lung abscess*, primary or secondary to bronchial obstruction by *new growth* or *foreign body*, or cavitating *pulmonary tuberculosis*. The *odour* of the sputum is important, a malodorous

sputum suggesting bronchiectasis, lung abscess, expectoration of a putrid empyema (generally secondary to a lung abscess), or sometimes anaerobic infection beyond bronchial obstruction, especially by a growth. The mode of production of sputum may be of importance. In bronchiectasis, lung abscess, and empyema with pleurobronchial fistula, the patient may be free from cough for long periods, and cough may be caused by changes of posture and then accompanied by expectoration of large amounts of sputum. The effect of posture on expectoration may have been noted only indirectly by the patient. Thus he may note that leaning forward to tie up his boot-lace, or adopting a certain position in bed makes him cough; and he may in fact have taken more note of the position which relieves him of his cough than of that which causes him to cough.

5. *The quality of the cough and the presence of associated changes in the voice* should be noted. Cough due to pressure on the trachea or main bronchi, as by an aneurysm, gives rise to a cough of a peculiar quality which is usually described as *brassy*. A cough which is accompanied by paralysis of a vocal cord, nearly always the left, as when it is due to primary or secondary new growth in the mediastinum, or to aneurysm of the transverse part of the aortic arch, may have a peculiar hoarse quality and be accompanied by hoarseness of the voice. The cough of laryngitis will be accompanied by changes in the voice, as will that of carcinoma, tuberculosis, or syphilis of the larynx.

CLASSIFICATION OF CAUSES OF COUGH

1. In the Larynx and Pharynx:
a. Acute and chronic laryngitis.
b. New growths of the larynx.
c. Tuberculosis of the larynx.
d. Syphilis of the larynx.

2. Affecting Trachea and Bronchi:
a. Acute tracheobronchitis, including those forms due to acute specific fevers, especially measles, pertussis, and enteric fever.
b. Chronic bronchitis, including that due to cigarette-smoking.
c. Exposure to irritant gases.
d. Foreign bodies.

e. Bronchiectasis (*Fig.* 198).
f. Pressure on trachea and bronchi from without due to the causes listed under **5**.
g. Carcinoma (*Figs.* 199–202) and other rarer tumours.
h. Cystic fibrosis (*see* p. 757).

3. In the Lungs:
a. Pneumonias (*Figs.* 203–205)—often associated with more or less bronchitis.
b. Pulmonary tuberculosis (*Figs.* 206, 207).
c. Pulmonary suppuration.
d. Pulmonary fibrosis.
e. Secondary new growths.
f. Hydatids—especially if complicated by rupture, infection, etc.
g. Changes in the lungs due to heart disease listed under **6**.

4. In the Pleura:
a. Pleural effusion.
b. Empyema, especially with pleurobronchial fistula.

5. In the Mediastinum (acting mainly through pressure on the trachea and bronchi, but also sometimes due to secondary inflammatory changes in the bronchi and lung):
a. Aortic aneurysm.
b. Enlarged lymph-nodes:
   i. Tuberculosis (*Fig.* 208).
   ii. Secondary malignant, especially from carcinoma of the bronchus.
   iii. Hodgkin's disease, lymphosarcoma, and other reticuloses.
   iv. Bilateral hilar lymphadenopathy of sarcoidosis.
c. Tumours:
   i. Dermoids and teratomata.
   ii. Neurofibromata and other tumours of neural origin.
   iii. Mediastinal goitre.
   iv. Thymomata.
   v. Foregut cysts.

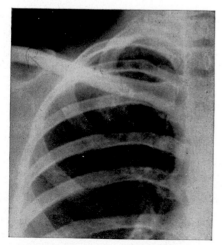

Fig. 207. Radiograph of chest showing upper part of right lung with a small area of tuberculous infiltration.

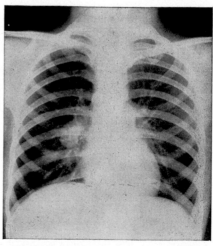

Fig. 208. Radiograph of the chest of a boy aged 11 years showing primary tuberculous complex in the right lung and hilar lymph-nodes with gross enlargement of the latter.

6. Due to Heart Disease:
  a. Pulmonary oedema due to left ventricular failure in hypertension, cardio-renal disease, and aortic incompetence.
  b. Pulmonary congestion in mitral stenosis.

7. Outside the Thorax:
  a. Psychological—as a habit spasm.
  b. Wax, foreign body, or inflammatory changes in the external auditory meatus.
  c. Due to subdiaphragmatic lesions (usually with secondary changes at the base of the lung and pleura):
    i. Subphrenic abscess with changes at the base of the lung, usually the right.
    ii. Hepatic abscess.

J. G. Scadding.

CRACKLING, EGG SHELL

This is a sign rarely seen today which can be elicited over an advanced giant-cell tumour

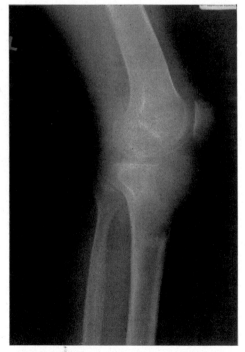

Fig. 209. X-ray of typical osteoclastoma of upper end of tibia. Note that the epiphysial part of the bone is involved. 'Soap bubble' appearance.

(osteoclastoma) of long bone; a thin cortex only of normal bone remains over the tumour mass and pressure imparts to the fingers sensation similar to crepitus (p. 193). There may be increased local heat and dilatation of the superficial veins over the massive swelling, which is likely to be around the knee, and the highly vascular mass may also give the sensation of pulsation. Diagnosis is confirmed by X-ray examination (*Fig.* 209)

which reveals the typical 'soap-bubble' appearance of a tumour which involves the adjacent epiphysis.

Harold Ellis.

CRAMPS

Cramps are involuntary muscular contractions accompanied by sharp pain in the voluntary muscles involved. They may arise in a variety of circumstances. In most instances cramps result from *over-exertion* of the affected muscles. The most striking example of this is *swimmer's cramp.* The victim is overtaken suddenly by painful spasm and paralysis of the muscles of a leg or arm; he is liable to drown unless help is speedily forthcoming. Similar but less extensive cramps may be experienced by persons taking part in the more strenuous of outdoor games— football, hockey, lacrosse—when some particularly sudden or violent effort may be followed by cramp in the thigh or calf muscles. Everybody has a proclivity to cramp during the night quite independently of activity; such cramps occur in perfectly normal people and in most cases are of no medical significance. The muscle is visibly and palpably taut and painful and is eased by getting out of bed and moving and massaging the affected area. The legs of stokers, iron-founders, and miners, who do heavy bodily work in a much overheated atmosphere, are liable to heat cramps, severely painful spasms in the muscles of the limbs and abdomen, in attacks lasting for many hours and followed by great weakness. In these, loss of sodium chloride in the sweat is the responsible factor. The diagnosis of cramps due to over-exertion, directly associated as they are with a definite history of muscular strain, should not be difficult. They rarely become so severe as to prevent their victims from continuing to take part in the occupations that provoke their occurrence.

It is quite otherwise, however, with patients who are afflicted with the *professional cramps* or *occupation neuroses* that result from chronic strain and over-use of certain groups of muscles. These occur in such persons as writers, typists, telegraph operators, compositors, painters, tailors, seamstresses, pianists, flute-players, violinists, 'cellists, drummers, blacksmiths, file-makers, watchmakers. In all these occupations, particular groups of muscles are in constant routine employment. If they are overworked they may become the seat of cramps and aching pains—professional cramps —as soon as they are used, their movements lose their delicacy and become incoordinated and spasmodic. A fine tremor is commonly to be observed in the affected limb. It is probable that over-use alone is not enough to set up these cramps. Anxiety, ill-health, local injury or disease, and mental (emotional) tension, all contribute to the establishment of professional cramps. The affected groups of muscles vary with the occupation of the patient. As a rule, the diagnosis of professional cramp is not difficult, but it is necessary to make sure that neither organic nervous affection nor local disorder is present. Thus underlying so-called writer's cramp may be early Parkinsonism, rheumatoid arthritis, or some other disorder. Affections of the joints or of the tendons at the wrists, such as rheumatoid arthritis, tenosynovitis, tuberculous infection, may all give rise to pain in, and interference with the movements of, the hand. Again, writer's cramp may be so much feared by nervous patients that the right hand may become so stiff, or weak, or painful as to prohibit its employment. Objective signs of the cramp, however, are lacking in such cases, which are cured by the re-establishment of the patient's self-confidence or the use of a typewriter!

Cramps are the main feature of *tetany*, a disease characterized by the occurrence of paroxysmal or continued tetanic spasms of the extremities and increased excitability of the nerves and muscles to electrical or mechanical stimulation. Tetany occurs in many different conditions, and at any age. It is often the result of decrease in the concentration of free calcium ions in the plasma and may be seen after accidental removal of parathyroids in thyroidectomy and also in aldosteronism, in alkalosis, in hypokalaemia, and in hypomagnesaemia. In infants and young children it is a complication of rickets, improper feeding, and gastro-intestinal disorders either with or without diarrhoea and vomiting, lack of or resistance to vitamin D being responsible. Tetany may also occur in renal tubular acidosis. Alkalosis may be the cause of tetany, by overbreathing, by persistent vomiting, hypokalaemia, or excessive consumption of alkali. When a patient under strict routine treatment for gastric ulcer becomes irritable, refuses food, and complains of headache, alkalosis is the probable cause (*see* p. 170 for the 'milk-alkali syndrome'). Twitchings may ensue, with a rise of blood-urea to even five times the normal. Epidemics of tetany in young adults, probably resulting from food-poisoning, have been described. In nursing women, tetany may follow prolonged lactation, or it may develop during pregnancy and recur in successive pregnancies. It may result from the operative removal of too much or all of the parathyroid glands. A few instances are on record in which tetany has followed the acute specific fevers, enteric fever, or poisoning by lead or ergot. The cramps of tetany are mainly in the extremities, and paroxysmal; they may continue for hours or days. During the spasms, the fingers are extended at the terminal, and flexed at the metacarpo-phalangeal joints and pressed together, while the thumb is adducted and flexed into the palm, so that the so-called 'accoucheur's hand' is produced. The wrist and elbow are flexed, the arms being usually folded over the chest; exceptionally the elbow may be extended stiffly. The toes are drawn together and flexed, the foot is arched and turned inwards, the ankles and knees are extended. As a rule the limbs only are involved, but in severe cases cramps occur in the face, neck, and even the trunk, when respiration may be seriously embarrassed. The rigid muscles are very tender to the touch. Three special signs are present in the intervals between the attacks of tetany and are of assistance in diagnosis: these are Trousseau's sign, or reproduction of the paroxysm by manual compression of the nerves or blood-vessels supplying the affected parts; Erb's sign, or hyperexcitability of the motor nerves to electrical currents (0·5–2 milliamperes); and Chvostek's sign, or reproduction of the spasm in the facial muscles by tapping either on the muscles themselves or on the branches of the facial nerve. Tetany must be diagnosed from *tetanus*, in which the spasms begin in the head and neck and trismus is an early symptom, and from *strychnine poisoning*, when the spasms are clonic rather than tetanic and affect the whole body and not the extremities primarily or principally. In the *carpo-pedal spasms* of rickety children or of infants with severe gastro-intestinal disease, the cramps are similar to those of tetany but are transient, and often affect the hands only, or the hands and arms. Such spasms may justly be regarded as identical with mild tetany. *Hysterical tetany* occurs, and is to be distinguished from true tetany by its association with other hysterical stigmata on the one hand, and by the absence of Trousseau's and Chvostek's signs on the other. Hysterical tetany may also be distinguished by associated sensory loss and by its failure to respond to the exhibition of calcium salts, since true tetany is the expression of hyperexcitability of the nerve-cells due to hypocalcaemia. Nevertheless, a hysterical patient may, by overbreathing, precipitate true tetany.

Reference may again be made to the fact that cramps are prone to occur in patients dehydrated by *acute fevers*; severe cramps in the legs and arms are often a highly troublesome feature of the convalescence from *cholera*. In many chronic diseases nocturnal cramps may give rise to considerable distress and may interfere seriously with sleep; in *uraemia, alcoholic neuritis*, and almost any chronic wasting disorder, complaint of cramp is not infrequent, but in such instances signs or symptoms of the responsible disease will be evident.

Intermittent claudication, a special variety of cramp-like pain in the legs due to arterial disease and induced by exertion, is described on p. 500. Here there is discomfort from inadequate arterial supply to the muscles, but no true muscle cramp or contraction. Similarly in spastic paralysis and myotonic conditions there is hypertonicity of muscles rather than involuntary muscle contraction.

F. Dudley Hart.

CREPITUS

Crepitus is a term generally used to denote the grating or crackling sensation and noise produced

7

when two rough substances rub together, as for instance the bony grating that can be felt and heard between the fractured ends of a bone. Articular crepitus arises most commonly from osteoarthrotic degenerative changes in joints, most commonly the knee, where subpatellar fine friction can be felt with the hands in many cases, often early in the degenerative process; the patient should be reassured that it is not a serious finding but is felt by most middle-aged or elderly persons at some time in their lives. Similarly, the awareness of a grating sensation in the neck, apparent to patient and clinician, is a common and usually a relatively unimportant finding. A coarser crepitation may be felt after trauma with subpatellar chondromalacia. Coarse crepitation or 'crackling' may be felt with the hands or heard with the ear wherever degenerative changes occur, for instance in the neck or shoulder, but is more common in the more mobile weight-bearing joints, where cartilage has become worn and degenerated, such as the ankle and, more commonly, the knee.

In rheumatoid arthritis a fine 'rubbing' crepitus occurs which can be felt over the joints in relatively early cases; this may become coarser as the cartilage becomes destroyed by the inflammatory process. At the shoulder inflammatory or degenerative processes may produce crepitus at scapulohumeral or acromioclavicular joints, and a peculiar sensation may be experienced with the hand over the scapular border as though the bone was moving over soft marbles; this again, is not a sign of serious disease and the patient can in most cases be fully reassured.

Crepitus from within a joint should be distinguished from sharp cracking sounds occurring in normal or abnormal joints after temporary immobility and from the slipping of tendons and ligaments over bone surfaces on movement.

On palpation of a joint with hydrarthrosis, the so-called 'silken crepitus' can occasionally be felt, as if two silken surfaces were being rubbed together by the examiner's hands. *Tenosynovitis*, especially around the flexor tendons at the wrist, can also produce a feeling of crepitus, to patient and examiner.

When there is an enlargement of a bone without fracture, and when on palpation a feeling of crepitus or egg-shell crackling is obtained, it indicates that some tumour is eroding the overlying cortex. A radiograph will be necessary to establish the diagnosis.

Rarefaction of the bones of the skull, either as the result of syphilitic lesions in adults, or of *hydrocephalus* or *craniotabes*, especially in the occipital region of congenitally syphilitic and rickety infants, may make the skull bones so thin that they bend readily on pressure, and sometimes the result is a sensation of crepitus. The diagnosis is generally obvious. The condition is very rare.

Apart from bony, arthritic, or synovial changes, a characteristic feeling of crepitus may be felt beneath the skin when gas or air has accumulated in the subcutaneous tissues as the result of SURGICAL EMPHYSEMA (p. 252). Occasionally a coarse pleural rub can be felt with the hand on the chest.

R. G. Beard.
F. Dudley Hart.

CYANOSIS

Cyanosis is seen whenever the red cells in the cutaneous and subcutaneous blood-vessels contain an excess of reduced haemoglobin; the blood in the subpapillary venous plexuses probably influences the colour of the skin more than that in the capillaries. The old dictum that there is a critical level of reduced haemoglobin, 5 g./dl., in capillary blood above which cyanosis appears is difficult to substantiate consistently. It does, however, explain the rarity of cyanosis if severe anaemia is present and the ease with which cyanosis appears in the presence of polycythaemia. In practice cyanosis is classified as central or peripheral. *Central cyanosis* is associated with arterial hypoxaemia and can usually be seen when the arterial oxygen saturation falls below 85 per cent (with a normal haemoglobin concentration). It is seen in all parts of the skin and mucous membranes, including the inner sides of the lips and the tongue. *Peripheral cyanosis* is due to a reduced rate of blood-flow through the skin allowing greater than normal extraction of oxygen; this may be due to a low cardiac output or to local vasoconstriction or to both factors. It is seen in the exposed areas such as fingers, ears, nose, and cheeks but not in the mucous membranes or in the warmer parts of the skin. Excessive amounts of methaemoglobin or sulphaemoglobin in the red cells causes *pigmentary cyanosis*. This is strictly a form of central cyanosis and it certainly enters into the differential diagnosis of that condition. It will be discussed separately, however, as it is of entirely different aetiology.

I. CENTRAL CYANOSIS

Arterial hypoxaemia can be due to one or more of four mechanisms. The most important is *unequal distribution of ventilation and perfusion* in the lungs. Alveoli which are poorly ventilated contain gas with a low P_{O_2} and hence the blood perfusing these alveoli is poorly saturated with oxygen; if this blood contributes largely to the pulmonary venous return arterial hypoxaemia and cyanosis will result. An extreme example of ventilation/perfusion imbalance is seen if totally unventilated alveoli are perfused as in collapse of a lobe or segment of a lobe. A *shunt* of blood occurs from pulmonary arteries to pulmonary veins without any gas exchange occurring. An exactly analogous situation is seen in the presence of a central veno-arterial shunt in cyanotic congenital heart disease. A third factor is general *alveolar hypoventilation* which is the mechanism of cyanosis in, for example, narcotic poisoning. Finally, *impairment of diffusion*—the transfer of oxygen from alveolar gas to capillary blood— may occur, particularly in the diffuse varieties of pulmonary fibrosis. The importance of this factor has been overemphasized in the past and 'alveolo-capillary block' is now regarded as, at most, a minor cause of cyanosis.

For clinical purposes the causes of central cyanosis can be classified as respiratory or cardiac. Whatever the cause, chronic hypoxaemia often causes secondary polycythaemia; this is due to a direct effect on the bone-marrow.

1. Respiratory Disease. Alveolar hypoventilation is the mechanism of cyanosis in obstruction of the upper airways. Thus, in the extreme example of total occlusion of the larynx by a foreign body, no ventilation is possible and alveolar and arterial

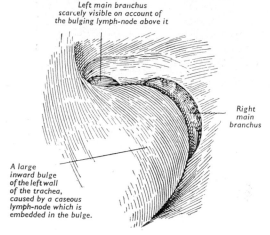

Fig. 210.—Bronchoscopic appearances of a case of tracheal compression from enlarged lymph-nodes. There was extreme dyspnoea and cyanosis in this case, relieved at once by the passage of the bronchoscope.

P_{O_2} rapidly fall to extremely low levels and the patient becomes deeply cyanosed. Lesser degrees of arterial hypoxaemia and cyanosis may be due to lesions such as retropharyngeal abscess, diphtheritic laryngitis, acute laryngeal oedema (which is often allergic in origin), and bilateral abductor paralysis such as may follow thyroidectomy. Tracheal obstruction is most commonly from without by such lesions as carcinoma of the thyroid, Riedel's thyroiditis, haemorrhage into a thyroid cyst, or neoplastic or, rarely, tuberculous lymph-nodes (*Fig.* 210). Primary carcinoma of the trachea, which is rare, and tumours of the main bronchi, growing upwards, may produce severe obstruction; tracheal stenosis following tracheostomy and subglottic stenosis after prolonged intubation (*Fig.* 211) are other possible causes.

Obstructive lesions of the main bronchi, such as, for example, bronchial carcinoma or, less commonly, tuberculous stenosis or adenoma,

may produce cyanosis if perfusion of the unventilated areas of lung continues. In practice there is often a considerable reduction in blood-flow in such cases and cyanosis is less intense than might have been expected. Similar considerations apply in massive collapse of the lung, a recognized complication of thoracic and upper abdominal surgery. The collapse of a lung which

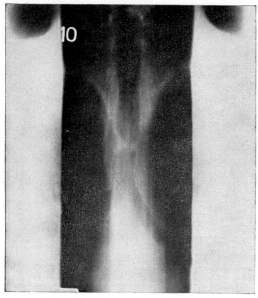

Fig. 211. Tomogram showing tracheal stenosis resulting from ulceration produced by an endotracheal tube. (*Film by courtesy of Dr. Basil Strickland.*)

can be caused by a badly introduced endotracheal tube must not be forgotten. If the tube is passed too far so that it enters a bronchus, usually the right, ventilation of the other lung ceases with, sometimes, dramatic effects (*Fig.* 212). Occlusion of a correctly sited tube by inspissated mucus can also produce severe hypoxaemia.

Of the diseases of the lungs themselves, there are hardly any in which cyanosis does not occur if the damage is severe and little purpose would be served by a comprehensive list. The major varieties of pulmonary disease are discussed in the section on DYSPNOEA (p. 236) where the importance of arterial hypoxaemia, itself due to ventilatory insufficiency, in causing increased exercise ventilation is emphasized. However, a few points relevant to cyanosis in lung disease should be discussed.

In chronic obstructive-airways disease, with varying combinations of chronic bronchitis and emphysema, the severity of the cyanosis turns to a considerable extent on the sensitivity of the respiratory centre to the raised arterial P_{CO_2}. In the so-called 'pink puffers' the respiratory centre retains its normal behaviour and responds to the hypercapnia by producing considerable hyperventilation. This maintains the arterial oxygen saturation at a near-normal level at the expense of severe dyspnoea. In the 'blue bloaters', on the other hand, the respiratory centre has lost its ability to respond to a rising P_{CO_2}; dyspnoea is less severe but hypoxaemia and cyanosis are marked and cardiac failure develops as a result.

In some varieties of restrictive lung disease, such as fibrosing alveolitis, cyanosis, particularly

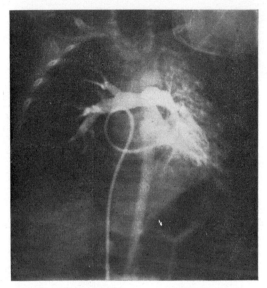

Fig. 212. Collapse of left lung as a result of faulty insertion of an endotracheal tube; angiocardiography was being performed under general anaesthesia. The tube can just be seen passing behind the right pulmonary artery to enter the right main bronchus. The contrast-filled right ventricle is displaced to the left. Continued perfusion of the airless left lung is demonstrated by the contrast medium within its vessels. (*Film by courtesy of Dr. Basil Strickland.*)

the eighteenth century and 'blue baby' in the twentieth testify further to the importance attached to cyanosis in this group of conditions although, in fact, rather less than a quarter of all cases of congenital heart disease are cyanosed.

An important point in the differentiation of cyanosis due to a central veno-arterial shunt from that due to primary lung disease is the

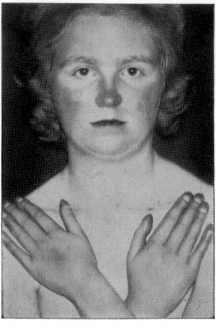

Fig. 213. Girl, aged 18, with Fallot's tetralogy. Central cyanosis and finger clubbing.

on exertion, is a prominent feature. It is possible that a diffusion defect, due to thickening of the alveolo-capillary membrane, plays some small part in this but it is now clear that disturbances in the ventilation/perfusion ratio are of much greater importance. The anatomical distortion of the smallest airways causes hypoventilation of many alveoli and, while the patient is breathing air, the alveolar P_{O_2} falls below normal as a result. The administration of oxygen raises the alveolar P_{O_2} despite hypoventilation and the hypoxaemia and cyanosis improve strikingly.

2. Heart Disease. Probably the commonest cause of hypoxaemia in heart disease is pulmonary venous hypertension in mitral valve disease and left ventricular failure. This is rarely severe enough to cause cyanosis except in attacks of acute pulmonary oedema.

Congenital heart disease is a numerically much less common but clinically more dramatic cause of cyanosis (*Fig.* 213). Graphic descriptions abound in the early literature as in the account by James Hope of the child who looked as if she had been eating blackberries, so blue were her lips. The emotive terms 'morbus caeruleus' in

response to oxygen. In the latter a considerable reduction in cyanosis can be expected to result from a rise in alveolar P_{O_2} unless many alveoli are completely unventilated, producing the effect of a shunt. In cyanotic congenital heart disease oxygen produces virtually no change in the arterial oxygen saturation as the veno-arterial mixing occurs down stream from the pulmonary vascular bed. Other features common to all types of cyanotic congenital heart disease are clubbing of the fingers and toes and polycythaemia, as in other conditions causing chronic arterial hypoxaemia. In severe cases the haemoglobin concentration may be well over 20 g./dl. and the finding of a 'normal' haemoglobin in such a case is tantamount to a diagnosis of anaemia.

Fallot's tetralogy is by far the most common congenital cardiac lesion to cause cyanosis. The four classic features are pulmonary stenosis, ventricular septal defect, over-riding aorta, and right ventricular hypertrophy; of these, the last is the direct haemodynamic consequence of the pulmonary stenosis; the over-riding aorta, although characteristic, is not a major factor in determining the presence or severity of cyanosis.

An associated anomaly in several cases is a right-sided aortic arch; this must not be confused with dextro-position of the aorta—a synonym for over-riding. Cyanosis is not often present at birth but develops, with clubbing, during the first year or two of life. The symptoms include dyspnoea, relieved by squatting, and syncope associated with deepening of the cyanosis (*see* DYSPNOEA and FAINTING, pp. 236, 283). The arterial and venous pulses are unremarkable except for, occasionally, a dominant a wave in the jugular venous pulse. The apex beat is little displaced and there may

pulmonary hypertension with reversed interventricular shunt. These conditions, and tricuspid atresia, another cause of cyanosis, are discussed in the section on DYSPNOEA (p. 236).

Transposition of the great arteries is a relatively common form of cyanotic congenital heart disease in infancy although few untreated patients survive. The aorta arises from the right ventricle and the pulmonary artery from the left and, clearly, communications betwen the two circulations, at atrial or ventricular level, must also be present if life is to be maintained. Pulmonary

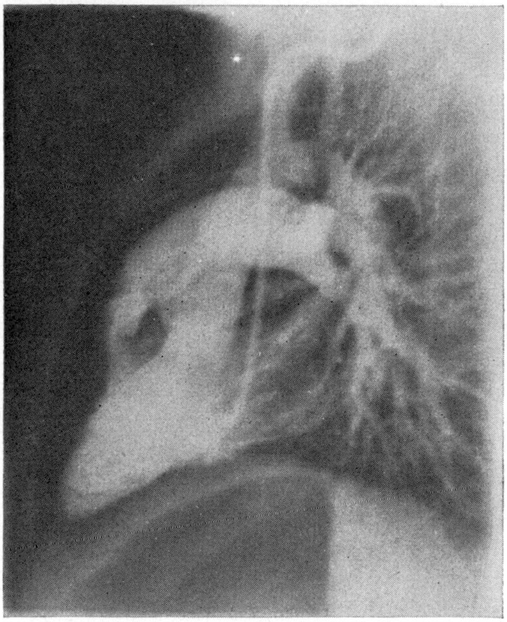

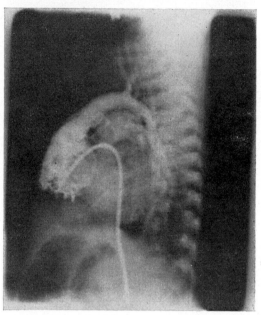

Fig. 214. Lateral view of angiocardiogram in Fallot's tetralogy. The contrast medium has been injected into the right ventricle and has passed both into the pulmonary artery via an infundibular stenosis and into the over-riding aorta via a large ventricular septal defect. The normal pulmonary valve can be seen just distal to the infundibular stenosis. (*Film by courtesy of Dr. Basil Strickland.*)

Fig. 215. Lateral view of angiocardiogram in transposition of the great arteries. The contrast medium has been injected into the right ventricle and has passed into the anteriorly placed aorta. The pulmonary artery, lying posteriorly, has been opacified via a ductus which is visible. (*Film by courtesy of Dr. Basil Strickland.*)

be a slight or moderate right ventricular impulse at the left sternal border. The systolic murmur is rather short and often loud enough to be accompanied by a thrill; the second sound is single. The X-ray and electrocardiograms are discussed in the section on DYSPNOEA (p. 236). The definitive diagnosis can be made by angiocardiography (*Fig.* 214).

Pulmonary atresia is embryologically related to Fallot's tetralogy and usually produces very severe cyanosis. The differentiation is easily made by the absence of the systolic murmur of pulmonary stenosis in atresia and its replacement by a subclavicular continuous murmur, usually bilateral, due to large anastomoses between the bronchial and pulmonary arteries. Other conditions which may be more difficult to distinguish clinically from Fallot's tetralogy are pulmonary stenosis with reversed interatrial shunt and Eisenmenger's complex, properly so called, that is

stenosis or pulmonary hypertension may also be present to complicate the haemodynamic situation. The physical signs vary with the associated abnormalities but the X-ray may be of diagnostic value. The vascular pedicle of the heart is rather narrow in the postero-anterior view and pulmonary plethora is nearly always present. As oligaemia of the lung fields is the rule in most types of cyanotic congenital heart disease, the association of cyanosis with plethora is very suggestive of transposition. Angiocardiography is diagnostic, showing, in the lateral view, the aorta arising anteriorly from the right ventricle and the pulmonary artery posteriorly from the left (*Fig.* 215).

Very rare types of cyanotic congenital heart disease include drainage of the superior or inferior vena cava into the left atrium and some cases of Ebstein's anomaly of the tricuspid valve with reversed interatrial shunt.

Congenital pulmonary arteriovenous aneurysm could perhaps have been classified under Respiratory Disease. However, as it produces a true veno-arterial shunt, from the pulmonary artery to a pulmonary vein, it can be considered here. It is frequently associated with cutaneous telangiectases and may occur in the familial condition, hereditary haemorrhagic telangiectasia. Continuous murmurs may be heard over the aneurysms, which may be multiple. In the X-ray

vasoconstriction of *acute left ventricular failure* can also cause peripheral cyanosis; in this condition, of course, central cyanosis may be present in addition, due to the pulmonary oedema. Peripheral cyanosis is also a feature of *mitral stenosis* in which the cardiac output is chronically reduced. The classic malar flush is no more than peripheral cyanosis localized, for no known reason, to that particular region. Cyanosis is also common following massive *pulmonary embolism*; this is partly peripheral in type but, in this condition, arterial hypoxaemia is also a factor.

There is a group of conditions in which peripheral cyanosis of the extremities occurs as a result of local arterial constriction. The best known is *Raynaud's disease* in which the digital arteries constrict tightly in response to cold or, less commonly, to emotional disturbances. The fingers and, sometimes, the toes are initially cold and pale but, later in the attack, as the minute

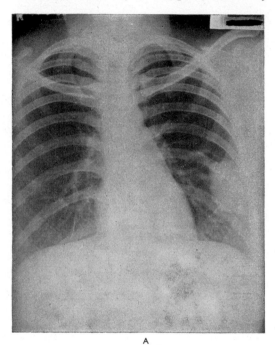
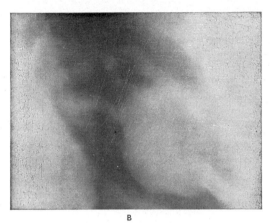

A   B

Fig. 216. Pulmonary haemangioma in a case of hereditary haemorrhagic telangiectasia. A, In the plain film large vessels can be seen passing to and from the tumour. B, These are shown more clearly in the tomogram. (*Films by courtesy of Dr. Basil Strickland.*)

one or more round opacities are visible and tomography will often reveal the feeding artery and draining vein (*Fig.* 216).

II. PERIPHERAL CYANOSIS

If, for any reason, red cells remain longer than usual in the capillaries, the continued tissue extraction of oxygen will reduce the oxygen saturation of the haemoglobin so that cyanosis appears. This may be due either to a reduced rate of inflow into the capillary bed as a result of a low cardiac output or local arterial disease, or to an obstruction to the venous drainage from the capillaries.

The ashen appearance of a patient in severe *shock* is a typical example of peripheral cyanosis due to a gross fall in cardiac output. This is so whether the shock is due to a fall in circulating blood-volume as, for example, in haemorrhage, severe diarrhoea, and vomiting, or to acute pancreatitis or to a primary fall in cardiac output as in the so-called cardiogenic shock following myocardial infarction. The low cardiac output and

cutaneous vessels relax, cyanosis appears. Pain is a prominent feature and, in severe cases, small patches of gangrene may appear on the fingers. *Raynaud's phenomenon*, producing similar manifestations, must be clearly distinguished from primary Raynaud's disease. It may be due to occlusive disease of the large arteries of the limbs, cervical rib and other similar lesions, systemic lupus erythematosus, or systemic sclerosis (scleroderma). Raynaud's phenomenon can also occur after severe cold injury and, as an occupational hazard, in workers with vibrating instruments such as pneumatic drills. *Acrocyanosis* is a relatively benign condition due to spasm of the smaller cutaneous arteries and arterioles. The hands and fingers are cold and mottled red and blue but pain is not a feature. Arteriolar spasm is also the mechanism of *erythrocyanosis*, a disease almost confined to young women in which cyanotic blotches which are virtually large chilblains are seen on the lower parts of the legs. It is invariably produced by exposure to cold and, as Sir Thomas Lewis said, 'it came in with short skirts and thin stockings and will go out with them'. That, of course, remains to be seen.

The cyanosis which may be a feature of *poly-cythaemia rubra vera* can conveniently be discussed here. In the past, an increase in the amount of reduced haemoglobin in the blood was postulated but it is now known that the arterial oxygen saturation is practically always normal. The cyanosis is probably caused by the reduced rate of blood-flow which results from the increased viscosity of the blood.

As the old name 'phlegmasia caerulea dolens' implies, cyanosis of the affected leg is common in *phlebothrombosis* if a large vein is involved and collateral channels are few. The cyanosis of the face which, together with gross venous engorgement and oedema, is a feature of *superior vena caval obstruction* is also peripheral in type and due to the failure of adequate drainage from the capillary bed. So-called *traumatic* cyanosis following crush injury to the chest is probably mainly peripheral in type and due to obstruction of the superior vena cava by mediastinal haemorrhage; in such cases intrapulmonary haemorrhage, causing central cyanosis, might well be present in addition.

Pigmentary Cyanosis. Cyanosis is a feature of a group of conditions in which methaemoglobin is present in a higher concentration than normal in the red cells; sulphaemoglobin is also often present in these conditions.

Haemoglobin can be readily converted to methaemoglobin by free oxygen *in vitro*, the ferrous (Fe^{++}) iron being oxidized to the ferric (Fe^{+++}) state. That this does not occur in the erythrocytes *in vivo* is due to the action of various intracellular enzymes. Hereditary deficiency of these enzymes or the formation of methaemoglobin which is abnormal in respect of its globin component are the bases of the *congenital methaemoglobinaemias*. The mode of inheritance is usually recessive but at least one type is believed to behave as a dominant characteristic.

Acquired methaemoglobinaemia can be produced by a large group of chemical substances some of which, such as nitrites and chlorates, are direct oxidizing agents; others, for example phenacetin, exert their effects indirectly. Nitrates can be converted to nitrites in the bowel and cyanosis has been reported in infants in association with a high nitrate content of drinking water. Poisoning with potassium chlorate can also produce methaemoglobinaemia apart from its more serious effects. Aniline derivatives, used in marking and dyeing textiles, have also been incriminated; these compounds can be absorbed through the intact skin. Phenacetin, also, can cause methaemoglobinaemia and cyanosis, more dramatic but less serious than the potentially lethal nephropathy. This is much less common than hitherto as phenacetin is no longer a constituent of many proprietary analgesic tablets; the same can be said of sulphaemoglobinaemia. As little as 1·5 g. methaemoglobin in 100 ml. blood will produce

clinical cyanosis: about 5 g. reduced haemoglobin must be present before a comparable degree of cyanosis is seen. Levels of less than 20 per cent methaemoglobin are usually symptomless. It is rapidly reversible on stopping the offending drug, unlike sulphaemoglobinaemia, which remains in the red cells until their death. Small amounts of sulphaemoglobin, such as 0·5 g., cause as much cyanosis as 1·5 g. methaemoglobin or 5 g. reduced haemoglobin.

The cyanosis of methaemoglobinaemia is said to be distinguishable from that of arterial hypoxaemia, by those who practised in what could be called the phenacetin (mixed analgesic) era. Such a cyanosis was relatively common then in the patients attending rheumatism units 25 or more years ago. The other symptoms, such as dyspnoea on exertion, dizziness, and headaches, are virtually those of severe anaemia to which the condition is closely analogous. The diagnosis can be confirmed by spectroscopic analysis of a 1 : 100 dilution of blood; in the presence of methaemoglobin a band is seen at 630 mμ which disappears on the addition of a reducing agent.

P. R. Fleming.

CYSTINURIA

This denotes the presence of cystine (di-β-thio-α-amino-propionic acid) in the urine in increased amounts. This is usually demonstrated by paper chromatography, when ornithine, lysine, and arginine are also found in typical cases of cystinuria. Cystine is a very insoluble amino-acid and typical hexagonal crystals of the compound may be seen on microscopy of a concentrated acidic urine specimen (*Fig.* 217). Cystinuria

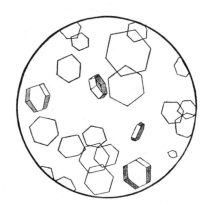

Fig. 217. Cystine crystals, as seen under the high-power microscope (⅙-in. objective): colourless flat hexagonal plates.

accounts for about 1 per cent of all urinary calculi, and a greater proportion in childhood and adolescence. The calculi are radio-opaque owing to the high sulphur content of the cystine molecule, but produce a much less dense shadow than calcium phosphate or calcium oxalate calculi of similar size. Accurate diagnosis of cystine calculi is important as methods of prevention of further stone formation are different from those used in other types of renal calculi. The nitroprusside test is useful; urine or a suspension of scrapings from a suspected calculus is treated with 5 per cent sodium cyanide solution for about 5 minutes, when cystine is reduced to cysteine. Drops of freshly prepared 5 per cent sodium nitroprusside solution are then added, and if cystine is present a reddish purple colour is produced. Confirmation of the diagnosis in positive cases by means of paper chromatography is obligatory.

Cystinuria is due to an autosomal recessive hereditary anomaly, and heterozygotes in some affected families, but not in all, show increased urinary excretion of cystine and lysine in amounts insufficient to cause cystine calculi.

Treatment is by surgical removal of large stones, and further calculus formation can often be prevented by a water diuresis, a urine volume of at least 3·5 l. per day being necessary in adult patients. It is especially important to maintain an adequate diuresis at night, as cystine crystallizes, particularly in the concentrated and acidic urine produced during sleep. If treatment by diuresis fails, oral penicillamine, 1·5–2·0 g. daily in adults may be useful, as the drug converts cystine to a more soluble mixed disulphide with consequent prevention of calculus formation. Unfortunately, penicillamine is both toxic and expensive, and cannot be tolerated by some patients.

M. D. Milne.

DEAFNESS

In considering the differential diagnosis of deafness it is necessary to establish first the degree of deafness present, secondly the site of the causative lesion, and thirdly the nature of the lesion.

But before this can be done it is essential to understand the basic classification of deafness, which is as follows. All cases of deafness can be classified in two main groups, *Conductive* or *Sensorineural*. The sensorineural group may be further subdivided into *cochlear* forms of deafness and *retrocochlear* forms, and the retrocochlear subgroup still further into *neural* and *central*.

Briefly, conductive deafness may be caused by an obstructive lesion of the external ear or some lesion of the tympanic membrane or ossicles whereby sound waves are prevented from reaching the inner ear. Sensorineural deafness, which in the past has often been referred to as 'perceptive' or 'nerve' deafness, comprises lesions of the cochlea (cochlear deafness), and auditory nerve or central connections (retrocochlear deafness).

HEARING TESTS

It is most useful, when investigating every case of deafness, to ascertain at the outset the extent of the hearing-loss by the use of the whispered and conversational voice.

The Spoken Word Test. The patient sits facing the wall at one end of the room and occludes the deafer ear by pressing a finger against the tragus. He is instructed to repeat after the examiner whatever the latter says.

The examiner, starting at the far end of the room, whispers test words and he approaches until the patient is able to repeat the words accurately. If the deafness is severe it may be necessary for the examiner to raise his voice to a 'conversational voice'. The distance from examiner to patient is now noted and might be expressed, for example in a slightly deaf person, as W.V. (whispered voice) at 6 ft, or in a case of severe deafness as C.V. (conversational voice) at 6 in.

Now the deafer ear is tested in the same way, the less deaf ear being occluded.

Care must be taken that lip-reading is avoided and it is possible in some cases, where a gross difference in the hearing acuity of the two ears is present, that a completely erroneous result may be obtained unless the better ear is masked with a Bárány noise apparatus whilst the more deaf ear is being tested.

Tuning-fork Tests. These have been employed for over a century for the purpose not of measuring the degree of deafness present but for the relegation of each case of deafness to its appropriate group in the classification. Nevertheless, great errors are made unless careful attention is paid to certain details. In the first place it is quite useless to attempt to carry out tuning-fork tests with the forks usually employed to confirm or exclude the presence of vibration-sense, e.g., a fork of 128 double vibrations; furthermore, a small fork which when struck produces a note that fades rapidly is equally inappropriate to the task. The tuning-fork of choice should have a frequency of 512 dB and should be massive enough for its note to last at least 60 seconds after being sounded, otherwise Rinne's test cannot be performed with accuracy.

Weber's Test. A vibrating tuning-fork placed on the head in the midline is normally heard equally in either ear, i.e., the sound cannot be lateralized by the patient; should one ear be affected by conductive deafness, the fork is heard better in that ear; in sensorineural deafness the sound is lateralized to the better hearing ear.

Rinne's Test. The base of a vibrating fork is held on the patient's mastoid process until he signifies that he can no longer hear the sound. The fork is then rapidly transferred until the prongs are close to the external auditory meatus and in the normal ear *or* in the ear afflicted by sensorineural deafness the sound can still be heard for some seconds. In other words, hearing by air-conduction is better than hearing by bone-conduction owing to the fact that the amplifying middle-ear apparatus is intact. On the other hand, if it is found that hearing by bone-conduction is better than by air-conduction a diagnosis of conductive deafness is made.

Absolute Bone-conduction Test. In this test the patient's ear is occluded by pressure on the tragus and the base of the vibrating fork is applied to the mastoid process. The patient signals as soon as the sound disappears and the examiner with one of his ears occluded immediately applies the fork to his own mastoid. If he can still hear the note it can be deduced that the patient has some degree of sensorineural hearing loss. This test presupposes that the examiner himself has good hearing.

Pure-tone Audiometry. The pure-tone audiometer produces tones of varying intensity (0–100 dB) and frequency (125 cps or Hz–8000 cps or 8 kHz), and by its application the examiner can detect the threshold of hearing for each frequency in each of the patient's ears. A graph is first plotted for air-conduction using headphones, and then for bone-conduction using an applicator in contact with the patient's mastoid process, and from the position of the lines on the graph can be deduced the degree of deafness and its place in the classification, i.e., conductive or sensorineural (*Fig.* 218).

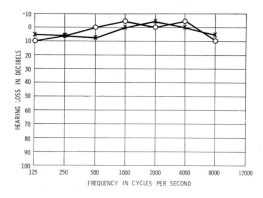

Fig. 218. Audiogram showing hearing that is within 'normal limits'. It is conventional to represent hearing by air-conduction in the right ear by O——O, and in the left ear by ×——×.

Békésy Audiometry. This machine is of value in distinguishing between cochlear and retro-cochlear deafness and demonstrates the presence or absence of what is known as *recruitment*. The latter is present in end-organ or cochlear deafness and is manifested in the patient by intolerance of amplification.

Speech Audiometry. In this test the examiner varies the loudness of a recorded list of test-words, noting the patient's 'score', and again the presence of loudness recruitment may be demonstrated.

Acoustic Impedance. The acoustic impedance meter is one of the most valuable tools of the audiologist and is used to show the degree of mobility of the tympanic membrane and to diagnose the presence of ossicular fixation or fluid in the middle ear. It is also employed to elicit the intratympanic muscle reflexes.

7*

In addition to the methods and tests mentioned, there are many others, such as Fowler's loudness balance test, the SISI test, and the tone decay test, and it is of interest to note that almost all these methods are subjective and depend on the co-operation of the patient. In recent years, however, two purely objective techniques have been evolved, that of evoked response audiometry and electrocochleography, and the reader is advised to consult the standard textbooks on otology and audiology for details.

CONDUCTIVE DEAFNESS

Efficient clinical examination of the ears will demonstrate the cause in most cases. The auricle, external auditory meatus, and tympanic membrane are examined for abnormalities, and the Eustachian tube is inflated to discover whether it allows the normal passage of air or is obstructed. The mouth, palate, fauces, tonsils, and nose are also examined and the nasopharynx is of particular importance.

There may be *blockage* of the *external auditory meatus* as a result of *congenital* or *traumatic stenosis*, a *furuncle*, or *otitis externa*, or by spread from an *inflamed auricle*. The lumen of the meatus may be occluded by *cerumen, foreign body, blood, exostoses*, or a *polypoidal growth*.

The tympanic membrane may be perforated as in *chronic suppurative otitis media*, active or quiescent, or it may be torn as in recent *trauma*. It may present an astonishing variety of appearances as a result of *quiescent otitis media*, thus it may seem atrophic and almost transparent or thickened and marked with white calcareous deposits. When inflamed, as in *acute otitis media*, the membrane loses its normal pearly colour and becomes pink and later deep red and bulging; later if pus forms in the tympanum it will burst and the discharge issues through the perforation formed.

In *secretory otitis*, a common cause of conductive deafness in childhood, the tympanic membrane loses its normal lustre and appears dull or even yellowish, and hairlines may signify the presence of fluid in the middle ear. The nasopharynx must be carefully examined in such cases for, in an adult, secretory otitis with conductive deafness may be the first sign of a *nasopharyngeal neoplasm*.

Otosclerosis causes, in the first intances, conductive and at a later stage mixed conductive and sensorineural hearing loss. Its onset is usually during the second and third decades and it is often accompanied by tinnitus. There may be a positive family history, and pregnancy may cause a marked worsening of the deafness. *Paracusis Willisii* or the hearing of conversation better in a noisy environment, e.g., bus, train, or factory, may be admitted to by the patient. On examination the tympanic membranes are intact and normal in appearance, though occasionally so much otosclerotic bone is present on the promontory that a pink tinge is seen through the membrane—Schwartze's sign. The diagnosis is confirmed by audiometry, tympanometry, and tympanotomy (*Fig.* 219).

SENSORINEURAL DEAFNESS

Under this heading will be included cochlear, neural, and central causes, for in some cases it is difficult to pinpoint the exact site of the lesion

a part. Tuning-fork tests and the pure-tone audiograms are diagnostic, the latter showing a symmetrical increase in hearing loss for the upper tones (*Fig.* 220).

Noise-induced hearing loss is another common cause of sensorineural deafness and is seen after exposure either to sudden very high intensity

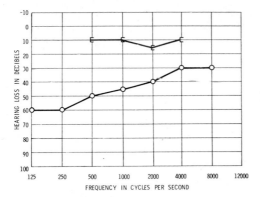

Fig. 219. Audiogram showing conductive deafness in the right ear in a case of otosclerosis. Hearing by air-conduction = ○——○. Hearing by bone-conduction = [——].

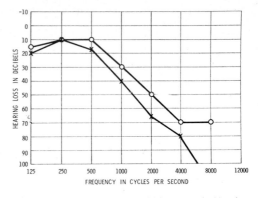

Fig. 220. Audiogram showing the fairly symmetrical hearing loss for high tones in presbyacusis.

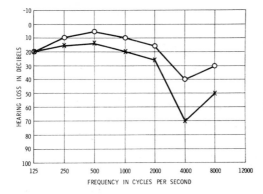

Fig. 221. Audiogram showing the typical findings in noise-induced hearing loss. In this case the patient had been shooting for some years with a 12-bore gun and the left ear, being nearer the muzzle, has sustained greater damage than the right.

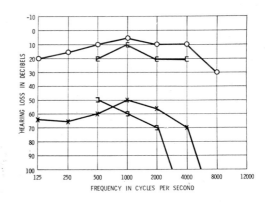

Fig. 222. Audiogram in a case of Ménière's disease affecting the left labyrinth. Careful investigations are required to exclude acoustic neuroma if unilateral sensorineural deafness such as this is found.

even with the sophistication of modern technology, and in others there may be a widespread disorder of the neural pathways.

By far the commonest cause of sensorineural deafness is *presbyacusis* or the deafness of increasing age, and as a rule both ears are affected to approximately the same extent. The upper tone limit of hearing begins to drop as we bid farewell to childhood and many persons between the ages of 50 and 60 years have difficulty in hearing door and telephone bells behind closed doors. There is widespread variation of individual susceptibility and numerous factors, e.g., heredity, arteriosclerosis, and varying exposure to noise in the lives of different individuals, play

sound or more prolonged exposure to gunfire, industrial noise, jet-engine noise, etc. It is of interest to note that most commonly the frequencies around 4 kHz are affected in noise-induced deafness; thus the audiogram is pathognomonic of the condition (*Fig.* 221). In late cases where, for example, there has been exposure to loud industrial noise for many years the adjoining regions of the basilar membrane become affected.

Labyrinthine hydrops causing *Ménière's disease* is characteristically associated with sensorineural hearing loss, tinnitus, and attacks of vertigo. It is of importance to note that the duration of the vertiginous attacks is measured in fractions or multiples of hours, not in seconds or weeks. Momentary or long-continued attacks of vertigo result from other causes. Other interesting features of the deafness are that it is liable to undergo fluctuations, whereas most forms of sensorineural hearing-loss are steadily progressive, and in some cases the low and medium tones are affected, thus producing a 'flat' type of audiogram—unusual in other forms of sensorineural deafness (*Fig.* 222). The diagnosis is confirmed by audiological investigations, caloric tests, and by carefully excluding other causes of deafness, e.g., *acoustic neuroma*.

Inner-ear deafness not infrequently arises from *vascular* causes. It may be gradual of onset and associated with *arteriosclerosis* or there may be definite evidence of *vertebrobasilar ischaemia*. On the other hand, vascular accidents may cause sudden deafness and these are regarded as being of the nature of spasm, or coagulation of the blood-vessels supplying the inner ear or even of haemorrhage in this region. *Hyperlipoproteinaemia* is undoubtedly associated with some cause of sensorineural hearing loss and is at present under investigation.

There are numerous less common causes of sensorineural deafness including the large group of *ototoxic drugs* of which neomycin, streptomycin, kanamycin, quinine, and alcohol (in excessive quantities) are only a few. Certain infections including *meningitis, mumps, influenza* (and other virus infections), and *enteric fever* are notorious and, of course, the infective process in *otitis media*, acute or chronic, may invade the inner ear causing *labyrinthitis* and severe deafness. *Syphilis* of congenital origin or, less commonly, late in the acquired form may cause serious and intractable deafness. Direct trauma, e.g., *fracture of the temporal bone*, can be responsible, also *Paget's disease*, *hypothyroidism*, and *avitaminosis*, and finally mention must be made of the various forms of *congenital* deafness dealt with in the following section.

The central connections of the neural pathways of hearing undergo such marked decussation and the auditory cortex is so extensive that widespread brain damage is necessary before central deafness becomes apparent. However, this may occur in *cerebral arteriosclerosis*, severe *cerebral trauma*, and *multiple sclerosis*. In the last condition the deafness may fluctuate.

DEAFNESS IN CHILDREN

Deafness in children is a matter of the utmost importance to the diagnostician for if it cannot be relieved it constitutes one of the most severe handicaps in life and its early recognition may in some cases do much to avert misery. In the first place it is necessary to realize what children may be 'at risk', and prenatal, perinatal, and postnatal causes have to be considered.

Some of the *prenatal causes* are familial in type, for example *Waardenburg's syndrome*, in which there is a white forelock, heterochromia iridum, and wide epicanthal folds, and the *Bing-Siebenmann, Scheibe, Mondini-Alexander* and *Michel* types in which there are varying degrees of development of the inner ear. In *Pendred's syndrome* a goitre and sensorineural deafness occur at birth, and in the *Usher syndrome* the deafness is associated with retinitis pigmentosa.

In addition to these familial causes of congenital sensorineural hearing loss, there are other causes of conductive deafness of familial type and associated with mandibulofacial dysostosis and varying degrees of abnormality of the middle-ear structures, tympanic membrane, and external ear. These are the *Treacher-Collins, Pierre Robin*, and *Franceschetti-Zwahlen* syndromes (*Figs.* 223, 224).

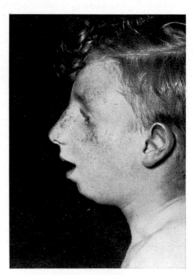

Fig. 223. Treacher-Collins syndrome, showing hypoplasia of the mandible and maxilla.

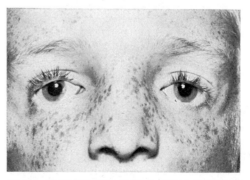

Fig. 224. Treacher-Collins syndrome, showing notching of the lower eyelid and deficient eyelashes.

Other prenatal causes of deafness are infections during the first trimester of pregnancy, the best known examples of which are *rubella* and *syphilis*. *Drugs* taken during pregnancy may also be responsible and *thalidomide* is of course well known in this connection. As a general rule, almost all drugs should remain suspect unless they have undergone, and passed, extensive trials of their potential teratogenicity.

Perinatal causes of congenital deafness are *haemolytic disease* or *kernicterus*, and *anoxia* associated with the delivery, and postnatal causes include such conditions as *meningitis* and *otitis media.*

Conductive deafness of onset during the first few years of life is most likely to be caused by *acute* or *chronic suppurative otitis media* or non-suppurative *secretory otitis* which is usually secondary to *tubal dysfunction.* Sensorineural deafness may make its appearance as a complication of the infectious diseases of childhood and the most common example of this is *mumps deafness* which is of interest inasmuch as it is usually unilateral.

As has already been stated, the recognition of any deafness in early childhood is a matter of supreme importance and any complaints from parents that their infant is inattentive or late in prattling must be taken seriously. Later, backwardness in speech or any disorder of speech should in the same way act as a warning sign to the medical attendant.

The accurate assessment of hearing loss in young children is a specialized technique and calls for experience, patience, and sophisticated equipment. In very young children drums, rattles, and pitch-pipes are employed and electro-cochleography and evoked response audiometry are now used for objective testing. Later the so-called 'show-me' tests are useful and towards the ages of 5–7 years pure tone and speech audiometry may be employed in assessment. The impedance audiometer in the assessment and differential diagnosis of deafness in children of all ages has proved invaluable.

Miles Foxen.

DELIRIUM

Delirium is a symptom of disordered function of all the highest cerebral centres. Its presence implies a depression of function short of coma; external and internal stimuli still reach the mind, but there is a failure of recognition, integration, and control, resulting in disordered thought and behaviour. The depression of function is not limited to any one function, although some aspects of intellectual activity may be more affected than others; it follows that delirium implies the presence of a diffuse cerebral disease or some general toxic factor rather than a localized cerebral lesion. An exception, apparent rather than real, is the occurrence of a delirium-like state in tumours of the third ventricle, but it is probable that the mental symptoms in such cases are due to the effect of raised intracranial pressure. The aberration of thought and conduct which occurs in the course of mental disease are not included in the term delirium, but they have to be considered in the differential diagnosis of the condition.

The range of aetiological possibilities is immense, and it is quite beyond the scope of this section to discuss the differential diagnosis in detail. Generally speaking, however, a carefully taken case-history, a thorough examination, and such laboratory procedures as may be suggested by the features of the case, will simplify what at first sight appears to be a very complex problem.

1. Delirium due to Toxaemia from Severe General Infections:

E.g., Septicaemia
    Typhus

2. Delirium due to Infections of the Nervous System:

Meningitis (any organism)	Trypanosomiasis
	Polio-encephalitis
Suppurative encephalitis	Cerebral malaria
Encephalomyelitis	Sydenham's chorea
Rabies	
Cerebral syphilis	

3. Delirium due to Non-infective Cerebral Disease:

Acute head injuries	Cerebral haemorrhage
Raised intracranial pressure	Subarachnoid haemorrhage
Diffuse cerebral tumour (primary)	Cerebral thrombosis
	Cerebral embolism
Carcinomatosis of brain and meninges	Arteriosclerotic cerebral degeneration
Pellagra (terminal stage)	Senile dementia
Terminal phase of cerebral degeneration, e.g., Schilder's disease	

4. Delirium due to Cerebral Anaemia:

Acute blood-loss	Severe primary anaemias
Carbon-monoxide poisoning	Terminal phase of heart failure

5. Delirium due to Exogenous Poisons and Drugs:

E.g., Alcohol
    Cannabis indica
    Spider and insect bites
    Mushroom poisoning

6. Delirium due to Endogenous Intoxications:

Uraemia	Cholaemia
Diabetic ketosis	Porphyria

7. Delirium due to Heat:

Heat-stroke (in the stage preceding coma)

8. Delirium due to Sudden Stoppage of a Drug Habit:

Alcohol	Cocaine
Opium and morphine	Heroin

9. Delirium mimicked by Psychological Illness.

The source of delirium due to *general infections* will usually be obvious, the mental symptoms being the result of severe toxaemia and of grave prognostic import. In a minority of cases, especially at the extremes of life and in debilitated or alcoholic subjects, the general reaction to infection is enfeebled and the evidences of infection may be slight, but delirium may be prominent. Pneumonia, bronchopneumonia, influenza, pyelitis, and perinephric abscesses are examples of infections which may behave in this way, but since it is the bodily reaction to infection rather than the nature of the infection which brings about this situation, the list might be extended.

Infections of the nervous system which are severe enough to cause delirium usually give other evidences of their presence—headache, photophobia, neck rigidity, cranial-nerve palsies, signs of implication of the long tracts, and so on. Examination of the spinal fluid will establish the presence of meningitis or syphilis, and may be of value in encephalomyelitis, polio-encephalitis, and brain abscess. Delirium occurring from seven to twenty days after one of the acute specific fevers of childhood, or after vaccination against smallpox or inoculation with antirabic vaccine, should always suggest the possibility of encephalomyelitis. Recent exposure to malarial infection is an indication for examination of a blood-slide. Delirium may initiate an attack of rabies, a condition which still occurs in India and Eastern Europe and is creeping across Western Europe, but the history of contact with a rabid animal will suggest the diagnosis. Sydenham's chorea causes no difficulty because the choreiform movements are usually well established by the time that delirium—a rare and grave symptom—appears.

The delirium which may occur during the course of *non-infective intracranial disease*, and during recovery from acute head injuries, is unlikely to cause difficulty inasmuch as there will be other and more definitive signs of the disease which is causing the mental symptoms. A rare exception to this generalization is seen in the case of slowly growing tumours of the frontal lobes and of the corpus callosum, which may cause mental symptoms amounting to delirium with very little in the way of either symptoms or signs of neoplasm. Another point of clinical interest is the circumstance that toxic factors—infections, renal insufficiency, sedatives given in normal therapeutic doses—which would not cause delirium in normal persons, may have this effect on persons with organic disease of the brain. This is often observed in early senile dementia, arteriosclerotic cerebral degeneration, general paralysis, and cerebral tumour. And a history of undue and unwonted intolerance to such factors should always suggest the possibility of a cerebral lesion.

Cerebral anaemia, whether the result of acute haemorrhage or of severe haemolytic or dys-haemopoietic anaemia, may cause delirium in enfeebled and arteriosclerotic subjects; sudden haemorrhage may induce the same symptoms even in youth. Carbon-monoxide poisoning may cause either coma or delirium owing to the replacement of oxyhaemoglobin by carboxyhaemoglobin, with consequent cerebral ischaemia.

Delirium due to exogenous poisons, including medicinal substances, is a vast subject. In some cases the mental symptoms are due to *idiosyncrasy* —as for instance to barbiturates, morphine and opium, quinine, salicylates. Cases of acute delirium can be caused by overdosage with phenobarbitone, and the same is true of the hydantoinates. The toxic encephalopathy due to poisoning with heavy metals, *lead, gold, arsenic,* and *manganese*, is accompanied by cerebral oedema, petechial haemorrhages, and cell changes which may be irreversible; early diagnosis is desirable, especially in the case of heavy metals, since it is now possible to accelerate the elimination of the poison by the use of dimercaprol or by chelating agents such as calcium edetate. In the case of chronic lead poisoning, with nephritis and hypertension, fits may replace delirium, the mechanism being similar to other forms of hypertensive encephalopathy rather than the direct toxic effect of lead on the brain, but the latter may also occur in the absence of hypertension. *Bromide intoxication* is rare today. Prolonged bromide therapy leads to the replacement of the chloride by the bromide radical in the tissue fluids—hence its sedative effect; but if the concentration of bromide in the blood exceeds 250 mg. per cent, confusion and delirium are apt to appear; dehydration from any cause may precipitate the condition, and it is not unknown for it to occur after vigorous and prolonged diuresis for cardiac oedema or in the course of prolonged illnesses in which fluids are not administered freely enough. Dehydration itself may lead to a mild delirium, especially in cases of pyloric stenosis with vomiting and incipient alkalosis; if bromide is given to such patients to quell nocturnal restlessness, it rapidly intoxicates the patient, who becomes still more noisy and 'requires' still bigger doses. The bites of adders, scorpions, hornets, wasps, and tarantula spiders, and the stings of certain rays and jelly-fish, are said to include delirium in their toxic effects. However unusual the form of intoxication may be in a given case, diagnosis is made easy by the fact that in the vast majority of cases there will be a history of having taken or been given the poison or drug; or, when there is no such history (as in many attempted suicides) there is usually a bottle or other container near the patient when he is found.

Delirium due to endogenous poisons is best exemplified by uraemia. This occurs as a result of bilateral renal disease, e.g., glomerulonephritis, bilateral pyonephrosis or hydronephrosis, polycystic kidney, lead nephritis, bilateral renal tuberculosis. The blood-urea is high, but while this serves as a useful indication of the state of affairs the urea itself is probably without much effect on cerebral function, symptoms being due to a mixture of high blood-pressure, acidaemia, alterations in the sodium-potassium ratio, and the retention of toxic products. Convulsions may interrupt the delirium; they are caused by a variety of factors—hypertensive encephalopathy, lowering of ionized calcium in the blood, acid-aemia, or vascular accidents. Mild delirium may also occur in *alkalaemia*, which is caused by excessive doses of alkalis given for peptic ulcer, or by excessive vomiting in pyloric stenosis and hyperemesis gravidarum. The blood-urea rises and the alkali reserve is reduced. Tetany is usually present in cases severe enough to exhibit delirium.

Cholaemia is the result of extensive liver damage in acute yellow atrophy, poisoning by phosphorus, antimony, aeroplane 'dope', arsenic, trinitrotoluol, etc., and diffuse infections of the liver and bile-ducts. Delirium due to this condition is almost invariably associated with deep jaundice, and the urine contains leucine and tyrosine crystals. In cirrhosis of the liver and after portacaval shunts, the products of normal protein digestion can give rise to a confusional state—'protein intoxication'—which responds rapidly to the withdrawal of protein from the food. *Diabetic ketosis* may cause either coma or delirium, usually the former. The essential factor in diagnosis is the discovery of sugar and ketones in the urine, but care must be taken to exclude poisoning by acetylsalicylic acid and its compounds, which can reduce Benedict's solution and produce a ketonuria; if the true diagnosis is not indicated by the circumstances of the case, or by satellite symptoms, blood-sugar estimation must be carried out as a matter of urgency.

Hyperinsulinism from a tumour of the islets of Langerhans gives rise to insulin coma and convulsions, rarely to delirium. Diagnosis depends on the history of similar attacks in the past, demonstration of a low blood-sugar (in the region of 50 mg. per cent) and relief of symptoms by giving glucose by mouth or intravenously.

Acute intermittent porphyria may be associated with an acute delirium, or with an ascending polyneuritis which is referred to elsewhere (p. 80). This condition occurs both as an idiopathic disease and also as a result of medication with drugs, especially barbiturates. It usually occurs in the third or fourth decade, and the nervous symptoms are preceded by abdominal colic and accompanied by the intermittent passage of urine which becomes burgundy-coloured on exposure to light. The delirium, which may be interrupted by convulsions and is sometimes associated with a transitory rise of blood-pressure, has no special features and the cause of the condition is unlikely to be recognized unless the colour of the urine is noticed, and porphyrins are found in it.

Heat-exhaustion is due to loss of fluid and chlorides by excessive sweating. This leads to exhaustion and collapse, with confusion and aberrations of conduct. *Heat-stroke*, on the other hand, is due to failure of sweating, with consequent hyperpyrexia. It gives rise to delirium, with or without convulsions, followed by coma.

Sudden stoppage of a drug habit induces restlessness and malaise, and in extreme cases, delirium. The best-known example is *delirium tremens* in alcoholism. The patient is confused, restless, and subject to visual hallucinations (the 'pink elephants' of the comedian), but he can often answer questions intelligently if held to the point. This condition is especially likely to occur when there is some other factor present, such as a lobar pneumonia, or a head injury, or a fractured leg. A similar state may develop when opium or cocaine is suddenly withdrawn; profuse scratch marks on the skin may be found in cocaine addicts, because the drug causes troublesome paraesthesiae and itch—the 'cocaine bug'.

Psychological illness may mimic delirium, as in manic states, catatonia, and severe emotional disturbances which paralyse the mind and interrupt normal thought. The past history of the case, the circumstances under which the 'delirium' commenced, and the absence of an organic cause provide assistance in what may prove an extremely difficult diagnostic problem.

Ian Mackenzie.

DELUSIONS

A delusion is a false belief, having no foundation in fact. It is incorrigible in that it fails to respond to any reasonable demonstration of its logical absurdity. It is also quite inappropriate to the sociocultural background of its possessor. On this account delusions may have to be distinguished from *superstitions* which are part of the cultural tradition and also from certain odd and *over-valued ideas*, often having a political, religious, or quasi-scientific basis, such as, for example, an intense but perhaps not, in the last resort, overwhelming belief in the reality of unidentified flying objects and many similar notions devised from studies of the occult and those which properly lie within the realms of science fiction. Apart from these, as some delusions may have a basis of truth it can sometimes be remarkably difficult to decide just how false are the allegations brought by a suspicious patient against his neighbours who, in their reaction to these, may further confuse the issue.

While such patients are commonly described as *paranoid* this term, strictly used, does not mean persecutory but refers to the patient's projections of his own ideas on to others or on to his environment so that such notions seem to come to him independently from without. However, because many paranoid beliefs or delusions do embody the notion of persecution, the patient often believes that a person or group of persons is in some way hostile to him; that they influence or persecute him; that they comment on him, watch him, or scheme against him; in general, that their attitude or behaviour signifies a threat to him. Many normal people have a disposition to entertain paranoid ideas about their fellows, to be touchy, jealous, or suspicious; if mental illness develops in such people, persecutory delusions are likely to appear. Thus the paranoid person is all too inclined to misinterpret what is said, and to pick up in ordinary conversation 'hints' that he is being tested or trapped.

In less fully developed cases the subject feels that the actions of others relate to him in some ill-defined way (*ideas of reference*), that they talk about him, cast 'meaningful' glances in his direction, and so on. In other instances he feels as if he is 'controlled' in some mysterious way; so that his thoughts, feelings, actions, etc. are no longer his own (*ideas of influence*; *passivity feelings*). Such symptoms are virtually pathognomonic of schizophrenia.

So are the so-called *primary delusions* of schizophrenia, i.e., delusions which are thought to emerge suddenly and without logically understandable antecedents. A patient sees a bus with the designation 'Newcastle'; this at once he construes with total conviction, as having something to do with the activities of his wife and family. Sometimes preceding this is a so-called *delusional mood*—a state best described as 'being about to become deluded' in which a distortion of symbolic meaning allows many impossibilities to become real to the patient. From this curious condition strange explanations, so-called *delusional ideas*, which, while although false explanations seem to bring with them a kind of security in a world which the patient finds all too threatening, are found as part of the clinical picture. Such paranoid ideas also occur in many other kinds of mental illness: in the disturbances associated with *organic brain disease*, in *mania* and *depression*, in a variety of neurotic or personality disorders in which they do not of course attain delusional strength and especially those in which guilt is prominent, and in some cases of *mental subnormality*.

Delusions that the *body* is in some way *disordered* or *diseased* are often seen in *schizophrenia*. These may be expressed in grotesque terms which betray a serious disturbance of thought; for example, a belief that the lungs are rotting away, or that part of the body has died or is dropping off. Alternatively, a patient may complain of a physical symptom which seems in itself unimportant, until it is found to be linked to a delusional system. Delusions having a sexual content are by no means uncommon. Thus, a patient may believe his sex is changing or that he is turning into a homosexual. In severe *depressive states*, the patient may believe that his bowels are stopped up, or his body is riddled with cancer; these beliefs (*holistic delusions*) are one aspect of the mood disorder and are consonant with it.

Delusions of guilt are not uncommon in *depressive states*; the patient may, for example, blame himself excessively for some trivial lapse, and expect to be put into prison or hanged on account of it. He may be convinced that he has committed an unspeakable crime and is being punished by his misery. A minor breach of good manners which happened twenty years before may in this way be invoked by the patient as an explanation of a depressive illness. *Grandiose delusions* are occasionally seen in *general paralysis*; thus, the patient may say he is the richest man in the world, and is about to marry the Prime Minister's daughter. Delusions of this type may also be seen in *mania* and in some cases of *paranoid schizophrenia*, also in *delirium*, though transiently.

The importance of a delusional belief must be assessed by the setting in which it occurs; it is an indication that other signs of mental disturbance are to be sought. False beliefs on a background of clear consciousness are of more grave significance than those occurring when consciousness is clouded, as in delirious states. As already indicated, the sudden emergence into the mind of a false belief, without discoverable external cause, often betokens the onset of a schizophrenic illness. Paranoid delusions, especially in older people, are of less weight than the other forms, and do not always point to the presence of serious mental illness. The patient does not always admit to delusional beliefs; their presence may have to be inferred from his behaviour. He may be found, for example, making preparations to counter an attack which he is expecting from an unknown assailant. Delusional beliefs are to be distinguished from the inventions of the pathological liar and also from the confabulations which may occur in *Korsakoff's syndrome* and in some cases in severe dementia. In the first instance the patient probably does not entirely believe in his own boastings, however much he would like others to do so; in the second the confabulations which occur are forgotten as soon as made.

W. H. Trethowan.

DEMENTIA

Given a state of clear consciousness, normal intellectual functioning—reasoning, memory, judgement, discrimination—appears to depend primarily, although not wholly, on the integrity of the cerebral cortex. Deterioration of mental ability which results from diffuse, usually irreversible damage to the higher centres is termed *dementia*, whereas failure of function due to interference with development is usually considered separately under the heading of 'mental subnormality' (*amentia*). In dementia, deterioration also shows itself in the emotional sphere where there is usually an initial increase in emotional lability so that the patient is more readily provoked to laughter, tears, or anger (*emotional incontinence*), although as the disorder progresses the capacity for emotional response may finally disappear. Early dementia may also be brought to the notice of the patient's friends and relatives by an alteration in his personality. Because disinhibition is an effect of the dementing process, undesirable personality traits, previously, perhaps, well controlled, may now become more evident so that, for example, a seemingly amiable and reasonably generous man may become, in the eyes of his friends, irritable, mean, and selfish.

Failure of memory, particularly for recent events, is also a common presenting symptom. The patient is forgetful; he cannot recall quickly and easily the names of those he has recently met, any unusual circumstances of his everyday life, or the tasks he has put aside to do later. In the case of those in whom dementia is due to *cerebral arteriopathy* these defects may also be noticed by the patient in himself so that he may become greatly concerned about what is happening to him. In dementia due to other causes there may, however, be little or no insight into the deterioration which, however, is soon obvious enough to others. Hand in hand with intellectual failure, there is a loss of emotional balance, manifested by general peevishness, unjustified despondency or elation, and sometimes by an ill-controlled uprush of sexual feeling. Pride in personal standards of appearance and cleanliness may deteriorate as may interpersonal relationships, leading the patient to become unexpectedly tactless or boorish.

There are a great many causes of dementia most of which are associated with advancing years. However, it has become customary to divide the disorder according to age of onset, i.e., before and after 65 into *presenile* and *senile* forms. Strictly, the term *presenile dementia* relates only to *Alzheimer's disease* which is fairly common, *Pick's disease* which is much less common and *Jakob-Creutzfeld's syndrome* (*spastic pseudosclerosis*) which is very uncommon indeed. The last is now thought to be due to a 'slow virus' and there is currently some conjecture as to whether Alzheimer's and Pick's diseases may not fall into the same category. There are also other forms of dementia which commonly make their appearance before 65, i.e., dementia due to *cerebral arteriopathy, Huntington's chorea, traumatic encephalopathy* following repeated head injury (i.e., in boxers, when it is known as 'punch-drunkenness'), *chronic alcoholism, epilepsy*, and a number of other conditions. So-called *senile dementia* is probably of mixed aetiology, including Alzheimer's disease of late onset (there are neuropathological features common to both, e.g., neurofibrillary tangles and argentophil plaques), together with changes due to generalized cerebral arteriopathy.

It is important to be aware, as in the case of delirious states, that mental manifestations of dementia give little clue as to its origin. The cause therefore can only be determined by the presence of associated findings, as in *general paralysis* (spastic quadriparesis, Argyll-Robertson pupils, positive C.S.F. Wassermann, etc.) or *Huntington's chorea* (choreiform movements, dominant heredity). In more obscure cases an ante-mortem diagnosis can only be made by brain biopsy which, however, is seldom justified. The most important diagnostic exercise is to separate from the rest those relatively few causes which, although not necessarily completely reversible, can be brought to a halt by appropriate treatment. Such causes include *myxoedema, pernicious anaemia, vitamin B-12, folic acid*, and other deficiencies; certain intracerebral disorders such as *subdural haematoma*, some *cerebral tumours*, e.g., *frontal meningioma* which may produce a degree of dementia which may possibly be relieved following operation; and even *general paralysis* (now very rare) in which a considerable degree of improvement may occur if the diagnosis is made early enough, i.e., by examination of the C.S.F., before gross neurological changes are evident, and if treatment with large doses of penicillin is promptly begun.

Dementia due to *cerebral arteriopathy* may be ushered in by a sudden attack of clouding of consciousness, with disorientation, restlessness, confusion, and perhaps hallucinations. Alternatively, the onset may be gradual, often in the late fifties or early sixties, although sometimes much earlier, with dizziness, headache, fatigue, disturbed sleep, increasing failure of memory, fits of depression, emotional outbursts, and hypochondriacal preoccupations. Fainting spells, or signs such as those of *hemiparesis* which point to a focal lesion, may precede or follow the other symptoms. Physical examination may show abnormal neurological signs resulting from such lesions, including *aphasia, tremor* of the hands, and *unsteadiness of gait*; occasionally epileptic seizures occur. Hypertension may be present but not necessarily so. The course of the condition is very variable; there may be much fluctuation in its general severity and in individual symptoms. Each focal attack cripples the patient further. In early cases, differentiation from simple depressive and anxiety states may be difficult; where there is definite dementia and objective signs of cerebral vascular disease, the diagnosis is more certain.

There is no sharp line between the mental changes usually associated with advancing old age and a state of *senile dementia*, though when the latter becomes gross it is readily recognizable. The old man has a less able and adaptable mind than the young; he keeps to the accustomed pattern of his daily life, *perseverates*, and tends to be anxious and confused if he has suddenly to cope with new conditions. His mental horizon contracts, his interest in the affairs of the world and of his own circle becomes less, and his concern for his own health and convenience more. His recollections of his youth remain bright, but events in the more immediate past are forgotten. Prolonged depression and, very much more rarely, *chronic mania* may occur. The patient's talk ranges over trivial personal affairs and his failure of memory may be covered by *confabulation*—the invention of imaginary happenings to a degree which may deceive the casual onlooker into believing that the patient may be more socially competent than he actually is (*presbyophrenia*). Alternatively, he may behave in a manner foreign to his normal character, for example, by the commission of delinquent acts, which bring him to the notice of the police. At night and in dark rooms he feels lost and may wander about; delirious states may occur. Paranoid states are very common, thus the senile patient may become secretive and take to hoarding, in the not always unfounded belief that his relatives are attempting to lay hold of his possessions.

Dementia is to be differentiated from transient *delirious states*; from *intoxication*, particularly by barbiturates and chronic overdosage with a wide range of psychotropic and antidepressive drugs, which may give a picture of confusion, failure to grasp, and memory disturbance resembling true dementia; and from the confusion which may accompany an *emotional crisis* in an elderly person. Because states of agitation and depression and paranoid conditions are not infrequent in the course of organic dementia, these may obscure the underlying condition. However, note should be taken of the fact that the same may be equally true the other way round if not more so. Thus, many old persons between 65 and 70 years of age who appear demented are often no more than depressed. If this is so and their condition is adequately treated all signs of mental abnormality may disappear. It is only over 75 that the prevalence of senile dementia exceeds that of depression.

W. H. Trethowan.

DEPERSONALIZATION

This is a peculiar condition which most patients find difficult to describe, so much so that it may sometimes be impossible to decide how much the experience of one sufferer is truly similar to that of another. Those features which most depersonalized subjects commonly experience include *a sense of unreality*, usually of sudden onset and which consists, in essence, of an unpleasant feeling of *estrangement* from the self, usually although not invariably accompanied by a degree of *derealization* in which the sense of estrangement also extends to the sufferer's immediate environment. Apart from its unpleasantness and quality of strangeness, a key feature in depersonalization appears to be a separation of feeling and intellect. The sufferer, while *knowing* what his reaction should be to others, who may be near and dear to him, or to various environmental happenings, nevertheless *feels* as if he is 'cut off' from his own emotional responses in an almost indescribable way, or that these no longer exist at all. This remarkable experience is best understood in terms of a *disorder of ego function* in which the concepts of 'I' and 'me' and 'I-ness' and 'my-ness', instead of remaining as indivisible parts of a whole, become, in some way, separated from one another.

Although the fundamental cause of *depersonalization* cannot yet be explained, the disorder occurs under a variety of circumstances. In otherwise normal persons depersonalization can occur under conditions which include *fatigue*, severe *physical deprivation*, *fever*, etc. Certain drugs such as *mescaline* and *lysergic acid diethylamide* (*LSD*) can produce a similar state. Some degree of depersonalization is present in most *depressive illnesses*, and in severe cases can give rise to *nihilistic delusions*, in which the patient may claim he is dead or may speak of himself in the third person in terms suggesting he is no more than an object and one of no consequence.

Depersonalization can also occur in almost 'pure forms', i.e. without any obvious accompanying mental disorder; although in such cases a degree of *obsessionalism* may be characteristic. Such depersonalized states tend not only to be of sudden onset but, once having made their appearance, may persist unremittingly for years, only occasionally being punctuated by short episodes of return to reality. In some patients whose personalities may also reveal *hysterical trends*, depersonalization can sometimes be construed as an attempt to escape from having to face unpleasant emotions in regard to a specific situation, a condition which, while bearing some resemblance to *dissociation*, nevertheless differs from it in several important respects. Dissociation is a state in which consciousness is clouded and which is usually transient. Depersonalization, on the other hand, occurs in a setting of clear consciousness and is remarkably persistent. One other variety of depersonalization which can occur in a neurotic setting is the so-called *phobic anxiety depersonalization syndrome* which may affect those with a variety of phobic states and which may accompany a rising sense of panic and loss of control. Under these conditions depersonalization is usually transient and resolves when the cause of the patient's phobic anxiety is removed. Depersonalization as a transient phenomenon may also occur as part of a *temporal lobe seizure*, in which strange feelings of change in the nature of self or of the world around are a feature.

Finally, similar but possibly not identical states of unreality can occur in *schizophrenia*, due once again to a disorder of ego function, which viewed in psychological terms is the central feature of this condition, accounting for most of the schizophrenic's disordered perceptions both of himself and of his own unreal world.

W. H. Trethowan.

DEPRESSION

It is important to note, at the outset, that *depression* is an ambiguous term, having at least two meanings. It is for this reason that some have suggested that the term *melancholia* is still to be preferred. Depression may refer to an appropriate, i.e., normal response, to a depressing situation, in which some kind of loss, e.g., *bereavement*, is a factor; or it may denote depression as an illness, in which the central and seemingly primary feature is a lowering of vital capacity which may affect any or virtually every sphere of a patient's activity. Apart from depressive reactions of proportions appropriate to the events which may evoke them, depression may be a symptom of almost every other kind of mental disorder; such as *schizophrenia*, most types of *neurotic illness*, and *organic*, notably *cerebral*, *disorders* of *arteriopathic origin*. Many physical illnesses, particularly *virus* infections, are prone to leave depression in their wake.

Although in primary depressive illnesses a depressed mood is usually to the forefront, in some patients this may be absent (*depression sine depressione*), leading them to smile, laugh, or even to crack jokes (*gallows humour*). Diagnostic error may be fostered by a patient refusing to admit that he is ill but insisting that his troubles are due to lack of will-power, poor moral fibre, and so on. To make it more difficult, depression and neurosis can be linked, for some patients develop *obsessive-compulsive* or *hysterical* illnesses only when depressed. It is, however, the circumscribed nature of these disorders which should point to the true diagnosis. Many patients who suffer from depressive illnesses are not markedly neurotic when well, whereas truly neurotic disorders extend as a rule back to childhood. In other cases a *depressive illness* may manifest itself in physical guise, thus depressed patients may believe they are physically ill and complain of a wide variety of symptoms: headache; facial pain; pain in the chest, back, and abdomen; digestive complaints, including constipation; and a variety of genito-urinary symptoms including menstrual irregularities.

As already emphasized, the key features of a primary depressive illness is a lowering of vitality and a general slowing down of activity even, in some cases, to the point of *stupor* (*see* p. 766). An early sign is impairment of mental agility together with *lack of concentration*. The patient finds it difficult to apply his mind efficiently even to the commonest affairs of everyday life, and constantly returns to his own problems. The content of his thoughts becomes increasingly gloomy. His spirits gradually lose their normal buoyancy, and a feeling of deepening unhappiness extends over his entire world. His capacity for sharing the experiences of others, his alertness, and his interest in outside affairs begin to wane. He takes longer and longer over accustomed tasks and is overcome by *indecision*. His usual degree of animation in walking and talking is damped down; gestures and accessory movements disappear. Sleep is broken and unsatisfying. He may suffer from disturbing dreams and tends to wake early. His appetite for food, drink, and sex is reduced. Characteristically, all those symptoms tend to be at their worst in the morning, and lighten somewhat towards evening. For this reason, when assessing the severity of a depressive illness account should always be taken of what time of day the patient is examined.

As the condition progresses there is still further limitation of activity, and the mood sinks to despair. Work becomes impossible. The sufferer's range of thought narrows to an intense preoccupation with disease, ruin, and death. *Suicidal ideas* may be prominent and are often openly expressed. These must be taken seriously; the patient may need to be placed under observation for his own protection. *Delusions* may appear. Thus a patient who has begun to suspect that he has cancer becomes convinced that this is so. An indiscretion of twenty years ago has, he believes, infected him with venereal disease, which now corrodes his vitals. He has made a mistake in his income-tax return and will be sentenced to life imprisonment. His property is worthless; he is ruined financially. The outlook is black, and the only reasonable course is to end it all. However, while he may prepare carefully for suicide he may sometimes deny that he has any such intention. While statements made by relatives may be useful in judging how severe depression is and how great the suicidal risk, not too much weight should be put on statements such as: 'He would never do a thing like that', which may be based upon false hopes rather than upon reality.

Depressive states may occur at any age but are rare in children. Although in adolescence they tend to become somewhat commoner they do not reach peak incidence until middle life. Usually some precipitating factor is present, a bereavement, a business reverse, or some failure of expectation. Other cases appear to develop for no good cause as far as can be seen. However, this does not mean that no good cause is present.

There are probably also several varieties of depressive illness, although it is not yet clear whether these can be regarded as distinct entities. In *manic-depressive* (*bipolar*) *depression* there is usually a strongly positive family history and there may well have been previous bouts either of depression or mania or both. There may also be a history of larval attacks in childhood or adolescence usually not recognized at the time but passed off as episodes of 'nervous debility' or something of the kind. In *unipolar depressions*, manic episodes do not occur nor do they occur in the so-called *involutional depressions* (*melancholia*) which occur for the first time in late middle life (45–65 years). These tend to affect those who are somewhat rigid, obsessional, and perfectionistic, who cannot accommodate themselves to growing old gracefully. Characteristically such depressive illnesses tend to be severe, accompanied by much agitation and by delusions of unworthiness, guilt, or a variety of hypochondriacal notions, and sometimes by frankly paranoid ideas. In those who are older and who suffer from *senile depression*, general slowing-down, together with a marked degree of functional intellectual impairment, may give a false impression of dementia which, however, resolves with treatment (*see* DEMENTIA, p. 207).

W. H. Trethowan.

DIAPHRAGMATIC HERNIA

1. Congenital. Failure of development of the diaphragm may lead to apertures allowing a communication between the abdominal and thoracic cavities. Because of the higher pressure in the abdomen, abdominal contents tend to pass into the chest and the commonest organs to behave in this way are the stomach and spleen. The site of the defect, however, determines which organs will be involved although, small defects being completely protected by the liver on the right side, these will occur more readily on the left. Defects may occur in the oesophageal hiatus, at the pleuro-peritoneal hiatus—the so-called foramen of Bochdalek—behind the medial lumbo-costal arch, through the foramina of Morgagni in front, and at the dome of the diaphragm, in that order of frequency. Once hollow viscera have passed into the thoracic cavity, they tend to become obstructed and may even strangulate.

Severe degrees of diaphragmatic hernia will be obvious in infancy because of obstructive symptoms or because the large bulk of viscera within the chest tends to embarrass either the heart or the left lung or both. Occasionally there is complete absence of one-half of the diaphragm, a condition which is hardly compatible with life. These conditions are diagnosed by radiograph when typical gaseous shadows of stomach or colon are seen within the chest (*Fig.* 225).

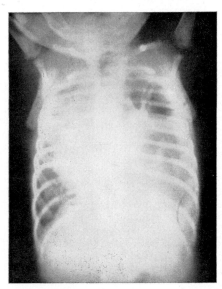

Fig. 225. Strangulated diaphragmatic hernia in infant, through hiatus of Bochdalek. Note mediastinal shift and gas and bowel shadows in left side of chest.

2. Acquired

a. TRAUMATIC. Severe penetrating or crushing injuries of the lower chest may lacerate the diaphragm or sever its attachments. Abdominal viscera will tend to pass into the chest and the diagnosis should always be thought of when there is a history of a likely predisposing injury.

b. NON-TRAUMATIC (HIATUS HERNIA) (*Fig.* 226).

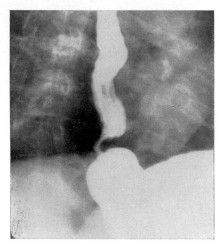

Fig. 226. Sliding hiatal hernia. (*Dr. John D. Dow.*)

i. *Oesophageal Hernia* (*Sliding Hernia*). In this type of hernia a weakness of the right crus of the diaphragm interferes with the snugness of fit around the oesophageal hiatus. As a result, particularly as years advance and increased deposits of fat raise the intra-abdominal pressure, or for the same reason, during pregnancy, the cardiac end of the stomach is thrust up into the chest through the lax hiatus. This disturbs the acute angle at which the oesophagus normally enters the stomach and allows reflux of gastric juice into the lower end of the oesophagus with a consequent oesophagitis. Fibrous contracture of this inflamed oesophagus may cause this organ to contract and draw more and more stomach into the chest. Very exceptionally, a congenitally short oesophagus will produce the same effect, but nearly all cases of short oesophagus are acquired as a result of reflux oesophagitis.

The symptoms are at first mild and consist of epigastric discomfort and a feeling of fullness with belching. Later, when oesophagitis develops, there is heartburn, acid regurgitation, especially when the patient is prone at night or on stooping, and often a severe anaemia due to the constant loss of small quantities of blood from the inflamed oesophagus. Dysphagia usually indicates stricture formation. Confirmation of this diagnosis which might suggest peptic ulceration or cholecystitis is obtained by X-ray of the stomach with the patient lying supine and the head tilted down, when the barium will be found to reflux above the diaphragm.

ii. *Para-oesophageal Hernia* (*Rolling Hernia*) (*Fig.* 227). Here, owing once more to raised intra-abdominal pressure, the fundus of the stomach rolls

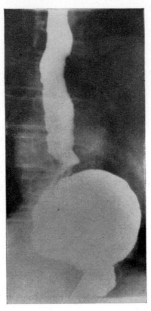

Fig. 227. Para-oesophageal hernia. (*Dr. John D. Dow.*)

up in front of the oesophagus and a pouch of this viscus protrudes into the thorax, either in front or to one side of the oesophagus. This pouch acts as a dilator to the defect and gradually more and more of the stomach passes up into the chest.

In this type of hernia, the angle of entry of the oesophagus is undisturbed and there is no reflux so that oesophagitis is not a complication. The symptoms depend upon the degree of visceral displacement into the thorax and the tightness of the neck. Usually there is a sense of fullness, eructation, and retro-sternal pain after meals. If the hernia is bulky it may impede the action of the left lung and lead to dyspnoea. Anaemia is common from the acute gastric erosions which are likely to occur in the congested, herniated stomach. This type of hernia may strangulate. Again, the diagnosis is confirmed by barium-meal X-ray with the patient in the 'head-down' position and with the application of manual pressure to the abdomen which will tend to drive the stomach up through the hiatus.

R. G. Beard.

DIARRHOEA

Diarrhoea (the too frequent evacuation of too loose faeces) is a symptom and not a disease in itself, so that in every case an attempt must be made to discover the underlying cause. In addition to routine history and physical examination (the latter including digital examination of the rectum) it may be necessary to employ sigmoidoscopy, examination of the stools by naked eye, by the microscope, and by bacteriological investigation, supplemented by a faecal fat estimation of the stool if indicated. Barium-enema X-ray examination of the large bowel and barium-meal follow-through studies of the small intestine may also be required. Most of these methods require no special description or are dealt with in other articles.

Although there is some overlap, it is convenient to consider the causes of diarrhoea grouped into those affecting infants and young children and those which occur in adult patients.

Diarrhoea in Infancy and Early Childhood. Diarrhoea, with or without vomiting, is a presenting feature of a wide variety of conditions occurring in infancy. The most important to be thought of are:

Infantile gastro-enteritis
Systemic infections, e.g., of the urinary tract or upper respiratory tract
Unsuitable feeds containing too much sugar
Hirschsprung's disease
Carbohydrate intolerance
Steatorrhoea, which in infants is likely to be due to fibrocystic disease of the pancreas, coeliac disease, or giardiasis
Protein-losing enteropathy
Drugs—antibiotics and iron
Ulcerative colitis and Crohn's disease, both rare in childhood.

Diarrhoea may be mimicked by the blood and slime associated with intussusception (red-currant-jelly stools) and by the pseudo-diarrhoea associated with constipation.

Infantile Gastro-enteritis, sometimes still termed summer or epidemic diarrhoea, is fortunately much less common in this country now than in previous times, thanks to improved social conditions, higher standards of hygiene, and generally healthier babies. In many parts of the world it remains a serious problem and a high source of mortality and morbidity in infants. The diarrhoea associated with systemic infections such as those of the urinary tract, the throat, or otitis media probably occurs because of the lowered resistance of the child to gastro-intestinal infection.

A wide variety of pathogenic organisms may be responsible for this condition, including *Shigella*, *Salmonella*, and enteropathogenic *E. coli* (especially in hospital epidemics). More rarely, staphylococci may be implicated.

In mild cases there may simply be diarrhoea without other systemic disturbances, but in fulminating examples the infant passes frequent watery green stools, may vomit, and soon passes into a state of shock due to extreme water- and electrolyte-loss.

Two serious conditions in children result in steatorrhoea:

Cystic Fibrosis is the commoner of the two and is estimated to occur in about 1 in 2000 births.

Meconium ileus may occur in the neonatal period but infants who survive this episode go on to develop steatorrhoea with pale, bulky, and offensive stools, fail to thrive, and show gross abdominal distension. The condition is associated with pulmonary fibrosis and the child is likely to succumb from respiratory infection.

Coeliac Disease, or gluten-induced enteropathy, becomes manifest after weaning when the child commences cereals. Steatorrhoea is accompanied by wasting and abdominal distension. Jejunal biopsy may show flattening of the jejunal villi and the child responds well to a gluten-free diet.

Diarrhoea in Adults. The following causes should be considered:

Specific bacterial infections, e.g., food-poisoning due to *Salmonella* gastro-enteritis, dysentery (either amoebic or bacillary), cholera

Inflamed or irritated intestine, e.g., ulcerative colitis, Crohn's disease, proliferative tumours of the large bowel, diverticular disease of the colon

Drugs, including antibiotics, abuse of purgatives, colchicine, mefenamic or flufenamic acids, magnesium-containing antacids, digitalis, arsenic, and other poisons

Loss of absorptive surface of the bowel following resection or short circuit, sprue, coeliac disease, idiopathic steatorrhoea, extensive Crohn's disease of the small bowel

Pancreatic dysfunction

Following gastrectomy and vagotomy (the reason for this is not fully understood)

Anxiety states

Associated with general diseases, e.g., thyrotoxicosis, uraemia, the carcinoid syndrome, and Zollinger-Ellison tumour of the pancreas.

Spurious Diarrhoea may be the blood and mucus discharging from a papilliferous growth of the rectum or liquid trickling around a mass of impacted faeces in the terminal bowel; a digital examination readily shows the presence of either of these two conditions.

ACUTE DIARRHOEA. Acute diarrhoea in an adult is likely to be due to bacterial infection, but inquiry may elicit some indiscretion of diet (the eating of unripe fruit, etc.), or the consumption of some toxic article of food ('food-poisoning'), or the ingestion of some drug which may be the responsible factor. Antibiotics may cause diarrhoea by changing the intestinal bacterial flora and the condition may be the result of excessive purgation.

In *dysentery* there will be tenesmus, with blood and mucus in the motions. In the amoebic variety, *Entamoeba histolytica* may be found in the stools and the character of the multiple, small, pitted ulcers seen through the sigmoidoscope (*Fig.* 70, p. 69) is almost pathognomonic. In the bacillary form (shigellosis) the bloodserum agglutinates Shiga's bacillus and this organism will be recovered from the stools. The incubation period is 1–5 days. *Salmonella* infection has a short incubation period of 8–24 hours or at the most 2 days and presents with acute vomiting and diarrhoea often associated with pyrexia.

'*Traveller's diarrhoea*', accompanied often by vomiting, which so frequently attacks visitors to foreign parts, especially where sanitary conditions are poor, may be due to specific *Salmonella* or dysenteric infections but is probably produced in most cases by alteration in the normal bacteria of the bowel. The widespread geographical distribution of this condition is indicated by the many slang terms applied to it such as 'Gippy tummy', 'Hong Kong dog', 'Simla trots', 'Normandy glide', and so on. In *cholera* the diarrhoea is extreme, to the extent of producing 'rice-water' stools. The diagnosis is generally suggested by geographical or epidemiological circumstances and can be confirmed by discovering the causal comma bacilli in the stools.

CHRONIC DIARRHOEA. This may be the manifestation of an extraordinary number of diseases of the bowel and of non-alimentary conditions which we have already enumerated above.

In *ulcerative colitis* the stools are frequent, blood is almost invariable, and mucus and pus often present. The diagnosis can be made in most cases by sigmoidoscopy which reveals a red oedematous friable mucosa. In tropical countries it may be necessary to differentiate *chronic dysentery* and this can be made by bacteriological examination of the stools. The barium-enema appearances show multiple minute ulcers which may be confined to the rectum (proctitis) or involve the whole large bowel. As the disease progresses the normal haustra are lost. Bouts of diarrhoea are frequent in *Crohn's disease* affecting either the small or large bowel and in *diverticular disease* of the colon. *Carcinoma of the large bowel* not uncommonly presents with diarrhoea and this is frequently accompanied by blood or slime. Apart from clinical examination, sigmoidoscopy may reveal the growth or, in higher lesions, its presence may be demonstrated by a barium-enema examination.

Pancreatic Disease, by interfering with lipase secretion, may produce steatorrhoea, although this is frequently overshadowed by the accompanying obstructive jaundice in tumours affecting the head of the pancreas.

Extensive Resection of the Small Intestine may result in the 'short-bowel syndrome'; an inadequate mucosal surface results in copious diarrhoea, steatorrhoea, and the inevitable consequences of malabsorption. It is interesting that a right hemicolectomy, by removing the ileocaecal valve, is often accompanied by some increased frequency of stool action.

Steatorrhoea may be *idiopathic* (the commonest cause in this country) with pale, frothy, and copious stools. There is usually a painful stomatitis involving the tongue and mouth. *Sprue* is seen in patients returning from overseas. The *blind-loop syndrome* may result not only from blind loops and culs-de-sac, resulting from surgical interventions, but is also seen in smallbowel strictures and jejunal diverticulosis. It may comprise some or all of the following features:

diarrhoea, steatorrhoea, anaemia, loss of weight, abdominal pain, and multiple vitamin deficiencies. Subacute degeneration of the cord may occur in association with a macrocytic anaemia. The condition is becoming less common now that tuberculous strictures of the intestine are unusual in civilized communities, and because extensive short circuits of intestine are now avoided by the surgeon if possible or taken down after the obstruction for which they were performed has been overcome.

Whipple's disease results from distension of the small-bowel villi with a glycoprotein material and presents with a triad of features: steatorrhoea, enlargement of lymph-nodes, and an arthropathy resembling rheumatoid arthritis.

Extensive infiltration of the small intestine by *lymphosarcoma* or the other reticuloses or widespread *Crohn's disease* also greatly reduces the available absorptive surface of the small bowel. The cause of the diarrhoea in the *Zollinger-Ellison syndrome* is not known for certain but may be associated with irritation of the small intestine by the enormous acid secretion induced by the gastrin-like material secreted by the tumour. Diarrhoea is a part of the *carcinoid syndrome* due to hepatic deposits of this serotonin-secreting tumour.

Anxiety states. If all the above causes of chronic or recurrent diarrhoea can be excluded and if there is an obvious emotional factor undoubtedly present then nervous diarrhoea may be diagnosed. It is, of course, essential that the history should be taken with particular care in such cases in order not to overlook a psychological precipitating factor.

Harold Ellis.

DIPLOPIA

Diplopia, or double vision, may be either uniocular or binocular; that is to say, an object may be seen double with one eye, or single with each eye separately and only double when both eyes are open. To distinguish between the two conditions it is necessary that each eye should be closed in turn. If with either eye the object is still seen double, the diplopia is uniocular and due to that eye alone; if, on the other hand, the object is seen double only when both eyes are open, the diplopia is binocular, and due to some disturbance of the balance of the two eyes.

Uniocular Diplopia is very rare, and may be due to dislocation of the lens (ectopia lentis) or a doubling of the pupil (congenitally), or after tears of the iris root. A distortion or replication of the image (but not a true diplopia) may be caused by early opacities of the lens or cornea, or facets of the corneal surface.

Binocular Diplopia may be either (1) Physiological, or (2) Pathological.

PHYSIOLOGICAL DIPLOPIA occurs unnoticed in all normal binocular vision. It is evident that as the two eyes view any given object from different standpoints, the retinal images must differ as do the two views taken by a stereoscopic camera. The diplopia is not apparent, however, as the two dissimilar images are combined by the higher visual centres of the brain to form a single solid conception of the object viewed. The amount of dissimilarity of the retinal images gives the impression of space and distance, near objects causing images more unlike than those formed by things remotely placed. The dissimilarity of the two retinal images in normal binocular vision, giving the idea of space, is termed in psychology 'disparateness'.

When, however, owing to some failure in the brain-centre which controls the mental fusion of the two ocular images, they are not combined (after drinking alcohol, for instance), or when some disturbance of the accurately balanced muscular mechanism upsets the automatic fixation of both eyes upon the same object, diplopia results.

Another important form of physiological diplopia which gives rise to complaint by some patients, and which, on the other hand, it is difficult even to demonstrate to others, arises from the fact that, when the two eyes are fixing an object at a certain distance, the images of objects which lie farther away from, or nearer to, the observer than the object fixed fall upon disparate retinal points and are thus seen double.

PATHOLOGICAL DIPLOPIA. Before discussing the various forms and causes of this condition it is necessary to have a clear idea of the visual process of localizing objects in space—projection, or orientation.

In normal binocular vision, looking at an object means that both eyes are so turned that the image of the particular object falls upon the central most sensitive area of the retina, the macula, in each eye, and objects other than that directly looked at form images upon the retina which are more or less peripheral. From our experience of such sensations and their locality on the retina we are able accurately to determine the relative positions of objects in space. The image of any object falls upon corresponding areas of the retinas of the two eyes. These areas, though always corresponding, are not in the true sense of the word symmetrical. The image of an object to the right of the eyes falls upon the nasal side of the right and the temporal side of the left retina; but the corresponding areas are in normal circumstances always stimulated simultaneously, and from these retinal images is derived the idea of the position of the object in space. If the normal relative position of the two eyes is upset in any way, the image of an object no longer falls upon two areas that usually correspond, erroneous ideas of projection are formed, with consequent diplopia, and it is from an examination of this diplopia that we can ascertain the displacement of the eye and its probable cause.

For example, *Fig.* 228 represents diagrammatically a condition in which the left eye is looking at or fixing the object O, while the right eye is pointing abnormally inwards—a convergent squint. In consequence of the abnormal position of the right eye, the image of the object O does not fall upon the yellow spot on the macula, f, but upon a point internal to it, a. In ordinary circumstances, with proper fixation of the two eyes, any object whose image fell upon a would be to the right of the object O, hence under the existing abnormal conditions the right eye erroneously projects the object O to the

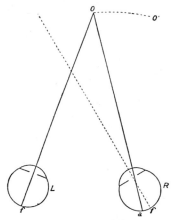

Fig. 228. Homonymous double images.

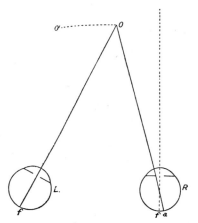

Fig. 229. Crossed images.

position O', and a diplopia results in which the right of the two images seen belongs to the right eye, and the left to the left eye. This is termed a homonymous diplopia. *Fig*. 229 shows in a similar manner the formation of a crossed diplopia in a divergent squint. These two figures illustrate the formation of a diplopia in lateral deviations of the eyes. A moment's consideration will show that deviation in a vertical or oblique plane will equally cause diplopia, owing to the disturbance of the normal corresponding areas of the two retinas.

It will be seen from the figures that, in horizontal deviations, a convergent squint causes homonymous, and a divergent squint, crossed diplopia. In ocular paralyses the separation will increase if the two eyes are carried in the direction of the usual action of the paralysed muscle. As an example, *Fig*. 228 may be chosen as a diagrammatic representation of a paralysis of the right lateral rectus muscle. The more the eyes are turned to the right the greater will be the convergence, owing to the inability of the right eye to turn to the right to the same extent as the left; the greater, therefore, will be the separation as the image of the object O falls farther and farther around on the nasal side of the right retina, the object being projected farther and farther to the right. It will also be seen from this consideration that in a case of diplopia from a muscular paralysis, when the eyes are carried as far as possible in the direction of the usual action of the paralysed muscle, the farthest displaced image always belongs to the paralysed eye.

The two images are not equally distinct; that in the unaffected eye falls upon the macula and is seen most distinctly—the *real image*; that falling upon the retina of the affected eye is more peripheral, and therefore not so definite; it is termed the *false image*.

Binocular diplopia may be caused by paralysis of any extra-ocular muscle, but it may also arise from the displacement of one eye from such causes as *orbital neoplasm, abscess, haemorrhage*, or *cavernous sinus thrombosis*; it may also occur after an operation involving the extra-ocular muscles, and when the excursion of one eye is limited mechanically, as, for instance, in cicatricial deformities. Diplopia occurs fairly commonly in the elderly, from localized cerebral haemorrhage or thrombosis. It may be unaccompanied by other signs, and is often only temporary.

Cases of displacement of the eye from local causes can usually be distinguished from those of ocular paralysis by the indeterminate character of the diplopia, which is accompanied by relative fixation of the eyeball, and sometimes by proptosis.

Diplopia may arise from the ocular palsies caused by many varieties of intracranial disease, such as syphilis, meningitis, tumours, multiple sclerosis, encephalitis lethargica, etc. It may occur as a manifestation of fatigue, as occurs in myasthenia gravis. Fractures of the skull may also give rise to diplopia, and so may toxins such as those of diphtheria, diabetes, and botulism.

Diplopia is a specific feature of pituitary exophthalmos. The onset of this disease is usually gradual and often unilateral; the lids swell and the conjunctiva becomes oedematous and brawny. The protrusion of the eye is axial and irreducible; ophthalmoplegia may precede the proptosis, the commonest and often the first movement to be affected being elevation. Lid retraction is usual, though ptosis may occur. Rarely there is papilloedema; central and peripheral field loss may ensue. The disorder is attributed to an 'exophthalmos-producing hormone' of the pituitary, and it often follows thyroidectomy; it generally affects middle-aged males. The disease tends to be self-limiting, though its course may cause considerable distress and discomfort. The ophthalmologist's main concern throughout is to protect the eye, for severe damage and even loss of the eye can occur from the exposure of the cornea, and tarsorrhaphy may be necessary.

Bacillus botulinis (*Clostridium botulinum*). The diplopia may be masked by ptosis, and is usually accompanied by mydriasis, dysphagia, dysphonia, vomiting, cramps in the limbs, and, especially in fatal cases, coma. The diagnosis generally depends on a history of one or more persons having partaken of a meal of some canned food and developing, at intervals varying from six to thirty-six hours, a combination of the

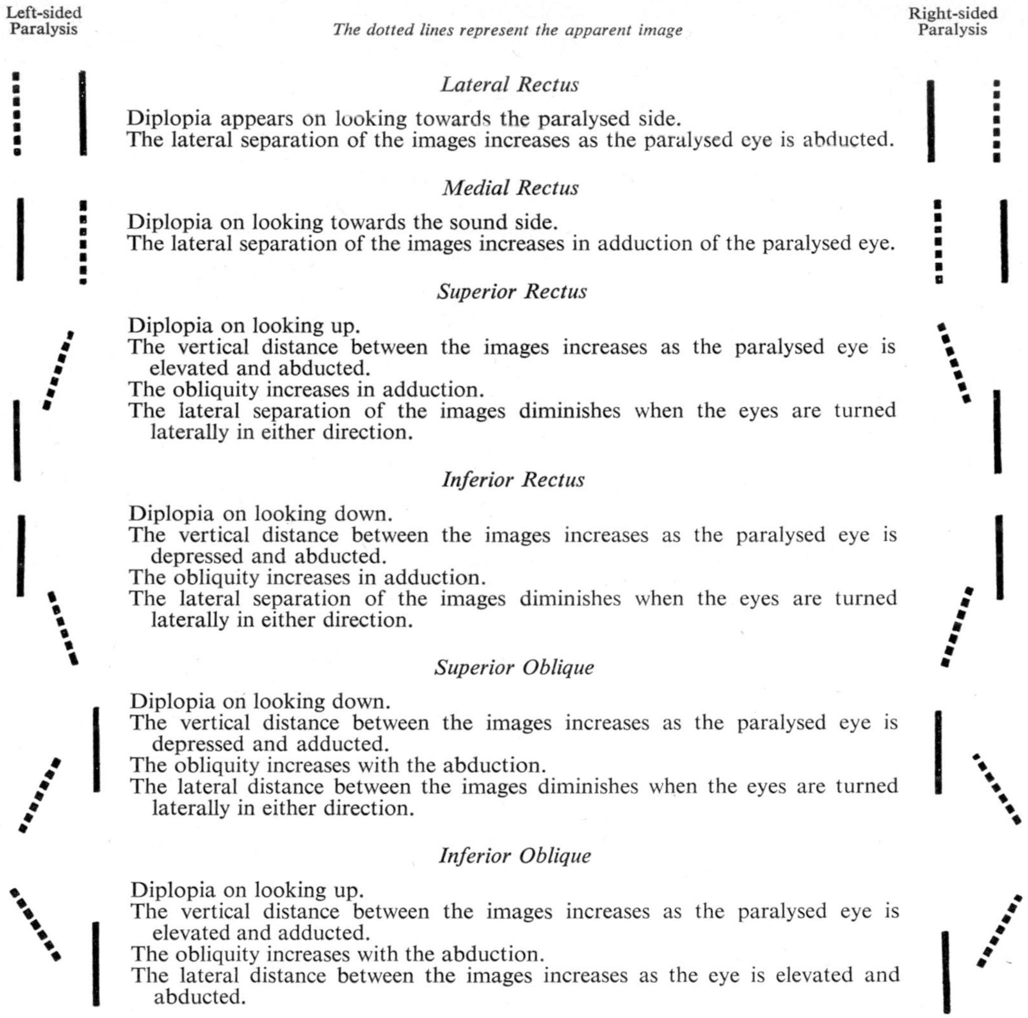

| Left-sided Paralysis | *The dotted lines represent the apparent image* | Right-sided Paralysis |

Lateral Rectus

Diplopia appears on looking towards the paralysed side.
The lateral separation of the images increases as the paralysed eye is abducted.

Medial Rectus

Diplopia on looking towards the sound side.
The lateral separation of the images increases in adduction of the paralysed eye.

Superior Rectus

Diplopia on looking up.
The vertical distance between the images increases as the paralysed eye is elevated and abducted.
The obliquity increases in adduction.
The lateral separation of the images diminishes when the eyes are turned laterally in either direction.

Inferior Rectus

Diplopia on looking down.
The vertical distance between the images increases as the paralysed eye is depressed and abducted.
The obliquity increases in adduction.
The lateral separation of the images diminishes when the eyes are turned laterally in either direction.

Superior Oblique

Diplopia on looking down.
The vertical distance between the images increases as the paralysed eye is depressed and adducted.
The obliquity increases with the abduction.
The lateral distance between the images diminishes when the eyes are turned laterally in either direction.

Inferior Oblique

Diplopia on looking up.
The vertical distance between the images increases as the paralysed eye is elevated and adducted.
The obliquity increases with the abduction.
The lateral distance between the images increases as the eye is elevated and abducted.

Fig. 230. To illustrate the behaviour of the double images in paralysis of the ocular muscles. The diagrams represent the patient's viewpoint.

In some rare cases of convergent or divergent squint with absence of binocular vision and good vision in each eye, there may be the power of alternate fixation with more or less evident diplopia. As a rule, however, the individual has the power of suppressing the image of the squinting eye, obtaining monocular vision.

Diplopia is a common symptom in the rare disease *botulism*, produced by the ingestion of the

symptoms just described. The disease generally occurs, therefore, in small epidemics, and the diagnosis may be suspected before it is possible to confirm it by cultivating the bacillus from the remnants of food. Should any of the infected food have been thrown out into the poultry yard, the rapid mortality amongst the fowls may afford another clue to the nature of the malady.

P. Trevor-Roper.

DISEASE, SMELL OF

Clinicians in the past, with fewer ancillary aids to diagnosis and more dependent on observation, recognized characteristic odours of many diseases to an extent almost entirely disregarded at the present day. Excellent though the modern clinician may be, if he is a regular heavy smoker he will be unlikely to detect anything through his olfactory sense.

It is sometimes maintained that everyone has an individual, natural body odour, the recognition of which is displayed by a comparative few. What is apparent to the dog is not so clear to the physician. Even skilled police dogs, however, err when it comes to identical twins.

The use of perfumes, cosmetics, and tobacco, and the taking of certain drugs (e.g., paraldehyde or alcohol) naturally introduce a complicating factor. In the case of disease bacterial decomposition in damaged tissues gives rise to typical pungent odours, as for instance an infected gangrenous foot in a diabetic. A faecal smell may be the sign of a fistula developing and the aroma of gas gangrene may fill a ward. This may be particularly and rapidly apparent when a lung abscess bursts into a bronchus and the abscess contents are expectorated. The sweet smell of acetone (keto-acetic acids) in an unbalanced diabetic is obvious to some clinicians and not apparent to others. It is present in the breath and is a good differentiating feature between diabetic and hypoglycaemic (treatment) coma, unless the patient has been vomiting, when it is often present. The unwashed-gentlemen's-lavatory smell of uraemia is characteristic, as may be the alcoholic aroma of the 'dead-drunk' unconscious patient or the more subtle, but still apparent, aroma of the alcoholic patient at his attendance next morning in the clinic. A peculiar odour in the sweat of schizophrenic patients is said to be due to the presence of trans-3-methyl-2-hexanoic acid.

F. Dudley Hart.

DROP ATTACKS

This term has now come into general usage to describe the usually elderly patient who, without warning, falls to the floor, his leg or legs giving way beneath him. There is no loss of consciousness, there is rapid recovery, and there are no residual neurological physical signs, the patient rising from the pavement shaken but intact. There is no warning or aura, as in epilepsy, and no residual neurological physical signs, as after a cerebral thrombosis. The long list of causes of fainting overlaps this syndrome, but the commonest type of faint, or vasovagal attack, is preceded by a short period of awareness of trouble-on-the-way, which is not the case in the drop attack: 'I was walking down the street, doctor, when suddenly my legs gave way beneath me and I found myself on the pavement.'

Drop attacks may be due to:

1. Transient cerebral ischaemia, usually in vessels of the brain-stem. The vertebral basilar artery may become narrowed, and possibly become kinked with certain movements of head and neck, leading to sudden weakness and loss of muscular tone in one or both legs. Diplopia may be present. The ischaemia here lies in the more ventral portions of the brain-stem supplied by the medial perforating arteries; ischaemia of the dorsal and lateral portions of the brain-stem supplied by the circumferential arteries tends to cause vertigo, ataxia, dysarthria, or dysphagia. Repeated attacks may occur. They point to underlying atherosclerotic disease of the cerebral vessels and the potential future dangers of major cerebrovascular episodes.

2. Loss of muscular tone in the legs, not uncommon in the elderly, where the legs literally give way from weakness of the quadriceps and other muscle groups, a transient hypotonus.

3. Coronary thrombosis may occur in the elderly without precordial pain, the condition presenting as a drop attack. Electrocardiographic and enzyme changes give the diagnosis.

4. Epileptic fits may be mild and transient but there is loss of consciousness, even if the patient is perhaps unaware of it. An unusual and interesting variant is that known as geloplegia, where the patient laughs at some amusing remark and falls onto the floor, recovering almost immediately.

F. Dudley Hart.

DWARFISM

Dwarfs are usually small in stature, often because their parents were also short, or because they themselves were genetically predestined to be undersized. Dwarfism may, however, be due to deformity of the limbs or spine, or to premature closure of the epiphyses associated with precocious sexual development. It may also be associated with infantilism, in which case failure of somatic growth is accompanied by gonadal deficiency. To label someone as a 'dwarf' is regarded by some people as a stigma and the expression 'short stature' is preferred.

Classification of Causes of Dwarfism:

1. DELAYED ADOLESCENCE.
2. GENETIC:
   a. Constitutional.
   b. Sporadic.
   c. Chromosomal.
      i. Gonadal dysgenesis: Turner's syndrome. (cf. Noonan's syndrome.)
      ii. Autosomal anomalies:
         Trisomy 21 (Down's syndrome).
         Trisomy 17 or 18 (Edwards' syndrome).
         Trisomy 13, 14 or 15 (Patau's syndrome).
3. SKELETAL:
   Congenital:
   a. Chondrodystrophy (Achondroplasia)

b. Chondro-osteo-dystrophy (Brailsford-Morquio disease).

c. Dysostosis multiplex (Gargoylism or Hurler's syndrome).

d. Chondrodystrophia calcificans congenita.

e. Epiphysial dysplasia multiplex.

f. Chondro-ectodermal dysplasia (Ellis-van Creveld syndrome).

g. Osteogenesis imperfecta.

Acquired:

a. Rickets: infantile, late, vitamin-D-resistant.

b. Spinal caries and deformities due to other causes, e.g., poliomyelitis.

4. NUTRITIONAL AND METABOLIC:
   a. Malnutrition.
   b. Malabsorption syndromes.
   c. Diabetes insipidus.
   d. Protein deficiency: kwashiorkor.
   e. Electrolyte imbalance.
   f. Glycogen storage disease.

5. INFECTIVE:
   Tuberculosis: malaria: congenital syphilis: hook-worm infestation.

6. SYSTEMIC:
   a. Renal.
   b. Coeliac.
   c. Fibrocystic disease of the pancreas.
   d. Hepatic.
   e. Circulatory.
   f. Congenital heart disease with cyanosis.
   g. Cerebral.

7. ENDOCRINE:
   a. Hypothyroid: cretinism.
   b. Precocious puberty.
   c. Sexual precocity of gonadal origin:
      i. Interstitial-cell tumour of the testis.
      ii. Granulosa-cell tumour of the ovary.
   d. Sexual precocity of adrenocortical origin:
      i. Congenital adrenal hyperplasia.
      ii. Adrenocortical tumour.
      iii. Cushing's syndrome.
   e. Hypopituitary:
      i. Congenital hypopituitary dwarfism: pituitary infantilism.
      ii. Isolated growth hormone deficiency.
      iii. Acquired hypopituitary dwarfism, e.g., tumour, etc.
   f. Pseudohypoparathyroidism and pseudo-pseudohypoparathyroidism.
   g. Xanthomatosis affecting the pituitary-hypothalamic region: Hand-Schüller-Christian syndrome.

8. HYPOTHALAMIC:
   a. Fröhlich's syndrome.
   b. Laurence-Moon-Biedl syndrome.

9. OTHER SYNDROMES OF UNKNOWN CAUSE:
   a. Progeria (Hutchinson-Gilford syndrome).
   b. Cockayne syndrome.
   c. Amsterdam dwarfism (de Lange syndrome).

1. DELAYED ADOLESCENT GROWTH AND DEVELOPMENT

This is probably the commonest cause of infantilism. The birth-weight and length are usually normal, but the child throughout infancy and childhood is up to two or three years behind his contemporaries in epiphysial, statural, muscular, sexual, and psychological development. A parent or some other member of the family may have exhibited a similar pattern of development. Puberty, though it may begin late—at the age of 16 or 17—does, however, leisurely appear and may be accompanied by a rapid spurt of growth, or may even then proceed so that final closure of the epiphyses is delayed. This may also happen in the case of the 'small-for-dates' foetus. Eventually, however, the individual becomes sexually mature and usually attains a normal adult stature. It is well to remember, before embarking officiously on endocrine therapy, that puberty varies considerably in its age of onset and its rate of development. Gonadotrophin levels after puberty are normal.

The presence of Human Growth Hormone (HGH) in the plasma may be demonstrated by radio-immunoassay either directly or after provocative tests such as the insulin tolerance test or after administration of arginine, Bovril, glucagon or levodopa. Growth hormone can be demonstrated in this type of infantilism and treatment with GH is not indicated.

2. GENETIC

a. The **Constitutional** type of dwarfism occurs in certain races (pygmies) and families which constantly breed individuals below the average height. In some cases the degree of dwarfism may be extreme and these 'midgets' may be found in circuses and fairs. Plasma GH is normal in African pygmies and it is to be presumed that there is an end-organ unresponsiveness to GH. There are examples of dwarf marriages producing both dwarf and normal offspring.

b. In the **Sporadic** type of primordial or genetic dwarfism, the child comes from a normal-sized family and is usually small at birth and grows slowly during infancy. There is normal epiphysial development and the bone age corresponds with the chronological age and plasma growth hormone can be demonstrated. Sexual development also occurs at the normal age and the features mature according to the natural age of the subject. The fact that these cases are resistant to all forms of treatment may be of diagnostic significance. The sporadic type may also be due to *intra-uterine growth retardation* if the mother was severely ill during the pregnancy or if there was placental deficiency.

c. **Chromosomal Gonadal Dysgenesis.** 'Gonadal dysgenesis' indicates that the gonads are represented by an undifferentiated primitive streak found in the broad ligament in the form of a thin strip of fibrous tissue. Examination of a buccal smear reveals in the majority of cases that the individual is chromatin negative. This is because the karyotype is 45/XO. Other chromosome patterns, however, do occur, such as the mosaics XO/XX and XO/XXX, which may give a chromatin-positive smear. The condition is almost invariably associated with dwarfism, which is a congenital defect and not an endocrine disorder, and a height of more than 5 ft. (152 cm.) is rarely achieved. Because of the lack of production of oestrogen there is complete failure of development of the breasts and labia minora, with an infantile uterus, an atrophic vaginal mucosa, and primary amenorrhoea. Another manifestation of oestrogen deficiency is osteoporosis which is typically found in the bones of the hands and feet and at the ends of the long bones. Pubic and axillary hair are scanty and late in appearing but they are usually present, in contrast to their complete absence in pituitary infantilism. Again, in contrast to the marked delay in epiphysial union found in hypopituitary dwarfism, the bone age is not markedly retarded. Furthermore, after the age of puberty the output of urinary gonadotrophin is abnormally high, whereas in cases of pituitary deficiency its presence cannot be demonstrated.

The most striking associated congenital abnormality is 'webbed neck' which is caused by triangular folds of skin running from the mastoid process to the tip of the acromion. When this is present the condition is referred to as *Turner's*

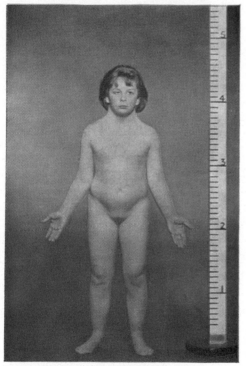

Fig. 231. Turner's syndrome in a patient aged 23. Note height is below 5 ft., typical facies, webbed neck, increased carrying angle, failure of breast development, and scanty growth of pubic hair. (*Courtesy of the Gordon Photographic Museum, Guy's Hospital.*)

syndrome (*Fig.* 231). The hair line extends downwards along the edges of the skin folds. In infancy there may be considerable lymphoedema of the lower limbs. Cases of Turner's syndrome are often accompanied by coarctation of the aorta, which is extremely rare in normal females and, indeed, all the cases of Turner's syndrome in

which it has been found have proved to be chromatin negative and therefore to have only one X in their sex chromosome pattern. Congenital renal abnormalities, such as horse-shoe kidney or double ureter, are also relatively common. A variety of bony deformities may occur, of which the most characteristic are cubitus valgus (increased 'carrying angle') and shortening of the fourth or fifth metacarpal. There may also be Madelung's deformity of the wrist. Owing to incomplete development of the nasal bones the bridge of the nose is flattened and there is an appearance of hypertelorism. There are also well-marked epicanthic folds. This produces a typical facies which is immediately recognized when it has been seen a few times. The skin of the body is unusually pale, and pigmented moles are found in almost every case.

Noonan's or *Ullrich's* syndrome. This condition, which in many respects resembles Turner's syndrome, may occur in males when the karyotype may be XO/XY mosaic or the normal male XY, or females with normal XX chromosome pattern. Pulmonary valve stenosis is the characteristic cardiac anomaly instead of coarctation of the aorta. Short stature is not invariable, though neck webbing is generally present. In males undescended testes are common. Autoimmune thyroiditis is also common, as it is in Turner's syndrome. The cause of Noonan's syndrome is unknown.

ii. Retardation of growth is a characteristic feature of various *autosomal abnormalities*, of which the commonest is trisomy 21 (Down's syndrome or Mongolism). Rarer conditions are trisomy 17 or 18 (Edwards' syndrome) and trisomy 13, 14, or 15 (Patau's syndrome) in which the infants, who die at the age of a few months, have grossly deformed ears and hands.

3. SKELETAL DISEASE

Congenital Skeletal Disease. *Chondrodystrophy, achondroplasia* (*Fig.* 232). The limbs are affected principally, being much shorter than normal. The long bones are commonly thickened, the humeri and femora showing expansion at the lower ends, and the tibiae are apt to be curved. The condition is due to a disturbance of endochondral ossification in which the growth cartilages are invaded by connective tissue. All the fingers are equal in length and the hands are small and stubby. Involvement of the bones at the base of the skull gives rise to a somewhat hydrocephalic appearance of the head. The nose is flattened and the lower jaw is unusually prominent. There is a marked lumbar lordosis with protruding buttocks. The condition is seldom associated with infantilism. Indeed there may actually be precocious development of the sex organs.

Chondro-osteo-dystrophy (Brailsford-Morquio disease) (*Fig.* 233) is a rare type of bony deformity, often familial, affecting chiefly the long bones and the spine (*see* p. 456). The epiphyses are deformed or fragmented, and a variety of deformities of the long bones have been described. The glenoid fossae and acetabula are poorly formed. The intervertebral spaces are increased, and, owing to the irregularity, flattening, or wedge-shaped deformity of the vertebral bodies; there is accentuated by limitation of extension of the hips and knees. The diagnosis can be made with certainty only by radiological examination (*Fig.* 234).

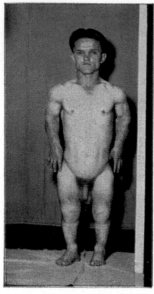

Fig. 232. An achondroplastic dwarf, showing large head and dwarfing due to shortness of the extremities. The proximal segments of the limbs are more affected than the distal, and there is some curving of the tibiae.

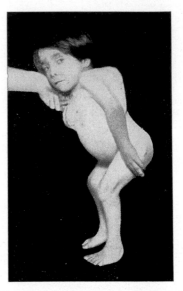

Fig. 233. Chondro-osteo-dystrophy. Dwarfism due to deformity; showing short neck, kyphosis, deformed sternum, and fixed flexion deformities of limbs. (*Mr. Fairbank's case.*)

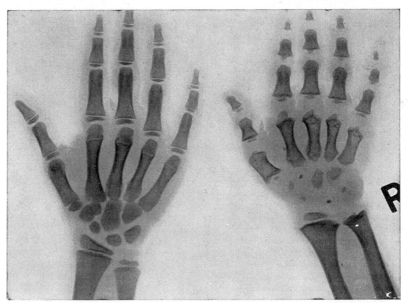

Fig. 234. Chondro-osteo-dystrophy: radiograph of hand on the right, showing wide joint spaces and deformity of epiphyses; on the left, a radiograph of a normal hand at the same age. (*Professor R. W. B. Ellis.*)

dorso-lumbar kyphosis and shortening of the neck, the head appearing to be pushed down on the shoulders. Many cases show a gross pigeon-breast deformity, and the dwarfism is further

In *dysostosis multiplex, gargoylism,* or *Hurler's syndrome* similar bone-changes occur, though a peculiar sabot-shaped deformity of the 2nd and 3rd lumbar vertebral body appears more constant, giving rise to angular kyphosis (*see* pp. 455, 529). The skull commonly shows oxycephaly or hydrocephalus and enlargement of the pituitary fossa. In addition, the syndrome is characterized by a

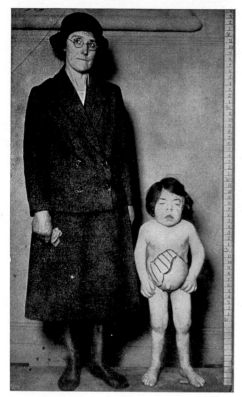

Fig. 235. Gargoylism. The patient, aged 18, with normal adult beside her, shows gross features, hepatosplenomegaly, umbilical hernia, and deformities of the extremities. In this case there is sexual infantilism. (*Professor R. W. B. Ellis.*)

peculiar grossness of the facies, enlargement of the spleen and liver, mental defect, and congenital corneal opacities. There is widespread deposition throughout the reticulo-endothelial system of a mucopolysaccharide, probably chondroitin sulphate. In the case illustrated (*Fig.* 235) infantilism was associated with the dwarfism, though this does not always occur.

Chondrodystrophia calcificans congenita is a rare condition in which the epiphysial centres of the long and small bones ossify and usually fuse into a single mass during early childhood. *Epiphysial dysplasia multiplex* occurs in older children in whom the long bones themselves are not affected but their epiphyses are 'stippled' or fragmented in a similar manner to those seen in hypothyroidism.

Chondro-ectodermal dysplasia (Ellis-van Creveld syndrome) is a type of chondrodystrophy in which there are also ectodermal deformities such as polydactyly, short tibia, dysplasia of the teeth, sparse hair growth, congenital malformations

of the heart, and inadequate function of the sweat glands leading to difficulties of temperature regulation.

Osteogenesis imperfecta, which is closely allied to, if not identical with, *fragilitas ossium,* is characterized by extreme brittleness of the bones; the multiple fractures which occur during intra-uterine life or in childhood, coupled with the fragility of the spine, result in gross deformity and dwarfism (*Fig.* 236). In familial cases, the diagnosis is confirmed by the occurrence of multiple

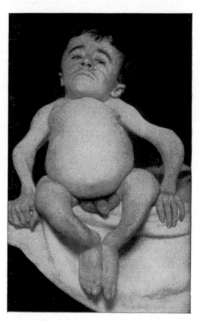

Fig. 236. Osteogenesis imperfecta. Age 18. Dwarfism without infantilism, due to deformities. Adult facies and genital development. (*Professor R. W. B. Ellis.*)

fractures or otosclerosis in other members of the family, or by the association with slaty-blue sclerotics. Radiographically the long bones are seen to be both shorter and more slender than normal, poorly calcified, with extreme thinning of the cortex. The appearances are quite distinct from those of rickets.

Acquired Skeletal Disease. This condition also produces dwarfism by virtue of the deformities of legs and spine. Thus in *infantile rickets* there is a general softening of the skeletal system in addition to the disorganization of ossification occurring at the ends of the long bones, resulting in bending of those bones subjected to weight-carrying or other pressure; in the severest cases, spontaneous fractures may add to the deformity, but this is less common; in infants who have begun to stand, the chief deformity is seen in the legs—genu valgum or varum, and acute bending of the tibiae, usually at the junction of the lower and middle thirds. General hypotonia may result in kyphosis or scoliosis.

The condition is recognized by the age incidence, commonly between 4 months and 3 years, a history of a deficient diet and of minimal exposure to sunlight, and the presence of other characteristic signs of rickets—enlarged or persistent anterior fontanelle, frontal bossing, delayed dentition, beading and flaring of the ribs, enlargement of epiphyses at wrists and ankles, and distended abdomen. In the acute stage a radiograph of the wrists shows a feathery, irregular line of ossification, with cupping of the lower end of the radius; as healing takes place, the line of ossification becomes regular and more densely calcified than normal. The biochemical changes in acute rickets are also characteristic; the blood phosphatase is consistently raised, and the plasma inorganic phosphorus is commonly reduced. The serum calcium is likewise below the average normal value, though the reduction is usually less marked than that of the phosphorus. It is generally true that a Ca × P product of under 30 (the two values being expressed in mg. per cent) indicates active rickets, and a value of over 40 excludes it. Estimation of the serum calcium serves to distinguish the rare condition of hyperparathyroidism causing osteoporosis, in which the serum calcium reaches high levels.

Late rickets, occurring in older children or adolescents, may be due either to the same causes as infantile rickets (juvenile osteomalacia) or to renal or coeliac disease.

Vitamin-D-resistant rickets is a hereditary disorder associated with short stature and low serum phosphorus, often without any skeletal deformities.

Spinal caries is recognized by pain and tenderness localized to one or more of the vertebrae, associated with angular kyphosis. Radiographs show destruction and collapse of the affected vertebral bodies, and serve to distinguish caries from congenital deformity of the vertebrae and kyphosis or scoliosis from other causes, e.g., poliomyelitis, in which an unrecognized paralysis of the muscles of the back is liable to result in a severe degree of postural deformity.

Still's disease. Rheumatoid arthritis in childhood (*see* p. 461) may give rise to early fusion of the epiphyses and stunting of growth.

4. NUTRITIONAL AND METABOLIC

Malnutrition. Inadequate intake of calories and of protein during childhood and adolescence will lead to progressive emaciation and retardation of growth. This is not uncommon in socially deprived families where the children are poorly fed and cared for. A child subject to severe emotional stress may also show grossly retarded growth and deficiency of growth hormone despite a sometimes voracious appetite. This may present as a social or psychiatric problem.

Malabsorption Syndromes may cause stunting of growth and should be excluded by faecal fat and other investigations.

Diabetes Insipidus leads to excessive fluid intake which is sometimes accompanied by impaired appetite and diminished growth.

Protein Deficiency, as in kwashiorkor, may give rise to considerable stunting of growth.

Electrolyte Imbalance giving rise to acidosis is sometimes found in children of short stature.

Glycogen-storage Disease (*Fig.* 237). This condition is due to an inborn error of metabolism

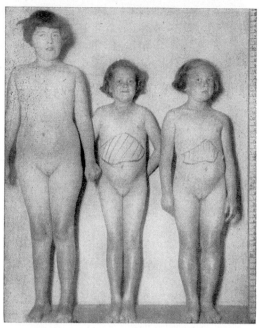

Fig. 237. Glycogen-storage disease in sisters aged 13½ and 10½, with normal control aged 10¼; infantilism and hepatomegaly.

as the result of which the liver, and in some cases the muscles, are unable to break down glycogen to glucose. There are various types with eponymous titles, such as 'von Gierke's disease'. Stunting of growth, when it occurs, seems to be caused by the excessive utilization of protein for conversion to sugar to meet the energy needs, so that there is no protein to spare for the growth process. There is gross hepatomegaly without enlargement of the spleen dating from infancy, particularly if this is familial.

5. INFECTIVE

Any chronic infection (e.g., bronchiectasis, malaria, or hookworm infestation) will be likely to retard normal growth and development. Syphilitic infection should be excluded in every doubtful case of infantilism.

6. SYSTEMIC

Renal Infantilism (*Fig.* 238). This condition is associated with chronic pyelonephritis occurring in childhood, the symptoms often dating from an early age. In many cases the nephritis is complicated by dilatation of the ureters and in some by infection of the urinary tract. There is seldom a clear history of a preceding attack of acute nephritis. The early symptoms are polyuria, polydipsia, and cessation of growth. Subsequently decalcification and rachitic deformities of the long bones are liable to occur. The condition may also be due to congenital malformations of the renal tract or disorders of tubular function, such as inability to retain potassium, giving rise to hyperkalaemic alkalosis.

and patent ductus arteriosus and severe pulmonary complaints such as asthma (especially if treated with corticosteroids), often cause marked retardation of growth. *Fibrocystic disease of the pancreas* with pulmonary and cardiac complications is another cause of stunted growth. Microcephaly, primary mental defect, and hydrocephalus following meningococcal meningitis, are

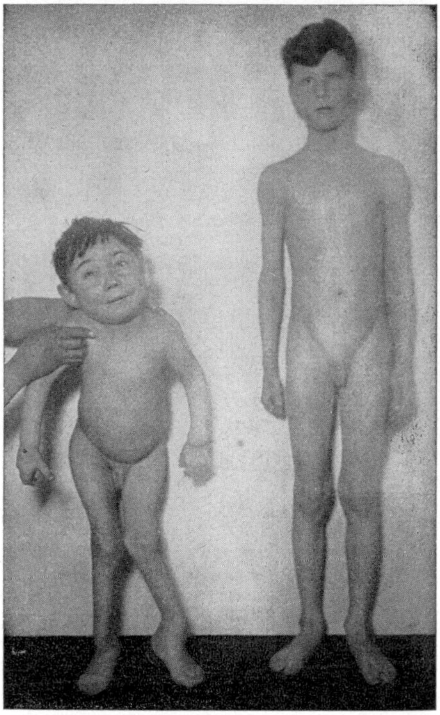

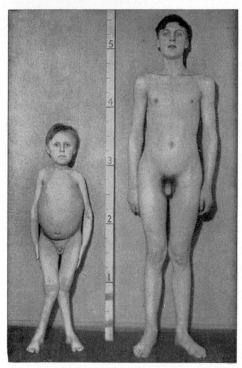

Fig. 238. On the left, a case of renal infantilism and rickets in a boy aged 9 years 10 months; the blood-urea was over 100 mg. per cent for more than 5 years; at autopsy, small sclerotic kidneys associated with dilated ureters were found. On the right, a normal boy of the same age. (*Professor R. W. B. Ellis.*)

Fig. 239. On the left, a case of coeliac infantilism in a boy aged 16, exhibiting infantile facies and genitalia, large abdomen and knock-knee. On the right, a normal boy of the same age. (*Dr. D. Hunter's case.*)

Coeliac Infantilism (*Fig.* 239). When there is a history of passage of large, pale, fatty, and offensive stools, associated with general wasting and distension of the abdomen, coeliac infantilism should be suspected. The condition is due to intolerance to wheat gluten leading to failure of fat absorption and steatorrhoea. Recurrent attacks of diarrhoea commonly begin between 6 months and 2 years of age, and some degree of fat intolerance persists.

Hepatic Infantilism. Occasionally, sporadic or familial cases of hepatic cirrhosis have been found to be affected with infantilism, accompanied by splenomegaly and evidence of portal obstruction (e.g., ascites, venous distension, and varices).

The remaining causes of systemic infantilism need not be considered in detail, since the other symptoms or signs will be more outstanding than the delay in development. Severe degrees of congenital heart disease, such as Fallot's tetralogy

also likely to be associated with some degree of interference with statural growth.

7. ENDOCRINE

Cretinism (*Fig.* 240) is usually recognized by the characteristic dull-looking facies, the general sluggishness of reaction, slow pulse-rate, constipation with distension of the abdomen and umbilical hernia, the presence of supraclavicular pads, and the yellowish pallor. The skin and hair often appear abnormally dry. The bodily proportions remain infantile in so far as the upper measurement (from the top of the head to the pubic spine) is significantly greater than the lower measurement (from the pubic spine to the floor). These measurements are equal in cases of hypopituitarism or simple retarded growth. Radiological studies show delayed epiphysial development, which is also found in pituitary infantilism. The presence, however, of the type of epiphysial dysgenesis referred to as 'stippled epiphyses' is especially characteristic of hypothyroidism, but is also found in epiphysial dysplasia multiplex. Retardation of dental development is characterized by delay in the formation of the tooth-buds.

Sexual precocity may result from either gonadal or adrenocortical over-activity. Gonadal precocity is due to an interstitial-cell tumour of the testis or a granulosa-cell tumour of the ovary. Adrenocortical precocity is confined to the male

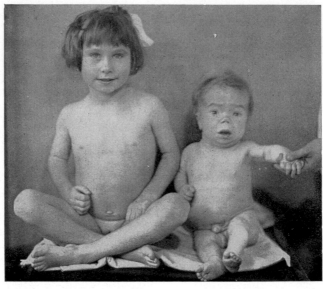

Fig. 240. Untreated cretin, aged 6, with normal child of the same age on the left. The cretin exhibits infantilism, characteristic facies, sparse hair, and umbilical hernia. (*Dr. Maitland-Jones's case.*)

Tests of thyroid function (p. 790) should be carried out to confirm the diagnosis.

The condition has to be distinguished from Down's syndrome (*Fig.* 241), in which the slanting eyes, brachycephalic skull, hypotonia, and the frequent association with congenital heart disease

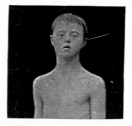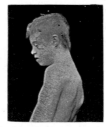

Fig. 241. Mongolism. Age 14. The general development is delayed. The physiognomy is undeveloped. The head is brachycephalic, the occipital region flat. The boy is an amiable imbecile. (*Professor R. W. B. Ellis.*)

form a picture which can be recognized at birth. The mongol, though mentally defective, does not show the sluggish reactions of the cretin and does not respond to thyroid administration.

Sexual Precocity with Early Epiphysial Closure. The differential diagnosis of sexual precocity is discussed on p. 722. Precocious puberty may be due to 'constitutional' or neurogenic causes or be associated with pigmentation and polyostotic fibrous dysplasia in girls (Albright's disease).

sex, being caused by excessive production of adrenal androgens. This may develop in foetal life giving rise to congenital adrenal hyperplasia which produces the clinical picture of macrogenitosomia precox: if it develops during the first decade it is almost always due to an adrenocortical tumour, whereas in the second decade the lesion may be either a tumour or adrenal hyperplasia.

Adrenal Virilism with Early Epiphysial Closure. Congenital adrenal hyperplasia or postnatal tumours or hyperplasia may also occur, of course, in girls. Indeed congenital adrenal hyperplasia is much more common in girls and gives rise to *female pseudohermaphroditism.* The clitoris is enlarged and may resemble a penis, except that its ventral aspect is anchored in a position of chordee. As the child gets older, hypertrophy of the clitoris increases and erections may become almost continuous. There is usually a single urethral orifice in the perineum. (Very rarely there are separate urethral and vaginal outlets.) The vagina opens into the urethra close to the external orifice. The rest of the female reproductive tract is entirely normal, so that if a urethroscope is introduced into the vagina, the cervix can be visualized and a ureteric catheter can be inserted into the uterus, and radio-opaque material will reveal a normal uterus and patent tubes. Under the influence of the excessive adrenal androgen output there is rapid skeletal growth, so that during the first decade the child is conspicuously taller than her contemporaries. Epiphysial union, however, occurs at an early age leading eventually to dwarfism with disproportionate skeletal development, the growth of the long bones being prematurely arrested, so that the span is significantly less than the height, and the lower measurement (pubis to floor) less than the upper measurement (head to pubis) (*Fig.* 242). Pubic hair appears at 4 years and is

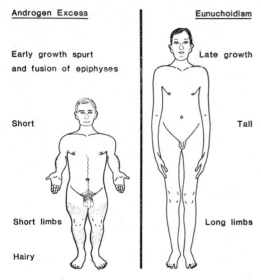

Androgen Excess	Eunuchoidism
Early growth spurt and fusion of epiphyses	Late growth
Short	Tall
Short limbs	Long limbs
Hairy	

Fig. 242. Comparison of short stature due to early closure of epiphyses and tall stature due to late closure of epiphyses in eunuchoidism with unimpaired growth hormone secretion. (*Courtesy of the Departments of Medical Illustration, Guy's and Westminster Hospitals.*)

soon followed by axillary hair growth. Acne and hypertrichosis with deepening of the voice and development of a muscular physique become evident at an early age. During the second half of the second decade the occurrence of amenorrhoea and the lack of mammary development are noticeable features. The condition is due to an enzymatic defect in the biosynthesis of the adrenocortical hormones belonging to the groups represented by cortisone and cortisol (glucocorticoids) and by aldosterone (mineralo-corticoids). The lack of cortisol releases excessive quantities of corticotrophin which are responsible for the bilateral adrenal hyperplasia, the excessive output of 17-oxosteroids, and the consequent virilism. In addition to the high levels of 17-oxosteroids (7–21 μmol/24 h during the first few months of life, 35–69 μmol/24 h by the age of 6 years, and 104–276 μmol/24 h at the age of 10 or 12) pregnanetriol may also be found in the urine and this is an important diagnostic feature of the hormonal analysis. Administration of corticosteroids will suppress the excessive

output of 17-oxosteroids and lead to successful feminization including breast development and the onset of regular, ovulatory, menstrual cycles in patients over the age of puberty. The possibility of such successful treatment emphasizes the desirability of early diagnosis.

If adrenal virilism develops during the first decade, it is nearly always due to an adrenocortical tumour. The picture of postnatal virilism is similar to that found in congenital adrenal hyperplasia, except that there are no congenital abnormalities of the reproductive tract and no excretion of pregnanetriol. After the first decade the lesion may be a tumour or hyperplasia. Distinction can be made between these two by means of the 'dexamethasone suppression' test. A dose of 0·5 mg. 6-hourly for 48 hours will depress the urinary 17-oxosteroid level by 50 per cent in the case of adrenal hyperplasia because of the suppression of corticotrophin output. A tumour, however, is 'autonomous' as far as corticotrophin is concerned and even 2 mg. dexamethasone q.d.s. will not suppress the androgen output. The finding of a high urinary level of dehydroepiandrosterone is strongly suggestive of a tumour.

Cushing's syndrome in children is always accompanied by short stature and retarded growth.

Hypopituitary. *Pituitary infantilism* is not easy to distinguish in the early stages from the sporadic type of primordial dwarfism mentioned above. The birth weight and growth during infancy may be normal, but gradually retardation of growth becomes evident, and marked delay in epiphysial development may be found. *Congenital hypopituitary dwarfism* is usually recognized a year or two after birth. During the normal phase of adolescence it is realized that sexual development is not taking place, and the features remain young and childish. During the third decade the skin loses its natural elasticity and the face becomes wizened, though still retaining its child-like characters. Further evidence of pituitary failure may be found in the tendency to hypoglycaemic attacks, often associated with an increased sugar tolerance. This lowered level of blood-sugar might of course result from a secondary adrenal cortical deficiency, due to lack of production of corticotrophin, though there is no evidence of disturbance of water and electrolyte balance or of lowered blood-pressure. The 17-oxosteroid figure is, however, abnormally low, indicating a failure of testicular and adrenal cortical androgen secretion. A valuable point of distinction between pituitary infantilism and primary gonadal failure is the degree of sexual hair growth. In the pituitary cases (*Fig.* 245), with secondary involvement of the adrenal cortex, there is no growth of pubic or axillary hair at all, whereas in primary gonadal failure a scanty growth of both usually occurs. Another method of locating the site of the deficiency is to estimate the urinary gonadotrophin level. In pituitary failure no gonadotrophin will be detected, whereas the figure will be abnormally high where the gonads are primarily at fault. In pituitary infantilism there is marked

Name............................ Date of Birth............ Reg.No..........

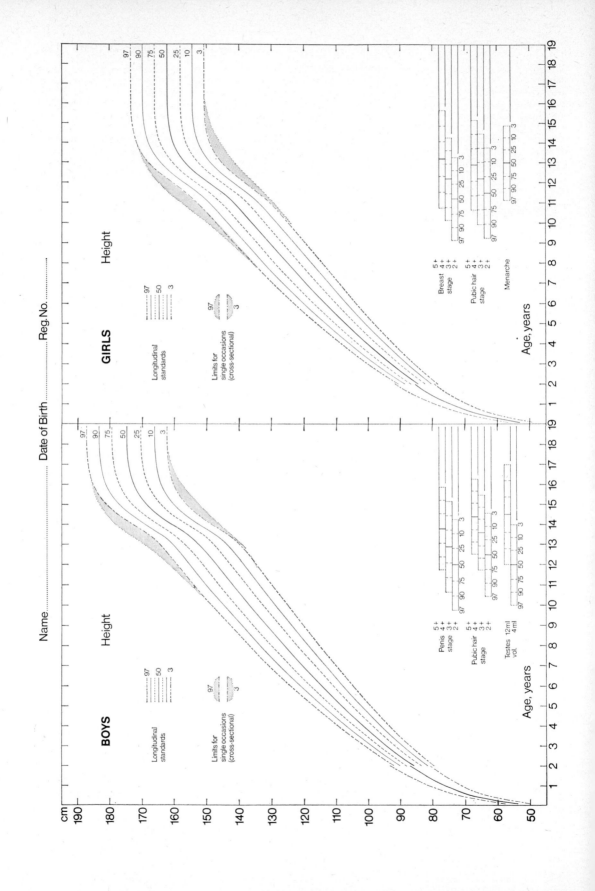

BOYS

Height

Longitudinal standards
97
50
3

Limits for single occasions (cross-sectional)
97
3

Penis stage 5+ 4+ 3+ 2+
Pubic hair stage 5+ 4+ 3+ 2+
Testes 12ml vol. 4ml

Age, years

GIRLS

Height

Longitudinal standards
97
50
3

Limits for single occasions (cross-sectional)
97
3

Breast stage 5+ 4+ 3+ 2+
Pubic hair stage 5+ 4+ 3+ 2+
Menarche

Age, years

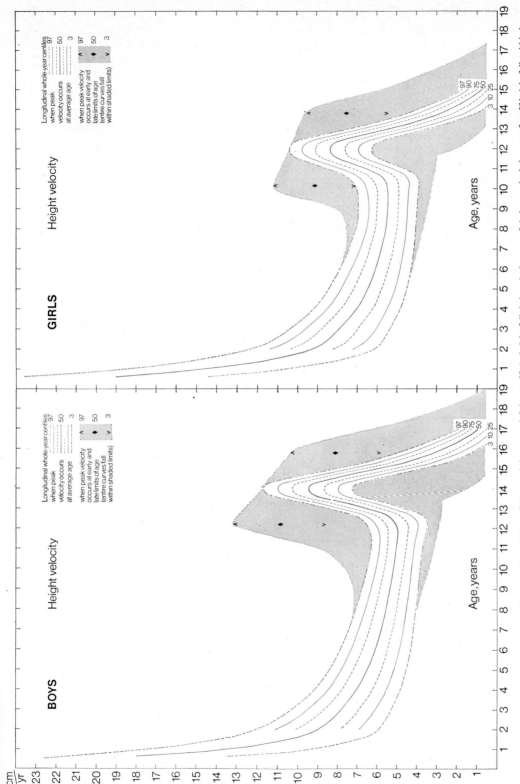

Figs. 243, 244. Height charts for use in identifying patients with possible growth hormone deficiency. If the height falls below the bottom of the lower shaded area, refer. If height falls within lower shaded area remeasure a year later; if the plot has progressed to nearer the lower border, refer. Velocity charts depict the individual rate of growth at different ages. *(Charts constructed by Professor J. M. Tanner and Mr. R. H. Whitehouse of the Department of Growth and Development, Institute of Child Health, London. Published with copyright by Castlemead Publications, Gascoyne Way, Herford, Herts.)*

retardation of epiphysial development throughout childhood and adolescence and epiphysial union never occurs, though there is no tendency to prolonged growth of the long bones owing to the deficiency of pituitary growth hormone. In dwarfism due to gonadal dysgenesis epiphysial development is only slightly retarded, if at all, though in eunuchoidism the late age of epiphysial fusion and the prolonged secretion of growth hormone leads to considerable, though disproportionate, increase in stature: the span is greater

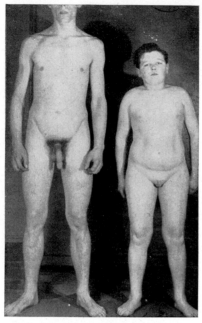

Fig. 245. Hypopituitarism. Obesity, stunting of growth; hypogonadism; absence of body and facial hair; youthful appearance. Age 23. Control, brother aged 18.

than the height, and the pubis-to-floor (lower) measurement is greater than the head-to-pubis (upper) measurement. In the normal infant the limbs are disproportionately short in comparison with the development of the head and trunk. The cretin retains these infantile proportions, whereas the child suffering from pituitary infantilism shows normal proportions, the limbs developing more rapidly than the head and trunk, so that by the age of 10 or 11 the height and span and the upper and lower measurements are equal.

In many cases of congenital pituitary deficiency most or all of the pituitary hormones fail to be secreted, but in about half the cases the short stature is due to *isolated growth hormone deficiency*. Plasma Human Growth Hormone (HGH) can be measured by radio-immunoassay and may be extracted from normal post-mortem pituitaries and used therapeutically in these cases, though it is completely ineffective in all other cases of short stature. From 100–200 pituitaries

are required for a year's treatment and will be supplied by the Medical Research Council for use in genuine cases. The earlier the treatment the better the chance of achieving normal adult height. The short height can sometimes be detected by the age of 2 and certainly before the child goes to school at 4 or 5. Height charts constructed by Professor J. M. Tanner may be obtained from Creaseys Ltd., Castlemead, Gascoyne Way, Hertford (*Figs.* 243, 244). These show the normal centile standards, the lowest being 3 centile. A shaded area is marked below this line, the bottom of this area being known as −3 SD (below the 3 centile standard deviation). Should the child's height lie within this shaded area he (or she) should be re-examined in a year's time. If the height has moved further down in the shaded area or even below it, the child requires immediate treatment with HGH. In isolated growth hormone deficiency children (much more commonly boys than girls) have a normal birth-weight and because growth hormone mobilizes fat they become fatter than normal. In boys the penis and scrotum are noticeably small though the testicles are usually normal in size. The bone age is retarded and the bones, especially of the hands, are thin. The condition may occur as an autosomal recessive and in more than one member of the family. Other cases of pituitary infantilism, with deficiency of thyroid-stimulating hormone and gonadotrophins, when puberty should develop should also be treated with growth hormone if this is shown to be deficient.

Acquired hypopituitary dwarfism may be due to a craniopharyngioma with X-ray evidence of calcification in or above the sella turcica, or more rarely to a chromophobe adenoma or eosinophilic granuloma, tuberculous meningitis, or trauma.

Pseudohypoparathyroidism and *pseudo-pseudo-hypoparathyroidism* are conditions associated with short stature, a rounded face, shortening of the fourth and fifth metacarpals, and ectopic bone formation. Hypoparathyroidism is due to loss of parathyroid tissue, for instance following thyroidectomy, giving rise to lack of calcium and tetany. In pseudo-hypoparathyroidism there is no lack of parathyroid tissue, though the clinical and biochemical signs are the same and the patient will not respond to parathyroid hormone. In pseudo-pseudo-hypoparathyroidism the biochemical signs are normal and there are adequate levels of calcium but the clinical signs are the same as in pseudo-hypoparathyroidism.

XANTHOMATOSIS AFFECTING THE PITUITARY HYPO-THALAMIC REGION: HAND-SCHÜLLER-CHRISTIAN SYNDROME. In this disease reticulo-endothelial cells are infiltrated with cholesterol and these xanthomatous deposits may invade the region of the pituitary and hypothalamus giving rise to pituitary dwarfism, obesity, or diabetes insipidus.

8. HYPOTHALAMIC

Fröhlich's Syndrome. This is a rare condition too commonly diagnosed. The classic triad of signs consists of obesity, genital hypoplasia, and stunting of growth. The vast majority of fat children show no true genital hypoplasia, though the envelopment of the shaft of the penis in the pubic 'sporran' and the normal prepubertal pea-like size of the testes convince the inexperienced observer of the lack of genital development: nor are such children undersized; indeed the overeating which produces the obesity also tends to increase somatic growth, and they are tall for their age. Fröhlich's patient was found to have a cystic tumour of the pituitary, but it was subsequently shown that the syndrome was produced only by tumours extending into the hypothalamic region, and that in some cases the pituitary itself was intact and unaffected. The clinical picture in these cases is due to the lack of the hypothalamic 'releasing' hormones—growth hormone-releasing hormone (GRH), thyroid-stimulating hormone-releasing hormone (TSHRH), and gonadotrophin-releasing hormone (FSH/LHRH).

Laurence-Moon-Biedl Syndrome. This is a rare condition in which dwarfism occurs in only 10 per cent of cases. The cardinal signs, which are all congenital abnormalities, are obesity (in 75 per cent of cases), retinitis pigmentosa (70 per cent), polydactyly or syndactyly (70 per cent), mental retardation (64 per cent), and genital hypoplasia (60 per cent). It is thought to be a recessively inherited condition involving the hypothalamus.

9. OTHER SYNDROMES OF UNKNOWN CAUSE

Progeria. In the *Hutchinson-Gilford syndrome* the patient becomes prematurely old and usually dies before the age of 20 (*see Fig.* 246). The infant is normal at birth but growth almost ceases within a few months to three years, and there is premature closure of the epiphyses. There is an almost complete absence of subcutaneous fat so that one can detect the bones, muscles, tendons, and vessels beneath the skin. It also accounts for the beaky nose, sharp retracted skin, and prominent ears. There is considerable muscular weakness. The premature old age is in some cases associated with an extreme degree of arteriosclerosis and there is usually a severe degree of mental deficiency.

The *Cockayne syndrome* is very similar to the Hutchinson-Gilford syndrome, though there appear to be familial influences, and it is regarded as being due to an autosomal recessive gene. The child is normal at birth but in the second year growth ceases and cerebral and other degenerative changes ensue. The clinical features are large hands and feet, large joints, kyphosis, a small skull with a narrow face, and closely spaced, sunken eyes. There is retinal degeneration, sometimes with optic atrophy, cataract, partial deafness, and low mentality.

Other somewhat similar syndromes have been described in which there is marked dwarfism, lack of subcutaneous fat, bird-headed features, sometimes with hypertelorism, large ears, and lanugo-type hirsutism (*leprechaunism*). The true cause

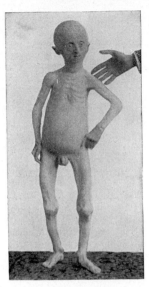

Fig. 246. Progeria. Age 15. The stature and proportions are childish, but the attitude, physiognomy, leanness, and baldness are elderly. The scalp is sparsely covered with grey hair. The ear lobule is absent, the nasal cartilages are conspicuous. The joints appear nodose owing to the wasting of the soft parts. (*Mr. Hastings Gilford's case.*)

of these various types of progenies is completely unknown, but at the moment it seems best to classify them under the heading of genetic abnormalities. *Amsterdam dwarfism* (the *de Lange syndrome*) has been referred to in the section on hirsutism (p. 396). The aetiology of this condition has still not been determined.

P. M. F. Bishop.

DYSMENORRHOEA

The causes may be tabulated as follows:

1. SPASMODIC OR PRIMARY:
   Uterine hypoplasia (small, acutely anteflexed uterus, long conical cervix, stenosed os)
   Congenital malformations
   Ovarian dysfunction
   Psychogenic

2. CONGESTIVE OR SECONDARY
   Arising from infection:
   Pelvic peritonitis, salpingo-oophoritis, parametritis, cervicitis
   Arising from endometriosis:
   Chocolate cysts of ovary, adenomyoma
   Retroversion of the uterus ⎱ if complicated by
   Uterine fibroids ⎰ pelvic infection or endometriosis
   Psychogenic

3. MEMBRANOUS.

The distribution of the cases into these three classes is often easy; in the first place, spasmodic cases are practically always *primary*, that is, they begin when ovulation first takes place, i.e., within two or three years of the onset of the periods; while congestive cases are *secondary*, that is, acquired later as a result of some definite lesion. Further, the nature of the pain is often characteristic of the type of case, for in spasmodic cases the pain begins with the flow or only just before it, is aching in character, often with griping or colicky exacerbations felt in the midline above the symphysis pubis and passing down the anterior aspect of the thighs. It is associated with prostration, pallor, headache, and vomiting. It usually continues for six to twelve hours until the menstrual flow is well established. In the congestive cases, on the other hand, the pain is continuous and aching, begins some hours or days before the flow, and in typical cases is relieved by the flow. In the membranous cases, which may complicate either primary or secondary dysmenorrhoea, the nature of the pain partakes of the characters of both the former types, being aching and continuous first, then becoming colicky and spasmodic when the uterus is attempting to expel the characteristic membrane or cast, and being finally relieved when this comes away. Many cases are met with in which the pain partakes of the nature of both the congestive and spasmodic types. This usually means that a woman who originally had spasmodic dysmenorrhoea acquires some lesion which in its turn gives rise also to the congestive type of pain.

Having settled that a case belongs to one of the three main types, it is possible to work out the actual causation. This is more difficult in the spasmodic cases than in the congestive, because the latter depend upon well-defined lesions, and the former do not.

1. Spasmodic Cases. The causation of the pain in this type of case is obscure because the physical signs are essentially normal. Not infrequently the uterus may be small with a long conical cervix and an exaggerated anterior bend (the 'cochleate' uterus of Pozzi). A sound may pass with difficulty into such a uterus giving rise to the suggestion that there is a stenosis of the internal os. These findings are common in young adult women, however, and are more likely to be a manifestation of their immaturity than a cause of the spasmodic dysmenorrhoea, because they are found just as often in girls of the same age who do not suffer from dysmenorrhoea. Many cases with spasmodic dysmenorrhoea, moreover, appear to have a normal uterus. In such cases evidence of degenerative or inflammatory changes in the presacral nerve have been described but their existence is very doubtful. The function of the ovarian hormones in causing spasmodic dysmenorrhoea is also not clear. For the first two or three years of anovular menstruation the periods do not as a rule cause pain. But when ovulation begins, a corpus luteum is formed and progesterone secreted and the periods become painful. Inhibition of ovulation by the use of the contraceptive pill usually renders the periods painless in such cases unless there is a large psychogenic element. It is tempting to explain spasmodic dysmenorrhoea by saying it is due to an ovarian dysfunction but if this is so its nature is unknown. The psychogenic factor is also emphasized and said to be increased by a doting mother who herself suffered from severe dysmenorrhoea. Marriage and child-bearing may improve or cure spasmodic dysmenorrhoea but this does not prove its psychogenic origin in the first place. Nevertheless, a healthy attitude by the patient to the condition and an assurance that it does not signify disease helps her to put up with it.

2. Congestive Cases. It is unnecessary to differentiate the congestive cases as tubal, ovarian, or uterine because the underlying cause in all is pelvic congestion accompanying such lesions as are shown in the table above. Their differential diagnosis is made by careful consideration of the history, combined with bimanual examination of the pelvic organs. Simple *retroversion and flexion* can be recognized on bimanual examination; the fundus will be felt posteriorly, the cervix looking directly down the vagina in a forward direction. Retroversion of the uterus by itself does not cause dysmenorrhoea and painful periods mean that either pelvic infection or endometriosis coexist. *Salpingo-oophoritis* in its typical chronic form gives rise to irregular tender swellings on either side and behind the uterus, sometimes forming definitely retort-shaped swellings, especially if pus is present in the tubes. Fixation of these swellings and of the uterus is a very definite sign of the disease; while the history of one or more attacks of acute illness, with pelvic pain, will assist to make the diagnosis certain. Small haemorrhagic cysts of the ovary, the contents of which may be 'tarry' or of chocolate-like consistence, are also important causes of premenstrual dysmenorrhoea; they are always fixed, and are of endometrial origin (*endometrioma of the ovary*). Adenomyosis may produce general enlargement of the uterus or there may be a localized adenomyoma in part of the uterus. Then an asymmetrical swelling can be felt in the uterus on bimanual vaginal examination, as in the case of a uterine fibroid.

Any psychogenic factor will naturally accentuate the pain. Often associated with this type of dysmenorrhoea is some constitutional disability, the result of anaemia, overwork, worry, anxiety or other conditions leading to a lowering of the pain threshold.

In nearly all cases of congestive dysmenorrhoea the underlying cause also produces other symptoms such as menorrhagia, dyspareunia, backache, and vaginal discharge. It is unusual to find congestive dysmenorrhoea as a symptom by itself.

3. Membranous Cases. A cast of uterine endometrium, complete or incomplete, may be passed in either spasmodic or congestive dysmenorrhoea. Its passage through the cervix is likely to cause spasmodic pain because of the colicky uterine contractions. The cast may have to be distinguished from a decidual cast passed following the rupture of an ectopic pregnancy or from the cast of an early miscarriage. In either of these conditions a careful review of the history should lead to the diagnosis but if there is doubt histology of the cast should settle it. In ectopic pregnancy the cast contains the decidua of pregnancy but no chorionic villi and in the case of an early miscarriage there are villi in the decidua.

Cases of dysmenorrhoea may be confused with those of abdominal pain due to other lesions unconnected with menstruation; and the differentiation of such cases may be a matter of considerable importance. It is conceivable that the following conditions may be mistaken for dysmenorrhoea:

Appendicitis
Colic: intestinal, renal, or hepatic
Perforated gastric ulcer
Ruptured tubal gestation
Torsion of an ovarian cyst pedicle
Haemorrhage from or into a Graafian follicle
Rupture of an ovarian cyst or pyosalpinx
Dyspepsia with flatulent distension
Threatened or actual abortion
Endometriosis.

Obviously, some of these lesions are dangerous to life, and therefore it is essential that they are not overlooked. The danger of this occurring is increased if any of these lesions start at or near the expected time of a menstrual period, and would hardly arise if a menstrual period had terminated recently, or was not expected for some days. It will be noted that all these lesions are accompanied by sudden abdominal pain, which might perhaps lead to a suspicion of spasmodic dysmenorrhoea, but hardly of congestive, owing to the character of the pain.

T. L. T. Lewis.

DYSPAREUNIA

Dyspareunia, or painful coitus, may depend on a variety of local lesions, or it may occur when no local lesion can be found. It is associated closely with vaginismus, or painful spasm of the levator ani muscle on attempts at coitus, and the same lesions which cause simple dyspareunia may also give rise to vaginismus; vaginismus is particularly likely to develop if the simple dyspareunia remains untreated for any length of time. In some women a local lesion produces no pain upon attempts at coitus which in others will cause pain accompanied by violent spasm of the levator ani. In some cases pain arises because there is a difficulty of penetration of the vaginal orifice, while in others there is no difficulty, but pain is caused on deep penetration—'deep dyspareunia'. The following lesions commonly give rise to dyspareunia:

Congenital absence of the lower part of the vagina
Unruptured hymen
Inflamed hymeneal orifice
Vulvitis
Bartholinitis

Disparity in size
Leucoplakic vulvitis
Kraurosis vulvae
Healed perineal lacerations giving rise to a narrow introitus
Urethral caruncle
Urethritis
Cystitis
Prolapsed tender ovaries with retroverted uterus
Salpingo-oophoritis
Anal fissure
Thrombosed piles
Endometriosis
Arthritis of the hips
'Functional' causes.

The lesions fall into natural groups, according as the situation of the lesion is at the vulva, the uterus and ovaries, the urinary passages, or at the anus and rectum; it is necessary to carry out a detailed examination of any case of dyspareunia in order to find out whether any of these well-defined lesions are present. The commonest is *inflamed hymeneal remains*, sometimes gonorrhoeal, accompanied by redness and swelling of the orifice of the duct of Bartholin's gland. The lesion is evident on inspection, and the parts are acutely sensitive to the least touch. *Leucoplakic vulvitis* is a lesion that is obvious from the white, sodden appearance of the labia, and causes pain on account of the sensitive cracks and fissures which accompany it. *Kraurosis vulvae* causes actual contraction of the vaginal orifice, and consequently penetration is difficult and causes pain. The red projecting growth from the urinary meatus, *caruncle*, is self-evident and acutely tender, while *urethritis* is diagnosed by the issue of pus on squeezing the urethra. *Cystitis* is diagnosed by the presence of pus and mucus in the urine, accompanied by frequency of micturition, and it causes pain because the bladder is painful and intolerant of the disturbance caused by coitus. *Prolapsed, tender ovaries* and *backward displacements of the uterus* cause no pain on penetration and no difficulty, but coitus with deep penetration gives acute pain at the time or a dull pelvic ache later; the condition is recognized by a bimanual examination, as is also *salpingo-oophoritis*, in connexion with which there is usually a history of some acute attack of pelvic peritonitis. Vaginitis due to a trichomonas infection, or a chronic endocervitis with or without erosion, may be responsible. Endometriosis in the pelvis is a common cause of deep dyspareunia. Ovarian and other neoplasms are hardly ever responsible; severe constipation is not an uncommon cause. Disproportion in size is rarely in itself of importance as the vagina is very distensile, but if in addition there is any local lesion the pain will be accentuated. *Anal fissure* and *thrombosed and inflamed piles* are recognized by careful examination of the anus and rectum by the finger or speculum. Arthritis of the hips or lumbar spine may cause dyspareunia.

In the cases which occur without local lesions the vaginal entrance will be found to be acutely hyperaesthetic and penetration difficult, and there is spasmodic vaginismus. Careful examination fails to demonstrate a lesion, and these cases are usually termed 'neurotic' or 'functional'; sexual desire is not necessarily absent; indeed many such patients are over-desirous of the consummation of marriage. Fear, arising from painful attempts at coitus, is often the cause of the condition. Enlarging the orifice by gradual dilatation, using vaginal dilators, or by a small plastic operation often leads to cure as the patient gains confidence. Childbearing also cures a case of this nature. These cases must be distinguished from those in which the underlying factor is absence of sexual desire and actual dislike of the sexual act, when the dysparcunia is merely a defence mechanism built up by the woman to avoid coitus. Unhappy and unsuitable marriages or fear of pregnancy conduce to this state of affairs, and the patient is prone to complain of pain when dislike is really what is meant. There is no difficulty in penetration in such cases.

T. L. T. Lewis.

DYSPHAGIA

Dysphagia means difficulty in swallowing. It may be (*a*) the consequence of mechanical obstruction, (*b*) of nervous origin, or (*c*) because of pain.

1. Dysphagia due to Mechanical Obstruction to the Oesophagus. Congenital stricture of the oesophagus is suspected if a newborn infant exhibits respiratory distress immediately on being fed. Passage of a soft rubber catheter reveals obstruction which will be confirmed by the instillation of a few drops of lipiodol and X-ray examination. Usually there is a fistulous communication between the lower oesophageal segment and the trachea. In adult life the usual history of progressive mechanical obstruction in the oesophagus is as follows: There is little or no pain, and difficulty in swallowing is experienced first only with the more solid kinds of food, such as meat, dry bread, and the coarser vegetables, so that the sufferer is obliged to live mainly upon pulpy foods, milk puddings, gruel, and the like. Later he can swallow only liquids and ultimately even liquids are regurgitated in consequence of a condition of complete obstruction at some point between the level of the cricoid cartilage and the lower end of the xiphisternum, which corresponds, as regards sensation, to the cardiac end of the oesophagus. When with such a history the patient gives an account of having, in the past, swallowed some strong irritant or corrosive substance such as a concentrated alkali or a mineral acid, the diagnosis of *fibrous stricture* from *corrosive* injury is highly probable. When similar obstruction succeeds the swallowing of a *foreign body*, such as a tooth-plate, a large piece of bone, or a coin, the diagnosis is also easy, though in some cases there may be doubt as to the existence of a foreign body in the oesophagus until the oesophagoscope is used, or X-rays employed with or without barium. Where the symptoms are not directly attributable to anything of this nature, but develop insidiously and progressively as described above, the diagnosis generally lies between *squamous-celled carcinoma* of the oesophagus, *carcinoma of the stomach* directly invading the lower end of the oesophagus, and *aortic aneurysm, mediastinal nodes,* or other tumour compressing the oesophagus from outside. There is danger in passing an oesophagoscope until aortic aneurysm has been excluded, a decision of difficulty when clinical grounds alone are available. For the aneurysm most liable to stenose the oesophagus is one affecting the descending thoracic aorta, behind the heart, where it can be neither heard nor felt, and in a situation unlikely to cause the conventional physical signs— inequality of the pulses, inequality of the pupils (from interference with the cervical sympathetic), paralysis of a vocal cord (from interference with the left recurrent laryngeal nerve), tracheal tugging, or pain down either arm. The only effects besides oesophageal obstruction likely to be due to an aneurysm in this position are: pain in the dorsal region of the spine, possibly radiating along the course of one or more of the intercostal nerves towards the left and simulating intercostal neuralgia, and perhaps obstruction to the lower part of the root of the left lung, causing impairment of note, of air-entry, or of voice-sounds, with or without some crackling râles over the left lower lobe behind. X-ray examination is essential. If the aneurysm cannot be seen in an anteroposterior view of the chest, owing to the heart shadow lying in front of it, it may be obvious in the left oblique position which is the best for viewing opacities in the posterior mediastinum.

The site of oesophageal obstruction may be demonstrated with the X-rays after the patient has swallowed barium sulphate (*Figs.* 247–249). The older the patient, the more likely is the obstruction to be due to carcinoma of the oesophagus. The differentiation between primary growth of the oesophagus and infiltration of the oesophagus by a growth starting at the cardiac end of the stomach is often impossible and is of academic interest rather than practical importance. Secondary nodules should be sought, especially in the liver or in the lymph-nodes in the lower part of the neck. A history of syphilis and evidence of syphilitic aortic regurgitation, especially in a man between the ages of 40 and 50, would render aneurysm likely.

When aortic aneurysm can be excluded, information as to the nature of an oesophageal obstruction may be obtained by oesophagoscopy, and this instrument can be employed at the same time in facilitating the removal of such things as a foreign body or lump of food that may have become impacted in the crater of an ulcerating stricture.

If a malignant stricture is encountered, a biopsy will enable differentiation to be made between a carcinoma of the lower oesophagus (squamous-cell tumour) and a carcinoma of the cardia (adenocarcinoma).

Dysphagia lusoria is a very rare condition due to compression of the oesophagus by an aberrant right subclavian artery, which arises from the aorta beyond the left subclavian and passes to the right side either in front of or behind the oesophagus; the diagnosis in such cases is difficult and indeed the condition may only be suspected on account of the coexistence of other congenital deformities, such as transposition of the viscera or *morbus caeruleus*. It may present itself as chronic superior mediastinal compression.

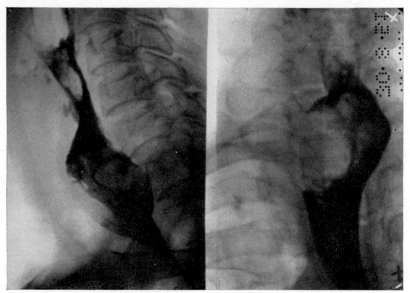

Fig. 247. Carcinoma of upper portion of oesophagus. (*Dr. Cochrane Shanks.*)

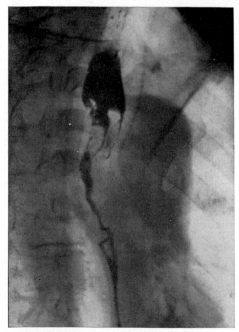

Fig. 248. Extensive carcinoma involving middle third of oesophagus showing gross irregularity of attacked portion and some dilatation of gullet above this. (*Dr. Cochrane Shanks.*)

8*

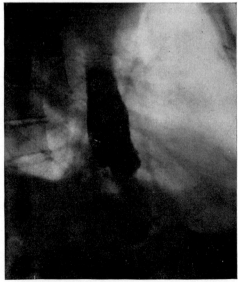

Fig. 249. Radiograph in a case of stenosis of the oesophagus by a carcinoma at the cardiac orifice. (*Dr. Cochrane Shanks.*)

Many cases of so-called 'globus hystericus' may have been mistakenly referred for psychological treatment when such a cause was actually present demanding surgical resection.

Pharyngeal pouches cause symptoms which can seldom be interpreted with certainty unless the patient is observed over some considerable time. As a rule the patient can swallow with ease on some days but with considerable difficulty on others. Aneurysm, new growth, and traumatic or corrosive obstructions will be excluded partly by the results of X-ray examination and partly by the age—the subjects with oesophageal pouch are relatively young. The particular feature that suggests the existence of a pouch is that the patient, who has been able to swallow perfectly well for a few days and then begins to experience difficulty in deglutition, finds relief presently through the regurgitation—clearly not from the stomach, but from some situation higher up—of a larger quantity of food material that had been recently swallowed, including perhaps articles recognizable as having been taken one or more days previously. The reason for these symptoms is that the pouch does not obstruct the oesophagus until it becomes much distended by the gradual accumulation in it of portions of the food swallowed, relief occurring when the greatly distended sac empties itself back into the oesophagus (*Fig.* 572, p. 569).

Peptic oesophagitis associated with hiatus hernia usually becomes evident in late middle life and may be responsible for dysphagia low down in the oesophagus, together with other features such as 'painful dyspepsia' and haematemesis. There is usually a typical history of heartburn and reflux on lying down and bending over. A barium swallow reveals a smooth stricture at the lower end of the oesophagus together with a hiatus hernia (*Fig.* 250). Differentiation from a carcinomatous stricture may be difficult since the latter may coexist with a hiatus hernia. If there is reasonable doubt, oesophagoscopy and biopsy of the stricture is indicated.

A simple but very troublesome mechanical cause of dysphagia is *xerostomia*; the lubricating value of saliva in the process of swallowing is not always adequately appreciated.

2. Dysphagia due to Nervous Causes without Obstruction.

Post-diphtheritic dysphagia, fortunately, has disappeared in the United Kingdom but may still be encountered in endemic areas. It is characterized by regurgitation of the food through the nose due to paralysis of the soft palate. There may be a history of sore throat and Klebs-Löffler bacilli may still be found in a swab from the patient's throat. There may or may not be paralysis of the ciliary muscles of the eyes or other signs of peripheral neuritis. In any case the development of regurgitation of food through the nose must always be strongly suspicious of an antecedent attack of diphtheria, possibly of a mild type that had been completely overlooked.

Hysteria as a cause for dysphagia is familiar as globus hystericus, the diagnosis of which is usually not difficult if the patient is a young woman who has suffered from other functional nervous affections, e.g., hysterical aphonia.

Less common varieties of dysphagia of nervous origin are as follows.

Bulbar paralysis, in which the progressive disability in the use of the lips, tongue, pharynx, and larynx points at once to the diagnosis; the only difficulty that may perhaps arise is to distinguish true bulbar paralysis, in which the lesion

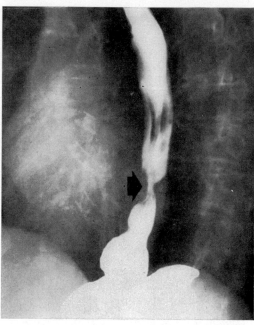

Fig. 250. Barium swallow demonstrating a benign stricture of the lower end of the oesophagus (arrowed) above a sliding hiatus hernia.

is in the motor nuclei of the medulla oblongata, from pseudobulbar paralysis, where the lesion is due to bilateral cortical softening. In the true form, but not in the pseudo variety, there is atrophy of the tongue.

Syphilitic degeneration of the medullary centres may produce symptoms not unlike those of ordinary bulbar paralysis but is generally differentiated by the simultaneous affection of other cranial nerves, particularly those of the eyeball, and there may also be evidence of a history of syphilis with or without a positive serological reaction in the blood or cerebrospinal fluid, which may exhibit cytological changes.

Lead poisoning and *alcoholism* may also be responsible for degenerative lesions which affect the nerves concerned in the process of swallowing.

General paralysis of the insane ultimately results in inability to swallow. The swallowing reflex is amongst the last to disappear so that the diagnosis should have been established earlier upon other grounds.

Spasm of the muscular coats of the oesophagus and pharynx is probably the cause of globus hystericus. Similar spasticity may occur in *hydrophobia* in which any effort to swallow liquids produces the symptom in extreme degree;

the history of a bite by a dog or other infected animal as a source of contagion is the chief point in arriving at the diagnosis. The spasm in *tetanus* may be recalled in this connexion. The symptoms of *acute encephalitis lethargica* are protean on account of the very variable distribution of the exudative lesions in the brain, midbrain, cerebellum, pons, and medulla. In most cases dysphagia is not pronounced, but in some, apparently when the medullary centres in particular are picked out, acute dysphagia may precede coma, and, the patient being in a state of active delirium at the same time, the disease may then simulate hydrophobia and the diagnosis may for some time be in doubt. A lesser degree of dysphagia may occur in the more chronic condition of *Parkinson's disease*.

Poisoning by *sodium fluoride*, which is used in solution for etching glass and as an insect and poultry-dusting powder, gives rise to dysphagia for a few hours after the drug is ingested, and the symptom persists for about a fortnight after a single poisonous non-fatal dose. Early symptoms will be vomiting, diarrhoea, cyanosis of lips, facial pallor, pain in limbs, drowsiness, and cranial nerve palsies.

Botulism—poisoning by the *Bacillus botulinus* —is uncommon, but instances occur from time to time and dysphagia is an early and pronounced symptom. The infection is generally caused by preserved foods. Potted meats have been responsible on occasion; more often, home-bottled fruits or vegetables which have not been re-cooked after the bottle has been opened. In a fairly typical case there is a latent period of from 6 to 24 hours. The patient then feels nauseated, vomits, and has difficulty in swallowing even water, the tongue feels stiff, the muscles of deglutition become ineffective, the voice becomes husky and weakens until there is complete aphonia with aphagia. The temperature is often subnormal, the pulse-rate raised. The eyes exhibit asymmetrical ptosis or strabismus. Vomiting may persist with headache and abdominal cramps, drowsiness supervenes, deepens into coma, and the patient dies of respiratory failure within a few days of the onset of the illness. *Bacillus botulinus* requires anaerobic methods for its culture.

Myasthenia gravis is a disease in which the affected muscles, although active, become fatigued with such rapidity that successive contractions become less and less effectual, until they cease, and can only resume work after a rest. The muscles of the neck, eye, larynx, and mouth become involved early (*Fig. 293, p. 275*), and difficulty in swallowing after the first few mouthfuls is sometimes a feature of the case. The myasthenic electrical reaction serves to distinguish these cases from those due to bulbar paralysis. The therapeutic test by neostigmine is diagnostic.

In *acute anterior poliomyelitis* dysphagia may occur from neuritis of the appropriate nerves.

Cases are encountered of uncertain pathology in which the oesophagus becomes enormously hypertrophied and dilated (oesophagectasis) and at times the patient cannot swallow though a mercury-loaded bougie passes perfectly well— *cardiospasm, achalasia of the cardia,* or *idiopathic dilatation and hypertrophy* of the oesophagus.

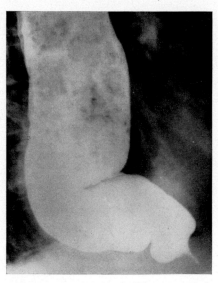

Fig. 251. Achalasia of the cardia showing great dilatation of the oesophagus, food retention, and characteristic 'candle-wick' lower end and absent gastric air-bubble. (*Dr. John Dow.*)

Whatever the pathology—which is probably related to the intrinsic nervous innervation of the muscular coat (Auerbach's plexus), an imbalance of the automatic nerve-supply—the oesophagus becomes more and more dilated and hypertrophied from the cardia upwards. The symptoms may extend over years, the diagnosis may have been one of chronic indigestion with recurrent bouts of vomiting, until the real nature of the trouble is demonstrated by a barium swallow (*Fig. 251*).

To some extent the same speculation may be applied to the achalasia at the pharyngo-oesophageal sphincter associated with iron-deficiency anaemia, known as the Plummer-Vinson syndrome. (The condition was described earlier by Paterson and Brown Kelly.) Although the dysphagia has apparently a neurogenic basis it is relieved by treatment of the anaemia with iron. In some cases there is an associated web stretched across the upper oesophagus. It is a precancerous condition and it is almost, if not entirely, restricted in its incidence to women.

3. Dysphagia due to Mechanical Defects of the Mouth or Pharynx, the Oesophagus being Normal. This group of cases includes patients suffering from such conditions as widely cleft palate, syphilitic stenosis of the pharynx, inability to use the tongue, either because it is acutely swollen from glossitis, bee-sting, or Ludwig's angina, or because it is fixed from carcinomatous infiltration, and so forth. There is little need to enter into the differential diagnosis of this variety of dysphagia for it can generally be determined by direct examination. Mumps, quinsy, tuberculous caries of the cervical spine, retropharyngeal abscess, and carcinoma of the hypopharynx (*Fig.* 252) belong

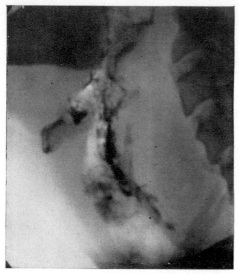

Fig. 252. Carcinoma of the hypopharynx after barium-swallow. Note the wide space between the spine and trachea. (*Dr. Cochrane Shanks.*)

to the same group, the last-named causing more dyspnoea than dysphagia and being confined to early childhood.

4. Dysphagia in which there is no Mechanical Obstruction, but in which, on account of the Pain incurred, the Patient refrains from Swallowing. The chief causes of dysphagia which come under this heading are: Inflammatory affections of the mouth or tongue, including the different varieties of *stomatitis* (p. 324); *pemphigus* or *erythema bullosum* of the buccal cavity, evidenced by similar eruption upon the skin (*see* BULLAE, p. 115); *ulcers of the tongue*, whether malignant, gummatous, tuberculous, actinomycotic, leprous, or due to chronic streptococcal glossitis (p. 799), or to erosion by a carious tooth or an ill-fitting tooth-plate; *sore throats* of various kinds (*see* THROAT, SORE, p. 784); pain in the mouth, pharynx, or oesophagus after swallowing acute irritants or liquids that are either extremely cold or hot; and *inflammatory affections of the larynx* and its immediate neighbourhood. The nature of the buccal lesions will generally be indicated by inspection followed by bacteriological or other special tests.

The laryngeal diseases that cause dysphagia are *acute laryngitis*, *tuberculous laryngitis* with or without ulcers, *carcinomatous ulceration* of the larynx, and *syphilis*. If tubercle bacilli can be found in the sputum, or if there are abnormal signs at the apices of the lungs, the diagnosis of tuberculous laryngitis is probable; pallid swelling of the aryteno-epiglottidean folds, multiple small ulcers of the edge or posterior surface of the epiglottis or of the free edges of the true or false vocal cords, or similar ulcers in other parts of the larynx, bilaterally situated, support the diagnosis (*Fig.* 253). Difficulty arises in chronic cases in which, after the larynx has become affected, the lung condition has improved, by which time bacilli may not be found in the sputum. Moreover, tuberculous ulceration of the larynx may occur as a primary condition in the absence of pulmonary

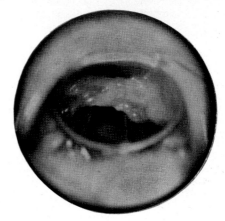

Fig. 253. Tuberculous ulceration of the epiglottis and one aryteno-epiglottidean fold.

involvement. Epitheliomatous ulceration of the larynx may be extensive yet for a long time remain confined to one side. This unilateral distribution of the infiltration is important in distinguishing epithelioma from syphilis of the larynx, in which another feature is the repair that may ensue even after extensive destruction of the tissues has led to much deformity of the parts. The influence of specific treatment may assist the diagnosis, and serological tests are, of course, employed. When it is very important to arrive at a certain diagnosis as soon as possible, a small portion of the affected tissue may be excised and examined microscopically. A papilloma of a vocal cord may have to be diagnosed from a malignant tumour. In all cases dysphagia will be accompanied by hoarseness or other alteration in the voice pointing to an affection of the larynx.

Harold Ellis.

DYSPNOEA

The term 'dyspnoea' does not admit of any precise definition, nor is it at all clear whether there is any qualitative difference between the breathlessness experienced by healthy subjects during vigorous exercise and that due to organic disease. In practice, however, this is of little importance and a suitable, though rather vague, definition might be 'awareness of the need for an increase in pulmonary ventilation', to which might be added some reference to increased *difficulty* in ventilation which must presumably play some part in the sensations experienced by, for example, an asthmatic.

Although dyspnoea may be present at rest, it is almost always aggravated by exertion and is likely to occur when the patient's ventilation is high in relation to his ability to breathe. The term 'dyspnoeic index' has been used to give some precision to this relationship. This is derived from the equation:

$$\text{Dyspnoeic index} = \frac{\text{exercise ventilation}}{\text{maximum breathing capacity}} \times 100.$$

The mathematical relationship is of less importance than the appreciation that dyspnoea may be due either to an abnormal increase in ventilation or to a reduction in ventilatory capacity. These two factors will be considered separately although, in practice, there is much overlap and interaction between them.

Increased (Exercise) Ventilation. This may be due to one or more of four factors. *Hypoxaemia* and *hypercapnia* both stimulate ventilation directly or indirectly and these states may, of course, be due to a primary disturbance of ventilatory capacity. *Acidosis* is another important ventilatory stimulant. This may be due to such conditions as renal failure or diabetic ketosis, but is more often due to a reduction in tissue blood-flow causing anaerobic metabolism and hence acidosis. The fourth factor is *pyrexia* which increases ventilation by a direct effect on the brain and also by producing some diversion of blood-flow to the skin; metabolism of the relatively ischaemic muscles may become anaerobic.

Reduced Ventilatory Capacity. This can be due to a large variety of diseases of the lung or the chest wall. Three main types of ventilatory disorder are recognized; these are (1) *obstructive airways disease* which can be reversible, as in asthma, or fixed, as in chronic bronchitis and emphysema; (2) *restrictive lung disease*, such as fibrosing alveolitis, in which it is the lung parenchyma rather than the airways which is predominantly affected; and (3) *hypoventilation* due to weakness of the respiratory muscles, as in anterior poliomyelitis. The clinical differentiation of these different types of ventilatory disorder is usually straightforward when the disease process is advanced. For the detection of less severe disease, however, and for the precise assessment of improvement or deterioration, tests of respiratory function are extremely valuable. Some of these are of some complexity, such as those involving the use of a body plethysmograph, but a great deal of useful information can be obtained from quite simple tests, of which a brief account will be given.

Respiratory function tests. The simplest and, in some ways, the most fundamental measurement is the vital capacity (VC)—the greatest

volume of gas which can be expired slowly after a full inspiration. There are three separate components of the vital capacity, the tidal volume (TV), inspiratory reserve volume (IRV), and expiratory reserve volume (ERV). The determination of these volumes by spirometry is not often clinically useful, but the measurement of the residual volume (RV) which is the volume of gas remaining in the lungs after a full expiration is of greater value; this is calculated by subtracting the vital capacity from the total lung capacity

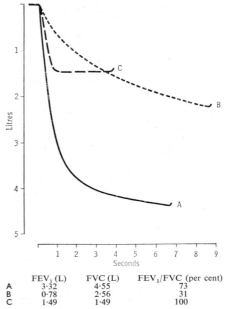

	FEV$_1$ (L)	FVC (L)	FEV$_1$/FVC (per cent)
A	3·32	4·55	73
B	0·78	2·56	31
C	1·49	1·49	100

Fig. 254. Superimposed tracings of expiratory spirograms in A, normal, B, obstructive airways disease, and C, restrictive lung disease. The measurements derived from these records are given in the table.

(TLC) measured by helium dilution. The latter two measurements can be usefully combined in the RV/TLC ratio, the proportion of the total volume of the lungs still containing gas at the end of a full expiration. Reduction of the total lung capacity is the hall-mark of restrictive lung disease and this is reflected in a, more easily measured, reduction in vital capacity; the latter, however, is not diagnostic of restriction on its own as it may be modified by airways obstruction, as described below. The static lung volumes described in this paragraph should therefore be supplemented by determination of the dynamic lung volumes.

The clinically relevant dynamic lung volumes are the forced vital capacity (FVC), measured during rapid expiration, the forced expiratory volume in one second (FEV$_1$), and the peak expiratory flow rate (PEFR). The first two and the ratio between them (FEV$_1$/FVC per cent) are very helpful in the differentiation of obstructive and restrictive lung disease (*Fig.* 254). The peak expiratory flow rate, recorded using a Wright peak flow meter, is a very convenient method of assessing airways obstruction. Although slightly less reliable than the FEV_1, it can be performed so quickly that it is often used for daily or twice daily recording to assess progress, for example in asthma.

Typical findings in obstructive airways disease are a reduction in FEV_1, FEV_1/FVC per cent, and PEFR. The RV/TLC is also reduced, particularly in emphysema and asthma, and this results in some reduction in vital capacity, although this is less abnormal than the forced vital capacity as air trapping is likely in the latter. In restrictive lung disease there is a marked reduction in vital capacity and the RV and TLC are about equally reduced so that the ratio RV/TLC is normal; the FEV_1/FVC is normal as is the PEFR unless the total volume expired is very low. Thus the two main varieties of ventilatory defect can usually be distinguished from each other by the measurement of static and dynamic lung volumes.

Further information about the state of the lungs can be obtained by studying the transfer of gas between alveoli and blood. The most sensitive measure of this is the transfer factor for carbon monoxide. This was previously regarded as a measure of diffusing capacity but it is now known that gas transport is markedly influenced by disorders of ventilation or of pulmonary blood flow or of the relationship between them —the ventilation-perfusion ratio—and the non-committal term 'transfer factor' is preferred. Transfer factor is reduced in emphysema and in pulmonary infarction, in both of which there is a significant loss of alveolocapillary membrane. It is also reduced in diffuse pulmonary fibrosis from any cause. In chronic bronchitis without significant emphysema, however, transfer factor is low only in the most advanced cases.

Measurement of arterial blood gases is a most important investigation in respiratory disease and provides information about both the severity and the aetiology. In general, a low Pao_2 and high $Paco_2$ are evidence of alveolar hypoventilation, either as a primary abnormality or, more often, due to chronic obstructive airways disease. In patients with pulmonary embolism and in fibrosing alveolitis and most other forms of restrictive lung disease a low Pao_2 is associated with a slight reduction in $Paco_2$ due to the hyperventilation induced by the hypoxaemia. In patients with cyanotic congenital heart disease and with intrapulmonary arteriovenous shunts, the Pao_2 is low and the $Paco_2$ about normal; in such patients little change occurs during oxygen breathing which can be expected to improve the hypoxaemia of obstructive or restrictive lung disease.

The causes of dyspnoea will be discussed under these major physiological headings, but it must again be emphasized that changes in both exercise ventilation and ventilatory capacity are seen in many cases; the classification is in terms of the primary factor only.

I. EXCESSIVE VENTILATION

The increase in exercise ventilation caused by hypoxaemia is seen most clearly in *cyanotic congenital heart disease*. In a condition such as Fallot's tetralogy, the mixed venous oxygen saturation falls on exercise as a result of the increased muscle metabolism; some of this blood passes directly to the aorta via the ventricular septal defect and a steep fall in arterial oxygen saturation results. This severe hypoxaemia and consequent dyspnoea can frequently be relieved somewhat by squatting, which is a prominent symptom in many cases of cyanotic congenital heart disease in childhood. The main effect of squatting is to produce partial obstruction of the venous return from the legs; the reduction in the volume of blood returning to the right side of the heart reduces the volume of the veno-arterial shunt. In addition to the effect of hypoxaemia on ventilation in cyanotic congenital heart disease, the metabolism of the tissues, supplied with poorly oxygenated blood, becomes anaerobic and metabolic acidosis results. This also causes an increase in ventilation.

Acidosis is also an important cause of increased ventilation in such conditions as *pulmonary stenosis* and *mitral stenosis* in which the cardiac output fails to rise normally with exercise with consequent tissue hypoxia. In mitral stenosis dyspnoea is also due to a diminution in ventilatory capacity; the work of breathing is increased by the reduced compliance of the lungs resulting from pulmonary venous hypertension. Similar considerations apply in left ventricular failure and these conditions are discussed more fully below.

Severe *anaemia* can cause dyspnoea and here also the mechanism is anaerobic muscle metabolism during exercise. The same may occur, to a smaller extent, in conditions such as *arteriovenous fistula* and *pregnancy* in which, although the cardiac output is normal or even high, it may be abnormally distributed and exercising muscles become selectively hypoxic. The dyspnoea of *mountaineers* is also mediated via hypoxia.

Arterial hypoxaemia is also an important cause of increased exercise ventilation in many varieties of lung disease. In most of these there is also a significant impairment of ventilatory capacity and they will be discussed in the next section. However, the effect of impaired gas transfer must be particularly mentioned here. The reduction in arterial oxygen saturation which occurs on exercise in many types of *parenchymal lung disease* causes a marked increase in ventilation which can be largely prevented by oxygen breathing. Collapse of a lobe, or of several segments, may also cause dyspnoea by virtue of an increase in exercise ventilation; in this situation perfusion of the unventilated part of the lung produces the effect of a veno-arterial shunt. It is important to remember that *carcinoma of the bronchus*, which is a common cause of lobar collapse, may be first manifest in this way.

It is convenient to discuss the dyspnoea of *pulmonary embolism* in this section. Effects vary with the size of the embolus but there is usually a striking increase in the minute volume of ventilation and the dyspnoea can be attributed to this. However, the cause of the increase in ventilation is not at all clear; arterial hypoxaemia is common but not invariable and is unlikely to be the only cause of the increased ventilation.

The *respiratory distress syndrome of the newborn* is another cause of severe hypoxaemia. This is seen in premature infants at, or shortly after, birth. Atelectasis and unequal alveolar expansion occur as a result of loss of pulmonary surfactant. The compliance is reduced and the work of breathing increased but more important is the hypoxaemia which causes pulmonary arterial hypertension and veno-arterial flow through the patent foramen ovale. This further aggravates the hyperventilation, and respiratory rates up to 100 per minute may be recorded.

Pyrexia is not a clinically important cause of increased ventilation but is a contributory factor in many patients. In addition, although the acidosis of *renal failure* or *diabetic ketosis* causes a striking increase in ventilation, this is more important as a physical sign and dyspnoea is not a prominent complaint in such patients.

II. REDUCED VENTILATORY CAPACITY

1. Airways Obstruction. Obstruction of the larynx or trachea, although an uncommon cause of dyspnoea, is nevertheless very important both because death may quickly occur and because relief can often be rapidly obtained by intubation or tracheostomy. Such obstruction may be due to severe *laryngitis*, particularly *diphtheritic*, or to laryngeal oedema of allergic aetiology. A *foreign body* may become impacted in the larynx or trachea or the obstruction may be due to the vocal cords themselves in *bilateral abductor paralysis*. Rare causes of laryngeal obstruction include the laryngeal crises of *tabes, laryngismus stridulus* due to hypocalcaemia, and *rheumatoid arthritis* of the crico-arytenoid joints with ankylosis in adduction. The trachea may be obstructed from without by *carcinoma of the thyroid* or haemorrhage into a *thyroid cyst*, by *neoplastic glands* in the neck or mediastinum, *aortic aneurysm*, or *dermoid tumour* of the mediastinum.

'Obstructive lung disease', as the term is usually understood, implies bronchial and bronchiolar narrowing and is extremely common. The term *chronic non-specific lung disease* has been used to cover all the major varieties of this condition and includes chronic bronchitis, bronchiectasis, emphysema, and asthma.

The diagnosis of *chronic bronchitis* is made on the history, the cardinal feature being cough productive of mucoid or purulent sputum for more than three months of each year. The most important aetiological factor is cigarette smoking; air pollution and other factors are also important. *Bronchiectasis* may or may not be associated with dyspnoea, depending on the extent of the disease and whether or not generalized bronchitis is also present. The production of copious purulent sputum and haemoptysis are well-recognized features and clubbing of the fingers is often present. The ventilatory effect is partly obstructive due to associated bronchitis and partly restrictive due to fibrosis (*Fig.* 255). *Emphysema* is a common association of chronic bronchitis but may occur in isolation. Aetiological factors which have

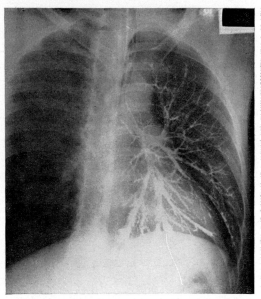

Fig. 255. Bronchogram showing bronchiectasis in the left lower lobe. (*Film by courtesy of Dr. Basil Strickland.*)

been identified include chronic cadmium intoxication and a congenital deficiency of α_1-antitrypsin. In uncomplicated emphysema cough is not prominent and the patient complains of progressive dyspnoea. The chest is overinflated, producing the typical 'barrel-chest', and the cardiac and much of the liver dullness is lost; the radiological appearances are obvious in a severe case (*Fig.* 256). The ventilatory defect is mainly obstructive in type due to collapse of the bronchi on expiration from loss of support by the interstitial tissue; a defect of gas transfer may also occur, due to loss of alveoli, causing hypoxaemia and increased exercise ventilation. Very large bullae may develop which act as space-occupying lesions and add a restrictive component to the ventilatory defect. Occasionally considerable relief of dyspnoea has resulted from resection of these bullae.

The clinical picture of advanced irreversible obstructive lung disease is only too well known. Dyspnoea with wheezing expiration and scattered sibilant rhonchi are cardinal features. Anoxaemia and hypercapnia develop and the pulmonary vascular resistance rises, partly due to the direct effects of hypoxia and partly on account of the involvement of the vessels in fibrosis. The rising pulmonary arterial pressure leads ultimately to right ventricular failure (cor pulmonale). Erythropoiesis is stimulated and gross cyanosis may be present. This clinical picture has been referred to as the 'blue bloater'. In most cases the respiratory centre has lost its responsiveness to a rising arterial P_{CO_2} but in a few cases this may be retained. In such cases dyspnoea is very severe due to the excessive ventilation produced by the

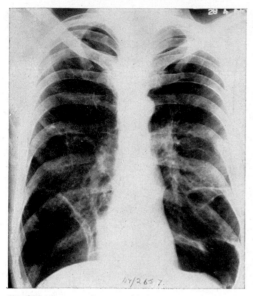

Fig. 256. Gross emphysema with large bullae at both lung bases.

high P_{CO_2}; anoxaemia is less severe and ventilatory and cardiac failure develop only when the airway obstruction is very severe. Patients with this clinical picture have been called 'pink puffers'.

This type of lung disease is usually seen in adults but may occur in children as a result of *cystic fibrosis* (*Fig.* 257).

Bronchial asthma produces an acute obstructive ventilatory defect which is usually partially or completely relieved by bronchodilators. In an attack the patient is extremely dyspnoeic with his chest held in inspiration; expiration is prolonged and wheezing. Tenacious mucus increases the obstruction of the airways and may be coughed up, with difficulty, as the attack subsides. *Bronchopulmonary aspergillosis* is also usually manifested by asthmatic attacks with cough and sputum. The chest X-ray may show transient pulmonary infiltrations and eosinophilia is common in the peripheral blood. A similar picture may be seen in a few cases of *polyarteritis nodosa* in whom asthma may be an early manifestation. Acute reversible airways' obstruction is also a feature of two varieties of industrial lung disease. *Byssinosis*, due to the inhalation of the dust of cotton, hemp, or flax, is characterized by bronchospasm with dyspnoea and wheezing which typically starts on Monday mornings and increases in severity during the

week only to subside during the week-end. Inhalation of *di-isocyanates*, used in the manufacture of polyurethane plastic materials, can also cause an acute obstructive ventilatory defect.

2. Restrictive Lung Disease. In its simplest form this is due to loss of functioning lung tissue. For example, *extensive pulmonary resection* can reduce the ventilatory capacity sufficiently to cause dyspnoea but, in practice, this is only likely to occur if the remaining lung tissue is diseased. Space-occupying lesions can produce a similar effect.

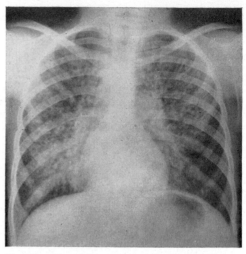

Fig. 257. Girl, aged 14, with cystic fibrosis (mucoviscidosis). Recurrent respiratory infections; cyanosed. Widespread inflammatory changes are seen throughout most of the lung fields. (*Film by courtesy of Dr. Basil Strickland.*)

Of these, two of the most important are *pleural effusion* and *spontaneous pneumothorax*. In an otherwise healthy young adult a pleural effusion, which in this context might well be tuberculous, is unlikely to cause significant dyspnoea unless it is very large. In an older patient, however, with, for example, left ventricular failure, quite a small effusion can cause a marked exacerbation of dyspnoea and aspiration may produce considerable relief. With a spontaneous pneumothorax, chest pain, which is sometimes but by no means always pleuritic in type, and mild dyspnoea on exertion, are common symptoms. Most of the so-called 'classic' physical signs are rather rare and the commonest findings are reduced movement and diminished breath-sounds on the affected side. Tension pneumothorax, on the other hand, by encroaching rapidly on functioning lung tissue, produces intolerable dyspnoea which demands immediate relief (*Fig.* 258). The possibility of bilateral pneumothorax must not be forgotten. Other space-occupying lesions which may cause dyspnoea are very large intrathoracic *tumours* and *hiatus hernia*, especially in children.

Conditions involving the thoracic cage can produce a similar ventilatory defect. The effects of extensive *thoracoplasty* are now rarely seen but severe *kyphoscoliosis* can cause serious impairment of ventilatory capacity; so also can *ankylosing spondylitis* although it is sometimes surprising how little disabled such patients may be even with extensive involvement of the costo-vertebral joints. *Sternal depression* (pectus ex-cavatum) is, on the other hand, almost never a cause of dyspnoea except of psychogenic origin.

In a large number of conditions diffuse pul-monary fibrosis produces a restrictive type of

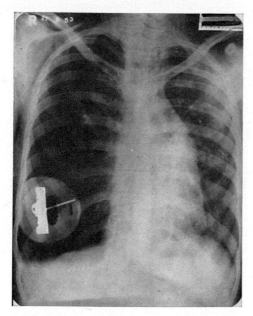

Fig. 258. Male, aged 20, with pulmonary tuberculosis. Ten-sion pneumothorax on right. Note the displacement of the heart to the left and an aspirating cannula in situ. (*Film by courtesy of Dr. Basil Strickland.*)

ventilatory defect. There is also, in many of these conditions, a defect of gas transfer produc-ing hypoxaemia; hyperventilation secondary to this frequently results in a slight reduction of the arterial P_{CO_2}. This situation has, in the past, been described as a 'diffusion defect' or 'alveolo-capillary block'. It is now clear, however, that changes in the alveolo-capillary membrane are of trivial importance and the most important cause of the hypoxaemia is simple reduction in the number of functioning alveoli.

Fibrosing alveolitis produces widespread fibrosis of the interstitial tissue of the lungs. The acute form, producing serious disability and death in a few weeks or months, is sometimes known as the Hamman-Rich syndrome. The more common chronic form presents with dyspnoea on exertion, unproductive cough, vague chest pains, and cyan-osis becoming much more marked on exertion. Clubbing of the fingers is common and coarse râles may be heard at the lung bases. Cor pul-monale is a common late complication. The chest X-ray shows a reticular pattern with some nodularity especially at the lung bases.

In most cases of fibrosing alveolitis no cause can be found but a very similar clinical picture can be produced by a group of allergens. These can produce a Type I allergic reaction, with early severe bronchospasm, in atopic subjects; in non-atopic subjects Type III allergic manifesta-tions predominate to produce the syndrome of *extrinsic allergic alveolitis.* This may be regarded as having the same relationship to fibrosing alveolitis as extrinsic allergic asthma has to intrinsic asthma.

Extrinsic allergic alveolitis is manifested by dyspnoea, cough, fever, and weight-loss, and closely simulates acute or chronic pulmonary infections. The ventilatory defect is predomi-nantly restrictive but an obstructive component may be present in a few cases. The diagnosis is suggested by a history of exposure to one of the allergens listed below and can be confirmed by finding a rising titre of precipitating antibodies to the appropriate antigen in the serum. Recovery is usual if the patient can avoid contact with the allergen but, in chronic cases, permanent diffuse fibrosis may result. Farmer's lung was one of the first types of extrinsic allergic alveolitis to be described. This is due to the inhalation of spores of the fungus *Microspora*, growing in mouldy hay. Fungal spores have also been incriminated as allergens in bagassosis, due to working with the residues of sugar-cane, in suberosis in cork-workers, sequoiosis in sawyers in the redwood forests of California, in wheat-weevil disease in workers with wheat-flour, and in lung disease in mushroom-workers, malt-workers, maple-bark strippers, and cheese-makers. A similar disease occurs in furriers, coffee-workers, and vineyard-sprayers but the causative allergen has not yet been identified. Hypersensitivity to avian pro-teins is the cause of bird-fancier's lung (which is not, of course, to be confused with ornithosis, a viral disease), and, in pituitary snuff-takers, bovine or porcine protein has been incriminated. The enzymes of *Bacillus subtilis* have also been shown to cause this condition. These are present in 'biological' washing powders and workers in this industry have been affected.

The dusts, which, when inhaled, cause allergic alveolitis, have no intrinsic irritant properties and thus differ from the agents responsible for the *pneumoconioses.* Silicosis is the most important and is often diagnosed radiologically before any symptoms are present. This is unlike other types of diffuse fibrosis and may be related to the fact that, in silicosis, the fibrosis is more nodular and thus more easily seen in the X-ray. Initially the nodules are small and discrete, not unlike those of miliary tuberculosis; they enlarge and coalesce as the disease progresses until eventually large masses of fibrosis may be present, particularly in the upper zones of the lung fields (*Fig.* 259). The main complaint is progressive dyspnoea and, later, symptoms of superadded bronchitis and emphysema appear so that the restrictive pattern of ventilatory defect is complicated by an obstruc-tive component. In asbestosis, dyspnoea develops more rapidly than in silicosis and is often worse than would have been suggested by the X-ray which shows a finely reticular pattern of fibrosis. The pleura is also often thickened with a rather 'shaggy' appearance; calcification, particularly of diaphragmatic pleura, is not uncommon. The finding of asbestos bodies in the sputum is evidence of exposure to asbestos but not necessarily of the disease asbestosis. An important complication of asbestosis is an increased incidence of

few physical signs unless severe localized fibrosis develops, in which case mediastinal displacement may be found. The diagnosis would usually be made, at this stage, by finding evidence of disease in other organs, such as iridocyclitis, swelling of the salivary and lacrimal glands, lymph-node enlargement, hepatosplenomegaly, and purplish nodules in the skin which may progress to scar formation. The sedimentation rate is raised; hypergammaglobulinaemia is common as is hypercalcaemia. The diagnosis can be confirmed by the Kveim test.

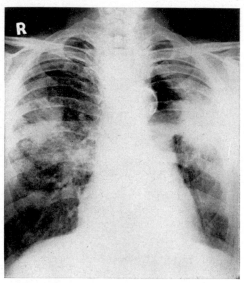

Fig. 259. Pneumoconiosis. Note diffuse fine mottling and massive fibrotic lesions in mid-zones of both lungs.

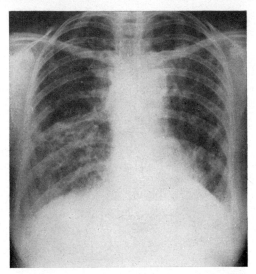

Fig. 260. Female, aged 46, with pulmonary sarcoidosis. Arterial oxygen saturation 80 per cent; pulmonary arterial pressure 55/19. Note nodular and fibrotic lesions especially in lower zones.

malignant pulmonary tumours, particularly pleural mesothelioma, which is a feature of this condition. Rarer industrial lung diseases include silo-filler's disease, due to the inhalation of nitric oxide. This is a form of obliterative bronchiolitis with the formation of fibrous nodules around the blocked bronchioles. Severe dyspnoea and cough are common and the finely nodular lesions are visible in the X-ray. Berylliosis may present as acute pneumonitis and pulmonary oedema or as diffuse fibrosis with progressive dyspnoea in a more chronic form.

The lesions of berylliosis very closely resemble those of *sarcoidosis*; indeed, if sarcoidosis is regarded as a type of tissue reaction rather than a disease entity, berylliosis is one of the causes of this reaction. The earliest pulmonary lesion of sarcoidosis is bilateral hilar lymph-node enlargement, often accompanied by fever, erythema nodosum, and arthralgia. There are no complaints referable to the lungs at this stage but, in some cases, granulomatous infiltration appears in the lungs, leading to an X-ray appearance of a fine nodularity with a reticular pattern of fibrosis throughout the lung fields (*Fig.* 260). Dyspnoea becomes progressively more severe, but there are

Pulmonary tuberculosis should, of course, be diagnosed long before dyspnoea becomes a significant symptom, and the clinical picture of chronic fibroid tuberculosis is becoming something of a rarity. Dyspnoea varies with the extent of the disease and is usually due to a restrictive ventilatory defect. The main symptom is a productive cough; the sputum is positive in untreated cases. The physical signs may include displacement of the mediastinum if fibrosis is predominantly unilateral, variations in percussion note, bronchial breathing, and râles, but it must be emphasized that clinical examination is unreliable and no substitute for radiography, often including tomography, in the assessment of the extent and progress of the disease.

Dyspnoea is not a common early symptom of *carcinoma of the lung*, unless bronchial occlusion by a primary tumour has caused extensive collapse. Later in the course widespread dissemination of a primary lung tumour or metastases from an extrathoracic tumour may cause breathlessness. This is particularly the case if the spread has been by lymphatic permeation to produce lymphangitis carcinomatosa which may be associated with intolerable dyspnoea. Unlike bronchial carcinoma, alveolar-cell tumours usually present with dyspnoea; this is due to the invasion of many alveoli producing a restrictive ventilatory defect and impairment of gas transfer with marked hypoxaemia especially on exertion.

The lungs can be affected in most of the generalized *connective-tissue diseases*. The asthma associated with some cases of polyarteritis nodosa has already been mentioned. In systemic lupus erythematosus, the commonest pulmonary manifestation is recurrent pleurisy with or without effusion. Intrapulmonary disease may be due to superadded bacterial infection or to a fine fibrosis, barely visible in the X-ray, which nevertheless

develop in the lung fields; these may calcify or cavitate (*Fig.* 261). Rheumatoid factor is present in high titre in the serum so that the condition can be diagnosed even if the lung disease develops before the arthritis, as may be the case.

Other diseases of the lung parenchyma which can produce a restrictive ventilatory defect include *schistosomiasis* (although in this condition most of the damage is to the pulmonary vessels), eosinophilic granuloma and other varieties of *histiocytosis* (*Fig.* 262), and a few cases of severe widespread *mycoplasma pneumonia*. *Alveolar proteinosis* produces progressive dyspnoea and a productive cough; the X-ray shows soft densities

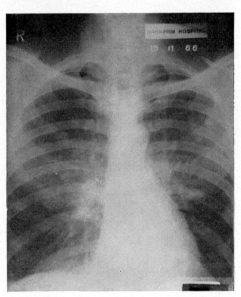

Fig. 261. Caplan's syndrome in a coal-miner, aged 51, suffering from rheumatoid arthritis. Note specially the nodular lesions in the left upper zone. (*Film by courtesy of Dr. Basil Strickland.*)

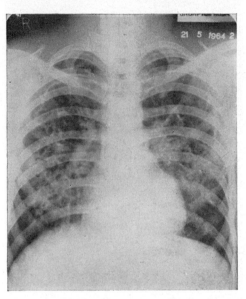

Fig. 262. Eosinophilic granuloma producing the appearance of 'honeycomb lung'. (*Film by courtesy of Dr. Basil Strickland.*)

produces a detectable ventilatory defect and impairment of gas transfer. Systemic sclerosis (scleroderma) produces a fairly typical diffuse interstitial pulmonary fibrosis. Cyst formation at the lung bases is common, producing the appearance of 'honeycomb' lung, and disseminated pulmonary calcification may also be seen in the X-ray. Pulmonary hypertension leading to cor pulmonale is partly due to hypoxia and partly to direct involvement of the pulmonary vessels by the disease. If the oesophagus is involved in systemic sclerosis the lungs are also affected by recurrent aspiration pneumonitis. Pulmonary involvement is very rare in rheumatoid disease but chronic interstitial fibrosis, like that in systemic sclerosis, can occur, more often in men. There is believed to be an increased risk of alveolar-cell carcinoma in both rheumatoid lung disease and systemic sclerosis. Caplan's syndrome is a variant of pneumoconiosis occurring in patients with rheumatoid arthritis. Multiple well-defined opacities up to 5 cm. in diameter

radiating from the hila which simulate pulmonary oedema. *Alveolar microlithiasis* and *pulmonary muscular hyperplasia* are other rare causes of chronic dyspnoea. Severe breathlessness occurs also in poisoning with the weed-killer *paraquat*; the lung lesions include striking proliferation of the epithelium of the terminal bronchioles and the damage is irreversible.

A most important group of conditions in which dyspnoea occurs by virtue of a restrictive ventilatory defect is that causing *pulmonary oedema*. The role of the low cardiac output of *left ventricular failure* and *mitral stenosis* in causing increased exercise ventilation has been discussed above. However, a much more important mechanism of dyspnoea in these conditions is the pulmonary venous hypertension they both produce. As the pulmonary venous and capillary pressures rise, the lungs become 'splinted' by their tense vasculature; the accumulation of fluid in the interstitial tissue and, later, in the alveoli, further increases the stiffness of the lungs. As the alveoli fill, gas transfer becomes progressively impaired and arterial hypoxaemia becomes more and more severe. Clinically, dyspnoea on exertion is accompanied by orthopnoea and paroxysms of nocturnal dyspnoea; the most dramatic manifestation of pulmonary venous hypertension is acute pulmonary oedema. The earliest feature is a dry cough which, over a few minutes, becomes much more troublesome and the patient rapidly becomes intolerably breathless. Râles develop throughout the lung fields with, often, much wheezing in addition. As respiration becomes more laboured the coughing produces the telltale fine pink froth which eventually, as the patient sinks back exhausted, may well from the mouth and nose spontaneously. In the earlier stages, or in milder cases, the differentiation from bronchial asthma may cause some difficulty but,

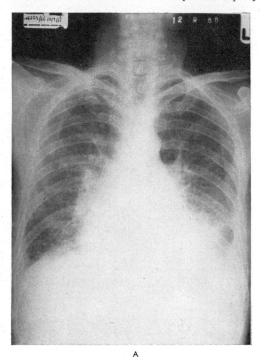
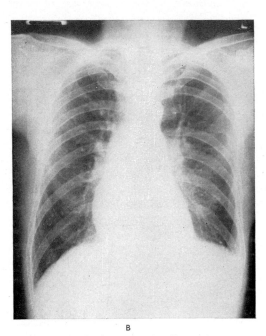

A   B

Fig. 263. Male, aged 58, with mitral stenosis. In A, gross pulmonary venous congestion is present and ossific nodules are seen at the lung bases. In B, after mitral valvotomy, all the congestive changes have cleared and the ossific nodules are more clearly visible.

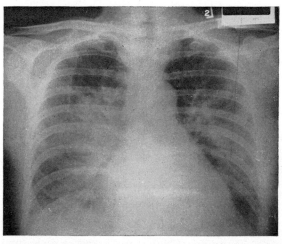

Fig. 264. Acute pulmonary oedema following myocardial infarction. The changes are more marked on the right where the fan-shaped opacity spreading out from the hilum is clearly visible. (*Film by courtesy of Dr. Basil Strickland.*)

in that condition, wheezing is much more prominent and the distinction is later obvious; the finding of mitral stenosis or a cause of left ventricular failure would, of course, favour pulmonary oedema. The radiological appearances of pulmonary venous hypertension are sometimes described as 'pulmonary venous congestion'. These include septal lymphatic lines and engorgement of the upper lobe veins in chronic cases (*Fig.* 263). In more acute cases, enlargement of the hilar shadows and haziness in the middle and lower zones progress to the fan-shaped mid-zone opacities of acute pulmonary oedema (*Fig.* 264).

Pulmonary oedema is a well-known hazard of over-enthusiastic infusion of saline. This is unlikely to occur if the heart is normal and renal function adequate; in oliguric renal failure, however, pulmonary oedema can be precipitated very readily. It also occurs occasionally after cerebral vascular accidents and is well recognized in salicylate poisoning in which it may be, partly at least, a hypersensitivity phenomenon. Hypersensitivity is also responsible for the pulmonary oedema which very occasionally complicates the injection of radiological contrast media.

Aspiration pneumonitis (Mendelson's syndrome) closely simulates acute pulmonary oedema. It is due to the aspiration of gastric acid into the airways and alveoli and is manifested by cyanosis, tachypnoea, tachycardia, hypotension, and cough with pink frothy sputum. Râles and rhonchi are heard throughout the lung fields.

3. Acute Pulmonary Infections. Many factors combine to produce breathlessness in acute infections of the lung and a brief discussion of these will serve as a summary of the mechanisms of dyspnoea outlined above. Acute inflammation of the bronchi, by causing vascular congestion and the accumulation of secretions, produces an increase in airway resistance. In patches of pneumonia vascular engorgement, interstitial oedema and inflammatory exudate in the alveoli add a restrictive component so that ventilatory capacity is reduced. Wide variations in the ventilation/perfusion ratio throughout the lungs cause more or less severe hypoxaemia; in lobar pneumonia continuing perfusion of the solid lung produces the effect of a veno-arterial shunt. Ventilation is therefore increased by the stimuli of hypoxia and hypercapnia to which pyrexia may add a further stimulus. If the infection is complicated by pleurisy, the vital capacity is further reduced as the breathing is restricted by pain and the impairment of coughing further encourages the accumulation of secretions.

4. Hypoventilation. Localized or generalized alveolar hypoventilation is, of course, the mechanism of respiratory failure in most types of lung disease. In this section attention will be directed to reduction of total ventilation, mainly by extrapulmonary factors. The concept of the 'dyspnoeic index' is less valid in this situation and the dyspnoea of which patients with hypoventilation will complain may be due to a disproportion between the drive to ventilation and the small minute volume produced. It may, indeed, be qualitatively different from the dyspnoea experienced by patients suffering from the many diseases already discussed.

Significant hypoventilation may be due to *weakness of the respiratory muscles* as in poliomyelitis, polyneuropathy, myasthenia gravis, motor neuron disease, muscular dystrophies, and potassium depletion. More rarely *lesions of the brain-stem* may produce a primary failure of the respiratory centre. Extreme *obesity* can produce the same effect by grossly increasing the work of moving the chest wall. This is known as the 'Pickwickian syndrome'. Cognoscenti of Dickens will, perhaps, pardon a digression to make it clear that it was not Mr. Pickwick himself who suffered from this condition but 'Mr. Wardle's favourite page, known . . . by the distinguishing appellation of the fat boy'. This obese youth found great difficulty in remaining awake—a clear case, some believe, of intermittent carbon-dioxide narcosis.

III. PSYCHOGENIC DYSPNOEA

Dyspnoea is one of the complaints in Da Costa's syndrome (*see also* CHEST, PAIN IN, p. 141). In such cases the underlying psychological disturbance is often *anxiety* and, in general, it is the tense, obsessional patient who may complain of dyspnoea without any organic basis. *Depression* also may lead to a complaint of breathlessness along with other somatic symptoms; the mental state may either be endogenous or it may be secondary to organic pulmonary disease, in which case the symptoms are out of proportion to the objective evidence of a ventilatory disorder or defect of gas transfer. In addition, it must be admitted that, in many cases, the most important psychological factor is *iatrogenic*.

The most significant finding is a gross irregularity of respiration. This may be seen in a spirogram especially during exercise and it may often be detected during conversation with the patient when he may be seen to sigh repeatedly. Indeed, a complaint of inability to take a deep enough breath is not uncommon. During an alleged attack of dyspnoea the breathing is rather shallow and the chest is held in inspiration; this may be demonstrated in a spirogram as a progressive increase in the end-expiratory level. Hyperventilation in such attacks may reduce the arterial Pco_2 below normal and the consequent symptoms such as paraesthesiae in the limbs and circumoral region, or even tetany, only serve to convince the patient more firmly that he has organic disease.

IV. DIFFERENTIAL DIAGNOSIS OF ACUTE DYSPNOEA

The sudden onset of breathlessness is a common and alarming emergency demanding energetic treatment. The urgency of the situation may be such that no time is available for radiography or other investigation and a diagnosis must be made on the basis of clinical examination. The differential diagnosis will be discussed in terms of the physical signs which may be elicited in such an examination.

Simple inspection may reveal much. The deeply cyanosed patient with engorged cervical veins, literally struggling for breath with violent excursions of the larynx, is probably suffering from *laryngeal or upper tracheal obstruction*. The stridor of upper airway obstruction with noisy inspiration and expiration must not be confused with the expiratory wheeze of bronchial constriction. Possible causes include laryngitis, laryngeal oedema, foreign body, and haemorrhage into a thyroid cyst. *Acute laryngo-tracheobronchitis* in children produces a similar picture. In less severely ill patients, more leisurely inspection may reveal pallor of the mucosae indicating severe *anaemia* as a possible cause of the dyspnoea; massive internal haemorrhage may present in this way.

Palpation of the arterial pulse might reveal uncontrolled *atrial fibrillation*, a most important cause of sudden, severe dyspnoea in mitral stenosis, or pulsus paradoxus suggesting *cardiac tamponade*, due, perhaps, to intrapericardial haemorrhage from malignant metastases. Tamponade also causes elevation of the jugular venous pressure with a paradoxical rise in pressure during inspiration. The venous pressure is also usually considerably elevated following a massive *pulmonary embolus*, another cause of acute dyspnoea.

Mediastinal displacement, as indicated by lateral displacement of the trachea, is a valuable sign in many cases of acute dyspnoea. *Massive collapse* of a lung, as may occur during the postoperative period, draws the mediastinum towards the affected side. Deviation of the trachea away from the lesion is a feature of *pleural effusion* and *tension pneumothorax*. The only fluid which is likely to accumulate very rapidly in the pleural cavity is blood, and *haemothorax* following pleural aspiration must be remembered as a cause of acute dyspnoea. A hyper-resonant percussion note will confirm a diagnosis of pneumothorax; in infancy a similar picture can be produced by *tension cyst* of the lung or *lobar emphysema*.

Examination of the heart will be informative in acute *pulmonary oedema* if the signs of tight *mitral stenosis* or gallop rhythm due to *left ventricular failure* are detected. It must be remembered that, occasionally, myocardial infarction may be virtually painless and present with acute left ventricular failure.

In the lungs themselves the prolonged wheezing expiration of *bronchial asthma* or the widespread râles of pulmonary oedema may be heard. Acute *pulmonary infections* do not often cause such severe dyspnoea unless there is underlying chronic lung disease; purulent sputum, pyrexia, and the signs of pulmonary consolidation or alveolar exudate will help to establish the diagnosis.

P. R. Fleming.

DYSTOCIA

Dystocia signifies difficult birth or labour. The difficulties of delivery show themselves by prolongation or delay in the completion of the stages into which labour is usually divided. Difficult labour is accompanied by progressive symptoms, objective and subjective, due to mental and physiological exhaustion, dehydration, and electrolyte imbalance. The results of difficult labour are of such importance, affecting, as they do, the life of the mother and child, that anticipation of it, and therefore early and appropriate treatment, are of paramount importance in scientific midwifery.

The causes may be tabulated according as they occur in the first, second, or third stage, the first series delaying the dilatation of the cervix, the second the expulsion of the child, the third difficulties in the separation and expulsion of the placenta, for delivery cannot be said to be complete until the placenta is expelled.

Successful delivery of the child under many of these conditions depends very much on their *anticipation*, rather than their recognition when delivery is already dangerously obstructed. Consequently, accurate diagnosis at the beginning of labour will often save much trouble to the practitioner, and danger to the mother and child. Indeed, some of the dangers of obstructed labour can only be avoided satisfactorily by repeated examination of the patient during pregnancy, from the 32nd week onwards. This applies especially to the recognition of contracted pelves, of pelvic tumours, of malpresentations and disproportion, and constitutes an important reason why every prospective mother should be examined weekly during the last month of pregnancy.

The routine method of examination of the pregnant woman, whether in labour or not, is the same, and the deductions to be made therefrom are identical. The examination is carried out as follows: first, by abdominal palpation; secondly, by vaginal examination.

Abdominal Palpation. First feel for the foetal head in the pelvis by the 'pelvic grip'. In a primigravida the head should be well down in the pelvis at the 36th week; not necessarily so in a multigravida. Failing to find the head in the pelvis, palpate for it at the fundus; failing to find it here, it will be found in one or the other lateral situation. If the head is in the pelvis, and fixed, there can be no pelvic contraction of importance, and tumours of the uterus or ovaries *below the brim* are quite unlikely. If, however, the head is above the brim and movable in a primigravida after the 36th week of gestation pelvic contraction must be suspected, while a tumour preventing entrance into the pelvis is a possibility. If the foetal head can be pushed down into the pelvis, there cannot be much disparity. It is most likely due to deficient flexion of the foetal head, as in occipito-posterior positions, or to poor tone in the abdominal and uterine muscle. Pelvic contraction may be verified by pelvimetry, for which *see below*. Abnormal presentations are recognized by abdominal palpation: breech and transverse by the actual position of the head: occipito-posterior by the presence of the 'small parts'—arms and legs—in front and felt on both sides of the mother's mid-abdominal line, and the absence of the back of the foetus in front; the position of maximum intensity of the foetal heart-sounds is also of value, being most distinctly heard farther out

with a powerfully acting levator ani muscle, the degree of descent into the pelvis of the foetal presenting part, and the *condition of the os*; note especially its consistence, whether the cervical canal is 'taken up', the degree of dilatation, whether the cervix fits the presenting part closely, and whether the membranes are intact. It may not be possible to recognize the presentation if this has not been made out by abdominal palpation unless the patient is in labour and the

CAUSES OF DELAY IN COMPLETION OF THE THREE STAGES OF LABOUR

FIRST STAGE	SECOND STAGE	THIRD STAGE
Weak uterine contractions—Primary inertia Incoordinate uterine action Rigidity of cervix: relative, spasmodic, cicatricial, new growths Pendulous belly, causing undue anteversion Malpresentations in general Anything which prevents the head entering the lower uterine segment Hydramnios Twins or triplets	Weak uterine contractions (threatened secondary uterine inertia) Absence of accessory muscular effort Contraction ring Rigidity of vagina and perineum Loaded rectum Distended bladder—cystocele Contracted pelvis Pelvic tumours: Fibromyoma, ovarian tumours, growths of the pelvic bones, haematoma, vaginal growths Malpresentations: Occipito-posterior, breech, face, brow, transverse (shoulder) Any abnormal enlargement of the child: Hydrocephalus, meningocele, ascites, cystic kidneys, tumours, double monsters, very large child Excessive ossification of head Short cord: absolute, relative Locked twins Large foetus	Weak uterine contractions Morbid adhesion of placenta Uterine spasm 'Hour-glass' contraction Adhesion of membranes Mismanagement of this stage of labour

laterally than in anterior positions. A face cannot be diagnosed absolutely except in mento-posterior cases, when the groove between the extended occiput and back will be felt in front while the head remains above the brim. *Hydramnios* may be recognized if there is fluctuation and thrill and the foetal parts can only be felt by deep dipping through the fluid. *Twins* may possibly be recognized by feeling two heads, many limbs or small parts, or hearing two foetal hearts beating with different rhythms. Confirm by X-rays.

Vaginal Examination. It is important to remember that if there has been any antepartum bleeding and the presenting foetal part is not engaged there may be a placenta praevia. In such a case a vaginal examination is strictly contra-indicated because if a finger is inserted through the cervix very severe bleeding may be precipitated. If there is no history of antepartum bleeding a vaginal examination should be done. The principles of surgical asepsis should be observed in the last week of pregnancy or during labour, the attendant wearing a mask and sterile gloves. The following should be noted: the *condition of the canal*, whether narrow or rigid,

cervix is dilating. If contracted pelvis is suspected, the important diameter, namely, the diagonal conjugate, should be measured with the fingers, and the true conjugate estimated by subtracting 1·5 cm. from this measurement. The anterior surface of the sacrum should be followed up by the finger and its concavity noted. The finger should not be able to reach the upper segment at all easily. The sacro-sciatic notch should accommodate the two fingers lying side by side. Follow the ileo-pectineal line round on each side with the first and second fingers. It should not be possible to follow the brim of the pelvis laterally for more than 7 cm. from the midline. If the lateral wall of the pelvis can be felt beyond this there is lateral contraction of the pelvic brim. Note the position and mobility of the coccyx, and the depth of the symphysis pubis. The subpubic angle should be at least a right angle, and the four knuckles of the closed fist should easily fit in between the tuber ischii. If this cannot be done the pelvic outlet is contracted. The amount by which the foetal head overlaps the pelvic brim may be assessed by combined abdominal and vaginal palpation (Munro-Kerr manœuvre) and hence the degree of disproportion estimated. External measurements are no longer considered to be of any importance. The internal measurements of the pelvis can now be deduced by means of radiographs. In any doubtful case X-ray examination should be done late in pregnancy to confirm the measurements. It also confirms the position of the foetus, and its maturity can be estimated. This method of examination does not directly affect the foetus and the risks of genetic damage or subsequent leukaemia are so small as to be outweighed by the advantage of the information gained. A lateral X-ray of the pelvis taken during labour is often most useful as an indication of the progress and probable termination of the labour in a case of 'trial labour'. The method is elaborate and has to be done by an expert. Cephalometry can be performed accurately by ultrasound; the biparietal diameter is measured and compared with the pelvic measurements.

Delay in the first stage of labour is most frequently due to primary inertia or incoordinate uterine action. In the former type the labour pains are weak and infrequent and short in duration. Palpation of the uterus reveals the feebleness of the contractions. In the second type the patient feels the pains acutely, the pains often being felt before the uterine contraction can be appreciated by the hand on the uterus. They are, moreover, irregular in frequency, duration, and intensity, being felt more acutely than in normal labour in the back or on one side of the abdomen. In this type of case deterioration in the woman's condition can take place early in labour unless the pains are relieved by an epidural anaesthetic block.

As soon as it becomes apparent that the cervix is failing to dilate and obstruction to delivery has been ruled out, labour should be accelerated by rupture of the membranes and an oxytocin drip. An epidural block will almost certainly be necessary and the foetal heart should be monitored continuously either by means of an external recorder or by attaching an electrode to the foetal scalp through the cervix. Uterine contractions are recorded also by means of an external or internal tokograph. Foetal distress is shown by slowing of the heart soon after the beginning of a contraction (type I dip) or late in relation to the contraction (type II dip). Type II dips are indicative of more severe foetal distress than type I dips. The distress is confirmed by foetal scalp puncture and measurement of the foetal blood pH on an Astrup machine. A pH of 7·25 or below is a sign of severe foetal distress.

When a difficulty arises during the course of labour accurate diagnosis is indispensable. The abdominal findings earlier in labour should be confirmed. If the head is engaged in the brim disproportion at that level in the pelvis can be excluded and is not likely to be serious at lower levels in the pelvis. A vaginal examination is most informative and should always be done unless a placenta praevia is suspected because of vaginal bleeding. The dilatation of the cervix should be noted and whether or not it is closely applied to the head. A loosely applied cervix and a large caput succedaneum suggest a degree of disproportion. If the cervix fails to dilate over some hours, inertia is present and disproportion as a contributory factor must be excluded. A standing lateral X-ray taken in labour is most helpful. Vaginal examination enables the presenting part to be felt and malpresentations can be accurately diagnosed. If a soft, irregular part presents that is not a hard rounded skull it may be a breech or a face or a shoulder or part of the trunk. If there is any doubt the examination should be performed under anaesthesia. Hydrocephalus may be recognized when the cervix is two fingers dilated. The foetal head will be above the brim and the sutures widely separated by membrane. Later in labour when the cervix is fully dilated, it may be necessary to insert the hand into the vagina to ascertain the cause of the obstruction if one is present. This is done under anaesthesia. The presenting part may then be grasped, and its true character determined. In this way occipito-posterior presentations (the commonest cause of difficult labour) can be diagnosed with certainty, and rectified. A contraction ring due to an irritable uterus as a result of attempts at forcible delivery will be felt gripping the foetus and preventing delivery. The hand may be pushed on above the head without danger in most cases, and the neck felt for coils of cord, and the body of the child palpated for the presence of tumours or enlargement by ascites. Tumours obstructing delivery are best felt from the vagina; they are usually wedged between the presenting part and the sacral promontory, partly below and partly above this prominence. If fluctuating and soft they are usually ovarian cysts; if hard and unyielding they may be fibro-myomata of the uterus, but these are apt to soften during pregnancy, and to feel like fluid tumours. Tumours of the pelvic bones are usually bony or cartilaginous; growths of the cervix may be fibroid, but occasionally are friable carcinomata, bleeding freely on examination. If there is no cause for an obstruction, the delay may be due to uncomplicated uterine inertia.

Only the method of examination can be indicated in a short article on the diagnosis of difficult labour; but too much stress cannot be laid on the value of abdominal examination and palpation and vaginal examination as the most important means of gaining information in any labour.

Delay in the Delivery of the Placenta, though not strictly a part of difficult labour, presents difficulties in the completion of delivery, and must not be overlooked. The placenta may be simply retained in utero, may be adherent to the uterus, totally or partially, or may be retained in the vagina. In the first case, if there is no haemorrhage, the placenta is likely to lie in the lower uterine segment and vagina, and is not expelled owing to weakness of the accessory muscles. Then the so-called signs of separation of the placenta are present: the cord has lengthened and a little bleeding has taken place, the uterus is small, contracted, relatively high in the abdomen and mobile from side to side. When, on the other hand, the placenta is still in the upper uterine segment, the uterus is large, soft, relatively low in the abdomen, and cannot be easily moved from side to side. Retention of the placenta within the uterus may be due to inertia of the uterine muscle, to a localized contraction of part of the uterus to form a *constriction ring*, or rarely to morbid adhesion of the placenta. If partially adherent, bleeding is certain to occur, whilst total adhesion does not permit of any bleeding. In any case of this kind, if after a sufficient time has elapsed the placenta cannot be delivered by the Brandt-Andrews method, the hand must be introduced into the uterus under a general anaesthetic in order to diagnose the condition and to remove the placenta. Haemorrhage always accompanies this operation if the placenta is partly separated. In some cases where concealed accidental haemorrhage has occurred, or when a dead foetus has been retained in utero for some weeks, the postpartum bleeding may be due to afibrinogenaemia. Then a few millilitres of venous blood stood in a test-tube will fail to clot and blood analysis will reveal a fibrinogen level of less than 100 mg. per 100 ml. or an excess of fibrinolysins.

The Symptoms of Exhaustion consequent upon Obstructed Labour need mention. They are seen only in neglected cases that are not properly supervised. The first are a drawn and anxious facial expression, rise of temperature, and increase in frequency of the pulse-rate. These afford very important indications of obstructed labour, and assist us to distinguish this from simple delay from weak uterine contractions, in which the pulse and temperature remain normal. The later symptoms of obstruction, if not relieved, are local and general. Locally, the vaginal secretions fail, the parts become hot, dry, and swollen. The uterus contracts powerfully, and may go into a tetanic condition, usually known as tonic contraction, in which case the uterus is hard, never relaxing, and is tender to the touch. The junction of the upper and lower uterine segments can be seen and felt as a circular depression around the uterus known as Brandl's retraction ring. Foetal distress is an early sign and unless it is relieved the foetus dies from asphyxia. It is recognized by slowing of the foetal heart-rate to less than 100 beats per minute and the passage of meconium in the liquor. In extreme cases the foetal heart-rate falls to less than 90 beats per minute and the rhythm becomes irregular due to dropped beats. Tumultuous foetal movements sometimes precede death of the foetus. The exact opposite occurs in uterine inertia, when the uterus remains flaccid, along with a normal pulse and temperature. Later still, vomiting may occur, signs of septic infection may appear, and rupture of the uterus may take place owing to the dangerous thinning of the lower segment when tonic contraction supervenes. Then the intermittent contractions of the uterus are replaced by continuous abdominal pain. The patient is invariably in a state of severe shock; she is pale and sweaty, her pulse is fast and thready and her blood-pressure falls. The abdomen is distended and very tender. Foetal parts may be felt separate from the contracted, empty, uterus and some vaginal bleeding takes place. This series of symptoms should never occur in properly conducted midwifery; their possible occurrence should always be anticipated by correct diagnosis early in labour, followed by immediate appropriate treatment, usually Caesarean section.

T. L. T. Lewis.

EARACHE (OTALGIA)

Earache denotes pain in or around the ear. It may be sharp and lancinating, dull and often graphically described by the patient as a sensation of 'boring'. Or it may be of a throbbing nature, in the rhythm of the heart-beat. It may imply serious disease and in any case it is difficult to endure with fortitude and cries out for relief.

Obviously many causes of earache are of aural origin, but it is seldom realized with what frequency *referred earache* occurs, and as a result of this lack of knowledge the diagnosis of relatively common conditions such as impacted third molars or Costen's syndrome may be long delayed.

AURAL CAUSES OF EARACHE

Causes arising in the *auricle* are obvious and embrace such conditions as *trauma*, *haematoma*, *frost bite*, *eczema*, *impetigo*, *insect-bite*, *perichondritis*, and *neoplasm*. *Chondrodermatitis chronicis helicis* is most common in elderly males and occurs as an exquisitely tender nodule of the helix. Gouty tophi are seldom painful and seldom cause earache unless they are traumatized or they become infected (*Fig.* 265).

Causes arising in the *meatus* are also numerous. *Boils* or *furuncles* can be exceedingly painful owing to the density of the meatal tissues, the lack of space for oedema, and the profuse sensory nerve supply. They are sometimes multiple and bilateral and may preclude a view of the tympanic membrane. Marked tenderness is noted on compression of the tragus and often severe pain by moving the auricle, and there may be tender swelling of the pre-auricular and upper deep cervical lymph-nodes. Diabetes must be excluded. Diffuse *otitis externa* is usually noted for discomfort, irritation, and discharge, but it can be very painful if associated with oedema, as can hard *impacted cerumen*. *Trauma* from either direct injury or a *foreign body* is also painful but as a rule the pain is short-lived unless the abrasion becomes infected. *Neoplasm* (*usually epithelioma*) of the meatal skin is a terrible affliction on account of the intractable pain which may occur during its relentless course (*Fig.* 266). Examination reveals an ulcer or friable mass, usually of the deep meatus, which is associated with blood-stained otorrhoea and later involvement of the regional lymph-nodes. Inspection under the microscope and biopsy confirms the diagnosis.

Causes arising in the *middle ear* include *acute otitis media*—one of the commonest of the numerous causes of earache and occurring predominantly in early childhood. The attack

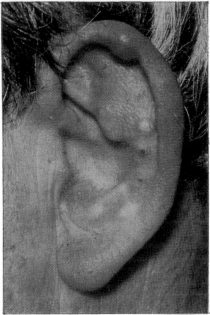

Fig. 265. Gouty tophi of the pinna.

usually follows an upper respiratory infection as coryza or influenza, or in association with the acute exanthemas. At first the pain is sharp and intermittent but later it becomes dull and throbbing. The temperature rises to 39 °C or more, deafness is present, and the appearance of the tympanic membrane varies according to the stage of the infection. At first it loses its lustre and is injected; later it becomes red and bulging and the familiar landmarks are lost. At a still later stage it ruptures and pulsating otorrhoea ensues (often sanguinous at first). When this occurs the pain usually disappears and the exhausted child falls into a fitful sleep. There is usually some tenderness over the mastoid process but the auricle can be grasped gently and moved without increasing the pain, a fact which serves to distinguish the condition from otitis externa and furunculosis.

Acute mastoiditis gives rise to severe pain in and behind the ear and extreme tenderness is present on pressure over the mastoid process. Oedema of the soft tissues covering the mastoid follows and if the infection spreads through the cortex to form a subperiosteal abscess there is considerable post-auricular swelling with displacement of the auricle forwards. Radiography is of value in confirming the diagnosis. In acute

otitis media the mastoid air-cells are often cloudy but in mastoiditis their outline is lost denoting that they have become confluent and form a homogenous mass.

In *chronic suppurative otitis media* (*Fig.* 267) pain occurs when there is an acute exacerbation of infection and it is of importance to note that these exacerbations are fraught with danger. The

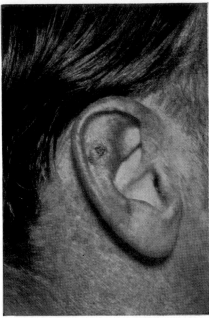

Fig. 266. Epithelioma of the pinna.

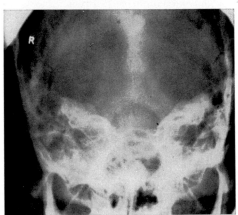

Fig. 267. Chronic suppurative otitis media with a large cholesteatoma of the right temporal bone. (*Dr. Lorna Davison.*)

pain may be associated with pyrexia and vertigo and may herald the onset of an intracranial infection such as meningitis or brain abscess.

Trauma in the form of direct injury of the tympanic membrane, e.g., a matchstick inserted by the patient, or more commonly caused by blast, e.g., a slap on the ear, causes intense pain of short duration—perhaps only a few seconds —and inspection may reveal a tear in the drum-head with a little bleeding. Probably the most common form of injury is *acute otitic barotrauma*, which takes place as a rule during aircraft descent. Factors which contribute to its occurrence are faulty cabin pressurization, too rapid descent, or the presence of tubal dysfunction, e.g., an upper respiratory infection. The earache may be severe and persist for some hours after landing, or longer if otitis media ensues. Examination will reveal an injected tympanic membrane, inter-stitial haemorrhages or, in extreme cases, a rupture. Barotrauma may also be caused by diving.

Secretory otitis, for example that which occurs in association with an upper respiratory infection but does not pass on to suppuration, is not as a rule associated with severe earache, but usually causes discomfort and crackling or gurgling noises in the ear in addition to the presenting symptom of deafness. Inspection reveals a dull yellowish drum, sometimes with hair-lines.

Malignant disease of the middle ear usually arises in cases of long-standing chronic suppurative otitis media or in a mastoidectomy cavity. It is characterized by severe and progressive pain of a boring nature and a bloodstained discharge.

Glomus tumour which is usually of extremely slow growth is not associated with severe pain until it is advanced. However, in its early stage discomfort and, often, pulsating tinnitus are present. Tumours of the middle ear spread to involve the labyrinth, causing vertigo, and also to the cranial nerves (5th–12th).

REFERRED EARACHE

Owing to the extensive nerve supply of the external and middle ear, drawn from the 5th, 9th, and 10th cranial nerves as well as from the 2nd and 3rd cervical nerves, pain may be referred to the ear from many other parts, a fact which often receives but scanty attention.

Pain Referred from the Region Supplied by the 5th Cranial Nerve:

Impacted lower third molars are a frequent cause of earache, particularly in females aged 15–25. The earache may in fact be the only symptom, and not infrequently these unfortunate young women pass through the hands of several advisers before the true nature of the trouble is discovered. Acute tenderness is elicited when forward pressure is applied above and behind the angle of the mandible, and in some cases trismus is present. The diagnosis is confirmed radiologically.

Caries and abscess of the lower molars are also likely to be responsible for referred earache.

Costen's syndrome of *temporomandibular dys-function* is another common condition which often escapes diagnosis for very long periods, as in many cases the only symptom for months or even years is earache. The condition usually arises as a result of malocclusion and is first noticed in middle age, perhaps after a number of molars have been removed and not replaced by a denture. Tinnitus and slight deafness may occur and there may be evidence of bruxism or grinding of the teeth, and clicking of the jaw. Examination almost always reveals acute tenderness over one or both temporomandibular joints together with limitation of movement.

Whilst considering the region supplied by the 5th cranial nerve it must be remembered that in some cases of *trigeminal neuralgia* the facial pain involves the ear and, rarely, it may be experienced exclusively in and around the ear.

Pain Referred from the 9th and 10th Cranial Nerves:

Lesions of the vallecula, the *posterior third of the tongue*, the *fauces* and *tonsil*, and the *larynx* and *hypopharynx* are often associated with severe earache, the pathways being via the 9th and 10th cranial nerves. Earache is found most constantly in *malignant disease* affecting these areas but may also occur in certain infections, e.g., in *quinsy*, *tonsillitis*, or in the first week after *tonsillectomy*. Sometimes very severe earache is present when an extensive *aphthous* ulcer affects the lateral pharyngeal wall or when an impacted *foreign body* is surrounded by infection, and in *laryngeal tuberculosis* earache is usually associated with the agonizing dysphagia. In the consideration of the 9th cranial nerve, *glossopharyngeal neuralgia* must be mentioned. Though rare, it is a definite clinical entity and is characterized by excruciating, lancinating pain in the tongue, jaw, and ear on the affected side. Its onset is sudden, during swallowing or talking, and occasionally a 'trigger area' is present in the region of the fauces.

Arnold's nerve, the auricular branch of the vagus, is part of the complex pathway whereby earache may be experienced in such diverse conditions as *cardiac disease, neoplasms of the oesophagus* and *mediastinum*, and lesions of the stomach.

Pain Referred from the C.2 and C.3 Region:

The commonest causes of referred earache from this region are *cervical osteoarthritis* and *cervical disk lesions*. Earache may also occur as a result of *wounds of the neck* or involvement of the *cervical lymph-nodes*, particularly in advanced *malignant disease. Herpes of the cervical nerves* is associated with vesicles of the skin of the neck and if the great auricular nerve is affected there may be complaint of great pain in or behind the ear.

THE RAMSEY HUNT SYNDROME (*Herpes zoster oticus*)

This is dealt with separately as the nervous pathways are not understood with certainty. It is characterized by very severe pain in one ear and this may last for several days before vesicles are noticed on and behind the auricle, in the meatus, and sometimes on the tympanic membrane itself. Occasionally vesicles are present on the palate and fauces. Concurrently with the appearance of the vesicles a complete lower motor neuron lesion of the facial nerve becomes apparent and there is a varying degree of pyrexia and constitutional disturbance and at times deafness, tinnitus, and vertigo, with nystagmus. Originally the condition was described as 'geniculate herpes', but clearly in many cases of the syndrome the 7th, 8th, and 9th cranial nerves may be involved.

Miles Foxen.

ELECTRODIAGNOSIS

Study of the electrical reactions of nerve-muscle units are of value in assessing the severity of damage to the lower motor neuron, in gauging the degree of recovery after such injury, in distinguishing between functional and organic paralysis, and in differentiating between paralysis due to muscular disease and paralysis which occurs with lesions of the lower motor neuron.

This is now best done by electromyography. The action potentials from affected muscles are directly recorded by means of needle electrodes inserted into them. If the muscle is completely denervated, action potentials will be absent, but the finer biphasic changes of potential caused by fibrillation are well marked. In favour of this method is the important fact that it enables the clinician to detect signs of either denervation or recovery at an earlier stage than is possible with other methods.

The demonstration of a slowed conduction time along a nerve may be of value in localizing the situation of a peripheral nerve lesion.

Ian Mackenzie.

EMPHYSEMA, SURGICAL

Surgical or subcutaneous emphysema is due to the escape of air into, or the development of gas in, the subcutaneous tissues. The crackling sensation on palpation is unmistakable. When escape of air is the cause, the commonest starting-place is some *injury to the lung*, for instance by a broken rib, a stab with a knife, a bullet wound, the rupture of alveoli due to excessive coughing, as in whooping-cough and bronchitis, during great strain, as in difficult labour, or after exploratory needling of the chest. Although the air escapes from within the lung to beneath the skin, traversing the punctured pleura, pneumothorax is seldom produced at the same time. The crepitus spreads rapidly, and may extend over a large area in a short time, disappearing in the course of a few days; in the neck it may result from the operation of *tracheotomy*.

The face may sometimes be almost suddenly involved unilaterally by the escape of air into the subcutaneous tissues from the upper part of the nose, after violent *sneezing* or energetic *blowing of the nose*.

Rarer causes for the escape of air into the subcutaneous tissues are *ulcerative* or *traumatic lesions* of the *oesophagus, stomach, duodenum,* *caecum,* or *rectum.* Air escaping into the areolar tissues around these parts may sometimes extend and become palpable as crepitus under the skin.

Quite another type is that in which the gas in the tissues is not air, but the result of *infection by gas-producing bacteria.* The three organisms likely to do this are the *Clostridium welchii, Cl. septique,* and *Cl. oedematiens.* Infection with gas-forming organisms is liable to follow heavily contaminated wounds of muscle, especially when the blood-supply to the part is cut off or reduced, the reason being that all these organisms are anaerobic and a free supply of well-oxygenated blood is inimical to their growth. Many septic wounds grow anaerobic gas-forming organisms, but serious consequences may then be expected only when gas forms within the tissue planes. This gas is detected by eliciting crepitations on palpation, or by hearing crepitations when pressure is made over the part with the stethoscope, and its presence can be confirmed radiologically. The skin around the wound and for some distance away may be brown or bruised in appearance. Two forms of infection are described: An anaerobic cellulitis where the infection is outside muscle; this form follows a benign course, is unassociated with pain or the sickly smell of muscle proteolysis, and is adequately treated by incising into the gas-filled tissue spaces together with the exhibition of penicillin.

The other is an anaerobic infection of muscle itself. In this type the general reaction is far more severe, there is pain and the part exudes a typical musty smell characteristic of 'gas gangrene'. In such cases, besides the exhibition of penicillin, radical surgery is usually indicated.

It should be observed that of the three causative organisms, *Cl. oedematiens* gives rise to minimal gas formation and but little pain, the diagnosis depending more upon the finding of swollen, paralysed muscles which become pale and slimy, and finally purple and deliquescent.

Very similar in its clinical presentation is the condition known as *anaerobic streptococcal myositis,* but here there is a well-marked skin erythema and the muscles, which are alive and react to stimuli, are copper-coloured. Furthermore, the smell is not so noticeable and culture of the wound gives a growth of anaerobic streptococci.

R. G. Beard.

ENOPHTHALMOS (OR RETRACTION OF THE EYEBALL)

This may occur: (1) In wasting diseases; (2) In paralysis of the cervical sympathetic; (3) In various congenital affections; (4) In phthisis (shrinkage) of the eyeball.

The enophthalmos in *wasting diseases* is due to the absorption of the orbital fat, and the diagnosis as regards the eye presents no difficulty.

Enophthalmos due to *paralysis of the cervical sympathetic* is never very gross, and is always associated with the other well-defined symptoms of this lesion, namely, diminution in the size of the palpebral aperture, constriction of the pupil, absence of sweating and blushing on the paralysed side. Occasionally it may be noticed that the hair over half the head on the affected side is behaving differently from that on the sound side—it may lie flatter, or may lack lustre to a degree that the patient observes. The pupil is constricted owing to the paralysis of the dilator fibres, the pupil therefore not dilating in a feeble light.

In certain *congenital cases* there is well-marked retraction associated with defective or irregular movements of the affected eyeball. Rarely, the condition is simulated by a maldevelopment of the globe, which has remained small and is usually extremely hypermetropic and poor-sighted.

P. Trevor-Roper.

ENURESIS

Enuresis occurs almost exclusively in children, and although most frequently confined to the night, it may occur in the day. It must be distinguished from incontinence of urine; the patient has usually full control of micturition during the day, although sometimes the desire to urinate must be satisfied quickly or a little dribbling may take place. The child completely empties the bladder, often without waking, once or several times during the night. The bladder need not be quite filled for micturition to occur, for it takes place in the early hours of the night.

Enuresis is often accompanied, and may be caused, by slight affections such as phimosis, balanitis, small urinary meatus, vulvitis, constipation, or intestinal worms, the correction of which remedies the trouble. However, there is no indication for wholesale circumcisions as cure for this common condition. Examination of the posterior urethra with a urethroscope may disclose inflammatory changes at the bladder neck, but in the vast majority of cases there seems nothing to promote the excitability of the detrusor muscle.

Neurogenic factors may be the cause, and a few children with enuresis are found to have congenital abnormalities of the spinal cord. If the bladder also shows the characteristic funnel-neck deformity on cystoscopy and possibly changes on cystometry the causal relationship is more certain. Sometimes there is a congenital lesion of the upper urinary tract, such as megaureter or hydronephrosis; this will be disclosed by intravenous urography (*see Figs.* 485, 496, pp. 476, 481). In most cases of enuresis the cause lies in the persistence of the infantile condition in which the normal adult cortical inhibition of the micturition centre in the cord via the pyramidal tracts has not fully developed. When the condition persists throughout childhood it may disappear at puberty.

It is important to exclude pyelitis, cystitis, diabetes mellitus, and diabetes insipidus before a diagnosis of simple enuresis is made. In each case nocturnal micturition may be the chief symptom; microscopical examination of the centrifugalized deposit will detect the pus cells or glycosuria may be found, and a bacteriological examination of a specimen of urine passed directly into a sterile bottle or obtained by a catheter should be made in order to diagnose or exclude coli bacilluria.

In many cases no source of irritation, alteration in the urine, or disease of the bladder can be found. The child is nervous and sensitive from a feeling of shame, but grows out of these troubles in time. In some the enuresis may accompany a minor epileptic attack, suggested perhaps by there being longer intervals between bedwettings than is usual in simple enuresis.

Harold Ellis.

EOSINOPHILIA

Eosinophilia denotes an increase in the number of eosinophil leucocytes in the blood. The upper limit of normal may be taken as about 50–400 per c.mm. The height of the normal count has a diurnal variation reaching the maximum between midnight and 3 a.m. and the lowest between 9 and 11 a.m. In asthmatics this is reversed. When properly stained they are unmistakable with their rather large, round, and bright pink granules all of uniform size. In addition the nucleus of the cell is usually characteristic, consisting of two large elliptical lobes connected on one side by a narrow band of chromatin.

Eosinophils appear to be principally concerned with the removal of antigen–antibody complexes from the tissues, and it is in disorders in which such complexes are found free in the circulation that eosinophilia predominates.

There are few conditions in which an eosinophilia is not occasionally found. Sometimes it is part of a general neutrophyl leucocytosis, but more commonly neutrophilia is associated with an eosinopenia, especially in infections. Most often an eosinophilia is found during a routine blood examination and the clinician is concerned whether this finding is compatible with the diagnosis based on other evidence, or whether it would suggest a careful search for some additional factor to account for it.

The conditions which most commonly are associated with an eosinophilia are undoubtedly those which can be classified under one of the following three headings:

Allergic diseases.
Skin diseases.
Parasitic infestations.

After dealing with these three main groups we shall consider the other conditions in which an eosinophilia is of common occurrence.

1. Allergic Diseases. *Bronchial asthma, hay fever, urticaria,* and *angioneurotic oedema.* In these the eosinophilia is generally between 400 and 1000 per c.mm. and only occasionally much higher; and it tends to increase during attacks and to diminish between them. The eosinophil cells are also to be found in the sputum, the nasal discharges, and in the fluid from the weals. An eosinophilia may be of help in distinguishing true asthma from cardiac asthma, and in deciding whether one is dealing with primary emphysema and bronchitis or whether these conditions have developed out of a primary asthma. It is important to remember that a moderate eosinophilia may be present in those who have inherited the allergic potentiality but have not yet developed any allergic manifestations: when an unexpected eosinophilia is discovered the patient should therefore be asked not only whether he himself suffers from any allergic disease, but also whether he has a family history of such diseases.

2. Skin Diseases. The highest and most constant eosinophilia in skin diseases is found in *pemphigus* and in *dermatitis herpetiformis,* in which it may occasionally be as high as 2000 per c.mm. It is less constant in *eczema, exfoliative dermatitis, mycosis fungoides, psoriasis, prurigo,* and many other dermatological conditions. The degree of eosinophilia often appears to be more closely dependent on the extent of the skin lesion than upon its precise nature.

3. Parasitic Infestations. Eosinophilia is common in cases infested with: *Taenia echinococcus (hydatid disease); Trichina spiralis; Bilharzia haematobia; Taenia solium; Taenia saginata; Strongyloides stercoralis;* Guinea worm; and *Ancylostoma duodenale.* It is less constant with *Filiaria sanguinis hominis, Ascaris lumbricoides,* and the parasite of *malaria.*

Eosinophilia is usually absent in cases infested with: *Oxyuris vermicularis; Trichocephalus dispar; Dibothriocephalus latus;* the *Amoebae; Trypanosoma gambiense; Acarus scabei;* and *Pediculus capitis, pubis,* and *corporis.*

In amoebic abscess of the liver eosinophilia is usually not present, though it may develop as a result of injections of emetine hydrochloride. On the other hand, a marked eosinophilia is common in hydatid disease of the liver, but when suppuration occurs the eosinophilia is replaced by a neutrophilia. When a patient is found to have a considerable eosinophilia of unexplained origin it is always advisable to make a careful examination of the faeces and urine for the parasites or their ova, if necessary before and after the administration of anthelminthic drugs.

4. Infections and Infestations. Eosinophilia is unusual in marked infections but may occasionally be present as the infection subsides. It is sometimes seen in the acute stages of childhood exanthemata. Eosinophilia may occur in polyarteritis nodosa. Mild eosinophilia is fairly common in many infections in childhood and especially during convalescence. In other infections it is a very inconstant finding.

'Pulmonary eosinophilia' is a term used to describe the appearance of transient radiological shadows in the lung associated with a marked eosinophilia. This condition is an allergic response to a number of factors amongst which the migrating larvae of ankylostoma and microfilaria, pulmonary aspergillosis, and certain drugs may be numbered.

5. Diseases of the Haemopoietic System. *Chronic myelogenous leukaemia; polycythaemia rubra vera; Hodgkin's disease; pernicious anaemia;* and following *splenectomy.* In leukaemia and polycythaemia the eosinophil cells are increased along with all the other granulocytes, but occasionally their percentage is also increased, and rarely, in the former condition, they may comprise the great majority of the cells present (*eosinophilic leukaemia*). Eosinophilia is seen in only about 20 per cent of the cases of Hodgkin's disease, usually when there is involvement of the skin. In pernicious anaemia an eosinophilia is a common occurrence during treatment with liver extracts. This is probably an allergic manifestation as it does not appear to happen when injections of vitamin B_{12} are used instead. After splenectomy the more common leucocytosis is sometimes replaced by eosinophilia and lymphocytosis.

6. Miscellaneous Conditions. In *polyarteritis nodosa* and *lupus erythematosus* a proportion of cases show an eosinophilia which may be very high. It also occurs in certain *neoplasms,* particularly of the ovary and those involving serous surfaces and bones; as a result of poisoning, particularly with *camphor, pilocarpine, phosphorus, hydrogen sulphide,* and *copper sulphate;* and following irradiation with *X-rays.* In ulcerative colitis, especially in relapse, eosinophilia may be seen, and in rare forms of gastritis.

7. Familial Eosinophilia. Several families have been reported in which the majority of members showed an eosinophilia which in some cases was very high. There have also been found a few individuals with an apparently persistently high eosinophilia but with no family history.

T. A. J. Prankerd.

EPIGASTRIUM, PAIN IN

Sudden Severe Epigastric Pain may result from the rupture of a gastric or duodenal ulcer, from a gangrenous appendix, or from acute pancreatitis. The pain in such a case is attended by severe shock and signs of collapse, and it is often impossible to decide which of the above causes is responsible. The past history of the patient and a careful study of the other signs present may guide one to a correct conclusion, but as all the conditions mentioned require immediate surgical treatment the differential diagnosis is of academic rather than practical importance, except perhaps in one instance. When the diagnosis of an abdominal emergency has to be considered, if the history, symptoms, and signs do not exactly fit acute intestinal obstruction, or stomach or duodenal perforation, perforating appendix, or acute cholecystitis, and yet have some resemblance to each of them, *acute haemorrhagic pancreatitis* is the most probable cause. Grey Turner's sign of blue discoloration, usually in the flanks, is a diagnostic but late feature. The site of the discoloration is in accordance with the nearest route of spread of pancreatic juice. The diagnosis is supported by a raised serum amylase and confirmed by finding fat-necrosis when the abdomen is opened, but the majority of surgeons are opposed to operating.

The pain of *acute intestinal obstruction* may be referred to the epigastrium. Vomiting is usually a prominent symptom in such a case.

During an attack of *biliary colic* the pain may be chiefly epigastric. The restlessness of the patient is often of diagnostic value. (*See* ABDOMINAL PAIN, ACUTE, LOCALIZED, p. 4.)

The pain of *coronary thrombosis* may be felt in the epigastrium and simulate an 'abdominal emergency' (*see* CHEST, PAIN IN, p. 133). Epigastric pain may be present in acute pericarditis, especially in children. Pain in Bornholm disease (epidemic myalgia), although more usually thoracic, may be epigastric in situation and sufficiently severe to encourage laparotomy. Acute porphyria also often causes such acute abdominal pain that laparotomy is contemplated (*see* p. 7).

Chronic or Recurrent Pain in the Epigastrium:
1. EXTRA-ABDOMINAL CAUSES must not be forgotten. Amongst these are *spinal caries* (especially to be thought of in children), other causes of nerve-root irritation, e.g., a spinal tumour, and *pleurisy*.

Small *epigastric herniae* may cause recurring attacks of severe epigastric pain. They are usually in the linea alba, and detected only by careful palpation. They are in fact protrusions of extraperitoneal fat.

Vascular or circulatory causes (*see* p. 133).

Affections of the abdominal muscles, e.g., strain from coughing, or rheumatism (especially in children), may also cause pain in the epigastrium.
2. Assuming these to be excluded, the cause of the pain should be looked for in the following organs:
a. STOMACH. The chief gastric causes of pain are carcinoma, ulcer, hiatus hernia, and pyloric stenosis. (*See* INDIGESTION, p. 422).

The pain in *carcinoma* is usually more or less continuous, although apt to be aggravated by food. A tumour may, but by no means always, be felt. Anorexia and nausea are usually present. The gastric contents in most but not in all cases show absence of free HCl and altered blood. X-ray examination if not conclusive is usually helpful.

In cases of *benign gastric ulcer* the pain usually occurs at a definite time after meals, and is generally but not always temporarily relieved by eating, though it may be aggravated by meals. The pain often wakes the victim at 1 or 2 in the morning. Vomiting, with or without haematemesis, is a variable feature. There may be localized deep tenderness on pressure, often over quite a small and well-defined area, and rigidity of the rectus muscle on one side; but physical examination is not on the whole of great assistance. The gastric contents usually show normal acidity; X-ray examination commonly reveals the ulcer. Gastroscopy together with biopsy may assist in the differentiation between a benign and a malignant gastric ulcer. The introduction of the fibre-optic gastroscope has rendered this procedure much safer and kinder than in the days of the rigid instrument.

Reflux oesophagitis associated with *hiatus hernia* may produce epigastric or retrosternal pain typically related to bending over or lying down. Certain drugs, such as aspirin, the corticosteroids, phenylbutazone, and indomethacin, may cause painful or painless gastric erosion. Indomethacin may cause a prepyloric ulcer which on X-rays may resemble a malignant condition.

Epigastric pain may also be felt to a greater or less degree in all conditions of the stomach associated with flatulence, in which case it is relieved by belching.

The *gastric crises* of tabes may be attended by severe epigastric pain, and as these may occur in the pre-ataxic stage of the disease, before other signs are present, the diagnosis is often in doubt and laparotomy has been mistakenly performed. The characteristic features are the sudden onset of the pain at irregular intervals accompanied by urgent and persistent vomiting. The abdomen is not rigid. Absence of the knee-jerk is not necessarily found, nor are the characteristic pupil signs of tabes. The Wassermann reaction in the blood or cerebrospinal fluid is in most cases positive.
b. DUODENUM. The characteristic 'hunger-pain' of duodenal ulcer is often referred to the epigastrium. It is quite impossible to differentiate between a gastric and a duodenal ulcer on the basis of relationship of the pain to meal-times. Duodenal diverticulum is considered on p. 336.
c. LIVER AND GALL-BLADDER. Epigastric pain may be produced by *congestion of the liver*, either active (hepatitis) or passive, as in mitral disease. It is also produced by such conditions as hepatic abscess and carcinoma (*see* LIVER, ENLARGEMENT OF, p. 503).

Gall-stones may sometimes be the cause of epigastric pain which may even be definitely related to meals, or to the taking of a particular article of food; the pain, however, is less 'punctual' than that of peptic ulcer. Pressure over the gall-bladder will often elicit tenderness, and if the patient is asked to take a deep breath whilst the pressure is applied there will be a painful catch in the breath as the diaphragm descends. An X-ray examination of both the stomach and gall-bladder will be of great help. Indeed these two common conditions often coexist.
d. PANCREAS. Pancreatic calculi, chronic pancreatitis, or new growth may all be causes of

epigastric and high lumbar pain. An accurate diagnosis of these conditions is difficult, often impossible, without laparotomy, but other signs of disturbed function of the pancreas may be present such as fatty diarrhoea. A tumour may be felt. Glycosuria may be present, but is not invariable. In cases of chronic pancreatitis there is usually a history of gall-stones, and transient periods of jaundice.

e. ABDOMINAL AORTA. An *abdominal aneurysm* may cause pain in the epigastrium, but the pain is more severe in the back. A pulsating expansile tumour may be felt on deep palpation. The X-rays may confirm the diagnosis, though an aneurysm may exist without radiographic abnormality.

Abdominal angina (*see* CHEST, PAIN IN, p. 133).

f. COLON. Spasmodic contraction of the intestine (enterospasm) may be a cause of epigastric pain, which may simulate gastric pain by being induced by the taking of food. Such pain, however, tends to be relieved by pressure, and by the passage of gas per anum. Obstinate constipation is usually a feature, and there are often mucus and shreds of membrane in the motions (mucomembranous colic). A similar pain may be due to *plumbism*, for the diagnosis of which *see* ANAEMIA, pp. 31, 53. The pain may be regarded as a substitute for the usual attack of headache.

Harold Ellis.

EPIPHORA

Epiphora, or overflow of the tears, may be due to: (1) *Increased secretion*; (2) *Imperfect apposition of the lacrimal puncta*; (3) *Obstruction of the lacrimal canaliculi or nasolacrimal duct.*

1. The most familiar cause of epiphora due to increased secretion of tears is the act of *weeping*, in which the flow is due to psychical stimuli. Epiphora may also occur in the lacrimation provoked by a *foreign body*, especially one which is lying in the longitudinal groove beneath the upper tarsal plate; in *conjunctivitis, corneal ulcers*, and other inflammatory affections of the eye (p. 263). It is sometimes a troublesome side-effect of certain drugs, particularly *iodides, bromides, arsenic*, and *mercury*, or certain vegetables and plants, notably *onions*.

2. Tears find their way down the canaliculi by capillary attraction, the lacrimal puncta being applied closely to the surface of the globe, aided by the movements of the lids. In *atonic ectropion*, following a laxity of the tissues in old age, and especially that due to *facial palsy* (owing to the failure of the orbicularis palpebrarum muscle), the lids are no longer braced up against the eye, and the lower lid droops away from the globe; tears collect in the sulcus thus formed, and run over on to the cheek; such an ectropion is usually aggravated by a chronic conjunctivitis (owing to the stagnant lake of tears). *Cicatricial ectropion*

from *burns, injury, scleroderma*, or *lupus* of the cheek may also result in epiphora.

3. Epiphora is sometimes produced by a *lacrimal calculus* in the canaliculus, formed by dense colonies of streptothrix. The calculi cause a swelling in the neighbourhood of the canaliculus, associated with the discharge of pus from the punctum. They may be mistaken for styes, but do not react to treatment unless the canaliculus is slit open and evacuated.

The nasolacrimal ducts may be obstructed from various causes. *Congenital obstruction* is usually unilateral and is due to imperfect canalization of the lower part of the duct; the epiphora is as a rule not evident till the seventh or eighth day, at which period the infant first begins to shed tears. The unilateral nature of the affection and the presence of tears or pus in the conjunctival sac are the diagnostic signs, and the obstruction may generally be cured by a single probing of the duct through the dilated canaliculus. Congenital absence of one or both canaliculi has been recorded. Stenosis of the lacrimal duct may also occur as the result of an ascending infection from the nasopharynx. The diagnosis is made by syringeing through the canaliculi; in catarrhal obstruction fluid can usually be forced into the nose, but, after some months, a fibrous stricture has usually formed, and the fluid will be returned through the other canaliculus; such cases may be relieved by the formation of a direct opening from the lacrimal sac into the middle meatus of the nasopharynx, a 'dacryocysto-rhinostomy'.

Excision of the lacrimal sac for chronic dacryocystitis cannot be expected to cure the epiphora which suppuration inevitably causes, but may reduce the epiphora, which has been augmented by the low-grade chronic conjunctivitis brought about by the constant presence of pus in the sac.

Injury to the duct or *canaliculus* may cause permanent epiphora.

The term 'crocodile tears' is applied to the phenomenon of profuse lacrimation occurring only when food is eaten. It generally follows a facial paralysis with misdirected nerve regeneration. Most cases respond to surgical severance of the efferent arc.

P. Trevor-Roper.

EPISTAXIS

Epistaxis, or bleeding from the nose, is a very common condition; it may be extremely serious and even fatal. It is of particular interest to the clinician as it may signify any one of numerous general disorders. It is in fact customary to classify the causes as *local* or *general*.

LOCAL CAUSES

By far the most common cause of nose-bleeding may be designated as '*spontaneous*' *epistaxis*, which arises from dilated blood-vessels of Kiesselbach's plexus on Little's area of the nasal septum, immediately posterior to the junction of the mucous membrane of the septum and the skin of the nasal vestibule. These fragile vessels often give rise to troublesome and recurrent epistaxis in childhood and in young adults and, although there may be aggravating factors such as minimal trauma or infection, most of the cases are truly spontaneous.

Trauma, for example a blow on the nose by a fist, cricket ball or the windscreen of a car, may

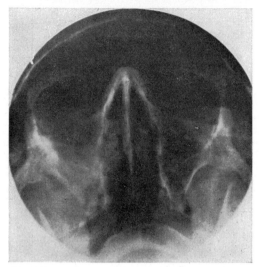

Fig. 268. Carcinoma of the antrum. Note the opaque antrum and dehiscent orbital floor. (*Dr. Lorna Davison.*)

result in extremely serious epistaxis, particularly if an artery is torn, in which case a pulsating jet of blood may spurt from the nose. Forms of trauma causing less violent bleeding are the presence of a *foreign body* and *nose picking*. *Infection* may account for some cases of slight bleeding if the mucous membrane of a deviated septum is impinged upon by the inhaled air column and ulceration ensues. In such cases, as in some perforations of the septum, a crust forms and when this separates the bleeding takes place. Other varieties of infection which may be associated with epistaxis are *syphilis, tuberculosis,* or secondary infections which may follow *operative intervention.* In *atrophic rhinitis* crusts form on the septum and turbinates and haemorrhage may follow if these are dislodged.

Neoplasm affecting the nasal cavities, paranasal sinuses, or nasopharynx are almost invariably associated with bloodstained nasal discharge and sometimes frank epistaxis (*Fig.* 268). A fairly frequent cause of persistent epistaxis is the *septal angioma* arising in Little's area and a much less common condition causing profuse epistaxis is the *nasopharyngeal angiofibroma.*

Non-healing granulomas of the *Wegener's* or *Stewart's type* cause similar presenting symptoms to those of malignant disease, inasmuch as a bloodstained discharge is more common than

profuse epistaxis. The differential diagnosis between non-healing granuloma is dealt with in the section on nasal obstruction.

Finally, attention must be drawn to the *Osler-Rendu-Weber disease* as a rare local cause of dramatic and recurrent epistaxis. The telangiectatic areas are multiple and distributed widely in the mucous membrane of the nose, lips, mouth, and tongue.

GENERAL CAUSES

These are very numerous and include *cardiovascular conditions* such as *hypertension*, and the high venous blood-pressure of *bronchitis, emphysema,* and *dilatation of the right heart. Abnormal conditions of the blood and capillaries* include such disorders as *haemophilia, von Willebrand's disease, anaemia, purpura, scurvy, leukaemia, jaundice, Hodgkin's disease, vitamin-K deficiency, thrombocytopenia,* and the use of *anticoagulants. Acute specific fevers* during their period of onset may be associated with epistaxis and the most notable of these are *enteric, influenza, scarlet fever,* and *smallpox.*

The diagnosis of the cause of epistaxis is elucidated by careful history taking, together with local and general examination. The history may throw light upon a tendency to epistaxis in the family and it is, of course, of great importance to determine whether previous attacks have occurred, and if so, which side of the nose has bled.

The local examination must be carried out with the aid of a head-mirror or lamp and nasal speculum, and in many cases the bleeding point will be seen or—as in one of the commonest varieties of epistaxis, 'spontaneous epistaxis'— a leash of engorged blood vessels can be clearly seen on Little's area.

Malignant tumours are usually apparent as friable granular masses, the diagnosis being confirmed by radiography and biopsy.

The general examination will be directed to the exclusion of cardiovascular disease and blood disorders, and may involve numerous special investigations.

Miles Foxen.

ERYTHEMA

Erythema is a reddening of the skin which disappears on pressure. It may be produced by external or internal causes and may be localized or generalized. The skin of certain individuals is more prone to become erythematous than others.

The list of substances that may produce a patch of localized erythema when applied to the skin is a formidable one and includes numerous drugs and many chemical substances, some of which are encountered in industry. It must be remembered, too, that erythema is the first stage of dermatitis and that a preliminary redness of an area of skin may be the beginning of a patch of localized dermatitis. Dermatitis of external origin may not progress to vesicle formation and in these cases erythema remains the principal sign (*Fig.* 269).

Localized erythema of internal origin is usually the result of some deeper-seated inflammatory process and may be the first sign of a boil or carbuncle, herpes simplex or zoster, impetigo, or erysipelas, and occurs over areas of venous thrombosis or lymphangitis and in gout. In

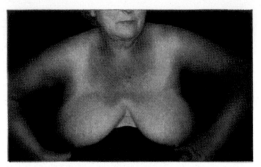

Fig. 269. Erythematous contact dermatitis caused by a black blouse. (*Dr. Peter Hansell.*)

these cases the diagnosis, if not at first obvious, soon becomes so. In localized erythema of external origin there will be a history of contact with, or the application of, known skin irritants.

Generalized erythema is never of external origin, although very large areas of the body may be involved in the first stage of extensive sunburn (erythema solare). It is usually toxic in origin due to ingested or injected substances or to bacterial toxaemia. Many food substances, not necessarily proteins, may cause generalized erythema, which is usually transient. The variety of foods which may so act is large owing to the great variation in personal idiosyncrasy. Common food factors producing erythema are shell-fish and fruits such as strawberries and raspberries, but in a given individual almost any food substance may act in this way. The history will give the answer to the problem. Drugs taken by the mouth or injected may cause erythema, notably belladonna, the sulphonamides, and penicillin. Enemata may cause a temporary erythema (enema rash); injected sera, particularly antitoxic sera, may cause generalized erythema either immediately or more commonly 8–10 days after administration. This is part of serum sickness in which there may be severe general illness with malaise, headache, stiffness and pains in the joints, nausea, and vomiting.

Generalized erythema is a minor symptom in cerebrospinal meningitis, typhoid fever, rheumatic fever, brucellosis, malaria, and in the early stage of leprosy.

Erythema is a major symptom in *scarlet fever*, in which it appears on the second or third day. It starts, usually at the height of the pyrexia, on the neck and behind the ears or on the upper part of the chest, and spreads rapidly over the whole body, leaving out the face, scalp, palms, and soles. It is a vivid red in colour and consists of bright punctate spots on an erythematous background. The rash lasts two or three days and is always followed by desquamation. Scarlet fever is usually easy to diagnose, as the early signs, vomiting, flushed cheeks with circumoral pallor, and strawberry tongue, and the later signs, namely the rash and raspberry tongue, are as a rule well defined. It must be distinguished from erythema scarlatiniform, which is a recurrent scarlatiniform rash associated with acute streptococcal tonsillitis. The other signs of scarlet fever are absent and pyrexia is only moderate. Further, scarlet fever never occurs more than once.

The erythema of *measles* is a characteristic one and unlikely to be mistaken for anything else. It is a blotchy erythema occurring on the fourth day and follows the early signs of coryza, moderate pyrexia, and Koplik's spots. In *rubella* the eruption is midway in appearance between that of scarlet fever and measles, but the other signs of those diseases are absent. *Fourth* or *Dukes's disease* is a mild exanthema which occurs in young children. The rash is a bright pink patchy erythema with some patches that may simulate the eruption of scarlet fever. It is associated with general adenopathy.

Fifth disease has an eruption similar to that of measles but more papular in character. There are practically no constitutional symptoms and the illness is over in four days.

Pink disease affects children of from six months to four years of age. It lasts from three to nine months and terminates by spontaneous recovery. It starts with coryza, general malaise, irritability, moderate pyrexia with profuse sweating and loss of muscle tone, appetite, and weight. The infant may be unable to walk. Later the hands, feet, and face become swollen, oedematous, and pink in colour. There is intense itching, especially of the hands and feet, and this, with the erythematous rash, may spread over the whole body. The loss of muscle tone persists, but there is no true paralysis. Before recovery takes place there may be profuse desquamation. The condition was usually due to mercury poisoning and has become rare since mercury has been excluded from teething powders.

Erythema multiforme (*Fig.* 270) is not a true erythema in that as a rule there are papular and vesicular elements present in the centre of the erythematous patches. It is usually of toxic origin but may occur spontaneously. It affects the limbs, more particularly the extremities, in the form of irregular circumscribed patches. In one common form known as *erythema iris* (*Fig.* 271) the lesions are round and target-like in appearance. In many cases erythema multiforme is precipitated by a virus infection, e.g., herpes simplex or vaccinia. *Hand-foot-and-mouth disease* or *Summer-term blains* is a similar condition occurring in small epidemics especially in girls' schools and affecting mainly the hands and feet with a few vesicles in the mouth. It is usually due to Coxsackie A 16 infection.

Erythema ab igne is a reticulated erythema which goes on to persistent pigmentation due to long continued exposure to heat. It is commonest on the legs of women, but also occurs in stokers. *Livedo reticularis* is a similar patterned erythema usually on the lower legs. It may be

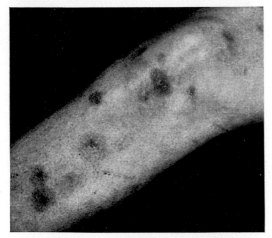

Fig. 270. Erythema multiforme. (Dr. Peter Hansell.)

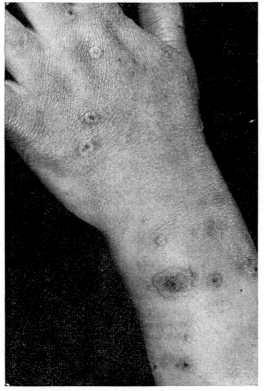

Fig. 271. Erythema iris. (Dr. Peter Hansell.)

due to one of several conditions including polyarteritis nodosa, rheumatoid arthritis, lupus erythematosus, and dermatomyositis. A physiological form called *cutis marmorata* is a reaction to cold and is seen especially in children.

There are a number of other erythematous conditions in which patches of erythema appear on the trunk and often in circular or gyrate patterns. Some of these are fixed, e.g., erythema annulare centrifugum, some are migratory, e.g., erythema chronicum migrans, and some are transitory, e.g., erythema marginatum, seen at times in rheumatic fever.

Rosacea: Erythema is a characteristic feature of rosacea. It may occur alone or in conjunction with papules or pustules. The erythema is due to flushing which for a time remits fairly quickly but later persists for long periods. It is most characteristically seen over the cheeks and nose but may also affect the forehead and upper part of the neck. Rosacea is more fully described under flushing (q.v.). (*See also Fig.* 637, p. 617.) Rosaceous (or perioral) dermatitis is very similar in appearance but found especially around the mouth. It is usually due to the use of fluorinated topical steroid applications for some other condition on the face.

Lupus erythematosus: This is probably the most important condition producing a fixed erythema. Two main varieties are recognized, the chronic discoid and disseminate (systemic) (S.L.E.).

Chronic discoid lupus erythematosus presents with patches of fixed erythema most often on the face, but also on the scalp, hands, or other areas of skin and less often on the mucous membranes In addition to the erythema there are scales which on removal may be seen to have small projections on their undersurface corresponding to dilated hair follicles in the area. Telangiectases and scarring are also important features of older lesions (*see Fig.* 701, p. 705). The scarred areas may lose their pigment while the surrounding area is more pigmented than normal. Without treatment the condition may gradually spread or remain static, but with treatment can usually be controlled and eventually the lesions may clear entirely and not recur. Possibly related to this is a condition called *lymphocytic infiltration of the skin* in which patches of erythema appear on the face or trunk and persist for weeks or months and then fade, only to return to the same site at a later date. There is no scaling or scarring. Patients with lupus erythematosus are usually sun-sensitive, but a few are sensitive to cold and the condition is largely restricted to the extremities. This variant is known as Hutchinson's chilblain lupus (*Fig.* 272).

Systemic lupus erythematosus is a much more serious condition than the chronic discoid form and often much more difficult to diagnose. Many cases will show no skin lesion at all and only a small minority have lesions resembling the chronic discoid form. A few cases of chronic discoid lupus erythematosus disseminate after exposure to ultraviolet light or after some surgical operation. Quite a high percentage of cases of chronic discoid lupus erythematosus will, however, show some evidence of dissemination without ever having symptoms of the more serious disease. The more thoroughly they are investigated the more often will some evidence of dissemination be found.

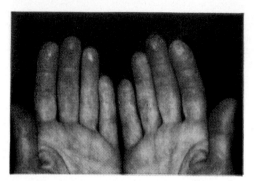

Fig. 272. Lupus erythematosus. (Hutchinson's chilblain lupus.) (*Dr. Peter Hansell.*)

When skin lesions occur in systemic lupus erythematosus they may be of many forms. The condition may present as an acute erythema of the butterfly area of the face, cheeks, and bridge of nose (*Fig.* 273); the mucous membranes of the

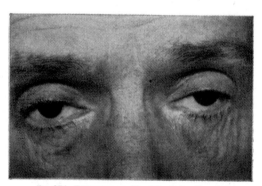

Fig. 274. Dermatomyositis. (*Dr. Peter Hansell.*)

lips and palate often show haemorrhagic erosions in these cases. Rosacea is the important differential diagnosis in these patients. A rather characteristic feature is erythema of the finger-tips and erythema and telangiectases on the dorsum of the fingers close to the cuticle. The cuticles may be broken or haemorrhagic. This type of erythema of the finger-tips is also seen in dermatomyositis, but in this condition patches of erythema are usually also present over the knuckles. Other sites where the skin may be involved in erythema are over pressure points, especially over the joints, whilst purpuric lesions or superficial erosions may occur anywhere.

Diagnosis of disseminate lupus erythematosus depends more upon the associated findings than upon the skin lesions themselves. Many patients

present with vague symptoms, especially a polyarthritis. Features of importance in the diagnosis are fever, leucopenia, raised E.S.R., biological false positive W.R., inversion of the albumin–globulin ratio with a raised gamma-globulin, and evidence of kidney damage. L.E.

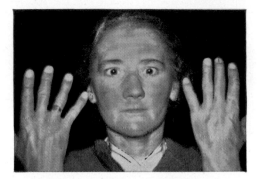

Fig. 273. Disseminate lupus erythematosus. (*Dr. Peter Hansell.*)

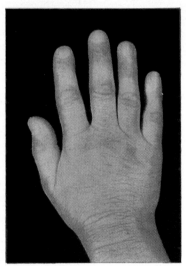

Fig. 275. Dermatomyositis. (*St. John's Hospital.*)

cells are found in the blood in about 80 per cent of cases, but they are also found occasionally in other disorders, such as chronic active hepatitis, rheumatoid arthritis, dermatomyositis, and scleroderma. These cells consist of leucocytes which have ingested a mass of nucleoprotein, derived from other leucocytes. There are many ways in which the L.E. test may be performed and some care is required in the interpretation of the result. The antinuclear factor (A.N.F.) test is positive in almost 100 per cent of cases of S.L.E. A high titre of antinuclear antibody is very suggestive of S.L.E. and is of more significance than the pattern of fluorescence.

Disseminate lupus erythematosus is considered to be an auto-immune process of the type in which the antigen is freely accessible, in contrast with Hashimoto's thyroiditis in which the antigen is inaccessible.

Dermatomyositis is another condition presenting with erythema. The muscle changes are described elsewhere (p. 180) so that only the skin lesions will be described here. The condition may occur at any age and may be acute, progressing rapidly downhill to death in a few months or chronic and persisting for years. Most cases are intermediate in type. The early lesions often consist of oedema of the eyelids and erythema around the eyes (*Fig.* 274). Patches of erythema may then appear on the upper chest and on pressure points over the back. Highly significant are patches of erythema of the finger-tips, bases of the nails, and linear erythematous patches over the knuckles (*Fig.* 275). These must be distinguished from similar lesions in disseminate lupus erythematosus. In the more chronic forms the erythema is less obvious, but there may be extensive oedema of the skin which is gradually replaced by a skin hardening very similar to scleroderma. The subacute type of dermatomyositis occurring in adults is an important disease as about half the cases are associated with carcinomata elsewhere in the body, breast, ovary, gut, larynx, and probably other regions also. Various auto-antibodies may be detected.

P. D. Samman.

EUPHORIA, EXCITEMENT, ELATION, AND ECSTASY

These conditions although distinct in several important respects have resemblances which suggest they may best be grouped together, in that they all relate to some extent to the subject's state of quality of mood. Thus the term *euphoria* is given to a particular quality of mood—well-being, cheerfulness, optimism, superficiality, and lack of seriousness—which is incongruous in respect of or unwarranted by the patient's actual situation. While the patient remains unworried about his actual condition, his friends, relatives, and indeed attendants may regard his situation as one deserving real concern.

Euphoria is an important symptom in some mental states associated with *organic cerebral disorders*, particularly those affecting the frontal lobes although, like other features of the *frontal lobe syndrome*, it may occur with focal brain lesions elsewhere. Characteristically there is a peculiar state of fatuousness combined with lack of insight and a marked tendency to make light of matters which should obviously be taken seriously (*witzelsucht*). Thus in some cases of *dementia* the mood may become shallow to the extent that the prevailing emotional state is one of constant fatuous euphoria unaffected by bad tidings or disturbing events, together with a defect of memory for recent events, failure of intellectual grasp, and deterioration of personal habits. Some patients with *multiple sclerosis*, in which the brain is affected, remain in a euphoric state although aware of their disease, although here, as in other instances, wish-fulfilment and denial probably play a considerable part. The same used to be seen before the days of modern antibiotic therapy in pulmonary tuberculosis in which false hopes of recovery were sometimes prominent (*spes phthisica*). Dementia in *general paralysis of the insane*, and more commonly following *head injury*, may also be associated with a euphoric mood.

States of *excitement* and *elation* often occur together, excitement referring primarily to activity and elation to mood. Excitement is a feature of several types of mental illness: *mania, catatonic schizophrenia, delirious states, drug intoxications*, etc. The patient in *manic excitement* has a greatly intensified feeling of power and importance; his mind seethes with ideas of every kind which, providing time allows, may sometimes be translated into action. He rides, as it were, on a wave of elation and undue energy. His talk flows with no constant direction and may be very difficult to follow. His attention is quickly distracted by any passing diversion but soon veers away. But to any obstruction of his activity, and to anything which he interprets as a slight, he responds with anger or even violence, which, however, usually lasts only a short time. Delusions and hallucinations are rare but grandiose ideas are common. Because of cheerfulness and apparent good feeling, it is easy to be momentarily in sympathy with him, though the impression may be gained that his gaiety is forced and that depression is very near the surface. Indeed it is startling to observe how, when frustrated, tears so easily break through. The impulsiveness of the manic patient often gets him into trouble. He may undertake impossible schemes, make false promises, start a task and abandon it lightheartedly on some whim halfway through; he may drink much more than is good for him, or indulge in scandalous behaviour often of a sexual kind. He may spontaneously or to some purpose compose himself for a brief spell so as to appear almost normal, and give a plausible account of his actions. For a time his energy seems inexhaustible, and he needs little sleep. He is not, as a rule, aware of being abnormal; his exuberance is felt by him as an intense *joie de vivre*. On one side, states of manic excitement shade off into a buoyant, talkative, energetic disposition (*hypomania*) which is within the limits of normal; on the other, into the more severe forms (*acute mania; delirious mania*). It should be noted, however, that mania does not necessarily bring elation in its wake. Some manic patients, although excited, are rude, irritable, sardonic and paranoid, and in no sense elated.

In *catatonic schizophrenia*, a phase of excitement with excessive activity is common and may appear with great suddenness. A pre-existing stuporous state may be interrupted without warning by a furious outburst of violence (*see* STUPOR,

p. 766). In *catatonic excitement* the patient's behaviour has that bizarre, incomprehensible quality that stamps the schizophrenic reaction; it lacks coherence. The patient appears to be in the grip of strong feelings of which his actions are the outcome, although these feelings do not communicate themselves to the observer, and seem foreign and strange. Delusional ideas may be expressed in speech and it may be possible to infer from these that the patient is hallucinated. Indeed his actions can at times only be interpreted as a response to hallucinatory perceptions. Apart from this, his activities may appear purposeless; he may adopt odd postures, laugh or mutter to himself, or exhibit repetitive movements or stereotyped behaviour such as pounding on the table, for hours at a time. He has no concern for his own well-being and may injure himself or, by his unpredictable violence, others may be injured. He may be extremely resistant to any attempts to subdue him. It may not be possible to hold his attention or to make any contact with him for more than a moment as he may be entirely engaged with his own bizarre thoughts and feelings.

States of excitement which show both manic and schizophrenic features may be encountered in association with certain forms of *drug addiction* or due, for example, to overdosage with drugs such as *mescaline, amphetamine* or *lysergic acid diethylamide* (*LSD*). In *delirious* states (e.g., *delirium tremens*) the patient may throw himself about and struggle with his attendants. In a phase of disordered consciousness apparently following an epileptic fit or as part of a prolonged temporal seizure—the so-called *twilight state*—or in acute epileptic delirium (*furor*), there may be overactivity and violence. Episodes of violence and destructiveness occur also in the *aggressive psychopath*, in whom an underlying cortical dysfunction, often influenced by alcohol, may bear a certain similarity to that of epilepsy (*see* ANTISOCIAL BEHAVIOUR, p. 60).

Finally, consideration may be given to so-called *ecstasy states*, which are very uncommon. They occur apparently only under two circumstances: in *cyclothymia*, which is that form of *manic-depressive* disorder characterized by mood swings from depression to mania without any intervening period of normality, and in *temporal lobe epilepsy*. In cyclothymia a state of ecstasy may be experienced as a transient phenomenon in the upswing from depression into mania, during which the patient feels an intense sense of 'at one-ness' with his environment so that the sky seems bluer than blue, the grass greener than green, bird-songs bolder and more beautiful than ever, etc. —a state which may be considered as the opposite to depersonalization (*see* p. 209) which could almost be described as 'hyper-personalization'. In temporal lobe epilepsy a somewhat similar state occurs, often associated with intensely religious feelings and sometimes with hallucinations of angels, the gates of heaven opening, etc.

W. H. Trethowan.

EXOPHTHALMOS (OR PROPTOSIS)

This may be bilateral or unilateral.

Bilateral Exophthalmos. The commonest cause of this condition is *Graves's disease*, in which the exophthalmos is associated with other general symptoms, such as tachycardia, swelling of the thyroid gland, fine tremors, and general nervousness. The eyes are pushed forward to a varying extent, in some cases the protrusion being so great that they cannot any longer be covered entirely by the lids. The protrusion causes the upper lid to be unusually raised, and the eyes look wide open, giving the patient an expression of alarm or astonishment (Stellwag's sign), due to spasm of the levator palpebrae superioris. When the eyes are lowered, the upper lids do not descend to the same extent as the cornea, but leave a broad portion of the sclera visible above the cornea (von Graefe's sign). Winking takes place less frequently, and convergence of the eyes is sometimes rendered difficult (the sign of Moebius). When the patient looks upwards, when the head is bent down with the chin towards the sternum, the forehead fails to wrinkle as it does in normal persons (Joffroy's sign).

The degree of exophthalmos in this condition may be unequal on the two sides, and in the early stages one eye may be prominent for some time before its fellow is affected.

Bilateral exophthalmos may also be caused by *thrombosis of the cavernous sinuses*. This condition is usually secondary to some furuncle or carbuncle of the skin of the face in the region of the eye, to orbital cellulitis, or suppuration in the accessory sinuses of the nose. It usually starts on one side, and invariably spreads to both in the later stages of the attack. The eyes are protruded, the eyelids are red and engorged, and the frontal and ophthalmic veins are dilated. Movements of the eyes are very limited, and there is much swelling and induration of the orbital tissues. In association with the orbital infiltration there is often some swelling in the region of the mastoid process, owing to the exit in this region of an emissary vein in connexion with the sinuses that communicate with the two cavernous sinuses. Further causes of bilateral exophthalmos are *empyema of the accessory nasal sinuses*, symmetrical *orbital tumours* (as lymphoma), *oxycephaly*, and *leontiasis ossium*.

Unilateral Exophthalmos may be due to:

Orbital cellulitis or granuloma
Thrombosis of the cavernous sinus
Thrombosis of the orbital veins
Orbital periostitis
Meningocele
Encephalocele
Neoplasm
Orbital haemorrhage
Orbital emphysema
Arteriovenous aneurysm
Distension of the accessory sinuses of the nose.

The diagnosis of *orbital cellulitis* and *thrombosis of the cavernous sinus* presents little difficulty, owing to the symptoms of acute inflammation that are present, orbital cellulitis being distinguished from cavernous sinus thrombosis by the fact that it is usually unilateral and there is no oedema in the mastoid region. In some cases a thrombosis of the orbital veins, causing unilateral exophthalmos, may exist before or without implication of the cavernous sinus.

Orbital periostitis, especially in more chronic cases, may give rise to varying degrees of proptosis, and in the absence of any obvious thickening of the orbital margins the diagnosis may be obscure. In any periosteal inflammation of long standing a radiograph will usually show a definite increase of density in the affected bone.

Meningocele and *encephalocele* may in some cases be difficult to diagnose from dermoid cysts. The latter are usually placed anteriorly in the orbit, and do not therefore cause proptosis, though they may displace the eyeball. A meningocele usually presents itself through a gap between

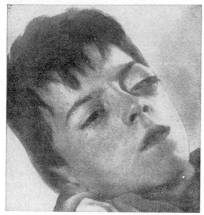

Fig. 276. Unilateral proptosis due to lymphosarcomatous deposits in the left orbit.

the ethmoid and the frontal bones, and is attached to the bone. An opening may sometimes be found through which the meningocele communicates with the cranial cavity. Meningoceles sometimes pulsate in association with the arterial and respiratory oscillations. They may also be diminished in size by pressure of the fingers, as the fluid can be squeezed into the cranial cavity. In many cases an exploratory puncture is the only means of making a certain diagnosis.

A *neoplasm of the orbit* (*Fig.* 276) has usually no distinctive feature, the exact nature of the trouble being verified as a rule by an exploratory operation and histological check. Radiography (including the use of tomography, constrast media, phlebography, and comparison of the optic foramina) will assist the diagnosis. *Ivory exostoses* or *osteomata* usually arise from the frontal bone and are attached by a broad base, so that their removal presents very great difficulty; the diagnosis depends on their slow growth and excessive hardness; a radiograph shows their presence with some certainty.

Orbital haemorrhage or *emphysema* may arise from trauma. The former may follow a sudden strain even in a healthy young adult and causes immediate protrusion of the globe, often accompanied by diplopia.

An *arteriovenous aneurysm* is nearly always associated with pulsating exophthalmos, in which there is protrusion of the eyeball and dilatation of the blood-vessels of the retina, lids, and conjunctiva. There may be orbital pulsation, and a loud blowing murmur on examination with the stethoscope. Compression of the carotid artery on the same side diminishes the pulsation and the sound. The usual cause of arteriovenous aneurysm is rupture of the carotid artery into the cavernous sinus as the result of an injury, most commonly a fracture of the base of the skull.

Rare cases are also seen of intermittent exophthalmos, which appears only at intervals or when the head is depressed; these are usually due to *varicose veins in the orbit*, not in communication with the artery.

The protrusion of the eyeball due to *dilatation of the accessory sinuses* of the nose is, as a rule, less an exophthalmos than a displacement of the eyeball downwards and outwards. A frontal sinus dilatation causes a displacement a little forwards and especially downwards and outwards. Ethmoidal and sphenoidal dilatation cause more proptosis than lateral displacement. With dilatation of the frontal sinus there may be some thickening and fullness of the supra-orbital ridge associated with pain and tenderness over the eyebrow; with dilatation of the ethmoidal cells there is usually a definite swelling to be felt at the inner side of the orbit, which is compressible though not distinctly fluid; dilatation of the sphenoidal sinus is sometimes accompanied by optic neuritis or atrophy; in all cases of proptosis due to sinus trouble of any duration there is evidence in the nose of inflammation of these cavities, the usual symptom being the existence of polypi or of definite swellings in the region of the infundibulum.

A growth of the superior maxilla causes displacement of the eye upwards. *Suppuration in the maxillary antrum* rarely causes proptosis or displacement of the eye.

P. Trevor-Roper.

EYE, INFLAMMATION OF

Inflammation of the eye is normally restricted to the conjunctiva (as a *conjunctivitis*), occasionally penetrating the cornea (a *keratitis*—usually in the form of a *corneal ulcer*), and less commonly affecting the interior of the eyeball (an *iritis*). Localized patches of *episcleritis* may superficially resemble conjunctivitis, and the dusky circumcorneal congestion in a strangulated eyeball (a *congestive glaucoma*) may simulate that from an iritis. The character of the inflammation varies with the type of the disease, but certain symptoms, such as *pain, photophobia,* and *lacrimation,* are common to all inflammatory conditions, and are by themselves of little value in differential diagnosis.

Conjunctivitis. In conjunctivitis the conjunctival vessels are dilated; they are freely movable over the subjacent sclera, and the conjunctival injection is most evident at a little distance from the corneal margin, the circumcorneal portion of the conjunctiva, owing to its firmer attachment to the sclera in this region, being relatively less injected. The cornea is clear and bright, if the condition is purely conjunctival; the anterior chamber and iris are normal in appearance, the pupil is black, and the iris active. Purulent discharge may collect at the inner angle of the palpebral aperture and on the edge of the lids,

pneumococcus or the Koch-Weeks bacillus may be found, and less often the streptococcus. When the infection is due to the Morax-Axenfeld diplobacillus, the condition is almost exclusively limited to the area of conjunctiva exposed in the palpebral fissure, especially towards the canthi (angular conjunctivitis).

Purulent conjunctivitis in adults may result from infection by the gonococcus. The reaction is intense; swelling of the lids and conjunctiva is extreme, and the discharge thick and profuse, though it may start by being serous and blood-stained. The condition is diagnosed by bacterio-logical tests of the discharge, but may be suggested by the existence of a concomitant urethritis.

Some particular forms of conjunctivitis deserve special mention. In *ophthalmia neonatorum* (acute

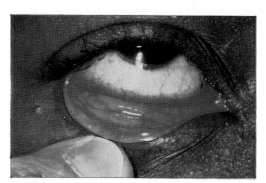

Fig. 277. Acute conjunctivitis. (*Institute of Ophthalmology.*)

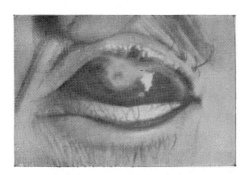

Fig. 278. Trachomatous scarring. (*Institute of Ophthalmology.*)

especially after sleep; there is often a feeling of grittiness as of sand or dust in the eye. A simple hyperaemia of the conjunctiva, possibly passing into a well-established conjunctivitis, may be a secondary condition; a foreign body on the cornea or in the fornix—or, more important still on account of the ease with which it is overlooked, in the subtarsal sulcus—may be the cause; or the lower lid may be turning inwards (an 'entropion'), causing trichiasis. There may be concretions in the palpebral conjunctiva which cause irritation, and inflammation of the conjunctiva through abrading the cornea; or the eye may be irritated allergically from the local use of drugs such as atropine or boracic acid, in which cases the skin of the lids usually shares in the reaction. Photophthalmia gives rise to similar appearances; the exciting agent may be any source of ultra-violet irradiation, such as strong sun-glare or the light reflected from snow. Conditions which may combine to cause similar hyperaemia are dusty, ill-ventilated atmospheres or errors of metabolism, such as gout.

Conjunctivitis may be *catarrhal, mucopurulent,* and *purulent.* In catarrhal conjunctivitis (*Fig.* 277) the lids may be stuck together after sleep, the pain is generally slight, and allayed by closing the eyes. Mucopurulent conjunctivitis is characterized by more profuse discharge and is frequently due to infection by the staphylococcus; or the

conjunctivitis of the newborn) there is often profuse mucopurulent discharge; the condition is diagnosed from imperfect canalization of the nasolacrimal ducts by the fact that in the latter the discharge is present without the accompanying inflammation. Ophthalmia neonatorum is, by statutory definition, purulent discharge from the eyes of an infant in the first twenty-one days of life, and is independent of the bacteriology of the condition; the gonococcal cases are in a minority; but the grave risks of secondary corneal ulceration call for urgent antibiotic therapy.

In *trachoma* (*Fig.* 278), a viral infection, endemic in the Middle East, but rare in England, the conjunctiva is studded with enlarged follicles, particularly on the under-surface of the upper lid and in the upper conjunctival fornix. The follicular enlargement is associated with thickening and oedema of the tissues of the upper lid causing partial ptosis, with lacrimation, and, in the later stages, vascular opacity (pannus) of that part of the cornea which is usually covered by the upper lid; in the later stages of trachoma the infiltration is followed by the formation of fibrous tissue, causing bending of the tarsal plate, entropion, and trichiasis.

Conjunctival *allergies* are characterized particularly by photophobia, oedema, and epiphora. They include non-specific responses to a wide miscellany of drugs, cosmetics, and other irritants, and three specific clinical forms: (1) *Hay fever*, from exogenous pollens, etc. (2) *Phlyctenular conjunctivitis* (due to an allergic reaction, usually to tuberculo-protein) featuring one or more round yellowish raised masses at the corneoscleral junction surrounded by a localized area of vascular conjunctiva; in some cases the phlyctenules encroach on the corneal surface, being followed by a trail or leash of conjunctival vessels. (3) *Spring catarrh*, which may usually be diagnosed from the history of its time of onset

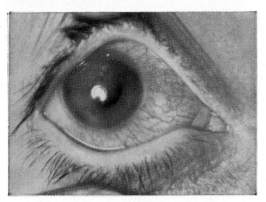

Fig. 279. Interstitial keratitis (*see* p. 185). (*Institute of Ophthalmology*.)

(spring or summer) and recurrent nature; it exists in a palpebral and a bulbar form, the former showing polygonal flat-topped conjunctival nodules, the latter gelatinous limbal thickening.

Tuberculous conjunctivitis, like its even rarer syphilitic counterpart, nearly always causes ulceration. There may be much formation of new tissue giving rise to 'cock's-comb' excrescences.

Corneal ulcers produce greyish or white opacities of the cornea over which the cornea has lost its polish. There may only be infiltration of the cornea, or in more serious cases actual

loss of substance, which may ultimately lead to perforation of the cornea; in some cases there may be pus in the anterior chamber—*hypopyon* (*see Fig.* 197, p. 185); the diagnosis presents no difficulty; the ulcers are obvious if the cornea is examined carefully, and stained with fluorescein. **Iritis.** In iritis the inflammation of the eye presents rather different characteristics, for the iris receives its blood-supply from the deeper ciliary vessels, and the dilatation of these shows a marked contrast to that of the conjunctival vessels. The injection is most evident in the circumcorneal region, the equatorial region of

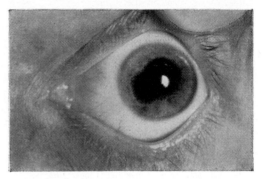

Fig. 280. Iridocyclitis synechiae. (*Institute of Ophthalmology*.)

the eyeball being paler, while the tarsal conjunctival is unaffected; and the colour of the injection is brick-red rather than pink (ciliary injection). The cornea retains it polish, but the aqueous may be turbid, and especially when the ciliary body is involved (iridocyclitis) there are punctate deposits of leucocytes on the posterior surface of the cornea (*keratic precipitates*), or rarely a hypopyon (*see Fig.* 197, p. 185). Owing to the increased vascularity of the iris, and to the exudation into its substance, its volume is increased and its mobility impaired; hence the

A SUMMARY OF THE POINTS OF DISTINCTION BETWEEN CONJUNCTIVITIS, IRITIS, AND ACUTE GLAUCOMA

	CONJUNCTIVITIS	IRITIS	ACUTE GLAUCOMA
Conjunctiva	Conjunctival vessels bright red and injected; movable over subjacent sclera; injection most marked away from corneoscleral margin; colour fades on pressure	Ciliary vessels injected, deep-red or bluish-red; most marked at corneoscleral margin; colour does not fade on pressure	Both conjunctival and ciliary vessels injected
Cornea	Clear, sensitive	Clear, sensitive	Steamy, hazy, insensitive
Anterior chamber	Clear; normal depth	Aqueous turbid; anterior chamber slightly shallow	Very shallow
Iris	Normal colour	Injected, swollen, adherent to lens, and muddy-coloured	Injected
Pupil	Black, active	May be filled with exudate, small, fixed	Dilated, fixed, oval
Intra-ocular tension	Normal	Normal	Raised

9*

pupil is small and sluggish. The presence of blood and exudate in the substance of the iris also changes its colour—a blue iris becoming greenish, and the fine detail of the iris structure is blurred and obliterated. Adhesions are apt to occur between the iris and the lens at the point of their immediate contact, the edge of the pupil; in the constricted state of the pupil these may not be seen, but on dilatation with atropine or homatropine these adhesions or *posterior synechiae* prevent the enlargement of the pupil at certain points, and it therefore becomes irregular in shape (*Fig.* 280). Small masses of iris pigment may also be seen on the anterior surface of the

the anterior chamber shallow, the iris discoloured, and the pupil dilated and fixed. The eye is hard to the touch and very tender. Vision fails rapidly, diminishing in a few hours from normal to the bare perception of light.

The distinction between subacute or acute glaucoma, as just described, and simple glaucoma cannot be too strongly emphasized. Simple glaucoma is a symptomless disease, and is usually discovered in the course of routine examination. No pain, obscuration of vision, haloes, or feeling of tension are complained of; and the visual-field loss which characterizes the disease is rarely noticed by the patient in the early stages.

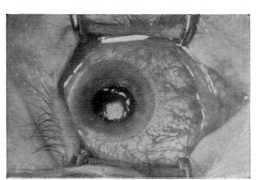

Fig. 281. Acute glaucoma. (*Institute of Ophthalmology.*)

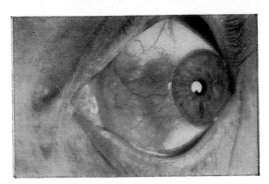

Fig. 282. Episcleritis.

lens where the mydriatic may have broken down some of the weaker adhesions. An exudate into the pupillary aperture may form a filmy grey membrane completely or partially blocking the pupil.

An important form of iritis (or, more properly, of 'uveitis', since the ciliary body and choroid normally share in any inflammation of the iris) may occur in the second eye following perforating injury in the first—'sympathetic ophthalmitis'. This possibility must always be borne in mind in cases of perforation of the globe, even operative; it is refractory to treatment (though systemic cortisone has revolutionized the outlook), and may demand removal of the injured eye in order to avoid the tragedy of functional loss of both from this relentless form of iridocyclitis.

Glaucoma. Congestive glaucoma is a disease of the later years of life, and of hypermetropes rather than myopes. It is precipitated by any of the factors that may provoke a dilatation of the pupil.

At first the chief complaint in subacute attacks is of temporary obscuration of vision and the appearance of haloes or rainbows around lights; there is often a feeling of tension in the eyes and a dull frontal headache in addition to the loss of vision. In severe attacks the pain is violent, radiating from the eye to the head, the ears, and the teeth, and is associated with sickness, a symptom that *may* lead to the mistaken diagnosis of migraine or sick headache. The lids may be oedematous and the conjunctiva injected (*Fig.* 281). The cornea is hazy and anaesthetic,

The importance of discriminating between iritis and congestive glaucoma cannot be overemphasized; the use of atropine or some similar mydriatic is the basic treatment of iritis, while in glaucoma it is disastrous.

Acute inflammation of the eye may be seen in *scleritis* and *episcleritis* (*Fig.* 282), which is frequently nodular, and is evidently due to a deeperseated lesion than conjunctivitis; the histology is essentially that of a rheumatic nodule, and the condition can normally be requited by topical hydrocortisone.

P. Trevor-Roper.

EYE, PAIN IN

Pain in the eye is not by itself pathognomonic of any particular lesion; but it may be noted in diverse circumstances, ranged into the following groups.

1. Pain associated with Visible Inflammatory Changes, due to:

Foreign body
Entropion or ingrowing lashes
Conjunctivitis
Keratitis
Iritis
Congestive glaucoma
Ocular herpes

The differential diagnosis between these is discussed in the article on EYE, INFLAMMATION OF (p. 263).

2. Pain without Visible Changes in the Eyeball, but with Acute Loss of Sight in one eye only, in both eyes together, or in one eye after the other: Retrobulbar neuritis.

The pain is generally referred to the back rather than to the front of the eye. The diagnosis is suggested at once if considerable loss of sight comes on suddenly in an eye which on examination proves not to be affected by intra-ocular haemorrhage, detachment of the retina, or any other visible lesion. After days or weeks, the pain may disappear and sight return to normal; on the other hand, in severer cases, the inflammation in the optic nerve may extend forward to the back of the eyeball and become visible as a papillitis. The cause of the mischief may be difficult to determine; most commonly it is due to multiple sclerosis; often it remains obscure; sometimes it is traced successfully to plumbism, syphilis, or to some acute infection such as influenza or a toxic-absorptive malady arising from septic teeth, intestinal toxaemia, septic tonsils, pelvic sepsis, and so on. It has been reported following the use of monoamine-oxidase inhibitors.

3. Pain without Inflammation and without Impaired Sight, but associated with errors of refraction: Eyestrain (the term is used in the colloquial sense: symptoms present but the eye is not 'strained').

The commonest cause of eyestrain or eye-fatigue is some error of refraction, especially hypermetropia, astigmatism, or presbyopia, and it arises mainly in persons whose occupation entails much reading of small print, fine needle-work, or close attention to minute details near to the eyes—as in microscopists; or in those whose work has to be carried on in too dim or too strong a light—especially electric or strong sunshine. The sensitivity of patients to such errors of refraction is very variable, and is largely conditioned by the neurotic tendencies of the individual, since the errors to which eyestrain is attributed are usually of very small degree. It should be emphasized that myopia does not cause eyestrain, but simply a blurring of distance vision, that presbyopes normally complain of having to hold the book far away, and that before the general availability of astigmatic lenses, a few decades ago, eyestrain was rarely mentioned—even among close workers, in (almost inevitably) poor illumination. A further occasional cause of eyestrain or ocular disability is an error of muscle balance, notably convergence insufficiency, which commonly responds to orthoptic exercises.

4. Pain in the Eyes due to Febrile or other Constitutional Causes. The most familiar example of cases which come under this heading is *influenza*. The pain is generally referred rather to the backs of the eyeballs than to the eyes themselves, but the complaint is one of pain in the eyes. The trouble occurs both as an early symptom of the disease and as a sequela when the fever has subsided. The diagnosis is made from the course of the pyrexia and the general symptoms. In a similar way pain in the eyes may form part of the clinical picture in other fevers, notably small-pox, typhus, typhoid fever, measles, secondary syphilis, and malaria. There may be coryza as well as pain, for instance in the early stages of measles. In other conditions, such as meningitis, there is PHOTOPHOBIA (p. 644) rather than pain in the eyes.

5. Pain in the Eyes due to Inflammation in Ethmoid, Sphenoid, or Frontal Air Sinuses. Sinusitis is probably the commonest cause of pain actually *in* the eye; the pain from ocular causes is frequently described as being around or behind the globe. It may be influenced by posture.

P. Trevor-Roper.

EYELIDS, AFFECTIONS OF

Apart from those conditions considered under EYE, INFLAMMATION OF (p. 263), there are various others of which the patient may complain that deserve mention.

Blepharitis, or inflammation of the lid margin, is normally a sequel to seborrhoea with an allergic aggravation; and, if secondarily infected with staphylococci, may become ulcerative. The margins are red, scales or crusts are found between the lashes, which are often small, distorted, or destroyed. Ectropion or trichiasis may result. The symptoms can normally be allayed by steroid/antibiotic applications.

External stye is a suppurative inflammation of an eyelash follicle. The condition is common and easily recognized; the general health and resistance to infection is often at fault.

An *Internal stye* is a similar infection of a Meibomian gland (in the posterior half of the eyelid margin). It does not normally clear spontaneously, but the inflammatory signs and symptoms recede, leaving a pea-sized swelling (which may develop without antecedent inflammatory signs), called a 'Meibomian cyst', a 'tarsal cyst', or a 'chalazion'.

Entropion, or rolling inwards of the lid margin, may be *spastic* or *cicatricial. Trichiasis,* or rubbing of the lashes on the eye, with consequent discomfort and inflammation, is a frequent result. The opposite condition of *ectropion* may also be *spastic* or *cicatricial,* but it also occurs as a *senile* and *paralytic* phenomenon.

Symblepharon, or adhesion of the conjunctival surface of the lids to the globe, usually results from caustic burns. *Ankyloblepharon* is the term applied to adhesion of the two lids to each other, and may be due to similar causes, or may be congenital.

Xanthelasma is a slightly raised plaque, yellowish in colour, found in the skin at the inner end of either lid, often symmetrical and multiple. It should be removed if sufficiently disfiguring.

A small clear cyst situated among the lashes is due to retention of secretion in a *gland of Moll.* Removal of the anterior wall results in its disappearance.

Molluscum contagiosum often chooses the lids as a site. The nodules are small, white, umbilicated, and characterized by the ease with which contact with another portion of skin (not infrequently during removal) causes the appearance of further nodules by transference of the causative virus.

Naevi or *moles* may occur on the lid, especially the margin, and involve the conjunctiva as well. They are usually pigmented. *Haemangioma* may be similarly situated, as may *papilloma*. The commonest malignant tumour of the lid is *epithelioma*; or a *rodent ulcer* may occur at the inner or outer canthus.

Congenital conditions of the lid already mentioned include ptosis, symblepharon, ankyloblepharon, ectropion, entropion, and trichiasis. *Coloboma* occurs as a notch in the lid margin, usually towards the nasal side in the upper lid. A double row of lashes (distichiasis) may be found as a congenital malformation, possibly causing trichiasis. A favourite site for a *dermoid cyst* is at the outer canthus; there is frequently a corresponding bony defect, and the condition needs careful distinction from *meningocele* before exploration. *Epicanthus* is a disfiguring semilunar fold of skin across the inner canthus, sometimes disappearing as the nose develops. *Plexiform neuroma* may cause a disfiguring drooping and distortion of the lids.

Though not primarily diseases of the lids, inflammatory affections of the lacrimal gland or sac cause swelling and oedema in this region. *Dacryo-adenitis* is rare; it causes a painful swelling in the outer end of the upper lid; a similarly situated though painless swelling is caused by tumours of the lacrimal gland, histologically resembling the mixed parotid tumours. In *Mikulicz's disease* there is enlargement of both lacrimal and salivary glands, probably lymphomatous in nature. *Acute dacryocystitis* causes a painful red swelling at the inner end of the lower lid; it should be treated conservatively as an abscess, and no attempt made to relieve the condition surgically until the inflammation has quite subsided. The abscess may rupture through the skin, or require incision. It is frequently preceded by chronic dacryocystitis and EPIPHORA (p. 256).

A disturbing symptom sometimes complained of, especially by elderly people, is 'flickering' of the lid—a periodic clonic spasm of the orbicularis, which may cause considerable distress and discomfort. The condition may respond to general sedatives, though novocain and even alcohol may have to be injected to arrest obstinate cases.

It is important to note that swelling and oedema of the lids, and oedema of the conjunctiva (*chemosis*) may be so intense as to suggest a far more serious state of affairs than the local inflammatory lesion which is its usual cause. Chemosis may occur from acute conjunctivitis, ocular inflammations, or orbital cellulitis; obstruction to the lymph-flow from an orbital tumour may be the cause; or general disorders, such as Bright's disease, anaemia, or angioneurotic oedema.

P. Trevor-Roper.

FACE, PAIN IN

Pain in the face may be due to: (1) Local disease of the eyes, sinuses, facial bones, nose, temporomandibular joint, teeth, or tongue; (2) Disease affecting the intracranial portion of the trigeminal nerve and its root; (3) Tic douloureux, an easily recognized condition of unknown aetiology, which may be more or less closely simulated by the conditions falling under (1) and (2) above; (4) Migraine.

Trigeminal Neuralgia (tic douloureux) is a distinct clinical entity, but its pathology is unknown. Beginning usually after 50 years of age it is a paroxysmal facial pain tending in the early stages to occur in bouts lasting days or weeks. The pain then recurs and as time goes on the periods of pain become longer and the periods of remission become shorter so that eventually, although still intermittent, the pain will occur at some time on most days. The pain is intense and usually described as 'shooting' or 'stabbing' and each series of stabs lasts a few seconds or a few minutes. It usually starts in the maxillary or mandibular division, rarely in the ophthalmic division to which it may later spread, and is provoked by touching the face as in washing the face or blowing the nose, or by a draught or by talking or eating. The severity of the pain often causes the patient to screw up the affected side of the face, hence the name *tic douloureux*. On examination there are no abnormal signs in the nervous system but the tongue may be furred on the affected side.

The pain may be relieved in more than half the patients by carbamazepine (Tegretol), but in those in whom the treatment is ineffective and in those who relapse *tic douloureux* can be relieved by numbing the face over the area where provoking factors cause pain. This can be done most simply by alcoholic injection of the maxillary or mandibular branches and the pain will be relieved as long as sensory loss persists. Although sensation will return within a few months pain will not necessarily reappear at the same time and this treatment may well be adequate in elderly patients. Other treatments are by alcoholic injection into the Gasserian ganglion, which will permanently destroy nerve cells, or by complete or partial section of the posterior root. With these procedures the cornea is rendered insensitive and thus becomes exposed to damage and possible ulceration so that glasses with a protective sidepiece must be worn. In order to obviate this and the discomfort arising from numbness (touch loss) over the face, the procedure of medullary tractomy was devised in which the spinothalamic tract (carrying only pain and temperature fibres) is divided in the medulla. This carries, however, a certain morbidity. More recently injection around the Gasserian ganglion with phenol rather than alcohol has been tried and this certainly reduces the numbness but carries with it a higher relapse rate.

Symptomatic Trigeminal Neuralgia. This is the name given to pain similar to tic douloureux but caused by disease of the sinuses, teeth, temporo-mandibular joint, and central nervous system. Although the quality and distribution of the pain may simulate the 'idiopathic' type, symptoms do not run the prolonged and intermittent course found in tic douloureux. This fact is clearly of no value in the diagnosis of a first attack, and identification of the source of the pain requires thorough clinical and radiological examination. In general, however, the evidence of disease is unequivocal in this symptomatic group, and it is a mistake to embark on extensive dental extractions or sinus operations unless the indications are clear. Active infection of the *frontal and maxillary sinuses, apical abscesses of the teeth, glaucoma and iritis, and malignant disease of the tongue* may simulate the pain of tic douloureux. The same is true of *disseminated sclerosis, gummatous meningitis, neuromas* and *meningiomas* in the posterior fossa, *naso-pharyngeal carcinomas, posterior fossa angioma*, and *tabes* (lightening pains). The neuralgia which follows *herpes zoster* of the Gasserian ganglion in elderly subjects is unlikely to cause confusion unless the history of herpetic eruption is missed. The possibility of diagnostic error emphasizes the need for a complete clinical, radiological, and serological examination in every case of trigeminal neuralgia.

Periodic Migrainous Neuralgia. This is a particular variety of paroxysmal headache and differs from migraine in that the headaches occur in bouts and are of greater frequency and shorter duration. The headache is sharply localized to one or other supraorbital region but may spread into the temple, eye, or cheek. Typically it wakens the patient from sleep every night an hour or two after he has gone to bed and is very intense. It lasts from 30 to 90 minutes and may be accompanied by watering of the eye and blocking of the nose on that side. There may also be a partial ptosis and smaller pupil on the affected side.

Such a headache may also occur irregularly, not necessarily at night or every day but sometimes two or three times in 24 hours. A bout of such headaches usually lasts for several weeks when there is spontaneous remission. There is, however, a tendency for the headache to recur, usually after an interval of months or years, sometimes with a seasonal incidence. It is commoner in men and may occur at any time in adult life. Its cause is unknown.

Treatment is preventive by subcutaneous injections of Ergotamine Tartrate 0·5 mg. or 0·25 mg. or by suppository containing 2 mg. If the attacks are occurring exclusively at night, this is given at bed-time. If, as usually happens, this brings freedom from attacks, the dose must be withheld every seventh night in order to see whether the

bout has come to an end. If the attacks are irregular or more frequent, it will be necessary to give such medication two or three times in 24 hours in order to ensure control of the headache. At the same time the patient may benefit from regular sedation with Amylobarbitone.

Frontal pain can be due to *upper cervical spondylosis* and also to *temporal arteritis*. Internal derangements of the temporomandibular joint, resulting as a rule from mal-occlusion of the teeth, can cause severe pain in the face and tongue on one side. The pain occurs only when the jaws are moved, as in speaking or in chewing, and its stabbing quality makes for confusion with tic douloureux. Temporomandibular pain of this type is one of the components of *Costen's syndrome*, which includes tinnitus and eustachian deafness in its rather confused symptomatology.

Ian Mackenzie.

FACE, PARALYSIS OF

Facial paralysis is seen in three clinical forms: (1) Upper-motor neuron paralysis, in which the lower half of the face is affected, and the upper half spared. (2) Lower-motor neuron paralysis, in which there is loss of movement in all the muscles on the affected side. (3) Myopathy.

Upper-motor Neuron Paralysis is due to a lesion of the corticopontine fibres of the pyramidal tract anywhere between the cortex and the middle of the pons. The eye can be closed and the forehead wrinkled, but the teeth cannot be bared on the affected side and there is weakness of the lips and buccinator muscles. In some cases involuntary emotional movements remain normal despite loss of purposive movements. In bilateral pyramidal lesions the upper part of the face is paralysed as well as the lower, and emotional movements are also involved. Rarely, emotional movements are lost and voluntary movements retained; this is occasionally seen in tumours or other lesions of the temporal lobe and premotor cortex.

Upper-motor neuron facial paralysis occurs in many conditions—vascular accidents, neoplasms, cerebral contusion, degenerative cerebral disease, and so on. It is usually associated with hemiparesis, or with weakness of the upper limb owing to the condensation of fibres which occur in the pyramidal tract in the internal capsule and below, but in cortical and subcortical lesions it may occur independently.

Lower-motor Neuron Paralysis occurs as a result of a lesion of the seventh nucleus or of the nerve itself. The upper and lower halves of the face are affected equally, and there is none of the dissociation of emotional and voluntary movements which may occur in upper-motor neuron paralysis. The reaction of degeneration appears after paralysis has been present for two or three weeks, and contractures may occur, the corners of the mouth being drawn to the affected side, thereby giving a false impression of weakness on the normal side. Fibrillation may be seen. Twitching movements are not uncommon in irritative lesions of the seventh nerve.

By far the most common form of peripheral facial palsy is *Bell's palsy* (*Fig.* 283), which appears to be due to an inflammatory lesion in the facial canal of the temporal bone near the stylomastoid foramen. The onset is rapid, the patient often waking up in the morning to find the face paralysed on one side; in other cases the condition takes a day or two to reach its climax.

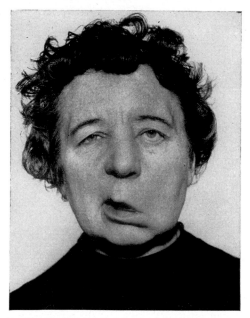

Fig. 283.—Paralysis of the left side of the face, the patient attempting to show her teeth. Note that the left palpebral fissure is wider than the right. (*Mr. Patrick Clarkson.*)

There is often slight pain just below the mastoid at the onset. The eye cannot be closed and is liable to injury by dust; slight ectropion of the lower lid leads to epiphora. Taste in the anterior two-thirds of the affected side of the tongue may be perverted or lost if the disease has spread up the Fallopian canal. At a still higher level, paralysis of the nerve to the stapedius may cause hyperacusis.

Other causes of facial paralysis are less common than Bell's palsy. *Trauma* stands relatively high on the list, whether it be due to stab wounds, gunshot wounds, surgical attacks on the parotid gland and mastoid, or fracture of the petrous portion of the temporal bone. Paralysis usually occurs immediately in fracture cases, but may appear for the first time a week or more after the injury, in which event the prognosis for recovery is good. Among infective causes are *poliomyelitis*, *polyneuritis cranialis*, *polyneuritis of Guillain Barré type*, *gummatous or other form of meningitis*, and *leprosy*. The swelling of the

parotid gland which occurs in *uveoparotid polyneuritis*, a form of sarcoidosis, is often associated with a bilateral facial paralysis. *Geniculate herpes*, in which herpes of the tonsil, soft palate, auditory meatus, and pinna is associated with facial paralysis, is so named from the belief that it is due to a zoster infection of the geniculate ganglion as suggested by Ramsey Hunt.

Neurofibroma of the 8th cranial nerve stretches the adjacent facial nerve and so adds facial palsy to the deafness, vertigo, and tinnitus which occur early in the condition. As the tumour grows it encroaches upon the trigeminal nerve above, with loss of the corneal reflex and sensory loss in the face, and causes cerebellar symptoms by

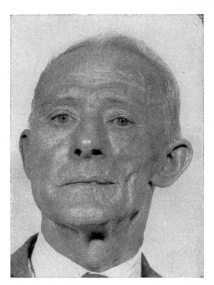

Fig. 284. Left facial hemiatrophy. (*Dr. Denis Williams.*)

posterolateral pressure on the cerebellum. A glioma of the pons may have a somewhat similar symptomatology, but if the nucleus of the facial nerve is involved by the growth the adjacent sixth nucleus is likely to be affected too. Primary and secondary *tumours of the petrous bone* are a rare cause of facial paralysis.

Congenital bilateral facial paralysis is due to absence of the facial nerves. The upper part of the face is sometimes affected alone, or the entire face may be affected. The condition is always bilateral and is then easy to distinguish from facial palsy due to birth injury.

Diseases of Muscle may cause facial weakness. This occurs in the heredofamilial dystrophies and in myotonic dystrophy, but in these conditions the affection is not limited to the face, the weakness is bilateral, and confusion is unlikely to occur. *Myasthenia gravis*, with its ptosis, diplopia, characteristic aggravation by exercise, and ready response to prostigmin, is easy to recognize. *Facial hemiatrophy* (*Fig.* 284) may, superficially, resemble unilateral facial paralysis (*Fig*. 283), but it is differentiated by the fact that the weakness is associated with an atrophy of all the tissues—skin, muscle, bone, nasal cartilage, and even the eye.

Ian Mackenzie.

FACE, SWELLING OF

In this article are included only swellings of the skin and subcutaneous tissues. Malignant and other diseases of the facial bones, etc., are considered under JAW, UPPER, SWELLING OF (p. 451), and BONE, SWELLING ON (p. 100). SALIVARY GLANDS, SWELLING OF, is discussed on page 697. It is necessary therefore to determine the anatomical site of the lesion before considering the pathology. Swellings of the parotid gland will lie below and in front of the ear, or in the anterior prolongation of the gland, the socia parotidis, lying on the outer surface of the masseter. Swelling of the lingual gland will be seen in the floor of the mouth close to the fraenum, while lateral to this will be felt the submaxillary gland, which is also palpable from outside in the submaxillary fossa.

Occasionally a patient may present himself with painless symmetrical *oedema of the face,* commonly of the eyelids where the tissues are loosest. This will almost certainly be of renal origin, cardiac oedema causing oedema primarily in the dependent parts. Another form of oedema which may involve the whole face, but chiefly the eyelids and lips, is angioneurotic oedema (p. 589). The recurrent attacks, each of sudden onset, the familial history, the associated symptoms of burning and irritation, and the presence of similar areas on other parts of the body should clinch the diagnosis.

Swelling of the face and neck is seen in Cushing's disease (p. 584), whether primary or secondary to corticosteroid therapy, and when there is obstruction to the venous return to the heart from the head and neck, as is seen with mediastinal and bronchial neoplasms. In trichiniasis oedema of the eyelids is common, though more diffuse oedema of the face may occur.

A well-defined *cystic swelling* on the face is most commonly a *sebaceous cyst*, a structure freely movable on the deeper tissues but attached to skin. *Dermoid cyst* is much rarer and occurs only at lines of suture, the commonest site being above the outer canthus of the eye. A cyst in this situation is strongly suggestive of dermoid origin, and the diagnosis is confirmed if there is attachment to bone but not to skin, and particularly if depression of the bone has occurred, as it does in long-standing cases, the edge of the depressed area being palpable. *Meningocele* may occur occasionally as a translucent swelling at the root of the nose. It will be present at birth and will exhibit an impulse on coughing or straining. *Haemangiomata* are frequently found on the face and may appear cystic on palpation, but their dusky colour and surrounding dilated vessels will give the clue to their identity. Pigmented naevi will be recognized on sight.

Solid tumours of the face are *lipomata* and *fibromata*. The latter are fairly common and include an important variety, the neurofibromata. These tumours vary in size from being quite minute to an inch or more in diameter, and may be hard or soft. Other stigmata of von Recklinghausen's disease such as pigmentation, either diffuse or in multiple café-au-lait spots, or a profusion of fibromata in other parts of the body, chiefly the trunk, help in the diagnosis. The condition sometimes runs in families.

Rodent ulcer is particularly common on the face and eyelids; it is the exception to find it elsewhere. It starts as a small nodule, often with a 'pearly' appearance, but soon breaks down to form the characteristic indurated ulcer with hard rolled edges (*Fig*. 285). *Epithelioma*, with its

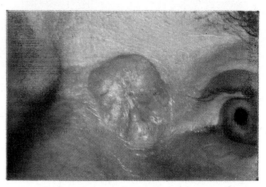

Fig. 285. Rodent ulcer.

raised everted margin and indurated base, and possibly secondary enlargement of regional glands, is another malignant condition found on the face, particularly the lips (*Fig*. 286). Confusion may arise in distinguishing epithelioma from the innocent condition molluscum sebaceum (contagiosum). However, molluscum runs a short course and the centre sloughs leaving an unsightly scar. Biopsy must be done early in any suspicious lesion.

Various inflammatory swellings are found on the face, of which the following are some of the more important:

BOILS and CARBUNCLES are common, particularly around the lips. They have the same character as elsewhere, except that oedema is more marked. ERYSIPELAS is prone to occur on the face. It is marked by a vivid red oedematous swelling associated with fever. The redness tends to spread, the edges being raised and well defined from the healthy skin. The oedema may be continuous, or it may disappear in one place and reappear in another. In very severe cases the fever is high, rigors occur, the cuticle may be raised in blebs, and sloughing may ensue.

ALVEOLAR ABSCESS and DENTAL CARIES are fertile sources of facial swelling, as is abscess in the nasal

sinuses. (*See* JAW, LOWER, SWELLING OF, p. 448.)
ANTHRAX chiefly affects operatives in wool and
horse-hair factories and workers of raw hides.
The disease is characterized by the formation of
a vesicle, which bursts, forms a scab, and then
becomes surrounded by a ring of vesicles around
which is an area of oedema. The diagnosis is
confirmed by discovering anthrax bacilli in the
discharge; a fluid prepared from a drop of fluid
from one of the vesicles contains long chains of

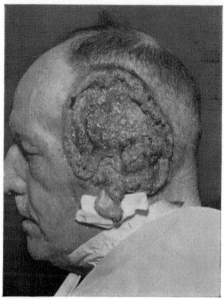

Fig. 286. Epithelioma of the scalp and pinna. (*Courtesy
of the Gordon Museum, Guy's Hospital.*)

large, square-ended, Gram-staining bacilli, which
have a characteristic growth on culture media.
VACCINIA. An accidental infection about the face
may be mistaken for an anthrax pustule. If
inquiry into the attendant circumstances is not
sufficient to exclude the graver disorder, a
bacteriological examination should be made.
PRIMARY SYPHILITIC SORE, if found on the face,
is generally situated on the upper lip, though it
may also occur upon an eyelid, the nose, or elsewhere. It is not so indurated as when on the glans
penis, but the surrounding oedema is more marked,
and the neighbouring lymphatic glands become
enlarged. The condition is often missed because
it is not expected. An absolute diagnosis can be
made by finding the spirochaetae in the serum
discharged from the ulcer, and by serological
tests, though the latter may not yet be positive if
the facial chancre is of recent date.

Unilateral periorbital swelling with diabetes
and signs of meningo-encephalitis in debilitated
patients of the Middle East and Africa may
suggest mucormycosis. A search should be made
for the fungus.

INSECT BITES OR STINGS—from mosquitoes, gnats,
bees, etc.—often cause large, lumpy, irritating

swellings. The only difficulty in diagnosis is
when the original bite or sting has become
indistinguishable owing to infection with pyogenic organisms.

The various skin diseases which may be associated with swelling of the face are considered under
PUSTULES (p. 677); VESICLES (p. 819); WEALS (p.
836); etc.

R. G. Beard.

FACE, ULCERATION OF

The ulcers most often met with on the face are
granulomatous, syphilitic, or malignant. In *lupus
vulgaris* (*see Fig.* 577, p. 574) (now rare) the ulceration is chronic. It begins as a deep-seated
nodule, which after a time breaks down to form
a granular ulcer covered with crusts. Around the
edge the characteristic 'apple jelly' nodules may
be seen. Necrosis of cartilage of the nose and

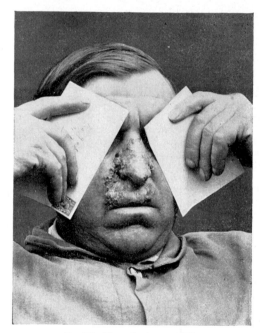

Fig. 287. Ulcerative late syphilide.

pinna is not uncommon, but bone is never attacked. This last fact is important in distinguishing lupus from syphilitic and cancerous ulceration. Lupus usually begins early in life. Other
mycobacteria can produce similar lesions but
they tend to progress more rapidly. *Mycobacteria
balnei* infection often follows a minor injury in
a swimming pool (*swimming pool granuloma*).
M. ulcerans is responsible for endemic ulceration
in Uganda and the Congo known as *Buruli* ulcer.
Although usually on the lower limbs, these ulcers
may occur on the face. The organisms may be
identified on culture. *Syphilitic chancre* may

occur anywhere on the face but especially on the lip. It develops rapidly from a small hard nodule to an indurated, painless ulcer with associated adenopathy. Its rapid growth should distinguish it from an epithelioma, and the *Treponema pallidum* should be found in large numbers on dark-field examination of serous exudate. The Wassermann reaction will be positive 10–14 days from the onset of the sore.

The cutaneous lesions of late syphilis (*Fig.* 287) tend to ulcerate rapidly and deeply, extending at the margins and healing in the centre. A positive Wassermann reaction proves the diagnosis.

Leishmaniasis may cause ulcers in the early stages of infection or later following the development of lupoid lesions. A history of travel in an area where the insect vector is present or the

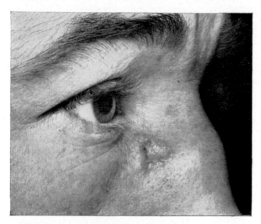

Fig. 288. Rodent ulcer in a man of twenty-one. This followed an injury with a broken bottle three years previously. (*Dr. Peter Hunsell.*)

finding of the causative organism in biopsy material should establish the diagnosis.

Rodent ulcer (*Fig.* 288) occurs most commonly on the face and is identified by its slow development and hard, rolled edge (*see also* p. 573). *Squamous-cell carcinoma*, except when it attacks the lip, is rare on the face. The non-malignant *molluscum sebaceum* (*see* p. 573) is more common.

The ulceration of *leprosy* and *actinomycosis* are rarities that must not be forgotten.

In all cases of ulceration of the face, where the diagnosis is obscure, the possibility of a self-produced lesion must be considered (*see Fig.* 696, p. 700).

P. D. Samman.

FACIES, ABNORMALITIES OF

The study of the face, while it cannot replace systematic examination of the body as a whole, may in many cases direct the observer's attention to the most likely field in which to find data for his diagnosis. Experience alone can teach the

student to detect all that is to be learned from the patient's facies. Photographs and drawings can only illustrate the coarse and obvious defects which are present when the face is at rest or when some particular movement is being sustained. The more subtle abnormalities of expression, the play of the emotions, and the response of the features to intelligence, are often too fleeting and too mobile to allow of reproduction on paper, and sometimes so intangible as to defy any attempt to describe them. Even if the brush of a skilled artist could succeed in portraying the passive vacant aspect of a chronic alcoholic, it must necessarily fail to depict the traitorous tremor which hovers about the corners of his mouth when he opens it to protest his temperance. The shifty eyes of the drug addict, the fatuous placidity of the patient with advanced disseminated sclerosis, the anxious look born of abdominal disease, the explosive suddenness with which the victim of hemiplegia bursts into laughter or tears, the vacant stare of the mentally defective child, the unsmiling sad appearance of the melancholic, the distant removed look of the schizoid personality, the excessive vivaciousness of the hypomaniac—these are a few of the many familiar and striking lessons of the face which must be seen in real life if they are to be learned and utilized. Indeed, the whole of clinical education and practice is concerned with training the eye (and to a lesser extent the other senses in their appropriate functions) to recognize the details of health and disease. It is a truism, almost a platitude, that it is upon the appearance of the face that people rely for the judgement of general health and well-being, for this is the only part of the body which everybody is habitually accustomed to see; and conclusion is based upon certain criteria which experience has led to association with good or bad health—plumpness or wasting, the complexion, the expression, the carriage of the head, for example. That appearances may be deceptive is another truism, indeed a platitude. Experience leads to caution: pallor is by no means the same thing as anaemia; a ruddy complexion is not necessarily a sign of rude health; it is often far from easy to distinguish the appearance of illness from the expression of unhappiness; it is only too easy to mistake for aggression what is really shyness.

The danger of jumping to conclusions and the ridicule that may follow on the revelations of ill-founded speculations are likely to shake faith and discourage an indulgence in the spectacular snap-shot diagnosis.

These warnings apart, the warmest approbation should be extended to the call to the use of observation in a proper clinical approach, as a revolt against the tendency towards the unrestricted, uncritical employment of accessory aids to diagnosis.

Cretinoid Facies. Compared with the general stunted growth of the rest of the body the head is relatively large. The expression is 'stupid' or stolid. The face is broad, and remarkable for thick eyelids, broad flat nose, thick lips (*Fig.* 299, p. 278), and large coarse ears. The mouth is usually open, the tongue may be more or less constantly protruded, and the chin is poorly developed. The hair is scanty and brittle, the skin coarse, dry or muddy, and often almost yellow. Confirmation of the diagnosis may be sought in the dwarfed size of the child, the pendulous 'frog-belly' (*Fig.* 289), and the thick pads of subcutaneous tissue especially frequent

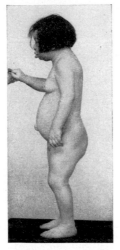

Fig. 289. A female cretin, to show the 'frog-belly'. (*Dr. R. G. Ollerenshaw, Manchester Royal Infirmary.*)

above the clavicles. The lack of mental development, the slow pulse, and subnormal temperature complete the clinical picture. Proof of diagnostic correctness is afforded by the improvement produced by adequate thyroid medication.

Myxoedematous Facies. The dulled intelligence of the patient is betrayed by the apathetic physiognomy (*Fig.* 290). The skin of the myxoedematous face is coarse, dry, sallow, pale, and waxy, with occasionally a tinted rose-purple flush over each cheek. The puffiness of the eyelids may suggest nephritis, but the subcutaneous tissue everywhere is of firm consistence, and doughy rather than oedematous. The tongue is enlarged. The nose is broadened, the ears are thickened, and the lips swollen. The hair is scanty, receding from the forehead, the eyebrows are thin and sparse (although the scantiness of the outer half often regarded as a diagnostic feature occurs too frequently in normal subjects for this to be reliable), the nails brittle and striated. Masses of fatty tissue may be found in the neck and trunk. The slow, husky speech, the expressionless face, and the general attitude of the patient may suggest Parkinsonism, but the diagnosis may be made by paying attention to the physical features just mentioned and by observing the slow pulse, subnormal temperature, and low basal metabolic rate. In hypopituitarism, the eyelids and nose, in contrast to myxoedema, are unaffected, and show no undue fatness. Another point of differentiation is that in pituitary disease complete loss of axillary and pubic hair is common, a feature that does not

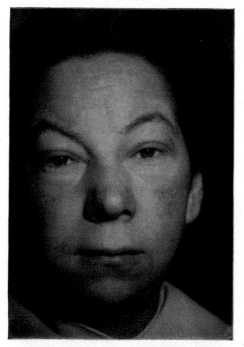
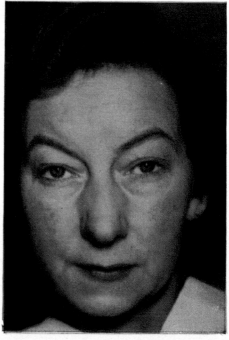

Fig. 290. Facies in myxoedema (left) before and (right) after treatment. (*Dr. P. M. F. Bishop.*)

always occur in myxoedema. In hypopituitarism the face is hairless in males or females and unduly wrinkled. The features are those of a middle-aged Peter (or Pauline) Pan. The skin is soft and smooth and the hair of soft texture, whilst in myxoedema hairs and skin are of coarser quality. The voice in myxoedema is a husky croak, in hypopituitarism normal.

Congenital Syphilitic Facies. The victims of congenital syphilis, after ten or twelve years of age, may present a facies which is unmistakable—an overhanging forehead, perhaps frontal bosses, a depressed nasal bridge (*Fig.* 291), striated scars

eyeballs. In other instances there is a droop of the upper eyelids rather than any tendency to exophthalmos. Inability of the patient to whistle or to blow out his cheek demonstrates the weakness of the orbicularis oris which is often rendered obvious by the large amount of labial mucous membrane exposed while the mouth is at rest.

Myasthenic Facies. In patients suffering from myasthenia gravis there are two types of facies which can hardly be reproduced by other diseases. The first illustrates the patient (*Fig.* 293) that cannot keep her eyes open. The second depends on the characteristic myasthenic smile, almost a sneer. This unfortunate and misleading facial expression is the result of deficient action on the part of the zygomatic and risorius muscles and exemplifies the curious way in which in this disease some muscles are affected and others escape, even when they derive their innervation from the same source.

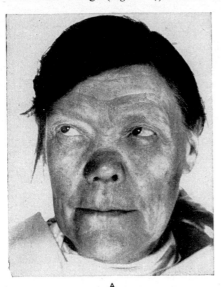

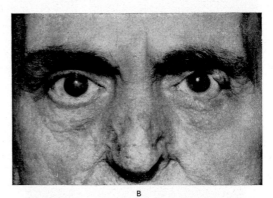

Fig. 291. A, Congenital syphilis, showing depressed nasal bridge and rhagades. (*Dr. J. C. Houston.*) B, Interstitial keratitis and nasal scarring in congenital syphilis. (*Mr. Rex Lawrie.*)

radiating from the corners and other parts of the lips, with a sallow, earthy complexion. Closer observation of the eyes and teeth may detect the opacities of old keratitis and the changes in the upper incisors which were stated by Jonathan Hutchinson to be pathognomonic (*Fig.* 292). These teeth are wide-gapped, irregular, and so deficient in enamel over the anterior and median parts of their cutting edges that the resulting crescentic notch imparts a striking appearance. Such a facies may be accompanied by deafness, mental deficiency, physical infantilism, tibial deformities, and chronic arthritis, especially of the knee-joints. The diagnosis may be clinched if the blood gives positive serological reactions.

Myopathic Facies. Many cases of myopathy show no characteristic facies; others are remarkable for the loose pout of their lips at rest and the 'transverse' character of their smile (*rire en travers*). These features are due to defective facial musculature, particularly to weakness of the orbicularis oris. Paresis of the orbiculares palpebrarum is only evident when an attempt is made to close the eyes, although it may sometimes lead to prominent and perhaps staring

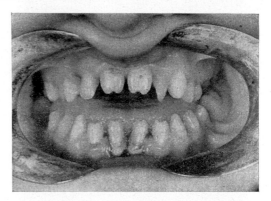

Fig. 292. Hutchinson's teeth in congenital syphilis. Note the upper central incisors which are peg-shaped and notched. (*Professor W. E. Herbert.*)

The *facies of exophthalmic goitre* depends chiefly upon the 'stare' (*Fig.* 294). Surprise or terror is suggested by the prominence of the eyeballs and the retraction of the eyelids. The degree of exophthalmos varies greatly and it may be completely absent; it is sometimes unilateral. The sclera is visible between the edge of the iris and the eyelids; the usual harmony of movement between the eyeball and the eyelid is lacking; normal blinking is much diminished or entirely in abeyance. The surface of the conjunctiva may be abnormally bright and glistening, and the secretion of tears may be

A moist skin and a readiness to flush may often be remarked in the face.

The Facies of Parkinsonism. In this disease a cardinal symptom is muscular rigidity which affects the skeletal muscles generally as well as those of the face. The ocular muscles, however,

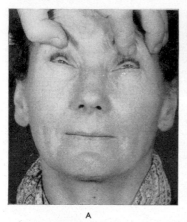 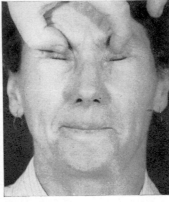 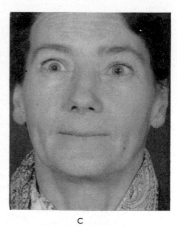

| A | B | C |

Fig. 293. Myasthenia gravis showing: **A**, Inability to keep eyes closed against light traction on upper eyelid; **B**, Effective resistance after prostigmin—note the return of power to the orbicularis oris; **C**, Normal facies under the influence of neostigmine. (*Dr. R. G. Ollerenshaw, Manchester Royal Infirmary.*)

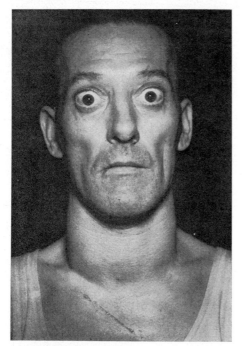

Fig. 294. Exophthalmic goitre. Note lid retraction and enlarged thyroid.

escape and, as a consequence, while the face as a whole is expressionless, 'starchy' or 'masked', the eyes appear to move with natural or even abnormal rapidity; for instance, they will turn in the direction to which the patient desires to look before the head has assumed a corresponding position. The face has often a staring expression, the eyelids being retracted by the tonic spasm of the orbiculares palpebrarum. An absence of normal blinking has been ascribed to the same cause (*Fig.* 537, p. 546). In contrast with the slow development of facial expression under the influence of emotion, there may be marked want of control over the fully developed emotional movement, and the patient protests that the exuberance of his laughter or tears is entirely out of proportion to his feelings of merriment or sorrow.

Parkinsonism may occur in patients who are suffering or have suffered from an attack of *encephalitis lethargica*. This syndrome, which includes the facies, stance, and gait of paralysis agitans, may develop rapidly during the acute stage of the encephalitis, and persist, perhaps in a modified form, for the remainder of the patient's life. In other instances it makes its appearance weeks, months, or years after the acute phase of the disease has subsided, and may progress slowly, so that the patient becomes gradually more and more disabled. In all cases, therefore, in which the syndrome is present it is important to elicit an exact history of the onset of the symptoms, and especially to inquire whether they coincided with or followed some transient illness which may have been wrongly and lightly diagnosed as 'influenza'. The post-encephalitic Parkinsonian syndrome may often be distinguished from that

excessive. In contrast with the white of the eyeballs, there is often considerable dark pigmentation of the eyelids which may also be the site of some oedema. The size of the pupils varies, undue dilatation occurring only in exceptional cases.

of paralysis agitans by the presence of disturbances in pupillary and other reflexes. The facies of Parkinsonism may also be caused by certain drugs, such as chlorpromazine, the picture reverting to normal after stopping the drug (*see* p. 545). *Tabetic Facies.* In a considerable number of cases of locomotor ataxy the appearance of the face is sufficiently striking to afford a clue to diagnosis. The small size or the inequality of the pupils may first attract attention. The drooping of the upper eyelids, combined with some wrinkling of the forehead produced by a compensating effort on the part of the frontalis muscle, imparts a sad expression. This drooping of the eyelid, which may be termed 'pseudo-ptosis' or 'hypotonic ptosis', is not due to any paresis of the

talk is not so noticeable as in the case of healthy individuals.

Facies of Acromegaly. In the course of acromegaly, changes in appearances frequently take place to such a degree that the patient becomes unrecognizable by friends who have known him only before the onset of his disease. These are

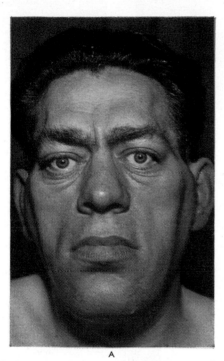 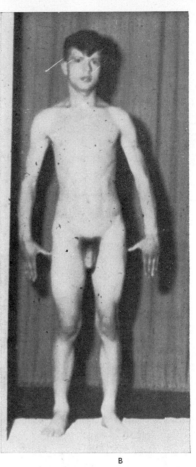

Fig. 295. A, A case of acromegaly, exemplifying the heavy enlargement of the front of the lower jaw. B, Tall acromegalic, originally a pituitary giant. (*Dr. P. M. F. Bishop's case.*)

levator palpebrae superioris, as may be shown by the raising of the lid when the patient is looking upwards, but depends on the fact that this muscle, like most of the muscles of the body, is in a condition of hypotonia so that under the influence of gravity the lid hangs like a half-raised curtain in front of the eyeball. In other respects the face may be normal, but the majority of tabetics have a sallow complexion and very little subcutaneous fat, two conditions which contribute to their generally unhealthy appearance. Many victims of this disease exhibit a deficiency of the emotional reflex movements of the facial muscles; during conversation the play of the features appropriate to the subject of their

the result of abnormal growth of the bony and subcutaneous tissues especially in the skull and extremities. The characteristic facies is brought about by osseous hyperplasia of the frontal ridges, the mastoid, zygomatic, malar, and nasal processes, while the lower jaw is usually enlarged in all directions. The prominent, arched brows, with retreating and wrinkled forehead, the massive nose, the long, thick upper lip, and the heavy chin (*Fig.* 295) form the most conspicuous features. The lower teeth are unduly wide apart and may project some distance in front of the upper. The tongue may be so enlarged as to keep the mouth open and to display many fissures and indentations as the result of its pressure against the teeth. In some cases the lower jaw is not affected, and the face may be described as abnormally square (*type carrée*).

Facies of Mongolian Idiocy (Down's syndrome). This facies is so distinctive that the diagnosis may often be made at a glance (*Fig.* 296). The head

in case of doubt the effect of thyroid treatment may clinch the diagnosis.

The Adenoid Facies is generally recognized in the child sufferer with the essential features of the wide open mouth in consequence of the oral breathing demanded by nasal obstruction, and

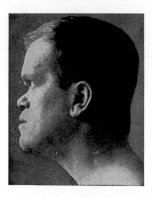

Fig. 296. Achondroplasia with Mongolian idiocy. (*Dr. S. A. K. Wilson.*)

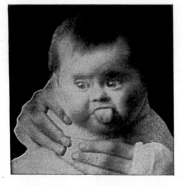

Fig. 297. A Mongolian idiot in infancy. The photograph shows the oblique palpebral fissures and the large protruding tongue.

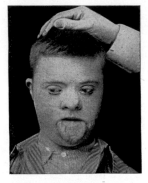

Fig. 298. A Mongolian idiot showing a large flabby tongue, which is deeply fissured. (*Dr. S. A. K. Wilson.*)

is brachycephalic; the palpebral fissures slant obliquely inwards and downwards towards a broad flat nose, rendered even broader by the presence of epicanthus; the eyelids show signs of chronic blepharitis; the ears are large and pitcher-shaped; the lips are fissured and often left open to allow a coarse tongue to protrude (*Figs.* 297, 298); the forehead is downy, and the hair of the scalp scanty, wiry, and frequently mouse-coloured; the complexion is florid and mottled. The almond-shaped eyes, the presence of epicanthus, the florid complexion, and the absence of fatty masses serve to distinguish the Mongolian from the cretinoid idiot (*Fig.* 299);

the overslung lower jaw and dental occlusion with consequent incomplete musculature of the mouth and receding cheeks. The expression is dull, listless, and vacant through inability to concentrate attention. In many cases deafness occurs.

Facies of Hepatolenticular Degeneration of Kinnier Wilson. The characteristic facies of this disease is seen only in advanced cases, and may be described as one of fixed emotion. The slightest attempt to engage in conversation may evoke a sustained expression of exaggerated mirth (*Fig.* 300), which is quite unlike that seen in other diseases of the nervous system. The accompanying photograph also illustrates the tendency to fall

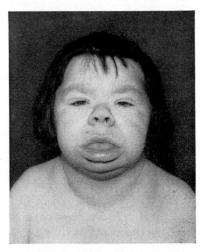

Fig. 299. Female cretin, showing half-closed eyes, thick nose, tongue and lips, fat chin, and squat neck. (*Dr. R. G. Ollerenshaw, Manchester Royal Infirmary.*)

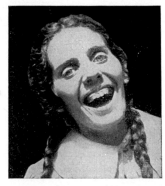

Fig. 300. Facies of familial lenticular degeneration.

to one side when in the sitting position. The malady is associated with bilateral degenerative changes in the lenticular nuclei together with cirrhosis of the liver, due to the excessive amounts of copper in the tissues. The most remarkable feature of the disease is the Kayser-Fleischer ring, a rusty-brown ring of pigment at the periphery of the cornea. In some instances azure blue coloration of the lunulae of the finger-nails has been observed (*Fig.* 301), the density of the colour increasing towards and being limited by

liver is in an early stage. Nor can one diagnose the existence of cirrhosis with certainty even when the facies is that of chronic alcoholism, with its telangiectases over the cheeks, coarsening of the tissues, especially on and around the nose and mouth, with purplish reddening in general. But

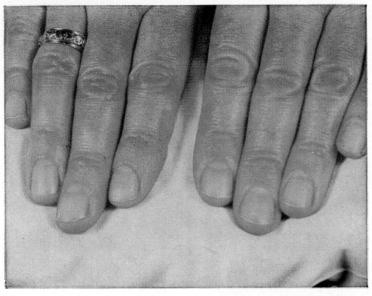

Fig. 301. Azure blue coloration of finger-nails in Kinnier Wilson's disease. (*By kind permission of Drs. Bearn and McKusick, from the 'Journal of the American Medical Association'.*)

the periphery of the lunula. Clinically the liver disease resembles chronic active hepatitis (*see* p. 440). The lenticular changes lead to choreiform or tetanoid tremors and spasticity in the limbs, slowly passing on to contractures and helplessness, now preventable by penicillamine therapy.
Facies of Mitral Stenosis. It is often possible to diagnose mitral stenosis at sight, on account of the remarkable malar hyperaemia and dark-crimson lips contrasting with the yellowish pallor of the forehead, peri-oral and perinasal skin. If one covers the malar regions and the lips the face looks sallow, yet the malar flush and the dark-crimson lips give a look almost of plethora (*Fig.* 302). When cardiac failure occurs and the liver becomes engorged, an element of icterus is added.
Facies of Splenomegalic Polycythaemia (Erythraemia). The coloration of the nose, lips, ears, and palpebral conjunctiva is the chief feature of the facies in this malady, presenting an appearance which may be described as a combination of weather-beatenness, plethora, and cyanosis. The diagnosis depends on discovering pronounced polycythaemia, and generally a large, firm spleen. Polycythaemia may also be secondary to other conditions, cardiac, pulmonary, or malignant disease (*Fig.* 303).
Facies of Cirrhosis of the Liver. There is nothing characteristic in the facies when cirrhosis of the

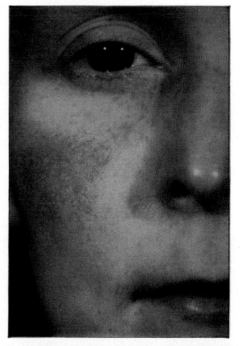

Fig. 302. The facies in mitral stenosis, showing the malar flush. (*Dr. R. G. Ollerenshaw, Manchester Royal Infirmary.*)

in the later stages of cirrhosis the sallow, dull, diffusely pigmented facies is often distinctive, though the actual peculiarities are not easily described.

Facies of Pernicious Anaemia. Though today rarely seen, the facies in Addisonian (pernicious) anaemia (untreated) may be absolutely characteristic in the later stages. There is no emaciation, but the colour is remarkable. Often described as lemon-yellow, it is more often a pale primrose yellow, with a peculiar delicacy in the yellowish tint that is unmistakable when it is fully developed.

Facies of Acute Nephritis. The generally swollen half-bloated look, the partial closing up of the eyes by oedema, are usually unmistakable, but a somewhat similar appearance may be presented by the effects of insect bites, of angioneurotic oedema, or after the administration of aspirin in those with an idiosyncrasy for this drug.

pigmentation only, without any suggestion at the time that there is malignant disease anywhere. It is probably an extreme degree of the liability to diffuse pigmentation of the skin that malignant disease in general tends to produce. It may also

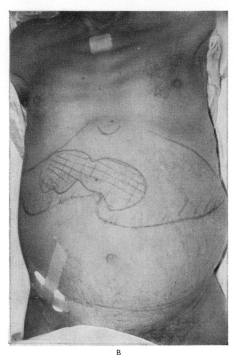

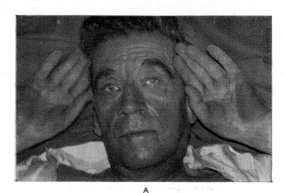

A   B

Fig. 303. Polycythaemia secondary to malignant hepatoma.

Facies of Dermatomyositis. In this rare malady many parts beside the face are involved; it is a collagen disease in which it is more or less fortuitous whether the skin, the muscles, the mucous membranes, or the subcutaneous tissues are most affected. The most characteristic rash consists of a dusky red eruption on the face, over nose and cheeks, periorbital regions, occasionally on forehead and on neck, shoulders, front, and back of chest and arms. The erythema may be mottled or diffuse and either intensely red or cyanotic or a mixture of both. Sometimes on the upper eyelids a dusky lilac hue is seen, the so-called heliotrope rash said to be typical of dermatomyositis.

Facies of Acanthosis Nigricans. The outstanding feature of this disease is the extreme pigmentation which develops in various parts of the body, as in the axillae, groin, nipples, and umbilicus, but also in the neck or face; the degree may be described as what would, more or less, result if a collier's hands were stroked over the skin, producing massive darkening, almost blackening, in the areas affected. Although the disease nearly always indicates abdominal carcinoma, especially carcinoma of the stomach, yet the patient may present himself for treatment on account of the

occur in Cushing's syndrome, acromegaly and the Stein-Leventhal syndrome.

Other colorations of diagnostic significance are those of *haemochromatosis*; the bluish tinge of the cartilage of the ears in *ochronosis*; the patchy pigmentation of the chloasma of pregnancy or that of vitiligo or albinism, and that resulting from prolonged administration of arsenic.

The usual skin lesion of *lupus erythematosus* has a butterfly distribution over the bridge of the nose and the cheeks. The facial skin lesion of *sarcoidosis* may have the same distribution but the eyelids and ears may be infiltrated with brownish nodules.

In *scleroderma* the parchment-like skin may be so tightly drawn over the underlying muscles that the face becomes completely expressionless (*Fig.* 304).

Facies of Addison's Disease. Generalized darkening of the skin of the face may be the first thing to attract attention in a case of Addison's disease, but the distinctive character of the pigmentation is that it occurs in the mucous membranes within the mouth (*Fig.* 536, p. 543), where it tends to be grey, as well as on the skin of the face and other parts of the body, where it is dark brown.

Facies in Cushing's Syndrome (see also Figs. 593, 595, pp. 584, 585) (OBESITY). The red 'moon face' and hirsutism (q.v.) are characteristic and often seen as the result of corticosteroid therapy (*Fig.* 305).

Facies of Argyria. This condition is rare nowadays. It may still be met with amongst workers in silver. The coloration is even and uniform, not patchy as in Addison's disease or acanthosis nigricans; it has a blue-grey appearance which persists when pressure is applied to the skin, and does not blanch as does a cyanotic skin. It is a subcutaneous rather than a dermal pigmentation.

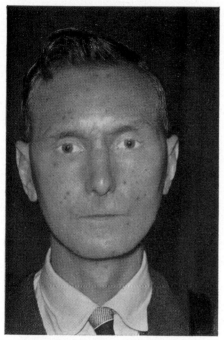

Fig. 304. Scleroderma, showing the pigmented, mask-like, smooth expressionless face.

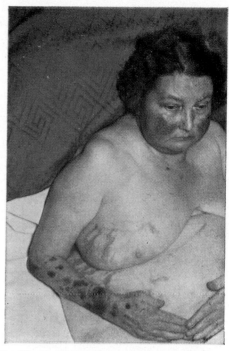

Fig. 305. The Cushingoid picture of corticosteroid therapy. Note also the striae and subcutaneous haemorrhages.

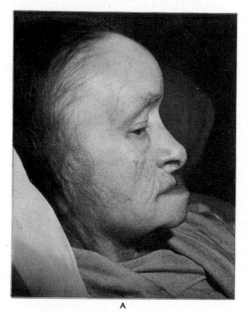

A

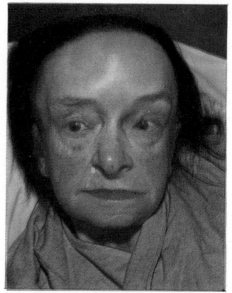

B

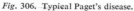

Fig. 306. Typical Paget's disease.

Facies of Acute Illness. Erysipelas, measles, scarlatina, and mumps often permit of immediate facial diagnosis. In lobar pneumonia the bright eyes, flushed cheeks, active alae nasi, and labial herpes constitute what may fairly be termed a typical picture. Respiratory distress advertises itself by expression of anxiety and fear in pulmonary and cardiac disease, although alterations in colour due to imperfect oxygenation are contributory to the appearance. Labial herpes (herpes febrilis) may also accompany many other febrile diseases, even a simple coryza, and may be due to sun sensitivity.

Alterations in Contour. In addition to those already described, some rarer conditions may be mentioned as generally identifiable at sight. In osteitis deformans (Paget's disease) the face has the shape of an inverted triangle and, in consequence of the prominence of the forehead, appears to be toppling forwards (*Fig.* 306). In leontiasis ossea there is progressive irregular enlargement of the bones of the cranium and face, with consequent asymmetry; the superior maxilla is particularly prominent. The rare condition of oxycephaly ('steeple head') need be seen only once to be subsequently recognizable. An opportunity to recognize leprosy rarely occurs in this country: illustrations in textbooks show the leonine face with superabundance of skin, bronzed and coloured patches, and complete disappearance of hair, eyebrows, and eyelashes.

The General Appearance of a face compounded of shape, colour, texture of the skin, and other contributions at once suggests such conditions as malignant disease and the tuberculous diathesis. The hectic flush, long eyelashes, and 'appealing expression', more familiar perhaps in the past than at the present day, were familiar expectations of *pulmonary tuberculosis*. The peculiar (*café au lait*) coloration in bacterial endocarditis may be recalled and the virile (hirsute) facies displayed by a woman suffering from a tumour of the suprarenal cortex or of the basophilic cells of the pituitary gland hardly requires description. The male eunuchoid presents a peculiar old-looking, wax-pale, hairless, wizened, wrinkled appearance.

The Eyes alone often provide diagnostic evidence of general as well as local disease. Pigmentation, oedema of the lids, and exophthalmos have been mentioned. A squint may demand a detailed consideration of the central nervous system, as will spontaneous nystagmus. Icterus of the conjunctiva may be early evidence of what will become generalized later, and the comparatively rare but striking appearance of blue sclerotics points to fragilitas ossium. 'Rings under the eyes' and bagginess of the tissues are generally devoid of any baleful significance but denote only lack of tone in the tissues.

Involuntary Movements besides the tremor of the head of old age and paralysis agitans may be due to alcohol, tobacco, or other drugs. The head-nodding of children may be mentioned in this connexion. Other involuntary movements point to chorea, habit spasms, or tics. In aortic insufficiency there may be a constant jerking of the head synchronous with the heart-beat (De Musset's syndrome). Facial paralysis and the peculiar condition of facial hemi-atrophy or hemi-hypertrophy are sometimes obvious, sometimes evident only on careful examination.

Expression. In the foregoing, many references have been made to expression. Differentiation of the emotional from the physical factors may be in many cases impossible. There may be an expression of melancholy or depression, of anxiety, nervous tension, or querulousness. In some cases depression hangs over the patient like a black cloud, the face being dull, expressionless, and uninterested in what is going on around her.

F. Dudley Hart.

FAECES, INCONTINENCE OF

Evacuation of the contents of the rectum without voluntary initiation is usually due to disease of the nervous system, but there are also some otherwise normal persons who find it difficult to withstand an imperative call to stool, as for instance in the course of diarrhoea or dysentery, and this is particularly common in children and old age. Mechanical incontinence is seen from time to time in patients whose sphincters have been injured by extensive perineal tears in childbirth or by local operations for fistulae, haemorrhoids, or fissure.

With regard to the nervous system, a distinction must be drawn between three groups of cases: (1) Patients with mental disease, who are apt to pass motions at inappropriate times and in unsuitable places, not because they are truly incontinent but because they are careless of social usages. This occurs in both organically determined psychoses and in the primary psychoses, and may be seen in persons with injuries to the frontal lobes, and during epileptic automatism. (2) Episodes of incontinence of urine and faeces during an epileptic fit, whether in idiopathic or symptomatic epilepsy. Faecal incontinence is rare in such cases, but it is apt to occur when the motions happen to be unduly soft. Fits in which there is isolated incontinence, without a convulsion or any considerable disturbance of consciousness, can be caused by a midline lesion (e.g., meningioma) involving both paracentral lobules on the inner aspect of the hemispheres. (3) Incontinence due to interruption of the pathway between the cerebrum and the rectum is the most common type, and is usually seen in affections of the spinal cord or cauda equina.

Unilateral lesions of the spinal cord seldom disturb the sphincters, but bilateral lesions involving the lateral columns cause, first, a precipitancy of defaecation, and later on, reflex evacuation which cannot be controlled by the will. There are usually, but not invariably, other signs of pyramidal tract involvement, and conversely there may be extensive pyramidal involvement with incontinence—a state of affairs often seen in disseminated sclerosis. The sphincter remains contracted in these cases unless there is a generalized depression of reflex activity, as in the presence of severe sepsis or shock. Where incontinence is due to an affection of the cauda equina, on the other hand, the sphincters are relaxed or weak and there is almost invariably some degree of sensory loss in the rectum and in the sacral dermatomes. If the faeces are very hard and bulky, they may be retained even though the neurological conditions for incontinence are present. It is therefore necessary to inquire as to the consistency of the motions when assessing sphincter functions.

Ian Mackenzie.

FAINTING

Attacks of transient loss of consciousness are common and the causes range from simple vasovagal attacks to epilepsy. Furthermore, a complaint of 'fainting' may not always imply actual loss of consciousness; some patients may mean no more than a feeling of unsteadiness or 'lightheadedness'. It is important, as always, to obtain from the patient and, whenever possible, from a witness a precise description of the nature of the attacks. The term 'syncope' has a more exact connotation and can be defined as 'transient loss of consciousness due to a reduction in the cerebral blood-flow'. It is this condition with which this discussion will be mainly concerned.

1. Vasomotor Syncope. This rather imprecise term will be taken to include the large group of conditions in which the cardiac output and blood-pressure fall as a result of a sudden fall in peripheral resistance and in the central venous pressure.

Vasovagal Attacks. These are extremely common and are almost always of no serious significance. Many predisposing factors are known including emotion, fatigue, prolonged standing, and chronic illness of almost any kind. There are other, more serious, conditions of which an apparently simple faint may be a manifestation. Haemorrhage causes syncope as a direct result of the fall in central venous pressure; if the bleeding is external no diagnostic difficulty arises, but, with internal bleeding as, for example, into the gastro-intestinal tract, syncope may occur before there is any direct evidence such as haematemesis or melaena. The mechanism whereby haemorrhage causes syncope can also operate in a few patients with very large varicose veins or angiomatous malformations in the legs in which the blood accumulates in the upright posture. Severe pain can also cause syncope as in dissecting aneurysm or myocardial infarction although, in the latter condition, there may also be a fall in cardiac output sufficient on its own to cause syncope. In elderly patients especially, syncope is quite commonly the presenting symptom of myocardial

infarction; on recovering consciousness the patient may not complain of chest pain, being perhaps more preoccupied with any trauma he may have suffered in his fall.

The clinical picture is well known, not least to the many medical students who have fainted at their first operation. The patient is nearly always in the upright position; indeed, a 'faint' occurring in the recumbent position is good evidence of some cause other than a vasovagal attack. A minor exception to this rule is the syncope experienced by some pregnant women while lying on their backs; this is probably due to pressure by the uterus on the inferior vena cava producing a fall in venous return. Prodromal symptoms include a feeling of weakness, nausea, sweating, and epigastric discomfort; within a few seconds or minutes the patient falls unconscious. The pulse is of small volume and slow and the blood-pressure very low; the face is pale and the skin cold and sweating. Incontinence of urine and muscular twitching are rare but can occur in transient loss of consciousness from any cause and do not necessarily imply that the attack is epileptic. Recovery is rapid as the cerebral blood-flow increases in the recumbent posture unless the patient is prevented from falling as in a crowd or by well-meaning bystanders. Weakness and nausea may persist for some time after recovery of consciousness.

The term 'vaso-vagal', which has been used to denote this type of vasomotor syncope, is now widely accepted. However, in the past, it was used, originally by Sir William Gowers, to describe curious 'seizures' which resembled the attacks described above in most respects. They differed only in that loss of consciousness was rare and, usually, no precipitating cause could be found. A theory that they represented a specific entity and were possibly epileptic in nature has now been discredited and it seems certain that these attacks were no more than a mild form of vasomotor syncope occurring in unusually susceptible subjects. All practising physicians have seen patients who faint not only from venepuncture but from a tourniquet or sphygmomanometer cuff being put around an arm.

Postural Hypotension. This condition overlaps with vasovagal syncope which, as has been said, almost always occurs when the patient is upright. It is, however, worth distinguishing a group of patients who have a steep fall in blood-pressure whenever they stand upright. In some of these patients a neurological cause for the failure of vasoconstriction and other compensatory mechanisms can be identified; to others the label 'idiopathic' has been applied but, in many of these, it is probable that detailed investigation would localize a neurological lesion.

Many drugs can cause a marked postural fall in blood-pressure. Among these are hypotensive agents such as ganglion-blocking drugs, guanethidine, and bethanidine; nitrites, phenothiazine derivatives, monoamine oxidase inhibitors, imipramine, barbiturates, amitriptyline, and other psychotherapeutic agents have also been incriminated. The hypotensive agent prazosin seems to be unusually liable to cause sudden loss of consciousness for periods of time ranging up to one hour. It is not known whether this is always due to postural hypotension and it may be a specific side-effect of this drug. Lesions of peripheral nervous pathways can produce a similar effect by interruption of the afferent or efferent pathways of reflex arcs. Thus postural hypotension is well known in tabes, diabetes, and acute polyneuritis, and has been described in alcoholic and carcinomatous neuropathy and in porphyria. Lesions of the central pathways are less easy to demonstrate but degeneration of the intermediolateral column in the spinal cord, vascular lesions of the brain-stem and craniopharyngioma, and other parasellar tumours, possibly involving the hypothalamus, have been demonstrated in some cases. Many of these neurological conditions have in common an abnormal response to the Valsalva manœuvre in that the blood-pressure continues to fall throughout the period of strain and no overshoot or reflex bradycardia occurs.

Carotid-sinus Syncope. In many subjects massage of a carotid sinus can cause bradycardia with some fall in blood-pressure. In some, mostly elderly patients, these changes may be more marked and this increased sensitivity of the carotid-sinus reflex can be produced by neoplastic or inflammatory lesions in the neck or by digitalis intoxication. In a few patients the haemodynamic changes may be so profound and the reflexes so easily elicited, as by a tight collar, shaving, or turning the head, that recurrent syncope occurs. Various types of carotid-sinus syncope have been described with or without bradycardia in addition to the hypotension but the distinction is largely of academic interest. The carotid sinus is innervated by the glossopharyngeal nerve, and a rare condition which may be related to carotid-sinus syncope is the fainting sometimes associated with glossopharyngeal neuralgia, a condition similar to trigeminal neuralgia but causing pain in the tongue, pharynx, and ear.

2. Cardiac Syncope. In this group of conditions the cardiac output falls as a result of a primary cardiac lesion. It differs from vasomotor syncope in that attacks are much less closely related to the upright posture.

Stokes-Adams Attacks. These are due to cardiac arrest usually in asystole but occasionally in ventricular fibrillation on a basis of atrioventricular block. Loss of consciousness can occur in any posture and is abrupt. The patient is pale and pulseless; respiration continues. After about 15–20 seconds twitching may begin due to cerebral anoxia. The attack usually lasts for about 30 seconds but may last longer and death may result. On recovery the patient becomes flushed; this is due to well-oxygenated blood which has been in the pulmonary capillaries during the period of circulatory arrest being flung into systemic capillaries which are widely dilated as a result of the accumulation of vasodilator metabolites. Occasionally, if the attacks occur when the patient is asleep, the only complaint may be of waking with the face feeling hot and flushed.

Paroxysmal Dysrhythmias. A paroxysm of tachycardia with a heart-rate much in excess of 200 per minute may cause syncope as diastolic filling of the heart is markedly reduced at these heart-rates.

Central Circulatory Obstruction. Syncope on effort and, more seriously, at rest is a well-recognized feature of aortic stenosis. The mechanism is not clear as this valve lesion is not associated with a low cardiac output unless failure has occurred. It may be that baroceptors within the left ventricular wall, stimulated by the very high pressure, are in some way responsible. Effort syncope is also not uncommon in other obstructive lesions such as pulmonary stenosis and severe pulmonary hypertension, but it is rare in mitral stenosis. The acute circulatory obstruction produced by massive pulmonary embolism or by the impaction of a left atrial thrombus or myxoma in the mitral orifice may also cause syncope. Obstruction to cardiac filling due to cardiac tamponade and constrictive pericarditis can have the same effect.

Cyanotic Attacks. Syncope in Fallot's tetralogy and other types of cyanotic congenital heart disease is due not so much to a fall in cardiac output as to a sudden increase in the veno-arterial shunt. This can be due to a fall in systemic resistance or to an increase in the severity of a muscular infundibular stenosis. There is little change in blood-pressure, but the patient becomes deeply cyanosed and the murmur of pulmonary stenosis becomes much softer as the greater part of the systemic venous return is shunted into the aorta via the ventricular septal defect.

Ischaemic Heart Disease. Syncope due to acute myocardial infarction has already been discussed under VASOMOTOR SYNCOPE, p. 283.

3. Syncope due to Cerebral Vascular Disease. Fainting is rare as a symptom of disease of the carotid arteries and their branches but is more common with stenosis or occlusion of the vertebral arterial system. Atherosclerosis of the vertebral or basilar arteries and external compression of the vertebral arteries by cervical spondylosis or in the Klippel-Feil syndrome can be responsible for syncopal attacks which may be induced by sudden rotatory movements of the neck.

4. Miscellaneous. There is a group of conditions in which syncope is associated with a rise in intrathoracic and intra-abdominal pressure. This includes *cough syncope* in which loss of consciousness occurs at the end of a violent paroxysm of coughing. A series of coughs produces the same circulatory effects as a Valsalva manœuvre and a marked fall in cardiac output and blood-pressure, probably combined with some degree of arterial hypoxaemia, is the mechanism of the syncope. The *breath-holding attacks* of early childhood producing syncope and cyanosis probably have a similar mechanism. The mechanism of *micturition syncope* is not fully understood.

It occurs typically when, after heavy beer-drinking, the subject rises in the middle of the night to pass urine. The sudden assumption of the upright posture and the vasodilatory action of alcohol are certainly relevant factors and this condition may be nothing more than a vasomotor syncope. However, it is possible that afferent impulses from the bladder may play some part.

Differential Diagnosis. The most important condition from which syncope must be distinguished is *epilepsy*. This can be very difficult but a careful history will usually resolve the problem. Epileptic attacks are characteristically stereotyped in their nature and duration and often occur without warning. Even if there is an aura it bears little resemblance to the prodromal symptoms of syncope except, possibly, in the case of temporal-lobe epilepsy. Most varieties of syncope, with the notable exception of cardiac syncope, occur almost exclusively in the upright posture whereas the onset of an epileptic fit is unrelated to posture. The typical tonic and clonic phases of major epilepsy should not be confused with the minor twitches which may occur in syncope if a history can be obtained from a reliable eyewitness. Urinary incontinence, a very common feature of epilepsy, is not a major differentiating factor as it can occur in severe or prolonged syncope. Electro-encephalography is certainly of value in some cases but, even with this aid, some doubt may remain.

Consciousness is not lost in *vertigo* so that a history from the patient himself should elicit an account of the typical sensation of rotation. However, the use by the patient of such terms as 'giddiness' to describe the premonitory symptoms of vasomotor syncope together with the nausea which is common to both conditions may confuse the unwary.

Hysterical attacks are nearly always described by the patients as 'faints' but the gracefully dramatic fall into a convenient armchair bears no resemblance to syncope in which the patient collapses like a house of cards. Swoons are out of fashion unless one includes the hysterical faints of teenage girls at 'pop' sessions. In the past, revivalist meetings had the same effect; the effects of the preaching of Wesley in the eighteenth century have been paralleled in the twentieth by the performances of Presley.

Hyperventilation is usually a hysterical phenomenon and the feeling of light-headedness induced may be described as faintness. Here, as always, a careful history will resolve the issue but it is worth recalling that hyperventilation followed by a Valsalva manœuvre will infallibly cause loss of consciousness. This is known variously as the 'mess trick' or the 'fainting lark'.

P. R. Fleming.

FATIGUE

Fatigue or excessive tiredness after exertion inadequate to cause it may occur in any condition of ill health, whether it be organic or psychogenic, which has lasted more than a few days or weeks. It may be caused by a deficiency state due to inadequacy of hormones, minerals, electrolytes, or vitamins necessary for the maintenance of normal health; to lack of or abnormality of blood; to chronic infection; new growth; lack of sleep; or states of anxiety, depression, unhappiness, or boredom. Examples of the more common causes are:

1. Continued unhappiness, boredom, or disappointment; overwork, lack of sleep.

2. Anxiety, tension, and depressive states.

3. Neoplasia, often but not always associated with loss of weight. Leukaemia. Hodgkin's disease.

4. Anaemia from any cause.

5. Chronic infection, e.g., tuberculosis, brucellosis, subacute bacterial endocarditis.

6. Connective-tissue inflammatory disorders such as rheumatoid arthritis or systemic lupus erythematosus.

7. Metabolic states, as in uraemia.

8. Endocrine disorder: e.g., hyper- or hypothyroidism, Addison's disease, or Simmonds's disease.

9. Malnutrition. Undernutrition. Avitaminosis. Colitis or Crohn's disease.

10. Electrolyte disturbances. Hyponatraemia, hypokalaemia, hyper- or hypocalcaemia.

11. Persistent chronic pain causing lack of sleep as in Paget's disease or metastatic disease of bone.

12. Chronic neurological disorders, e.g., myasthenia gravis, Parkinson's disease.

13. Chronic drug intoxication, e.g., alcoholism, barbiturates.

There is no end to the medical disorders which may cause fatigue. Loss of weight may suggest neoplasia, undernutrition, hypermetabolic states, or chronic infective and/or inflammatory conditions. Anaemia is a common cause and is usually readily investigated and treated. States of unhappiness, anxiety, or depression may not initially be evident but are common causes and may co-exist with organic disease. Anything which interferes with natural sleep at night contributes to fatigue in the day, good examples being ankylosing spondylitis, simple insomnia, or anxiety or depressive states. So wide is the reference that there is little point in extending a classification which would inevitably cover most of the conditions in medicine.

F. Dudley Hart.

FEMORAL SWELLING

By a femoral swelling is meant a swelling in Scarpa's triangle. The boundaries of this triangle are definite on paper, but in a fat patient they may be difficult to identify. Nevertheless two landmarks, the spine of the pubis and the anterior superior spine of the ileum, can always be made out, however fat the patient, the former being identified by tracing upwards the readily felt tendon of the adductor longus muscle, and a line joining these two points and curved slightly downwards can be taken to indicate the site of Poupart's ligament, and to separate the inguinal from the femoral region. Mistakes are often made, especially in fat people, because a horizontal crease in the thigh which lies below— sometimes as much as five cm.—is mistaken for the ligament. The first point in making the diagnosis is to decide definitely that the swelling is femoral, the next to determine its nature.

In many instances the diagnosis is obvious. A well-marked acute adenitis with redness and oedema of the skin, and an undoubted source of infection such as a sore toe or other septic lesion in the territory drained by the infected glands, can hardly be mistaken for anything else. An aneurysm of the femoral artery showing expansile pulsation is equally unmistakable. Supposing, however, the signs are not so clear, then the various conditions may be classed broadly under two heads: (1) Swellings that are reducible and give an impulse on coughing; (2) Swellings that are irreducible and do not give an impulse on coughing.

1. Reducible Swellings with an Impulse are: (*a*) Femoral hernia (reducible); (*b*) Saphena varix; (*c*) Psoas abscess. All these give an impulse on coughing; are reducible on pressure; may disappear on lying down and reappear on standing. How then is one to distinguish between them?

a. FEMORAL HERNIA (REDUCIBLE). The sex of the patient is no real guide, for though it is more usual to find a femoral hernia in a woman than in a man, this is not sufficient to base the diagnosis on. Before puberty it is rare in either sex. A femoral hernia leaves the abdomen through the femoral canal and turns directly forward, forming a tumour in the upper and inner part of the femoral region; then, finding the line of least resistance, it turns upwards, extending often above Poupart's ligament, thus simulating an inguinal hernia. More rarely, the hernia extends downwards along the femoral vessels. Its course must be remembered in attempting to discover whether the swelling is reducible. If it is large and contains intestine it will be resonant, and a gurgling may be heard or felt on reduction, distinguishing it at once from all other femoral swellings. If it is reduced and the finger held over the femoral aperture, the hernia will be felt projected forcibly against the finger when the patient is asked to cough. If a swelling is complained of, and none is found even on standing and straining, it is suggestive of femoral hernia with only occasional descent, and the patient should be examined at another time after exercise.

b. SAPHENA VARIX is a localized dilatation of the saphenous vein at the saphenous opening, immediately before it joins the femoral vein. It may easily be confounded with a femoral hernia, but it forms a swelling just below the position of a femoral hernia, it disappears on lying down, reappears on standing, and gives an impulse on coughing. A little care, however, should suffice to distinguish the two. The impulse is quite different—in a saphena varix it is more in the nature of a thrill, such as may be felt in a varicocele or in big varicose veins in the leg. If, while the patient is standing, a finger is pressed on the swelling, it collapses gradually, and as the finger is withdrawn the swelling follows, regaining its shape like an air-ball, whereas a hernia comes out with a pop. A saphena varix is almost always associated with varicose veins in the leg, though none may show between the knee and Scarpa's triangle.

c. PSOAS ABSCESS. The need to differentiate between this and the two conditions mentioned above exists only when the abscess has extended from the iliac region, has passed under Poupart's ligament and the femoral vessels, and is pointing in the inner part of Scarpa's triangle. There is an impulse on coughing and the swelling is reducible; but another swelling is to be found above Poupart's ligament, and fluctuation is to be obtained between the two. Conclusive proof can be found by an examination of the back. This should be made with the patient standing and the whole length of the back and the hips exposed. An angular kyphotic curve may be seen at once, or, if that is not present, there may be rigidity and impaired movement denoting some disease on the anterior surfaces of the bodies of the vertebrae. The spine should be radiographed.

2. Irreducible Swellings without Impulse: (*a*) Femoral hernia (irreducible); (*b*) Lymphatic glands—inflammatory or malignant; (*c*) Primary tumours—lipoma, fibroma, sarcoma; (*d*) Ectopic testis.

a. FEMORAL HERNIA (IRREDUCIBLE). An irreducible femoral hernia which presents itself as a rounded elastic swelling in Scarpa's triangle is commoner than one with the classic characters of a hernia. The irreducibility may be accounted for in four ways: (i) Strangulation; (ii) A piece of omentum adherent to and plugging the neck; (iii) An empty sac but a mass of extraperitoneal fat around it; (iv) A hydrocele of the sac.

If strangulation has occurred there will be the signs of intestinal obstruction, and the hernia will be tender. It must be remembered that the swelling may be but a small one, and when the patient is very fat it may be missed.

It is usual to find around the sac of a femoral hernia a quantity of extraperitoneal fat, even in a thin person, and it is quite impossible to say without dissection whether the swelling is due to a plug of omentum inside the sac or to a collection of fat outside it.

A hydrocele may be formed as a result of a long-standing hernia into which there has been no descent of bowel or omentum, and in which the communication with the general peritoneal cavity has become constricted or closed. The sac may then become cystic and filled with fluid. Fluctuation may be obtained in the swelling, though it is often only on dissection that the exact nature of the condition is revealed. A hernial swelling is single, and though it may be movable in some directions it is always tied down by its neck to the aperture of the femoral canal.

b. ENLARGED GLANDS may be: (i) Inflammatory; (ii) Malignant (*see* p. 517).

Chronically inflamed glands may be hard to differentiate from a small irreducible femoral hernia. A gland is usually ovoid and firm, while the hernia is globular and elastic. The whole limb is to be examined to see whether there is any possible source of infection, and the whole patient to see whether there is a general enlargement of the glands, as in lymphadenoma. The chief distinguishing feature between the two conditions is that femoral hernia forms only one swelling, whilst it is rare for only one gland in its group to be picked out by an infecting agent. Therefore, if there is more than one swelling the chances are that these are glands. Perchance both conditions are present, a femoral hernia and enlarged glands—a very difficult combination unless the femoral hernia happens to be reducible or gives an impulse on coughing. In such a case an attempt should be made to feel the neck of the sac running up to the femoral canal.

c. PRIMARY NEW GROWTHS. A lipoma is relatively common in the subcutaneous tissues over Scarpa's triangle. It has the characteristic soft texture and lobulated outline, and can be felt to lie outside the fascial envelope of the thigh with no deep connexions. Fibroma and sarcoma are rare in this situation.

d. ECTOPIC TESTIS. One of the places into which a testis may be drawn abnormally is Scarpa's triangle, which it reaches by passing over Poupart's ligament. The facts that the swelling has the shape of the testis, though generally smaller than normal, and that the corresponding half of the scrotum is empty, make the diagnosis easy.

Certain swellings are neither truly femoral nor truly inguinal, but betwixt and between, bulging Poupart's ligament forwards. They are generally deep, and on that account obscure. They may be due to:

1. Distension of the hip-joint, as in tuberculous disease of the hip.

2. Distension of the bursa between the tendon of the ilio-psoas muscle and the capsule of the hip-joint. This condition is often difficult to distinguish from psoas abscess or from distension of the hip-joint, with which, indeed, it often communicates. Diagnosis may be aided by puncturing the swelling with an aspirating needle.

3. Osteophytic outgrowths from the acetabulum in osteo-arthritis of the hip-joint.

R. G. Beard.

FEVER, PROLONGED (PROLONGED PYREXIA)

A fever may be described as prolonged if it persists beyond 3 weeks. In some instances there are signs or symptoms or facts in the history which lead to an explanation, in others the cause of the pyrexia may remain uncertain for weeks, and elucidation may necessitate resorting to more than one special method of diagnosis from amongst the following:

Blood-counts to see if there is leucocytosis, and, if so, whether there is a relative polymorphonuclear increase suggestive of purulent infection and to see if any abnormal cells are present.

Serum agglutination tests, for typhoid fever, paratyphoid fever, abortus fever.

Blood-cultures, positive in some cases of streptococcal, staphylococcal, or meningococcal septicaemia or infective endocarditis, and in the first week of typhoid or paratyphoid fever.

Urine-cultures, yielding evidence not only when the urinary tracts are themselves involved, as in coliform infections, but sometimes also when the kidneys although healthy are eliminating living organisms from the septicaemic blood-stream, as, for instance, in typhoid fever, pneumococcal, streptococcal, or staphylococcal septicaemia.

Bacterial swabs if appropriate and smears for malignant cells.

Lumbar puncture, revealing for example unexpected meningococcal or tuberculous meningitis.

X-ray examination of the thorax, kidney, colon, and elsewhere, to identify or exclude infection or neoplasm.

Rectal and vaginal examination, for the possibility of prostatic or pelvic lesions.

Tissue cultures, e.g., from bone, spleen, or liver biopsy.

Animal inoculations with blood, sputum or urine, for instance in spirochaetosis icterohaemorrhagica or tuberculosis.

CAUSES OF PROLONGED PYREXIA

The list of conditions that may cause prolonged pyrexia is lengthy. The relative frequency of the different causes varies greatly from country to country and, to a less extent, from time to time. The more common conditions to consider are:

1. Specific Fevers:
Viral:
    Infectious mononucleosis
    Coxsackie B diseases
Salmonella:
    Typhoid
    Paratyphoid
    Typhimurium
Rickettsia:
    Epidemic and scrub typhus
    Rocky Mountain spotted fever
    Q fever
    Trench fever
Chlamydia
Psittacosis
Fungus:
    Coccidioidomycosis
    Histoplasmosis
Spirochaete:
    Syphilis
    Rat bite fever
Brucella:
    Abortus and melitensis fever
Tuberculous disease

Acute and subacute bacterial endocarditis
Tularaemia.

2. Bacteraemia:

Staphylococcal
Streptococcal
Meningococcal
Gonococcal (rarely)
Coliforms.

3. Localized Infection:

Prostatic abscess
Ischiorectal abscess
Pyosalpinx
Suppurating ovarian cyst
Parametritic abscess
Empyema of the maxillary antrum
Frontal sinus or ethmoidal air cells
Osteomyelitis
Suppurating lymph-nodes in neck, axilla, groin
Mammary or submammary abscess
Empyema thoracis
Lung abscess
Hepatic abscess
Renal abscess
Splenic abscess
Empyema of gall-bladder
Suppurative cholangitis
Suppurative pyelephlebitis
Subdiaphragmatic abscess
Bronchiectasis
Appendicular abscess
Perinephric abscess
Diverticulitis
Lumbar and iliac retroperitoneal abscess
Psoas abscess
Actinomycosis of jaw, cheek, neck, lung, liver, spine, or caecum.

4. Infective and Inflammatory Conditions:

Pyelonephritis and other urinary infections
Papillary necrosis
Chronic cystitis
Chronic cholecystitis
Phlebitis
Thyroiditis
Pneumonia and pneumonitis
Bronchopneumonia
Parametritis
Vesiculitis
Dysenteric colitis, bacillary or amoebic
Ulcerative colitis
Crohn's disease (regional enteritis)
Pancreatitis
Familial Mediterranean fever
Sarcoidosis.

5. Non-purulent Hepatic Affections:

Cirrhosis
Secondary carcinoma
Hepatitis, subacute and chronic

6. The Connective-tissue Disorders:

Rheumatoid arthritis
Rheumatic fever
Systemic lupus erythematosus
Polyarteritis nodosa and other arteriopathies
Polymyositis and dermatomyositis
Giant cell arteritis
Scleroderma, rarely

7. Blood Diseases:

Aplastic anaemia
Agranulocytosis
Lymphatic myeloid or monocytic leukaemia, acute or chronic
Haemolytic anaemias

8. Diseases of Tropics and Subtropics:

Malaria
Trypanosomiasis
Kala-azar
Plague
Relapsing fever
Filariasis
Leprosy
Schistosomiasis

9. Meningeal and Cerebral Haemorrhage.

10. Skin Conditions:

Pemphigus
Severe or exfoliative dermatitis
Bullous pemphigoid

11. Malignancy:

Lymphoma (Hodgkin's disease, Lymphosarcoma)
Sarcoma
Carcinoma

12. Allergic (Antigen-antibody Reactive) Conditions, e.g.:

Anaphylactoid purpura
Allergic skin rashes
Post-cardiac injury syndrome

13. Fictitious Pyrexia produced by Malingerers.

14. Drug Reactions, e.g.:

Sulpha drugs
Antibiotics
Arsenicals
Iodides
Barbiturates, etc.

Such a list is bound to be incomplete and cannot be comprehensive. Space does not permit a full description of each of the diseases mentioned, but the following are some of the salient points:

1. Specific Fevers

Infectious mononucleosis is today one of the commonest causes of prolonged fever in children and young adults, and diagnosis is often difficult. Paul-Bunnell or 'Monospot' tests are useful after the first 2 weeks or so in diagnosis.

Typhoid fever suggests itself when a patient, previously in good health, suffers from a progressive fever of considerable and increasing degree with a pulse-rate that is relatively slow in relation to the temperature, the illness starting with headache and malaise but without any conspicuously abnormal signs. During the first week, the temperature rises each night to a slightly higher level than that of the previous night until a maximum is attained and maintained during the second week, after which there is a progressive diminution during the third week until normal is reached again (*Fig.* 307). Diarrhoea may occur with foul-smelling stools of pea-soup consistency, but constipation is more usual. The headache, which is in most cases a conspicuous feature, persists for about a week when it almost invariably ceases, thus contrasting with the headache of tuberculous meningitis. Blood-cultures are positive in the first 10 days and in acute relapse, similar cultures later on proving negative although urine and faecal cultures may by then be positive. The spleen becomes palpable early in the disease and remains so until defervescence; it enlarges again in a relapse. Typical typhoid rose spots appear —chiefly on the abdomen, less often on the

animals, and cattle. In the history of Mankind they rank high as a cause of epidemic disease causing great suffering and death.

Abortus fever is a not uncommon cause for prolonged unexplained pyrexia, lasting usually for several months and occasionally for years. It is due to infection by *Brucella abortus*. This organism causes fatal abortion in cows, and apart from the geographical circumstances the fever is identical with Mediterranean fever in which the

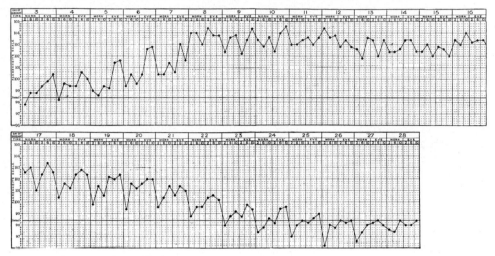

Fig. 307. Temperature chart of a typical case of typhoid fever.

chest or back, and seldom on the limbs—from the seventh day onwards and in successive crops. They are the size of a pin's head, that is about two or three millimetres in diameter, rose red, fading on pressure, and without a central punctum. The majority of patients, but not all, develop a rise in agglutinins against the O antigens of the typhoid bacillus during the course of the disease. Another help in diagnosis is the absence of leucocytosis, and in the differential leucocyte count the lymphocytes are relatively increased, the polymorphonuclear cells being absolutely reduced. The leucocyte count may, however, be influenced by complications. Rigors are exceptional, a fact which sometimes helps in diagnosis from septicaemia, pylephlebitis, and malaria.

Some difficulty arises in the diagnosis of those cases in which there has been previous immunization of the patient by antityphoid inoculations; the fever is then of shorter duration and the illness relatively mild.

Of a large number of *Salmonella* serotypes recovered from humans the commonest is at present *S. typhimurium*. Infection with *S. typhimurium* is often mild but may on occasion be lethal.

The Rickettsial disorders are numerous, ranging from epidemic typhus to trench fever. Different rickettsiae are transmitted by lice, fleas, ticks, and mites via man, wild rodents, domestic

disease is communicated by goat's milk. Infection may arise from ingestion of milk or the handling of infected animals or excreta. This infection may underlie obscure, long-continued febrile illness either in children or in adults. There are no characteristic symptoms, although arthritis is a frequent accompaniment. Diagnosis is usually by agglutination tests, rarely by blood-cultures. Rarely it causes bacterial endocarditis, sometimes fatal. Cultures taken from bone-marrow or liver may be positive when blood-cultures are negative. Brucellar infections are particularly persistent, probably due to the intracellular location of the organism in the reticulo-endothelial tissues.

Melitensis, Mediterranean, or *Malta fever* is one of the most prolonged of the fevers due to a known specific organism, in this case *Brucella melitensis*. In the undulant form of the disease successive exacerbations of pyrexia may prolong the illness into the sixteenth, eighteenth, or twentieth week or longer (*Fig.* 308). It may simulate typhoid fever, including the enlargement of the spleen and the paucity of abnormal physical signs, but there are no rose spots or other eruption. The diagnosis may be suggested by geographical factors—recent residence, for instance, in some part of the Mediterranean coast or islands, or Spain, Portugal, the Canary Islands, or parts of South America, especially if the patient has been taking goat's milk, the medium by which the infection is transmitted. The diagnosis is established by serum-agglutination tests, which may be positive from the fifth day onwards, the patient's diluted blood-serum agglutinating cultures of the *Br. melitensis*. Blood-cultures should be done. *Brucella suis* infections, contracted from pigs, are also diagnosed by agglutination tests and blood-cultures.

Secondary syphilis may be a febrile illness to such an extent that it may be mistaken for small-pox during an epidemic. The diagnosis becomes

suggest that the pyrexia and the abdominal symptoms have a tuberculous basis. The presence of enlarged cervical lymph-nodes is in support of this diagnosis.

Rat-bite fever. (*See* p. 696.)

Psittacosis or *Ornithosis* is transmitted to man from parrots and the parrot family, pigeons, and a number of other birds, including ducks, turkeys, and chickens. It is due to a Gram-negative obligate intracellular parasite, *Chlamydia psittaci*, formerly classified as a virus. The illness may be transmitted from the patient to others in contact

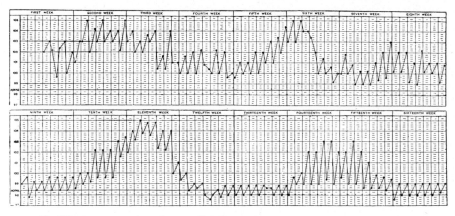

Fig. 308. Temperature chart of a case of Mediterranean fever of undulant type (*Br. melitensis*).

obvious, however, when the roseola is carefully examined, and when it is associated with a fading primary sore, typical snail-track ulcers of tonsils, fauces, and pharynx, and generalized enlargement of most of the palpable lymph-nodes. Spirochaetes may be isolated from the skin lesions.

Tuberculosis. Tuberculous lesions often occur without pyrexia. On the other hand, the occurrence of some degree of fever without any apparent cause may be the sole evidence of such disease, especially the miliary form. Pulmonary tuberculosis is almost invariably pyrexial but in an earlier stage there are often long periods of apyrexia even when the tuberculous process is active, with brief febrile spells. Tuberculous arthritis is often apyrexial unless secondarily infected. Glandular tuberculosis is less likely to be pyrexial when the nodes involved are cervical or bronchial than when the mesenteric and other abdominal nodes are caseous and softening ('tabes mesenterica'), when there may be, and usually is, prolonged pyrexia. The diagnosis may be easy if there is ascites in a child or if there are palpable abdominal masses, but it may be difficult in the absence of lumps and ascites in a condition of ill health with pyrexia and with vague abdominal pains which may be mistaken for some other non-tuberculous abdominal disease. The patient is usually young, often a little child, and the general look of the facies may

with him. Clinically the illness is similar to typhoid fever, with liability to considerable pulmonary complications. The fever lasts about three weeks, tending to end abruptly followed by slow convalescence, but may last for as long as three months. When the disease is contracted from parrots or parakeets it tends to be more severe and prolonged. The diagnosis is suggested in a patient with an illness that bears a general resemblance to typhoid fever but whose blood does not give the agglutination test and especially if there has been contact with a recently imported parrot, budgerigar, or pigeon. The organism may be isolated from the blood or sputum. A rising titre of complement-fixing antibody in the patient's blood is useful in diagnosis.

Tularaemia is uncommon in England, but cases have occurred amongst those who have had the handling of live rabbits—for instance, in connexion with bacteriological laboratories. It is a specific infectious disease due to *Pasteurella tularensis*, transmitted from rodents by ticks, flies, or mosquitoes, although there is some reason to believe that infection may be acquired from the excreta of diseased rodents and other animals. It is not transmitted directly from human to human. A sore place on a finger is commonly the start, the sore becoming a small ulcer in a day or two, with associated enlargement of the epitrochlear and axillary lymph-nodes; a chill or rigor is usual, and pyrexia continues for two or three weeks with marked prostration followed by slow convalescence. There may be erythematous blotches on the skin, or even purpura. The diagnosis can be confirmed by a skin test which becomes positive in the first week, or the causal organism can be recovered from mucocutaneous ulcer or regional lymph-node and occasionally from sputum and gastric washings, on appropriate cultures or on animal inoculation. The illness is severe and prolonged, but the prognosis is good.

2. Bacteraemia

Disseminated infection may occur in association with a local lesion and metastasize to new areas. This may occur with many organisms. As an example, in *meningococcal infection* meningitis is not always present. In the early stages patients are acutely ill, with fever, chills, arthralgia, and myalgia, particularly severe in the legs and back. They are very prostrated, hypotensive, and 70 per cent develop a characteristic petechial rash. (*Fig.* 309.) Meningococci are cultured from the blood and sometimes from scrapings from the skin lesions, and from the cerebrospinal fluid in cases with meningitis. A rare form of chronic meningococcaemia occurs which lasts for weeks or months and is characterized by fever, rash, and arthritis or arthralgia.

Infective or bacterial endocarditis. The comparatively rare acute or malignant endocarditis is

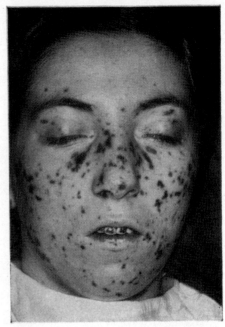

Fig. 309. Meningococcal septicaemia which presented as subarachnoid haemorrhage and purpuric rash.

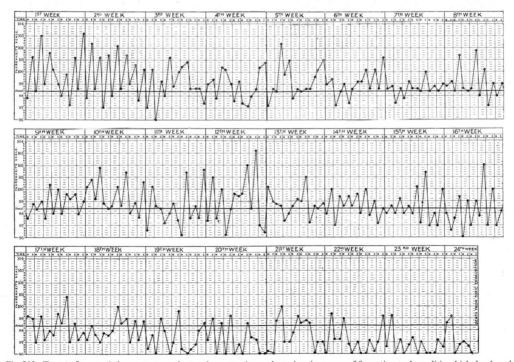

Fig. 310. Twenty-four weeks' temperature chart, taken morning and evening, in a case of fungating endocarditis which developed in the days before sulpha drugs and antibiotics in connexion with post-rheumatic mitral stenosis. The liability to hypothermia is pronounced in the later stages of the malady, as the patient became more and more toxic and asthenic.

due to infection by one of the pyogenic bacteria, such as the *Streptococcus haemolyticus*, the *pneumococcus*, the *gonococcus*, and the *staphylococcus*. Many other organisms may cause endocarditis: *Corynebacterium diphtheriae*, Brucella, and numerous others. Pseudomonal endocarditis may follow open-heart surgery. The type termed the 'subacute' variety, nowadays more frequently seen, occurs in a subject of chronic valvular disease of congenital or rheumatic origin when the organism in question is usually *Streptococcus*

over middle age, if not immediately treated, may be cured of the infection but die of cardiac failure due to the damage to the myocardium.

3. Localized Infection

Many cases of continued fever are due to localized infection, i.e., abscess formation. Elicitation of local signs, in addition to pyrexia and other evidence of generalized systemic illness, will give the diagnosis, but it may be long delayed.

Rectal or vaginal examination should serve to detect *prostatic abscess*, *periproctal abscess*,

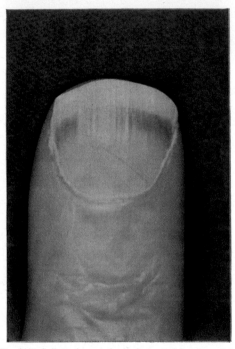

Fig. 311. Splinter haemorrhages in bacterial endocarditis. (*Dr. R. G. Ollerenshaw, Manchester Royal Infirmary.*)

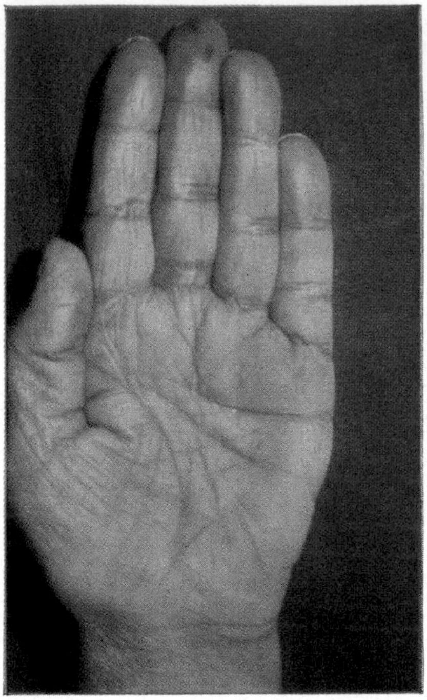

Fig. 312. Embolism affecting tip of middle finger in a case of infective endocarditis. (*Dr. R. G. Ollerenshaw, Manchester Royal Infirmary.*)

viridans. Patients present themselves with cardiac symptoms, with anaemia, with cerebral vascular lesions, or most commonly with pyrexia of unknown origin (*Fig.* 310), a feature which arouses suspicion when progressive anaemia of normocytic and orthochromic type develops. The white cell-count is variable, a polymorphonuclear leucocytosis up to about 9–12,000 per c.mm. is common. Other diagnostic features are an enlarged spleen, clubbing of the fingers in half the subacute cases, rarely in the malignant type, petechial haemorrhages under the nails (*Fig.* 311), and in the retina and conjunctiva, and Osler's nodes which are infected cutaneous emboli (*Fig.* 312). Emboli may occur in other situations.

Red blood-cells in the urine are invariable in greater or less degree.

Blood-cultures should be done immediately as treatment must not be delayed. The patient, if

ischiorectal abscess, pyosalpinx, suppurating ovarian cyst, or *parametritic abscess*, all of which are likely to cause local pain in the perineum, anal region, sacral region, back, or lower abdomen.

Empyema of the maxillary antrum, when acute, causes pain and tenderness over the affected maxilla with oedematous swelling of that side of the face, but in chronic cases the symptoms may be much less definite. The diagnosis may be suggested by face-ache, local swelling, and perhaps an intermittent discharge of pus from one nostril. Confirmation may be afforded by transillumination, X-rays, and antral aspiration.

Empyema of a frontal sinus may be acute or chronic, causing pyrexia in either case. The diagnosis may be suggested by complaint of local headache above the eyes, generally on one or other side of the midline rather than central, especially if such headache is associated with local tenderness to percussion. Identification becomes easy if the abscess points above the inner canthus of the orbit near the root of the nose; but doubt may persist for a long time. Difficulty in diagnosis applies still more to *empyema of the ethmoidal sinuses* or to *empyema of the sphenoidal sinuses* in which few objective signs are to be expected. The patient may complain of severe frontal headaches, often worse in the morning and passing off later in the day, and a purulent nasal discharge may be present; pyrexia may be only slight, but is generally persistent.

Suppurating lymph-nodes will be diagnosed from the character of the tender swellings that precede the skin-reddening and the actual formation of an abscess; the site is likely to be neck, axilla, or groin, and there will usually be an indication of the source of the trouble in the form of a septic focus in the skin corresponding to the lymph-drainage of the node concerned— impetigo, a septic cut or wound, or a whitlow. One source of trouble that may be overlooked is *pediculosis* of the scalp; it should be suspected if there is irritation of the back of the neck at the roots of the hair in association with enlargement of the occipital as well as of the cervical lymph-nodes.

Mammary and *submammary abscess* may be of chronic type and cause pyrexia without much pain.

Empyema thoracis is generally easy of diagnosis. The abnormal physical signs at the base of one lung suggest the presence of fluid; on needling the chest pus will be found. The condition may be simulated by subdiaphragmatic abscess, but X-ray examination will usually help in distinguishing the two. In some cases both conditions are present. Difficulty in diagnosis may on occasion be considerable when the empyema is interlobar, or between the pericardium and the pleura, or between the diaphragm and the lower lobe.

Lung abscesses may be single or multiple, and may be part of a blood-borne or local infection or be associated with a bronchial neoplasm. Much of the fever and acute systemic upset in the last case is due to infection rather than the primary neoplasm. X-rays and tomograms will help in the differential diagnosis.

Hepatic abscess, especially the type following amoebic dysentery, may be a subacute or chronic rather than an acute condition, with fluctuating pyrexia persisting for months. The diagnosis may be suggested by complaint of pain or tenderness over the lower part of the right chest in front or behind, by dome-shaped dullness at the base of the right lung, or by friction sounds over the liver. A history of amoebic dysentery is not always forthcoming. Pain is in some instances referred to the right shoulder. When pyrexia and rigors are the only objective features malaria is simulated, but a high polymorphonuclear leucocytosis is against this diagnosis. The diagnosis of hepatic abscess is clinched by needling the liver and finding pus, often chocolate coloured or resembling anchovy paste; on occasions the pus is coughed up as the result of its ulceration through the diaphragm and pleura into a bronchus.

Empyema of the gall-bladder. Jaundice is generally absent. Pyrexia may be considerable and prolonged, and rigors are to be expected. The diagnosis depends largely upon the patient's complaint of pain in the right hypochondrium associated either with enlarged gall-bladder or with acute pain and tenderness on palpation of the gall-bladder region below the tip of the right ninth rib cartilage.

Suppurative cholangitis is the result of extension of pyogenic infection up the hepatic ducts into the biliary canals within the liver. It generally is associated with obstruction in the bile-duct by stone or growth. When the infection has extended to become suppurative cholangitis the patient becomes increasingly ill. The supervention of cholangitis may be indicated by progressive, soft, uniform, and tender enlargement of the liver, associated as a rule with jaundice. Recurrent rigors are almost invariable.

Suppurative pylephlebitis arises from infection somewhere in the periphery of the portal area— for example, previous appendicitis. It is often fatal. The liver becomes studded with multiple small abscesses around the intrahepatic subdivisions of the portal vein. The liver becomes progressively, smoothly, and uniformly enlarged, and generally tender; jaundice is present in less than half the cases. The high degree of pyrexia, the rigors, the asthenia and wasting all indicate that the patient has developed some form of septic extension from his original disease. There is a high degree of leucocytosis.

Subdiaphragmatic abscess is often difficult to diagnose even with full X-ray examination. Since the pus is often spread in a thin layer between the liver and the diaphragm or between the spleen and the diaphragm, attempts to locate it by needling are frequently unsuccessful. There may be no abnormal physical signs, but more usually infection of the pleura through the diaphragm leads to impaired percussion note at the base of one lung accompanied by pleuritic friction and râles.

Bronchiectasis may be responsible for prolonged periods of pyrexia with afebrile intervals of varying length. The pyrexial bouts are due either to invasion of the pus-containing cavities by fresh organisms or to recrudescences in the activity of infection already present, possibly brought about by impaired bronchial drainage. The abnormal physical signs in the lungs, the abundant foul sputum, and the clubbed fingers indicate the diagnosis. Not infrequently there is considerable inflammation in the lung tissues around the area of bronchiectasis, the so-called 'peribronchiectatic pneumonitis'. In any patient where consolidation, often with pleurisy, recurs repeatedly in one area of the lung this condition should be suspected.

Appendicular abscess may be easy of diagnosis on palpating the tender swelling in the right iliac fossa. In other situations of the abscess identification may be difficult; rectal examination leads to the detection of the abscess when it descends into the pelvis. Pyrexia ceases as a rule when the pus obtains free drainage, so that it is exceptional for appendicular abscess to be the cause of prolonged pyrexia.

Perinephric abscess may cause pyrexia of considerable degree, possibly lasting for several weeks. Pain in the loin is almost always present, eventually with tenderness to palpation in both the loin and the lumbar region, but it is often absent in the early stages, and may not appear until the patient has been febrile for some weeks. There may be no defined tumour but only a sense of resistance evident when, with the patient recumbent, the examiner places one hand behind each loin with the finger-tips external to the erector spinae muscles, and then makes as if to raise the patient from the bed though without actually lifting him: the fingers on the affected side will not feel the hollow of the loin clearly as will those on the sound side. The signs may be yet more striking if the patient lies prone. If the patient is well enough to sit up in bed with the back bared and the observer then looks down his spine from above, it may often be apparent that, whereas the loin on the sound side is slightly concave, that of the perinephric abscess side is either flat or slightly convex; only in pronounced cases does the loin show a distinct convexity. Perinephric abscess is generally the result of pyogenic infection within the kidney; or it may be due to pus tracking up behind the colon from appendicitis or it may be a delayed result of a loin injury, a haematoma due to the injury becoming infected and slowly forming a perinephric abscess weeks or months after the trauma. In many cases the history is obtainable of a suppurative process a short time previously. Pre-existing neutropenia, or corticosteroid therapy, will in these cases, as in all infective processes, predispose to abscess formation.

Diverticulitis abscess may be subacute and yet causative of prolonged pyrexia. It is generally situated in the left lower part of the abdomen producing a tender tumour that may simulate carcinoma. It is preceded by chronic bowel symptoms, constipation, and colic. Haemorrhage may occur, sometimes profusely. It is a disease of the second half of life.

Psoas abscess results from tuberculous spinal disease; the condition may be apyrexial, but, like any other form of tubercle, it may cause protracted irregular pyrexia. Pain localized to some part of the back and stiffness of the corresponding part of the spine in a child are suggestive features. X-rays must be performed (*Fig.* 642, p. 621). On the other hand, the diagnosis may remain unsuspected until a tender swelling appears above or below one groin as the abscess tracks down from the spine along the course of the psoas muscle ultimately giving fluctuation from above to below the inguinal ligament.

Actinomycosis is diagnosed by the discovery of the organism. It may be in the discharge issuing from a sinus communicating with the focus infected, generally the cheek, jaw, neck, lung, liver, caecum, or spine. It may, however, occur anywhere in the skin or viscera, and the true nature of the disease is only too likely to be missed if bacterial investigation is not undertaken. An actinomycotic ischiorectal abscess, for instance, may be regarded as of merely pyogenic origin. There is diffuse infiltration of deep as well as superficial parts, liability to discharge through one or more sinuses, and a suggestive purplish-red colour of the skin adherent to the lesion. The course is chronic, often apyrexial, but frequently there are periods of pyrexia.

4. Infective and Inflammatory Conditions

Coliform infection of the urinary tract may be chronic and apyrexial but is liable to exacerbations with prolonged pyrexia, aching or pain in one or both loins, frequency of micturition, pain during micturition. It may exist, however, especially in children, with so few symptoms of urinary disease that its responsibility for continued pyrexia may be missed.

Chronic or recurring pyelonephritis is more common in women than men but may be associated with an enlarged prostate, or urethral stricture. The patient is ill, with rigors and high, long-continued pyrexia; the urine is purulent and yields a positive culture of the causative organism or organisms. In papillary necrosis the renal calices become clubbed and pyuria is common even when urine cultures are sterile. Prolonged fever is not uncommon. It may be due to prolonged taking of compound analgesic tablets or diabetes mellitus.

Gall-stones may be silent causing no symptoms or they may be associated with irregular and sometimes prolonged pyrexia (Charcot's fever), and with bouts of pyrexia in attacks of biliary colic.

Phlebitis in a superficial vein is indicated by tenderness, with or without redness and swelling along the course of the vein; pyrexia of variable degree and duration accompanies the disorder in the earlier stages, but usually subsides in a few days. The diagnosis is much more difficult when the inflamed vein is deeply situated. Intra-abdominal phlebitis may be responsible for both continued pyrexia and vague but possibly severe abdominal pain in certain cases for which no explanation is forthcoming. *Thrombophlebitis migrans* occurs uncommonly. Venous thrombosis in the pelvis, not necessarily associated with obvious femoral or popliteal thrombosis, may account for pyrexia after childbirth.

Thyroiditis, an inflammatory but non-infective condition, may truly cause the complaint of sore throat, the thyroid itself being painful and tender.

Parametritis is diagnosed by pelvic examination. It is likely to be the after-effect of recent labour and is often associated with continued pyrexia, pain in the pelvis and lower part of the back. Abscess formation may occur. Elderly women are apt to develop a purulent form of endometritis, sometimes pyrexial, with pelvic pain, bearing-down pain, pain in the back, a foul vaginal discharge often blood-stained, the condition simulating advanced carcinoma of the body of the uterus.

Vesiculitis, though it may be of septic origin, is generally due to gonococcal infection of the seminal vesicles. The complaint is mainly of hot burning pain in the rectum aggravated by defaecation; proctitis, or carcinoma of the rectum or acute prostatitis are simulated. Diagnosis is established by rectal examination, the finger locating a tender swelling in the vesicles.

Colitis, whether infective or ulcerative, will be suggested by a history of diarrhoea with the passage of blood and mucus associated with more or less pain along the course of the colon, particularly the descending colon; carcinoma, or diverticulitis, may be simulated. The diagnosis is confirmed by endoscopy, barium enema, and/or bacteriological studies.

Crohn's disease (regional enteritis) should be suspected when there is a history of chronic intermittent diarrhoea, fever, loss of weight, and abdominal pains or distension. Barium studies are necessary. Intermittent small-bowel obstruction is common. Amyloidosis may occur.

Pancreatitis, when subacute or chronic, is very difficult to diagnose. It is sometimes but not always pyrexial. It may simulate other abdominal lesions such as gall-stones. Glycosuria in association with pyrexia and a dull aching pain in the abdomen across the site of the pancreas may be suggestive, but the symptoms are generally too vague to be characteristic. There is often a curious dull-brown pigmentation of the skin. Chronic pancreatitis should be suspected in a patient with recurrent abdominal pain, particularly if the pain or tenderness extends to the left of the midline, if gall-stones are present, and if there have been bouts of overconsumption of alcohol. X-rays may show pancreatic calcification. Repeated serum or urine amylase estimations taken within 12 hours of an acute episode are elevated in most cases, but as more acinar and ductal cells are destroyed these become less evident. After acute pancreatitis suppurative pancreatitis may occur in the second or third week with return of fever.

Sarcoidosis, a chronic granulomatous inflammatory condition, may cause prolonged fever, sometimes with relatively little systemic upset. Hilar glandular enlargement in X-rays, erythema nodosum, a weakly positive or negative tuberculin test, and a positive Kveim test are diagnostic findings.

5. Non-purulent Hepatic Affections. Quite apart from fever that occurs in obviously infective lesions of the liver, such as hepatic abscess, infective and serum hepatitis, cholangitis, and pylephlebitis, pyrexia, generally without the ordinary concomitants of fever, often occurs when the liver tissue is affected by lesions which are not obviously pyogenic, particularly *cirrhosis* and *carcinoma*. Laennec's (alcoholic) cirrhosis, postnecrotic, and biliary cirrhosis may all be accompanied by prolonged fever as may chronic active hepatitis (lupoid hepatitis), a disorder largely of young women, in which hypergammaglobulinaemia is a striking feature and arthritis or arthralgia occurs in over half the cases. Rapidly growing neoplasms are sometimes accompanied by essential pyrexia. The appetite may be fairly good, and the patient may even be carrying on his ordinary work although his health is failing.

6. The Connective-tissue Disorders

Rheumatoid Arthritis. In some cases prolonged fever is a part of the clinical picture of rheumatoid arthritis.

Systemic Lupus Erythematosus may for many months present as pyrexia, often accompanied by skin rashes, albuminuria, and L.E. cells in the blood. The high E.S.R. and joint pains may lead to confusion with rheumatoid arthritis (*Fig.* 313).

Polyarteritis nodosa and other arteriopathies, such as giant cell arteritis or Wegener's granulomatosis, may cause prolonged fever, though the latter is usually rapidly fatal in a few weeks or sometimes less. *Polymyositis* and *dermatomyositis* may also be associated with fever, as may *scleroderma*.

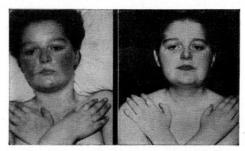

Fig. 313. Female patient with prolonged fever and flitting joint pains due to systemic lupus erythematosus. The contrast is striking between the red butterfly rash of the disorder and the Cushingoid appearance on full steroid therapy 1 month later.

7. Blood Diseases. Any one of the severe blood diseases may be associated with prolonged pyrexia: diagnosis depends upon other factors, particularly the blood-count, as in *leukaemia* (p. 54 et seq.). In agranulocytosis and aplastic anaemia infection is responsible for the fever, but in any severe prolonged anaemia, particularly in childhood, prolonged pyrexia may be seen. In previous times, for instance, untreated Addisonian anaemia was a febrile disease. Febrile episodes occur also in haemolytic anaemias.

8. Diseases of Tropics and Subtropics. Trypanosomiasis is a parasitic infection occurring particularly in Africa where *Glossina palpalis*, the tsetse fly, abounds; the bite of this insect spreads the disease, sleeping sickness, by invasion of the central nervous system. It is not always pyrexial and at times malaria may be simulated. The trypanosoma may be identified in blood-films, lymph-node aspirates, more rarely bone-marrow, or, in the final sleeping stage, in the cerebrospinal fluid. There is no distinctive feature on the temperature chart.

Malaria. The two main types are the tertian (*Plasmodium vivax* or *Plasmodium ovale*), in which rigors occur on alternate days with a maximum temperature of 103–104° F. (*Fig.* 314) and

larly, infection by two lots of parasites might result in a complicated clinical picture in which the attacks of pyrexia might be irregular or almost continuous. As a rule, a paroxysm with its various cold, hot, and sweating stages lasts about eight hours. The diagnosis of malaria will be rendered certain by the discovery of parasites in the blood (*Figs.* 317–319).

One remarkable feature is that malaria may remain latent for many years, particularly with

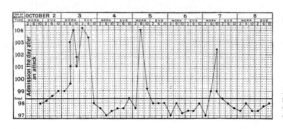

Fig. 314. Case of simple tertian malaria, showing the attacks occurring every third day. (*Figs.* 314–6 *from the London School of Tropical Medicine.*)

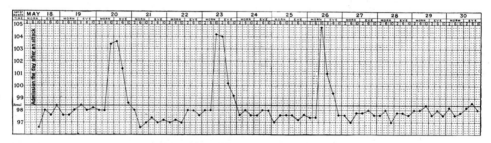

Fig. 315. Temperature chart from a case of quartan malarial fever, the attacks recurring every fourth day.

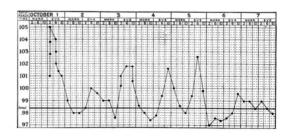

Fig. 316. Temperature chart from a case of malaria to illustrate quotidian fever due to double tertian infection.

complete freedom on the intermediate days, and the quartan (*Plasmodium malariae*) in which there are 2-day intervals so that the paroxysms occur every fourth day (*Fig.* 315). The intervals between the attacks of fever vary in accordance with the time that successive generations of the various strains of parasites take to mature. A patient may be infected by one set of bites by a mosquito with a tertian or quartan ague and become subsequently infected by other mosquitoes with either tertian or quartan parasites so that there is a mingling together of the effects of different broods of *Plasmodium* and the patient would have a daily (quotidian) paroxysm (*Fig.* 316). Simi-

P. malariae. Considering the large number of serving men infected in the last war, however, relapses of malaria 1 year after returning home have been rare. Reappearance is brought about by cold, general depression of health, or through some intercurrent malady.

Kala-azar. There is no characteristic chart, the pyrexia, often extreme, being of a swinging but continued type. Great enlargement of the spleen with continued pyrexia would suggest the diagnosis, which is confirmed by discovering Leishman-Donovan bodies from material obtained by splenic or sternal puncture. It is not uncommon on the Spanish coast and Mediterranean littoral and may be acquired on a short Continental holiday.

Plague is also epidemic; its types are various, the two best known being the bubonic and the pneumonic. The diagnosis depends on discovering plague bacilli (*Pasteurella pestis*) in fluid obtained by puncturing a bubo or from the sputum

Relapsing fever was at one time prevalent in Great Britain and acquired the name 'famine fever' from the circumstances of its occurrence. It is due to infection with *Spirochaeta recurrentis* (*Borrelia recurrentis*) introduced by an infected louse being crushed against an abrasion or wound. Many strains are also conveyed by

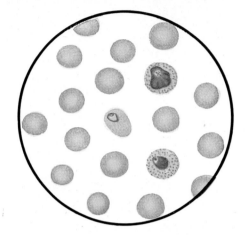

Fig. 317. *Plasmodium vivax*: causing benign tertian malaria. Three stages of development of the ring-parasite (schizont) are shown: as the ring grows it expands the red corpuscle, and produces multiple small dots of dark pigment which distinguish it from the *Plasmodium malariae* of quartan fever, in which case the pigment is in larger spots, few in number. No crescents are formed. (Stained by the Wright-Romanowsky method, and viewed under the ¹/₁₂-in. oil-immersion lens.)

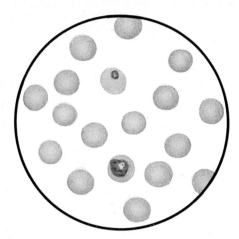

Fig. 318. *Plasmodium malariae*: causing benign quartan malaria. Two stages of development of the ring-parasite (schizont) are shown; as the ring grows it does not expand the red corpuscle as does that of benign tertian (*Plasmodium vivax*), and the pigment particles are in the form of relatively large dots, few in number, instead of the multiple tiny dots of *Plasmodium vivax*. Crescents are not formed. (Stained by the Wright-Romanowsky method, and viewed under the ¹/₁₂-in. oil-immersion lens.)

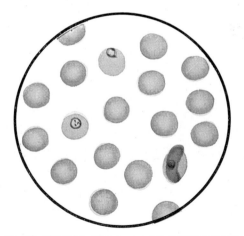

Fig. 319. *Plasmodium falciparum*: causing malignant malaria. Two stages of the ring-parasite (schizont) and one crescent (gametocyte) are shown. (Stained by the Wright-Romanowsky method, and viewed under the ¹/₁₂-in. oil-immersion lens.)

by special bacteriological methods. The pneumonic form is the more acute and it may simulate lobar pneumonia; the bubonic form is of longer duration with a lower grade of pyrexia. Both cholera and plague when they occur in England tend to be in persons coming from India or the East, particularly members of ships' crews.

ticks and the disease transmitted by their bites. The course of the disease is characteristic. There are outbreaks of high pyrexia (*Fig.* 320) associated with extreme prostration and severe illness lasting five or six days, alternating with complete intermission of about the same duration. There may be an indefinite number of relapses before death or recovery. The spirochaete may be identified in a blood-film shortly before the febrile paroxysm, but not in the intervals.

Schistosomiasis is widely spread through Egypt, Rhodesia, and certain other parts of Africa. Involvement of the urinary tract with *S. haematobium* is extremely common in these countries. *S. mansoni* affects the colon more and is associated with splenomegaly. Pyrexia over long periods is not uncommon with either type of infection.

9. Meningeal and Cerebral Haemorrhage. Almost any malady that interferes radically with the heat-regulating centres in the brain may cause pyrexia, often without the other symptoms usually associated with fever. As a rule death or recovery renders such types of pyrexia of short duration, for instance in cases of pontine haemorrhage (*Fig.* 179, p. 168). Sometimes, however, the patient may survive long enough to come into the category of cases of prolonged pyrexia.

10*

10. Skin Conditions. These are discussed in the article on BULLAE (p. 115); there is less tendency to pyrexia in dermatitis herpetiformis, herpes gestationis, and erythema iris, than in acute and subacute pemphigus. Pemphigus is always a serious and often a fatal malady, the skin blebs being but a local manifestation of some severe but ill-defined systemic infection. Eosinophilia is usual. Any diffuse inflammation of the skin, from acute psoriasis to a gold dermatitis, may be accompanied by fever.

pyrexia, but the cause is self-evident. The post-cardiac injury syndrome may occur after any injury to the heart, whether it be an operation, stab-wound, or a coronary occlusion (Dressler's syndrome). Fever, pericarditis, pleurisy, and pneumonitis may occur 2 or more weeks after the injury and recurrences are common.

13. Fictitious Pyrexia produced by Malingerers. From time to time one meets with cases in which illness is simulated by a patient who deliberately deceives by one or other of various devices, such

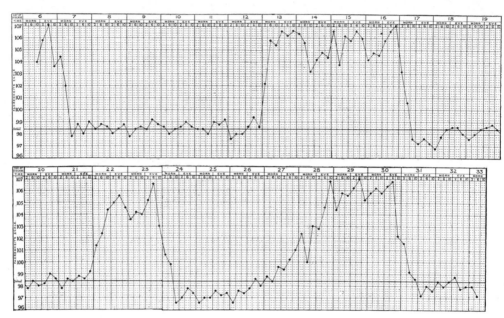

Fig. 320. Four-hourly temperature chart in a case of severe relapsing fever.

11. Malignancy. Lymphomata, of different kinds, including Hodgkin's disease, may be associated with prolonged fever, the Pel-Ebstein type depicted in *Figs.* 321, 322 being seen typically in this condition though not confined to it. Lymphosarcoma may be associated with prolonged pyrexia, as may carcinoma, particularly if associated with sepsis, as is seen not infrequently in the bronchus and large intestine. Infection is not necessary for pyrexia to be present; high fevers are occasionally seen in primary and secondary carcinoma where no sepsis exists, and a low-grade pyrexia is common.

12. Allergic (Antigen–Antibody Reactive) Conditions, being inflammatory disorders, are often pyrexial. This is seen, for example, in anaphylactoid purpura (which includes Henoch's and Schönlein's), and various skin allergies. Any diffuse inflammation of the skin, whatever the cause, may be accompanied by considerable

as dipping the thermometer bulb in a cup of tea, holding it against a hot-water bottle, or rubbing it violently against the blankets. It is said that some have the art of squeezing the bulb between the fingers or between the teeth with just sufficient force to raise the temperature, but without breaking the glass; on suspicion of such a possibility the temperature is taken under careful scrutiny preferably per rectum.

14. Drug Reactions. In any persistent unexplained fever where drug treatment is being given the possibility of therapy being the cause should be considered. Fever occurring in the treatment of pulmonary tuberculosis, for instance, may be due to isoniazid, aminosalicylate, streptomycin, or all three drugs. Antibiotics, sulpha drugs, arsenicals, iodides, barbiturates, and many others may be responsible. When in doubt the motto should be, if possible, 'Stop treatment'.

F. Dudley Hart.

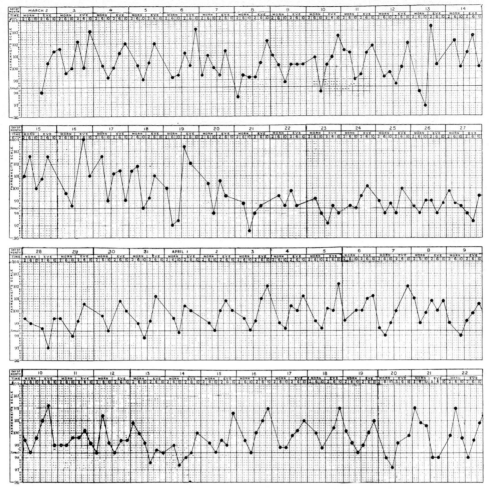

Fig. 321. Prolonged pyrexia in a case of Hodgkin's disease. The fever is irregular without indications of the periodicity of the pyrexia seen in the Pel-Ebstein type of this disease.

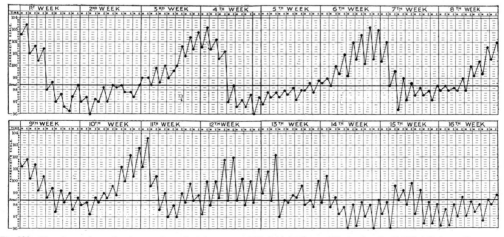

Fig. 322. Morning and evening temperature chart in a case of Hodgkin's disease, illustrating the Pel-Ebstein type of recurrent or periodic pyrexia that may occur in this disease.

FEVER WITHOUT OBVIOUS CAUSE

1. FEVER IN CHILDREN

The heat-regulating mechanism takes time for its stable and complete development and is apt to be disturbed in children by causes that would not produce pyrexia in an adult; hence transient, irregular, or recurrent rises of temperature in a child may often be of but little significance. *Excitement* is apt to produce transient pyrexia in this way; the influence of visiting day at a hospital is well recognized. A bout of *bad temper, coughing*, or *crying* may have a similar result and so may any *gastro-intestinal upset*. In none of these is it necessary to implicate an infective process.

Nevertheless, if such rises of temperature, even in a child, should prove otherwise than transient, it is unwise to regard them as purely trivial; there are four conditions in particular that need to be specially borne in mind: (1) *Urinary infection*; (2) *Upper-respiratory-tract infection*; (3) *Exanthemata and the infectious diseases of childhood* before their specific rashes or other clinical features appear; and more rarely (4) *Tuberculous disease*.

Urinary Infection, usually due to *E. coli*, is only too easily missed in a child, for there may be no symptoms attracting attention to the urinary system. The presence in the urine of leucocytes with perhaps just a trace of protein makes the diagnosis likely, though it needs culture of a clean specimen of urine to establish it.

Upper-respiratory-tract Infections include tonsillitis, acute pharyngitis and rhinitis, and otitis media. Although symptoms usually point to the cause of the fever in a small child this is not always so; the child has fever, is distressed, and apparently in pain, but cannot indicate to the parents where the trouble lies.

Tuberculous Disease may exist in children without production of symptoms, and though the condition is much less common than it was a few years ago it must still be kept in mind. It is from tuberculous mesenteric nodes that tuberculous peritonitis develops, and previous to the true nature of the trouble becoming obvious there may be no other clinical evidence than bouts of pyrexia of obscure origin. There may possibly be vague abdominal pains, described as one manifestation of 'periodic disease', simulating appendicitis or coliform urinary infection; or cough without abnormal physical signs in the chest. Suspicious lymph-nodes may sometimes be palpated in the neck and X-rays of the chest (*Fig.* 208, p. 191) show glandular enlargement and sometimes collapse of a lobe or segment of a lobe. The tuberculin test is strongly positive and should only be done initially, if at all, in high dilutions.

2. PYREXIA IN ADULTS

The types of obscure pyrexia in adults fall into two main groups: (1) *Transient or short pyrexia*; (2) *Continued pyrexia*.

Transient or Short Pyrexia. This is usually due to one of a number of mild viral or bacterial infections, the common cold, sinusitis, nasopharyngitis, mild pyelonephritis, and a host of others. It is as well to remember that drugs may themselves cause fever, and that the curative drug may sometimes maintain the fever, it was used to cure. It is also as well to remember that products of tissue death may cause fever, as after myocardial infarction, pulmonary infarction, gangrene and tissue necrosis, and accumulation of blood in body cavities, gut, joints, or elsewhere.

Continued Pyrexia. This may occur in any of the large number of conditions listed under FEVER, PROLONGED (p. 287). In Great Britain today one thinks primarily of the more common conditions: coliform infections of the urinary tract, infectious mononucleosis, carcinoma (particularly of the bronchus), tuberculous disease, chronic sepsis (as in sinusitis), abortus infections, and so on. With air travel readily available, malaria, kala-azar, or any other tropical disease may be imported overnight, and with a large immigrant population from overseas conditions such as schistosomiasis and leprosy may be encountered in the ordinary out-patient clinic.

F. Dudley Hart.

FINGERS, CLUBBED

Clubbing of the fingers consists in increase in volume of the soft tissues around the terminal phalanges and increased curvature of the nails, especially longitudinally. When both these features are well marked (*Fig.* 323), the appearance of the fingers with their swollen rounded ends has been likened, rather fancifully, to that of a drumstick, and can hardly be missed. But there is every gradation between this and normality; the two features, swelling of the soft tissues and excessive curvature of the nails, may be present in different degree, and in some instances it is difficult to be certain whether the finger-ends are to be regarded as clubbed. Certain other features should be sought in such instances. The skin-fold around the nail is hyperaemic and swollen, and the nail 'rocks' more than usual on the swollen nail-bed. In profile (*Fig.* 324), the swelling of the end of the finger and the curvature of the nail are evident, and the angle between the skin on the dorsal surface of the terminal phalanx and the nail, normally rather less than 180°, is increased, sometimes to more than 180°. It has been shown by plethysmography that the swelling of the soft tissues is accompanied by increase in blood-flow. If the appearances are equivocal, it is best to record them in detail, feature by feature, rather than as an arbitrary decision as to whether clubbing is present or absent. Clubbing affects the toes as well as the fingers, but is generally less easily detected in them.

Hippocrates noted that the nails of the hand might be bent in empyema thoracis, and this is generally quoted as the first reference to the association of clubbing of the fingers with lung disease. For this reason, clubbed fingers are sometimes called 'Hippocratic fingers', especially in France. Clubbing may be observed in certain diseases of the lungs, bronchi, and pleurae; in cyanotic congenital heart disease; in infective

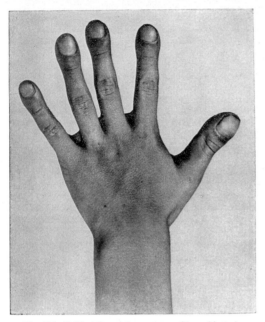

Fig. 323. Clubbed fingers from a case of bronchiectasis.

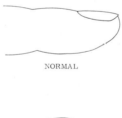

NORMAL

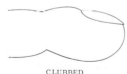

CLUBBED

Fig. 324. Profiles of normal and clubbed fingers.

endocarditis; in liver disease; in ulcerative colitis and Crohn's disease; in carcinoma of the lung and, much more rarely, tumours of other organs; and, rarely, as a familial disorder without evidence of any associated disease.

Among *diseases of the lungs, bronchi, and pleura*, bronchial carcinoma and intrathoracic suppuration are the leading causes of clubbing of the fingers. In Great Britain, bronchiectasis, lung abscess, and chronic empyema are no longer common diseases, whereas the incidence of bronchial carcinoma continues to increase; bronchial carcinoma has therefore become the commonest acquired disease associated with clubbing of the fingers. A few cases of secondary malignant disease in the lung, especially those presenting as large tumour masses, show clubbing of the fingers. Pulmonary tuberculosis is not associated with clubbing unless there is secondary pyogenic infection of fibrotic and bronchiectatic lung. Similarly, chronic bronchitis and emphysema are associated with clubbing only in the presence of pyogenic infection, generally in dilated bronchi. Widespread fibrosis of the lung may be associated with clubbing, but different types of fibrosis vary widely in their liability to be so associated. Cryptogenic fibrosing alveolitis (diffuse interstitial fibrosis of unknown cause) is commonly accompanied by clubbing early in its course, whereas the widespread fibrosis consequent upon extrinsic allergic alveolitis (farmer's lung, bird-fancier's lung, etc.) gives rise to clubbing, if at all, only late in its course. Other forms of widespread non-industrial fibrosis of the lung (e.g., sarcoidosis, honeycomb lung due to histiocytosis X) are rarely associated with clubbing, except in the presence of secondary bacterial infection. Among pneumoconioses, asbestosis is especially liable to be associated with clubbing; uncomplicated coal-miner's pneumoconiosis shows no such liability. Occasionally, a benign intrathoracic tumour may cause clubbing: a remarkable example of this is the very rare fibroma of the pleura, in which clubbing, often with pulmonary osteo-arthropathy, may be a presenting feature.

Even among those pulmonary diseases in which clubbing is frequent, its incidence is variable; it may be observed to develop early in one case, but not in another apparently similar in other respects. In a few cases, especially of bronchial carcinoma and of cryptogenic fibrosing alveolitis, clubbing appears before any other symptom.

Among *diseases of the cardiovascular system*, cyanotic congenital heart disease is constantly associated with fully developed 'drumstick' clubbing of the fingers in patients who survive infancy. On the other hand, clubbing does not occur in non-cyanotic congenital cardiovascular malformations, such as uncomplicated atrial or ventricular septal defects, persistent ductus arteriosus, or coarctation of the aorta. Patients with subacute bacterial endocarditis may develop clubbing in 3–6 weeks if untreated. Rarer cardiovascular causes of clubbing include pulmonary arteriovenous aneurysms and atrial myxoma. Unilateral clubbing of the fingers has been reported in association with subclavian aneurysm.

Clubbing, usually of mild to moderate degree, develops late in some cases of *cirrhosis of the liver*, especially in biliary cirrhosis; in *coeliac disease* and other intestinal malabsorption syndromes; and rarely in ulcerative colitis and Crohn's disease.

Pseudohypertrophic pulmonary osteo-arthropathy (p. 467) includes clubbing of the fingers as one of its features, but only a small minority of patients with clubbing develop osteo-arthropathy. Malignant disease of the lung and, less frequently, bronchiectasis and other forms of intrathoracic suppuration are the usual underlying causes. In such cases, in addition to clubbing, there is swelling of the soft tissues around wrists, ankles, and sometimes other joints, notably the knees, sometimes with effusion into the joints. Radiologically, periosteal new bone formation can be seen, especially at the distal ends of the long bones adjoining the affected joints, and in the metacarpals, metatarsals, and phalanges. The causative factors in clubbing and pulmonary osteo-arthropathy are probably not identical, since arthropathy is very rare in cyanotic congenital heart disease, in which severe drumstick clubbing is common.

Familial forms of clubbing (hereditary acropachy) and of pseudohypertrophic osteo-arthropathy, which are not associated with any pulmonary, cardiac, or other disease, are rare, but well documented. The absence of associated disease and the occurrence of a similar condition in other members of the family should lead to correct diagnosis. Hereditary osteo-arthropathy is associated with thickening of the skin of the hands and of the face, the latter giving rise to a characteristic appearance with large features and coarse skin with deep creases; this very rare familial condition has been called 'pachydermoperiostosis'.

Finally, it is of interest to note how rarely patients observe even the most gross clubbing in their own fingers, and often state there is no change whatsoever in fingers which have only recently become markedly clubbed due to the development of serious underlying disease. Their own statement that there has been no change should not be taken, therefore, as evidence of the disorder being congenital.

J. G. Scadding.

FINGERS, DEAD

Digital arteries normally react to cold by constriction. In the majority of subjects no symptoms result from this but, in quite a large minority, the fingers become pale and numb or, in lay parlance, 'dead'. Such a reaction, seen for example after bathing, may be thought to be evidence of a 'bad circulation', but it is compatible with perfect health in all other respects and it is rarely of any serious significance. This phenomenon, which is equally common in the two sexes, represents one end of a spectrum at the other end of which is florid Raynaud's disease. (*Fig.* 325.)

In *Raynaud's disease*, which is very much commoner in females, the attacks are much more easily provoked, occurring both in summer and in winter, and are more frequent and prolonged. Initially the affected fingers—usually of both hands—become pale as the circulation is halted. Subsequently the capillary bed reopens, the digital arteries remaining constricted, and the fingers become blue. Short attacks may pass

unnoticed but these are rare and, if the attack lasts for more than half an hour, the patient will complain of numbness, progressing to pain which may be very severe. With recovery the fingers gradually become bright red, beginning at the bases; the red and blue areas are sharply demarcated from each other. In very severe cases recovery may be incomplete with patches of red and blue alternating and changing one into the other as the digital arteries relax slightly only to

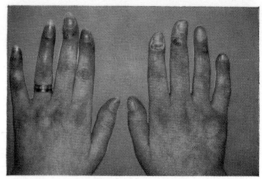

Fig. 325. Typical cold blue fingers of Raynaud's disease in a young woman. Notice the ulceration on the right side typical of severe disease. (*Professor Harold Ellis.*)

constrict once more. In long-standing cases the soft tissues become atrophic so that the fingers taper to their ends and the nails become curved. Resorption of terminal phalanges may occur and the skin becomes bound down to the subjacent tissues, losing its natural wrinkles and becoming shiny and hard. The term 'sclerodactyly' is applied to this condition; this is acceptable as a descriptive term, provided that it is not confused with scleroderma (*see below*). Gangrene of a whole finger is rare but minute painful areas of necrosis can develop on the finger-tips.

There are several groups of conditions in which some or all of the manifestations of Raynaud's disease may occur. In such cases a diagnosis of Raynaud's *phenomenon* should be made. The distinction from primary Raynaud's *disease* is important as the treatment should clearly be that of any underlying cause. It follows also that a diagnosis of Raynaud's disease should not be made until the conditions to be discussed below have been excluded. *Occlusion of a subclavian or brachial artery* will cause the fingers of the affected hand to become cold, together with other evidence of ischaemia; in a few cases a complete Raynaud's phenomenon develops with exposure to cold. The occlusion may be due to athero-sclerosis, arterial thrombosis, or, rather frequently, cervical rib. The chronic intermittent occlusion of the axillary artery produced by an old-fashioned crutch may also cause Raynaud's phenomenon. This reaction may also follow *trauma* to the fingers. Rarely, an injury to a single finger may leave that finger alone subject to the typical attacks. More commonly they occur in workers whose fingers regularly suffer minor trauma from holding vibrating instruments such as pneumatic drills. Typical attacks of Raynaud's phenomenon may also occur in some *connective-tissue diseases*, such as Sjögren's syndrome, rheumatoid arthritis, polymyositis, systemic lupus erythematosus, and systemic sclerosis (scleroderma). It is particularly characteristic of the last named condition of which, as also of the other disorders, it may be the presenting manifestation. Certain drugs, ergot and methysergide, for instance, may cause the phenomenon. Finally, there is a group of conditions in which abnormal reactions occur in the blood itself as a result of exposure to cold. These include *cryoglobulinaemia* in which proteins which precipitate in the cold, *in vitro* and *in vivo*, are found in the serum. This condition is most often a complication of diseases of the reticulo-endothelial system, particularly myelomatosis. Raynaud's phenomenon may also occur in the rare variety of auto-immune *haemolytic anaemia* in which haemolysins active only in the cold are found; this is sometimes a rare complication of congenital syphilis.

P. R. Fleming.

FINGERS, SORE

Digital lesions may be erythematous, papular, vesicular, bullous, pustular, squamous, or ulcerative, representing a long list of cutaneous affections. The *erythematous* affections which may attack the fingers are erythema multiforme, lupus erythematosus, dermatitis, urticaria, chilblains, frost-bite; the *papular*, lichen planus and granuloma annulare, pityriasis rubra pilaris, angiokeratoma, dermatitis, and papular syphilides;

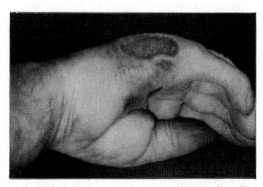

Fig. 326. Tertiary syphilis (gumma). (*Dr. Peter Hansell.*)

the *vesicular*, scabies, cheiropompholyx (dyshidrosis), dermatitis, chilblains, dermatitis caused by handling skin irritants, notably occupational dermatitis; the *bullous*, epidermolysis bullosa, scabies, leprosy, herpes simplex; the *pustular*, scabies, boils, whitlow, impetigo contagiosa, dermatitis, and pustular syphilides; the *squamous*, psoriasis, dermatitis, ichthyosis, lichen planus, syphilis, and verruca necrogenica; the *ulcerative*, chilblains and frost-bite, X-ray ulcer,

dissection wounds, lupus vulgaris, lupus erythematosus, leprosy, chancre and syphilitic ulcer (*Fig.* 326), epithelioma, Raynaud's disease, diabetic gangrene, trophic ulcer, sclerodactylia, and bed-sore. Persons working with chromium salts may develop ulcers on the fingers (*Fig.* 327) or in the nose.

In the majority of these conditions lesions typical of the disease in question occur on other parts of the body so that the diagnosis may present no real difficulty.

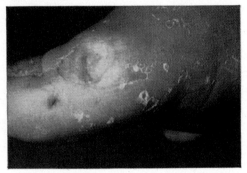

Fig. 327. Chrome ulcer. (*Dr. Peter Hansell.*)

Syphilitic chancre of the finger may be overlooked, but the presence of a painless ulcer at the lateral margin of the nailfold, frequently of the index finger, should arouse suspicion, especially if it does not yield to the usual treatment for a septic infection within a short time. Positive serological tests after the tenth to fourteenth day or the development of a secondary rash after from two to three weeks will clinch the diagnosis.

P. D. Samman.

FLATULENCE

It is necessary to distinguish between (1) gastric flatulence in which wind is eructated and (2) intestinal flatulence in which it is passed per anum.

Gastric Flatulence. This is usually due to air swallowing (aerophagy). The belching is violent and odourless; the patient can belch 'to order' and observation will reveal the gulping down of air which precedes it. This may be merely a habit in otherwise normal healthy individuals, may occur in neurotic subjects, or may be associated with almost any form of gastric or biliary disorder in which the patient attempts to relieve the abdominal discomfort by swallowing air and then belching it again. This must be distinguished from cases in which gas is produced by fermentation in stagnating gastric contents associated with pyloric obstruction or which may follow a vagotomy operation in which the surgeon has failed to drain the atonic stomach adequately. In these cases the eructations are offensive due to the presence of methane and hydrogen sulphide; it should be noted that this gas mixture is inflammable and several examples of explosions have been recorded when such patients indulge in cigarette-smoking. There are usually the other features of gastric dilatation, including projectile vomiting of large amounts of fluid containing stale food and the presence of a gastric splash or visible gastric peristalsis. X-ray examination will confirm the dilatation, obstruction, and delayed emptying of the stomach.

Intestinal Flatulence is often associated with aerophagy, the excessive amounts of swallowed air passing rapidly along the alimentary canal and passing per anum half to one hour later. Less commonly intestinal flatulence is due to partial intestinal obstruction or to abnormal fermentation which may occur in some patients with steatorrhoea. Increased gas production may occur after large meals or certain foodstuffs, such as cabbage, cauliflower, peas, beans, and sauerkraut, and soup made of root (Jerusalem) artichokes.

Harold Ellis.

FLUSHING

Flushing is a slowly spreading erythema of the skin due to a temporary dilatation of the capillaries, and differs only from blushing in that whereas the latter is invariably caused by emotional disturbances, occurs rapidly, and is confined to face, neck, and the upper anterior part of the chest, flushing may be caused by a number of conditions of which emotional disturbance is one. It may be accompanied or followed by nausea, vomiting, fainting, a sense of suffocation, numbness of the affected areas, tremors, tinnitus, giddiness, and tachycardia, and may even be painful.

The physical states from which flushing arises include menstruation and menstrual irregularities, the climacteric, pregnancy, and febrile states, in scarlet fever, for instance, where it precedes the rash; it may also be an expression of emotion, may be caused by alcoholic indulgence, or may be a part of an epileptic aura. It is the commonest clinical feature of the carcinoid syndrome, affecting head and neck (the blush area). In general, flushing is commoner in women than in men. It may also occur in diabetics under insulin as a symptom of both hypo- and hyperglycaemia, usually the latter. Post-prandial flushing of the face, especially the middle third, is a characteristic of *rosacea* (*see Fig.* 637, p. 617). In this disease the reddening later becomes permanent, with dilatation of the superficial vessels. This is followed by papule formation as a result of inflammation of the sebaceous glands and follicles. In some cases these papules become secondarily infected and pustulation takes place; in others there is hypertrophic thickening of the skin of the nose, with eventual lobulation (*rhinophyma*).

Rosacea is distinguished from acne vulgaris by the absence of comedones, the redness of the affected surface, the limitations of the eruption to the face, especially the nose and cheeks, the dilated capillaries, the nasal hypertrophy, and by its being an affection of middle life rather than of puberty. It differs from *lupus erythematosus* by the absence of scaliness and of atrophy, in its border, which is not raised and shows no signs of active spreading, and by its fluctuations.

Seborrhoeic dermatitis may be met with in the flush area of the face when there is considerable scaliness; the skin around the eyes is usually involved as well. From *tertiary syphilides* rosacea is distinguished by its slow course, its symmetry, the dilatation of blood-vessels, and the absence of any tendency to ulceration and scarring, or to atrophy. In syphilis, further, there will be the remains or the history of earlier lesions; and, of course, positive serological tests.

P. D. Samman.
F. Dudley Hart.

FOOT, ULCERATION OF

Perforating ulcer of the foot (*Fig.* 328) usually occurs under the ball of the great toe, but may appear on the outer side of the sole. Pressure associated with local vascular changes, disorders of the central nervous system which cause analgesia of the part, and trophic changes are the cause. Thus it occurs in diabetes mellitus, tabes

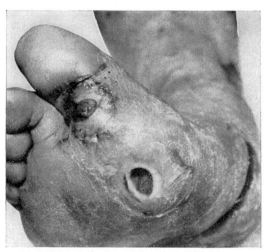

Fig. 328. Perforating ulcer of foot in a case of thrombo-angiitis obliterans.

dorsalis, leprosy, paraplegia, Raynaud's disease, and thrombo-angiitis obliterans. At first there is a dry hyperkeratosis. This becomes soft, moist, painful, purulent, and foul-smelling; finally a painful indolent ulcer results. It may bear a slight resemblance to the ulceration following a septic corn, but the latter is a more rapid process.

The so-called *phagedaena* or phagedaenic ulcer is a chronic ulcer in feet or legs caused by mixed bacteria in persons suffering from starvation and neglect (*Fig.* 329).

Ulcers of the sole are not uncommon when plantar warts have been over-treated with X-rays or radium. They also occur in severe chilblains, burns, frost-bite, and as a result of trauma.

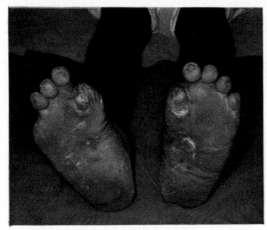

Fig. 329. Sporadic ulcero-osteolytic condition in itinerant Bantu, the result of alcoholic peripheral neuropathy, malnutrition, and trauma. (*Courtesy of Dr. Ingram Anderson.*)

In *fungous infections of the feet*, particularly between the toes, there may be deep and painful ulceration. Very severe and painful ulceration of the feet may occur in blastomycosis, sporotrichosis, and maduromycosis.

P. D. Samman.

FOREHEAD, ENLARGEMENT OF

Many individuals who have passed middle age —males more so than females—tend to develop an increasing prominence of that part of the forehead which corresponds with the outer casing of the frontal air sinuses; with the result that their eyebrows seem to overhang the eyes more and more, and the countenance looks different from that of ten or fifteen years before. This is due to slow enlargement of the air cells of the frontal sinuses, and is not pathological. This normal enlargement of the forehead has to be distinguished from two diseases which, though rare, are generally recognizable with ease if the patient is watched over a period of months or years— namely, *leontiasis ossea* and *acromegaly*.

Leontiasis ossea is a generic term applied to many different pathological conditions having the common property of thickening the bones of the skull, especially the frontal bones and the maxillae, and giving to the patient a leonine aspect. All these conditions are relatively benign and slow-growing, so that the patient may live for many years with no other disability than disfigurement, though this may be severe and terrible. The pathological conditions concerned are fibrous dysplasia, craniometaphyseal dysplasia, hyperphosphatasia, and Paget's disease. Syphilis is now a very rare cause of this appearance. Fibrous dysplasia may start in childhood or in early adolescence and is relatively slowly progressive. When it occurs in young girls it may be associated with patchy brown skin pigmentation and precocious pubity (Albright's syndrome). Bony lesions frequently coexist elsewhere, in the femur and pelvis, as well as in the skull, which gives similar radiological appearances. Hyperparathyroidism may co-exist with fibrous dysplasia. Very occasionally malignant neoplasm of the maxilla mimics for a short time leontiasis ossea, but the rapid progress soon betrays the true nature of the lesion.

Paget's disease is a not uncommon cause of enlargement of the forehead in adults (*see Fig.* 306, p. 281); enlargement of the skull may lead to the patient wearing larger hats, and may be associated with headaches and nerve deafness. The alkaline phosphatase is invariably considerably raised in the serum of such patients. Rare under the age of 40 years, its incidence increases steadily thereafter.

In acromegaly it rarely happens that the frontal bone is affected alone; more often the affection of the forehead is much slighter than the increase in size of the lower jaw (p. 450) and of the phalanges of the hands and feet. If, however, the changes were more marked in the frontal bone or in the bones of the skull generally than in those elsewhere, a case of acromegaly might be diagnosed as one of leontiasis ossea. Whereas in acromegaly the bigness of the lower jaw makes the characteristic facies, in leontiasis ossea the prominence of the forehead and maxilla gives the face that leonine character from which the name of the disease is taken. If the temporal halves of the fields of vision were contracted, and still more if there were bilateral temporal hemianopia, the diagnosis is acromegaly and not leontiasis ossea. In case of doubt a radiograph of the skull would be taken laterally to see the size of the sella turcica, which might be of normal dimensions in a case of leontiasis ossea, whereas in acromegaly the sella would be enlarged by hypertrophy of the pituitary body to which this disease is due.

No other maladies in adults are likely to cause uniform increase in the size of the forehead, but occasionally one meets with tumours of the frontal bone which cause an asymmetrical enlargement of the forehead, the most important of these being the *ivory exostosis*—a non-malignant tumour which may arise from any of the flat bones of the skull; it grows very slowly but enlarges progressively, and in so doing is apt to displace anything which comes in its way, and in the course of many years great deformity of the eye or nose may thus result. The slowness of the growth, and its very hard character generally, point to the diagnosis at once, and a radiographic examination may help to confirm it.

Other asymmetrical enlargements of the forehead may result from *syphilitic nodes* caused by gummatous periostitis terminating in bony organizations; *sarcoma of the periosteum*, a very rare primary growth in this region, but when met with, suggested by the relative softness of the mass, its rapid increase in size, and possibly eggshell crackling on palpation; *secondary malignant disease*, likely to be mistaken for primary sarcoma if no primary growth elsewhere is known, but uniform stretching such as hydrocephalus gives rise to (*Fig.* 330), or whether there are not some parts which are enlarged and other parts which are more or less normal. Both congenital syphilis and rickets are apt to produce diffuse round prominences of the parietal regions as well as of the frontal regions, so that there are four main bulges with an anteroposterior and a transverse groove between them, constituting the hot-cross-bun-shaped head; the difficulty of excluding

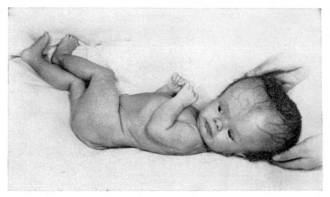

Fig. 330. Hydrocephalus, showing the huge head and bulging forehead. (*Dr. R. MacKeith.*)

diagnosed readily if the existence, now or formerly, of a carcinoma of the breast, thyroid gland, or other part is known.

Any other tumours in connexion with the frontal bone are exceedingly rare. The very extensive disease of the frontal as of any other cranial bone which used to be met with in syphilitic subjects is now practically unknown on account of the greater adequacy of the treatment of syphilis in its earlier stages.

Leprosy may be mentioned as a cause of enlargement of the forehead, for in the nodular form any part may be affected, but it must be very rare for leprosy to affect the forehead region only, and the diagnosis will be suggested by the lesions elsewhere and by the history of the case.

In children other causes will suggest themselves, the four most important being: (1) *Hydrocephalus*; (2) *Rickets*; (3) *Congenital syphilis*; (4) *Haematoma*.

It happens not infrequently that a child's forehead enlarges very considerably, and bulges with much convexity to such an extent as to raise a fear of hydrocephalus when the child is suffering from nothing more serious than rickets. The diagnosis may be in doubt for months if there are not at the same time the other familiar signs of rickets mentioned on pp. 130, 222. The same applies to the swelling of the frontal bone that may result from congenital syphilis. In the case of both rickets and congenital syphilis one will examine the whole of the head carefully, and try to make up one's mind whether the enlargement, which usually affects not only the forehead but also other parts of the skull, is a more or less

hydrocephalus is greater when, as sometimes happens, there is such thinning of the bones in the occipital regions from craniotabes that the bones can be dented inwards like stiff parchment; such craniotabes may result either from rickets or from congenital syphilis. One would then pay special attention to the regions of the sutures; if these are obviously stretched asunder the condition is almost certainly hydrocephalus, and not rickets or congenital syphilis. One would also be able to draw a conclusion from the appearance of the eyes, for the eyeballs will be in normal position when the cause of the forehead enlargement is rickets or congenital syphilis, whilst with hydrocephalus the eyes give the impression of being depressed as the result of the downward pressure exerted by the excess of fluid upon the roofs of the orbits. If the enlargement and prominence of the forehead date from birth or soon afterwards, the argument is in favour of hydrocephalus; if the change develops later in the child's life, the history will be of importance, because the commonest cause of acquired hydrocephalus is a preceding attack of meningococcal meningitis from which the child has recovered. The optic disk should also be examined, for in some cases of acquired hydrocephalus there is optic atrophy (*Fig.* 619, p. 605), and this is practically never met with as the result of rickets, and very seldom as the result of congenital syphilis. It is only when the degree of hydrocephalus is moderate that it is difficult to distinguish it from forehead enlargements due to rickets or congenital syphilis. Major degrees of hydrocephalus cause such extreme enlargement of the whole head, coupled with such thinning of the bones and stretching of the sutures, that the diagnosis is almost unmistakable.

Simple or malignant tumours affecting the frontal bones in an infant are rare; they should be diagnosed in the same way as similar tumours in adults. *Chloroma* may perhaps be mentioned specially, rare though it is. The growths in such a case are never single, but as they may develop upon bones they sometimes attract notice first in connexion with the cranial bones, and thus perhaps a local enlargement of the forehead may be the first symptom in the case. There is a tendency for the lymphatic glands generally to become enlarged and sometimes the spleen also, and in some respects the malady simulates lymphatic leukaemia; but there are no characteristic blood changes. Neoplasm of some kind will be an early suspicion, and the nature of the growth is suggested by the greenish colour of the excised tumour. The diagnosis is made more often post mortem than during life.

The commonest local swelling of the forehead in a child is a *haematoma* resulting from injury, and as the blood-clot is often deep-seated there is sometimes no discoloration of the skin, and some more serious tumour may be thought of until the disappearance of the mass in the course of a week or two proves its simple character. Such a haematoma softens in the middle in a remarkable way after a day or two, leaving hard raised edges and a soft centre; on palpation it feels almost as if there were a hard bony ring with an absence of any bone at all within it; the first time such a softening haematoma of the scalp is felt one can hardly believe that it is only a haematoma and not an actual hole in the bone covered merely by scalp and skin. This apprehension is justifiable in a child where a depressed fracture of the vertex of the skull may occur with an intact scalp. In the adult, however, a force sufficient to fracture the vertex of the skull with indentation of the bone will almost invariably split the scalp. An intact scalp, therefore, in an adult patient giving the crateriform swelling described above argues that the condition is one of simple haematoma. In any event a radiograph of the skull is highly desirable.

R. G. Beard.

FRACTURE, SPONTANEOUS

Spontaneous fracture signifies fracture of a bone from causes which ordinarily would be inadequate. Tremendous muscular efforts sometimes lead to the breaking of a bone without any external violence, but this would not constitute spontaneous fracture if the degree of muscular effort seemed adequate. A man may, for instance, dive into shallow water, and, to prevent his head from striking the bottom, use his neck muscles so strenuously in bending his head back as actually to fracture his vertebrae. This fracture is not spontaneous, but due to excessive muscular exertion. There are five main groups of causes for true spontaneous fracture, namely, excessive brittleness—*fragilitas ossium*; conditions associated with crippling and prolonged immobility; osteomalacia and osteoporosis; parathyroid tumour; and unsuspected inflammatory or neoplastic lesions of the bones.

Fragilitas Ossium (Osteogenesis Imperfecta). When the first fracture occurs in such a patient, there may be doubt as to the diagnosis; but when repeated breaking of different bones occurs, in each case from apparently trivial causes, the diagnosis becomes clear. The undue fragility may show itself in early life, but more often not until the patient has reached adult stature and weight.

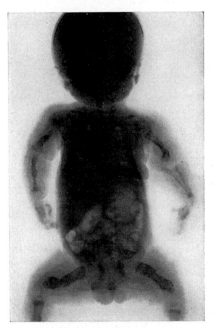

Fig. 331. Osteogenesis imperfecta. Every long bone in the body has been fractured. (*Dr. T. H. Hills.*)

There is a familial type of the disease, in which successive generations contain members who have fragile bones amongst others who are healthy; the latter have white sclerotics; those exhibiting fragilitas ossium have blue sclerotics. Both bones and sclerotics lack part of their proper matrix; the diagnosis is easy, though the condition, 'blue sclerotics with brittle bones', is rare.

The history of spontaneous fractures may not be true. The clinician should always be aware of 'battered babies', where the injuries have been inflicted by parents.

Two maladies which differ from fragilitas ossium, and yet which may cause undue bending, or partial or green-stick fracture of bones, are *rickets* in children, in which disease, for a time at least, there is excess of preparation for bone formation, but deficiency in completing the ossifying process, so that the bones, being unduly soft, not only bend, but also give way as a green stick would, causing the partial or green-stick fracture; and *osteomalacia* in adults. This is seen in conditions characterized by chronic intestinal malabsorption and steatorrhoea. Complete or incomplete fractures may occur in extremities and in vertebral bodies. *Osteoporosis* increases gradually with age and is more common in elderly females. In such patients fractures, particularly of vertebral bodies, occur with minimal trauma, especially if the patient is relatively or absolutely immobile. Corticosteroid therapy adds to the risk.

Spontaneous fractures in conditions associated with crippling and prolonged immobility are not uncommon. Rheumatoid arthritics, particularly if on prolonged corticosteroid therapy, are an example. Patients with dementia paralytica (general paralysis of the insane) are today rarely seen.

Hyperparathyroidism. Some cases of spontaneous fracture are associated with a greater or less degree of rarefaction of the whole skeleton and with the excretion of large amounts of calcium in the urine. The serum calcium is usually raised in these patients. Bilateral or unilateral kidney stones may complicate this condition which is due to an innocent adenoma of one (or rarely more than one) of the four parathyroid glands. The adenoma is often so small that it cannot be felt and, if the calcium balance studies indicate it, the neck should be explored and an adenoma, sometimes no more than a centimetre in diameter, but sometimes larger, will be found in one of the four classic sites of the parathyroid or in an ectopic position almost anywhere within the neck or superior mediastinum. The surgeon may be guided to an abnormally situated parathyroid tumour by a slender twig arising from the inferior thyroid artery and leading to the lesion. Removal of the adenoma corrects the metabolic abnormality; the bones recover their strength and no fresh calculi are formed.

Before concluding that spontaneous fracture of a bone is due either to neurotrophic causes, to parathyroid tumour, or to fragilitas ossium, it is important to exclude the possibility of primary or secondary *new growth* in the affected bone, or *tuberculous caries.* It may be that the patient is already suffering from a bony swelling before the fracture takes place, or it may be known that there is, or has been, a primary growth elsewhere; for instance, in the breast, kidney, prostate, bronchus, testis, or thyroid gland. The chief difficulties arise, first, when there are no symptoms of the primary growth itself, for instance in the case of a small, hidden, malignant neoplasm of the thyroid; secondly, today much less common, when the patient is suffering from tuberculosis caries whose existence has been unsuspected. Multiple myelomatosis is a not uncommon cause. Radiographs may be of value in detecting a neoplasm or a tuberculous focus in the affected bone (*see* BONE, SWELLING ON, p. 100).

A rare cause of brittle bones is chronic fluoride poisoning. It may occur amongst glass-etchers and workers with insect powders.

R. G. Beard.

FRIGIDITY

Frigidity, like impotence (*see* p. 420), is due to a wide variety of causes, by far the most important of which are psychogenic. However, severe physical malformations of the genital tract whether congenital or acquired can, of course, interfere with sexual intercourse or lead to a failure to achieve orgasm. The same may also be an outcome of *dyspareunia*, due also to some physical lesion.

Quite a substantial proportion of women appear to be *constitutionally frigid*. This implies that there seem to be no good physical or psychological reasons for their inability to achieve orgasm. This may, however, be more apparent than real and, in the case of many women, be related to a lack of knowledge of what is to be expected from sexual intercourse. However, with increasing sophistication, in part the outcome of better sex education, the level of expectation among women appears to be rising, which in turn may have led to a fall in the number of those who might once have been regarded as constitutionally frigid. Nonetheless, there remains an unknown number of women who, while they insist on superficial questioning that their sex lives are satisfactory, may, when pressed, reveal that they have never actually obtained full sexual satisfaction. Such women have often been brought up to believe that sexual intercourse is something to be endured rather than enjoyed.

Before considering what may be pathological, two other relevant factors need consideration. One is that the achievement of sexual satisfaction by women appears to be more closely bound up with an affectionate or loving relationship than is the case with men, to whom mere physical satisfaction may be sufficient. The second is that women are slower to arouse sexually than are men. This means that if the male partner lacks technique, hurries the proceedings unduly, or, being partially impotent, suffers from premature ejaculation, with loss of tumescence, the woman concerned may not have sufficient time in which to achieve orgasm. If she is herself inexperienced and does not understand the reason for this, she may come to regard herself as frigid.

This type of difficulty may be regarded as *pseudofrigidity*, a state in which potential ability to achieve orgasm is present but, owing to unpropitious circumstances, may not be realized. Other circumstances which may likewise lead to failure of orgasm may be *fear of pregnancy*— some women deliberately suppress orgasm in the belief that this may prevent pregnancy occurring —sleeping in the same house as parents or in-laws, or sharing a bedroom with children, etc. *Alcoholism* in the marital partner may also be a source of difficulty, the inconsideration of a partly intoxicated spouse tending in due course to bring about an intense revulsion for sexual intercourse.

Like impotence, frigidity may arise out of *inexperience* or be due to *simple anxiety*. It may also be an outcome of *emotional immaturity*, a state often reflected by the inability of a young bride to live a separate existence independent of her parents. Frigidity is a common affliction among neurotic women who are either over-attached to their fathers or have a poor relationship with their parents which may be the outcome of cruelty in marriage, alcoholism, etc. *Sexual interference* in childhood or adolescence by either a male relative or some other person may also later impair a normal capacity for satisfactory intercourse.

In the case of *female homosexuals* (*Lesbians*) frigidity in a heterosexual relationship is common though not apparently invariable. Some basically homosexual women marry and make a success of it sometimes by arranging a *ménage à trois*. Many professional *prostitutes* are said to be frigid and many are probably homosexual also. The same, paradoxically, applies to *nymphomania* in which state, although there is an apparently intense desire for sexual relationships, sometimes with any available male partner, satisfaction is never achieved. It has also been suggested that nymphomania represents an attempt by the female to denigrate male sexuality.

Certain matters pertaining to childbirth may be important. In some women an *abortion* may occasionally give rise to frigidity though the vast majority remain unaffected by this event. Fear of pregnancy has already been mentioned but, even in the absence of this and where satisfactory contraceptive methods are employed, some women tend to become frigid after the birth of a second or third child when no more children are desired, which may be a reflection of the more intimate relationship between child-bearing and sex which exists in women as opposed to their husbands. Likewise, and sometimes surprisingly, a loss of libido quite often appears to follow sterilization—for whatever reason. Loss of sexual desire is not necessarily a sequel to the menopause; indeed, a capacity to enjoy sexual relationships may persist in some women to a relatively advanced age although there is naturally a wide variation.

Finally, as in the case of the male, loss of libido may occur in women due to a *depressive illness*. Following treatment and satisfactory resolution of the illness sexual function may be restored once again to normal.

W. H. Trethowan.

GAIT, ABNORMALITIES OF

Gait may be disturbed by: (1) Mechanical defects in the lower limbs and pelvis. (2) Pain in the legs, pelvis, or lower lumbar spine.

The way in which the patient spares the painful joint or joints as much as possible is characteristic. The tender heels of Reiter's disease, for instance, make the patient walk in a particularly careful apprehensive manner (the 'pussyfoot' gait). (3) Disease of muscles. (4) Disease of the nervous system: (*a*) Increased tone, either striatal or pyramidal; (*b*) Weakness, either pyramidal or peripheral; (*c*) Ataxia, either sensory or cerebellar. (5) Disease of the vestibular apparatus. (6) Hysteria.

1. Mechanical Defects. Inequality in the length of the legs, congenital dislocation of the hips, ankylosis of the knee or hip joints, and deformities of the feet give rise to a characteristic bold, painless limp, the source of which is readily found on examination of the limbs.

Coxa vara and coxa valga may lead to characteristic gaits. Painless ankylosis of both hips leads to all movements being made at knees, ankles, and feet giving a short-stepping smooth gait, almost as if the patient was on roller-skates. This is seen, for instance, in cases of ankylosing spondylitis.

2. Painful Limp, due to pain in the pelvis or lower limb, is easily recognized by the manner in which the patient puts the weight on the sound leg and hurries off the affected one. The source of the pain may be in the limb itself, or it may be referred from disease in the pelvis, lumbar spine, or cauda equina. Localized pain usually means localized disease at that site, referred pain tending to have a more diffuse and linear distribution, but many exceptions occur. The pain referred from a diseased hip may be felt only in the knee—an important feature in children with tuberculosis of the hip, and occasionally a root pain is limited to a small area in the foot (S. 1) or the lateral border of the leg (L. 5). Local tenderness at the site of the pain often indicates local disease, but it may equally well be present in referred pain. On the other hand, local deformity or swelling always means disease at that point. The more important causes of a painful limp are enumerated in the following list:

THE JOINTS:
  Injuries
  Arthritis or arthrosis of lumbar spine, or of hip, knee, ankle, and/or foot on one or both sides
THE BONES:
  Injuries
  Neoplastic, congenital, or metabolic disease
  Inflammatory and/or infective disease
THE MUSCLES:
  Injury
  Wasting and weakness
THE BLOOD-VESSELS:
  Intermittent claudication from arterial disease or embolism
  Phlebitis
THE LUMBOSACRAL ROOTS:
  Prolapse of intervertebral disk
  Lesions of cauda equina
  Lesions of lumbar vertebrae
  Pelvic masses

OTHER TISSUES:
  Foreign body in foot (children)
  Bursitis (gluteal, patella and tendo Achillis)
  Corns and bunions
  Flat feet
  Chilblains

3. Diseases of Muscles are rare, and are therefore seldom responsible for disturbances of gait. In the heredofamilial *myopathies*, usually seen in early life, the gait is waddling, the muscles weak and either hypertrophied or atrophied, and sensation is normal. In *myotonia congenita* members of affected families experience from birth a peculiar difficulty in relaxing muscles after voluntary contraction. Thus on attempting to walk, the muscles go into a tonic spasm, but this can be worked off by continued exercise. If called upon to change the tempo, direction, or size of the step, the patient is at once seized with myotonia and may fall to the ground. Diagnosis is made on the family history, the presence of prolonged contraction after voluntary effort, the production of a persistent localized contraction on percussion of the affected muscles, and high-frequency discharges in the electromyogram, likened on the loudspeaker to the noise of a dive-bomber. A similar myotonia is seen in *dystrophia myotonica*, a familial disease of adult life; the gait is disturbed by myotonia, but weakness and atrophy of the quadriceps and of the dorsiflexors of the feet are a further embarrassment to walking. The presence of wasting and myotonia in the face, sternomastoids, and forearm, and the frequent presence of premature baldness, cataracts, and testicular atrophy, indicate the correct diagnosis. In *myasthenia gravis*, the legs, in common with the rest of the musculature, fatigue rapidly: the gait is normal after rest, but as fatigue supervenes it becomes shuffling, unsteady, and weak. The weakness and extreme hypotonia of the muscles in *amyotonia congenita* interfere with gait in those children who survive the first critical years of infancy. They learn to walk later, and they then present the unsteadiness of weakness, but even this incapacity may be outgrown.

4. Disease of the Nervous System

  a. Spasticity due to bilateral pyramidal disease will affect both legs, as in congenital spastic diplegia, spinal compression, disseminated sclerosis, subacute combined degeneration of the cord, intramedullary tumours, syringomyelia, etc. Tone is increased in the extensors and adductors, so that the limb is held in extension, with plantar flexion of the foot, and some degree of adduction. Gait is stiff, the toes scrape the ground, and if the adduction and spasticity are severe, there is a 'scissors gait'. Weakness increases the disability. A unilateral pyramidal lesion gives rise to a similar stiff, extended limb, which is dragged around its normal fellow by tilting the pelvis, thus overcoming the adduction and allowing the extended foot to clear the ground.

  The rigidity of *extrapyramidal disease* affects extensors and flexors equally, but the legs are held slightly flexed at the hip and knee because the flexors are more powerful than the extensors. Steps are short, shuffling, and crabbed. The patient tends to walk faster and faster, as if chasing his centre of gravity. If pushed backwards, he tends to run backwards with short, hasty steps. Fixity of expression, flexion of the neck and trunk, adduction of the arm with flexion of the elbows, and the characteristic rhythmic tremor of the forearms, hands, and fingers afford diagnostic assistance when the extrapyramidal lesions are due to Parkinson's disease, one of the earliest signs being a failure to swing the arm on walking. A similar gait results from extrapyramidal lesions due to encephalitis lethargica, arteriopathic cerebral degeneration, carbon monoxide poisoning, hepatolenticular degeneration, and (rarely) after severe head injuries.

  b. Weakness plays a part in pyramidal lesions, but it is often difficult to distinguish the relative importance of this weakness and the associated spasticity in the disturbances of gait which are described above. On the other hand, weakness due to disease of the anterior horn cells or of the peripheral nerves to the legs gives rise to abnormal gaits, the features of which depend on the distribution of the weak or paralysed muscles. Where there is foot-drop, as in any form of polyneuritis, injuries to the common peroneal nerve, poliomyelitis, or a lesion of the cauda equina, there is a high-stepping gait, in which the foot is lifted high and then slapped down on the ground as if walking in long grass or over heather. If the calf muscles are paralysed, as in a lesion of the posterior tibial nerve, the gait loses its natural spring. Furthermore, disease affecting the motor fibres often attacks the sensory fibres too; proprioceptive sensory loss then adds a sensory ataxic element to the gait, which becomes clumsy, unsteady, irregular, and broad based, as in tabes, many types of polyneuritis (*see* p. 718), and gross disease of the cauda equina. When sensory ataxia thus complicates muscular weakness, balance is worse in the dark or when the eyes are shut.

  c. Sensory *ataxia* has been mentioned as a factor in the clumsy, incoordinated, noisy, wide-based gait of polyneuritis, tabes, lesions of the cauda equina, and some cases of subacute combined degeneration of the cord. A second form of ataxic gait is seen as a result of disease or injury of the cerebellar system and the cerebellum, the cerebellar peduncles, and the spinocerebellar tracts. The gait is wide-based and clumsy, but it is little aggravated by darkness or by closing the eyes. There is a tendency to deviate towards the side of the lesion, but overcompensation may occur, with consequent deviation to both sides in an irregular, staggering, and drunken manner. The normal 'swing' of the arm on the affected side may be diminished or lost, but this feature is often absent. 'Cerebellar' ataxia is seen in disseminated sclerosis, the heredofamilial ataxias, occasional cases of tabes without proprioceptive sensory loss, and in inflammatory, neoplastic, degenerative, traumatic, and vascular lesions of the cerebellum.

5. Vestibular Ataxia. Disease of the labyrinth, the vestibular nerve, or the vestibular nucleus in the pons can give rise to disturbances of gait. Vertigo makes the patient feel disorientated; the gait is unsteady and there is a tendency to deviate to the affected side. This occurs in acute phases of Menière's disease, acute labyrinthitis, and vascular lesions of the pons.

6. Hysteria is sometimes responsible for abnormal gaits. There is no set pattern, but, however bizarre hysterical gaits may be, they have in common a certain improbability and flamboyance; a tendency to subside gracefully and safely on the floor, and to stagger in the direction of objects upon which to lean. 'Astasia abasia' is a term which was formerly used for inability to stand or walk despite normal movements of the limbs when recumbent, but it is desirable to recall that in hereditary spinocerebellar ataxia, and in affections of the flocculo-nodular lobe and the vermis of the cerebellum, a gross ataxia of gait may be found despite good performance in all tests of co-ordination when in bed. This is due to the fact that these functions, of balance and co-ordination, are subserved by different regions of the cerebellum which can be involved separately in disease processes, co-ordination depending on the integrity of the lateral lobes of the cerebellum and balance on the midline structures. Hysterical gaits are recognized by their inconsistencies, and by a quality which can best be described as insincerity; confirmation is to be found in the presence of psychoneurosis and the absence of organic disease. Unlike organic disorders of gait, they can be cured by suggestion.

Ian Mackenzie.

GALL-BLADDER ENLARGEMENT

Physical Signs. On occasions a grossly distended gall-bladder in a thin subject may be visible as a distinct globular swelling in the right upper abdomen. However, palpation is the physical method of examination in detecting enlargement of the gall-bladder. One may feel an oval, smooth swelling moving downwards close behind the anterior abdominal wall when the patient inspires, descending either from beneath the right costal margin near the tip of the 9th rib, or attached to the undersurface of a palpable liver in the right nipple line. As it enlarges, the tumour generally extends inwards as well as downwards so that it may ultimately cross the midline below the level of the umbilicus. It may be large enough to be palpable bimanually in a thin patient but it does not fill out the loin in a way that a renal tumour may do. It may or may not be tender, depending on whether the cause of the enlargement is or is not associated with inflammation. It feels firm and tense rather than hard. An impaired but not quite dull note is obtained on percussion.

Diagnosis from other Swellings. It has to be distinguished particularly from four groups of conditions: (1) From *carcinoma* arising in the bile-ducts or gall-bladder itself; (2) From *tumours* in or attached to the liver in the neighbourhood of the gall-bladder—secondary new growth, primary hepatoma, or more rarely gumma, abscess, or hydatid cyst; (3) From *mobile kidney, hydronephrosis,* or *renal tumour;* (4) From *tumours in the neighbouring organs,* such as carcinoma of the pylorus or the right suprarenal.

1. CARCINOMA OF THE GALL-BLADDER. It is often difficult to decide whether a tumour is merely an enlarged gall-bladder or a growth infiltrating and replacing it, since in either case there may be a history extending over years of gall-stones, with biliary colic, pyrexia, and even jaundice, and primary new growth of the gall-bladder is often associated with gall-stones. The rapidity of the enlargement in the absence of any definite cause will suggest growth, particularly in a person of the cancer age; careful palpation may show that the mass is not smooth as in the case of most simple gall-bladder enlargements, but more or less nodulated or covered with bosses or irregularities, which in themselves suggest new growth. In some cases there may be secondary deposits in the liver, ascites, and sometimes the enlargement of the left supraclavicular lymph-node points to malignant disease with metastasis. Notwithstanding these points, however, the differential diagnosis may be so difficult that laparotomy will be necessary for decision.

2. THE TUMOURS ATTACHED TO OR IN THE LIVER. Those most likely to be mistaken for enlargement of the gall-bladder are Riedel's lobe, secondary carcinoma of the liver, and, much more rarely, hepatoma, gumma, abscess, or hydatid cyst. It may, by physical examination, be impossible to distinguish a *Riedel's lobe* (p. 504) from an enlarged gall-bladder or from a mobile kidney. Owing to the absence of symptoms there is seldom need for laparotomy, but occasionally the fear of some more serious condition encourages this procedure to verify the diagnosis. Speaking generally, a Riedel's lobe usually descends from the liver farther to the right than does a gall-bladder, and it is more apt to simulate an enlarged or a mobile kidney.

Secondary new growth in the liver nearly always causes considerable and sometimes enormous enlargement and great hardness of the organ, not infrequently associated with JAUNDICE (p. 433), ASCITES (p. 75), or both. The diagnosis depends, first, upon the discovery of a primary growth, which in the case of carcinoma is likely to be in the stomach, duodenum, pancreas, colon, or rectum, or, in the case of melanoma, the eye; and secondly, on the discovery in the liver of several separate nodules, some of which may be felt to be umbilicated, that is to say depressed in their central part and raised around the edges.

Hepatoma, although rare in this country, occasionally occurs in cirrhotics and may be multifocal. In the Far East and in eastern Africa it is far more common and, in patients from those areas, is an important condition to consider in differential diagnosis.

Gumma of the liver is rarely encountered nowadays, and when it occurs is usually mistaken for new growth unless there is a convincing history of syphilis or the effects of tertiary lesions are visible elsewhere, especially gummatous lesions of the skin or leucoplakia of the tongue. The diagnosis may be confirmed by obtaining a positive serological reaction, or by the beneficial effects of antisyphilitic treatment, though this does not always lead to rapid disappearance of a gumma of the liver. Even when the liver is inspected at laparotomy the diagnosis between gumma and new growth is not always easy.

Abscess of the liver (p. 504), if it is to simulate an enlargement of the gall-bladder, is likely to be a single large one which, if it has not arisen in some pre-existent mass, such as a gumma, new growth, or hydatid cyst, is almost certain to have been acquired in a tropical country where the patient has suffered from amoebic dysentery. The diagnosis may not be evident until laparotomy is undertaken or the mass is punctured with an exploring needle.

Hydatid cyst of the liver is seldom situated in such a position as to cause difficulty of diagnosis from gall-bladder enlargement; more usually the cyst is embedded in the liver substance, or projects from its upper surface. The diagnosis might be entertained if the patient were known to have hydatid cysts elsewhere; but in most cases it is determined only when laparotomy has been performed. It might have been suggested by the discovery of eosinophilia, and also by the specific hydatid serum reaction if the hydatid cyst is alive and active. But latent or obsolete hydatid cysts cause no symptoms, do not produce an eosinophilia, and are not associated with a positive hydatid blood-serum reaction. Their walls, if calcified, can be seen on X-rays of the region.

3. THE DISTINCTION BETWEEN AN ENLARGED GALL-BLADDER AND A MOBILE KIDNEY OR HYDRONEPHROSIS. There may be no jaundice to suggest gall-bladder trouble, nor need there be any urinary changes to suggest kidney, so that the diagnosis may have to be made chiefly by palpation. Facts to stress are that a gall-bladder is more easily felt anteriorly than posteriorly, whilst the reverse is the case with the kidney; that the kidney is, as a rule, the more freely movable of the two; that it is seldom possible to demarcate the upper pole of an enlarged gall-bladder in the way that the top of a movable kidney can sometimes be defined; that with kidney tumour the loin is dull, whilst with gall-bladder enlargement it is resonant; and that, on rather firm bimanual palpation, the patient may experience a peculiar sickening sensation which is characteristic of kidney. In cases of doubt, an intravenous pyelogram will demonstrate whether or not the right kidney is normal. (*See also* KIDNEY, ENLARGEMENT OF, p. 470.)

4. TUMOURS OF OTHER ORGANS SIMULATING ENLARGEMENT OF THE GALL-BLADDER may be distinguished to some extent by the fact that new growths of the pylorus, transverse colon, or suprarenal big enough to simulate an enlargement of the gall-bladder seldom have the smooth oval outline that the gall-bladder nearly always possesses. In addition, there may have been symptoms attributable to the primary growth, such as dilatation of the stomach, coffee-ground vomit, or evidence of secondary deposits in the liver, in the left supraclavicular lymph-node, or elsewhere, to indicate the diagnosis. Nevertheless in some of these cases it is impossible to exclude enlargement of the gall-bladder without resorting to laparotomy.

The Causes of Enlargement of the Gall-bladder:

Empyema of the gall-bladder.
Chronic pancreatitis.
Carcinoma of the head of the pancreas.
Cholecystitis from: (1) Gall-stones; (2) New growth.
Typhoid fever.
Obstruction of the common bile-duct by a gall-stone.
Obstruction of the cystic duct by a gall-stone.
Simple mucocele.

It is noteworthy that *gall-stones* comparatively seldom lead to enlargement of the gall-bladder. If the associated inflammation does not progress to empyema, the gall-bladder usually becomes thick-walled, contracted, and embedded in dense adhesions which prevent it from dilating even when the cystic or common bile-ducts become obstructed by a stone. Indeed, in a middle-aged patient in whom there has not been any very definite attack of biliary colic, the occurrence of progressive and considerable enlargement of the gall-bladder, associated with a deepening jaundice and without ascites, arouses serious suspicion of a *lesion of the head of the pancreas* which has extended along the pancreatic duct so as gradually to occlude the common bile-duct, the commonest cause of these symptoms being either *chronic pancreatitis* or *carcinoma* of the head of the pancreas. In obstruction of the common bile-duct due to gall-stones, the gall-bladder is as a rule not palpable: in obstruction due to carcinoma of the head of the pancreas it is usually distended and is palpable in about 50 per cent of patients (Courvoisier's law, *Fig.* 332). Painless progressive jaundice suggests a carcinoma arising at the ampulla of Vater and, if this ulcerates, the stools may be positive for occult blood. Jaundice preceded by epigastric or upper lumbar pain is more likely to be due to carcinoma or chronic pancreatitis of the body of the pancreas. Sometimes sloughing of part of the tumour allows the pent-up bile to escape into the duodenum with puzzling temporary remission or even disappearance of the jaundice. In cases in which gall-stones are the cause of the enlargement there is nearly always tenderness over the gall-bladder and pain when it is palpated firmly, associated with a rise of temperature, possibly with rigors, especially if the inflammation has spread to the bile-ducts (infective or suppurative cholangitis). Leucocytosis, with a relative increase in the polymorphonuclear cells, would indicate that in addition to gall-stones there is *empyema of the gall-bladder* demanding urgent surgical treatment.

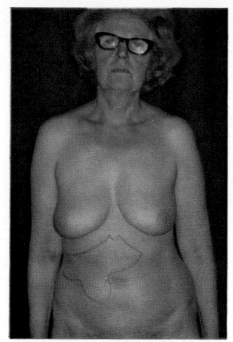

Fig. 332. Courvoisier's law. Obstructive jaundice due to a carcinoma of the head of the pancreas. The liver is smoothly enlarged due to biliary obstruction. The gall-bladder forms a globular palpable mass at its lower border.

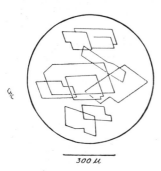

300 μ

Fig. 333. Cholesterol crystals; flat parallelograms with notched corner. (High power.)

Another cause of empyema of the gall-bladder is *typhoid fever*. The diagnosis is not difficult as a rule, for in most of the cases there will be no question of new growth or of gall-stones and the patient will have been suffering from a prolonged asthenic fever already diagnosed serologically. In some typhoid patients bacillary infection of the gall-bladder causes it to enlarge rapidly even

to the extent of rupturing spontaneously and causing general peritonitis. In less severe cases, the inflammatory products discharge themselves naturally by the bile-passages.

Simple mucocele of the gall-bladder is a relatively unusual event which results from impaction of a gall-stone at the outlet of the gall-bladder when it happens to be empty. The walls of this organ continue to secrete mucus so that it becomes greatly distended with perfectly colourless mucoid liquid, free from bile-pigment though sometimes containing crystals of cholesterol (*Fig.* 333). The fluid is sterile. There are usually no symptoms. Such a mucocele may be mistaken for a mobile kidney and the diagnosis of the nature of the mass is sometimes obscure until revealed by operation.

Harold Ellis.

GANGRENE

Gangrene means death of a part of the body from deprivation of its blood-supply. This obstruction to the blood-vessels may be mechanical, infective, degenerative, spasmodic, or neoplastic.

COMMON CAUSES OF GANGRENE

Trauma:

Division of the main artery to a limb, or pressure by splints or plaster-of-Paris. The effect of extreme heat or cold—frost-bite, etc.

Diseases of the Blood-vessels:

Embolism, thrombosis, Buerger's disease (thromboangiitis obliterans), Raynaud's disease, arteriosclerosis (atheroma, Mönckeberg's calcification), venous gangrene.

Infection:

Carbuncle, 'gas gangrene', etc. (Both arteriosclerotic and infective gangrene are common in diabetes mellitus.)

LESS COMMON CAUSES:

Traumatic: Electric shock, chemical burns.
Infective: Septic wounds, erysipelas, anthrax, cancrum oris.
Complicating the following Diseases and due to Slight Trauma: The typhoids, typhus, smallpox, measles, marasmus, cholera, plague, yellow-fever, malaria, poisoning by snake-venom, leukaemias.
Neuropathic: Peripheral neuritis, syringomyelia, tabes dorsalis, leprosy, myelitis, meningomyelitis, lesions of the medulla spinalis.
Circulatory: Rheumatoid arteritis, syphilitic endarteritis, ergotism, erythromelalgia, carbolic dressings, aneurysm, polyarteritis nodosa, systemic lupus erythematosus, intra-arterial injection of pentothal sodium, obstruction by new growth, following carbon-monoxide poisoning.

Gangrene is classically referred to as 'dry' or 'wet' and attempts to relate these two manifestations to different mechanical factors have exercised the minds of pathologists for many years. Here we need not go into the still unsettled question as to whether the type of gangrene depends upon how the vascular supply is cut off, or whether the concomitant veins are also obstructed; suffice it to say that where infection complicates gangrene this becomes wet whatever the underlying pathology.

The clinical picture of gangrene is exemplified best in the extremities. Here the failing blood-supply is often first manifest by cramps in the muscles on exercise (intermittent claudication), and lividity of the toes or fingers, which may be colder than normal. Later, in the case of the

difficulty in that the history will betray the cause. Nevertheless, it may be important to ascertain *where* the vascular obstruction has occurred, and, although there are exceptions, it may be stated that where the distal half of the foot becomes gangrenous the obstruction is probably in the region of the popliteal artery; when the gangrene affects the lower half of the leg, the obstruction is at about the level of the bifurcation of the common femoral artery, observations which hold good whatever may have been the cause of the obstruction.

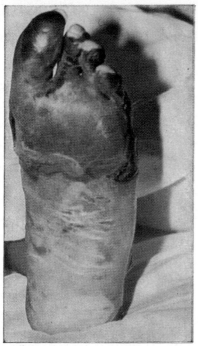

Fig. 334. Gangrene of the foot, due to arteriosclerotic arterial obliteration. (*Courtesy of the Gordon Museum, Guy's Hospital.*)

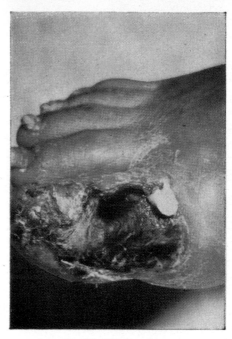

Fig. 335. Diabetic gangrene.

legs, there is pain at rest, especially in bed at night when the warm environment raises the metabolic requirements of the part beyond that with which the inadequate circulation is able to cope. Finally the extremities become purple and then black and mummified, or in the case of 'wet' gangrene, black and deliquescent. Adjacent to the dead area there is a zone of inflammatory hyperaemia (*Fig.* 336) distal to which a definite line of demarcation eventually develops. This classic picture is modified in different sites, and dependent upon the presence and degree of infection, so that it will be necessary now to examine the individual causes of gangrene and see how these may be differentiated according to the clinical picture presented.

It is of paramount importance to exclude diabetes mellitus in all cases of gangrene. It is common particularly in the elderly and the gangrene is often 'wet'. (*Fig.* 335.)

Trauma. The diagnosis of the pathology of traumatic gangrene can rarely give rise to any

Diseases of the Blood-vessels

EMBOLUS. Gangrene due to embolism will be sudden in its inception and rapid in its onset. The embolus is commonly from vegetations on cardiac valves from a thrombus within the left atrium associated with mitral stenosis and atrial fibrillation, and occasionally from thrombi forming on the wall of the left ventricle after a coronary thrombosis, or from atheromatous plaques detached from large-bore vessels proximal to the site of the obstruction. The condition must be differentiated from acute thrombosis because the treatment of early embolism is by embolectomy, and the treatment of acute thrombosis is generally by heparinization and encouragement of the collateral circulation by conservative treatment or sympathectomy.

If, in a case of acute onset, the heart is known to be diseased and the valves known to have vegetations, while the peripheral vascular system is normal, the diagnosis of embolism may be made with confidence and the only problem of diagnosis is to ascertain precisely where the embolus has lodged. If, on the other hand, the patient is known, or can be shown, to have atheromatous disease of the peripheral vessels then the case may be one of embolism or acute thrombosis, and arteriography is necessary to differentiate between the two, the filling defect in an embolism showing a smooth, rounded outline like a cigar butt, that of acute thrombosis being irregular and merging indefinitely with the jagged outline of the locally diseased vessels.

The diagnosis as to *where* the embolism has lodged depends partly on clinical signs and symptoms, but in the last analysis upon arteriography which, if the limb is to be saved, should be performed upon these cases of acute vascular obstruction, in the first place to exclude acute thrombosis, and in the second to localize the obstruction with precision. Nevertheless, the level of the developing gangrene (*see above*) will be of some help, particularly if it be remembered that emboli commonly ride astride a vessel at its point of bifurcation. The site of the initial pain may be misleading and attempts should always be made, by palpating along the course of a vessel, to find at what point the pulse is lost.

THROMBOSIS. Gangrene from this cause is usually of slow onset and always accompanies localized arterial disease, which latter may of itself have already obstructed the blood-supply to a considerable extent; in fact the final occlusion, whatever the underlying pathology, is almost invariably due to thrombosis. Cases of acute thrombosis can only be diagnosed from embolism by arteriography (*see above*).

Venous gangrene is rare but is seen occasionally in the foot in severe cases of iliofemoral venous thrombosis.

BUERGER'S DISEASE (THROMBO-ANGIITIS OBLITERANS). This disease affects the medium-sized arteries, chiefly of the lower extremity, and usually in men under the age of 45. The first symptom of vascular insufficiency is generally intermittent claudication and later rest pain at night in bed. There are often minor attacks of superficial thrombophlebitis. Examination of the affected leg may show absence of pulsations in the line of the dorsalis pedis, medial malleolar, and posterior tibial arteries. In advanced cases the popliteal pulse is also absent, but femoral pulsations usually persist indefinitely. The affected foot and toes are at first livid and cold; later gangrene of one or more toes ensues.

This syndrome is due partly to irreversible changes in the walls of the affected vessels—both arteries and veins, and partly to an abnormal degree of sympathetic stimulation giving rise to spasm of the collaterals. Some idea of the improvement likely to be obtained by sympathectomy can be gained by paralysing the sympathetic supply temporarily and measuring the rise in skin temperature of the extremity. The sympathetic can be paralysed by spinal anaesthesia (the most readily available method), by raising the environmental temperature (the best method, but one

requiring suitable apparatus), or by paravertebral injection of the sympathetic fibres with local anaesthetic (a method which has the peculiar advantage that the patient can walk about immediately afterwards so that the effect on intermittent claudication can be gauged; but a method requiring some dexterity and practice before accurate results can be guaranteed). Methods depending upon raising the internal environmental temperature by injection of T.A.B. or other vaccines are contra-indicated, as they

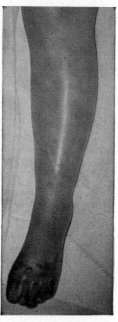

Fig. 336. Gangrene secondary to iliofemoral venous thrombosis. Case of widespread carcinoma of the gall-bladder.

may produce a thrombosis. With all these methods a really satisfactory result should show a rise in skin temperature of 6° C. to 7° C. as a result of sympathetic block, and the maximum skin temperature should reach 34° C. to 35° C. Nevertheless the operation of lumbar sympathectomy is so simple and the consequences of arterial deprivation so grave that most authorities now advise lumbar sympathectomy in this condition whatever the results of the preliminary tests, which are now altogether reliable and are now often omitted. The completeness of the sympathectomy is best assessed postoperatively by measuring the dampness of the normally innervated skin as compared with the dryness of the denervated skin by means of the conductivity of the respective parts to an electric current; where sympathectomy has been complete, the dry skin will show a high resistance, elsewhere the moist skin lowers resistance to the passage of a current.

Buerger's disease usually affects both legs eventually, although, one being slightly worse than the other, the intermittent claudication in the more advanced leg brings the patient to a halt and masks the symptoms which would otherwise soon develop on the other side. In very advanced cases the upper limbs are also affected and very occasionally the upper limbs may be the first to suffer. Smoking is absolutely forbidden in these cases as nicotine aggravates the condition. RAYNAUD'S DISEASE, or as it is more commonly referred to nowadays, in a somewhat strained endeavour to be precise, *Raynaud's phenomenon*, affects the terminal or digital vessels usually of the upper limb and generally in women between 25 and 40.

As a result of exposure to cold the fingers become white and later slate blue. As they are 'thawed out' they change from a livid purple to deep red, this cycle being readily precipitated by plunging the hands into a basin of cold water. Because the disease affects only the terminal vessels, the radial pulse is normal and, in those cases where the toes are affected, the dorsalis pedis and medial malleolar pulsations are not lost. The disease, as might be expected, is subject to exacerbations in the winter and remissions in the summer, but at least for some years is gradually progressive so that, in a severe case, the tips of the fingers become gangrenous (*Fig.* 337).

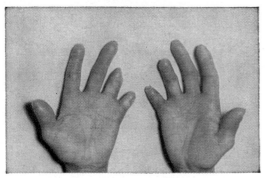

Fig. 337. Raynaud's disease. Note loss of pulp and parts of fingers.

Raynaud's disease is commonly associated with scleroderma, in which the skin over the fingers becomes thickened and stiff so that they are held immobile in a position of semiflexion; and microstomia, a similar condition affecting the skin of the face and causing, as the name implies, a contraction of the mouth with radiating creases at the corners, together with pinching of the nostrils. Disappearance of the distal half of the distal phalanges causes shortening of the fingers and this effect is well demonstrated radiologically. In addition there may be calcinosis, or the deposit of calcium salts in the subcutaneous tissues.

Tests of the effect of paralysis of the sympathetic are best made with a stellate ganglion block using local anaesthetic and testing the skin temperatures of the hand and fingers. As in the case of thrombo-angiitis obliterans, where the disease is severe and the alternative is gangrene, most patients would wish sympathectomy to be performed if there is any chance of success in preventing or even postponing these crippling manifestations.

ARTERIOSCLEROSIS. This term is used here to cover a variety of degenerative processes, including atheroma, Mönckeberg's calcification, and medial sclerosis, which affect the arteries with age. In a proportion of cases the arterial deprivation is sufficiently severe to produce gangrene, and in this event it is usually the lower limb which is affected, and the stages of intermittent claudication and rest pain are passed through just as in Buerger's disease. In fact the condition mimics Buerger's disease very closely apart from the age of onset, which is usually over 50, the presence of calcification in the arteries which may be shown up by X-rays, and other evidences of vascular degeneration as revealed by palpation of the brachial artery or by retinoscopy. Just as in Buerger's disease, too, the peripheral pulsations are lost progressively in the leg, but the femoral pulses are usually retained. Sooner or later an embolus or thrombus (*see above*) may completely occlude the already constricted vessel and gangrene will rapidly ensue. In relatively young patients (up to the age of 65) contracting this disease and faced with the desperate necessity for eventual amputation, it is justifiable to consider sympathectomy as a palliative measure and even, if arteriography shows a local block, excision of the blocked segment with insertion of a graft or the operation of endarterectomy. In this the short length of diseased artery is incised between clamps and the block is removed by dissecting in a plane of cleavage which runs through the media; after which the artery is repaired by stitching up the remains of the wall of the media.

Ergotism. This now rare cause of gangrene arises from frequent ingestion of rye bread made from infected grain attacked by *Claviceps purpura*. The fingers are affected more frequently than the toes. Early signs of gangrene have been reported following excessive use of ergotamine for migraine.

Infective Gangrene. The inclusion of carbuncle, cancrum oris, and 'gas-gangrene' together with the causes of gangrene hitherto described is such a well-established convention that no account of this syndrome is held to be complete without mentioning them. Nevertheless, carbuncle, cancrum oris, 'gas-gangrene' (*see* EMPHYSEMA, SURGICAL, p. 252), and other acute infections with thrombosis of the surrounding vessels are distinct clinical entities and are hardly likely to be confused with other types of gangrene.

Listed above, under the heading 'Less Common Causes' are mostly those conditions in which gangrene is an incidental complication of a clinical picture otherwise coloured by the primary condition; or, on the other hand, local causes, such as carbolic acid dressings and the injection of pentothal sodium into an artery, where the diagnosis is clear cut. Finally, it may be explained that a degree of trauma, which under normal conditions would produce little in the way of tissue damage, may, where the body is wearied by infection or racked by the torments of an unsuitable environment, lead to widespread gangrene. In this connexion one may recall the fate of the slight injury to the finger of Evans on Captain Scott's second polar expedition, or the high incidence of *sphacelatio* which complicated the epidemics (? typhoid, ? typhus) ravaging the armies of Rome in their North African campaigns against the Numidians, or later, the similar fate which befell the invading French Armies of 1848, when the conditions in Algeria so decimated their ranks and gangrene was so common that the whole venture nearly ended in catastrophe.

R. G. Beard.

GIGANTISM (TALL STATURE)

The present tendency is to refer to 'tall stature' rather than gigantism, which is reminiscent of circuses, and since the introduction of Tanner's centile height tables and their almost universal use this refers to individuals whose height is above the 97th centile, which in adult life reaches 6 ft. 6 in. (195 cm.). Cases of giants of 8 ft. 6 in. (255 cm.) and more, however, have been recorded.

CLASSIFICATION

1. Simple.
2. Endocrine
    Hyperpituitary
        Excessive Human Growth Hormone (HGH) production without detectable tumour
        Excessive HGH production from a pituitary tumour.
    Cerebral gigantism
    Hypogonadal
        Sexual precocity (early stage)
        Infantile thyrotoxicosis.
3. Foetal. High birth weight.
4. Nutritional—childhood obesity
5. Chromosomal—XXY or XYY syndrome.
6. Local.
    Acromegaly, e.g. Big toe.
    Arachnodactyly
    Big toe.
7. Unknown aetiology
    Lipodystrophy
    Soto's syndrome.

1. Simple Excessive Height. This may be racial or familial or simply sporadic. It is more usually found in men than in women. These giants are well proportioned and their strength is commensurate with their height. When girls become excessively tall it may be embarrassing and oestrogens are sometimes used before the epiphyses of the knee joints have united. This accelerates epiphyseal closure. Progestogens should also be administered at regular monthly intervals to prevent heavy metropathic bleeding. The

plasma growth hormone concentration and the bone age are normal.

2. Endocrine
Hyperpituitary Gigantism
    Without detectable tumour. This may be associated with hyperplasia of the eosinophil cells of the anterior lobe of the pituitary which secrete growth hormone under the influence of the growth hormone releasing hormone (GRH) of the hypothalamus. The plasma growth hormone level which in normal men may be as high as 5 ng. per ml. and 30 ng. per ml. in women,

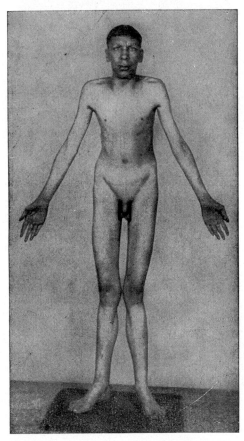

Fig. 338. Hypogonadal or eunuchoid gigantism. Long-limbed skeleton. (*Dr. H. Gardiner-Hill's case.*)

though it may be above this figure in children and relatively quite high in the new born, may reach 1000 ng. per ml. in hyperpituitary giants and acromegalics. Furthermore, in normal health the GH level may drop below 5 ng. during a glucose tolerance test, whereas in gigantism and acromegaly this fall does not take place and there may even be a rise.

With a pituitary adenoma. Whereas GH is normally produced by eosinophil cells of the pituitary, the tumour may be a chromophobe adenoma or one of mixed histological appearance because these cells are unable to store GH and it is consequently rapidly secreted from them.

Acromegaly. If fusion of the epiphyses has already taken place simple gigantism is unlikely to occur and the clinical picture is one of acromegaly. Indeed, acromegalic features may often develop in hyperpituitary giants during adolescence. An adenoma almost always gives rise to acromegaly rather than to simple gigantism and is always situated within the gland. This gives

may be increased. Upward extension of the tumour may stretch and even rupture the diaphragma sellae and may account for some of the quite severe headaches complained of by about a third of the patients. Neighbourhood symptoms, as opposed to endocrine disturbances, mainly consist of visual disorders, of which the most classic though not necessarily the commonest is bitemporal hemianopia (p. 387). Oc-

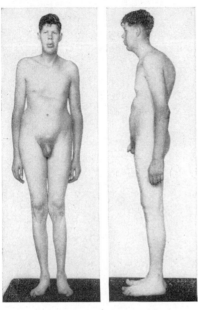

Fig. 339. Pituitary giant aged 19 years, height 7ft. 1½in.
(*Dr. R. G. Ollerenshaw, Manchester Royal Infirmary.*)

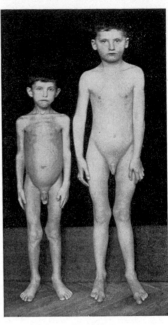

Fig. 340. Hyperpituitary gigantism in a boy of 6 years, with normal control; associated with local gigantism of great toes. (*Dr. R. Traub's case, by kind permission of 'Archives of Diseases in Childhood'.*)

rise to enlargement of the pituitary fossa and sometimes erosion of its bony structure which can be demonstrated radiologically. Acromegaly means enlargement of the extremities and not only do the bones of the hands and feet enlarge but there are characteristic changes in the facial bones (*see* p. 277), such as enlargement of the frontal sinuses and hyperostosis frontalis interna. The thorax is barrel-shaped and there is marked kyphosis and scoliosis. 'Tufting' of the terminal phalanges of the fingers can be demonstrated radiographically and is a diagnostic sign. Not only does the excessive growth hormone affect the bones but also all the internal organs (splanchnomegaly) and integumental tissues, with large coarse heel and finger pads, which partly accounts for the need to wear larger shoes and gloves. Constriction of the carpal tunnel with consequent tingling in the fingers may be an early sign. Excessive sweating is a tiresome symptom. Cardiomegaly and myopathy are often accompanied by hypertension, and death from cardiovascular disease at a relatively early age commonly occurs. Loss of libido and impotence are often late sequelae though in earlier stages sexual activity

casionally galactorrhoea occurs, presumably because of excessive output of prolactin which is secreted by the eosinophil cells of the pituitary. Because of the effect of growth hormone on glucose metabolism many acromegalics are diabetic. The thyroid is enlarged in many cases but is rarely associated with thyrotoxicosis. The adrenal cortex is sometimes enlarged and adenomata may develop. Hirsutism and virilism are common but excessive production of corticosteroids is rare.

Cerebral Gigantism. This is a rare condition that occurs in infancy, sometimes with normal levels of plasma GH, when it may be assumed that the foetus or infant is unduly sensitive to GH. On the other hand, there may be neurological signs and mental retardation, perhaps suggesting a hypothalamic origin with excessive production of GRH (growth-hormone releasing hormone).

Hypogonadal Gigantism (Fig. 338). Primary atrophy of the gonads, castration, or destruction of the gonads by tumours or other disease occurring during childhood lead to late closure of the epiphyses and will result in a characteristic type of long-limbed, eunuchoid gigantism. The height may be as much as 6 in. less than the span, and the measurement from the pubic bone to the floor ('lower measurement') is greater than that from the crown of the head to the pubic bone ('upper measurement'). The patients remain sexually infantile and the voice unbroken; secondary sexual characters do not appear. Whilst eunuchs are usually either of the tall, lanky type described above, or are shorter and obese, the hypogonadal

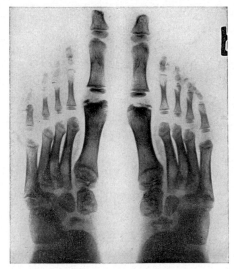

Fig. 341. Local gigantism of great toes with fragmentation of scaphoids. (Same case as *Fig.* 340.)

giant may show increasing obesity with age, the fat having a femine distribution in the male. Plasma GH levels are normal in this type of gigantism.

Sexual Precocity. This induces increased height in the early stages, but premature closure of the epiphyses eventually stunts the child's growth.

Infantile Thyrotoxicosis. This usually leads to rapid growth and the child becomes tall.

3. Foetal Gigantism. This term may be applied to infants weighing more than 15 lb. at birth. The causes of foetal overgrowth are: (*a*) Simple gigantism (*see above*); (*b*) Hormonal dysfunction of mother or foetus; and (*c*) Post-maturity.

The maternal endocrine disturbance most likely to produce foetal gigantism is diabetes mellitus. It has been shown that the diabetogenic factor of the anterior pituitary is identical with the growth hormone, which is producing diabetes in the mother and excessive growth in the foetus. It is not uncommon for diabetic mothers to give a history of having given birth to more than one overweight infant before the disease became manifest.

Hyperpituitary gigantism of the infant may date from foetal life, though in many instances hyperpituitary giants have been of normal size at birth. (*Fig.* 340.)

Post-maturity can usually be diagnosed from the history, and the size of the foetus confirmed by radiological examination before birth.

4. Nutritional. Children who tend to be overweight from birth tend to be excessively tall.

5. Chromosomal. Males with an XXY (Klinefelter) sex chromosome pattern and men with an XYY pattern tend to be abnormally tall.

6. Local Gigantism. Varieties of local gigantism, or hypertrophy of one or more organs, are so numerous that only the main types affecting the skeletal system will be referred to.

Acromegaly. This type, in which hypertrophy due to hyperpituitarism affects the extremities, jaw, nose, and tongue, has already been discussed (p. 277).

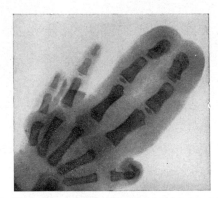

Fig. 342. Local gigantism and syndactyly of 2nd and 3rd fingers, in an infant. (*Mr. D. Levi's case.*)

Arachnodactyly (*Marfan's Syndrome*). This is characterized by the extreme length and slenderness of the fingers and toes and increased length of the legs. The condition is congenital, and is frequently associated with other congenital defects, e.g., bilateral dislocation of the lens, laxity of ligaments, congenital morbus cordis, high arched palate, and mental defect (*see* p. 456).

Local Gigantism of Individual Limbs or Digits (*Figs.* 341, 342). This occurs as a congenital abnormality, either alone or in association with generalized gigantism or with other congenital abnormalities. In some instances it is possibly due to partial constriction of the affected organ by bands in utero.

7. Soto's Syndrome. A condition associated with lipodystrophy which shows a tendency to tall stature.

P. M. F. Bishop.

GIRDLE PAIN

This is a pain passing around the trunk bilaterally or, with a permissible extension of the definition, unilaterally, indicating the involvement of a thoracic root on one or both sides. The pain is thus intermittent, liable to be provoked or aggravated by movement, straining, coughing, or sneezing, and has a radicular distribution which, over the trunk, readily indicates the root involved, the distribution being intercostal. The likely cause is compression of the root by neoplasm or, less likely in this region, a disk. Pain in this distribution due to herpes zoster should provide

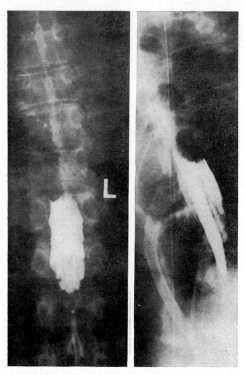

Fig. 343. Myelogram showing opaque medium arrested in its caudal flow by a spinal tumour. (*Dr. R. D. Hoare.*)

no diagnostic difficulty on account of the eruption. A similar sensation may be simply one of constriction, which may also occur in the legs and gives the feeling of the part being held in a vice or tightly bandaged. This occurs in lesions involving the posterior columns of the spinal cord, and is common in disseminated sclerosis. It may also occur with neoplasms, subacute combined degeneration of the cord, tabes dorsalis, and other conditions. It is not an accurate localizing symptom and more accurate localization must depend on elicitation of motor, reflex, and sensory signs with the addition of contrast myelography if this seems indicated. (*Fig.* 343.)

Ian Mackenzie.

GLYCOSURIA

The term 'glycosuria' implies the presence in the urine of a substance reducing alkaline copper solution on heating. The substance most likely to do this is of course glucose, but there are a number of other substances which must be considered. The classic tests are those of Fehling and Benedict, and of these Benedict's is to be preferred as it is more stable and less reactive with non-sugar reducing substances, such as uric acid. The same principles are employed in the convenient 'Clinitest' tablets. The glucose oxidase tests ('Clinistix and Test Tape') are specific for glucose but give little or no information as to the amount of sugar present.

Benedict's Test. In this test 10 vol. of reagent (5 ml. or $1\frac{1}{2}$ in. in an ordinary test-tube) are mixed with 1 vol. of urine (0·5 ml. or 8 drops) and, after shaking, the mixture is boiled on the flame for two minutes or placed in the boiling-water bath for five minutes. A positive result is shown by a green or brown colour. If there is any doubt in interpreting a green tinge the mixture should be allowed to stand for fifteen minutes and the bottom of the tube inspected without disturbing the solution. The test should not be reported positive unless a definite brown deposit of cuprous oxide is seen on the bottom of the tube.

Reducing Substances other than Glucose. Positive urine tests for reducing substances using copper reagents, e.g., Benedict's test, are due to glucose in about 90 per cent of cases. Other compounds giving a positive reaction in the remaining 10 per cent are other carbohydrates, e.g., lactose, pentoses, fructose, and galactose, and drugs excreted as glucuronides, e.g., salicylate and chloral, and also some unusual metabolite such as homogentisic acid. Only glucose itself will give a positive reaction with 'Clinistix' (*see above*). With the single exception of galactose these other reducing substances are of little clinical importance. If necessary, other carbohydrates can be characterized by paper chromatography. The effect of drugs can be recognized by temporarily stopping the suspected medicament.

A diagnosis of galactosuria is of great importance in the newly born child or infant, as hereditary galactosaemia is a serious and indeed fatal disease easily treatable by a lactose- and galactose-free diet. It should be suspected if a reducing test, e.g., Benedict's test, is positive and the 'Clinistix' test is negative. The presence of galactose in the urine can then be confirmed by paper chromatography.

Glucose-tolerance Test. Assuming that the reducing substance has been identified as glucose, or is thought to be glucose, the next step will usually consist of some type of blood-sugar examination and in most cases a glucose-tolerance test will be desirable. Of course this investigation may be superfluous in some cases; for example, in patients with repeatedly high fasting blood-sugar values (over 150 mg. per 100 ml.) and other clinical manifestations of diabetes. In such cases the full test is unnecessary as the diagnosis can be made from the fasting results. However, a large proportion of cases will require this further procedure to elucidate the diagnosis.

The glucose-tolerance test is performed on the patient after a twelve hours' fast. In addition it is desirable that there should have been no drastic restriction of carbohydrates in the diet during the previous week. The test is best performed first thing in the morning and is begun by collecting blood for the fasting blood-sugar estimation and getting the patient to empty the bladder. The patient then drinks 50 g. of glucose dissolved in a glass of water and blood is collected at half-hourly intervals for the next two hours, further urine specimens being collected at one and two

the end of two hours. The urine specimens contain large amounts of sugar and usually acetone.
3. MILD DIABETES. The fasting blood-sugar level is either normal or slightly increased. The blood-sugar rises above 180 mg. per 100 ml. and has not returned to a normal fasting value by two hours. Sugar will probably be present in the urine at one and two hours.
4. LAG-STORAGE CURVE. Fasting conditions are normal, the blood-sugar rises above 180 at about

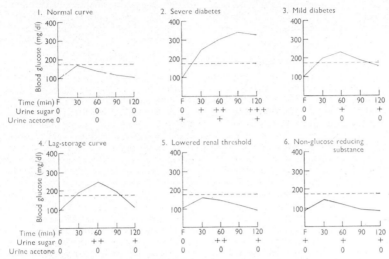

Fig. 344. Glucose-tolerance tests, showing varying responses. Broken line represents the mean renal threshold above which glycosuria normally occurs. In diabetes mellitus in all but mild cases fasting blood sugars are also elevated above 100 mg/dl, normal fasting (non-diabetic) figures being below this figure.

hours after the dose of glucose. The blood should preferably be capillary blood collected from the finger or ear. Any standard method of estimation may be employed, although the normal range of values is slightly different with the different methods. Methods depending on copper or ferricyanide reduction (e.g., Auto-analyser) give results about 20 mg. per 100 ml. higher than the true glucose, which can be estimated by glucose oxidase procedures.

Typical normal and abnormal results for the blood-sugar estimation in glucose-tolerance tests are shown in *Fig.* 344. The following points should be noted.
1. NORMAL CURVES. Normally the fasting value should fall between 80 mg. and 120 mg. per 100 ml. (ferricyanide reduction). The blood-sugar reaches a peak at the half-hour specimen, which should not exceed 180 mg. per 100 ml. This value applies to capillary blood, and the appropriate normal limit for venous blood would be about 160 mg. per 100 ml. The blood-sugar reaches a normal fasting value at two hours. No sugar appears in the urine.
2. SEVERE DIABETES. The fasting value is grossly abnormal and sugar and acetone are likely to be present in the fasting urine. The blood-sugar continues to rise throughout the test, still rising at

one hour, but returns to a normal fasting value at two hours. Sugar is probably present in the urine at one and two hours. Although lag-storage curves may at times be seen without any obvious pathology, most cases are due to one of three causes—gross liver damage, hyperthyroidism, or operations on the upper alimentary tract (gastrectomy, gastro-enterostomy). It will be seen that all these conditions depend either upon liver damage or increased intestinal absorption of sugar, or both (*see below*).
5. LOWERED RENAL THRESHOLD. The blood-sugars are all within normal limits but sugar appears in the urine between one and two hours. In this case the renal threshold is evidently somewhere between 100 and 160 mg. per 100 ml. In extreme degrees of lowered renal threshold sugar may be constantly present in the urine irrespective of the blood-sugar level, which tends in this case to be in the low normal range.

Lowered renal threshold is probably the commonest cause of symptomless glycosuria. It is usually a harmless inherited anomaly, but also occurs in renal acidosis (Fanconi syndrome, *see* AMINO-ACIDURIA, p. 23). The common type does not appear to depend upon any structural abnormality of the kidney and the condition is rarely seen in gross renal diseases, such as nephritis, etc. A temporary lowering of the renal threshold may be seen during pregnancy.

6. NON-GLUCOSE REDUCING SUBSTANCES. The curve shown here is from a case of pentosuria and illustrates a type of curve likely to be seen when the reducing substance in the urine is not glucose. Note the normal blood-sugar levels, the lack of correlation between the blood-sugar level, and the low concentration of urinary reducing substance. This curve should be compared with the previous one for lowered renal threshold in which sugar is absent from the fasting urine and in which the degree of glycosuria bears a relationship to the height of the blood-sugar.

INTERPRETATION OF RESULTS

The results described here are those of average or typical cases and slight deviations may be seen, particularly with abnormally high or low renal thresholds in diabetic subjects. It will be seen that the principles underlying the interpretation of the curves may be summarized as follows.

In the first place the blood-sugar either rises above normal or it does not. If it does not, any glycosuria can usually be safely attributed to lowered renal threshold. Secondly, if the blood-sugar rises above normal it either returns to a normal level at two hours or it does not. If it does the curve is described as a lag-storage curve; if it does not, as diabetic. Finally it must be emphasized that the occurrence of a diabetic glucose-tolerance test is not synonymous with a diagnosis of diabetes mellitus. A diabetic blood-sugar curve, with or without ketosis, implies the existence of a particular type of biochemical disturbance, which although most frequently due to diabetes mellitus may be caused by other conditions as noted below. The diagnosis of diabetes mellitus therefore depends upon combining the glucose-tolerance test with clinical data, and in particular implies that various conditions such as acromegaly, basophilism, and thyrotoxicosis have been excluded. This subject is dealt with in detail in the next section.

Causes of impaired glucose tolerance other than diabetes mellitus: Any of these conditions may cause the appearance of glucose in the urine. They may be classified as follows:

1. Endocrine Disturbances

a. Pancreatic Conditions. Gross pancreatic destruction from any cause can produce diabetic manifestations. These are particularly likely in cases of pancreatic calculi, but occur rarely with pancreatic carcinoma and chronic pancreatitis. The fibrosis of the pancreas associated with haemochromatosis (bronze diabetes) is a well-recognized rare cause of diabetes. This condition is commoner in males. In addition to the usual diabetic symptoms a bronze pigmentation of the skin will usually be present, the liver will be enlarged, and the pubic and axillary hair is likely to be absent or diminished.

b. Pituitary Conditions. Diabetes is a well-recognized complication of acromegaly which may terminate in diabetic coma. Basophilic adenoma of the pituitary (Cushing's syndrome) may also cause glycosuria, although the impairment of sugar-tolerance here is usually less extreme.

c. Hyperthyroidism. Glycosuria in hyperthyroidism is not uncommon and is usually associated with a lag-storage type of curve. True diabetes mellitus may, however, coexist and patients with thyrotoxicosis have a slightly increased chance of developing diabetes.

d. Adrenal Conditions. Emotional glycosuria may be placed in this group, being due to oversecretion of adrenaline. Any type of fear or excitement may produce this effect, which may sometimes cause an initial glycosuria when an anxious patient is examined for the first time. Severe muscular exercise may also produce glycosuria in this way. There is in addition a rare type of adrenal tumour (the phaeochromocytoma) which gives rise to attacks of faintness and giddiness due to adrenaline secretion. In such cases the blood-pressure will be raised during the attack and paroxysmal tachycardia may be present. Phaeochromocytoma may also cause sustained hypertension; the urinary catecholamine estimation is a useful diagnostic aid. Glycosuria may also be caused by oversecretion of the adrenocortical hormones, as in Cushing's syndrome or during corticosteroid therapy.

2. Cerebral Conditions. Glycosuria with hyperglycaemia may occur with any gross cerebral catastrophe such as fractured skull, cerebral haemorrhage, etc. The mechanism of this effect is similar to that of the 'Piqûre diabetes' of Claude Bernard, and depends upon the stimulation of hepatic glycogenolysis via the splanchnic nerves. The clinical importance of this syndrome is obvious, since the finding of glycosuria in an unconscious patient might lead to an incorrect diagnosis of diabetic coma if this alternative possibility were not considered. There will, of course, usually be neurological signs in these conditions and the degree of ketosis will be much less intense than that seen in diabetic coma.

3. Diseases of the Liver. Gross hepatic destruction tends to produce hypoglycaemia rather than hyperglycaemia but may also produce a lag-storage curve with glycosuria as an accompaniment. This occurs mainly in cases of advanced cirrhosis or carcinomatosis and is due to a failure of the storage mechanism.

4. Gastro-intestinal Diseases. Gross alterations in the mechanics of the upper intestinal tract can also produce glycosuria due to a lag-storage effect, in this case owing to ultra-rapid absorption of sugar from the upper small intestine. This is seen particularly after gastrectomy or gastro-enterostomy and in such cases a postprandial glycosuria may be associated with some degree of hypoglycaemia between meals (dumping syndrome).

5. Fevers and Infections. Any acute infection may cause a temporary impairment of glucose tolerance, and this is particularly marked with staphylococcal infections. This may lead to the appearance of glycosuria in a previously normal subject or may call for an increase in the insulin dosage of a known diabetic. Glycosuria with boils and carbuncles may raise difficulties in diagnosis in cases where there is no previous diabetic history. In such cases the best course is to treat the patient expectantly, with insulin if necessary, until the infection has been cleared up. A glucose-tolerance test may then be performed. It is of little value to do the tolerance test at the height of infection since some type of diabetic curve will probably be present in any event.

SCHEME FOR INVESTIGATING A CASE OF GLYCOSURIA

The following scheme of investigation makes use of the principles discussed above.

1. Confirm the presence of reducing substance with Benedict's reagent, using measured quantities of urine and reagent. A darkening of the mixture during heating may indicate the existence of rarities such as alkaptonuria, melanuria, or tyrosinosis.

2. Consider the question of non-glucose reducing substances, particularly if any special indication is present (*see above*). The glucose oxidase test should be used to confirm the presence of glucose, and if this is negative other investigations will be indicated as noted above.

3. The presence of acetone together with sugar is very suggestive of diabetes mellitus. The history and clinical signs may also strongly suggest such a diagnosis at this stage.

4. Repeat observation of glycosuria on more than one occasion to eliminate emotional glycosuria.

5. If the diagnosis is still in doubt a glucose-tolerance test is probably indicated. This will decide between 'diabetic' and 'non-diabetic' conditions.

6. Reconsideration of the clinical picture should now be undertaken in the light of the considerations outlined above. This will usually enable the case to be allotted to one or other of the conditions listed. Supplementary investigations such as radiography of the skull for pituitary tumour and basal metabolic rate estimations for hyperthyroidism, etc., may now be indicated in special cases.

M. D. Milne.

GUMS, BLEEDING

A spongy, bleeding condition of the gums, attaining such a degree that the teeth become covered by the exuberant blood-oozing tissues, was a prominent feature of *scurvy*. Although nowadays rarely encountered in its full development, it may still be found in a mild form amongst children—infantile scurvy, or Barlow's disease—as the result of long-continued feeding with tinned milk or other food deficient in ascorbic acid. Its chief features are anaemia,

and tenderness of the long bones due to haemorrhages under the periosteum; in severer cases, besides sponginess and bleeding of the gums with more or less general stomatitis, there may be purpura and other haemorrhages. The diagnosis is suggested by the dietetic history, and confirmed by the benefit that follows the addition of fresh milk and, in older children, fresh vegetables. A similar condition may arise in adults whose circumstances compel them to live on tinned foods, appropriately termed 'bachelor's scurvy'. It is also seen from time to time in patients with peptic ulcer existing on a diet of milk and slops and in cranks who have invented bizarre diets for themselves deficient in fruit and vegetables. It may also occur in chronic alcoholics who drink excessively but eat little fresh foods. Apart from scurvy there are many other more common causes of bleeding of the gums, some in which it is due to local changes only, some in which it is part of a more general condition.

1. Bleeding Gums due to General Conditions or preceded by Lesions elsewhere than in the Mouth:

Scurvy
The blood dyscrasias (e.g., acute leukaemia, aplastic anaemia, thrombocytopenia, haemophilia)
Purpura
Syphilis
Febrile or asthenic states.
Hodgkin's disease (rarely).

2. Bleeding Gums due to purely Local Conditions:

Injury, e.g., by toothbrush
Dental caries
Tartar
Pyorrhoea alveolaris
Papilloma
Epulis
Myeloma
Epithelioma
Actinomycosis
Acute or chronic stomatitis not obviously due to any of the causes already mentioned, e.g.: aphthous stomatitis, ulcerative stomatitis, Vincent's angina, gangrenous stomatitis (cancrum oris, phagedaena oris, noma oris)
Tuberculous gingivitis
Erythema bullosum, dermatitis herpetiformis, pemphigus, affecting the mouth as well as the epidermis.

1. BLEEDING GUMS DUE TO GENERAL CONDITIONS

Many of the above conditions are discussed under other and more prominent symptoms, so that here we need to refer to them but briefly (*see* SPLEEN, ENLARGEMENT OF, p. 746; ANAEMIA, p. 25; PURPURA, p. 669; etc.). A blood-count will generally diagnose or exclude *leukaemia, thrombocytopenia* or *aplastic anaemia*. The history may suggest *haemophilia. Hodgkin's disease* may attract attention more on account of the enlargement of the spleen or of the lymph-nodes (p. 513), or of the anaemia, than because of spongy gums. *Purpura* is itself a symptom and not a disease (p. 669).

Syphilis, particularly in its secondary stage, may produce stomatitis, pharyngitis, laryngitis, and gingivitis with bleeding.

Mercury is apt to cause profuse salivation and acute stomatitis, with distressing and painful swelling of lips, gums, tongue, and cheeks, the glairy saliva hangs in strings from the protruding tongue and bulging lips, the mucosa bleeds on the slightest touch. Some persons are especially intolerant of mercury, but its worst effects have occurred when the teeth are carious or the mouth is unclean. The diagnosis depends upon a knowledge of the drugs that are being given or, in occupational cases, of the chemicals employed in the patient's work. The so-called 'Pink disease', once not uncommon in small children, has disappeared since teething powders containing mercury have been discontinued.

Phosphorus was at one time responsible for severe stomatitis, going on to necrosis of the jaw—'phossy jaw'—not infrequently ending in death as the result of fatty degeneration of the liver and heart. Since restrictions are now laid upon the use of crude yellow phosphorus in the manufacture of matches it is almost unknown. Apart from occupation, the patient may, with suicidal intent, have been taking a rat paste or other vermin-killer containing phosphorus.

Arsenic and *lead* are rare causes of bleeding gums; occupation, or medical prescription, habits as regards drinking, or the possibility of arsenical administration in the form of weed-killer with homicidal intent, may suggest the diagnosis, and there may be other signs of the poisoning, particularly pigmentation of the skin, vomiting, diarrhoea, hyperkeratosis of the soles and palms, and generalized peripheral neuritis in the case of arsenic, and the symptoms given under ANAEMIA in the case of lead. Arsenic may be found in excess in the hair, or lead may be detected in the faeces or in the residue from a bulk of urine.

Phenytoin, used in the treatment of epilepsy, may produce hypertrophic gingival changes rendering the gums more liable to trauma.

Febrile and *asthenic states* cause sordes and bleeding gums only when the patient has already been ill some while, or when the nursing has been inefficient.

2. BLEEDING GUMS DUE TO LOCAL CONDITIONS

When care has been taken to exclude general causes of bleeding of the gums, differentiation between the various local causes is not difficult. Some patients are alarmed by the symptom when its cause is nothing more serious than the use of a *new toothbrush* whose hard bristles have lacerated gums that are accustomed to a softer brush. In such cases, however, gingivitis is usually present. The history will indicate other forms of local injury—an ill-fitting tooth-plate, perhaps. Haemoptysis may be simulated.

Dental caries may be obvious or it may be hidden away between adjacent teeth and yet be irritating the gum sufficiently to cause it to bleed with undue readiness when the teeth are brushed. *Tartar* is usually evident on inspection. *Pyorrhoea alveolaris*, also known as *suppurative gingivitis* or *Rigg's disease*, is the result of septic infection extending down into the sockets, loosening the teeth, causing the gum margins to recede by erosion, and leading to a purulent discharge from between the gums and the teeth. This condition may be present even when the external aspect of the teeth seems perfect. An X-ray examination may be required to determine the condition of the submucosal portions of the teeth. In severe cases the gums bleed on the slightest touch, the breath is foul, and the constant swallowing of pyogenic organisms and their products may be credited to dyspepsia, with the causation of a variety of conditions causing ill health.

The diagnosis of *alveolar abscess* is generally obvious, though infection of a benign or *malignant new growth* may simulate it for a time. Microscopical examination of the excised tumour is the only certain way of diagnosing the nature of an odontome, papilloma, simple epulis, myeloid sarcomatous epulis, or epithelioma of the gum.

In *actinomycosis* the jaw, gum, and cheek are sometimes affected. The diagnosis is confirmed by finding ray fungi in the purulent discharge, or in sections from parts excised.

Stomatitis in its various degrees may have a general cause, such as mercurialism (*see above*), or it may be due to purely local infection with micro-organisms. It may be classified bacteriologically—the variety spoken of as 'thrush' being due to *Monilia albicans*, for instance; other cases are due to organisms such as *Streptococcus haemolyticus*, *Streptococcus viridans*, the *Spirilla* and *Bacilli fusiforms* of Vincent, the *pneumococcus*, Friedländer's *pneumobacillus*, *Staphylococcus aureus*, Pfeiffer's *Haemophilus influenzae*. While periodontal disease (gingivitis) is the commonest cause of spongy bleeding gums, in severe cases of acute necrotizing ulcerative gingivitis Vincent's angina ('Trench mouth') should be suspected. Clinically, stomatitis is classified by its degree as acute catarrhal, ulcerative, and gangrenous. All these affect the mucosa of the cheeks, tongue, and palate in addition to the gums, and any of the inflamed parts bleed readily. The first degree is characterized by redness, swelling, tenderness, and pain with inability to move the tongue, swelling and protrusion of the lips, foulness of the breath, and generally salivation. There may or may not be localized greyish or white aphthous patches; these are commoner in children. When ulcers occur, these are generally multiple and shallow, very painful, with more or less glazing of the ulcerated surface, and acute hyperaemia of the margins. The gangrenous form is known as *cancrum oris*, a condition nowadays exceedingly rare in this country but not in underdeveloped parts of the world, though sometimes seen in ill-cared-for children with measles or some other acute debilitating fever. The cheek is affected first, a dusky red or black spot appearing within and without, spreading rapidly and leading to sloughing and perforation, gangrene of the gums and jaw, falling out of the teeth, and a very foul nauseating odour of the breath. It frequently results in death from exhaustion. (*See also* p. 661.)

Tuberculous gingivitis is rare. The nature of the bleeding gums will be suggested by the coexistence of phthisis, and tubercle bacilli may abound in smears from the gum.

Erythema multiforme (Stevens-Johnson syndrome), Reiter's disease, Behçet's disease, *dermatitis herpetiformis*, and *pemphigus*—particularly the first—may affect mucous membranes as well as the skin, especially the mouth, colon, and vagina. The result as regards the mouth is very distressing; the crusts and resultant inflammation of lips, gums, tongue, cheeks, palate, fauces, and pharynx may make mastication impossible, rapid loss of weight and severe pyrexial illness ensue. The mucous membrane bleeds on the slightest touch. The mucous membranes are, however, seldom attacked unless the skin is also affected (*see* BULLAE, p. 115, and EOSINOPHILIA, p. 253).

Harold Ellis.

GUMS, RETRACTION OF

Retraction of the gums is rarely a symptom of which complaint is made. In most cases it results from a local infective process, periodontal disease, beginning as a gingivitis and spreading to involve the adjacent tissues, and also dental caries. These conditions are discussed under the heading of GUMS, BLEEDING (p. 323), though retraction may be considerable without bleeding.

Harold Ellis.

GYNAECOMASTIA

Gynaecomastia is enlargement of the male breast due to development of its glandular components. Prominence of the mammary tissue due to deposition of fat may be referred to as pseudo-gynaecomastia.

Causes of Gynaecomastia

PHYSIOLOGICAL:
1. Neonatal
2. Pubertal
3. Involutional.

PATHOLOGICAL:
Endocrine:
  Testis:
    Prepubertal testicular failure.
    Tumours. Teratoma. Chorion epithelioma. Seminoma. Interstitial-cell tumour. Sertoli cell tumour
    Leprosy
    Mumps orchitis.
  Thyroid:
    Hyperthyroidism.

Adrenal:
  Adrenocortical tumour.
Disorders of sex:
  True hermaphroditism
  Testicular feminization.
Pituitary:
  Acromegaly
  Chromophobe adenoma.
Miscellaneous:
  After prostatectomy
  Albright's syndrome.
Liver disease:
  Cirrhosis.
Renutrition.

SEX CHROMOSOMAL ANOMALY:
  Klinefelter's syndrome.

DISEASES OF THE C.N.S.:
  Traumatic paraplegia
  Friedreich's ataxia
  Syringomyelia
  Myotonica congenita.

DISEASES OF THE RESPIRATORY SYSTEM:
  Bronchogenic carcinoma.

DRUGS:
  Oestrogens
  Androgens
  Chorionic gonadotrophin
  Digitalis
  Chlorpromazine
  Isoniazid
  Tricyclic antidepressants
  Spironolactone
  α-Methyl dopa
  Meprobamate
  Reserpine
  Radioactive iodine.

Neonatal Gynaecomastia. Seventy per cent of male infants have some degree of enlargement of the mammary glands, and in these fluid can be expressed from the breasts in 60 per cent ('witch's milk'). The condition may be caused by maternal chorionic gonadotrophin stimulating the Leydig cells of the testis (which immediately after birth are found to be relatively abundant) to secrete oestrogen which produces the gynaecomastia. On the other hand, it has been suggested that it is due to the hang-over influence of the high concentration of maternal oestrogen. Or yet again it may not be due to maternal chorionic gonadotrophin, but to prolactin, though prolactin is not found in adult cases unless they are associated with galactorrhoea. On histological examination these breasts are found to be miniature lactating glands.

Pubertal Gynaecomastia. The great majority of adolescent boys develop a 'puberty node' (a small, hard, subareolar plaque) which may be tender, but which always disappears in due course and does not require treatment. (This may be classified as Grade I, *Fig.* 345.) A number of boys have been studied—beginning actually before the gynaecomastia became evident there was a slight but significant increase in plasma oestradiol concentration before the plasma testosterone concentration rose. The plasma prolactin levels were also higher than normal in the pre-gynaecomastia stage but fell to normal when the breasts began to swell. These changes did not take place in boys who did not subsequently develop gynaecomastia. In a few cases the gynaecomastia is more extensive (Grade II, *Fig.* 345) and may even lead to the appearance of the normal adult female breast (Grade III, *Fig.* 345).

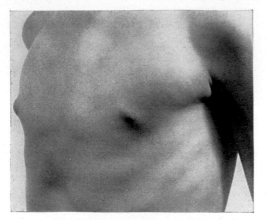

Fig. 345 A, Gynaecomastia Grade I.

It should be pointed out that the natural progress of biosynthesis of the sex hormone steroids is progesterone→androgen→oestrogen and the degree of conversion from androgen to oestrogen depends on the activity of the appropriate enzyme system. If mammary-gland tissue has developed (Grades II and III) spontaneous remission is unlikely and it will probably be necessary, therefore, to remove the excessive mammary tissue by plastic surgery. In order to save the boy from embarrassment this should not be too long delayed. It is important to be certain that the boy is not taking any drugs which might possibly cause gynaecomastia. Very rarely a teratoma of the testis may develop at this adolescent age and even more rarely give rise to gynaecomastia. The testes should therefore be palpated in all cases.

Involutional Gynaecomastia. Very rarely gynaecomastia develops in men in the sixth decade or later associated with loss of libido and a raised urinary output of gonadotrophins and sometimes with hot flushes. It is essential that organic conditions such as liver disease, bronchogenic carcinoma, etc., should be excluded before assuming the gynaecomastia to be due to the male climacteric.

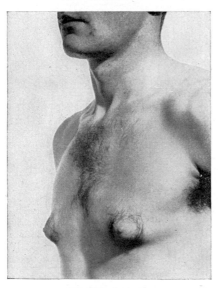

Fig. 345 B, Grade II.

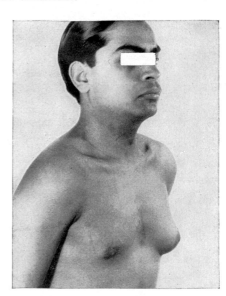

Fig. 345 C, Grade III.

Often the condition occurs in one breast only, or gynaecomastia develops in one breast some weeks or months before it appears in the other. Occasionally fluid can be expressed. In an appreciable number of cases there is a history of neonatal gynaecomastia, or even a family history, suggesting that the mammary glands are constitutionally excessively sensitive to the oestrogen secreted by the Leydig cells. At puberty the Leydig cells, which have regressed since the neonatal period, reappear and become functionally active, secreting both androgen and oestrogen.

Disorders of the Testes

1. HYPOGONADISM. It is important to note that gynaecomastia is not encountered in hypogonadism due to pituitary deficiency and is usually not seen in cases of testicular failure developing in adult men. There are, in fact, only two types of hypogonadism with which it is commonly associated, namely, prepubertal testicular failure and Klinefelter's syndrome (*see* p. 328). *Prepubertal Testicular Failure.* In this condition no testicular tissue can be found in the scrotum which contains, however, remnants of Wolffian

duct derivatives such as epididymis and vas deferens. This is associated with signs of androgenic deficiency which may appear even before puberty, the eunuchoidism becoming more marked during adolescent years. Usually the patients are not seen before the normal age of puberty and after this age they have high urinary gonadotrophin titres. Gynaecomastia is usually present, though it may not reach more than Grade I. Because of the absence of testicular elements it is difficult to suggest a cause for the gynaecomastia. One can only suppose that it is due to oestrogens secreted by the adrenal cortex.

2. TUMOURS.

a. Chorion Epithelioma. Gynaecomastia, pigmentation of the nipples and areolae, often with secretion of a white fluid from the nipples, are commonly found in cases of chorionic carcinoma of the testis, as well as in extragenital chorionic carcinoma and teratoma of the testis with chorionic carcinoma in metastases. Chorionic gonadotrophin is present in large quantities in the urine and stimulates the production of oestrogen by the interstitial cells. Often gynaecomastia is the only clinical manifestation of chorion epithelioma of the testis and the tumour in the early stages may be impalpable. A quantitative estimation of urinary chorionic gonadotrophin should therefore be made in cases of otherwise inexplicable gynaecomastia. Chorion epithelioma is by far the commonest testicular tumour to produce gynaecomastia.

b. Seminoma. It is rare for seminoma to be associated with gynaecomastia, but it has been recorded.

c. Interstitial-cell Tumour. When this tumour occurs in an adult it does not usually give rise to endocrine features but when it does, gynaecomastia is usually present. The condition is extremely rare before puberty, and gynaecomastia has seldom been a feature, though when it has occurred the boys have also shown signs of male sexual precocity. The gynaecomastia is probably due to the excessive production of oestrogen, as well as androgen, by the interstitial cells of the tumour. It regresses when the tumour is removed. Tumours may develop in the testis from adrenocortical rests and are very hard to distinguish from true interstitial-cell tumours. Gynaecomastia is more likely to occur with this type of tumour.

d. Sertoli-cell Tumour. This is the rarest of all the testicular tumours in man. It occurs less rarely in dogs in which it usually gives rise to feminization and swelling of the nipples. Gynaecomastia has been reported among the rare human cases, possibly because of the conversion of testicular androgen to oestrogen, and was associated with loss of libido and impotence.

3. LEPROUS ORCHITIS. The microscopical appearance of the testis is similar to that found in Klinefelter's syndrome, namely clumps of Leydig cells, absence of spermatogenesis, intact Sertoli cells, and in addition peritubular fibrosis. This picture is accompanied by raised urinary gonadotrophin levels and sometimes by gynaecomastia.

4. MUMPS ORCHITIS. Rarely gynaecomastia has developed 6 to 12 months after an attack of mumps orchitis which has caused atrophy of the testicles. This atrophy gives rise to the characteristic picture of testicular histology found in leprous orchitis.

To summarize, gynaecomastia associated with testicular lesions is probably brought about in the following way: Damage to or degeneration of the germinal epithelium leads to release of increased amounts of gonadotrophin by the pituitary, as evidenced by the high urinary gonadotrophin levels. The augmented gonadotrophic stimulus causes hyperplasia of the interstitial cells which secrete both androgen and oestrogen, depending on the activity of the enzyme system responsible for the conversion of androgens to oestrogens. If the output of oestrogen is relatively high, and if the mammary tissues of that individual are sufficiently sensitive, gynaecomastia will occur.

Disorders of the Thyroid. A few cases of thyrotoxicosis have been described in association with gynaecomastia. Not all have been submitted to testicular biopsy which has usually shown normal findings and hormone assays within the normal range, though the gynaecomastia, which was accompanied by loss of libido and potency, subsided when the thyrotoxicosis was treated. However, changes similar to those found in Klinefelter's syndrome have been observed.

Diseases of the Adrenal Cortex. Adrenal cortical tumours or hyperplasia are rare in males. Some cases give rise to no endocrine manifestations and it is possible that in others signs of super-masculinization are overlooked. The typical endocrine picture is one of feminization, occasionally occurring during the first decade. Gynaecomastia is often the first sign. It may be accompanied by pigmentation of the nipples, and occasionally clear or milky fluid can be expressed from the nipples. Libido and potency progressively diminish. Aspermia is usual and the testes may be palpably atrophied. Testicular biopsy shows hypoplasia of interstitial cells. The urinary 17-oxosteroid output is considerably raised in some of the cases in which it has been reported, though in others it has been within normal limits. Oestrogen levels have been raised in some cases. Sometimes a tumour is large enough to be palpable, but in most cases tumour or bilateral hyperplasia can be identified. The tumours are usually malignant, so that early diagnosis is important. Hyperplasia is very rare in the cases giving rise to feminization reported up to date. It is interesting to note that the testicular histology is completely different from that encountered in the majority of cases in which gynaecomastia is associated with testicular disorders. Adrenocortical feminization is due to excessive oestrogen produced by the adrenocortical tumour or hyperplasia, and the interstial cells of the testis actually undergo hypoplasia.

Disorders of Sex:

1. TRUE HERMAPHRODITISM. In this rare condition gynaecomastia frequently develops. One case has been described in which the right side of the body showed normal female configuration and 'gynaecomastia' (or rather, normal female breast development) and the left side was typically male. There was a right ovary and a left testis.

2. TESTICULAR FEMINIZATION. This is a type of male pseudohermaphroditism, and studies of the nuclear chromatin pattern indicate that the patients are genetic males. The gonads are testes and are found to consist of small tubules containing Sertoli cells but no germinal elements, or at the best undifferentiated spermatogonia, and hyperplasia of the interstitial cells. These testicles are secreting normal amounts of androgen and

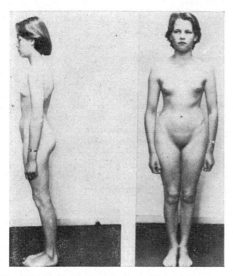

Fig. 346. Testicular feminization. Normal female configuration. Note absence of pubic hair. (*Courtesy of the Gordon Photographic Museum, Guy's Hospital.*)

oestrogen but all the tissues of the body are unable to respond to androgen and therefore assume female physical characters. The external genitalia are those of a normal female, but the vagina ends as a blind pouch, and the uterus is either vestigial or absent. The bodily configuration is that of a normal female and the breasts are of normal size though the nipples and areolae are sometimes small. The individual, therefore, cannot strictly be said to be suffering from gynaecomastia. Pubic and axillary hair are absent. There is a strong familial incidence, the condition occurring not only in siblings but in members of three or more generations. (*Fig.* 346).

Diseases of the Pituitary Gland:

1. ACROMEGALY. Since prolactin and the growth hormone are both secreted by the eosinophil cells, milk secretion might be expected to be an occasional accompaniment of acromegaly and indeed galactorrhoea has been described. Gynaecomastia,

however, has only very rarely been reported in association with acromegaly.

2. CHROMOPHOBE ADENOMA. It is established that certain chromophobe cells are pre-eosinophil cells and some cases of acromegaly are found to be associated with chromophobe adenomata. Very occasionally a case of chromophobe adenoma accompanied by impotence, atrophy of the testes, and gynaecomastia has been described.

Miscellaneous Endocrine Disorders:

1. FOLLOWING PROSTATECTOMY. A very few cases of gynaecomastia following prostatectomy and in some instances subsequently subsiding have been described. It is difficult to suggest what the pathogenesis may be, if indeed the association is not coincidental.

2. ALBRIGHT'S SYNDROME. This consists of precocious puberty, polyostotic fibrous dysplasia, and patchy pigmentation of the skin. It usually occurs in girls but has been described in boys and occasionally gynaecomastia occurs.

Disease of the Liver. It is established that 'free' oestrogens circulating in the systemic bloodstream are 'conjugated' in the liver. Severe damage to the liver cells might therefore be expected to lead to failure to inactivate oestrogen and the appearance of manifestations of feminization. Thus it is not surprising that gynaecomastia occurs in many cases of cirrhosis with severe liver damage in which other obvious signs were prominent. However, though it may be prudent to perform routine liver-function tests in cases of gynaecomastia of unknown origin in adult men, it is seldom that one will incriminate the liver. It is interesting that haemochromatosis has not so far been accompanied by gynaecomastia.

Renutrition. Gynaecomastia was a fairly common feature in prisoner-of-war and concentration camps and was usually associated with renutrition following the arrival of food parcels or on the voyage home after release, and with reawakening of libido. It is probably associated with a resurgence of pituitary activity with secretion and release of gonadotrophins such as occurs at the time of puberty.

Klinefelter's Syndrome. This condition is due to the abnormal sex chromosome pattern 47-XXY. The presence of the Y chromosome is responsible for the development of testes, but in Klinefelter's syndrome it has to compete with two instead of one X chromosome. Consequently no germinal epithelium develops and most of the seminiferous tubules disappear. The testes are therefore very small, but of firm consistency. Interstitial cells, however, are increased in number and presumably produce androgens and oestrogens in varying proportions. If the conversion of androgen to oestrogen is abnormally high gynaecomastia may develop, and in some cases signs of androgenic deficiency may be evident.

Diseases of the Central Nervous System:

TRAUMATIC PARAPLEGIA. About 20 per cent of patients with paraplegia develop gynaecomastia. In the cases in which the testicular histology has been studied the picture is similar to that found in Klinefelter's syndrome. Traumatic paraplegia is followed by a period of catabolism with marked loss of protein. Furthermore abnormal brom-sulphthalein retention is found in some cases. It is possible that this phase of malnutrition and mild liver deficiency may account for the testicular changes.

SYRINGOMYELIA AND FRIEDREICH'S ATAXIA are also sometimes associated with gynaecomastia, when disturbances of metabolism and nutrition have been recorded. In these cases the testicular histology resembles that found in Klinefelter's syndrome.

DYSTROPHIA MYOTONICA. Gynaecomastia has, very rarely, been found in this condition, sometimes accompanied by a state of extreme debility. The changes in the testes are similar to those found in Klinefelter's syndrome.

Diseases of the Respiratory System:

BRONCHOGENIC CARCINOMA. The association of this condition with gynaecomastia is rare but interesting. Most of the cases have also shown osteo-arthropathy. In one instance the nipples were deeply pigmented which suggests that the gynaecomastia was due to excess of oestrogen. In another the gynaecomastia disappeared rapidly on removal of the tumour, suggesting that the tumour itself was secreting something that caused the gynaecomastia.

Drugs:

OESTROGENS. When oestrogens are administered therapeutically to men one must expect gynaecomastia. When the oestrogen administered is stilboestrol a deep-brown or black pigmentation of the nipples and areolae develops (*Fig.* 347) which scales off when the effect of the oestrogen begins to subside. In every case of gynaecomastia in which the cause is not obvious, one should inquire about any pills or ointments which the patient has recently been taking. Men who worked in pharmaceutical factories packaging oestrogen preparations used often to develop gynaecomastia.

ANDROGENS. These very seldom give rise to gynaecomastia (the incidence in a series of 101 cases was 3. It seems possible that methyl testosterone may lead to gynaecomastia, whereas other androgens probably do not.

CHORIONIC GONADOTROPHIN. It has already been pointed out that 'witch's milk' and 'puberty mastitis' are probably due to the influence of chorionic gonadotrophin on the neonatal testis and of pituitary gonadotrophins on the adolescent testis. Administration of chorionic gonadotrophins to normal adult men leads to an increased production of oestrogen and the Klinefelter picture of testicular histology. Gynaecomastia occasionally develops when chorionic gonadotrophin is administered in the treatment of undescended testicles.

DIGITALIS. The occurrence of gynaecomastia in patients treated with digitalis is occasionally reported. Whether it is fortuitous, or whether it is related to a significant improvement in the

patient's health and is therefore reminiscent of the gynaecomastia of renutrition, is at the moment a matter of speculation.

CHLORPROMAZINE and RESERPINE have been reported as giving rise to gynaecomastia on rare

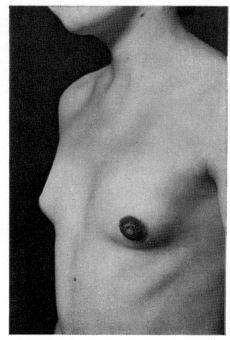

Fig. 347. Black pigmentation of the nipples in a man to whom stilboestrol has been administered. (*Courtesy of the Gordon Photographic Museum, Guy's Hospital.*)

occasions. Isoniazid, tricyclic antidepressants, spironolactone, α-methyl dopa, and meprobamate are other drugs which occasionally give rise to gynaecomastia.

P. M. F. Bishop.

HAEMATEMESIS

Haematemesis (vomiting of blood) has often to be distinguished from HAEMOPTYSIS: the distinction is based upon points discussed on p. 352.

CAUSES OF HAEMATEMESIS

1. Swallowed Blood:
  Epistaxis
  Haemoptysis
  Bleeding from the mouth and throat
  Malingering.

2. Diseases of the Oesophagus:
  Reflux oesophagitis (associated with hiatus hernia)
  Simple ulcer
  Epithelioma
  Aortic aneurysm rupturing into the oesophagus
  Rupture of varicose oesophageal veins
  Rupture or laceration of oesophageal wall in vomiting (Mallory-Weiss syndrome)

11*

Mediastinal new growth perforating the oesophagus and aorta

Foreign body perforating the oesophagus and aorta.

3. Diseases of the Stomach:

Acute gastritis

Chronic gastritis

Drugs, such as strong acids or alkalis, arsenic, phosphorus, antimony, aspirin, phenylbutazone, cortisone, indomethacin, alcohol

Ulcer

Haemorrhagic erosions

Pseudoxanthoma elasticum

Carcinoma

Multiple telangiectasis

Haemangioma

Leiomyosarcoma

Mallory-Weiss syndrome.

Telangiectasia (Osler-Rendu-Weber)

4. Diseases of the Duodenum:

Ulcer

Carcinoma, either primary or invasion from pancreas

Diverticula

Gall-stone ulcerating into the duodenum.

5. Portal Obstruction:

Cirrhosis of the liver

Portal vein thrombosis.

6. Acute Febrile Diseases:

Malignant variola

Malignant scarlet fever

Malignant measles

Blackwater fever

Anthrax

Malaria

Yellow fever

Dengue

Cholera

Acute yellow atrophy

Bacterial endocarditis

Leptospirosis icterohaemorrhagica (Weil's disease).

7. Blood Diseases:

Purpura

Scurvy

Polycythaemia

Haemophilia and allied disorders

Leukaemia

Aplastic anaemia with thrombocytopenia

Malarial cachexia

Von Willebrand's disease.

8. Miscellaneous:

Abdominal aneurysm opening into the stomach

Chronic nephritis: uraemia

Anticoagulant therapy

Following abdominal operation, trauma, and burns (Curling's ulcer)

Prolonged jaundice

Polyarteritis nodosa

Excessive strain on the stomach, e.g., in severe sea-sickness

Abdominal injury

Malignant hypertension.

There are only four *common* causes of *profuse* haematemesis—namely, *acute gastric erosion, gastric ulcer, duodenal ulcer,* and *cirrhosis of the liver.* The differential diagnosis between these is not always easy. A history of alcoholism may point to cirrhosis of the liver; at this stage of the malady there may be neither jaundice nor ascites, but the liver may be enlarged and firm and the spleen may be palpable. The term *gastrostaxis* was originally applied to the haemorrhage which appeared to occur in the absence of any lesion of the stomach, but gastroscopy and open gastrotomy at the time of surgical exploration have proved the presence in such cases of single or multiple erosions of acute ulcers. Acute erosions are especially common in patients who have recently ingested aspirin, butazolidin, indomethacin, or steroids, and may follow an alcoholic debauch. A long history of typical peptic ulcer symptoms is frequently elicited in patients bleeding from a gastric or duodenal ulcer. It must, of course, be remembered that cirrhosis of the liver and peptic ulcer may coexist.

1. SWALLOWED BLOOD

EPISTAXIS. If obvious bleeding from the nose is followed by haematemesis, the probability is that blood from the nares has been swallowed and then vomited. When nasal bleeding has taken place during the night, blood may have been swallowed unconsciously.

HAEMOPTYSIS. Blood coming from the lungs may be swallowed, especially if haemorrhage occurs during sleep. If the patient has a cough, or expectorates blood-stained sputum and presents physical signs of lung disease the possibility of swallowed blood must be considered as a cause of the haematemesis, though difficulties may arise in forming a correct conclusion, for cirrhosis of the liver, for instance, may be complicated by pulmonary tuberculosis.

BLEEDING FROM THE MOUTH AND THROAT. The gums, tongue, and fauces should be examined carefully, as blood from any of these sources may be swallowed and subsequently vomited. Bleeding from the gums is most likely to occur when they are spongy, as in scurvy or mercurial stomatitis. The amount of haematemesis due to blood swallowed from these sources is seldom great.

MALINGERING. The possibility of (animal) blood having been drunk in secret and afterwards vomited with intent to deceive must be considered in some cases when no cause can be found to account for its occurrence. The red corpuscles should be examined microscopically since their shape and size may supply a clue to an extraneous source. It must also be remembered that the vomiting of coloured liquid or of material which has a superficial resemblance to blood may supply an erroneous diagnosis of haematemesis to both patient and doctor.

2. DISEASES OF THE OESOPHAGUS

AN OESOPHAGEAL ULCER is a comparatively rare condition, usually existing as an ulceration in a peptic-lined oesophagus. Bleeding is more likely to be from *reflux oesophagitis* associated with hiatus hernia. (*See* p. 234 and *Figs.* 348, 349.) Haematemesis may on occasion be of considerable degree, although more usually it is occult.

EPITHELIOMA. Haemorrhage is rare in the commonest form of epithelioma of the oesophagus, which leads to an annular stricture, but it may occur from erosion of small blood-vessels as the result of ulceration, the amount of blood brought up being small. When the ulceration is deep and

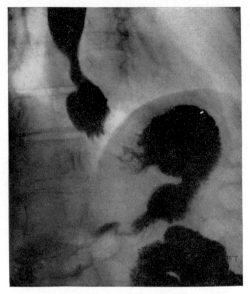

Fig. 348. Hiatus hernia with narrowing of oesophagus immediately above it as the result of oesophagitis and secondary fibrosis. (*Dr. H. W. A. Post.*)

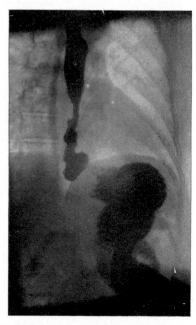

Fig. 349. Radiograph showing short oesophagus with simple ulcer causing distortion of lower third. The bulbous portion above the diaphragm is stomach herniated into the thorax. (*Dr. T. H. Hills.*)

extensive a larger vessel, even the aorta, may be opened, with the occurrence of sudden, profuse, and rapidly fatal haemorrhage. The diagnosis of this cause does not, as a rule, give rise to much difficulty; in nearly all the cases dysphagia is the earliest symptom (*see* p. 232).

AN ANEURYSM OF THE THORACIC AORTA compressing the oesophagus may finally erode and open into it, with profuse and fatal haematemesis.

RUPTURE OF VARICOSE OESOPHAGEAL VEINS. Varicose veins occur in the lower end of the oesophagus as a result of portal obstruction, especially that form which is due to cirrhosis of the liver, and the rupture of such veins is often followed by profuse haematemesis. It is rarely possible even by oesophagoscopy to determine whether the blood comes from the lower end of the oesophagus or from the stomach, so that the diagnosis resolves itself into one of whether the patient has cirrhosis of the liver or not.

RUPTURE OR LACERATION OF THE OESOPHAGEAL WALL. Massive painless haematemesis results from lacerations that traverse the gastro-oesophageal junction from forced vomiting or from severe coughing bouts. The history is one of repeated vomiting *followed* by haematemesis (Mallory-Weiss syndrome). The lacerations extend into the submucosa but do not rupture through the entire thickness of the wall.

MEDIASTINAL GROWTH PERFORATING THE OESOPHAGUS AND AORTA. Vomiting of blood is an infrequent complication of mediastinal growth, but it may occur if the growth erodes the oesophagus. It is most likely to be mistaken for thoracic aneurysm or epithelioma of the oesophagus. The tendency of new growth to compress and invade the large veins, leading to oedema of the neck and upper extremities, cyanosis, and dilated superficial veins, is generally characteristic, and serves to distinguish it from aneurysm, from which severe venous obstruction is much rarer.

FOREIGN BODY PERFORATING THE OESOPHAGUS AND AORTA. Copious fatal haemorrhage may be produced as a result of a foreign body, such as a pin, fishbone, or tooth-plate, perforating both the oesophagus and some large vessel or the aorta. A history of such a foreign body being swallowed, followed by a feeling of discomfort in the oesophagus, would suggest such a condition, which might be confirmed by the use of X rays or the oesophagoscope. Rarely a foreign body penetrates a vessel in the stomach wall; we have reported a fatal example due to a fragment of chicken bone.

3. DISEASES OF THE STOMACH

ACUTE GASTRITIS. The mucous membrane of the stomach in this condition is congested, and small haemorrhages and erosions are visible through the gastroscope (*Fig.* 350). The haemorrhage which occurs is slight unless the lesion is unusually serious, when it may be profuse; more often there are merely streaks of blood mixed with mucus in the vomit. Acute gastritis is caused by irritating foods, alcohol, or corrosive or irritant poisons. The chief symptoms arc a feeling of discomfort and tenderness in the epigastrium, nausea, eructations, vomiting, constipation—or in children diarrhoea. *Anthrax* in its septicaemic stage causes haemorrhagic ulcerative gastritis and haematemesis.

CHRONIC GASTRITIS. The mucous membrane of the stomach may be thickened and congested (*see Fig.* 351 B) sometimes with scattered haemorrhagic erosions. The vomit usually consists

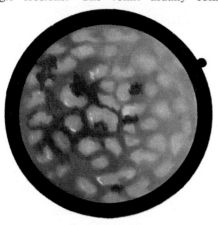

Fig. 350. Hypertrophic gastritis as seen through the gastroscope, the appearances being somewhat similar to those of the surface of the scars. Note the submucous haemorrhages.

mainly of mucus with occasionally a little blood. Chronic gastritis may follow acute gastritis but it is most frequently caused by continued excessive ingestion of alcohol or of tobacco or irritating and indigestible articles of diet. Chronic congestion due to diseases of the heart, lungs, or liver may be responsible. The main symptoms are tenderness in the epigastrium aggravated by the taking of food, nausea, vomiting—especially in the early morning if due to alcohol—flatulence, foul breath, a furred tooth-indented tongue, constipation, concentrated urine, and slight pyrexia. Atrophic gastritis may be associated with typical gastroscopic appearances (*Fig.* 352). The term 'gastritis' is frequently employed as a convenient name for any form of dyspepsia whether attributable to organic disease or functional disorder.

GASTRITIS DUE TO DRUGS AND CORROSIVE POISONS. Strong acids or alkalis destroy the surface tissues of the mouth, throat, oesophagus, and stomach, and cause intense pain in the mouth, throat, and abdomen, dysphagia, pain and tenderness behind the lower end of the sternum or in the epigastrium, distension of the abdomen, collapse, a rapid feeble pulse, and vomiting of blood and blood-stained mucus. Damage in the mouth and pharynx with sloughing suggest corrosion; chemical examination of the vomit furnishes evidence of the nature of the poison.

In *arsenic* poisoning the mucous membrane of the stomach is red, inflamed, partly detached,

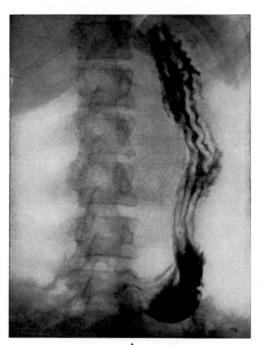

A

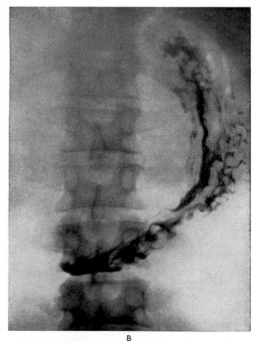

B

Fig. 351. A, A radiograph, after a barium meal, showing the normal mucosal relief of the stomach. B, A radiograph, after a barium meal, showing the mucosal relief of the stomach in a case of gastritis; these features are coarsening in calibre and irregularity in pattern of the rugae. (*Dr. G. T. Calthrop.*)

and covered with blood-stained mucus. The chief symptoms are nausea, violent and incessant sickness, burning pain in the epigastrium, diarrhoea, faintness, and depression. The vomit is usually a brownish, turbid fluid mixed with mucus and streaks of blood in which arsenic may be detected by appropriate tests. Later, there may be severe diarrhoea. *Phosphorus*, antimony, and other irritant poisons may also cause haematemesis, and in many instances the symptom has been shown to be due to *aspirin* or, more rarely, *indomethacin* or *phenylbutazone*.

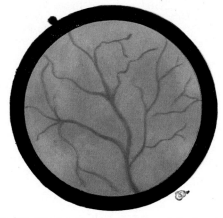

Fig. 352. Pale atrophic gastric mucosa rendering branching vessels clearly visible through the gastroscope. This appearance may arise from atrophic gastritis or from non-inflammatory atrophy.

Cortisone is not a gastric irritant but may activate a quiescent ulcer. Iron-containing tablets such as ferrous sulphate or carbonate may produce gastric erosion in children and in some adults.
GASTRIC ULCER. Haematemesis, although an important symptom of gastric ulcer, occurs in less than 20 per cent of cases both in the acute and chronic forms of the disease, being due in the former to erosion of small vessels and in the latter to the ulcerative process extending to and opening up larger vessels. The amount of blood varies within wide limits. If the quantity is small, or if it is gradually poured out into the stomach, it may remain there a sufficient time for the acid gastric juice to convert the haemoglobin into haematin which gives to the vomit a dark-brown 'coffee-grounds' appearance. In some cases the blood is not vomited but appears in the stools as melaena (p. 523). If a medium-sized or large vessel is eroded, the bleeding may be very copious, a quart or more of blood being vomited, either liquid and arterial in colour or as large red clots. A profuse haemorrhage causes sudden pallor, a feeling of faintness, restlessness, syncope, and a rapid feeble pulse. Occasionally haematemesis is the first intimation of the presence of a gastric ulcer, particularly of the acute type, but in the majority of cases other symptoms and signs have preceded it. In addition to haematemesis, the features most characteristic of gastric ulcer are

abdominal pain, nausea, vomiting, and melaena. Pain is felt in the epigastrium, either just below the xiphoid cartilage or at a point an inch or two lower than this, often quite localized; and either in the midline or to the left of the midline, less often to

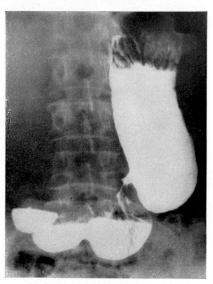

Fig. 353. Hour-glass stomach caused by chronic benign gastric ulcer visible on the lesser curvature. (*Dr. Keith Jefferson.*)

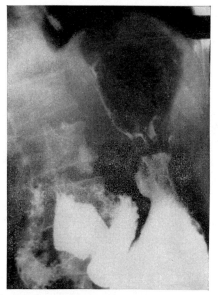

Fig. 354. Large benign gastric ulcer on lesser curvature. (*Dr. Keith Jefferson.*)

the right. It usually begins within an hour of the ingestion of food and is relieved by vomiting and by alkalis. Characteristically, the pain awakes the patient at 1 or 2 in the morning and he gets into the habit of taking milk or an alkali to bed with him in order to relieve this pain. It should be noted that it is quite impossible, on the history of the pain alone, to distinguish between gastric and duodenal ulcer. Pain may also be felt in the back between the 10th dorsal and 1st lumbar spines; its character and intensity are variable but it is usually severe and fairly localized. Tenderness on pressure in the epigastrium may also be present. Melaena, whether or not accompanied by haematemesis, is invariable.

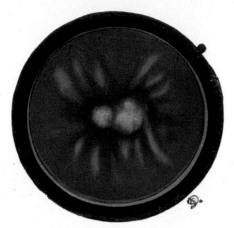

Fig. 355. A simple gastric ulcer in the process of healing, as seen through the gastroscope. Note the convergence of rugae due to scarring in and around the base of the ulcer. The central yellow area is due to slough.

There is more or less anaemia, according to the extent of the blood-loss.

Simple ulcer is often difficult to differentiate from cirrhosis of the liver or carcinoma of the stomach. Although examination of the stomach with X-rays after a barium meal often affords positive evidence of the nature of the lesion (*Fig.* 353), it is possible for the radiographic appearances to be those of a normal stomach even when an active ulcer is present (*Fig.* 354). An ulcer can usually be seen through the gastroscope (*Fig.* 355).

Haemorrhagic erosions are virtually minute ulcers; indeed the distinctions between haemorrhagic erosions and multiple small gastric ulcers are differences of degree and not of kind. There are certain conditions, however, especially specific fevers of malignant severity, purpura, infective endocarditis, septic states, yellow fever, black-water fever, and anthrax, in which a general tendency to subcutaneous and submucous haemorrhages may be associated with multiple small gastric erosions which produce haematemesis that may be as severe as is that of ordinary gastric ulcer.

PSEUDOXANTHOMA ELASTICUM (Grönblad-Strandberg Syndrome) is a disease of hereditary predisposition characterized by widespread abiotrophy of elastic tissue throughout the body. Massive gastric haemorrhage is a prominent visceral symptom, evidently due to disintegration of the elastica of the submucosal arteries.

The condition *multiple telangiectasis* is a hereditary affection in which numerous minute dilatations of the capillaries on the face (*Fig.* 50, p. 40) and mucous membranes occur, with persistent and often uncontrollable haemorrhage from the corresponding areas, including the stomach.

CARCINOMA. Frank haematemesis is a comparatively rare feature in carcinoma of the stomach and gastric cancer accounts for less than 5 per cent of all cases of this emergency. The familiar 'coffee-grounds' appearance is more usual than bright red blood, since a slight degree of bleeding in the form of a slow ooze from the ulcerated surface of the growth is a common occurrence. Although examples earlier in life, even in adolescents, have been noted, the majority occur between the ages of forty and sixty. The chief symptoms and signs of the disease are pain in the epigastric region, nausea, vomiting, anorexia, loss of weight and strength, pyrexia, anaemia, cachexia, and the presence of an abdominal tumour. In some instances a growth may remain completely silent and the sufferer complain of vague ill-health or even only of loss of weight. Pain varies considerably in degree and position and indeed may be completely absent. It is referred most frequently to the epigastrium but may be in the back or elsewhere especially when penetration occurs into adjacent structures. Vomiting is another symptom which varies in frequency and character according to the position of the growth. When the pylorus is involved (*Fig.* 356) and stenosed the stomach dilates but generally to a less extent than when similar pyloric stenosis results from the healing of a simple ulcer. The patient, instead of vomiting at intervals of several days large quantities of frothy brownish fluid, is more inclined to be sick every day and sometimes more than once a day, the amount brought up corresponding with that of the last meal and discoloured by altered blood of 'coffee-grounds' type. When the growth is at the cardiac orifice the symptoms resemble those of epithelioma of the oesophagus, the food meeting with obstruction so that after a few minutes some or all of it is returned—by regurgitation rather than by true vomiting. In a case of growth which involves neither of the orifices the greater curvature is usually the site of an ulcerating mass (*Fig.* 357), there may be no vomiting, or if present it may have no special characteristics, the symptoms being mainly those of dyspepsia or gastritis; whilst with diffuse carcinoma of the stomach, 'leather-bottle' stomach, fibrous growth may almost entirely replace the muscular tissue so that vomiting is impossible, bleeding is absent, no tumour is felt, and the diagnosis may be arrived at unexpectedly on an X-ray examination after a barium meal carried out because the patient has been able to eat so little food at a time.

Chemical analysis of the gastric juice after a test-meal may show deficiency of free hydrochloric acid but the value of this test is limited:

first, because about 3 per cent of perfectly healthy adults have no free hydrochloric acid in their gastric contents, apparently as a normal idiosyncrasy; secondly, because there are other pathological conditions besides carcinoma of

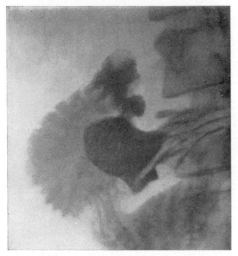

Fig. 356. Carcinoma involving distal third of stomach showing narrowing and rigidity common in the leather-bottle variety. (*Dr. T. H. Hills.*)

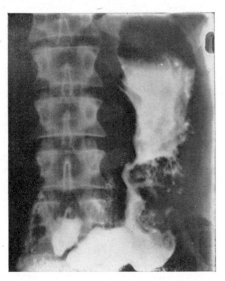

Fig. 357. Hour-glass deformity of the stomach due to carcinoma of the greater curvature. Compare with *Fig.* 353. (*Dr. Keith Jefferson.*)

the stomach in which there is deficiency or absence of free HCl in the gastric contents—cachexia of any kind, cirrhosis of the liver, heart disease with failing compensation, pneumonia, enteric and other fevers, achylia gastrica, combined scleroses of the spinal cord, Addisonian (pernicious) anaemia—as well as other conditions

in which the patient is ill enough for all his secretions to be reduced or suspended, amongst them the gastric juice. Today gastric analysis plays virtually no part in the diagnosis of stomach cancer.

A growth in the stomach may be seen with the aid of the gastroscope. The modern fibre-optic machine has the added advantage that a biopsy can be taken of the lesion for microscopic examination.

Loss of weight and strength is usually progressive, and is amongst the most constant signs of the disease, always meriting early attention in a patient of middle age who has never, until the last month or two, complained of any gastric symptoms. Anaemia of hypochromic type, with a low colour-index, may be so pronounced that a primary blood disease may be suspected. Palpation of the abdomen may reveal an ill-defined epigastric tumour. The position and character of the tumour vary according to the part of the stomach which is affected. Pyloric growth may cause the abdomen to be distended as a result of gastric dilatation and a movable tumour may be felt above the umbilicus, near the middle line and to the right of it. When the cardiac orifice is involved there may be no palpable tumour, and the same applies to the small 'leather-bottle' stomach of diffuse carcinoma ventriculi. A tumour of the body of the stomach may be felt in the epigastrium, or below the left costal margin. It may be necessary to examine under a general anaesthetic, and even laparotomy may be advisable as a diagnostic measure.

Troisier's sign—enlargement of the left supra-clavicular lymph-node—whilst indicative of abdominal (less frequently thoracic) malignant disease—is not a feature in the majority of cases.

Haemangioma is a benign tumour made up of newly-formed blood-vessels.

Leiomyosarcoma is a sarcoma containing large spindle cells of unstriped muscle. This, and the benign leiomyoma, are unusual but both have a high propensity to ulcerate and bleed, both in the stomach and elsewhere along the length of the alimentary tract.

INJURIES. Haematemesis may follow blows, stabs, or gunshot wounds in the epigastric region, or the passage into the stomach of instruments or foreign bodies such as a broken thermometer.

ABDOMINAL ANEURYSM OPENING INTO THE STOMACH. Rupture of the sac may lead to a sudden, profuse, and fatal attack of haematemesis. The condition may have been previously known by reason of there having been an epigastric tumour with distinct expansile pulsation, and severe pain both in the abdomen and in the back over the site of the bulge in a male arteriosclerotic patient; abdominal aneurysm in a woman is of very rare occurrence.

In these days of sophisticated vascular surgery, rupture of an infected Dacron replacement graft into the adjacent gut is being reported with increasing frequency.

4. DISEASES OF THE DUODENUM

DUODENAL ULCER. Haematemesis results when a duodenal ulcer opens a blood-vessel in its base and some of the blood regurgitates through the pylorus into the stomach to be vomited, the rest passing down the intestines to produce melaena. The condition is commoner in men. As in the case of gastric ulcer, melaena may occur independently of haematemesis. In acute ulceration a copious intestinal haemorrhage may occur in

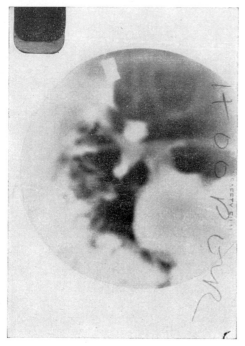

Fig. 358. Trefoil deformity of the duodenal cap and large ulcer. (*Dr. Keith Jefferson.*)

the stomach itself being of relatively small transverse type with active peristalsis, and emptying itself so rapidly that all the barium may have passed on after even so short an interval as two hours (*Fig.* 358). The transverse type of stomach emptying with undue rapidity is not necessarily associated with ulcer; but when found in conjunction with clinical symptoms suggestive of duodenal ulcer it provides presumptive evidence of that condition.

A test-meal, whether fractional or otherwise, will sometimes assist the diagnosis; there is no character of a fractional test-meal result that

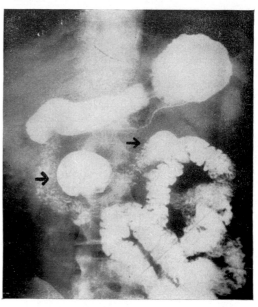

Fig. 359. Large duodenal and jejunal diverticula which gave rise to repeated upper abdominal colic. (*Dr. Cochrane Shanks.*)

an apparently healthy person, accompanied by acute pallor and faintness, followed by the evacuation per rectum of a mixture of black altered blood and bright arterial blood. The more profuse the bleeding, the greater the tendency for part of the blood so passed to remain red. Pain, although often severe and considerable, may be entirely absent. It is generally deep-seated in the upper part of the abdomen; its onset is usually two or three hours after the ingestion of food although the time relationships are variable and do not allow differentiation from gastric ulceration. One almost pathognomonic feature is of the relief of pain on taking food. Vomiting may occur though in many cases it is entirely absent; it is usual when the ulcer is of chronic fibrosing type, interfering with the proper emptying of the stomach and leading to pyloric stenosis. In such a case the X-rays show a large gastric shadow, and much barium may be evident in the stomach after eight hours. In many cases of duodenal ulcer quite the reverse type of radiograph may be found,

can be called pathognomonic of duodenal ulcer, but in the majority of cases of duodenal ulcer hyperchlorhydria is present; in the case of gastric ulcer a total acidity and a free acidity which are not abnormally high are more usual.

DUODENAL DIVERTICULA are in the majority of cases asymptomatic unless very large, or unless inflammation arises when food accumulates within. The symptoms may resemble those of duodenal ulcer but there is not the regular food relationship, although a coexisting ulcer is sometimes present which is responsible for the more conventional symptoms including haematemesis. Patients are as a rule over the age of 50; the diverticulum is always on the inner (pancreatic) side of the duodenum. (*Fig.* 359.)

CARCINOMA OF THE DUODENUM is very rare. Most examples prove to arise in the ampulla of Vater and thus are apt to cause jaundice and pale or 'silvery' stools.

GALL-STONES ULCERATING THROUGH FROM THE GALL-BLADDER INTO THE DUODENUM may rarely cause haematemesis and melaena. Previous attacks of pain occasioned by the gall-stone might lead to a diagnosis of gastric or duodenal ulcer; but if the pain were colicky in character, associated with tenderness below the tip of the ninth right rib and with jaundice, a gall-stone would be suggested. In some instances there is no jaundice and the symptoms closely simulate those of duodenal ulcer. The diagnosis might be confirmed by discovery of the stone in the faeces or as a result of direct X-ray examination or, in the case of a very large calculus, by the occurrence of acute intestinal obstruction from its impaction in the small intestine.

5. PORTAL OBSTRUCTION

Obstruction to the flow of blood through the portal vein may lead to portal hypertension and varicosity of the gastric and oesophageal veins, rupture of which may cause severe haematemesis. The chief cause is *cirrhosis of the liver*. Haematemesis may be the earliest symptom, and the hepatic cause may remain in doubt until, years later, ascites and cholaemia supervene. There may be a history and the signs and symptoms of chronic alcoholism, but cirrhosis can occur in lifelong total abstainers. The liver may be enlarged and firm, but its surface at this stage is generally smooth and its edge as yet neither irregular nor beaded. The spleen may be enlarged as a result of the portal obstruction, but in adults rarely attains the enormous size of the spleno-megalic variety of cirrhosis in children and young adults.

Non-suppurative thrombosis of the portal vein is rare. It may, however, give rise to sudden and profuse haematemesis. It may result from umbilical neonatal infection, abdominal trauma, pancreatitis, and polycythaemia. It is distinguished from other forms of portal obstruction by the relatively sudden onset of ascites, haematemesis, melaena, and enlargement of the spleen, and by absence of signs and symptoms of cirrhosis of the liver and other causes of portal obstruction.

PRESSURE ON THE PORTAL VEIN. Haematemesis when due to this cause is generally associated with ascites and jaundice, the common bile-duct as well as the portal vein being compressed on account of their close proximity to each other. (*See* JAUNDICE, p. 433.)

6. ACUTE FEBRILE DISEASES

MALIGNANT VARIOLA. Haematemesis occurs in about a third of the cases of haemorrhagic smallpox. It is associated with cutaneous, sub-cutaneous, and submucous haemorrhages, haematuria, epistaxis, melaena, and bleeding from the gums. The sudden initial rigor, intense backache and headache, severe vomiting, epigastric pain, cutaneous haemorrhages, and the diffuse hyper-aemic rash with small punctiform haemorrhages appearing first on the groins and lower part of the abdomen, would point to a diagnosis of haemorrhagic or black smallpox if such a case occurred during an epidemic of the disease.

MALIGNANT SCARLET FEVER. In the haemorrhagic form of scarlet fever—nowadays exceedingly rare—haematemesis may occur; but haematuria, epistaxis, and cutaneous haemorrhages are more frequent. The sudden and severe onset, the very high temperature, the rapid and feeble pulse, the headache and delirium, and the appearance of the rash on the second day would point to scarlet fever.

MALIGNANT MEASLES, or black measles, is extremely rare in Western countries but it is met with in areas where measles has been recently introduced. The haematemesis is less prominent than is the generalized purpura, and the diagnosis is indicated by the nature of the general epidemic.

In *Blackwater Fever* and in *Anthrax*, haematemesis may occur without purpura, though there is a tendency to all kinds of haemorrhages.

YELLOW FEVER. 'Black vomit' due to the presence of altered blood is a characteristic feature of this disease. Hyperaemia and catarrhal swelling of the mucous membrane is the only change which is found in the stomach. It is essentially a disease of tropical and sub-tropical countries. The onset is sudden, with a chill, headache, and severe pain in the back and limbs. The face is flushed, and jaundice very soon appears. After the first day of illness the pulse-rate drops, so that with a temperature of 103° or 104° the rate may be only 70 or 80. In addition to the black vomit there may be cutaneous petechiae and bleeding from the gums. It may be difficult to distinguish from malignant malaria; moreover the two diseases may coexist.

CHOLERA may be associated with haematemesis. The sudden onset of acute gastro-intestinal symptoms, the frequent rice-water stools, and the epidemic nature of the malady, point to the diagnosis, which may be confirmed by recovering the causal *Vibrio cholerae* from the motions.

ACUTE MASSIVE LIVER NECROSIS. Haematemesis is the commonest form of haemorrhage in this rare disorder. Women between twenty and thirty are affected more frequently than men, especially during and just after pregnancy. It may result from the effects of industrial chemicals such as T.N.T., yellow phosphorus, or benzole, and as a sequel of infective hepatitis. The first symptoms are indistinguishable from those of infective hepatitis—viz., malaise, loss of appetite, nausea, vomiting, and jaundice. Vomiting soon becomes intractable, jaundice increases, and drowsiness, restlessness, and delirium supervene. The vomit is black from altered blood, and may resemble unrefined treacle. Melaena, epistaxis, and subcutaneous petechiae may be observed. The tongue becomes dry and brown; the liver dullness diminishes, and the urine shows considerable diminution in the amount of urea and bile-pigment.

LEPTOSPIROSIS. Severe haemorrhagic manifestations occur in very ill patients but some bleeding is present in about 40 per cent of all cases, haematemesis and haemoptysis being the most common.

7. BLOOD DISEASES

PURPURA HAEMORRHAGICA. Haematemesis may occur either as a result of swallowing blood derived from the mucous membrane of the nose or mouth, or by reason of superficial erosions of the gastric mucosa itself. There will generally be haemorrhages from other mucous membranes— epistaxis, oral bleeding, haematemesis, uterine or vaginal haemorrhage, blood per rectum. Before making a diagnosis of purpura haemorrhagica various examinations of the blood will be necessary to exclude conditions in which purpura may be a feature (see PURPURA, p. 669).

SCURVY. Haematemesis occurs in severe cases. The swollen, spongy gums, anaemia, cutaneous haemorrhages, and subcutaneous indurations, in a patient who has been living on a diet deficient in fresh vegetables, would point to scurvy. Confirmation is accorded by response to administration of ascorbic acid.

HAEMOPHILIA AND ALLIED DISORDERS. Excessive bleeding from slight cuts or after tooth extraction, epistaxis, bleeding from the mouth, and haemorrhage into the joints are the earliest and the commonest manifestations of the disease. The association of haematemesis with haemorrhage from other parts and with haemorrhage into joints in particular, in a patient whose near male relations show a tendency to bleed on the slightest provocation, is the diagnostic feature. In the hereditary coagulation disorders in general, gastro-intestinal bleeding, when persistent or recurrent, is based on a local organic lesion, for instance gastritis or a peptic ulcer.

LEUKAEMIA. Haemorrhages from and into various parts, especially epistaxis, are common in this disease; haematemesis may be severe and even fatal. Gastric haemorrhage in association with enormous enlargement of the spleen is not pathognomonic of leukaemia, for the two conditions may be present in chronic malaria, splenic anaemia, and splenomegalic cirrhosis. Diagnosis is established by an examination of the blood. (See ANAEMIA, p. 25.)

HODGKIN'S DISEASE. In the late stages of this malady there is a tendency to haemorrhage from and into various parts of the body, e.g., epistaxis, bleeding from the mouth, cerebral haemorrhage, and rarely haematemesis. The last-named is seldom an early symptom and the disease will have been recognized previously from its characters described on p. 513.

MALARIAL CACHEXIA. Anaemia and splenic enlargement may follow repeated attacks of malaria and severe haematemesis may occur. (See p. 296.)

8. MISCELLANEOUS

CHRONIC NEPHRITIS. Haematemesis occasionally occurs in this disease. Its association with high blood-pressure, hypertrophy of the heart, retinopathy, polyuria, and urine of low specific gravity containing albumin and renal tube-casts, would point to chronic nephritis as the cause.

FOLLOWING ABDOMINAL OPERATIONS. Haematemesis may occur after severe abdominal operations, independently of injury to the stomach or duodenum; it may follow any other stress, e.g., trauma or severe burns, and is due to the development of acute ulcers, usually of the duodenum (Curling's ulcer).

PROLONGED JAUNDICE. The importance of jaundice as a cause of almost any variety of bleeding by oozing lies chiefly in the added danger attending operations in such cases.

SEA-SICKNESS, AEROPLANE-SICKNESS, and allied conditions may produce such violent strain on the stomach from retching and vomiting, that small gastric vessels may rupture and lead to haematemesis. (See MALLORY-WEISS SYNDROME, p. 331.) The amount of blood brought up is generally not large, but occasionally it has led to the fear that a gastric ulcer may be responsible.

INJURY TO THE EPIGASTRIUM, for instance by a kick, by a punch, or by the steering-wheel in a motor-car accident, may be followed by haematemesis from direct injury to the stomach.

Harold Ellis.

HAEMATURIA

Blood may appear in the urine as the result of injury, of disease in some portion of the urinary tract or of other organs involving the urinary apparatus, or of a few general diseases. The blood may be present in large, small, or microscopic amounts, it may continue for days or weeks, or, appearing suddenly and without apparent cause, may disappear completely for a variable period. It may be present in the urine either as corpuscles or as haemoglobin; in haemoglobinuria the urine is dark brown from the presence of methaemoglobin, and any deposit consists of brownish debris in which no red blood-corpuscles can be found (see HAEMO-GLOBINURIA, p. 350). Occasionally the colouring matter of the blood may escape from the corpuscles if the urine has been retained for long in the bladder, when crenated or disintegrated corpuscles will be found on microscopical examination of the sediment. The following list gives the chief causes of haematuria.

I. HAEMATURIA FROM AFFECTION OF SOME PART OF THE URINARY TRACT:

A. Renal Causes:
Malignant tumours of kidney:
  Carcinoma
  Nephroblastoma (Wilms's tumour)
  Carcinoma of the renal pelvis
    Transitional-cell (papillary or solid)
    Squamous-cell
Innocent tumours:
  Angioma
  Adenoma
  Papilloma of pelvis, etc.
Injury of the kidney

Calculus
Tuberculosis
'Essential' haematuria
Hydronephrosis
Hydrocalicosis
Polycystic disease
Aneurysm of the renal artery
Renal arterial occlusion
Polyarteritis nodosa
Papillary necrosis
Intrarenal arteriovenous fistula
Acute pyelonephritis
Oxaluria
Nephritis, acute and subacute
Hereditary (Alport's syndrome)
Medullary sponge kidney
Chronic renal failure
Hydatid disease of the kidney
Drugs: anticoagulants, turpentine, carbolic acid, cantharides, potassium chlorate, hexamine, sulphonamides
Relief of tension by sudden decompression
Renal purpura.

B. Ureteric Causes:

Calculus
Carcinoma or papilloma
Ureterocoele.

C. Vesical Causes:

Papilloma
Carcinoma, papillary, nodular, ulcerative, or adenocarcinoma
Sarcoma
Haemangioma
Enlarged prostate ('prostatic varices')
Carcinoma of prostate
Tuberculosis of bladder or prostate
Calculus
Acute cystitis
Chronic interstitial cystitis (Hunner's ulcer)
Radiation cystitis
Purpura
Injury
Bilharzia haematobia (schistosomiasis)
Foreign body.

D. Urethral Causes:

Acute urethritis, impaction of calculus, injury
Papilloma or carcinoma
Angioma
Foreign bodies
Caruncle.

II. Haematuria from Disease of the Neighbouring Viscera involving the Urinary Organs:

Carcinoma of the uterus, vagina, or colon
Acute appendicitis
Acute salpingitis
Pelvic abscess
Dysenteric or tuberculous ulceration of the intestine
Diverticulitis of the colon.

III. Haematuria in General Diseases:

Renal infarction in endocarditis
Arteriosclerosis
Leukaemia
Purpura
Scurvy or avitaminosis C
Haemophilia and other bleeding diatheses (including anticoagulants)

Acute fevers: Malaria, smallpox, yellow fever, blackwater fever
Excessive exercise
Sickle-cell trait or disease.

In considering the diagnosis of a case presenting haematuria as a symptom there may be other symptoms present, such as pain, tumour, or increased frequency of micturition, which will point to one or other organ as the source of the bleeding, but in some cases haematuria may be the only symptom. The following points will often help in the differential diagnosis.

The Colour of the Urine. If the urine is bright red the haemorrhage is most likely to arise from the bladder or lower urinary tract. Dark-coloured blood in the urine may, however, be due to the retention of blood in the bladder for some time, or from the large amount present in the urine.

The Distribution of the Blood in the Urine during Micturition. Terminal: If the urine during micturition is only tinged with blood during the final expulsive efforts, or the terminal urine is stained more deeply than the rest, the source of the haematuria is almost certainly in the bladder. *Initial*: If the first urine passed is blood-stained and the remainder clear, the bleeding is probably from the urethra or prostate. *Total*: If the urine is evenly stained with blood throughout it suggests that the source of haemorrhage is in the kidneys or ureter, or is pre-renal in origin, although a vesical lesion which causes more than a slight haemorrhage may also give rise to a deeply blood-stained urine throughout micturition.

The Quantity of Blood present in the Urine. A large quantity of blood in the urine in the absence of trauma suggests some form of growth in the bladder or kidney. Papillomata and papillary carcinomata in the bladder may cause sudden profuse haemorrhage without pain or other symptom, whilst equally profuse haemorrhage may arise from a malignant tumour in the kidney which has invaded the renal pelvis. Enlargement of the prostate often causes fairly profuse haematuria, especially in hypertensive men. Examination of any clots of blood passed may occasionally afford information in determining the seat of haemorrhage. The urine should be poured into a large flat tray containing water, and the clots floated out, when some may show the triangular or pyramidal shape indicating their formation in the renal pelvis, or others the thin, worm-like form with tapering or decolorized ends from their formation in the ureter; the passage of clots down the ureter is accompanied by the same acute colic that is caused by renal calculus ('clot colic'). Clots formed in the bladder are flat and disk-like, but often broken up in their passage through the urethra.

If the quantity of blood is increased by movement or exercise, suspicion of renal stone or growth will arise. In one case profuse haematuria occurred after three successive railway journeys, when the lesion found at operation was an early carcinoma of one kidney which had recently invaded the renal pelvis.

The Association of Other Elements from the Urinary Organs with Blood in the Urine. Microscopical examination of the deposit obtained by centrifuging the urine may reveal cellular elements distinctive of the renal pelvis or vesical mucous membrane, or epithelial, granular, and blood-casts from the renal tubules, which may help in the diagnosis in a case of haematuria. The presence of a number of urinary crystals in a urine of acid reaction will point to renal calculus. Occasionally, small pieces of growth may be passed in the urine from the delicate villous papilloma or villous-covered carcinoma of the bladder, and more rarely plugs of mucopus from a caseous tuberculous cavity in the kidney may

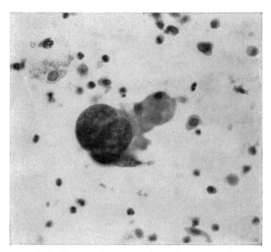

Fig. 360. Clumps of transitional carcinoma cells in the urine in a case of carcinoma of the bladder. (*Dr. J. O. W. Beilby, Middlesex Hospital.*)

be found. The presence of a villous tuft in the urine may give some indication whether it is derived from an innocent papilloma or a villous-covered carcinoma; although it becomes detached only from the surface of the growth, an expert pathologist may be able to distinguish between benign and malignant cells by modern methods of staining. The cells in the centrifuged deposit of the urine should be stained by the Papanicolaou method; the science of *exfoliative cytology* is now sufficiently advanced to enable the recognition of cells from a tumour of the renal pelvis, ureter, or bladder to be made (*Fig. 360*). Cells from a carcinoma of the renal parenchyma do not exfoliate so freely and cannot at present be detected with so much certainty.

The association of pus with blood in the urine does not give much assistance in determining the seat of the bleeding. Both pus and blood will often be present with either calculus or tuberculosis of the kidney or bladder, and they may both be present with vesical growth, prostatic enlargement, or pyelitis.

The Amount of Protein. If the amount of protein in the urine is in excess of that which

would be due to the amount of blood present, the bleeding is probably renal in origin.

The Reaction of the Urine is of very slight assistance in determining the source of bleeding. Generally speaking, blood in an acid urine is more likely to be derived from the kidney than from the bladder; this, however, is no universal rule, for blood may be present in an acid urine in a case of vesical calculus or growth; whereas, on the other hand, there may be blood in alkaline urine in a case of phosphatic renal calculus as well as in pathological conditions of the bladder.

The association of *unilateral lumbar pain*, situated in the angle between the last rib and the border of the erector spinae muscle, passing forwards above the iliac crest into the groin, with occasional attacks of colic, would suggest a renal lesion; while haematuria accompanied by *increased frequency of micturition*, or by *penile pain* immediately following micturition, would indicate vesical disease; *sacral pain* with haematuria suggests malignant disease in the bladder or prostate. This statement must be taken in only a general sense, for exceptions to it are frequent. Thus a vesical tumour causing haematuria may implicate a ureteric orifice sufficiently to cause increased intrarenal tension on that side with lumbar aching or even hydronephrotic enlargement of the kidney; or a tuberculous lesion in the kidney, with descending ureteritis, may cause increased frequency of micturition before there is vesical infection. It is important to take into consideration the *age of the patient*. Thus, in a young adult, continued slight haematuria with increased frequency of micturition is highly suggestive of tuberculous disease of the kidney, transient episodes of haematuria in a young woman with associated dysuria and frequency are probably due to cystitis, whereas slight haematuria in a more elderly patient suggests vesical carcinoma or calculus. At any age, severe haematuria may be present with a villous tumour of the bladder, or in a patient more advanced in years with renal growth or prostatic enlargement.

Further evidence of the source of the haemorrhage may be obtained upon the *physical examination of the patient*. This should be carried out systematically, and not only should the urinary organs be examined, but any evidence of disease elsewhere in the body, particularly the heart, lungs, blood, liver, or pelvic organs, sought for also. Each kidney should be examined bimanually, one hand being placed in the angle made by the last rib and the margin of the erector spinae muscle, and the other in front, immediately below the costal margin. The patient is then directed to breathe deeply while pressure is maintained by the two hands, when an enlarged or unduly mobile kidney may be felt to descend, or may be grasped on deep inspiration. Any pain or undue tenderness on either side should be noted, especially any sharp, pricking pain experienced by the patient if the anterior hand is depressed suddenly, a sign indicative of renal stone.

Examination of the bladder by palpation in the suprapubic area may elicit pain in acute inflammatory conditions, or may give evidence of a distended bladder in a case of haematuria from prostatic obstruction; but much more knowledge may be gained by a thorough *rectal examination*. For this purpose the patient should assume the knee–elbow position, or the recumbent position with the hips and knees flexed, when the examining finger can explore not only the prostate, but the vesiculae seminales, the lower end of each ureter, and the bladder base, as well as the lateral pelvic space. The prostate may show the uniform, elastic, and movable characteristics of the adenomatous enlargement, or may be infiltrated with primary carcinoma— far from uncommon—when the gland presents marked firm, rounded nodules, is inelastic, loses it median vertical groove which demarcates the lateral lobes from each other, and is often immovable in the surrounding tissues. Search should be made for any nodules in the prostate or vesicles, or thickening of the lower end of the ureter, suggestive of tuberculous disease, or thickening or infiltration in the bladder base, which may often be felt in a case of vesical carcinoma. Examination in the lateral pelvic space may show thickening due to lymphatic spread in the extravesical tissues in a case of carcinoma of the bladder or prostate. *Examination of the testes* should always be made. A nodule in either epididymis may indicate tuberculous disease which may have spread from the urinary organs, but care must be taken not to mistake a nodule dating from a gonorrhoeal epididymitis for one due to tuberculous disease. Vaginal examination similarly may show thickening in the vesical base or in the lateral lymphatic areas with carcinoma of the bladder, or may give evidence of disease in the pelvic organs. The lower end of each ureter can sometimes be palpated in the fornices if it is diseased or contains a calculus.

The greatest assistance may be obtained by the use of the *cystoscope* (*Figs.* 365–370, p. 346; *Figs.* 682–685, p. 680). Great gentleness must be used in carrying out instrumentation to avoid further haemorrhage which would obscure a view by the cystoscope, and if any bleeding is present an attempt should be made to arrest it by irrigation of the bladder. If the bleeding is profuse it may be difficult to obtain a satisfactory view of the interior of the bladder, but with slighter haemorrhage rapid distension of the bladder may produce a medium clear enough to obtain a view of the seat of bleeding. Thus in renal haematuria blood-stained urine may be seen to be emitted from one ureteric orifice (*Fig.* 370, p. 346), and clear urine from the other before the medium is too obscured; or with vesical haemorrhage a vesical tumour may be seen. Even slight haemorrhage will, however, rapidly render the medium in the bladder too hazy for a satisfactory examination of any minute changes in the vesical wall to be obtained—tuberculous disease, for example. In cases in which the bladder is found to be healthy, changes in the appearance of the ureteric orifice of one side, oedema, ulceration, or ecchymosis may indicate the side of the bleeding. Blood in small quantity in the efflux from a ureteric orifice may be difficult to detect; in these cases a ureteric catheter may be passed into each ureter and the urine from each kidney compared, though it must be remembered that haemorrhage may be caused by the trauma of the passage of the catheter along the ureter.

In every case of haematuria a cystoscopic examination should be insisted upon, and it is frequently a distinct advantage to carry out the examination while the bleeding is going on. Should the haemorrhage be arrested, a cystoscopic examination would show any vesical lesion, but if the bladder is normal it may be impossible to determine whether the bleeding has come from one or other kidney. Further assistance may be obtained by *radiographic examination* combined with *pyelography* or *excretion urography* (*see* p. 474).

I. HAEMATURIA FROM AFFECTION OF SOME PART OF THE URINARY TRACT

A. Renal Causes

The Malignant Tumours of the Kidney—carcinoma and nephroblastoma to a lesser extent— are all associated with profuse haematuria at intervals. Carcinomata are the most common; they arise in the parenchyma of the kidney, and vary in their rate of growth. The nephroblastomata (Wilms's tumours) occur mainly in children and are extremely malignant, while carcinoma of the renal pelvis, either in the papillary form or as a squamous-cell carcinoma, is less common. These tumours cause aching in the loin, and may, especially in children, lead to considerable enlargement of the kidney before haematuria occurs. In the progressive growth of the tumour the renal pelvis or calices are involved gradually and haematuria is evoked. This is usually severe, so that clots may be formed in the calices of the renal pelvis or in the ureter, and cause the typical pain of colic in their descent of the latter. Attacks of pain in the loin result from the increasing tension in the tumour and also from areas of localized haemorrhage in the tumour mass. The renal tumour usually maintains the shape of the kidney, but in some cases may present a nodular form. Hence profuse intermittent haematuria, with clots of pyramidal or worm-like shape, associated with renal enlargement, is strongly suggestive of a renal malignant growth. A pyelogram will show deformity of the renal pelvis or calices (*Figs.* 501, 502, pp. 484, 485).

An *adenoma* of the kidney, forming a small tumour in the renal tissues, or an *angioma* developing at or near the apex of a renal papilla, may cause profuse haematuria; these are rare conditions which are not generally diagnosed until the kidney is operated upon or is seen post mortem. The pyelogram is normal and the only hope of preoperative diagnosis is the presence of a tumour blush on renal angiography.

A *papilloma of the renal pelvis* is an uncommon form of innocent tumour, and may give rise to profuse intermittent haematuria and to renal enlargement which in this instance is due to hydro- or haematonephrosis from the obstruction to the ureter by the papillary growth or by blood-clot. Thus the renal tumour may vary in size and consistence. Papillomata of the mucous membrane of the renal pelvis are accompanied occasionally by similar growths in the ureter, and may also show a similar growth at the ureteric orifice upon inspection of the bladder. Pyelography may show a filling defect in the renal pelvis.

The *papillary carcinoma* of the renal pelvis causes very similar symptoms, and cannot be diagnosed from the innocent papilloma until a histological examination is made after removal; the older the patient the more likely is the growth to be malignant. *Squamous-cell carcinoma* of the renal pelvis is a rare disease, sometimes associated with renal calculus, giving rise to haematuria that is seldom profuse.

Injuries to the Kidney may cause haematuria; the diagnosis is usually obvious. The history of the accident, a blow or kick, or severe squeeze to the lumbar region, associated with haematuria, would point to an injury to the kidney. There may be renal enlargement, but this must be diagnosed from an extravasation of blood in the perinephric tissues from rupture of the renal cortex. Comparatively slight injury to the loin may produce haematuria from a small lesion in the renal tissues, while in some cases there is no sign or recollection of external violence. In any case of haematuria following trauma it is essential to diagnose an injury to the kidney from injury to the *urethra* or *bladder*. In urethral injury the canal may be merely contused, or partially or wholly ruptured; blood may be found at the urethral meatus, or may be marked in the first portion of any urine that may be passed, while if the urethra is entirely divided, signs of extravasation of urine, with inability to micturate, will appear. If the bladder is injured blood may be present in any urine drawn off; or after rupture of the bladder involving the peritoneal coat fluid may be found in the abdominal cavity, with increasing signs of peritoneal irritation. At the same time, a thorough examination of the bony pelvis (including radiography) should be made for any sign of fracture, which is frequently the cause of direct injury to the bladder or urethra.

With Renal Calculus the bleeding is seldom profuse, is usually associated with a small amount of pus, and frequently is increased after exercise or the jolting of a journey. The subject of a renal stone will usually complain of aching pain in one loin, which will remain of this character so long as the stone remains fixed, in which condition slight haematuria is often present.

When, however, the calculus projects into or is free in the renal pelvis the urine also contains a small quantity of pus, and attacks of colic come on, characterized by very acute pain in the loin, passing forwards and downwards to the groin, upper part of the thigh, and testicle of the same side, and accompanied by frequent desire to pass urine. The calculus may be passed into the bladder along the ureter, may become impacted in the course of the ureter, or may remain in the renal pelvis, in which case successive attacks of renal colic may occur. The previous passage of a small calculus per urethram, following an attack of renal colic, is an important point in the history of such a patient, but in any case an examination by radiography should be carried out, when a calculus may be proved present in the kidney or ureter (*see* p. 474). A calculus in the kidney may attain a size too large to become engaged in the upper end of the ureter, when renal colic will be absent; or it may cause hydronephrosis, renal abscess, or pyonephrosis, with corresponding additional symptoms.

Renal Tuberculosis, apart from the miliary form of children, is the usual primary manifestation of tuberculous disease in the urinary tract, although evidence of former tuberculous infection may be present in the lungs, joints, and lymphatic glands. The patients affected are usually young adults, who complain of a slight aching in one loin with occasional attacks of more acute pain resembling renal colic. At the onset of the disease, when the foci are limited to the renal tissues, there is no change in the urine beyond the presence of albumin; but as it advances the foci coalesce and form a softened area which opens into the renal pelvis, when there is a constant or intermittent discharge of small quantities of pus and blood in the urine. The liberation of tuberculous material into the renal pelvis and ureter causes infection of the mucous lining of these passages, and is marked almost constantly by increased frequency of micturition during both day and night, even before any tuberculous infection has occurred in the bladder. These cases are often mistaken for renal calculus or for pyelonephritis, but in any case of persistent slight haematuria or pyuria, particularly in a young adult, a careful search should be made for tubercle bacilli in the urine. A radiograph may in late cases show a shadow produced by a tuberculous focus in the kidney (*Fig.* 361), but this generally differs from that due to a calculus in its less definite border and by variations in the density. In renal tuberculosis the haematuria is rarely increased by exertion on the part of the patient, as is frequently the case with calculus, and pain in the loin is less mitigated by rest in bed. In renal tuberculosis the lower end of the ureter of the affected side may be felt to be thickened on examination per vaginam, or per rectum, while in the male tuberculous nodules may be felt in the prostate or seminal vesicles, and in either sex the cystoscopic appearances of the vesical end of the tuberculous ureter may be distinctive. In tuberculous disease of the kidney the excretion of the indigocarmine after intravenous injection is considerably delayed or even absent, and a pyelogram shows that some of the calices are irregular and lose their definition. Intravenous pyelography may fail to show a shadow of the renal pelvis or calices owing to the loss of functional efficiency of the kidney, but in an early case will show a 'moth-eaten appearance' of the affected area. (*Fig.* 362.)

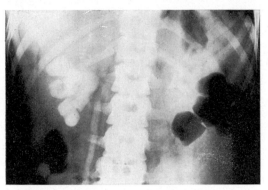

Fig. 361. Pyelogram of tuberculous right kidney. Note the fine scattered calcification in the upper pole. The calices are dilated and clubbed.

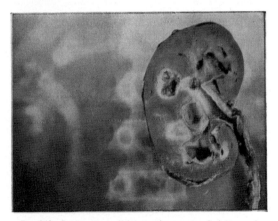

Fig. 362. Intravenous pyelogram in a case of right renal tuberculosis; all the calices are irregular and clubbed and the ureter is dilated. The superimposed kidney shows the extent of the cavitation.

Essential Renal Haematuria is the name given to a group of cases in which definite unilateral haematuria is present, but in which examination of the kidney on exploration or pyelography has failed to show the cause of the haemorrhage. The bleeding may be profuse, and comes on suddenly without any apparent cause; it is intermittent, and may be accompanied by lumbar aching, but there is no tenderness and enlargement of the kidney and on cystoscopic examination it is proved to be unilateral. In the intervals of haematuria there may be no albuminuria. The kidney on exploration appears to be normal;

but in some of these cases there is a small papilloma, adenoma, or angioma, non-malignant, undiagnosable except by surmise unless shown by very careful selective renal angiography. Areas of focal nephritis, thickening of the peripelvic fat, and vascular congestion have also been found. The condition should not be diagnosed unless a complete urological and general examination has proved negative.

Hydronephrosis occasionally gives rise to haematuria, and the combination of renal tumour and haematuria would suggest a growth in the kidney. The blood from a hydronephrotic kidney, however, is very rarely copious, and the other symptoms of hydronephrosis would distinguish the two, in particular intermittency with corresponding changes in the amount of the urine.

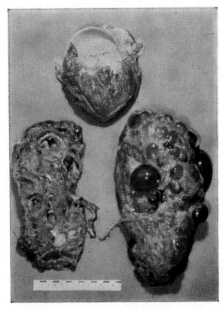

Fig. 363. Bilateral grossly enlarged polycystic kidneys. Note the associated hypertensive cardiomegaly.

Much assistance may be obtained in the examination of a suspected renal swelling by *pyelography* (*Fig.* 478, p. 472).

In Hydrocalicosis the dilatation affects one calix only owing to constriction of its outlet into the pelvis; the dilated calix may contain stones.

Polycystic Disease of the kidneys is commonly accompanied by haematuria in the later stages of the disease. It occurs in childhood or in adult life, and is most commonly bilateral (*Fig.* 363), forming an enlargement of each kidney which may reach large dimensions, although, on the other hand, a tumour may only be felt on one side. In the early stages the diagnosis is difficult; there is polyuria with a low-specific-gravity urine, and, later, pain, bilateral tumour, haematuria, and signs of renal insufficiency and hypertension will be present. The renal tumour caused by polycystic disease is smooth and rounded or sometimes lobulated, but differs from hydronephrosis in that fluctuation can seldom be obtained. Bilateral hydronephrosis may be diagnosed from polycystic disease by the finding of some lesion obstructing the normal urinary flow, such as stricture of the urethra, prostatic or vesical disease, or carcinoma of the pelvic organs invading the ureters. Polycystic disease of the kidney gives a characteristic pyelographic picture in which the renal calices are much elongated and drawn out (*Fig.* 504, p. 486), without the large rounded areas shown by the cavitation of the kidney in hydronephrosis.

Aneurysm of the Renal Artery is a rare condition which may follow injury or arise spontaneously. It usually causes haematuria from renal congestion before a swelling is palpable. There may be a bruit on auscultation and hypertension is present. Plain radiography sometimes shows a ring shadow but aortography is diagnostic.

Renal Arterial Occlusion (arterial infarction) is usually accompanied by sudden, sharp, continuous pain in the flank or upper abdomen, the common cause being an embolus. Microscopic haematuria is present in about half the cases and gross haematuria may occur. There is usually some source for the embolus—atrial fibrillation or subacute bacterial endocarditis, for example.

Polyarteritis Nodosa may also cause haematuria, as may *papillary necrosis*, whether due to diabetes mellitus, analgesic therapy (especially phenacetin) sickle-cell disease, chronic alcoholism, or urinary-tract obstruction. Haematuria may be accompanied by fever, pains in the flank, and shivering turns.

Intrarenal arteriovenous fistula may arise from trauma but is more often due to a new growth; it causes hypertension and is usually accompanied by haematuria.

Acute Pyelonephritis, due to infection with *B. coli* and other organisms, may give rise to haematuria. The acute onset of the disease, accompanied by rigors, pyrexia, and frequency of micturition, with the presence of organisms and a small amount of albumin and pus in the urine and the absence of epithelial and blood casts, will serve to diagnose it from acute nephritis.

Oxaluria (p. 610) may give rise to slight haematuria. The passage of large numbers of oxalate crystals in the urine occurs in some patients, especially after a diet containing rhubarb, gooseberries, tomatoes, strawberries, or spinach, and is often accompanied by dyspepsia. Examination of the urine on successive days will demonstrate the condition. The aching in one loin, and the envelope crystals (*Fig.* 627, p. 611) in the urine, may simulate renal stone, but the absence of a shadow in the radiograph will disprove a stone.

Acute Nephritis is accompanied by haematuria, but is usually obvious by the rapid onset of the disease, by the history of some specific fever or of a chill, and by the subcutaneous oedema of legs, back, and eyelids. The urine is scanty and of high specific gravity, and contains, in addition to blood disks, hyaline and epithelial tube-casts, many renal epithelial cells, and abundant albumin. There are some cases of acute nephritis in which no oedema occurs, and then the abundance of renal tube-casts in the urine affords the main evidence as to the diagnosis.

Hereditary Nephritis with Deafness (*Alport's Syndrome*). This is a familial disease characterized by a renal disorder, an auditory disorder, and ophthalmic defects. It is transmitted as a partially sex-linked dominant trait and has a serious prognosis in males but is less severe in females. The renal disorder is shown by symptomless haematuria and albuminuria occurring in the first weeks of life; in males it proceeds to chronic nephritis with death before the age of 30. The auditory disorder is a perceptive deafness of gradual onset but usually apparent by the age of 10; it affects boys more often than girls. The ophthalmic defects are less constant and include cataracts and spherophakia.

Haematuria may be microscopic or macroscopic; it is often heavy for some years before gradually diminishing. It increases during any virus infection and these are frequent. The diagnosis is made mainly from the family history; the mother may have had albuminuria during pregnancy and brothers or sisters may be affected. The blood-urea is normal in the early stages, but the serum α_2 globulin may be increased and the γ globulin depressed. The haematuria is unaffected by bed rest; the blood-pressure gradually rises and the male patients die from renal failure. Histologically there are the changes of chronic glomerulo-nephritis.

Chronic Renal Failure in its terminal stages may be associated with profuse haematuria.

Hydatid Disease of the kidney is rare in England. The cases are characterized by attacks of renal colic with haematuria and the appearance of hydatid hooklets (*Fig.* 74, p. 79) and remains of daughter cysts in the urine. Before the cyst has ruptured into the pelvis the only evidence of its presence may be a renal swelling. The Casoni test and the complement-fixation test may be positive.

Drugs taken by the mouth may in certain patients cause haematuria. In the treatment of disease by anticoagulants, hexamine, etc., blood may be passed in the urine, and cases have been recorded in which haematuria occurred during treatment with sulphonamides, especially if the urine was not kept alkaline.

Relief of tension by the sudden emptying of the bladder in a case of chronic retention of urine may produce haematuria; in a mild case the blood comes from vessels in the bladder, but in a more severe case there is renal bleeding. Such patients usually die from suppression of urine (*Fig.* 364).

Renal Purpura may occur without evidence of the generalized disease; such a kidney shows pelvic submucous areas of haemorrhage.

B. Ureteric Causes

Ureteric Calculus may cause haematuria, either during the descent of the stone or when the latter becomes arrested in the duct without causing complete obstruction to the flow of urine. The diagnosis is usually easy from the history and the character of the pain, accompanied by the increased desire to micturate; but in some cases on the right side it may be mistaken for appendicitis. The previous history of the passage of a calculus or of symptoms of renal stone may be elicited. A calculus may become obstructed in any part of the ureter, though most commonly in the pelvic portion. Cystoscopic examination

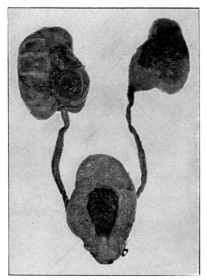

Fig. 364. Kidneys, ureters, and bladder filled with blood-clot following sudden emptying of the bladder in a case of chronic retention. (*From 'Proceedings of the Royal Society of Medicine'.*)

may show swelling and ecchymosis of one ureteric orifice if the stone is near the bladder or occasionally it may be seen partly projecting from the orifice. Radiographic examination may show a shadow in the line of the ureter, but this should always be confirmed by a stereoscopic radiograph taken with an opaque bougie passed into the ureter or by excretion urography. Shadows very similar to calculi may be caused by phleboliths or by calcareous glands; these are frequently multiple and calcified glands show variations in density with indistinct outline, but if single and in the apparent line of the ureter, may cause trouble in diagnosis unless a stereoscopic radiograph with an opaque bougie is obtained (*see* p. 476).

Papilloma in the Ureter may cause haematuria even after the removal of the primary disease in the renal pelvis by nephrectomy. For this reason it is usual to carry out complete ureterectomy at the same time as the nephrectomy, if this cause is suspected.

Primary Carcinoma of the Ureter is rare; it is diagnosed by the filling defect of the ureter with dilatation above, on ureterography, and by the brisk bleeding which occurs when a ureteric catheter is passed. A negative shadow in the ureterogram can be produced by a new growth, a non-opaque calculus, or an air bubble.

C. Vesical Causes

The profuse haematuria due to a *Papilloma*, or a *Papillary Carcinoma* of the bladder, frequently occurs without any other symptom, coming on suddenly without any exciting cause; it may last a variable time, and then disappear entirely, to reappear after a varying interval. With the carcinomatous form there may be some increased frequency of micturition in the absence of bleeding, but in either variety the clotting of blood in the bladder may cause urgent desire to micturate, or even retention of urine. A bimanual pelvic examination under general anaesthesia may give evidence of infiltration of the base of the bladder or of the pelvic lymphatics in the malignant form, but it is only rarely that an innocent tumour is hard enough to be felt per rectum, although occasionally it may be large enough to be palpable as a soft mobile swelling. In the intervals between haemorrhages, a cystoscopic examination will demonstrate the presence of vesical growth (*Figs.* 365, 366). The common situation for a vesical tumour is at the base of the bladder, above and outside the ureteric orifice of one side; the latter may be obstructed, or dragged upon by the growth in such manner as to cause renal distension or hydronephrosis, so that a malignant vesical tumour may give rise to renal pain and tumour, and in this way be mistaken for a renal growth. This difficulty will be overcome by a cystoscopic examination of the bladder. A papilloma of the bladder may occur at any age, though it is infrequent under the age of 25 years, whereas a papillary carcinoma is unusual before 45 years. Papillomata may be multiple from direct implantation or from the inherent tendency of the particular vesical mucous membrane to produce them from multicentric foci of origin.

Nodular and Ulcerative Carcinomata occur in elderly patients, and cause slight but fairly constant haematuria. For haemorrhage to take place from a vesical carcinoma there must be ulceration of the surface of the growth, and other symptoms will be present, namely, increased frequency of micturition both day and night, penile pain following the act of micturition, and pyuria. The blood often occurs as a few drops at the termination of urination, or may be mixed throughout the act. Usually the tumour is situated on the base of the bladder, and may be felt as a distinct infiltration per rectum, but there is a form of adenocarcinoma which may arise in the urachus which occurs in the dome of the bladder.

Sarcoma is a rare form of malignant disease in the bladder which occurs in children, or occasionally in adults, as a rapidly growing tumour mass, sometimes resembling a bunch of grapes (sarcoma botryoides).

Haemangioma may occur as a spider naevus of the mucous membrane or as a solid tumour of considerable size.

Prostatic Enlargement of the adenomatous or of the carcinomatous variety may cause haematuria, though, contrary to what might be expected, it is more common with the former. The age of the patient (50 or more), the increased frequency and difficulty in micturition, and the evidence obtained by rectal examination suffice to diagnose the disease. The haematuria of prostatic enlargement is often profuse, and may occur early; but on careful inquiry it will usually be found that there has been for some months a

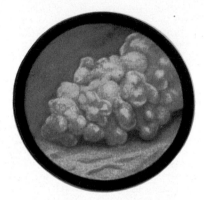

Fig. 365. Pedunculated papillary carcinoma of bladder.

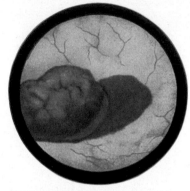

Fig. 366. **Nodular** carcinoma of bladder.

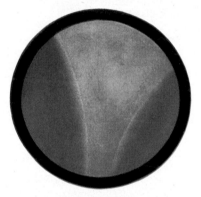

Fig. 367. Appearance at the urethral orifice in adenomatous enlargement of both lateral lobes of the prostate.

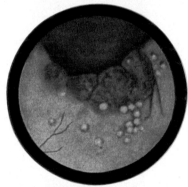

Fig. 368. *Schistosoma haematobia* (schistosomiasis) of the bladder wall.

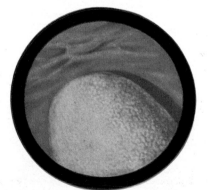

Fig. 369. Uric acid calculus in bladder.

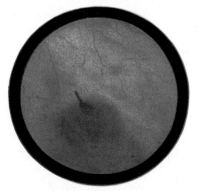

Fig. 370. Blood-stained urine issuing from the ureter.

Figs. 365–370. Bladder appearances seen through the cystoscope.

gradually increasing frequency of micturition. The diagnosis is made at cystoscopy. The bleeding can be observed to come from the surface of the enlarged prostate over which distended veins may be visible ('prostatic varices'). The patient is often a hypertensive subject.

Vesical Tuberculosis occurs commonly in young adults. Persistent frequency, slight haematuria, and acid pyuria in a young patient will always suggest tuberculous disease, and a very careful search should be made in the centrifugalized urine for tubercle bacilli; it should be supplemented by guinea-pig inoculation and culture on Lowenstein's medium, and other evidence of tuberculous disease, especially in the kidneys, testes, vesiculae seminales, and prostate, should be looked for. Tuberculous disease of the urinary organs rarely occurs as a primary disease, and usually there is evidence of former tuberculous disease in the chest, joints, or other sites. Apart from an infection secondary to disease in the generative organs, tuberculosis in the urinary organs almost always starts in one kidney, in an area which softens and opens into the renal pelvis. Infection then occurs in the mucous and submucous coats of the pelvis and ureter, as well as in the peri-ureteric lymphatics, and spreads to the bladder. Even before there is any visible infection of the latter there is persistent pyuria, haematuria, and increased frequency of micturition, so that vesical disease may be thought to have started while the infection is limited to the kidney. Cystoscopic examination may reveal changes in the ureteric orifice of the affected side, or evidence of vesical infection (*Figs.* 684, 685, p. 680). A careful rectal or vaginal examination may show an enlarged and thickened ureter. When tuberculous disease spreads to the bladder from the direct ulceration of a prostatic or vesicular focus, haematuria is usually present. Examination of the testes and of the prostate and vesicles will reveal the nature of the infection.

Vesical Calculus also causes slight haematuria, usually as a few drops in the terminal urine. The subject of a calculus in the bladder unaccompanied by cystitis will complain of increased frequency of micturition during the day or during exercise, but may be free during the night. There is pain of a pricking character in the glans penis after micturition, and there may be a history of sudden stoppage of the stream during the act. The patients are usually men, and there may be a history of previous calculi in the bladder or of attacks of renal colic with the descent of a renal calculus which has not been passed per urethram, but which has increased in size since it entered the bladder. The stone if large may sometimes be felt on pelvic examination but it can be seen with a cystoscope (*Fig.* 369). Radiographs are also useful in detecting the stone (*Fig.* 371), although a urate stone may be of such low density that it forms no shadow on an X-ray film. Haematuria is more likely to be associated with oxalate stones, which are sharp and spikey, than with

the smooth urate or phosphate calculi. If the calculus has caused cystitis, there will be in addition pyuria and nocturnal micturition.

Acute Cystitis is accompanied by haematuria; but the other symptoms, such as vesical tenesmus, suprapubic pain, and pyrexia, together with pyuria and a cause for the condition, will point to the disease. There is a form of haemorrhagic cystitis in which bleeding predominates over other symptoms; cystoscopy shows multiple patches of submucous haemorrhage not unlike

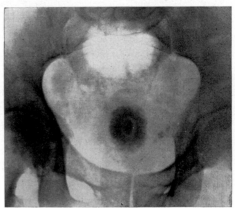

Fig. 371. Radiograph of a composite (oxalate and phosphate) vesical calculus.

those seen in purpura of the bladder but without the cutaneous manifestations of that disease.

Simple Ulcer of the bladder may be found as a result of severe localized inflammation in acute cystitis.

Chronic Interstitial Cystitis (Hunner's ulcer) is often associated with painful haematuria and increased frequency of micturition from a small contracted bladder.

Radiation Cystitis. After X-ray therapy for carcinoma of the bladder or of the uterus there may be multiple telangiectases in the vesical mucosa or areas of necrosis which continue to bleed even if the original tumour has been controlled. This may indeed be so severe and persistent that total cystectomy becomes mandatory.

Bilharzia Haematobia (*Schistosomiasis*) causes slight haematuria, and gives rise to symptoms very similar to vesical tuberculosis. The discovery of the typical ova in the urine, together with a history of residence in an affected district, notably Iraq, Egypt, or certain parts of Central and South Africa, will make the diagnosis clear. The cystoscopic appearance in the bladder of small, glistening yellow nodules and small areas of raised granulation tissue is distinctive of the disease (*Fig.* 368).

Foreign bodies may be introduced by design or accident. Their presence will be shown by cystoscopy and radiography.

D. Urethral Causes

Acute Urethritis, whether gonococcal or septic, may cause blood in the urine from the acute congestion of the urethral mucous membrane. The history and the presence of an acute urethral discharge make the diagnosis evident.

The Impaction of a Calculus in the urethra causes some bleeding from direct injury to the urethral mucous membrane. There is usually retention of urine, so that true haematuria may not occur; but the history of sudden stoppage of the stream of urine during micturition, with acute penile pain, together with the previous history of renal or vesical stone, will usually make the diagnosis clear. It was formerly not uncommon in male children. The calculus may be felt from the outside in the course of the urethra, often at or near the meatus, or seen by an endoscopic examination or by radiography (*Fig.* 372).

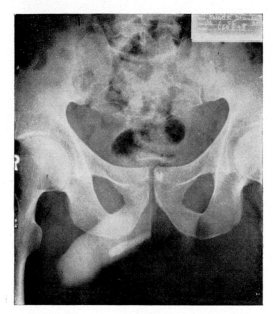

Fig. 372. Elongated urethral calculus which caused retention of urine.

Papillomata of the urethra may occur just within the external meatus in conjunction with papillomata of the glans penis, or in the prostatic urethra. They give rise to initial haematuria, or to spontaneous bleeding from the urethra not associated with micturition. They can be recognized with the urethroscope or by direct inspection (*Fig.* 373).

Carcinoma is rare, but may supervene on a longstanding urethral stricture; it is therefore usually situated in the bulb. A spreading induration combined with more frequent bleeding should arouse suspicion in such a case. The diagnosis can be made by urethroscopy and urethrography (*Fig.* 374).

Angioma of the urethral mucous membrane is a rare but important cause of severe and recurrent haematuria, the patient generally presenting no other symptoms beyond the spontaneous bleeding

and serious anaemia resulting from it. The blood is passed both with and apart from micturition. There may or may not be bleeding naevi elsewhere; but the condition is precisely analogous to the small bleeding naevi of the tongue and mouth that have been described in conjunction with naevi of the skin by Osler and others. The

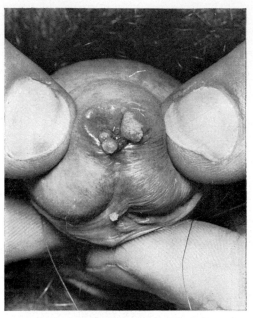

Fig. 373. Papillomata of the urethra projecting from the external urinary meatus.

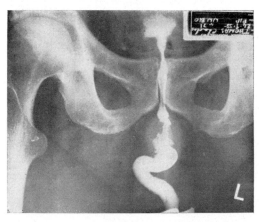

Fig. 374. Irregular filling defect in a urethrogram caused by carcinoma of the urethra which supervened on a longstanding stricture.

diagnosis of a urethral angioma could scarcely be made with certainty except by urethroscopy.

Foreign Bodies, other than fragments of bone or missile resulting from fractures or gunshot wounds, are sometimes introduced into the urethra as a form of sexual excitement, under the influence of alcohol or to maintain an erection. Pencils, glass rods, grasses. and hairpins are amongst the many objects which have been found. They may produce haematuria, urethral bleeding, or retention of urine (*see also* p. 807). A *Caruncle* at the external urethral orifice in the female may occasionally give rise to blood in the urine; it will be readily diagnosed on inspection.

II. HAEMATURIA FROM DISEASE OF THE NEIGHBOURING VISCERA INVOLVING THE URINARY ORGANS

The direct spread of *carcinoma* of the pelvic organs may in its progress involve the bladder, as is not uncommon in the later stages of carcinoma of the uterus, vagina, rectum, or pelvic colon. The infiltration of the bladder wall before actual ulceration has occurred is usually indicated by vesical irritability, followed by ulceration and haematuria, together with the passage of urine by the vagina or faecal matter or fat in the urine. Occurring as a late stage of carcinomatous disease there is usually little difficulty in the diagnosis.

Haematuria may occur during an attack of *acute appendicitis* from the direct spread of the inflammatory process to the vesical wall. In some cases in which the inflamed appendix turns downwards over the pelvic brim it may become adherent to the bladder, or an abscess may form in immediate relation to the bladder wall. The localized inflammation of the vesical mucous membrane causes haematuria, while the sudden appearance of a quantity of pus in the urine has been noticed when an appendicular abscess has ruptured into the bladder. The history of acute pain low down in the right iliac fossa, the pyrexia, and general symptoms of peritoneal inflammation before any urinary symptom was noted, will point to the disease; a rectal examination may reveal the inflammatory process in the right pelvic region.

Acute Salpingitis or *Pelvic Abscess* may similarly cause haematuria from direct inflammatory extension to the vesical wall, but this is rarer than in appendicitis.

Tuberculous and *Dysenteric Ulceration of the Intestine* have both caused haematuria by the adhesion of the bowel to the fundus of the bladder and the subsequent inflammatory condition of the mucous membrane. In a case of slight haematuria a cystoscopic examination showed a localized area of intense congestion at the fundus of the bladder without any other vesical lesion, and on opening the abdomen a coil of small intestine, obviously ulcerated by tubercle, was found adherent to the peritoneal aspect of the bladder. A similar congested area in the bladder causing haematuria has been seen in a case of tuberculous endometritis where the uterus was in contact with the bladder.

Diverticulitis of the colon occasionally results in a pelvic abscess which may ulcerate into the bladder, giving rise to haematuria, and to an intestino-vesical fistula. The preceding history of attacks of intestinal colic, of the passage of blood and mucus per rectum, and of irregularity of the bowels is very similar to that of colonic carcinoma, and the diagnosis is seldom certain until laparotomy has been performed, though the radiographic appearances after a barium meal, with the dotted residua of the barium in the diverticula of the bowel, may be suggestive.

III. HAEMATURIA IN GENERAL DISEASES

The sudden plugging of a renal vessel by embolism (*renal infarction*) is not uncommon in cases of endocarditis, and may be accompanied by haematuria. Embolism is seen most commonly in infective endocarditis; it is indicated by sudden pain in the loin, followed by haematuria. The occurrence of acute endocarditis in the course of acute septic processes, such as acute osteomyelitis, is not uncommon, and it will usually be diagnosed before there is any evidence of renal embolism. On the other hand, there are certain cases of chronic heart disease in which the first evidence of infective endocarditis having become superadded may be the occurrence of sudden haematuria. In some such cases there may be difficulty in excluding acute glomerulonephritis, because around each infarct there is local acute inflammation, and therefore the urine will contain tube-casts as well as blood. The other signs of infective endocarditis (p. 291) should be watched for.

Leukaemia may be accompanied by haematuria; but enlargement of the spleen, general symptoms of anaemia, and the total and differential blood-counts (p. 36) will point to the diagnosis.

Scurvy and the various forms of PURPURA (p. 669) may be accompanied by haematuria, but the general symptoms of each disease are usually well marked before this occurs. Subclinical scurvy due to deficiency of vitamin C in the diet has been known to cause haematuria which was relieved on the addition of adequate amounts of the vitamin.

Haematuria occurs sometimes after *excessive exercise* and is seen occasionally in long-distance runners without evidence of any pathological lesion.

Conditions simulating Haematuria. Haemoglobinuria is considered in the next section. *Beeturia* is the name applied to the passage of red or pink urine after beetroot has been eaten, usually in large quantities. It is due to the absorption of a pigment, betacyanin, a type of alkaloid. It occurs in a small number of normal individuals, estimated at 13·8 per cent, but is commoner in those with pernicious anaemia or with iron deficiency anaemia who have not been given oral iron. It can be recognized from the history and the absence of any appreciable number of red blood cells in the urine. The colour disappears on alkalization but reappears on reacidification.

Harold Ellis.

HAEMOGLOBINURIA

Haemoglobinuria means the passage of urine containing free haemoglobin in solution. It must be distinguished from the much commoner condition of haematuria, in which the urine contains intact red cells so that the haemoglobin is confined within the cell envelope. When, as often happens in haematuria, the red cells are uniformly mixed with urine, the freshly passed specimens in the two conditions will present essentially similar appearances to the naked eye. If, however, the two fresh specimens be immediately centrifuged the distinction between them becomes obvious: in that from the case of haematuria the red cells fall to the bottom of the tube and can be seen microscopically in the sediment, leaving a practically normal coloured urine on top; while that from the case of haemoglobinuria will appear to the eye practically unchanged after centrifuging, retaining the uniform blood-tint throughout the fluid, while the microscope reveals few, if any, red cells in the sediment. The colour of the urine in a case of haemoglobinuria may range from slight smokiness, through pink, red, and brown, to black. With the spectroscope, if necessary after suitable dilution of the centrifuged urine, the characteristic bands of oxyhaemoglobin will be seen and generally those of methaemoglobin as well. These should be distinguished from those of myoglobin by precipitation with ammonium sulphide. The ordinary chemical tests for blood will also be positive. Since haemolysis may take place in the urine both while it is in the bladder and after it has been passed, centrifuging a specimen from a case of haematuria does not necessarily remove *all* traces of blood-pigment: the essential point is that the pigment will be very much less in the spun than in the unspun specimen. Moreover, the confusion on this point will be less likely to arise if the urine is examined as soon as possible after it is passed.

Haemoglobinuria results from an intravascular haemolysis which is sufficiently rapid for the free haemoglobin to reach about 140 mg. per 100 ml. of plasma, at which critical level it exceeds the binding capacity of plasma haptoglobin. This is a β-globulin which binds haemoglobin and, because of its larger molecule, prevents the smaller haemoglobin molecule from passing across the renal glomeruli into the urine. Once, however, haemoglobinuria has begun it may persist until the plasma-haemoglobin has dropped to the much lower level of about 40 mg. per 100 ml. This is because the haptoglobin level in the blood is rapidly depleted by the continual liberation of haemoglobin from the haemolytic process. In the majority of haemolytic conditions the process is not usually sufficiently rapid to result in haemoglobinuria; instead the plasma-haemoglobin, before it has time to reach the critical level, is converted into billirubin, and this latter pigment, by its accumulation in the plasma, gives rise to the more common haemolytic manifestation of icterus.

Cases of haemoglobinuria may be classified under the following headings:

1. Occurring as an essential feature of the specific clinical conditions known respectively as (*a*) paroxysmal, (*b*) nocturnal, and (*c*) march.

2. Due to haemolytic crises in patients with intracorpuscular defects such as sickle-cell disease and hereditary spherocytosis.

3. Due to transfusions of incompatible blood or of blood which has been stored for too long.

4. Due to many chemical and other poisons particularly in patients whose red cells have a deficiency of glucose-6-phosphate dehydrogenase (*see the* Table *on* p. 52). Other chemicals such as lead, benzene, phenylhydrazine, chlorates, methyl chloride, arsenuretted hydrogen, and organic arsenicals may produce acute haemolysis and haemoglobinuria in normal individuals exposed to sufficiently high concentrations of these chemicals. Certain drugs, such as stibophen, quinine, quinidine, para-amino-salicylic acid, penicillin, and methyldopa, may produce haemolysis and haemoglobinuria in particular individuals as the result of the formation of a red-cell antibody.

5. Due to infective and toxic processes, particularly malaria, and during pregnancy and the puerperium.

6. Due to extensive burns.

7. In acute haemolytic anaemias due to unclassified haemolysins, and red-cell antibodies.

PAROXYSMAL COLD HAEMOGLOBINURIA, which is rare, affects both sexes, children, adolescents, or grown-ups; and in some cases the patient has syphilis, which is more often of the congenital type. It is characterized by sudden attacks of haemoglobinuria, which may persist for a day or two and usually follow exposure to cold. The exposure may be of the body generally or only part of the body, such as the immersion of the hands in cold water. There may be no other symptoms, but often an attack is ushered in by shivering or an actual rigor, with feelings of malaise, with pain in the back or legs, or headache. If repeated attacks occur at short intervals anaemia will develop. Vasomotor disturbances, particularly Raynaud's disease, are sometimes found, but they are much more likely to be associated with the haemoglobinuria due to cold agglutinins. The disease is due to a haemolysin which unites with the red cells at a low temperature, and destroys them when the temperature subsequently rises. A rough form of the Donáth-Landsteiner reaction for the demonstration of the haemolysin is done as follows: a few ml. of venous blood from the patient and a normal person are placed respectively in two tubes and allowed to clot. They are then placed in iced water for ten minutes and subsequently warmed in a water-bath at 37° C. for thirty minutes. If the test is positive the serum from the patient will be blood-stained, while that from the control will be clear. The diagnosis depends on the demonstration of haemoglobinuria, the history of paroxysmal attacks, the test just described, and the finding in many of the cases of a positive Wassermann reaction, but the proportion of cases associated with syphilis is probably less than with viral diseases and the positive Wassermann reaction may be non-specific.

NOCTURNAL HAEMOGLOBINURIA (*Marchiafava-Micheli syndrome*) is a very rare condition occurring in either sex, generally between the ages of 20 and 50, and characterized by attacks of haemoglobinuria taking place at night. The first specimen passed on waking may be a deep red, while subsequent specimens passed during the day become less and less coloured or completely colourless, the phenomenon being repeated on successive days. Haemoglobinuria will also appear when the patient wakes up after a long sleep in the middle of the day. The attacks usually last for several weeks, and are separated by intervals of months which tend to grow shorter. There is an anaemia of haemolytic type, which though mild at first is gradually progressive; the indirect van den Bergh reaction is positive and there is usually a greater or less degree of icterus. Unlike most haemolytic anaemias the blood may show a marked leucopenia. Blood transfusions tend to precipitate severe haemolytic crises and washed red cells may be required to avoid this. Most patients die within three to six years either from anaemia or from portal or systemic thromboses which are common complications. The Donáth-Landsteiner reaction is negative. Ham's test is positive and consists of demonstrating lysis of red cells in their own plasma at a pH of 6·9, but this does not occur if complement has been inactivated. The cause of the condition is an abnormality of the red cells which results in their being haemolysed by the action of complement. Thrombin and other unknown factors are involved in initiating this haemolytic process. Although acidity is a factor *in vitro* there is no evidence that this is so *in vivo*. Haemolysis may be precipitated by infections, some drugs, and even by blood transfusion. Unlike other patients with haemolytic anaemias, these patients may develop iron deficiency.

MARCH HAEMOGLOBINURIA, another very rare condition, occurs in healthy soldiers and athletes, following strenuous exercise in the upright position, such as prolonged marching or running. The passage of blood-stained urine is transitory and there are usually no other symptoms. The recognition of the condition and of its harmlessness is, however, of importance in view of the alarm it may cause in affected subjects. In marathon runners haemoglobinaemia is common, but the plasma-haemoglobin does not reach the renal threshold value. The haemolytic process may sometimes be prevented by the use of soft insoles in the shoes.

MYOGLOBINURIA may mimic haemoglobinuria but they can be differentiated by the spectroscopic character of the two pigments. Paralytic myoglobinuria very occasionally occurs in man but is well recognized in horses who have been taken out to exercise after prolonged rest. Myoglobinuria may be seen in the 'crush syndrome' developing after severe crushing injuries to muscles, and rarely as a condition known as 'paroxysmal myoglobinuria' in which episodes of acute muscle pain and weakness are associated with the appearance of this pigment in the urine; the aetiology is unknown.

During or after BLOOD TRANSFUSIONS haemoglobinuria may occur if the blood given is incompatible with that of the recipient, on account of the AB or occasionally the Rh and other factors; it is then a sign of serious import. In both instances there is hypotension and frequently oliguria and/or anuria which may be fatal. Occasionally haemoglobinuria and rapidly developing jaundice may follow the transfusion of compatible blood which has been stored too long, especially if a large volume of it has been given. Provided the blood was not infected, no serious symptoms are likely to develop and the haemoglobinuria and jaundice rapidly subside. After incompatible blood tranfusions the absence of any oliguria is a very hopeful sign.

In addition to the chemical and other poisons already mentioned haemoglobinuria may sometimes occur as a result of any of the following: the oral administration of potassium chlorate, turpentine, ether, carbon bisulphide, pyrogallic acid, naphthol, carbolic, hydrochloric, sulphuric, nitric, oxalic and chromic acids, glycerin, chloroform, sulphonal, veronal, trional, tannin, saponin, strychnine, and hexamine; the inhalation of carbon monoxide, naphtha vapour, arseniuretted, antimoniuretted, phosphuretted, or sulphuretted hydrogen; the eating of various poisonous fungi; the ingestion of ricin, abrin, robin, crotin, phallin; and the introduction of the poisons of certain snakes, venomous toads, and spiders. It has also occurred after the intravenous injection of normal horse serum, and of antitetanic, antimeningococcal, antidysenteric, antidiphtheritic, antistreptococcal, antipneumococcal, and antianthrax sera.

The severe form of haemoglobinuria known as BLACKWATER FEVER, occurring in malarial patients, is a manifestation of the disease, although it is probable that quinine and other antimalarial drugs and glucose-6-phosphate-dehydrogenase deficiency may play a part in precipitating the attack. Other infections which occasionally give rise to haemoglobinuria include: syphilis (*see above under* PAROXYSMAL HAEMOGLOBINURIA), typhoid, gas gangrene, generalized anthrax, and yellow fever.

FAVISM (or *Fabism*) is due to eating raw or imperfectly cooked broad beans by a patient who suffers from glucose-6-phosphate dehydrogenase deficiency and produces haemoglobinuria and jaundice. It occurs in Sardinia and other parts of Italy and also in Greece and North Africa. A few instances have been reported in the United States, but it is unusual in Negroes.

It is thought that the haemolysis and consequent haemoglobinuria following extensive *burns* is due to direct damage to the red cells by the heating of the blood.

Haemoglobinuria occasionally occurs in chronic haemolytic anaemias especially in the crises that may accompany hereditary spherocytosis and sickle-cell disease. It may also be associated with the idiopathic auto-immune haemolytic anaemias which may be associated with either warm- or cold-reacting antibodies.

Occasionally the cause of the haemolytic process is unknown and, when short lived and self-terminating, the disease is sometimes known as 'Lederer's haemolytic anaemia'.

It will be seen from the above that though the causes of haemoglobinuria are numerous, the conditions which give rise to it are either themselves rare, or only rarely give rise to haemoglobinuria.

T. A. J. Prankerd.

HAEMOPTYSIS

'Haemoptysis' means blood-spitting. By a widely accepted convention, it is generally used to refer specifically to the expectoration of blood from the bronchi or lungs. The blood, either alone or mixed with sputum (p. 753), is nearly always produced by coughing, but rarely may trickle past the larynx and be spat out without exciting cough.

Bleeding from the nose, mouth, pharynx, or larynx may lead to the spitting of blood or blood-stained secretions. This is sometimes called

In rare instances, sudden massive bleeding into the lungs causes death before the blood can be coughed up; thus haemoptysis is not synonymous with bleeding from the lower respiratory tract.

HAEMOPTYSIS AND HAEMATEMESIS

Haemoptysis is usually distinguishable without difficulty from the vomiting of blood (HAEMATEMESIS, p. 329), especially if the incident is observed. The principal differences about which inquiry should be made in doubtful cases, such as those in which the patient's account of the incident is the only available evidence, are listed in *Table I*. If, after assessment of these, doubt remains, the oesophagus and upper gastro-intestinal tract should be considered with the respiratory system as possible sources of the bleeding.

SOURCES OF HAEMOPTYSIS

The diseases in which haemoptysis is a recognized symptom are listed in *Table II*. Since this symptom may be the first that draws attention to serious disease—e.g., bronchial carcinoma in middle-aged or older, and pulmonary tuberculosis in younger patients—it is essential that it should be properly investigated. As a generality it is perhaps true to say that an effortless haemoptysis of 1–2 ml. blood or more is much more likely to prove of serious diagnostic and prognostic importance than small 'streaky' haemoptyses resulting from much repeated coughing and respiratory effort. Physical examination, with special attention to the respiratory and

Table I. HAEMOPTYSIS AND HAEMATEMESIS: DISTINGUISHING FEATURES

	Suggesting Haemoptysis	Suggesting Haematemesis
Previous history	Respiratory symptoms	Dyspepsia
Immediately before the episode	Tickle or gurgle in the throat; cough	Faintness; abdominal pain; nausea
Characteristics of the episode	Blood produced by repeated acts of coughing, may be mixed with sputum	Blood produced by isolated acts of vomiting, may be mixed with food debris
	Usually bright red, may be frothy, reaction on alkaline side	Usually dark in colour, may resemble coffee-grounds, and usually acid in reaction
	(Rapid bleeding either from lungs or from upper alimentary tract produces only slightly altered blood, with or without clots)	
After the episode	Bloodstained sputum may be produced for several days. Stools usually normal in appearance; may contain occult blood; rarely, after severe haemoptysis, melaena	Stools often dark and tarry (melaena) and always give positive test for occult blood

'spurious haemoptysis', since the blood is not in the strict sense expectorated, i.e., raised from the chest. This verbal distinction may be difficult to apply, e.g. when blood from a site above the larynx trickles down into the bronchi and is subsequently coughed up. Irrespective of verbal usages, bleeding from the upper respiratory tract must be included in the differential diagnosis of haemoptysis.

cardiovascular systems and to the mouth and nasopharynx, and a chest radiograph are obligatory. If there is sputum, it should be examined microscopically for acid-fast bacilli and for malignant cells and by culture for mycobacteria. If the source of true haemoptysis is not otherwise established, bronchoscopy will be indicated. These procedures often provide either a definitive diagnosis, or clear indications for further

Table II. Sources of Haemoptysis

Mouth:
  See Gums, bleeding, p. 323
Nose:
  See Epistaxis, p. 256
Larynx:
  Carcinoma
Trachea:
  Carcinoma
  Foreign body
Bronchus:
  Carcinoma
  Adenoma
  Bronchiectasis
  Foreign body
  (Chronic bronchitis: *see text*)
Lung:
  Tuberculosis
  Other infective granulomatoses
  Pneumonia
  Lung abscess
  Parasitic infestations
  Infarction
  Arteriovenous aneurysm
  Idiopathic haemosiderosis
  Goodpasture's syndrome
  Trauma
Cardiovascular:
  Mitral stenosis
  Left ventricular failure
  Aortic aneurysm
Bleeding states:
  Thrombocytopenia
  Henoch-Schönlein purpura
  Leukaemia
  Scurvy

investigations. Nevertheless, it must be recognized that in practice haemoptysis, especially isolated incidents of bloodstaining of sputum, often remains unexplained even after competent investigation; some careful observers have reported inability to identify its source in as many as half the patients presenting with a history of this symptom, even after repeated investigation.

The need for further action after initially negative investigation in such cases must be assessed individually; as a general rule, patients can truthfully be told that the risk of undetected serious disease is small, but instructed to return for review after an interval of 6–8 weeks. If the initial investigation was unequivocally negative, the haemoptysis has not recurred, no other symptom has arisen, and clinical examination and chest radiograph remain normal, no further action is required.

Upper Respiratory Tract. Bleeding from the upper respiratory tract usually presents as evident bleeding from the gums (p. 323) or from the nose (Epistaxis, p. 256). But, as noted above, it may give rise to haemoptysis, because blood can trickle down past the larynx, especially during sleep, and subsequently be expectorated, possibly mixed with bronchial secretions. The nose, the mouth, and the pharynx should therefore be examined in all cases of haemoptysis; but it is unwise to conclude that the upper respiratory tract is the source of bleeding unless an abnormality causing it can be confidently recognized, and investigation has failed to demonstrate a source in the bronchi or lungs.

Lower Respiratory Tract. The initial probability about the source of haemoptysis is greatly influenced by the prevalence of diseases in the population and age-group from which the patient comes. Where tuberculosis is a common disease, haemoptysis must always give rise to suspicion of *pulmonary tuberculosis*, especially in younger patients; and with the increasing incidence of *bronchial carcinoma* in the cigarette-smoking populations of 'developed' countries, this disease has become a frequent cause of haemoptysis in middle-aged or older patients. With either of these diseases there may be a history of ill-health with banal respiratory symptoms, such as cough, expectoration, chest pain, and dyspnoea preceding the haemoptysis for a few weeks or months; but an incident of blood-spitting is often the first event that induces the patient to seek medical advice.

Haemoptysis may occur at various stages of *pulmonary tuberculosis*. It may be the initial or an early symptom, as noted above. At this stage, it is unlikely that physical examination will show abnormal signs, but radiographic changes are to be expected, and may be obvious, consisting in localized mottled shadowing or consolidation, possibly with cavitation. Rarely, haemoptysis may arise from disease so localized that it is difficult to detect on a posterior-anterior radiograph, being hidden by the shadows of ribs or clavicle; or behind the hilar shadow in the apical segment of a lower lobe; lateral, apical, or olique views or tomography may then be required to resolve doubt. Haemoptysis in patients with active tuberculosis varies in severity from blood-staining of sputum to profuse expectoration of unmixed blood. In chronic cavitated disease, severe haemoptysis may arise from rupture of an aneurysmal dilatation of an artery, which exceptionally remains patent in a strand of tissue traversing the cavity—the so-called 'aneurysm of Rasmussen'. In chronic tuberculosis with much fibrosis secondary bronchiectasis may develop and be the source of haemoptysis, even after the tuberculosis has become inactive. Haemoptysis is sometimes associated with multiple calcified foci in the lungs, perhaps with some other evidence of old-standing, possibly healed, tuberculosis such as apical fibrosis. Thus haemoptysis in patients with old-standing fibrosis is not necessarily evidence of activity of tuberculosis.

Especially after effective antituberculosis chemotherapy, some patients with cavitated pulmonary tuberculosis are left with residual cavities, even though bacteriological cure appears to have been attained. Such cavities may both become colonized by the common mould *Aspergillus fumigatus* and be the source of haemoptysis. Cavities containing a *fungus ball*, or *aspergilloma*, are thus a recognized source of haemoptysis, which may be profuse.

Investigation of all cases in which there is radiological evidence suggesting tuberculosis, active or inactive, must include search for tubercle bacilli by microscopy and by culture, in sputum, if produced, or in fasting gastric contents. Where diagnosis is in doubt, and bronchoscopy is undertaken, e.g., to detect a possible bronchial carcinoma, bronchial secretions or material obtained by bronchial lavage should be examined similarly for mycobacteria. In the presence of radiological and other signs of active tuberculosis, the finding of tubercle bacilli is final confirmation of the diagnosis of disease requiring specific chemotherapy. In cases where haemoptysis is associated with radiological and other findings compatible with apparently inactive old tuberculosis, careful clinical assessment for evidence of activity—weight loss, lassitude, fever, raised sedimentation rate—must be accompanied by examination of at least three samples of sputum or gastric contents for tubercle bacilli by microscopy and culture. It is frequently advisable in such cases to repeat the radiological and bacteriological assessment after an interval of 3–6 months. In some instances, changes in radiological appearances provide evidence of activity; in some, the finding of tubercle bacilli is the only evidence of active disease requiring treatment.

In areas where these diseases are prevalent, *histoplasmosis*, *coccidioidomycosis* and *blastomycosis* must be considered in the differential diagnosis of haemoptysis associated with abnormal radiological appearances in the lungs, when commoner diseases such as tuberculosis have been exluded. Diagnosis depends upon isolation of the causal organism, and may be aided by skin and serological tests. Other rare infections that must be similarly considered when tuberculosis has been excluded include *actinomycosis*, *nocardiasis*, and *cryptococcosis*; diagnosis of these depends upon isolation of the causal organism.

In *bronchial carcinoma*, haemoptysis as an early symptom usually takes the form of blood-streaking of sputum or possibly small free haemoptysis, often repeated over days or weeks. Later more severe bleeding may occur, from erosion of larger vessels either by the tumour or by the suppuration which often results from bacterial infection beyond it. Bronchial carcinoma must be suspected especially in cigarette-smokers at or past middle age, but may occur in younger individuals. Radiologically, the more common findings are of two sorts. The first is associated with tumours originating in large bronchi; air-absorption collapse or consolidation of a segment, a lobe (*Fig.* 375), or even a whole lung beyond a complete obstruction, or patchy inflammatory consolidation beyond a partial obstruction. The second consists of localized, usually rounded shadows in the lung fields, produced by tumours originating more peripherally; in some cases with squamous-cell carcinoma, a rounded shadow of this sort may show a central transradiant area, due to necrosis of the central part of the tumour. Appearances of these sorts must lead to a provisional diagnosis of bronchial carcinoma. In occasional cases, a bronchial

carcinoma arising in a large bronchus causes haemoptysis before it has obstructed the bronchus, and therefore before radiographic changes are present. In such cases diagnosis can be made only by bronchoscopy or sputum cytology. In all cases, bronchoscopy is advisable to confirm the diagnosis and to obtain samples of tissue for biopsy to ascertain the cell type, which affects prognosis and decisions about treatment, and

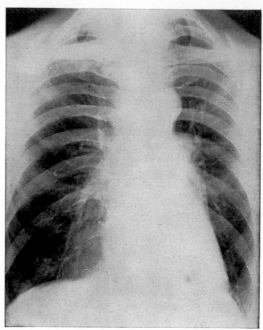

Fig. 375. Radiograph of chest showing atelectasis of the left lower lobe due to carcinoma of the bronchus. Note the displacement of the heart to the left, the slight raising of the left diaphragm, and slight narrowing of the spaces between the left lower ribs; the displaced heart almost hides the characteristic triangular shadow of the collapsed lobe itself.

to assess operability. With fibre-optic instruments, tumours in fairly peripheral bronchi can be seen and submitted to biopsy. With more peripheral tumours, it may be necessary to perform needle biopsy, either transbronchially at bronchoscopy or percutaneously under radiographic control to obtain histological confirmation.

Haemoptysis is an important symptom in *bronchial adenoma*, since these tumours may be very vascular. Episodes of haemoptysis may occur over several years, and there may also be a history of recurrent attacks of pneumonia involving always the same lobe. There may be clinical and radiological evidence of lobar atelectasis or consolidation, possibly with abscess-formation, but an adenoma in a central bronchus, not causing obstruction, may be difficult to detect radiologically. Since most of these tumours arise in large bronchi, bronchoscopic diagnosis is usually easy.

An acute illness in which haemoptysis accompanies fever, chest pain, and cough suggests *pneumonia* or *pulmonary infarction*. In pneumonia, there may have been a preceding upper respiratory tract infection; and the severe illness sometimes starts with a rigor. Haemoptysis rarely amounts to more than blood-staining; the rusty sputum associated especially with pneumococcal pneumonia usually does not appear until several days after the beginning of the illness. If the sputum is or becomes frankly purulent, the possibility of a suppurative pneumonia or *lung abscess* must be considered, and may be confirmed by radiography. Haemoptysis associated with lung abscess may be profuse. Either pneumonia or lung abscess may be secondary to bronchial obstruction, e.g., by a carcinoma, especially in middle-aged or older smokers, more rarely by an adenoma or a foreign body. An acute bacterial infection causing pneumonia may precede haemoptysis in bronchiectasis, chronic pulmonary tuberculosis, and other chronic broncho-pulmonary disease (*see below*).

Pulmonary infarction occurs as the result of embolism in peripheral pulmonary arteries, either in association with heart disease or secondary to thrombophlebitis, generally of veins in the leg or pelvis, especially postoperatively or during an illness leading to prolonged rest in bed. The diagnosis is simple if haemoptysis is preceded or accompanied by pleuritic pain of sudden onset and possibly by slight fever, with or without dyspnoea, in a patient with heart disease, especially if there is atrial fibrillation, or with peripheral venous thrombosis. But symptoms are variable, being dependent upon the size of the vessels embolized, and upon the number and timing of episodes of embolization. Haemoptysis, being a symptom of infarction, occurs at an interval after the actual embolism. Occasionally, a large embolism in a central pulmonary artery (p. 139) giving rise immediately to the syndrome of acute cor pulmonale—central chest pain, dyspnoea and hyperpnoea, cyanosis, tachycardia with evidence of right ventricular strain and acute pulmonary hypertension, and raised jugular venous pressure—is followed after the acute symptoms have subsided by haemoptysis from infarction by lodgement of a detached fragment in a peripheral vessel; this sequence of events also can leave little doubt of the diagnosis. But a small peripheral pulmonary embolism may cause infarction with haemoptysis as the only obvious symptom.

Thus in all cases in which the cause of haemoptysis is not immediately evident, the possibility of pulmonary embolism must be considered and lead to careful examination for evidence of heart disease and of peripheral venous thrombosis. The clinical signs of thrombosis in the veins of the lower leg may become evident only after those of the consequent pulmonary infarction, and thus provide retrospective confirmation of this diagnosis.

Haemoptysis in a patient with a long history of cough and persistently or intermittently purulent sputum, possibly with episodes of increased volume and purulence and fever, suggests *bronchiectasis*. Localized crepitations may be found persistently over the affected part of the lung, and clubbing of the fingers may be present, particularly in those with long-standing persistently purulent infection; but in some cases, physical examination is non-contributory. Bleeding probably arises from the large pulmonary-systemic arterial anastomoses that develop in long-standing cases. It may be the principal symptom, and severe even with bronchiectasis of limited extent. Bronchography may be required to establish the diagnosis in such cases.

Haemoptysis occurring in patients with the varying combinations of chronic cough, expectoration, and dyspnoea which are frequent in a cigarette-smoking, town-dwelling population (chronic obstructive bronchitis, with or without emphysema) presents special problems. It is doubtful whether it should be attributed to *chronic obstructive bronchitis* alone. Among those suffering from these common symptoms, at least the usual prevalence of diseases known to be associated with haemoptysis must be expected. Indeed, one of them, bronchial carcinoma, is especially frequent among heavy cigarette-smokers, who are also especially liable to chronic bronchitis. Some chronic bronchitics become liable to recurrent purulent bronchial infections; these may lead to localized bronchopulmonary damage, including fibrotic scars and bronchiectasis, which may be associated with the changes in the vascularization of the lung noted above and thus be a possible source of haemoptysis, especially in association with episodes of acute infection. In practice, patients with chronic bronchitis who suffer haemoptysis must be investigated to exclude known causes of bronchopulmonary bleeding, especially bronchial carcinoma and chronic pulmonary tuberculosis; but especially in those who have persistent or recurrent bacterial infections (chronic mucopurulent bronchitis) with or without evidence of localized bronchopulmonary damage, it may be necessary, after proper investigation, to accept that the haemoptysis was associated with these changes.

Foreign bodies in the tracheobronchial tree can give rise to haemoptysis in two ways. Soon after lodgement, a hard foreign body with sharp edges may lacerate the mucosa or cause local ulceration, and lead to bleeding, usually slight, with no more than blood-streaked sputum. Later, infection beyond a foreign body obstructing a bronchus can cause pneumonia, abscess formation, and, if neglected, eventually bronchiectasis, all of which are possible causes of haemoptysis. If it is not radio-opaque or if it is lodged centrally where it may be hidden in the mediastinal shadow, a foreign body will be radiologically inapparent, and cause no radiological evidence of its presence until the secondary changes arising from bronchial obstruction appear. A non-occluding foreign body of metal, bone or plastic material often produces no immediate irritative symptoms, and occasionally haemoptysis is the symptom that first draws attention to its presence. The diagnosis will be made or confirmed at bronchoscopy.

Parasitic infestations may cause haemoptysis either as parasites pass through or when they finally settle in the lungs. Most of them have fairly well-defined geographic distributions, and are likely to affect only those who are or have been resident in endemic areas. Among parasites whose passage through the lungs may cause haemoptysis are *Ascaris lumbricoides*, which is world-wide, but causes pulmonary symptoms, among which haemoptysis is not prominent, only in exceptionally heavy infestation; *Schistosoma*, of which various species have different, mainly tropical, distributions, and which may cause haemoptysis during the passage of larvae through the lungs, but of which the principal pulmonary manifestation, obliterative arteriolitis with granuloma formation, arises later and is not specially associated with haemoptysis; and *Dirofilaria immitis*, the heart-worm of dogs in Australia, which may cause haemoptysis and radiologically detectable lesions in the lungs of man.

Hydatid cysts are endemic wherever dogs and sheep are closely associated with man. Haemoptysis is not a common symptom, and usually no more than streaking of mucoid sputum; when the cyst has ruptured, infection often complicates the picture, with all the possible consequence of pulmonary suppuration, including more severe haemoptysis. The diagnosis will be suggested by the chest radiograph, which will show one or more rounded shadows; rupture of cysts and added infection will, of course, affect the appearances. Complement fixation and Casoni skin tests may be helpful in diagnosis (p. 10).

Haemoptysis is a leading feature of infestation with the lung fluke, *Paragonimus westermani*. This occurs principally in Japan, China, Korea, and Formosa. In addition to haemoptysis, cough and chest pain occur; chest radiography shows varying shadows, and diagnosis finally depends upon the finding of ova in sputum or stool.

Goodpasture's syndrome consists in haemoptysis, usually recurrent and not severe, followed by or associated with glomerulonephritis. It has aptly been called *lung purpura with nephritis*. It is rare, but its occurrence is a reminder of the importance of examining the urine repeatedly in all cases of unexplained haemoptysis, since the haemoptysis may precede the appearance of clinical signs of nephritis by weeks or months. There may be no abnormality, or only transient changes after episodes of haemoptysis, in the chest radiograph.

Idiopathic pulmonary haemosiderosis is characterized by recurrent episodes of bleeding into the lung, apparently from pulmonary capillaries. These may or may not give rise to haemoptysis, but are associated with constitutional symptoms of varying severity, and widespread fine mottling in the lung fields in the chest radiograph, appearing or becoming more extensive and denser during each episode, and clearing partially or completely afterwards; there is often an iron-deficiency anaemia. In children, the course is less episodic, haemoptysis not a constant feature, and anaemia more prominent than in adults, in whom episodes of haemoptysis, accompanied by transient radiographic shadows are the leading feature. The similarity of the pulmonary changes to those of Goodpasture's syndrome is evident; in practice the only distinguishing feature is the absence of evidence of renal involvement in the cases categorized as idiopathic pulmonary haemosiderosis.

In the rare cases of *polyarteritis nodosa* in which pulmonary arteries are involved, with consequent small infarctions of lung, haemoptysis may occur. Diagnosis depends upon the recognition of the concurrence of a combination of clinical features suggesting this diagnosis, leading to biopsy of an affected tissue; the lung is not a favourable site for biopsy in this disease, as the characteristic vascular changes, even when present in pulmonary arteries, may be missed in the small sample obtained. Haemoptysis may also occur in *Wegener's granulomatosis*, in which granulomatosis with vasculitis affecting small arteries and veins with consequent necrosis affects the lungs and upper respiratory tract (nose and sinuses, pharynx, middle ear). Renal involvement may occur at any stage. Diagnosis is easy by biopsy if the upper respiratory tract is involved. The lungs may be the first site of clinically evident lesions, and in such instances open lung biopsy may be required to establish the diagnosis.

Arteriovenous aneurysm of the lung (p. 198) usually causes symptoms and signs arising from shunting of mixed venous blood directly from pulmonary artery into pulmonary vein, effectively a 'right-to-left' shunt. Haemoptysis occurs in only a minority of cases. About half are associated with hereditary haemorrhagic telangiectasia (p. 198), of which epistaxis is a frequent symptom.

Trauma may lead to haemoptysis, not only when the lung is directly penetrated or lacerated by fractured ribs, but also in non-penetrating injuries. These may be associated with contusion of the lung, even without rib fractures. Exposure to blast from explosions may cause haemorrhagic consolidation of the lung (blast injury) with haemoptysis.

Among cardiovascular diseases, *mitral stenosis* is especially associated with haemoptysis. Pulmonary embolism leading to infarcts, especially in patients with atrial fibrillation, is a frequent cause. Less severe bleeding leading to blood-stained sputum may be associated with the high pulmonary venous pressure. *Left ventricular failure* associated with hypertension or aortic valve disease may give rise to similar haemoptysis, and the thin frothy sputum produced in pulmonary oedema is frequently tinged pink with blood. Diagnosis depends upon the recognition of the underlying cardiac disease. *Aortic aneurysm* may erode into a bronchus, leading to rapidly fatal haemorrhage with massive haemoptysis; in such cases, there may be smaller haemoptyses before the final catastrophe. The underlying aneurysm, even if not diagnosable on clinical grounds, is likely to be evident radiographically.

In diseases associated with disturbances of haemostasis and clotting, such as *thrombocytopenia, Henoch-Schönlein purpura, scurvy, leukaemias*, and *aplastic anaemia*, haemoptysis may occur, but as a minor feature of a generalized bleeding tendency in which epistaxis and bleeding from the gums are more prominent. These may be accompanied by bleeding from the alimentary or urinary tracts, or by purpura (p. 669), leading to appropriate haematological investigations. Haemoptysis is virtually never the sole clinically evident presenting feature of these diseases.

Factitious 'haemoptysis'. When a patient presents with a history of haemoptysis as the sole symptom, and investigation has shown no evidence of its source, nor of any organic disease, it must be remembered that single episodes of unexplained haemoptysis are not uncommon. Moreover, the patient may have come for investigation because he wanted reassurance; for instance, he may have a friend who has been found to be suffering from tuberculosis or bronchial carcinoma with haemoptysis as an initial symptom, and become alarmed lest the streaks of blood he notices after cleaning his teeth are the first sign of the same thing in himself. Very occasionally, a patient returns with recurrent complaints of haemoptysis, the blood being deliberately produced by various forms of trauma in the mouth or pharynx. Usually the motivation underlying this is fairly easily apparent, and combined with the discovery of the site of trauma enables the situation to be recognized.

J. G. Scadding.

HALLUCINATIONS

A hallucination is a sensory perception which occurs without any external stimulus whatsoever. An exception to this general rule are so-called *functional hallucinations*, in which a patient hearing, for example, a dripping tap or an aeroplane flying overhead also hears voices addressing him. These, while bearing no relation to the actual stimulus, cannot be considered merely as illusions despite the fact that they disappear when the sound source also vanishes. Such hallucinatory experiences may, however, be related to synaesthesiae (the illusory experience in one sense modality of a stimulus in another), which may be produced by drugs such as lysergic acid diethylamide (LSD-25). Otherwise schizophrenia is the most likely cause. Apart from these, true hallucinations may occur in any sense modality, i.e., auditory, visual, olfactory, gustatory, tactile, visceral, and vestibular. Hallucinatory sensations of movement or of heat or cold may also be perceived.

Delirious states, in which a patient's thinking and grasp of reality are grossly disturbed, are frequently accompanied by visual, auditory, and tactile hallucinations. Such hallucinatory experiences dissolve and change from moment to moment; their general nature is unpleasant and threatening, as in *delirium tremens*. In this state and in kindred disorders the differential diagnosis is that of the primary condition (*see* DELIRIUM, p. 204). Visual hallucinations in particular are indicative of an organic disturbance of brain function of an acute kind, e.g., due to drugs or alcohol, rather than in schizophrenia where except in very acute cases their occurrence should always render this diagnosis suspect.

In schizophrenia the commonest hallucinations are auditory although all other sensory modalities may be affected. Schizophrenic auditory hallucinations usually take the form of a voice or several voices, which give orders, ask questions, or make comments about the patient. The voices may be heard within his head, or may appear to issue from some other part of his body, such as his genitals. They may be heard as emanating from objects or people in his environment. He may also hear his own thoughts spoken aloud (*echo de la pensée*). The content of the hallucinations—what the voices say—may sometimes be understood in terms of the patient's mental state in that it may represent a thought or impulse of his own which is not acceptable to his conscious mind and is 'projected' on to the outside world. For example, a patient in whom homosexual desires are present but repressed may hear a voice accusing him of homosexual activities. An apparently senseless action, in a hallucinated patient, may be a response to such an accusation, or to a hallucinatory command.

In schizophrenia occurring in middle and later life, systematized auditory hallucinations and florid paranoid delusions are prominent (*paraphrenia*). These, unlike the schizophrenic illnesses from which younger patients suffer, may be unaccompanied by gross thought disorder or intellectual deterioration so that the patient appears alert and well orientated. Other forms of hallucinations—visual, tactile, olfactory, visceral—also occur in schizophrenic reactions, but are rarer. They are to be distinguished from the hallucinations of organic disease by their bizarre character. The patient may hear the voices of others speaking about him, or plotting to injure him. On inquiry it may be found that he believes himself to be the object of some malevolent influence, applied via the television or radioactivity.

In severe *depressive reactions*, hallucinations of one or of several senses may form part of the clinical picture; the content of these is in keeping with the patient's mood. However, these, which usually occur when the patient's state of consciousness is somewhat 'clouded', are more likely to be illusions experienced under strong emotion rather than true hallucinations. The patient may not actually hear voices accusing him but may mistake what others say as an accusation. True hallucinations only occur very rarely, if at all, in depression.

Stimulation of certain areas of the cerebral cortex can give rise to sensations which are interpreted as coming from without; thus, a lesion in the posterior part of the occipital lobe, such as a tumour, may cause the patient to see bright flashes or coloured spots (*elementary hallucinations*). Temporal lobe lesions may give rise to much more elaborate visual hallucinations of objects, human beings, or extensive scenes which may accompany and form part of an attack of temporal lobe epilepsy (*complex hallucinations*). Such attacks are usually accompanied by a state of altered consciousness accompanied by a strange dream-like state and a sensation of false familiarity (*déjà vu*) or less commonly by perception of an environment which should be familiar as strange and unknown (*jamais vu*). Micropsia or macropsia may occur, musical hallucinations or strange hallucinations of taste and smell (uncinate attacks). The variations of these phenomena, when associated with temporal lobe disturbances, appear to be endless. In lesions of the *parietal cortex* the patient may experience tingling, numbness, or a sensation of movement, usually spreading from the periphery towards the head. All these types of sensory and sometimes motor phenomena (*Jacksonian attacks*) may occur in isolation or may progress to a major epileptiform seizure.

Very many normal people, during the process of falling asleep, experience vivid sensory impressions which have the character of hallucinations of sight or of hearing; these are termed *hypnagogic* or, when awakening after a period of sleep, *hypnopompic* hallucinations. Such experiences occur both in health and in states of emotional tension; in the latter, the content of the hallucinations may be an indication of the source of the tension. Hypnagogic hallucinations are also particularly common in *narcolepsy* in which the patient who sleeps lightly is often to be found in the half-waking state.

Although *true* hallucinations probably do not occur in neurotic states, *pseudo-hallucinations* are sometimes present, particularly in those suffering from a mixture of *hysterical* and *obsessional* personality traits. They also commonly occur in *grief reactions* where the bereaved seems to hear or see a phantom of a dear-departed one, as if still alive. Pseudo-hallucinations lack the objectivity of true hallucinations, lying somewhere half-way between true hallucinations, which are as objective as are real perceptions and images, which, while having existence in the mind's eye, are, as it were, only partially projected and not into 'real' space. They sometimes occur in more than one sensory modality at once, e.g., the ghostly vision of one who speaks. True hallucinations never, however, occur in more than one modality other than independently of one another where content is concerned.

W. H. Trethowan.

HEAD, RETRACTION OF

Is usually the result of severe meningitis, but it can also occur in children as the result of asphyxia. Intermittent spasms of retraction occur in tetanus, strychnine poisoning, rabies, torsion spasm, and spasmodic torticollis. Stiffness of the neck, short of actual retraction, will also be considered in this section; it can be due to meningism, meningitis, subarachnoid haemorrhage, meningeal carcinomatosis, and pressure cones resulting from increased intracranial pressure. Stiffness due to disease of the cervical spine and paraspinal tissues is dealt with separately on page 744.

CAUSES OF RETRACTION OF THE HEAD
(including stiffness of the neck)

1. MENINGISM.

2. BACTERIAL MENINGITIS:

Meningococcus	*B. anthracis*
Pneumococcus	*H. influenzae*
Streptococcus	*A. aerogenes*
Staphylococcus	*P. vulgaris*
Gonococcus	*Salmonella*
Enterococcus	*A. foecalis*
M. tuberculosis	*P. tularensis*
E. coli	*B. melitensis*
B. pyocyaneus	*P. pestis*
Pseudomonas	*Listeria*

VIRUS MENINGITIS:

Poliomyelitis	Glandular fever
Lymphocytic	Herpes zoster
choriomeningitis	Virus encephalitis
Mumps	(various)

SPIROCHAETAL MENINGITIS:

T. pallidum	*L. ictero-haemorrhagica*
T. recurrentis	*L. canicola*

'MENINGITIS', VARIOUS:

Fungal infections	Carcinomatosis
(e.g., candidosis	Sarcoidosis
(thrush)	

3. SUBARACHNOID HAEMORRHAGE:

Aneurysm	Head injury
Angioma	Purpura
Hypertension	Cerebral tumour

4. PRESSURE CONES:

Intracranial tumour	Extradural
Intracranial abscess	haematoma
Subdural haematoma	Cerebral oedema
	Hydrocephalus

5. ASPHYXIA:

Bronchopneumonia	Laryngeal foreign body
Capillary bronchitis	Retropharyngeal
Laryngeal diphtheria	abscess

6. INTERMITTENT RETRACTION:

Tetanus (p. 193)	Torsion spasm
Strychnine poisoning	Spasmodic torticollis
(p. 193)	(p. 551)
Rabies	

7. SPINAL AND PARASPINAL DISEASE (p. 744).

The term *meningism* is applied to the headache, photophobia, and stiff neck which occur, as a rule in children, in the course of general infections such as tonsillitis, pneumonia, and pyelitis. The pressure of the spinal fluid is raised, but its contents are normal.

Meningitis causes resistance to forward flexion of the neck, but this may be absent in very mild cases and also in fulminating infections. Actual retraction of the head is best seen in tuberculous meningitis and in meningococcal meningitis; it has become rare since the introduction of antibiotics. Inflammation of the leptomeninges is caused by many organisms—bacteria, viruses, spirochaetes, and yeasts—and a low grade 'meningitis' can occur when the meninges are invaded by secondary carcinomatosis and sarcoidosis. It is sometimes possible to guess the identity of the agent from a consideration of the clinical features of the case, but examination of the spinal fluid is always essential for confirmation.

Features common to most cases of meningitis are headache, photophobia, vomiting, giddiness, and fever. There may be a rigor, or a convulsion, at the onset of the more virulent types, especially in children. There is stiffness of the neck, spinal muscles, and hamstrings. Thus, forward flexion of the neck is resisted, and it may evoke flexion of the hips and knees (Brudzinski's sign). There is resistance to extension of the knee on the flexed thigh (Kernig's sign), because this movement pulls on the roots of the cauda equina. There may or may not be evidence of focal damage to the brain and cranial nerves. The latter are involved as they traverse the subarachnoid space, and the brain itself can be damaged by spread of the infection along the meningeal sheaths which cover the vessels as they penetrate the surface of the brain. Moreover, thrombosis both of arteries and of veins can occur, with infarction, oedema, or brain abscess as a result. Thrombosis of the dural sinuses is an important event, the results of which depend on which sinus is involved. It is especially likely to occur as a complication of infection in the middle ear, the mastoid, and the paranasal sinuses. Thrombosis of the superior longitudinal sinus interferes with the venous return from the cerebral veins and with the absorption of cerebrospinal fluid, so leading to cerebral oedema, a rise of intracranial pressure, and softening of the brain on either side. A similar train of events follows the spread of a thrombus from the lateral sinus to the torcula. If the sigmoid sinus thromboses, clot will spread thence to the internal jugular vein. There are two further factors which can raise intracranial pressure in meningitis: the presence of inflammatory exudate itself, and hydrocephalus caused by interference with the free passage of spinal fluid from the fourth ventricle to the convexity of the brain, where it is absorbed. Finally, intracranial pressure may be raised by the presence of subdural collections of fluid (subdural hygroma), which are not infrequent after meningococcal meningitis in young children.

Infection can gain access to the meninges by several routes. In most cases it is blood-borne, and in an important minority it spreads from local infections in the ear, accessory nasal sinuses, face, and scalp. The existence of this second group emphasizes the need to seek for evidence in the history and on physical examination as to the possibility of local infection in every case. Points to be looked for are the presence of otitis, mastoiditis, or sinusitis. Moreover, a history of head injury, whether recent or remote, may mean that there is a fracture and a dural tear leading into an air sinus, thereby providing a path for the entry of micro-organisms. In such cases, meningitis is apt to be associated with an abscess, whether extradural, intradural, or intracerebral, along the track of entry. Sepsis in the face or scalp, such as furunculosis, erysipelas, infected scalp wounds, or herpes, can lead to meningitis in debilitated persons. Infection may also enter via a meningocele, or a congenital dermal sinus at the base of the spine, and these must be looked for in unexplained meningitis in infants. Yet another manner of infection is following lumbar puncture or spinal anaesthesia; in such cases low grade infection is usual, e.g., by *Bacillus pyocyaneus*.

Meningococcal meningitis (syn. spotted fever, cerebrospinal fever) usually occurs in epidemics which are initiated by droplet infection from healthy carriers. A bacteriaemia precedes the meningitis by hours, days, or even weeks. Occasionally there is a *chronic meningococcal septicaemia* with fever, purpura, and transient pain, and swelling in the joints, and a proportion of these will end up with meningitis. In another small group, the patient is overwhelmed by a fulminating septicaemia within a few hours of the onset; some pass rapidly into coma, without a significant fall of blood-pressure, while others remain clear of mind but suffer a drastic fall of pressure due to circulatory collapse, and these cases usually present a diffuse purpuric rash on the skin (the *Waterhouse-Friderichsen syndrome*, which is also seen in other severe infections and can result from overdosage of anticoagulants). In the usual type of meningococcal meningitis, however, there is fever, meningeal irritation, severe headache, and sometimes a purpuric or macular rash. Convulsions may occur at the onset. Transient cranial nerve palsies and papilloedema may be found, and delirium is common. Tendon reflexes are reduced, and extensor plantar responses are common in the more severe cases. The condition is one of meningo-encephalitis, and this explains the intellectual and emotional changes which may be present in survivors. These symptoms are not unlike those which often follow cerebral contusion, and like them, they may be complicated by an anxiety state in persons who find themselves unable to cope with life as a result of the mental incapacity caused by the meningo-encephalitis. The spinal fluid in meningitis usually contains a polymorph pleocytosis, with a rise of protein and a fall of glucose. Both intra- and extra-cellular diplococci are to be found in the pus.

In some cases of *meningococcal meningitis*, the exudate is largely confined to the base of the brain, thereby leading to an obstructive hydro-cephalus. There is mild fever, vomiting, papill-oedema, and head retraction. In infants—the usual victims—the head enlarges, and there is a slow downward course with emaciation, vomiting, and increasing stupor. In the first few days of the illness the changes in the spinal fluid are the same as in the ordinary type of meningococcal menin-gitis, but thereafter the meningococci disappear and there is merely a lymphocytic pleocytosis, a rise of protein, and rather a low sugar content. In such cases ventricular tap may produce the diplococcus.

Further sequels of meningococcal meningitis are the subdural hygroma referred to above, cranial nerve palsies, and disabilities arising from the formation of scar tissue around the spinal cord. These include a lower-motor neuron paralysis of muscles in the limbs, and occasionally an incomplete transverse lesion of the cord with paraplegia, sensory impairment, and sphincter disturbances.

Other forms of pyogenic meningitis are sporadic rather than epidemic in incidence, do not as a rule produce a rash, and are usually derived from a more or less obvious source of infection. Thus *pneumococcal cases* commonly arise from infection in the ears or sinuses, or from pneumococcal pneumonia. *Streptococcal meningitis* is rarer than the pneumococcal form but occurs in similar circumstances; in a propor-tion of cases, however, there is a cerebral abscess in addition to the meningitis, and this must always be looked for, if necessary by angiography, brain scan, or ventriculography. *H. influenzae*—(Pfeiffer)—is an important cause of meningitis in infants, and may cause the disease in adults; it may or may not be preceded by upper respiratory infection or by pneumonia. The signs of meningeal irritation may be slight. The other organisms listed on p. 358 are rare causes of meningitis, and they will be identified by culture of the spinal fluid. Some of them occur as a result of lumbar puncture, or spinal anaesthesia, or penetrating wounds of the brain, or intracranial operations, while others, such as anthrax, plague, melitensis, and infection by *P. tularensis*, occasionally complicate those diseases.

Meningitis with a predominantly lymphocytic response in the cerebrospinal fluid occurs in infec-tion by tuberculosis, viruses, yeasts, and spiro-chaetes. Of these, tuberculosis is the most important. The meningitis is secondary to tuber-culosis elsewhere, although the source may not be clinically apparent. It rarely occurs before the age of 6 months and is most common in children and young adults. The onset is commonly insidious, with malaise and occasional headaches which may precede the signs of meningitis for days, weeks, or even months. The meningeal phase includes headaches, signs of meningeal

irritation, and retraction of the head. Epileptic attacks—whether focal or general—and sudden hemi- or monoplegia, aphasia or cranial nerve palsies, mental changes, and papilloedema with visual loss, are common; hydrocephalus tends to increase, leading in untreated cases to stupor, incontinence, a rise in pulse, and medullary failure. Choroidal tubercles may be found on examination of the retina, and the Mantoux test is positive in the majority of cases. The spinal fluid is under increased pressure, and may be either clear or opalescent; a fibrin clot forms on standing for some hours. There is an excess of lymphocytes and there may be a few polymorphs. The protein is raised, and the chloride is reduced *in the later stages of the disease*; the sugar content falls at an early stage. The definitive test is the demonstration of the organism in the fluid, whether by direct smear, culture, or guinea-pig inoculation; if the evidence in favour of the disease is good, treatment by streptomycin should not be withheld until the organism is found. In the early stages of the disease the conditions which may cause difficulty in diagnosis are acute lymphocytic choriomeningitis and other virus infections of the meninges in which, however, the sugar and chloride content of the cerebrospinal fluid is normal, and the clinical course quite different, with rapid recovery in most cases. In acute syphilitic meningitis the Wassermann reaction is positive, while in meningitis associated with aural and sinus infections there may be both lymphocytes and polymorphs present, with negative culture and a normal sugar content in some cases (*aseptic meningitis*).

Meningitis can complicate *Weil's disease* (*spiro-chaetosis icterohaemorrhagica*), but an acute and predominantly lymphocytic meningitis can also occur without jaundice, renal damage, or haemor-rhagic symptoms, and this is called *meningitis leptospirosa*. It occurs in persons who have been in contact with rats, e.g., canal bathers, sewage workers, etc., and the spinal fluid is sterile if ordinary culture media are used. Sugar and chloride contents are normal. A benign menin-gitis can also be caused by *L. canicola*, which is carried by dogs. There may be conjunctival suffusion, and a rash which may resemble erythema nodosum. The spinal fluid contains an excess of lymphocytes, while the chloride and sugar content is normal, and the fluid is sterile in ordinary culture media. Diagnosis is confirmed, as in Weil's disease, by guinea-pig inoculation and by the detection of antibodies in the blood.

Lymphocytic meningitis may also occur with *tick-borne relapsing fever* (*T. recurrentis*), either during the first attack of fever, or more often in subsequent bouts. There is severe headache, neck stiffness, and slight papilloedema. Cranial nerve palsies, notably the seventh, are not un-common. There is increase of protein and lymphocytes in the spinal fluid, and the organ-ism can be identified by dark ground illumination, or by inoculation of the spinal fluid into a suit-able animal.

A well-marked lymphocytic meningitis can be caused by the viruses of acute choriomeningitis, mumps, and glandular fever, whereas the meningeal reaction of poliomyelitis, zoster, and arthropod-borne encephalitis is usually less obtrusive. A specific virus is responsible for acute *lymphocytic choriomeningitis*, a benign disease characterized by a prodromal period of malaise, headaches, muscle pains, pyrexia, and upper respiratory catarrh; this is followed after a week or two by severe headache, photophobia, neck stiffness, and a positive Kernig sign. In a minority of cases transverse myelitis, facial palsy, or temporary mental and emotional changes may occur. In the cerebrospinal fluid the protein is raised, and there may be from 50 to 3000 cells, of which at least 95 per cent are usually lymphocytes. Chlorides and sugar are normal, and the virus can sometimes be got from the fluid. *Mumps meningitis* usually starts on the fifth to the tenth day of the illness, but meningeal symptoms may precede the parotitis, or they may occur with orchitis but without parotitis. The meningitis may be accompanied by encephalitis with disturbances of consciousness and, rarely, focal cerebral and cerebellar signs. Cranial nerve palsies and myelitis have been described. Sudden permanent deafness, in one or both ears, with or without vertigo and vomiting, may occur in mumps without evidence of meningo-encephalitis. In *glandular fever* there may be a well-marked lymphocytic meningitis of sudden onset, with enlargement of glands, increase of the mononuclears in the blood, and an increasing titre in the Paul Bunnell test. Acute polyneuritis may complicate the disease, or may occur in glandular fever without meningitis. Of the *arthropod-borne forms of virus encephalitis*, *Louping-ill* is an epidemic disease of sheep, found in the northern parts of the British Isles, which is sometimes transmitted to sheep farmers and laboratory workers. It is carried by a tick. A phase of malaise and headache for a few days is followed by apparent recovery, and then illness characterized by fever, meningeal irritation, drowsiness, and cerebellar or other focal signs. There is a lymphocytosis in the cerebrospinal fluid. The prognosis is good. *Japanese B. encephalitis* occurs in Japan and China, and a celebrated outbreak occurred in Okinawa. The virus is spread by mosquitoes. There are meningeal signs, drowsiness, stupor, signs of diffuse cerebral involvement, convulsions, and tremors. There is a lymphocytosis in the spinal fluid, the sugar remaining normal. The mortality in this disease can be over 50 per cent. Moreover, both mental impairment and change of personality may occur in the survivors. *St. Louis encephalitis* occurs in the U.S.A. and is transmitted by mosquitoes. It is a summer disease, with fever, headache, meningeal signs, tremor, ataxia, and difficulty in speech, and these are sometimes preceded by pain in the muscles, sore throat, and malaise. There is usually a lymphocytosis and increase of protein in the spinal fluid, but no fall in the sugar content. *Equine encephalomyelitis* is a disease of horses in North and South America, but has been transmitted to humans, probably by mosquitoes. It is a feverish illness with meningeal signs and convulsions. In the early stages the cerebrospinal fluid may contain 1000 or more cells per cubic millimetre, polymorphs predominating at first. Cases of lymphocytic meningitis have occasionally appeared during *epidemics* of *pleurodynia* (Bornholm disease), but there is no really good evidence that the meningitis in such cases is caused by the coxsackie virus.

Infection by yeasts has been uncommon in the past, but it appears to be on the increase since the advent of antibiotics. *Cryptococcosis* (*Torula histolytica*) involves the subcutaneous tissues, the lungs, and the central nervous system, alone, or in combination, or in series. Subcutaneous granulomata break down to form abscesses and ulcers. Pulmonary lesions may mimic either chronic tuberculosis or carcinoma. The cerebral type usually starts insidiously with headaches, dizziness, and stiffness of the neck, but it may commence suddenly. There is little or no fever, but gradually the cerebrospinal pressure rises, producing papilloedema, and there may be cranial nerve palsies, hemiparesis, or ataxia. Large granulomata may, in fact, cause symptoms of a cerebral tumour. The patient eventually sinks into coma. There is a marked mononuclear pleocytosis in the spinal fluid, and the protein is raised. The glucose content is reduced, and cryptococci—which are readily mistaken for erythrocytes or lymphocytes—can be found in small numbers in the fluid.

Sarcoidosis, which causes uveoparotid polyneuritis, can also give rise to a low grade meningitis with headaches, slight stiffness of the neck, and a rise of lymphocytes and protein in the spinal fluid. It can pass on to cause an obstructive hydrocephalus, with papilloedema and optic atrophy. Cranial nerve palsies and diabetes insipidus have been described. The diagnosis can only be inferred by the presence of typical lesions in other areas, e.g., skin, liver, lungs, and eyes.

Subarachnoid haemorrhage is usually due to rupture of a saccular aneurysm, or of an atheromatous aneurysm. Less common causes are hypertension, angiomatous malformations, mycotic and syphilitic aneurysms, and purpura. An abrupt onset, early loss of consciousness in most cases, and the presence of blood in the spinal fluid distinguish the average case from meningitis. When the leak is slow, however, the severe headache, stiffness of the neck, slight pyrexia, ocular palsies, and positive Kernig sign may simulate meningitis, and it is only the blood in the spinal fluid which clinches the diagnosis. If the lumbar puncture is delayed for a day or two, the fluid may be found to be yellowish in colour (xanthochromia), and not blood-stained. Rarely, pain starts in the lumbar region and gradually spreads down the back of the legs and up to the neck. Another unusual form is sudden coma, and there

12*

may, in such a case, be a history of former attacks of unexplained coma with neck stiffness.

Pressure cones at the tentorial hiatus and at the foramen magnum can cause stiffness of the neck. They occur as a result of space-occupying lesions and, occasionally, from cerebral oedema. The local rise of pressure from an expanding mass in the head, or from hydrocephalus, dislocates and displaces brain substance. Thus a mass in the middle fossa, e.g., tumour or extradural haematoma, can dislocate part of the temporal lobe into the posterior fossa, with the result that the midbrain and the displaced tissue are tightly wedged in the dural ring. This may obstruct the aqueduct, thus aggravating the situation by causing internal hydrocephalus. In posterior fossa tumours, the reverse is seen: oedematous brainstem and cerebellar tissue is displaced upwards through the tentorial notch. Downward herniation of the medulla and cerebellar tonsils through the foramen also occurs, and will also give rise to rigidity of the neck.

Pressure cones can arise as the result of intracranial space-occupying lesions: tumour, abscess, haematoma, internal hydrocephalus, and occasionally from cerebral oedema due to vascular lesions. All these conditions may therefore cause stiffness of the neck. It is important to recognize the presence of a pressure cone, because the removal of even a small quantity of spinal fluid by lumbar puncture may cause collapse and death.

Asphyxia can cause retraction of the head, or stiffness of the neck. The more striking examples are usually seen in children with bronchopneumonia, or capillary bronchitis, or foreign body in the larynx. It has also sometimes been noted in retropharyngeal abscess. Even in adults with severe bronchopneumonia there may be stiffness of the neck, though retraction is rare. That asphyxia without cerebral oedema can cause retraction of the head is well illustrated by the retraction which is seen during the administration of pure nitrous oxide, e.g., for the extraction of teeth, but this may not be the whole explanation in the diseases mentioned.

Ian Mackenzie.

HEADACHE

Headache is of minor significance in the majority of cases but it may be the first, indeed the only, symptom of grave disease. Symptomatic treatment of a headache should never precede careful examination and possibly investigation with the object either of excluding or of recognizing one or other of its more serious causes.

The explanation of the mode of production of the pain known as *headache* is not easy. It is generally agreed that the principal pain structures of the head are extracranial, especially the arteries, though some intracranial structures, such as the venous sinuses, parts of the dura mater at the base of the brain, the dural arteries, the cerebral arteries at the base, the 5th, 7th, 9th and 10th cranial and upper three cervical nerves may play a part in some cases. To arrive at the diagnosis of the cause in a particular case, attention should be paid to the character, situation, and time of occurrence of the pain, to its constancy, intermissions, or paroxysmal exacerbations, to circumstances which alleviate or aggravate it, and also to accompanying symptoms.

CHARACTER. Diagnostic assistance may be afforded by such descriptions as throbbing, paroxysmal, or as being affected by movement or alterations of position.

SITUATION. This may be frontal, vertical, occipital, or unilateral, and in cases of organic disease of the cerebrum may occasionally aid in localizing the situation of the lesion. It may be unilateral in migraine, tumour, abscess, middle-ear disease, or occipital in cerebellar disease. Occipital headache spreading to the vertex and even to the forehead may be produced by cervical spondylosis, although a similar headache may occur in basal subarachnoid haemorrhage, in some cases of tumour in the posterior fossa, and in meningitis. Purely frontal headache is suggestive of frontal sinusitis though it is also familiar as a sequel of malaria—*brow ague*. Headaches over the vertex associated with other bizarre symptoms, such as a sensation of the skull closing and opening, are usually manifestations of psychoneurosis.

TIME OF OCCURRENCE. Headache associated with organic disease of the brain or its meninges often persists or becomes worse at night and may wake the patient from his sleep, whereas that due to toxic and functional causes is relieved by rest in a horizontal position. Grave suspicion should be entertained of an organic nature of the headache which disturbs the patient's sleep at night. A headache experienced on rising in the morning may be due to a stuffy ill-ventilated room, to the effects of coal-gas leaking perhaps imperceptibly from the pipe, to the fumes of a coke stove or gas fire, to excessive smoking or consumption of alcohol, or to cervical spondylosis. Persistent morning headache may be associated with chronic nephritis, or with chronic purulent sinusitis; such a headache tends to disappear during the day. In antritis and sinusitis frontal and facial headache may come on after breakfast, persist most unpleasantly through the day, and pass off in the late afternoon. Evening headaches are often due to mental stress or eyestrain. Even a normal eye can exhibit the condition of strain if work is excessive, the light bad, or the general health poor. True ocular headache is, however, relatively infrequent, apart from glaucoma and acute inflammatory states of the eye. It is more common with hypermetropia and astigmatism than myopia.

For the purposes of classification it is convenient to divide the causes of headache into three main groups: (*A*) *Local organic disease* (brain, intracranial vessels, meninges, skull, special sense organs); (*B*) *Toxic states*; (*C*) *Functional conditions*.

A. Causes due to Local Organic Disease:

These may be classified anatomically as follows:

1. DISEASES OF THE BRAIN:

   Post-concussional
   Tumour
   Abscess
   Cyst
   Encephalitis
   Polio-encephalitis
   Hydrocephaly
   Tumours of the pituitary gland.

2. DISEASES OF INTRACRANIAL VESSELS:

   Haemorrhage
   Thrombosis
   Embolism
   Aneurysm

3. DISEASES OF THE MENINGES:

   Meningitis, various forms—localized or diffuse
   Pachymeningitis
   Syphilis—meningeal type
   Tumour
   Cyst
   Following lumbar puncture.
   Chronic subdural haematoma.

4. DISEASES OF THE SKULL:

   Tumours $\begin{cases} \text{Innocent} \\ \text{Malignant} \end{cases} \begin{cases} \text{Primary} \\ \text{Secondary} \end{cases}$

   Suppuration or new growth in frontal, antral, sphenoidal or ethmoidal sinuses
   Mastoiditis
   Dental diseases
   Paget's disease.
   Tertiary syphilis

5. EXTRACRANIAL DISEASES:

   Cervical spondylosis. Emotional states. Trigeminal, sphenopalatine, and occipital neuralgias. Herpes supra-orbitalis. Cranial (giant-cell) arteritis. Rheumatoid arthritis or ankylosing spondylitis.

6. DISEASES OF SPECIAL SENSE ORGANS:

   Eye—errors of refraction, iritis, glaucoma, conjunctivitis, melanotic sarcoma.
   Ear—middle-ear disease.
   New growth.

Headache in Organic Cerebral Disease. Although headache is the presenting symptom in 90 per cent of patients with tumours of the posterior fossa, it occurs in only about 33 per cent of supratentorial tumours. Headache from intracranial sources is due to traction and displacement of venous sinuses, middle meningeal arteries, large arteries at the base of the brain, and dilatation and distension of intracranial arteries. Inflammation or pressure on pain-sensitive structures may cause headaches.

TIME OF OCCURRENCE. Organic cerebral disease should be suspected when there is a history of recurrent nocturnal or morning headaches.

SEVERITY. The pain is often intense and sometimes paroxysmal in character, but seldom interferes with sleep. In cases of brain tumour rarely is it as bad as a severe migraine.

SITUATION. This may give some clue to the existence and localization of an organic lesion. In cases of cerebral tumour the pain may be unilateral or frontal, with a cerebellar lesion it is more often occipital. About one-third of all headaches roughly overlie the tumour, and if there is no raised intracranial pressure about two-thirds. In middle-ear and mastoid disease headache is unilateral with localized tenderness. Occipital headache may be one of the earliest symptoms of meningitis.

ASSOCIATED SIGNS AND SYMPTOMS. One or more of the following signs and symptoms may present themselves at an early period in cases of headache due to organic cerebral disease, so that their prompt recognition is important:

   Vomiting of the 'cerebral type' (*see* VOMITING, p. 829): it usually bears no relation to food. There is usually no preceding nausea
   Inequality of the pupils
   Squint
   Papilloedema
   Drowsiness
   Twitchings
   Convulsions.

Tapping the skull over the site of the pain may reveal local tenderness.

The presence of any of these signs associated with headache would point to the existence of one or other of the organic lesions enumerated above. Ophthalmoscopic examination is essential. Lumbar puncture and investigation of the cerebrospinal fluid is often desirable (*see* p. 123) but development of a pressure cone is a very real danger in cases with increased intracranial pressure and fresh symptoms may be precipitated by this investigation. X-rays of the skull, and in some cases brain scanning, may be of value.

Cerebral haemorrhage, thrombosis, and *embolism* are often followed by headache of varying severity. With *cerebral aneurysm* complaint may be made of a rhythmic beating or pulsation and rushing noises, but such throbbings are commoner as the result of *arteriosclerosis* and *high blood-pressure.* Similar rhythmic beatings or noises in the head are not unusual in many anaemic and nervous introspective persons.

In cranial (giant-cell) arteritis severe headache may occur when the temporal vessels are involved.

In *meningitis,* especially in the epidemic cerebrospinal and the post-basal varieties, the character of the headache is significant. It is intense, occipital, and even at an early stage attended by stiffness of the neck and retraction of the head. Examination of the cerebrospinal fluid (*see* p. 123) clinches the diagnosis.

Lumbar puncture may be followed by severe headache which is usually relieved by absolute rest in the recumbent position without pillows.

Diseases of the skull are revealed by clinical and radiological examination as is also the case with headache due to spondylosis and arthritis of the cervical spine.

SPECIAL SENSE ORGANS: EYE. Headaches due to astigmatism, hypermetropia, cataract, glaucoma, iritis, are generally frontal or temporal. An error of refraction may cause what appears to be a disproportionately severe headache, particularly in children. This headache is frontal, occurs mostly in the evening or after school hours, is increased by close work, or by reading in artificial light that is either too dim or too bright, and it is often attended by a burning, pricking, or watering of the eyes. Correction of the defect by suitable glasses may by curing the headache confirm the diagnosis. The warning may be repeated that the significance of minor errors of refraction is exaggerated and as a consequence other causal circumstances are overlooked. Myopia as a cause of headache is relatively rare.

The headache of sinusitis is really of infective origin. A 'vacuum headache' is due to obstruction to drainage of a sinus as from the congestion of rhinitis and is not necessarily purulent in nature: even the absorption of air in a blocked sinus is sufficient to produce it.

B. Toxic Causes:

These may be subdivided into two groups: (1) Those in which the cause lies initially outside the body, *exogenous*; (2) Those in which it is within, *endogenous*.

1. OF EXOGENOUS ORIGIN:

Foul air, as in close, ill-ventilated rooms, exhaust gases from motor-cars
Poisonous gases, CO_2, CO, chloroform, ether, coal-gas, acetone, etc.
Drugs, e.g., quinine, iron in some individuals, salicylates, opium, barbiturates indomethacin
Alcohol
Tobacco
Lead poisoning.

2. OF ENDOGENOUS ORIGIN:

Uraemia
Gastro-intestinal disturbances: rarely constipation, acidosis, alkalosis
Toxaemias: acute infections, high fevers from any cause.

Of the endogenous causes, *uraemia* is one of the most important. Uraemic headaches may be of all degrees of severity, from a slight frontal headache felt on rising in the morning to an intense vertical or general cephalalgia. Other uraemic manifestations may be present, such as vomiting, drowsiness, dyspnoea, affections of vision, and retinal changes.

C. Other Miscellaneous Causes:

Migraine
Hypertension
Venous congestion
Mental strain
Emotional disturbances
Persistent noises—'gun headache'
Menstruation
Post-epileptic
Sunstroke
Insufficient sleep
Psychoneurosis
Psychoses
Exhaustion states
Following head injuries—compensation headache
'Cough headache'.

The *migrainous* headache is recurring and paroxysmal, generally although not always unilateral. It is accompanied by nausea, vomiting, and dizziness and frequently preceded by disturbances of vision or other sensations or motor aurae. There is complete freedom between attacks. Migraine also appears to bear some relation to water retention. Attacks are more common premenstrually, preceded by oliguria and followed by polyuria. Onset is often in childhood or adolescence and in girls may start at the menarché. A positive family history is common. It should be added that the onset after the age of 40 should arouse suspicion of organic intracranial disease.

Hypertension is a not very common cause of headache, usually of a throbbing character, accompanied by a sense of fullness of the head. The headache tends to come on when stooping. The headache associated with malignant hypertension may be particularly severe.

The headache familiarly associated with menstruation is due to many factors, one of which is water retention.

In *epilepsy*, headache is frequent in the post-epileptic state, and it may also follow the slighter manifestations of *petit mal*.

After *sunstroke*, chronic headache, usually vertical, may persist for months, and the same applies to the after-effects of head injuries: a subdural haematoma must not be overlooked. Psychogenic headache is common, nervous tension and anxiety states being relatively common causes. In compensation cases the post-traumatic headache may persist until the legal aspect is settled for or against the patient. The act of *coughing* may aggravate any headache but rarely produces it. Attacks of transient pain in the head may be precipitated by coughing in intracranial tumour, but cases have been described of 'benign cough-headache' which rarely appears apart from coughing or similar procedure, e.g., straining at stool. The majority of sufferers are males. Headache due entirely to emotional cause is not usually aggravated by coughing, straining, or physical exertion.

Some people have such a remarkable susceptibility to headache that the slightest provocation can produce it. This is particularly true of migrainous subjects, but headaches may also be used by the patient for a variety of social and other reasons, what might be truly called a 'sick-headache evasion syndrome'.

It is sometimes difficult to distinguish between *headache*, which implies pain inside the skull, and *neuralgia*, which is pain felt in the peripheral course of a nerve trunk (*see* FACE, PAIN IN, p. 268). Neuralgia, if of wide distribution, may simulate headache. The local distribution, the often intense and paroxysmal character of the pain, the presence of 'tender spots', the existence of some definite exciting cause such as dental caries, should point to the diagnosis of neuralgia.

There are, therefore, almost as many causes for headache in medicine as there are disorders. The most common are tension and anxiety states, sinusitis, migraine, cervical spondylosis, eyestrain, and states of fatigue.

F. Dudley Hart.

HEART, ENLARGEMENT OF

For the purposes of this discussion enlargement of the heart will be taken to mean either dilatation of the cavities due to an increase in the volume of blood contained therein, or an increased muscular mass due to hypertrophy or, as is commonly the case, a combination of both conditions.

Clinically cardiac enlargement is detected by determining the position of the apex beat. This is normally in the fifth left intercostal space within the mid-clavicular line; in young children it may be in the fourth space and a little further to the left. Displacement of the apex beat either laterally or downwards is good evidence of cardiac enlargement provided that displacement of the heart as a whole by such conditions as pectus excavatum, pleural effusion, and pulmonary fibrosis can be excluded (see HEART IMPULSE, DISPLACED, p. 378). There is a general tendency for the apex beat to be displaced more downwards than laterally in left ventricular enlargement and more laterally than downwards in right ventricular enlargement, but these findings are too inconstant to be of much diagnostic value. There are, in any case, better ways of distinguishing enlargement of the two ventricles. Clinically this can be done by the detection of a powerful impulse felt, reasonably enough, over the appropriate ventricle. Thus, if such an impulse is felt at the apex beat, left ventricular hypertrophy is likely; right ventricular hypertrophy produces an impulse at the left sternal border and in the epigastrium. Radiography and, especially, electrocardiography are also valuable in making this distinction.

Percussion of the area of cardiac dullness is of very limited value. It may be of some value in outlining the left border of the heart if the apical impulse is impalpable; dullness in the second right intercostal space can be detected with an aneurysm of the ascending aorta. The value of percussion has declined with the ready availability of radiography which is the best method of determining the size of the heart. There is, however, one condition in which percussion may be superior to radiography, namely pericardial effusion. The enlarged cardiac silhouette in the radiograph may be difficult to distinguish from enlargement of the heart itself, but the finding of the apex beat well within the left border of cardiac dullness is a useful sign of pericardial effusion.

In a 6-foot postero-anterior chest film, cardiac enlargement can be diagnosed if the transverse diameter of the heart exceeds half that of the bony thorax. The only exception to this rule is in the case of pectus excavatum in which the heart, being compressed anteroposteriorly, is expanded laterally. This condition is, of course, obvious on clinical examination.

Radiography is less reliable than electrocardiography in the distinction between left and right ventricular enlargement. For example, in aortic stenosis, there may be little or no enlargement of the heart shown in the radiograph but clear evidence of left ventricular hypertrophy in the electrocardiogram.

I. ENLARGEMENT OF THE LEFT VENTRICLE

Hypertrophy of the left ventricle occurs whenever its work, in terms of pressure generated or volume ejected, is increased. Dilatation is a feature of an increase in volume load only; this may be seen in such conditions as aortic incompetence and persistent ductus arteriosus. Dilatation also occurs when the ventricle fails, whatever the cause. Thus, in aortic stenosis, if the left ventricle is markedly enlarged in the radiograph and there is no evidence of a lesion such as aortic or mitral incompetence which can cause dilatation, left ventricular failure is likely to be present (*Fig.* 376).

1. AORTIC VALVE DISEASE

Aortic Stenosis is about four times as common in men as in women and, as seen clinically, occurs in two distinct age-groups. Children and adolescents are seen with *congenital* stenosis of the valve or of the left ventricular outflow tract. Over the age of 40 *calcific* aortic stenosis occurs. This is a heterogeneous group consisting of a few cases of congenital valve stenosis, calcified congenitally bicuspid valves, and, most commonly, rheumatic or degenerative valve disease. It is very difficult to identify the different causes even at autopsy and quite impossible to do so clinically.

The cardinal symptoms of aortic stenosis are angina, syncope, and dyspnoea. Angina may occur even if the coronary arteries are quite healthy but associated coronary artery disease is common and the old teaching that aortic stenosis 'protects' the coronary arteries is quite wrong. Syncope on exertion or, more ominously, at rest usually implies tight stenosis, and dyspnoea suggests that left ventricular failure has occurred.

The pulse is characteristically small in volume and slow-rising often with an anacrotic inflection on the upstroke; it is often rather slow, around 60 per minute. The apex beat is not much displaced unless failure has occurred and the impulse is powerful and sustained due to the prolonged left ventricular ejection. An atrial impulse may be palpable, and an atrial sound heard, at the apex. The aortic second sound is usually soft or absent in adults but in children, with valve stenosis, it is frequently loud and there is, in addition, an ejection sound heard at the apex or aortic area. Paradoxical splitting of the second sound may occur (*see* HEART-SOUNDS, SPLITTING; TRIPLE RHYTIIM, p. 383). If the stenosis is due to a subvalvular membrane the ejection sound is not heard and the second sound is soft. The characteristic mid-systolic murmur, which is often loud enough to be accompanied by a thrill, is heard in the second right interspace and radiates to the neck; it may also be well heard at the apex.

in men as in women and it is seen at almost any age. The commonest cause is previous *rheumatic* affection; the diastolic murmur may be heard at the time of the acute attack although without any peripheral manifestations. The recognition of the aetiology as rheumatic depends on a suitable history or on the association with mitral stenosis. In this connexion the Austin Flint murmur may

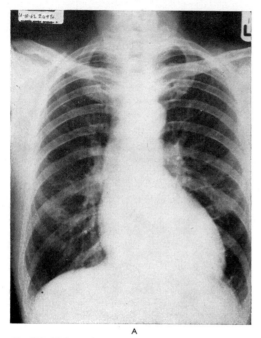
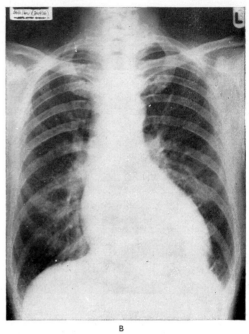

A   B

Fig. 376. Male, aged 48, with aortic stenosis. A, The enlarged left ventricle and dilated ascending aorta should be noted; at that time his main complaint was angina, and dyspnoea was not severe. B, Six weeks later, the left ventricle has enlarged further and pulmonary venous congestion is present; by this time he was extremely breathless.

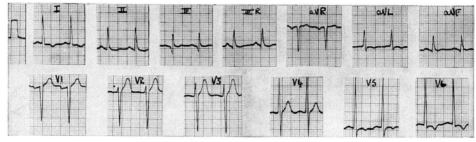

Fig. 377. Electrocardiogram of a man, aged 56, with aortic stenosis. The gradient across the aortic valve was 50 mm. Hg. Tall R waves are present in Leads V5 and 6 with T inversion; no Q waves are visible in these leads.

In the chest radiograph there may be little enlargement of the cardiac shadow but post-stenotic dilatation of the ascending aorta is often striking (*Fig.* 376). In severe aortic stenosis the electrocardiogram almost always shows clear evidence of left ventricular hypertrophy, with small or absent Q waves in the left ventricular leads (*Fig.* 377).

Aortic Incompetence is a good deal more common than aortic stenosis; it is about twice as common

cause some confusion. This is a presystolic or delayed diastolic murmur at the apex heard in cases of aortic incompetence in whom no organic disease of the mitral valve is present. In practice the Austin Flint murmur should only be diagnosed if it is virtually certain, on other grounds, that the aortic lesion is not rheumatic. *Syphilis*, a less common cause of aortic incompetence than it used to be, affects a somewhat older age-group than rheumatism. The lesion is primarily one of dilatation of the valve ring with little damage to the cusps. The diagnosis can be made on the basis of positive serological tests and on the presence of other signs of late syphilis such as pigmented scars on the limbs and leucoplakia. In the radiograph calcification of the ascending aorta is a useful sign of syphilitic aortitis provided that it is confined to that region; the aorta may be irregularly dilated or an aneurysm may be present. *Athero-sclerotic* changes in the valve are another important cause of aortic incompetence, especially in the elderly. Other causes include *infective endocarditis* and *dissecting aneurysm*, in both of which the incompetence is of relatively sudden onset. Bacterial infection of a previously stenosed or bicuspid valve may cause regurgitation either by gross destruction of the cusp or by causing a discrete perforation. In dissecting aneurysm disruption of the valve ring is the mechanism of the valvular incompetence. Less common causes include *ankylosing spondylitis*, *Reiter's syndrome*, *rheumatoid heart disease*, and *systemic lupus erythematosus*. Occasionally *hypertension* seems to be an important factor but this is probably always associated with atherosclerotic valve damage; it is doubtful whether a high systemic blood-pressure can cause a normal aortic valve to become incompetent. As an isolated lesion aortic incompetence is almost never congenital in origin, but it is well recognized as occurring with *hypoplastic aortic valves*, for example in Marfan's syndrome, in *osteogenesis imperfecta*, *mucopolysaccharidosis*, and in association with *coarctation of the aorta* and *ventricular septal defect*. An aortic diastolic murmur is heard in many cases of membranous *subvalvular aortic stenosis* and this may be a point in differentiation from congenital valvular stenosis, in which incompetence is rare.

Many patients with aortic incompetence remain symptom-free for many years but palpitations, due to the vigorous action of the left ventricle, are quite a common early, benign symptom. Angina is common particularly if the lesion is syphilitic, in which case involvement of the coronary ostia may play an important part. Syncope can also occur although less commonly than in aortic stenosis, and dyspnoea with orthopnoea and paroxysmal dyspnoea indicate the presence of left ventricular failure.

The pulse is typically large in volume and collapsing in quality; this is best felt by raising the patient's arm and feeling the radial pulse with the palmar surface of the fingers rather than with the finger-tips. It must be distinguished from the large volume pulse without any collapsing quality found in arteriosclerosis and with bradycardia from any cause. Also in many conditions such as cor pulmonale, severe anaemia, arteriovenous fistula, persistent ductus arteriosus, and hepatic failure something approaching a collapsing pulse may be felt; the pulse-volume may certainly be large in these conditions but only with a large persistent ductus in childhood does the pulse have the classic 'water-hammer'

quality of aortic incompetence. The typical arterial pulse is also easily visible in the neck; it was this feature and not the palpable pulse that was described by Corrigan in 1832. Related to the collapsing pulse and due to the associated vasodilatation is the capillary pulsation which may be seen in aortic incompetence. This is most conveniently demonstrated in the nail-beds. Gentle pressure on the centre of a finger-nail produces an area of blanching into which the surrounding normally pink colour encroaches with each beat of the heart. The double intermittent murmur of Duroziez which may be heard over the femoral or other large artery is of interest but of little diagnostic value. The systolic pressure is high and the diastolic low on sphygmomanometry; sounds may be heard down to zero pressure. If left ventricular failure develops the diastolic pressure may rise towards normal, demonstrating that the wide pulse-pressure of aortic incompetence is partly due to vasodilatation which is abolished by failure.

The apex beat is markedly displaced to the left in the presence of aortic incompetence of any severity; this is the case whether or not failure is present. The impulse is powerful and thrusting, the large amplitude being related to the very high velocity of left ventricular ejection, and is of relatively brief duration unlike the sustained impulse of aortic stenosis. An atrial impulse may be palpable. The definitive diagnosis is made by the finding of the typical immediate diastolic murmur starting at the second sound and continuing in a diminuendo fashion for a greater or lesser part of diastole. Generally speaking, the more severe the incompetence the shorter the murmur (*see* CARDIAC MURMURS, p. 119). The murmur is well heard in the aortic area and in the third left interspace; it is frequently audible at the apex but radiates hardly at all into the neck. In most cases there is, in addition, a mid-systolic murmur producing the typical to-and-fro cadence; it is important to recognize that this does not necessarily imply associated aortic stenosis. The systolic murmur is usually due to the large left ventricular stroke volume. The Austin Flint murmur which is not, in fact, very common has been discussed above (p. 366). Sometimes the aortic diastolic murmur may be difficult to hear; it can often be more easily detected at the left sternal border with the patient leaning forward and holding his breath in expiration.

Left ventricular enlargement is usually obvious in the chest radiograph and both the ascending aorta and aortic arch are dilated (*Fig.* 378). The electrocardiogram shows evidence of left ventricular hypertrophy with prominent Q waves; these are, however, neither so wide nor so deep as to suggest myocardial infarction.

Aortic Stenosis and Incompetence frequently coexist. The cause is usually rheumatic or degenerative valve disease and the physical signs vary depending on which lesion is dominant. In the truly mixed lesion the pulsus bisferiens may be present; this has a well-marked notch on the apex of the pulse wave and two impulses can be felt with each heart-beat. The bisferiens pulse must not be confused with the apparent double impulse which can be produced, particularly in the brachial pulse, if a collapsing pulse is partially occluded by the palpating finger.

common and the systolic murmur is best heard between the lower left sternal border and the apex; it is rather late in onset. Mitral incompetence is a common complication; regurgitation into the left atrium does not begin until the middle of systole and the mitral systolic murmur is superimposed on the ejection murmur.

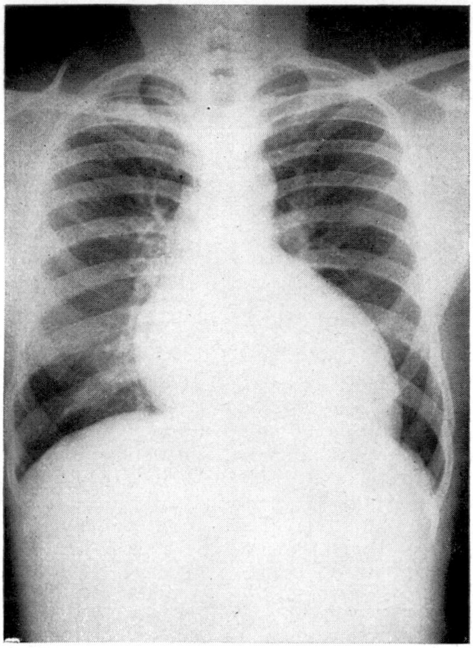

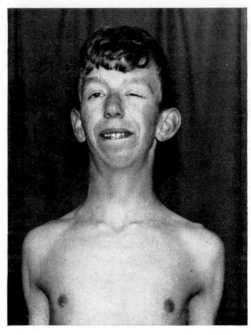

Fig. 378. Male, aged 23, with aortic incompetence. The left ventricle is greatly enlarged but the aorta is rather less prominent than is often the case in this condition.

Fig. 379. Boy, aged 15, with supravalvular aortic stenosis. Note the heavy cheeks, rather thick lips, and large ears.

2. OTHER FORMS OF LEFT VENTRICULAR OUTFLOW TRACT OBSTRUCTION

The differentiation of aortic valve stenosis from *membranous subvalvular* stenosis has been considered above; an ejection sound and a loud second sound favour stenosis at the valve and an immediate diastolic murmur is to be expected in most cases of subvalvular stenosis.

Hypertrophic Obstructive Cardiomyopathy can also cause a significant obstruction to left ventricular outflow. The degree of obstruction is characteristically variable, being increased by factors which reduce the volume of the left ventricle; these include positive inotropic agents such as isoprenaline and hypovolaemia from any cause. A striking rise in the pressure gradient across the outflow tract, with a fall in the aortic systolic pressure, is also seen in the beat following an extrasystole and this feature may be helpful in making the diagnosis during left-heart catheterization. The typical physical signs of this condition include a jerky pulse which may have a bisferiens quality, a prominent a wave in the jugular venous pulse, and a double impulse at the apex beat. On auscultation an atrial sound is

Supravalvular Aortic Stenosis is very rare. It is associated with a characteristic facies (*Fig.* 379) and mental subnormality with, often, a history of hypercalcaemia in infancy. The radial pulses may be unequal and the blood-pressure in the right arm usually higher than that in the left.

3. MITRAL INCOMPETENCE

Compared with the relative simplicity of the structure and function of the aortic valve, the mitral valve with its attached chordae tendineae and papillary muscles is a much more complex mechanism. Incompetence can result from lesions of the valve cusps themselves, from damage to the subvalvular mechanism, and from dilatation of the left ventricle. Not infrequently these lesions are combined.

Valvular incompetence is most commonly *rheumatic* in origin. Its significance ranges from a trivial accompaniment of dominant mitral stenosis through a combination of stenosis and incompetence of about equal severity to the, rather unusual, pure incompetence. The latter occurs more frequently in men than in women in a ratio of 3 : 2, thus contrasting sharply with mitral stenosis in which females predominate 4 : 1 over males. Thickening and shortening of the cusps are complicated by a subvalvular component with shortening and matting of the chordae. *Congenital* mitral incompetence is also nearly always valvular, occurring in association with the ostium primum type of atrial septal defect, occasionally with other congenital lesions and, very rarely, as an isolated anomaly. *Infective endocarditis* can also cause, or aggravate, mitral incompetence by destruction or perforation of the cusps; in addition, rupture of one or more chordae may occur.

There are numerous causes of subvalvular mitral incompetence. The commonest is ischaemic damage to a papillary muscle; infarction of this muscle can cause rupture with the sudden development of severe regurgitation and pulmonary oedema. More often a severely ischaemic papillary muscle, failing to contract and becoming fibrous, allows rather less severe regurgitation to occur. This situation is called *papillary muscle dysfunction* and a similar lesion may result from infiltration of the papillary muscles by, for example, sarcoid. Subvalvular regurgitation may also occur in *hypertrophic obstructive cardiomyopathy* and, less often, in other varieties of left ventricular outflow tract obstruction, in *endomyocardial fibrosis, endocardial fibro-elastosis,* and rare congenital lesions of the valve mechanism such as *parachute deformity* of the mitral valve, *subvalvular aneurysm,* and *idiopathic prolapse* of the posterior cusp, a benign familial condition. *Infective endocarditis* has already been mentioned in this connexion.

It was previously believed that the mitral incompetence associated with dilatation of the left ventricle was due to concomitant dilatation of the mitral annulus. It is now thought that it is due to distortion and malfunction of the subvalvular apparatus. The regurgitation, although usually not severe, may be a serious burden to a failing ventricle. It may be reversible if the failure is brought under control.

Serious symptoms appear late in the natural history of mitral incompetence but a complaint of palpitations is quite common earlier. Effort dyspnoea is mainly due to left ventricular failure although the direct effect of the regurgitation in elevating left atrial pressure plays some part. Atrial fibrillation is a common complication, bringing with it the risk of systemic embolism, although this is rather less common than in mitral stenosis.

The pulse is of small volume and often rises so sharply as to be justifiably called collapsing; it is frequently irregular due to atrial fibrillation. The apex beat is displaced and the impulse is thrusting in quality and of brief duration, not unlike that found in aortic incompetence. A left parasternal impulse suggesting right ventricular enlargement may be present, but confusion sometimes arises if the left atrium is very large and thrusts the whole ventricular mass against the anterior chest wall to produce an impulse in the left parasternal region.

The diagnostic sign is a pansystolic murmur maximal at the apex and typically radiating to the axilla and even to the back. This murmur may be modified in various ways. In some, particularly elderly, patients with mild or moderate mitral incompetence only a late systolic murmur is heard; this has, in the past, been regarded as innocent but is now known to signify organic regurgitation. In papillary muscle insufficiency, particularly when the posterior papillary muscle is affected, the murmur may be shorter and may radiate medially from the apex so that it may be confused with that of aortic stenosis. A third sound is commonly present which, in this context, does not imply left ventricular failure, and a short delayed diastolic murmur may be heard and must not be regarded as evidence of associated mitral stenosis. An opening snap is rarely heard in pure mitral incompetence but may be present if one or other cusp, usually the anterior, remains pliable.

Left ventricular and left atrial enlargement are seen in the chest radiograph (*Fig.* 380) and the electrocardiogram shows evidence of left ventricular hypertrophy which is usually less gross than that seen in aortic valve disease.

4. HYPERTENSIVE HEART DISEASE

Although clearly left ventricular work is increased in all cases of systemic hypertension, clinically manifest hypertensive heart disease varies considerably in severity. In some patients symptoms and signs of left ventricular hypertrophy and failure may appear quite early; in others, particularly elderly women, a similar hypertensive burden may be tolerated with very few overt manifestations.

Common symptoms of hypertensive heart disease are dyspnoea on exertion with, later, orthopnoea and paroxysmal dyspnoea implying left ventricular failure, and angina of effort. The last may be due to associated coronary artery disease but this is not always severe and the angina may be mainly due to the overwork of the left ventricle and respond to hypotensive therapy.

The pulse is usually regular but atrial fibrillation occurs in about 10 per cent of cases and has an unfavourable prognostic significance. Displacement of the apex beat is commensurate with the degree of left ventricular enlargement; the impulse is heaving and fairly well sustained but much less strikingly abnormal than in aortic valve disease. An atrial sound is not uncommon, implying severe left ventricular overload; a third sound is evidence of failure. The typically loud aortic second sound is of no great importance, implying only that the blood-pressure is raised. An aortic ejection sound may also be heard but this too is of no great moment. Pulsus alternans, if present, is a most important sign as it is unequivocal evidence of left ventricular failure.

Electrocardiography confirms left ventricular hypertrophy and the chest X-ray demonstrates enlargement of the heart shadow if the hypertension has been present for a considerable time.

If the heart is not much enlarged it is likely that the hypertension is of recent onset.

5. CONGENITAL HEART DISEASE

Certain types of congenital heart disease can cause dominant enlargement of the left ventricle; of these aortic valve disease has already been discussed. The other conditions are those in which the left ventricle receives a greater than normal volume of blood from the left atrium. Of these one of the commonest is *persistent ductus arteriosus* in which the increased burden falls exclusively on the left ventricle unless significant pulmonary hypertension develops. This lesion

if pulmonary hypertension develops. The arterial pulse is unremarkable and the venous pressure normal unless failure occurs. In the cases with large shunts the apical impulse is vigorous and there is also usually an impulse at the left sternal border over the right ventricle. The typical murmur is pansystolic and is often loud enough to

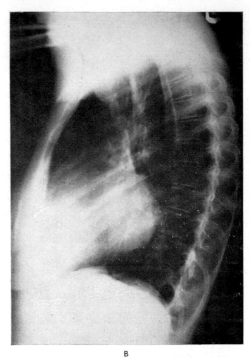

Fig. 380. Female, aged 45, with severe mitral incompetence. A, There is considerable cardiac enlargement. The straight left border of the heart and the vertical course of the right upper pulmonary vein (just below the right pulmonary artery) suggest left atrial enlargement. B, This is seen to be gross in the lateral film.

occurs about twice as often in women as in men and is often relatively benign, the diagnosis being made on routine examination. A large ductus may, however, cause cardiac failure in infancy. The pulse is of large volume and may be collapsing if the shunt is large. At the apex which may or may not be displaced depending on the size of the shunt, a vigorous thrusting impulse may be felt. The diagnostic sign, which may be the only abnormality if the ductus is small, is the classic continuous, machinery murmur heard best in the second or third left interspace and loudest towards the end of systole. In the presence of a large shunt a delayed diastolic murmur is heard at the apex due to the very large flow through the mitral orifice. The electrocardiogram may be normal but shows left ventricular hypertrophy if the shunt is large; in the radiograph left ventricular enlargement, dilatation of the main pulmonary artery and aorta, and pulmonary plethora are seen.

The left ventricle is also enlarged in the presence of a *ventricular septal defect* (*Fig.* 381); the right ventricle may also be enlarged particularly

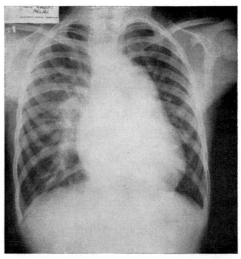

Fig. 381. Boy, aged 9, with a large ventricular septal defect. The heart is considerably enlarged, the main pulmonary artery is dilated, and there is marked pulmonary plethora.

be accompanied by a thrill; it is best heard at the left sternal border in the third and fourth interspaces, and a mitral diastolic murmur may also be heard as in persistent ductus. If the defect is small the only abnormality is the systolic murmur, and it is in this situation only that the term 'maladie de Roger' should be used. Pulmonary hypertension modifies the findings by reducing the size of the shunt; the mitral diastolic murmur disappears and the murmur produced at the defect becomes mid-systolic in timing.

Cyanotic congenital heart disease is nearly always associated with enlargement of the right ventricle but *tricuspid atresia* is an exception. In this condition the left ventricle receives the reduced pulmonary blood-flow and, in addition, all of the systemic venous return via an atrial septal defect. Blood reaches the lungs via a ventricular septal defect, a ductus, or bronchial arteries. The electrocardiogram shows the unusual and, in this clinical context, virtually diagnostic pattern of right atrial and left ventricular hypertrophy.

II. ENLARGEMENT OF THE RIGHT VENTRICLE

As in the case of the left ventricle, hypertrophy and dilatation of the right ventricle occur whenever its work is increased by a pressure or volume load. Thus right ventricular enlargement may be due to pulmonary arterial hypertension, of which there are numerous causes, to disease of the pulmonary valve, or to intracardiac arteriovenous shunts.

1. MITRAL STENOSIS

In this condition the rise in pressure in the left atrium is transmitted to the pulmonary veins and capillaries where it is the cause of the typical symptoms. Dyspnoea with orthopnoea and paroxysmal nocturnal dyspnoea are the commonest complaints and haemoptysis is also frequent. Further retrograde transmission of the rise in pressure to the pulmonary artery produces 'passive' pulmonary hypertension of a degree commensurate with the rise in left atrial pressure. This, in itself, produces a slight increase in right ventricular work but much more important is the disproportionately large rise in pulmonary arterial pressure which occurs in some cases. This is due to changes in the smallest arteries in the lungs which can be quantified as the pulmonary vascular resistance; this can be calculated from the expression:

Pulmonary vascular resistance (units)=

$$\frac{\text{mean pulmonary arterial} - \text{mean left atrial pressure (mm. Hg)}}{\text{pulmonary blood-flow (litres/min.)}}.$$

From the normal value of 1–3 units, the resistance may rise to well over 10 units in some cases of severe mitral stenosis.

Mitral stenosis occurs about four times as often in women as in men and patients present most commonly between the ages of 20 and 40. Some of the symptoms have been mentioned above (*see also under* DYSPNOEA, p. 236); others include recurrent winter bronchitis, probably due to the engorged bronchial mucosa, and systemic embolism. The latter is often, but not always, associated with atrial fibrillation which occurs sooner or later in most cases of mitral valve disease.

The characteristic malar flush is a reflection of the low cardiac output causing peripheral cyanosis; the fingers also may be cold and blue. The malar flush is of some small diagnostic significance, but it must be remembered that a very similar appearance can be seen in myxoedema. The pulse is of small volume and regular until atrial fibrillation occurs. In the jugular venous pulse a tall a wave is seen in the presence of severe pulmonary hypertension if sinus rhythm persists; elevation of the mean jugular venous pressure implies right ventricular failure. The apex beat is usually little, if at all, displaced and frequently a tapping impulse is felt, due to the loud first sound. Thrills may be palpable in association with the murmurs which are described below. Over the right ventricle, that is along the left sternal border, a heaving impulse may be felt and, in addition, it may be possible to feel a sharp tap in the second left interspace immediately after the main impulse; this is due to a loud pulmonary second sound. Right ventricular pulsation may also be felt in the epigastrium. On auscultation at the apex the loud first sound is preceded by a presystolic murmur if the patient is in normal rhythm. Shortly following the second sound the high-pitched opening snap immediately precedes a delayed diastolic murmur of which the length is some measure of the severity of the stenosis. In the presence of severe pulmonary hypertension the Graham Steell murmur of pulmonary incompetence may occasionally be audible at the left sternal border; in the context of rheumatic heart disease it may be very difficult to distinguish this from the murmur of aortic incompetence.

The radiographic appearances are often diagnostic (*Fig.* 382) and the severity of the pulmonary venous congestion is a reliable objective measure of the severity of the stenosis. In the electrocardiogram the degree of right ventricular hypertrophy reflects the rise in pulmonary vascular resistance; in patients with 'passive' pulmonary hypertension only very little evidence of right ventricular hypertrophy may be seen. In sinus rhythm left atrial hypertrophy can be diagnosed from the typically abnormal configuration of the P wave (*Fig.* 383).

2. CHRONIC LEFT VENTRICULAR FAILURE

The left atrial hypertension of left ventricular failure can produce haemodynamic changes on the right side of the heart similar to those produced by mitral stenosis. Pulmonary hypertension severe enough to cause right ventricular hypertrophy will develop if the left ventricular failure is long-continued. This does not, in the nature of things, occur very often. Bernheim's syndrome should be mentioned here as this may simulate right ventricular failure secondary to a left-sided lesion. Gross hypertrophy of the left ventricle, particularly of the interventricular septum, can, by encroaching on the right ventricle,

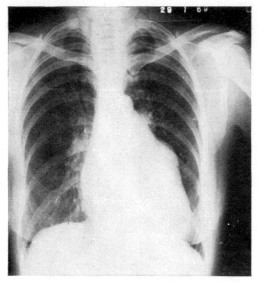

Fig. 382. Female, aged 50, with mitral stenosis. The left atrial appendage forms a prominent bulge on the left border of the heart. The aorta is rather small as is often the case in mitral stenosis.

of the infradiaphragmatic type, can also cause serious pulmonary hypertension.

4. COR PULMONALE

Among various definitions of this condition, one of the most comprehensive is that proposed by an Expert Committee of the World Health Organization. This reads 'hypertrophy of the right ventricle resulting from disease affecting the function and/or the structure of the lungs except when these pulmonary alterations are the result of diseases that primarily affect the left side of the heart or of congenital heart diseases'. This definition includes affections of the pulmonary vessels as well as of the lung parenchyma.

Massive pulmonary embolism can cause acute dilatation of the right ventricle with a high jugular venous pressure. The diagnosis is discussed under CHEST, PAIN IN (p. 133). Recurrent pulmonary emboli which may be very small may produce the condition known as *thrombo-embolic pulmonary hypertension*. This presents with the insidious development of right ventricular failure and may be seen in young women after childbirth or in any other situation in which recurrent phlebothrombosis of the legs occurs. On examination the pulse is small, peripheral cyanosis is common, and the jugular venous pulse shows a tall a wave with which is associated a right atrial gallop rhythm. The right ventricle is much hypertrophied and a heaving impulse extends from the left sternal border to the apex beat which may be formed by the right ventricle. The pulmonary component of the second sound is loud and a Graham Steell murmur may be heard. A chest

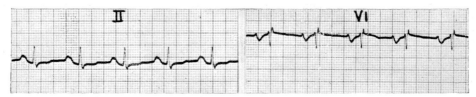

Fig. 383. Left atrial hypertrophy in mitral stenosis (P mitrale). In Lead II the P wave is abnormally broad and there is a suggestion of a notch on its peak. The biphasic P wave in Lead VI, with a prominent negative left atrial component, is very characteristic.

impair the filling of that chamber and cause elevation of the jugular venous pressure. The pulmonary arterial pressure is normal in such cases who are not in right ventricular failure.

3. OTHER CAUSES OF PULMONARY VENOUS HYPERTENSION

Left atrial myxoma can mimic mitral stenosis in some respects and pulmonary arterial hypertension occurs occasionally. Systemic embolism and recurrent syncope are important features and constitutional effects such as fever, anaemia, and increased sedimentation-rate are also seen. In children *cor triatriatum*, in which a perforated septum stretches across the left atrium between the pulmonary veins and the mitral valve, and in infants *total anomalous pulmonary venous drainage*

radiograph shows a large right ventricle, dilated pulmonary arteries, and markedly attenuated pulmonary vascular markings. Right ventricular and right atrial hypertrophy are seen in the electrocardiogram. In *primary pulmonary hypertension* an identical clinical picture is seen without, of course, any history suggesting multiple emboli; in practice the diagnosis can only be made after all other causes of pulmonary hypertension have been excluded. Other causes of this type of pulmonary hypertension include *polyarteritis nodosa, systemic lupus erythematosus*, pulmonary *schistosomiasis*, and *systemic sclerosis*.

Disease of the pulmonary airways and parenchyma can produce pulmonary hypertension by various mechanisms. These include direct involvement of the pulmonary vessels by fibrosis and constriction of the pulmonary arterioles as a result of hypoxia. Cor pulmonale can therefore occur in almost all of the chronic pulmonary diseases which are described in detail in the section on DYSPNOEA (p. 236); in Britain much the commonest causes are chronic bronchitis and emphysema. The signs of pulmonary hypertension outlined above may be present but are usually much less florid than in thrombo-embolic pulmonary hypertension. Superimposed on the cardiac signs may be evidence of an increased cardiac output and peripheral vasodilatation; the extremities may be warm, the pulse quite

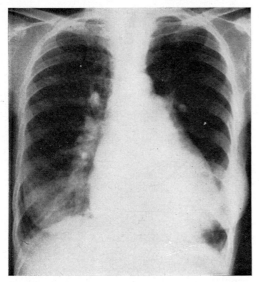

Fig. 384. Female, aged 56, with a history of bronchitis for many years, who had recently developed congestive heart failure. A diagnosis of cor pulmonale was confirmed by finding severe airways obstruction, arterial hypoxaemia and hypercapnia, and pulmonary hypertension. The heart is enlarged and the larger pulmonary arteries are dilated.

large in volume with a collapsing quality, and throbbing may be felt in the fingers. These features are at least partly due to the raised arterial PCO_2. Detection of cardiac enlargement may be difficult clinically as the apex beat may be hidden by the overinflated lung, but gallop rhythm may be heard over the right ventricle. X-ray shows the changes of the causative pulmonary disease with enlargement of the right ventricle and dilatation of the pulmonary arteries (Fig. 384). The electrocardiogram confirms the diagnosis of right ventricular hypertrophy. Right ventricular failure is commonly precipitated by a respiratory infection and cardiac function may improve markedly with antibiotics and other treatment.

5. CONGENITAL HEART DISEASE

Right ventricular hypertrophy is a feature of many varieties of congenital heart disease and may be due either to an increase in the volume work of the ventricle or to a rise in right ventricular pressure as a result of pulmonary

hypertension or pulmonary stenosis. Various combinations of these factors frequently occur.

The ostium secundum type of *atrial septal defect* is usually in the region of the fossa ovalis but may be higher or lower in the septum, overriding the superior or inferior vena cava. The shunt from left to right atrium can be very large so that the pulmonary blood-flow may be four or more times the systemic. The pulmonary vessels dilate to accommodate this huge flow so that the pulmonary arterial pressure is usually normal. The condition may present in childhood but, because the patients often remain symptom-free for many years and the physical signs are less obtrusive than those of other defects, it is not infrequently first diagnosed in adults. Older patients may complain of slight dyspnoea on exertion which becomes worse if atrial fibrillation

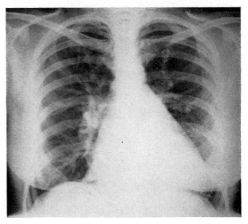

Fig. 385. Female, aged 44, with ostium secundum atrial septal defect. There is well-marked pulmonary plethora and the aorta is small but the main pulmonary artery is not as dilated as is sometimes the case in this condition.

develops; atrial septal defect is one of the very few congenital lesions of which atrial fibrillation is a common complication. The arterial pulse may be small in volume and the venous pulse is unremarkable. Pulsation can be felt over an area extending laterally from the left sternal border towards the apex; pulsation may also be felt in the second left intercostal space over the pulmonary artery. A moderately loud mid-systolic murmur is heard in the pulmonary area in most cases and the second sound is widely split with little change during respiration. In addition, if the shunt is large, a delayed diastolic murmur is heard in the tricuspid area. Both the murmurs are due to the large volume of blood passing through valve orifices which themselves are normal. In the chest X-ray the most obvious abnormality is gross dilatation of the main pulmonary artery and its branches which pulsate vigorously on fluoroscopy; the right ventricle and right atrium are also dilated and the aorta is rather small (Fig. 385). In Lutembacher's syndrome, in which the septal defect is complicated by mitral stenosis, the left atrium may also be enlarged; this condition is very rare. The electrocardiogram shows an RR′ pattern in Lead VI or right bundle branch block (*Fig.* 386). *Anomalous pulmonary venous drainage* into the right atrium can produce a picture very similar to that of atrial septal defect.

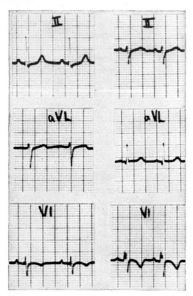

Fig. 386. Electrocardiograms in atrial septal defect. The record on the left is from a girl, aged 8, with ostium secundum defect. In VI an rR′S pattern is seen and there is right-axis deviation, shown by the dominant negative deflexion in aVL and positive deflexion in Lead II. On the right is a record from a girl, aged 6, with ostium primum defect (atrioventricular defect). The pattern in Lead VI is similar to the other record but marked left-axis deviation is present.

The ostium primum type of atrial septal defect, situated low in the septum, is one of the types of atrioventricular defect. In this group of conditions there are, in addition, a high ventricular septal defect and clefts in the septal cusp of the tricuspid and anterior cusp of the mitral valves. This type of defect, which has already been discussed as a cause of mitral incompetence, produces symptoms much earlier than the secundum defect and is distinguished from it by the associated mitral and tricuspid systolic murmurs and by the electrocardiogram which shows left axis deviation in addition to the RR′ pattern in Lead VI (*Fig.* 386).

Ventricular septal defect and persistent ductus arteriosus have been discussed as causes of left ventricular enlargement; in the former there is some enlargement of the right ventricle also. These conditions must be considered further here, however, as they cause a large increase in pulmonary blood-flow which may lead to a rise in the pulmonary vascular resistance so that severe pulmonary hypertension may develop. In that case the volume of the shunt becomes less as the pulmonary arterial and right ventricular pressures approach those in the aorta and left ventricle.

Finally, the shunt may reverse so that the patient becomes cyanosed. It is to this condition, that is a veno-arterial shunt due to pulmonary hypertension, that the term *Eisenmenger's syndrome* is applied. Eisenmenger's original description referred to ventricular septal defect with pulmonary hypertension only and this is sometimes designated 'Eisenmenger's complex'. However, this phenomenon can occur with a shunt at any level, although it is unusual with atrial septal defect, and the terms 'Eisenmenger's syndrome' or 'reaction' are used to cover all such cases. The signs are those of pulmonary hypertension which have been outlined above, with central cyanosis. In the case of a persistent ductus the cyanosis may be more marked, or only present, in the lower limbs but, on the whole, once the shunt has reversed it may be very difficult to identify its site except by catheterization and angiocardiography.

Pulmonary stenosis is the commonest form of congenital heart disease. Two main types can be distinguished depending on the position of the aortic root. If this is normally placed the pulmonary stenosis is usually at valve level and is frequently the only abnormality. Dextroposition of the aorta, with an associated ventricular septal defect, is combined with pulmonary stenosis in Fallot's tetralogy; in this condition the obstruction to right ventricular outflow is frequently in the infundibulum.

The symptoms and signs of isolated pulmonary stenosis vary with the severity of the lesion. In severe cases effort dyspnoea, syncope, and, occasionally, angina are common; less severe cases may be symptom-free. The main sign is a long, loud systolic murmur in the pulmonary area often accompanied by a thrill. In mild or moderately severe cases this is preceded by an ejection sound, which, unlike most right-sided sounds and murmurs, is louder on expiration, and the pulmonary component of the second sound is loud and a little delayed. In more severe cases evidence of right ventricular hypertrophy is present, including a powerful left parasternal heave, a giant a wave in the venous pulse, and a right atrial sound; the pulmonary second sound becomes very soft or inaudible.

If an atrial or ventricular septal defect is present in addition reversal of the shunt can readily occur. More common is the veno-arterial shunt which may be found in infants with severe pulmonary stenosis and a patent foramen ovale. The radiograph shows post-stenotic dilatation of the pulmonary artery and, in severe cases, enlargement of the right ventricle and right atrium (*Fig.* 387). These changes are also reflected in the electrocardiogram.

Right ventricular hypertrophy is also present in Fallot's tetralogy. The patients are usually cyanosed and finger-clubbing is common. Effort dyspnoea is the main complaint and in children is relieved somewhat by squatting. This reduces the venous return from the legs and, therefore, the volume of the veno-arterial shunt. Adults with Fallot's tetralogy rarely squat, presumably because it is socially unacceptable; there is no haemodynamic reason why it should not produce as much relief in them as in children. Syncope on exertion is another common complaint. The physical signs differ from those of pure pulmonary stenosis in that the jugular a wave is rarely very large and the right ventricular heave is much less impressive. The systolic murmur is produced by

ventricular hypertrophy is usually seen in the electrocardiogram but the changes are less florid than in pure pulmonary stenosis (*Fig.* 389).

Tricuspid Valve Disease. This is not, of course, a cause of right ventricular enlargement but may be conveniently discussed here as it frequently complicates several of the conditions which have already been mentioned and may markedly increase the degree of cardiac enlargement.

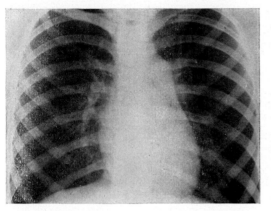

Fig. 387. Pulmonary valve stenosis. The gradient across the pulmonary valve was 75 mm. Hg. Note the post-stenotic dilatation of the main pulmonary artery and the somewhat oligaemic lung fields. (*Film by courtesy of Dr. Basil Strickland.*)

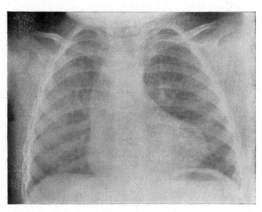

Fig. 388. Fallot's tetralogy. The uptilted apex of the heart and the prominent concavity on the left border of the heart have produced the typical 'cœur en sabot' appearance. (*Film by courtesy of Dr. Basil Strickland.*)

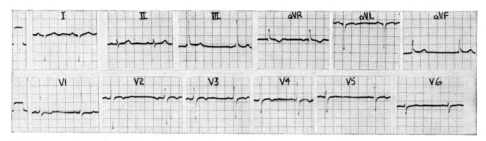

Fig. 389. Electrocardiogram in Fallot's tetralogy. Considerable right ventricular hypertrophy is present, manifested by right-axis deviation (axis + 150°) and the dominant R wave in Lead V1. The T wave is inverted in Leads V1–4 and there is considerable clockwise rotation. Note the half-standardization in the chest leads.

the pulmonary stenosis and not, or hardly at all, by the ventricular septal defect. This is proved by the disappearance of the murmur in cases of infundibular stenosis in which the degree of obstruction may suddenly increase with a reduction in pulmonary blood-flow, increase in the veno-arterial shunt, and deepening of cyanosis. The murmur is heard in the pulmonary area and differs from that of pure pulmonary stenosis only in that it is a good deal shorter. The second sound is single and an ejection sound which probably arises from the overriding aorta is often present.

The radiograph often shows the classic 'cœur en sabot' appearance with the apex of the heart appearing to be tilted upwards. There is a concavity in the region of the main pulmonary artery and the lung fields are oligaemic (*Fig.* 388). Right

Tricuspid incompetence is most often due to dilatation of the valve ring secondary to severe pulmonary hypertension or stenosis. It is often seen, transiently or permanently, in cases of chronic rheumatic heart disease with mitral and aortic valve disease. The jugular venous pulse shows a tall systolic wave in severe cases and a pansystolic murmur may be heard at the lower left sternal edge. This murmur may become louder during inspiration but this feature is not easy to elicit. Tricuspid stenosis is nearly always rheumatic and is often accompanied by some incompetence. In sinus rhythm a tall a wave is seen in the venous pulse and tricuspid presystolic and delayed diastolic murmurs with an opening snap may be heard. In practice it is often difficult to identify these if, as is commonly the case, mitral valve disease is present as well, and it may be necessary to perform cardiac catheterization to demonstrate a gradient across the tricuspid valve.

A rare cause of tricuspid, and also of pulmonary, valve lesions is *carcinoid heart disease*. This occurs in association with large hepatic metastases from a carcinoid tumour of the small bowel. A layer of fibrous tissue is laid down over the endocardium of the right atrium and ventricle and over the tricuspid and pulmonary valves. Whether this is due directly to the excess of circulating 5-hydroxytryptamine is not clear. Another rare cause of acquired pulmonary stenosis is compression of the pulmonary artery or right ventricular outflow tract by a tumour.

III. GENERALIZED ENLARGEMENT OF THE HEART

Any of the causes of left ventricular enlargement may, in time, cause enlargement of the right ventricle also to produce generalized cardiac enlargement. This is, perhaps, most striking in chronic rheumatic heart disease, the components and complications of which have already been discussed. It must be remembered that in such cases, in severe failure, the murmurs of valvular disease may be unobtrusive and it is, for example, quite possible to miss severe aortic stenosis in a large failing heart; a loud murmur may have become almost inaudible as a result of the markedly reduced stroke volume. This section will be concerned with conditions which, by involving the myocardium as a whole, cause generalized cardiac enlargement *ab initio*.

By far the most important disorder of the myocardium is *ischaemia*. The brunt falls on the left ventricle on account of the greater pressure it must generate; indeed significant ischaemia of the right ventricle is almost unknown unless its work load has been increased by severe pulmonary hypertension or stenosis. The diagnosis will usually be clear as most patients will have had a history of angina with or without one or more attacks of myocardial infarction. Rarely no such history is given and chronic ischaemic fibrosis, progressing insidiously, may cause cardiac failure as the first clear manifestation. The symptoms are such as might be expected; progressive dyspnoea, perhaps with orthopnoea, and, later, congestive heart failure are common. The impulse at the apex, which is displaced, is unremarkable and gallop rhythm is common. A systolic murmur of mitral incompetence, due either to dilatation of the ventricle or to papillary muscle insufficiency, may be heard. The chest radiograph shows cardiac enlargement and evidence of pulmonary venous congestion only and is of little value in differential diagnosis unless there is evidence of a left ventricular aneurysm. The electrocardiogram is also not as helpful as might have been expected, as it may be very difficult to distinguish ischaemic changes in the RS–T segment and T wave from those due to other myocardial diseases. Even the pathological Q wave of infarction is not completely reliable as a similar appearance can be seen in some types of cardiomyopathy. If an aetiological diagnosis must be made, and this would rarely be the case in this clinical situation, there may be no alternative to coronary angiography.

Thyrotoxicosis can cause generalized cardiac enlargement but this is rarely a prominent feature in primary Graves's disease in young people. In such cases the diagnosis is usually straightforward, being made on such clinical features as heat intolerance, weight-loss despite a good appetite, sweating, tachycardia, tremor, and exophthalmos. A more difficult diagnostic problem is posed in the older patient in whom the symptoms and signs are much less florid. Not infrequently such patients present with unexplained cardiac failure and no other clinical evidence of thyrotoxicosis. Almost always they have atrial fibrillation and, in this situation, estimation of serum thyroxine and other investigations are essential as this is one of the few varieties of reversible myocardial disease.

The cardiac enlargement produced by *myxoedema*, which may be partly due to a pericardial effusion, is also reversible to some extent. The diagnosis is made either immediately or only after a long delay and it is important to bear this possibility in mind. Suggestive physical signs include a dry, cold skin, bradycardia, and a strikingly slow relaxation of the tendon reflexes. The electrocardiogram shows low-voltage complexes and flat or inverted T waves in all leads. The changes are quickly reversed with thyroxine, the heart size and the electrocardiogram returning to normal (*Fig. 390*).

The development of *atrial fibrillation*, which is common in many varieties of heart disease, often causes the heart to enlarge or any pre-existing enlargement to increase. Occasionally 'lone' atrial fibrillation with no known aetiology can, after many years, cause, or at least be associated with, cardiac enlargement which may be gross.

There are numerous types of congestive cardiomyopathy, nearly all of which cause cardiac enlargement. The term 'congestive' is used to distinguish them from the obstructive variety which has been described above. The heart is usually very large with gallop rhythm. Arrhythmias are common and the electrocardiogram usually shows non-specific changes in the RS–T segment and T wave associated with intraventricular conduction defects. Almost all are irreversible with the exception of that due to vitamin-B_1 deficiency (*beriberi*); the dramatic response to aneurin in this condition is the definitive diagnostic test. The cardiac enlargement of severe *anaemia* is also reversible with treatment, and in *alcoholic* cardiomyopathy some reduction in heart size may occur with total abstention. Space does not permit a full list of the types of cardiomyopathy but a somewhat loose classification into broad groups is possible. *Familial* cardiomyopathy may be non-specific but within this group can be included cardiac involvement in *Friedreich's ataxia*, various *muscular dystrophies*, and *mucopolysaccharidoses.* A *metabolic* group overlaps with the familial types to include infiltration of the myocardium in *haemochromatosis,* type II *glycogenosis* (Pompe's disease), and cardiac *amyloidosis.* Alcoholic cardiomyopathy and beriberi to many agents ranging from emetine and antimony to such exotic poisons as *Argemone mexicana* and the sting of *Tityrus trinitatis,* a West Indian scorpion. Within the *endocrine* group, thyrotoxicosis and myxoedema have already been

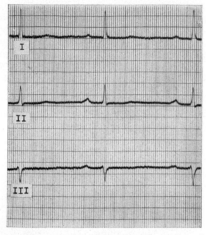 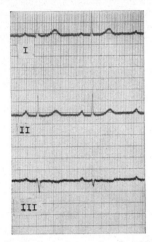

Fig. 390. Electrocardiogram in myxoedema. Note the bradycardia and low or flat T waves in the record on the left. The record on the right, 3 weeks after beginning treatment with thyroid extract, has reverted to normal. Time marker 0·1 and 0·02 second.

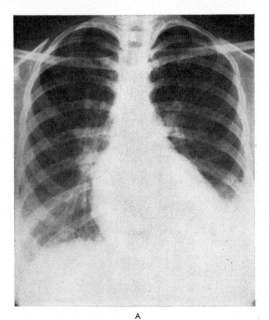

discussed and *acromegaly* should be added. *Endomyocardial fibrosis,* already mentioned as a cause of mitral incompetence, is difficult to classify but is an important cause of cardiac enlargement and failure in parts of Africa. It must not be confused with the similarly named *endocardial fibroelastosis,* a disease seen throughout the world, particularly in infants and children but occasionally also in adults (*Fig.* 391). Finally, it must be

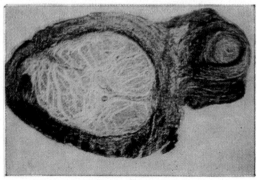

A   B

Fig. 391. Female, aged 35, with severe congestive cardiac failure. No cause for the failure could be found clinically. A, The radiograph shows no diagnostic features. At autopsy endocardial fibro-elastosis was found. B, A cross-section of a left ventricular trabecula is shown; the endocardium is grossly thickened and contains much elastic tissue (stained black).

have been mentioned and can be included with the myocardial lesion of potassium depletion in a *nutritional* type. The *toxic* group includes myocardial damage by a wide variety of drugs and poisons. The lesion may be due to a specific hypersensitivity, for example to sulphonamides, or the damage may be dose-dependent and due admitted that the largest group is one in which no definite aetiology can be found and to which the unsatisfactory label *non-specific non-familial cardiomyopathy* is applied.

Myocarditis would be included, by some authorities, as an inflammatory type of cardiomyopathy. Within this group are such conditions as the cardiac lesions of *systemic lupus erythematosus* and *rheumatoid* disease, *granulomatous* or giant-cell myocarditis which is possibly an allergic manifestation, and the inflammatory infiltration and necrosis of the myocardium seen in a few cases of *myasthenia gravis*, often in association with a malignant thymoma. Myocarditis can also be caused by a large variety of organisms. Protozoa include *Trypanosoma cruzi*, the cause of Chagas' disease, a common variety of heart disease in parts of South America, and *Toxoplasma gondii*. Myocarditis is probably not uncommon as a relatively benign complication of viral infections. Occasionally, however, especially in infancy, serious, even lethal, myocardial damage may occur. In man the viruses known definitely to cause myocarditis are Coxsackie B and some strains of poliovirus. Bacterial and rickettsial myocarditis can also occur.

IV. PERICARDIAL DISEASE

Pericardial disease *per se* does not cause cardiac enlargement but the enlarged heart shadow in the radiograph produced by a pericardial effusion may be confused with that due to enlargement of the heart itself (*Fig*. 392). The clinical differentiation has been discussed above (pp. 137, 365) and depends on the delineation of the cardiac outline

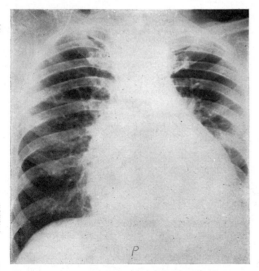

Fig. 392. Large pericardial and left pleural effusions due to carcinoma of the bronchus. The rather clear outline of the heart shadow is suggestive of effusion but the diagnosis cannot be made for certain on the evidence of this radiograph. (*Film by courtesy of Dr. Basil Strickland.*)

by percussion. A definitive diagnosis can almost always be made by echocardiography. If the effusion is under a low pressure there are no other signs. A high-pressure effusion produces cardiac tamponade with a small paradoxical arterial pulse, a low blood-pressure, and a raised venous pressure which rises further on inspiration (Kussmaul's sign). Similar signs are also seen in constrictive pericarditis, with the addition

of a rather high-pitched third sound at the lower left sternal border; hepatomegaly, dependent oedema, and ascites are also common. The differentiation from congestive cardiac failure and hepatic cirrhosis may be difficult. One point of value in the diagnosis of constrictive pericarditis is the normal or near-normal heart size; in cardiac failure the heart is almost always enlarged. A definite diagnosis can be made if pericardial calcification is seen in the radiograph. A syndrome resembling constrictive pericarditis may be seen in some varieties of cardiomyopathy such as that due to amyloid infiltration in which the constrictive process, preventing adequate ventricular filling, occurs within the myocardium itself. This type of cardiomyopathy is sometimes referred to as 'restrictive'.

P. R. Fleming.

HEART IMPULSE, DISPLACED

The most important cause of displacement of the apex beat is cardiac enlargement which has been discussed in the section on HEART, ENLARGEMENT OF (p. 365). The normal position of the apex beat and the method of localization are also described in that section. Marked displacement to the left implies ventricular dilatation due either to a lesion which increases the stroke volume of one or both ventricles or to cardiac failure from any cause. This section will be concerned with displacement of the apex beat due to displacement of the heart as a whole.

The heart may be displaced by skeletal deformities. In *pectus excavatum* the anteroposterior diameter of the thorax is reduced so that the heart, compressed between the sternum and the spine, is expanded laterally; in gross cases the heart moves, as a whole, to the left. In either case the cause is obvious clinically (*Fig*. 393). Cardiac function is almost always normal with pectus excavatum. This is not the case with *kyphoscoliosis*, another skeletal cause of displacement of the heart, in which respiratory insufficiency may cause sufficient hypoxia to lead to cor pulmonale. The displacement of the heart in this condition is usually into the concavity of the scoliosis (*Fig*. 394).

Displacement of the apex beat is a feature of some diagnostic importance in four important pathological processes which may affect the lungs; deviation of the trachea is often present in addition. *Collapse* of a lobe or, more dramatically, of a whole lung reduces the volume of the tissues on that side of the chest so that the heart is drawn towards the lesion (*Figs*. 395, 396). Collapse of a lobe, implying occlusion of a bronchus, should always suggest the possibility of carcinoma of the bronchus. Supporting evidence might be provided by a history of cigarette-smoking, cough with, frequently, haemoptysis, and finger-clubbing. Bronchoscopy is mandatory and, if the occlusion is of a major bronchus, will often confirm the diagnosis. However, it must be emphasized that a negative bronchoscopy does not exclude a carcinoma. Collapse may also be due to other bronchial tumours such as adenoma; haemoptysis is common in this condition also. Intrabronchial foreign body must not be forgotten as a cause of bronchial occlusion and lobar collapse. The paroxysm of coughing which must have occurred at the time the foreign body was inhaled is forgotten by a surprisingly large number of patients and absence of such a history by no means excludes the diagnosis. Following

abdominal or thoracic surgery, respiration is inhibited by pain and a bronchus may become occluded by a plug of mucus to produce collapse of a lobe or of the whole lung (*Fig.* 397). The diagnosis should present little difficulty as the

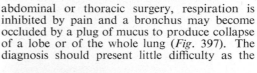

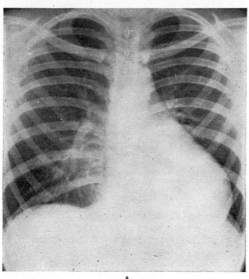

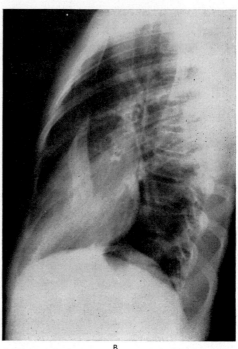

<table>
<tr><td>A</td><td>B</td></tr>
</table>

Fig. 393. Pectus excavatum. A, The heart is compressed anteroposteriorly so that it appears to be enlarged in the posteroanterior film. B, The sternal depression is clearly visible in the lateral film. (*Films by courtesy of Dr. Basil Strickland.*)

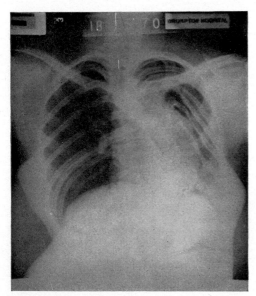

Fig. 394. Gross scoliosis. The heart is displaced to the right, into the concavity of the scoliosis. (*Film by courtesy of Dr. Basil Strickland.*)

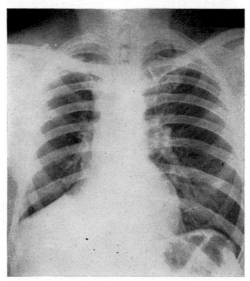

Fig. 395. Collapse of right, middle, and lower lobes with slight, but definite, displacement of the heart to the right. (*Film by courtesy of Dr. Basil Strickland.*)

displacement of the apex beat, and of the trachea, is considerable. Breath-sounds on the affected side are either absent or, more often, reduced; herniation of the opposite lung is responsible for such breath-sounds as may be heard.

The traction exerted by *fibrosis* of the lung may also cause mediastinal displacement. Fibrosis may be due to chronic tuberculosis or occur in association with bronchiectasis or chronic lung abscess. Bilateral fibrosis, as in pneumoconiosis, is unlikely to produce displacement of the apex beat unless it is much more marked on one side. Lesser degrees of fibrosis produce no detectable mediastinal displacement but may distort

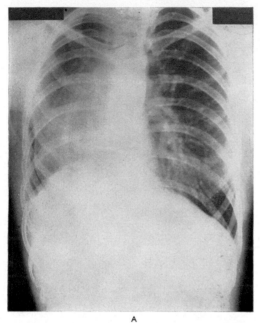

A

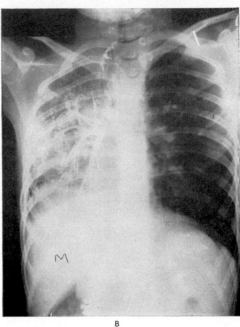

B

Fig. 396. A, Gross displacement of heart to the right as a result of collapse of right upper lobe; this was due to tuberculous bronchial stenosis. B, In the bronchogram only the lower and middle lobe bronchi are filled and are displaced upwards as these lobes have expanded to occupy the whole right hemithorax. (*Films by courtesy of Dr. Basil Strickland.*)

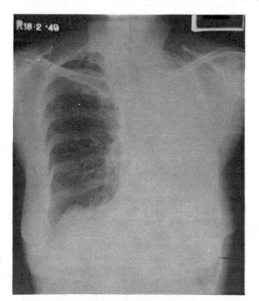

Fig. 397. Collapse of the whole of the left lung, as a result of an intrabronchial mucous plug, in an asthmatic. (*Film by courtesy of Dr. Basil Strickland.*)

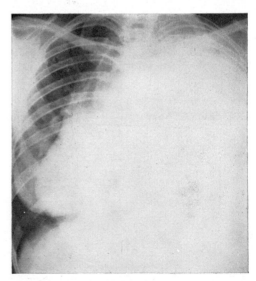

Fig. 398. Very large left pleural effusion causing gross displacement of the heart and trachea to the right. (*Film by courtesy of Dr. Basil Strickland.*)

mediastinal structures such as the pulmonary arteries; this may be visible in the X-ray.

Displacement of the heart away from the affected side occurs with *pneumothorax*. This is not very marked unless the pneumothorax is under tension due to a valvular mechanism at the pleural leak (*Fig.* 258, p. 241). Associated cardiac failure and the nephrotic syndrome, pleural effusion is common but, as it is nearly always bilateral, mediastinal displacement does not occur.

Less common causes of displacement of the apex beat include *hypoplasia of the lung* (*Fig.* 399)

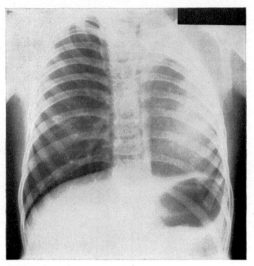

Fig. 399. Agenesis of left lung. The radiolucent area on the left is due to herniated right lung. The heart is markedly displaced to the left. (*Film by courtesy of Dr. Basil Strickland.*)

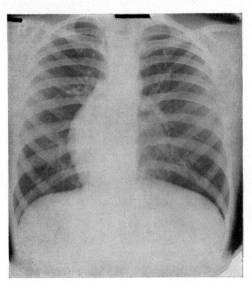

Fig. 400. Rotation of heart around its vertical axis—pivotal dextrocardia—in association with multiple congenital cardiac anomalies. (*Film by courtesy of Dr. Basil Strickland.*)

physical signs include a hyper-resonant percussion note, diminution in breath-sounds and in vocal fremitus and resonance, and, very occasionally, the 'coin' sound or 'bruit d'airain'. In young adults, among whom males predominate, the cause is usually rupture of a small subpleural bleb. Over the age of 40 spontaneous pneumothorax is more often due to emphysema or to one of the numerous varieties of localized or generalized pulmonary fibrosis. The only pulmonary tumours to cause a pneumothorax at all commonly are metastases from osteogenic sarcoma or other connective-tissue tumour. In infancy the thin-walled abscesses of staphylococcal pneumonia may rupture into the pleura or the clinical picture of a tension pneumothorax may be simulated by distension of one of the cavities to form a *tension cyst*.

The fourth common condition in which the apex beat may be displaced is *pleural effusion*; as in pneumothorax the displacement is away from the side of the lesion. Stony dullness with absent breath-sounds and, perhaps, aegophony at the upper level of dullness will confirm the diagnosis (*Fig.* 398). Among the numerous causes of pleural effusion are bacterial, but not mycoplasmal, pneumonia, pulmonary infarction, primary or secondary tumours of the lung, tuberculosis, lung abscess, and connective-tissue diseases such as systemic lupus erythematosus. In conditions causing generalized fluid retention, such as

and large *diaphragmatic hernia*. Very little acumen is required to recognize massive *ascites* or abdominal swelling from other causes and previous *pneumonectomy* as causes of displacement of the apex beat.

The apex beat may be impalpable due to gross obesity, to emphysema, or to pericardial effusion. Before concluding that one of these conditions is the cause of one's inability to feel the cardiac impulse, it is wise to palpate the right side of the chest. *Dextrocardia* is rare and, usually, unimportant but it is embarrassing to miss it. Mirror-image dextrocardia is nearly always associated with total situs inversus and the heart is normal; Kartagener's syndrome, consisting of bronchiectasis, rudimentary or absent frontal sinuses, and situs inversus, is worth remembering in this context. If the abdominal viscera are normally located in the presence of dextrocardia (isolated dextrocardia), congenital heart disease is nearly always present, most commonly transposition of the great arteries. The other viscera are normal also in pivotal dextrocardia in which the heart is rotated around its vertical axis; the heart is usually abnormal in other respects (*Fig.* 400).

A rare congenital lesion causing displacement of the apex beat is *congenital absence of the pericardium*. The heart is abnormally mobile and the position of the apex beat varies markedly with the position of the patient.

P. R. Fleming.

HEART-SOUNDS, ACCENTUATION AND DIMINUTION OF

The first heart-sound is produced by closure of the mitral and tricuspid valves. The tricuspid component is softer than the mitral and is barely audible at the apex. The second sound, due to aortic and pulmonary valve closure, is best heard in the second right and left intercostal spaces close to the sternum. At the apex only the aortic sound is normally audible. The two components of the second sound are identified not only by the areas in which they are best heard but also by their relationship to each other and changes in this due to respiration (*see* HEART-SOUNDS, SPLITTING; TRIPLE RHYTHM, p. 383).

Too much emphasis has been placed in the past on soft heart-sounds, and the term 'poor quality' applied to the heart-sounds, carrying with it the implication of a poor-quality myocardium, cannot be too strongly condemned. Much the commonest cause of heart-sounds which are softer than normal is the interposition of a thick layer of tissue between the heart and the stethoscope. Thus, all the heart-sounds are soft in obesity and emphysema; another, less common but more serious, cause of heart-sounds of reduced intensity is pericardial effusion.

The intensity of the *Mitral First Sound*, at the apex, is related to the position of the valve cusps at the onset of left ventricular systole. The farther the cusps are apart at this time the louder the sound produced. Thus, if atrial systole precedes ventricular by a short interval only, as when the P–R interval is short or as may happen by chance frequently if complete heart-block is present, the cusps have no sooner been flung wide apart by atrial systole than they are closed again by the contraction of the ventricle and a loud first sound is heard. If the interval between atrial and ventricular systole is long, as in first-degree heart block or, as a random occurrence, in complete heart block, the cusps of the valve will have floated towards a mid-position after having been wide open during rapid ventricular filling and the first sound will be soft. In high-output states such as thyrotoxicosis, severe anaemia, fever, and anxiety, the first sound is loud and this is probably due to the cusps being held open by the large atrioventricular flow continuing throughout diastole, which is itself abbreviated by the associated tachycardia. In contrast, in hypovolaemic states with, necessarily, a low cardiac output, atrioventricular filling is over very early in diastole and a soft first heart-sound is common. Also, if the heart-rate is very slow for any reason, ventricular filling may be over long before the end of the long diastole and the first heart-sound may be rather soft. The first sound is strikingly loud in mitral stenosis, in which the pressure gradient across the mitral valve may persist throughout diastole and the cusps be held apart until the onset of ventricular systole. Another factor of importance in increasing the intensity of the first sound in mitral stenosis is the structure of the stenosed valve itself; a loud sound generally implies that the substance of the cusps has remained fairly pliable. In mitral stenosis complicated by atrial fibrillation the first sound is usually louder after the shorter diastoles, at the end of which the atrioventricular pressure gradient is still considerable; this is not, however, always the case. The first sound in mitral stenosis, apart from being loud, is rather characteristically short and high-pitched and slightly delayed; it has much the same quality as the opening snap which also is related to the anatomical state of the valve cusps. Indeed, the first sound in mitral stenosis has sometimes been called a 'closing snap'. While not in itself diagnostic, a first sound of this intensity and quality should prompt a more than usually careful search for other evidence of mitral stenosis.

The *Aortic Second Sound* is heard best in the second right interspace close to the sternum but is also easily audible elsewhere in the precordium. The commonest cause of accentuation of this sound is systemic hypertension in which it is, of course, of no diagnostic importance; hypertension may be suspected on hearing a loud aortic second sound but the diagnosis can only be made by sphygmomanometry. Dilatation of the ascending aorta, even in the absence of hypertension and whether aneurysmal or not, can also cause accentuation of the second sound; the sound has a rather striking ringing quality and has been called the *bruit de tabourka*—a tabourka being an Algerian drum. Hypovolaemia, or hypotension from any cause, can produce diminution in the intensity of the aortic second sound. The aortic second sound is also characteristically soft in calcific aortic stenosis and may indeed be absent in severe cases. This does not apply in congenital aortic valve stenosis when the aortic valve has not yet begun to thicken or calcify; in this condition aortic valve closure is well heard. The second sound is rather soft, however, in membranous subvalvular aortic stenosis. In mitral incompetence it may be extremely difficult to hear the second (aortic) sound at the apex as the pansystolic murmur runs up to and past it; it is clearly audible, however, at the base of the heart in such cases.

The *Pulmonary Second Sound* is heard best in the second and third left interspaces close to the sternum and accentuation of this sound is a feature of pulmonary hypertension from any cause. As pulmonary valve closure is normally inaudible at the apex beat the pulmonary component is certainly accentuated if two second sounds can be heard at this site. As the pulmonary artery is closely related to the anterior chest wall an accentuated pulmonary second sound may be palpable in the second left interspace as a soft tap immediately succeeding right ventricular systole which, in the presence of pulmonary hypertension, is itself palpable as a left parasternal heave. It is therefore sometimes possible to conclude, from palpation alone, not only that right ventricular hypertrophy is present but that it is probably due to pulmonary hypertension. The causes of pulmonary hypertension include mitral stenosis, cor pulmonale, and congenital arteriovenous shunts, and are discussed in detail in the section on HEART, ENLARGEMENT OF (p. 365). The pulmonary artery is partly covered by the upper lobe of the left lung and fibrosis with contraction of this region may occasionally uncover the pulmonary artery so that the second sound is heard more clearly. Diminution in the intensity of the pulmonary second sound is a feature of severe pulmonary valve stenosis. In Fallot's tetralogy and pulmonary atresia the pulmonary second sound is absent.

Both components of the second sound are rather loud in children in the second and third left interspaces. This is probably due only to the rather thin chest wall.

P. R. Fleming.

HEART-SOUNDS, SPLITTING; TRIPLE RHYTHM

Some definitions of the terms to be used in this section are necessary. The term 'splitting' refers to the first and second heart-sounds. Each has two components, from the left and right sides of the heart, and when both of these components—for example the sounds of aortic and pulmonary valve closure—are clearly audible, that sound is said to be split. The smallest degree of splitting which is detectable by the trained observer is about 0·01 second. 'Triple rhythm' is sometimes used as if it were synonymous with 'gallop rhythm', but this practice is not recommended as the term 'gallop rhythm' has acquired a special significance of its own and, to many physicians, implies serious ventricular disease. In clinical practice there is little need to use the term 'triple rhythm' but it is convenient, if only for classification purposes, to have a term which covers all situations in which three separate sounds can be heard in each cardiac cycle. It is in that sense that 'triple rhythm' is used here.

Sounds are normally produced by the heart valves when they close; in certain pathological states sounds may also be heard at the time of valve-opening. In addition, sounds may be produced at the two moments in the cycle at which atrioventricular flow is rapid, that is during atrial systole and just after the opening of the atrioventricular valves. These sounds probably arise mainly from vibrations in the cusps of the atrioventricular valves and in their attached chordae tendineae and papillary muscles, although other structures may also be involved (*Fig.* 401).

The mitral valve closes fractionally before the tricuspid and both components of the first sound can be heard normally, particularly in the tricuspid area. Wide splitting might have been expected in right bundle branch block but this is, in fact, not common except in the rare Ebstein's syndrome. Splitting of the first sound must be distinguished from two other situations in which added sounds are present close to the first sound in time. These are the ejection clicks and atrial sounds.

The commonest source of confusion is an ejection sound or click, produced at the time of semilunar-valve opening. This follows the first sound by about 0·07 second and can arise from either side of the heart (*Fig.* 401 b). An aortic ejection click is well heard at the apex, at the left border of the sternum, and in the aortic area, and is present most often in association with dilatation of the ascending aorta, although the mechanism is not clear. Thus it is a feature of hypertension and coarctation of the aorta. In congenital aortic valve stenosis a loud ejection click is also common and, in this case, it is due to vibrations of the valve itself; this is confirmed by the fact that the click is not heard if the valve is calcified. Similar considerations apply to the pulmonary ejection click which is loudest in the second and third left interspaces near the sternum and is common in pulmonary hypertension and in mild pulmonary valve stenosis. A pulmonary ejection click is not common in atrial septal defect despite marked dilatation of the pulmonary artery but it may appear after closure of the defect. Systolic clicks may also be heard well after semilunar-valve opening; the mechanism is not clear. They are usually benign but a click may sometimes be audible just before the late systolic murmur occasionally heard in mitral incompetence.

An atrial sound, preceding the first sound, implies a powerful atrial systole and rapid ventricular filling resulting therefrom (*Fig.* 401a). This sound is also called the fourth heart-sound but this seems a rather inappropriate term as it is, in fact, the earliest sound in the cycle. Atrial systole is more than normally powerful if the corresponding ventricle is burdened by a large work load; the increased end-diastolic stretch of the ventricular fibres increases the force of ventricular contraction. A left atrial sound is heard therefore, at the apex, in hypertensive heart disease and aortic valve disease. It is also a well-recognized feature of ischaemic heart disease, especially after myocardial infarction; there is no absolute increase in left ventricular work in this situation but rather a reduced amount of myocardium striving to maintain a normal cardiac output. A right atrial sound may be heard at the lower end of the sternum in pulmonary hypertension and pulmonary stenosis. Atrial 'sounds' are often easily palpable and may, in fact, be more easily felt than heard. The term 'gallop rhythm' is appropriate here and an atrial gallop implies severe ventricular overload but not failure, in the strict sense of the word. An atrial sound is also heard if the P–R interval is prolonged but this, of course, is of much less serious significance and it is inadvisable to use the term 'gallop' in this situation.

Closure of the aortic and pulmonary valves signals the end of ventricular ejection, and the timing of the two components of the second heart-sound is therefore a reliable clinical measure of the duration of left and right ventricular systole. Ventricular systole is prolonged by a large stroke volume, by outflow tract obstruction, and by failure; both the onset and the end of ventricular systole are delayed in bundle branch block.

Aortic valve closure normally precedes pulmonary by a brief interval; this interval is longer

branch block causes very wide splitting of the second sound with further widening on inspiration (*Fig.* 402 c). In pulmonary hypertension right ventricular systole is not prolonged unless right ventricular failure occurs, so that wide splitting is not a feature of this condition until late in the course of the disease.

Delay in aortic valve closure may cause the aortic second sound to follow the pulmonary. If this is the case, the normal behaviour of the

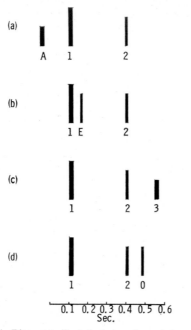

Fig. 401. Diagram to illustrate timing of sounds in cardiac cycle. I and 2, First and second heart-sounds; A, Atrial sound; E, Ejection sound or click; 3, Third sound; O, Opening snap.

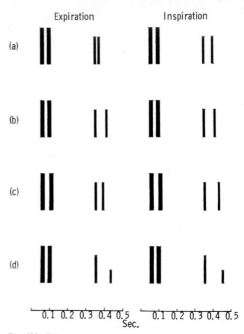

Fig. 402. Diagram to illustrate the behaviour of the second heart-sound during respiration. a, The normal increased splitting on inspiration is shown. b, The wide, fixed splitting found in atrial septal defect is illustrated. c, The wide splitting, with further widening on inspiration, found in right bundle branch block is shown; the slight increase in the splitting of the first heart-sound should also be noted. d, The behaviour of the second sound in pulmonary stenosis is shown; the wide splitting is due to the late pulmonary component which is diminished in intensity.

during inspiration when the fall in intrathoracic pressure increases the venous return and hence the right ventricular stroke volume. Splitting of the second sound which is more marked on inspiration is, therefore, a normal finding, well heard in the second and third left interspaces; it is particularly obvious in children (*Fig.* 402 a). If the right ventricular stroke volume is very much increased, compared with the left, as with an atrial septal defect, wide splitting of the second sound results. Inspiration increases left ventricular filling by reducing the flow across the defect; hence right and left ventricular systole are affected equally by respiration and the splitting is 'fixed' (*Fig.* 402 b). The prolongation of right ventricular systole due to pulmonary stenosis also delays pulmonary valve closure so that wide splitting of the second sound is a feature of this condition; as the pulmonary second sound becomes very soft or inaudible with severe pulmonary stenosis the sign can only be elicited in cases of not more than moderate severity (*Fig.* 402 d). The delay in right ventricular activation due to right bundle

pulmonary second sound with inspiration will cause the two components to become closer together. Splitting of the second sound which is more marked during *expiration*, known as 'paradoxical' or 'reversed splitting', is, therefore, a sign of delayed aortic valve closure. Thus paradoxical splitting is a feature of left ventricular outflow tract obstruction as in aortic stenosis and hypertrophic obstructive cardiomyopathy (*Fig.* 403 c), of left bundle branch block (*Fig.* 403 b), and of persistent ductus arteriosus in which the left ventricular stroke volume greatly exceeds that of the right ventricle. It is also found in left ventricular failure from any cause. Abnormalities in the second heart-sound, particularly paradoxical splitting, may be difficult to elicit with certainty and a well-known author has described the pulmonary area, where splitting is best heard, as 'the area of auscultatory romance'.

There is enough truth in this to emphasize the need for great caution in the interpretation of these auscultatory findings.

In mitral incompetence the behaviour of the second sound varies with the state of the left ventricle. Aortic valve closure may be abnormally early, producing wider than normal splitting

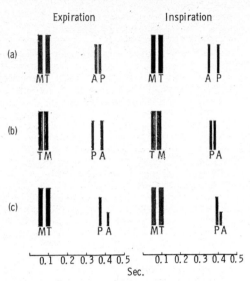

Fig. 403. Diagram to illustrate paradoxical splitting of the second heart-sound. M, T, A, and P refer to closure of the mitral, tricuspid, aortic, and pulmonary valves respectively. a, The normal situation is shown. b, The delay in mitral and aortic valve closure is due to left bundle branch block. c, The soft, delayed, aortic second sound of aortic stenosis is shown. In b and c the normal prolongation of right ventricular systole during inspiration causes the second sound to be less widely split at this time.

but, if left ventricular systole is prolonged by failure, the splitting may become normal or even paradoxical. Early aortic valve closure with wide splitting of the second sound is also a feature of ventricular septal defect.

The opening snap of the mitral valve is occasionally confused with wide splitting of the second sound if, as is sometimes the case, it is well heard in the third left interspace (*Fig.* 401 d). It is, however, appreciably later than a delayed component of the second sound and is usually most easily heard at, and just medial to, the apex. Its presence suggests that one at least of the mitral cusps is pliable and it is often associated with a loud first sound. The closer the snap is to the second sound the higher the pressure in the left atrium at the time of mitral opening and the more severe the stenosis. The presence of a snap does not exclude mitral incompetence and it may be audible, though rarely, even when the latter lesion is dominant. Tricuspid stenosis may be associated with an opening snap heard at the tricuspid area and a little to the right of the xiphoid.

A third heart-sound, occurring at the time of rapid atrioventricular flow following mitral- and tricuspid-valve opening, is commonly heard in

normal children and adolescents and in a few young adults (*Fig.* 401 c). In such cases it is of no significance. In older patients its presence at the apex implies that left atrial pressure is high at this time due either to a large atrioventricular flow as in mitral incompetence, ventricular septal defect, persistent ductus, and high-output states, or, if these conditions can be excluded, to left ventricular failure. In that case the term 'diastolic gallop rhythm' may be used; in the other situations the simple expression 'third heart-sound' is to be preferred. A diastolic gallop may be heard over the right ventricle if that chamber is failing; in constrictive pericarditis also a rather characteristically high-pitched third sound is heard over the right ventricle.

The term 'summation gallop' is used when the heart-rate is so rapid that an added sound in diastole cannot be certainly identified as either a diastolic or an atrial gallop sound. It nearly always implies severe heart failure.

P. R. Fleming.

HEARTBURN

In Hebrew, Greek, and other ancient languages, the same word was used both for the stomach and for the heart. Thus the Greek word 'cardialgia' appears to have referred both to precordial pain and to gastric disorders. This double meaning has been perpetuated in the use, by some writers, of 'cardialgia' as a synonym for 'heartburn', which is thus regarded as a sensation felt in the region of the cardia (heart) as a result of a disorder of the cardia (stomach). In practice the term 'heartburn' has come to be applied to one of a group of symptoms collectively referred to by patients as 'indigestion'. Such a complaint requires detailed and precise analysis as, apart from heartburn, it may include epigastric discomfort or pain, eructation of gas, nausea, and vomiting.

Most often a complaint of heartburn implies a burning, tight sensation felt in the region of the xiphisternum and radiating upwards to the neck. This sensation is intermittent over a period of several minutes and varies in severity from a mild feeling of warmth to a discomfort severe enough to be described as pain. Excessive salivation may occur in association with heartburn, but this must not be confused with water-brash which is the sudden accumulation of large amounts of clear, watery saliva in the mouth; this occurs, rather uncommonly, in association with duodenal ulcer.

It seems certain that the sensation of heartburn always originates in the lower oesophagus and that it is due to the regurgitation of gastric contents; whether it is due to the effect of acid on the oesophageal mucosa or to muscular spasm, or to both, is not clear. Heartburn may be confused with angina if only on account of its localization but, in typical cases, the accounts of the two sensations are very different. Other varieties

13

of oesophageal pain, however, may simulate angina more closely.

The most clearly identified, but by no means the most common, cause of heartburn is reflux oesophagitis due to hiatus hernia of the sliding type. Initially the discomfort is felt only after heavy meals and is brought on by lying down or bending forward; relief may be obtained by sitting or standing up, by drinking any bland fluid, or by antacids. Later, when the oesophagitis is established, the pain is more easily provoked, lasts longer, and dysphagia may develop. At this stage it is no longer possible to describe the sensation as heartburn. Haemorrhage from the inflamed oesophageal mucosa or from the herniated stomach is common and severe hypochromic anaemia may result. It must be remembered, however, that hiatus hernia is frequently demonstrated radiologically as an incidental finding and gastro-intestinal haemorrhage should not be attributed to this cause until all other possibilities have been excluded.

Heartburn may occur in healthy individuals as a result of dietary indiscretions or of overindulgence in tobacco or alcohol. It is also a feature of many other varieties of indigestion and, by itself, is of no differential diagnostic significance. Patients with duodenal ulcer commonly complain of heartburn and it may occur in association with gall-bladder disease, as a result of gastric irritation by various drugs, or in psychogenic dyspepsia, especially when it is associated with aerophagy.

See also CHEST, PAIN IN (p. 133).

P. R. Fleming.

HEEL, PAIN IN

Pain in the heel may be troublesome and persistent without any adequate cause for it being found; children often limp from it and yet one may find little wrong; the cause is then usually either the effect of some forgotten injury or strain or else a thorn or other foreign body; in older people a cause that needs bearing in mind is calcification of the posterior end of the long plantar ligament forming a spine on the undersurface of the calcaneus, productive of continued and troublesome pain in the centre of the under part of the heel, the diagnosis depending on detection of this spine with radiographs (*Fig.* 515, p. 499). There are other causes, however, the chief of which are as follows:

The effect of constant jarring of the heel, as from walking on hard roads
Cornification of the skin
Chilblain of the heel
Pressure soreness over the tendo Achillis from boot, shoe, or legging
Bursitis between the tendo Achillis and the calcaneus
Injury:
    Tearing of ligament fibres below the internal or external malleolus, or of the long plantar ligament

    Tearing of ligament fibres near the insertion of the tendo Achillis
    Cracking or fracture of calcaneus
    Detachment of hinder end of the astragalus
    Bruising of periosteum of the calcaneus
Fasciitis
Periostitis of the calcaneus
Ankylosing spondylitis
Reiter's disease
Tuberculous caries of the calcaneus
Foreign body, such as pin, needle, thorn
Sarcoma of the calcaneus.

The differential diagnosis depends on obtaining a clear history of how the pain began, exactly where it is, and what produces it; on inspection of the part for local discoloration or swelling; on palpation, to locate the precise site of the pain, and particularly of any tenderness, especially if the latter is increased by movement; and on the results of radiographic examination of the part for fracture, caries, foreign body, or spine.

Constant *jarring* of the heel such as may be produced by walking in thin shoes on hard roads, or by occupations which involve the use of the foot on vibrating surfaces or instruments, may cause pain in the heel resulting partly from periostitis of the calcaneus, partly from thickening of the soft parts involving the nerves; the thickening may affect the skin and produce *cornification* in the form of a diffuse rather than a localized corn, though localized corns may sometimes be found on the heel just as they are on the toes.

Chilblain of the heel is commoner on the posterior than it is on the under aspect, particularly over the tendo Achillis above the top of the back of the shoe. The trouble is apt to be bilateral, and is indicated by its occurrence in cold weather, by the purplish discoloration of the skin, and by the way the skin and soft parts are thickened and tender. The liability to chilblain is increased by the effects of *pressure over the tendo Achillis*, not only by boots or shoes, but by the lower edges of leggings, and drivers of motor-cars are apt to be afflicted in this way as the result of pressure of footwear on the tendo Achillis owing to plantar-flexion of the foot in using clutch-pedal, accelerator, and brake.

Bursitis of the bursa lying between the tendo Achillis and the calcaneus may be very painful without obvious swelling or discoloration; or there may be local swelling on either side of the lower part of the tendo Achillis. The diagnosis depends on accurate localization of the site of the tenderness and pain. The trouble may be associated with chilblain and pressure effects or may result from local injury; or, again, it may be purely inflammatory.

Injury is a common cause of pain in the heel, often persisting long after the injury occurred. It may be difficult to decide just what form the effects of the injury have taken; radiographic examination will be needed to diagnose or exclude *cracking* or *fracture of the calcaneus* or *astragalus*; if there is no proof of bone affection, the trouble will probably be in connexion with either ligamentous fibres or the periosteum, and the further diagnosis depends on what spot is found to be most tender on palpation and manipulation; tearing of the ligamentous fibres attached to the internal malleolus causes local, and possibly acute, tenderness below the ankle on the inner aspect of the heel; of the similar fibres from the external malleolus, on the outer aspect; of the tendo Achillis, behind and to one or other or both sides of the posterior aspect of the heel; of the long plantar fascia, often resulting from a stumble or from a jump from a height, infero-posteriorly.

Fasciitis of the soft parts of the heel, or *peri-ostitis* of the calcaneus, may simulate the effects of injury; indeed, injury may be but a factor bringing out the effects. No local examination will settle which is which; the diagnosis depends upon col-lateral evidence of causes elsewhere—ankylosing spondylitis, Reiter's disease, and, more rarely, rheumatoid arthritis. Periostitis is distinguishable from inflammatory affections of the other soft parts only by the locality of the tenderness and by the depth at which the tenderest part seems to be.

Tuberculous caries of the calcaneus is rare; in the earlier stages it simulates the effects of injury, strain, or sprain.

Foreign body in the heel is not uncommon; if it is a metal body, such as a pin, a needle, part of a nail or tin-tack, diagnosis with radiographs is easy; commonly, however, especially in children, or in adults who have been walking barefoot, a thorn not demonstrable with the radiographs may have penetrated without certain knowledge on the patient's part. A local corn with a tender, open centre may develop, and it may be weeks before the true nature of the trouble becomes manifest through this corn festering and the thorn coming out.

Sarcoma of the calcaneus is rare; it causes pro-gressive swelling of the heel before pain, and the diagnosis is made by radiographic examination followed by operation.

Spur on the under-surface of the calcaneus is quite a common lesion, but it is often forgotten, and many a patient suffering from the pain in the heel due to it is treated for arthritis or injury because no radiograph is taken. Radiographs make the diagnosis obvious (*Fig.* 515, p. 499). It is a malady of the second half of life, and is suggested when the spot tender to deep palpation is on the under-surface of the heel, in the middle line, about 2·5 cm. or a little more from the back of the foot. Such spurs or spines may, how-ever, be seen in younger, usually male, patients suffering from Reiter's disease or ankylosing spondylitis.

R. G. Beard.

HEMIANOPIA

Hemianopia, or hemianopsia, means inability to see objects in one-half of the field of vision.

In the majority of cases both eyes are affected: in bitemporal hemianopia there is loss of both temporal fields (*Figs.* 405, 406), and in homony-mous hemianopia the loss affects the right or left halves of each field (*Figs.* 407, 409). Quadrantic hemianopia refers to loss in one-quarter of one field, but it is usually found in both eyes as a homonymous defect affecting the upper or lower quadrants. It must be emphasized that the visual loss indicated by these terms need not be absolute. Indeed, the earliest sign of a hemianopia may be a relative defect known as an 'attention hemi-anopia': if the affected eye is confronted simul-taneously with two objects, one in either field, the object in front of the affected field will not be noticed although it will be clearly seen if it is presented by itself, i.e., if visual attention is not distracted by the other, more easily seen, object. Such attention hemianopia is relative, not absolute, and its recognition affords a valuable clue in early diagnosis. At a later stage, vision for large objects may be retained in the affected fields, but small objects, which reflect less light, are missed. Quantitative perimetry, which con-sists in field testing with objects of graduated size and different colours, is thus an essential method of determining the presence or absence of early field changes. Without it, early field defects resulting from pituitary tumours and disease of the optic radiation are easily missed, with unfortunate results.

Bitemporal Hemianopia. There is only one situa-tion in which a single lesion can produce this condition, viz., at the chiasma. The fibres from the nasal side of the retinae, which serve the temporal field of vision, run in the medial portion of the optic nerves, and after decussating in the centre of the chiasma, they still remain on the medial side of the optic tracts (*Fig.* 404). There-fore a lesion immediately in front of or just behind the chiasma is liable to produce bi-temporal field defects; these may or may not be symmetrical in extent and degree, depending on whether the interference with the two sides is equal or not. The usual cause of bitemporal hemianopia, whether symmetrical or not, is pitui-tary tumour (*Figs.* 405, 406). Less common causes are suprasellar cysts, aneurysm of the anterior communicating artery, meningiomata in the region of the tuberculum sellae, and pressure upon the chiasma from hydrocephalic distension of the third ventricle (e.g., in cerebellar tumours).

While it is true that the field defects which result from a lesion in the region of the chiasma usually appear first in the periphery of the field, cases are not rare in which the earliest changes are found in the central area of the field and not at the periphery. In such a case, the perimeter may show a normal peripheral field, while testing on the screen will reveal a temporal indentation of the normal field for small objects. Similar bitemporal depression of the internal isopters occasionally occurs in gummatous meningitis, and as a result of a plaque of demyelinization in the chiasma in disseminated sclerosis. Chronic arachnoiditis around the chiasma has been credited with similar effects, but the pathological reality of this condition is open to question.

It might be supposed that bitemporal field changes, whether peripheral or central, would appear first in the lower fields in pressure from above, and in the upper quadrants in pressure from below, but this expectation is occasionally proved wrong in the event, and the origin of the lesion is more accurately determined from other considerations. Field changes due to a tumour

of the pituitary are usually accompanied by radiological evidence of expansion of the sella; a normal pituitary fossa indicates that the lesion is extrasellar. (*Figs.* 410, 411.) The distinction between disease of the chiasma, and pressure from above, will depend more upon satellite symptoms and signs than upon the nature of the field defects. **Homonymous Hemianopia** is usually due to disease of the suprageniculate pathway, i.e., between

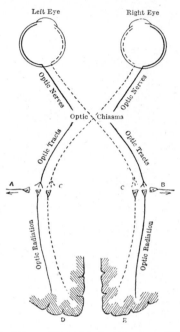

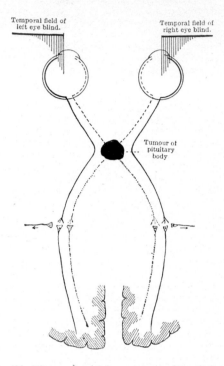

Fig. 404. Diagram illustrating the connexions of the optic nerves and tracts, the 3rd cranial nerves, and the occipital cortex. A, 3rd nerve going to left eye; B, Ditto to right eye; C, Relay of cells in optic thalamus and superior corpus quadrigeminum; D, The left occipital cortex, which sees objects in the right half of the field of vision; E, Right occipital cortex, which sees objects in the left half of the field of vision.

Fig. 405. Diagram showing how a tumour of the pituitary body affecting the decussating fibres at the optic chiasma prevents impulses passing from the nasal half of either retina to the corresponding cortex or to the corresponding 3rd nucleus. Hence bilateral temporal hemianopia and absence of pupil reaction to light thrown on the nasal half of either retina.

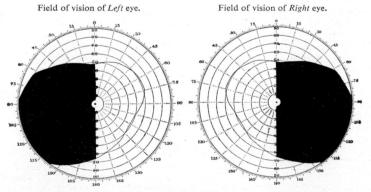

Field of vision of *Left* eye.   Field of vision of *Right* eye.

Fig. 406. Perimeter chart showing bilateral temporal hemianopia due to enlargement of the pituitary body in acromegaly. The blackened areas indicate the parts of the field of vision that had become blind (compare *Fig.* 405). The eccentric line indicates the average normal field of indirect vision. Note that central vision remains good. The black areas of the fields are blind.

the geniculate body and the visual cortex (*Fig.* 408). It is due to a lesion of the optic tract in very few cases, because there are comparatively few diseases which involve it. In most cases it will be possible to distinguish between the hemianopia of tract lesions and the more common is in the optic radiation. Consequently, a lesion of the tract may affect the fibres from the two eyes to an unequal degree, producing asymmetry of the field defects and inequality in the depth of visual loss (*Fig.* 409, bilateral homonymous hemianopia). This asymmetry in extent and degree

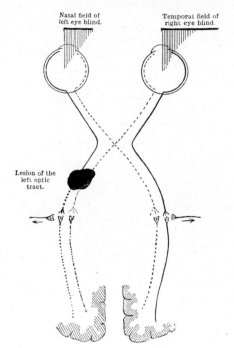

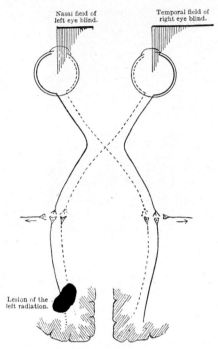

Fig. 407. Diagram showing how a lesion of the left optic tract causes blindness of the right half of the field of vision of each eye, and also prevents the left pupil from reacting in response to a ray of light falling on the blind half of either retina.

Fig. 408. Diagram showing how a lesion of the left optic radiation or of the visual portion of the left occipital cortex causes blindness of the right half of the field of vision of each eye, but does not prevent the pupils from reacting in response to a ray of light falling on the blind half of either retina.

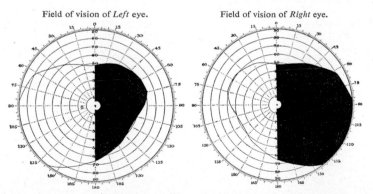

Fig. 409. Perimeter chart showing bilateral homonymous hemianopia resulting from left-sided embolism of the optic radiations (compare *Fig.* 408). The black areas of the field are blind.

variety by a study of other symptoms and signs, but when no assistance is forthcoming from these sources, help may be got from a study of the field changes themselves. In the optic tracts, the intermingling of fibres from the homonymous halves of the two retinae is not as complete as it of the field changes is spoken of as 'incongruity'. In radiation lesions, however, it is the rule for the field defects to be congruous, i.e., identical in shape and in degree. A further point of importance is that in hemianopia due to cortical lesions macular vision is sometimes spared, i.e., the straight line which divides the blind from the seeing half of each field is deviated at the fixation point so that the dividing line spares the macula, whereas in complete interruption of the optic tract the dividing line goes through the fixation point. This 'sparing of the macula', typical of

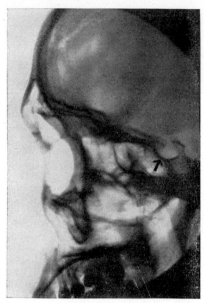

Fig. 410. Normal pituitary fossa in an adult.
(*Dr. Cochrane Shanks.*)

cortical lesions, is not, however, constant in disease of the radiation itself. Homonymous hemianopia, like the bitemporal form, may start as an indentation of the peripheral field which works inwards, or as a central or paracentral scotoma which ultimately spreads outwards to involve the entire half-field. The nature of the field defect will clearly depend on the size, situation, and progress of the lesion. Thus a gunshot wound which involves the tip of an occipital lobe will produce a homonymous hemiscotoma in the opposite half-fields of vision in both eyes, whereas a lesion of the anterior part of the calcarine sulcus will give rise to a homonymous loss in the peripheral part of the opposite half-fields. In practice, the peripheral and total forms of defect are more common than the scotomatous, but both must always be looked for. Visual defect is usually obvious to the patient with the central scotomatous type of homonymous hemianopia, but in the peripheral type this is not so, and he may be completely unaware of a complete homonymous hemianopia.

It has already been noted that the field changes of homonymous hemianopia due to *tract lesions* are incongruous unless section of the fibres is complete, and that they may be scotomatous or non-scotomatous in form. They are rare, because the tract is seldom the seat of primary disease. The least uncommon cause is pressure upon the

tract from a tumour in a nearby structure— the pituitary, the temporal lobe, the postero-inferior part of the frontal lobe, the thalamus, the corpora quadrigemina. Berry aneurysms, gummatous meningitis, gunshot wounds, and closed head injuries are rare causes. Disseminated sclerosis is occasionally the cause of a transient tract hemianopia.

Lesions of the *optic radiation* and visual cortex are much more common than diseases of the optic tract. The field defects may be central, or

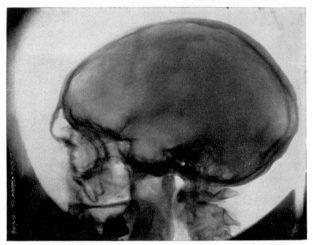

Fig. 411. Pituitary fossa widened by tumour. Note destruction of posterior clinoid processes. (*Dr. R. D. Hoare.*)

peripheral, or total, and they may affect one or both quadrants of the half-fields, but they are congruous in extent and density. There is one exception to this congruity of extent which must be mentioned. A homonymous hemianopia involves the nasal field of one eye and the temporal field of the other but since the nasal field is smaller than the temporal, the extent of the field defect is greater on one side than the other. This asymmetry is sometimes of practical importance, for a lesion which is limited to the anterior end of the calcarine fissure may involve the fibres from the periphery of the retinae, with the production of a peripheral crescentic loss in the opposite temporal field only. The earliest sign of a developing homonymous hemianopia may thus be a crescentic temporal loss limited to the opposite eye (*Fig.* 412 C).

The extent of a homonymous hemianopia varies with the size of the lesion. Complete hemianopia is to be expected as a result of a thrombosis affecting the posterior limb of the internal capsule, but from this point the radiation probably fans out, the fibres representing the upper quadrants of the opposite half-field passing laterally into the temporal lobe before curving back to the occipital cortex. This anatomical separation of the upper and lower fibres has been finally established by the fact that amputations of the anterior pole of the temporal lobe, as for example in the surgical treatment of 'temporal lobe epilepsy', may cause a sharply demarcated upper quadrantic hemianopic defect (*Fig.* 412 A).

The first part of the optic radiation lies behind the portion of the internal capsule which conveys common sensation to the cortex, and medial to the auditory radiation. Any considerable lesion at this point, such as a vascular accident, is likely

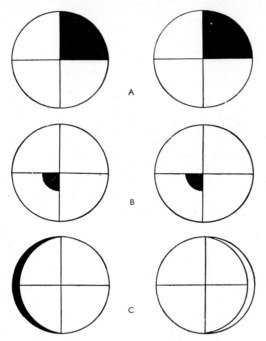

Fig. 412. A, Homonymous quadrantic hemianopia (upper). B, Homonymous quadrantic hemiscotoma. C, Showing unpaired temporal crescent of visual loss due to a lesion at the anterior end of the calcarine fissure.

to produce hemianaesthesia as well as hemianopia, but auditory loss does not occur in a unilateral lesion at this point; if, however, the lesion extends to the superior temporal convolution, sensory aphasia may appear. Localization depends on the nature of the field changes determined by perimetry and on satellite symptoms and signs. The distinction between tract and radiation lesions depends more on these factors than on the hemianopic pupillary reaction described by Wernicke and credited with a usefulness which it does not possess. Theoretically, the pupillary reflex to light should be lost in tract lesions if the blind side of either retina be illuminated by a thin pencil of light, whereas the reflex should be retained when this procedure is carried out in hemianopia due to a lesion of the supra-geniculate pathway (*Figs.* 407, 408). In practice, it is difficult to confine the illumination to only one side of the retina because of the diffusion of light within the eye, and the test is correspondingly fallacious.

Ian Mackenzie.

HEMIPLEGIA

DEFINITION. Hemiplegia means paralysis of one side of the body, but conventional usage has limited its application to cases in which the paralysis is due to disease of the upper motor neuron. It is not used for unilateral Parkinsonism or for paralysis of an arm and leg by poliomyelitis, or for the apparent paralysis of hemichorea. Neurologists customarily speak of hemiplegia when paralysis is severe, and of hemiparesis when it is slight, a distinction which is useful and deserves wider adoption. They are usually caused by intracranial disease, but can be the result of a high cervical lesion, in which event the face is spared and there is usually some degree of sensory loss in the non-paralysed side of the body.

Clinical Forms of Hemiplegia and Hemiparesis. In complete hemiplegia due to a lesion of the internal capsule, the contralateral arm and leg are paralysed and spastic. The leg is held in an attitude of extension at the hip, knee, and ankle, and the arm is adducted at the shoulder, and semiflexed at the elbow. The muscles of the trunk are affected, but less severely: on attempting to sit up, the umbilicus shifts towards the sound side, and the respiratory excursion of the chest is reduced on the affected side—so much so that it may lead to a suspicion of pulmonary disease. Of course there may be a lesion in the lung, such as a bronchogenic carcinoma or pulmonary fibrosis, but the relative immobility of the chest is more often due to the hemiplegia itself. The lower half of the face is weak in both voluntary and involuntary movements; but the orbicularis oculi and the frontalis are either normal or but slightly affected. The muscles of articulation and deglutition are seldom affected by a unilateral pyramidal lesion, but transient disturbance may occur in the early or acute phase of a complete hemiplegia. Speech may be slurred by weakness of the lips on the affected side. Ocular movements are spared in unilateral lesions.

Immediately after the onset of an acute hemiplegia, as for instance in cerebral thrombosis, the affected limbs may be limp, atonic, and show a depression or absence of all reflex activity, but as the stage of shock passes off the tendon reflexes are exaggerated, the plantar response is extensor, and clonus may be elicited at the ankle and knee. The abdominal reflexes and the cremasteric reflex are lost on the side of the paralysis. It will be appreciated that each of these reflexes depends upon its own especial pathway, and whether it is affected in the manner described will depend on whether the lesion has interrupted that pathway. Thus a flexor plantar response is quite compatible with a pyramidal lesion which is confined to the corticospinal fibres to the face and upper limb. A lesion limited to the motor cortex proper can give rise to a hemiplegia which remains flaccid but, exhibits the reflex changes appropriate to pyramidal dysfunction.

Atrophy of muscles is not prominent in hemiplegia, but contractures of muscles and adhesions around joints are common. If paralysis occurs in infancy or childhood, the affected limbs do not grow as fast as those on the normal side, and they therefore appear wasted, shortened, and deformed by contractures.

Topical Diagnosis in Hemiplegia. *Cortical hemiplegia* is often confined to the lower leg, or the upper limb, or the face and upper limb; complete hemiplegia requires an extensive lesion at this site. Lesions limited to the anterior half of the *internal capsule* are more likely to produce a complete hemiplegia, and if they extend backwards into the sensory portion of the capsule the paralysis is accompanied by sensory loss and, in extreme cases, by homonymous hemianopia. A *thalamic lesion* may involve the adjacent internal capsule, and the hemiplegia or hemiparesis is then accompanied by the thalamic syndrome (*see* p. 716) and by ataxia; athetosis may develop in chronic cases.

THE CAUSES OF HEMIPLEGIA

1. Congenital:

Atrophic lobar sclerosis
Porencephaly
Cerebral agenesia
Cerebral angioma
Sturge-Weber syndrome

2. Head Injury:

Birth injury
Cerebral contusion
Late traumatic apoplexy

3. Vascular Accidents:

Cerebral thrombosis
Hypertensive encephalopathy
Cerebral haemorrhage
Subarachnoid haemorrhage
Cerebral embolism
Softening without thrombosis

4. Neoplasms:

Primary neoplasms
Secondary neoplasms

5. Infection:

Meningitis (various)
Cerebral abscess
Cysticercosis
Cortical thrombo-phlebitis
Thrombosis of sagittal sinus
Hydatid cyst
Encephalitis lethargica
Encephalomyelitis
Polio-encephalitis

6. Miscellaneous Conditions:

Disseminated sclerosis
Schilder's disease
Epiloia
Pick's disease

7. Hysteria.

A lesion in the crus cerebri (cerebral peduncle) in the brain-stem involves the issuing fibres of the third nerve as they pass through the still uncrossed pyramidal tract and thus causes an ipsilateral third nerve palsy and a contralateral hemiplegia (Weber's syndrome). If a lesion involves the tegmentum and thus the red nucleus, the ipsilateral third nerve palsy will be accompanied by a contralateral tremor of the so-called cerebellar type but possibly more violent (Benedikt's syndrome).

In the Millard-Gubler syndrome a lateral rectus palsy is accompanied by an ipsilateral facial paralysis and a contralateral hemiplegia due to involvement of the still uncrossed pyramidal tract. In the Foville syndrome a facial paralysis is accompanied by an ipsilateral paralysis of conjugate gaze and a contralateral hemiplegia.

Bilateral pyramidal lesions *in the medulla*, or at a higher level, cause double hemiplegia and spastic palsy of bulbar function. Bilateral affections of the pyramidal fibres destined for the third, fourth, and sixth cranial nuclei give rise to paralysis of conjugate movements of the eyes in one or more directions. Disease of or injury to the *upper cervical cord* on one side can cause hemiplegia; the cranial nerves are spared, but atrophy of the small muscles of the hand is an interesting feature of some of these cases.

The causes of hemiplegia are many. Classification according to the mode of onset has a limited usefulness, because while it is true that an abrupt onset usually signifies a vascular accident, the catastrophe may be a complication of a cerebral neoplasm. Moreover, disseminated sclerosis may be gradual in onset, but the patient may equally well wake up one morning to find himself the victim of a hemiparesis due to the same condition. These considerations make an aetiological classification preferable.

Congenital Hemiplegia may be due to cerebral agenesia or to the prenatal toxic-infective process which has been designated 'atrophic lobar sclerosis'. In either case there may be mental defect, athetosis, and epilepsy. But there is general agreement that hemiplegia dating from birth is more often due to birth injury than to the foregoing. Porencephalic cysts are probably the end-result of intracerebral venous haemorrhage occurring during prolonged labour, and therefore belong to the group of birth injuries. The distinction between natal and prenatal forms of hemiplegia is not wholly academic, for the former are less likely to be associated with mental deficiency and epilepsy than the latter, and the prognosis is brighter. Occasionally, however, hemiparesis due to porencephaly rapidly grows worse in adolescence or early adult life; the cause thereof is not known, but its occurrence is apt to lead to a mistaken diagnosis of neoplasm.

Head Injuries occurring at birth are mentioned above. In later life, closed head injuries and penetrating wounds are also a common cause of hemiparesis and hemiplegia. Diagnosis is obvious, but occasionally cases are encountered in which a head injury is followed some days later by the abrupt occurrence of hemiplegia due to a cerebral haemorrhage or a carotid thrombosis. The former is usually fatal unless the blood-clot is evacuated at once; the latter may cause permanent hemiplegia, with or without additional symptoms such as aphasia, sensory loss, or homonymous hemianopia. Where the head injury has been severe and the post-traumatic amnesia prolonged, these focal deficiencies may be aggravated by a general loss of intellectual capacity and a deterioration of the personality, which may prove a greater handicap than the hemiplegia.

Chronic subdural haematoma is not a common or important cause of post-traumatic hemiplegia. Transient hemiparesis may occur, either on the same side as the haematoma or on the opposite side, but severe permanent paralysis following a subdural haematoma is more likely to be due to a complicating cerebral contusion or cerebral thrombosis. The occasional occurrence of syphilitic cerebral thrombosis after head injuries is a reminder of the need for examination of the blood and spinal fluid (*see* p. 125).

Vascular Accidents are the most common cause of hemiplegia in adults. Cerebral haemorrhage is abrupt in onset and usually proceeds rapidly to a fatal termination within 24 hours; a few recover. It occurs in atheroma, with or without arterial hypertension; less often, as a haemorrhage into a glioma or secondary tumour, or from an angioma or congenital berry aneurysm within the substance of the brain; rarely, as a result of diseases characterized by or associated with purpura. If blood escapes into the ventricular system, the neck may be stiff and the temperature high. The distinction from *cerebral thrombosis* is made with difficulty, if at all. Free blood in the spinal fluid is diagnostic, but is often absent in haemorrhage. In general, recovery favours thrombosis rather than haemorrhage. If syphilis be present, thrombosis is likely, and a vascular accident which comes on during sleep is unlikely to be due to haemorrhage. Recurrent hemiparesis of increasing severity can be caused by atheromatous stenosis of the internal carotid artery giving rise to emboli in the neck. It may be associated with a systolic bruit, and diagnosis is confirmed by arteriography. *Cerebral embolism* from other sources is more common in young adults than in the later decades. The onset is abrupt, and—as in a small thrombosis there may be no loss of consciousness. Convulsions, either generalized or Jacksonian, may occur in all forms of vascular accident. Embolism is to be considered if there is a source of emboli—bronchiectasis, mitral stenosis, auricular fibrillation, coronary thrombosis with a mural clot, infective endocarditis, atheroma of the extracranial arteries, caisson disease, or multiple fractures of bones with resulting fat embolism.

Subarachnoid haemorrhage occasionally results from rupture of an atheromatous blood-vessel at the base of the brain. More important is its occurrence from a congenital berry aneurysm on the circle of Willis or one of its branches. Hemiplegia may result either from the blood tearing into the brain substance or from softening of the brain distal to the point of rupture, due to spasm of cerebral vessels. This has now been frequently demonstrated by angiography which at first shows the cerebral vessels to be narrowed but later shows them to be of normal calibre. The sudden headache, unconsciousness, and blood-stained spinal fluid provide a guide to diagnosis. It should be noted, however, that hemiplegia is a rare sequel to subarachnoid haemorrhage.

13*

Cerebral Neoplasms usually cause slowly oncoming symptoms, of which hemiparesis is one. Headache and papilloedema may or may not be present, depending on the rapidity with which the tumour grows and the stage at which it is seen. Secondary metastases often cause hemiplegia without these features of increased intracranial pressure. *Any slowly developing hemiplegia in adults or children should suggest the possibility of a cerebral tumour, whether there are symptoms of raised intracranial pressure or not.*

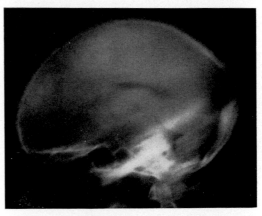

Fig. 413. Normal air encephalogram showing third ventricle, aqueduct, and fourth ventricle.

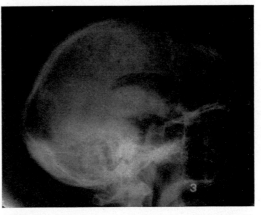

Fig. 414. Normal air encephalogram showing anterior part of ventricular system.

X-ray examination of the skull may show changes in the bone overlying a meningioma; if the pineal gland is calcified, it may be seen to be pushed to one side by an invisible tumour of the opposite hemisphere; slowly growing gliomata (e.g., oligodendrogliomata and some astrocytomata) may show calcification within their substance; separation of the sutures and a 'beaten silver' appearance of the skull indicate a high intracranial pressure; calcification may reveal the presence of capillary angiomatosis of one hemisphere, the calcification being not in the angioma but in one of the cortical layers—this being associated sometimes with a cutaneous naevus on the upper part of the face on the same side (Sturge-Weber syndrome). Many cases require further investigation, by gamma scan (*Fig.* 417) or by further radiology as by an EMI-scan,

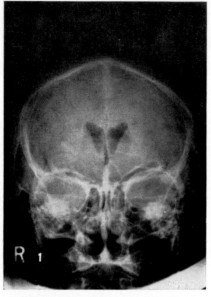

Fig. 415. Normal air encephalogram in anteroposterior view.

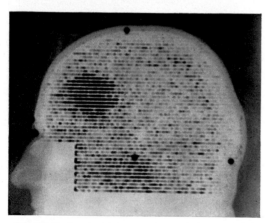

Fig. 417. Gamma scan in same patient as in the ventriculo-gram (*Fig.* 416) showing increased uptake in left frontal area. The lesion proved to be a metastatic tumour.

or by positive contrast radiology by angiography or (*Figs.* 413–416) ventriculography. Electro-encephalography may help to localize a cortical or subcortical growth, but this evidence is obscured if the intracranial pressure is much raised. Every case of suspected cerebral tumour should be carefully examined, both clinically and radiologically, to exclude the possibility of a primary growth elsewhere in the body, but despite every

precaution a small carcinoma of the lung may easily be missed.

Infections of the Nervous System are an uncommon cause of hemiplegia. *Metastatic cerebral abscess*, the result of blood-borne infection, may cause it. Any form of *meningitis* may be

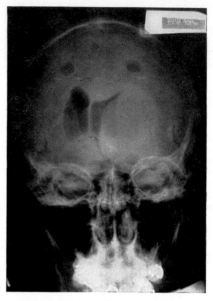

Fig. 416. Ventriculogram showing large left frontal expanding lesion.

complicated by hemiplegia, mostly due to haemorrhagic softening or frank cerebral thrombosis. Hemiplegia occurs in *encephalitis lethargica*, in *encephalomyelitis* following specific fevers and vaccination, and in rare cases of *polio-encephalitis* during an epidemic of poliomyelitis. The hemiplegia which sometimes occurs without other neurological symptoms *during* the course of general infections is due to cerebral thrombosis and not to encephalomyelitis. *Phlebitis of the cortical veins*, with or without *thrombosis of the superior sagittal sinus*, is more likely to cause bilateral symptoms (e.g., crural paraplegia) than a hemiplegia, but the latter does occur; it is usually associated with Jacksonian fits in the affected limbs, and the pressure of the spinal fluid is raised; there is usually an increase of the cells, and sometimes of the protein content. Cortical thrombophlebitis is an infective condition which occurs as a result of infected wounds of the head, furunculosis (the nose and face especially), and rarely as a complication of pyaemia. *Cysticercosis* may give rise to a transient hemiparesis at the time of invasion, but it clears up and is not a feature of the phase of calcification which causes epileptic fits. *Hydatid cysts* present the features of a rapidly growing space-occupying lesion, with localizing signs which may include hemiplegia if the cyst is appropriately placed.

Miscellaneous Lesions. *Disseminated sclerosis,* the aetiology of which is unknown, is characterized by repeated attacks of transient neurological symptoms—diplopia, retrobulbar neuritis, sudden weakness of a limb, attacks of 'numbness' in the extremities, cerebellar ataxia of gait, speech, and hands, and so on. Occasionally there is a transient hemiparesis as part of this changing and intermittent picture, and rarely, in older patients, there is simply a slowly progressive hemiplegia. Usually, however, there are indications from the past history and from the examination of the nervous system which show that there are, or have been, lesions other than that which is the cause of the hemiplegia.

Epiloia (syn. tuberous sclerosis) is a disease, often heredofamilial, characterized pathologically by the presence of large nodules of glial tissue in the cortical grey matter and to a lesser extent elsewhere in the brain. These may be associated with adenoma sebaceum and other congenital cutaneous lesions, and skeletal malformations are common. Mental deficiency and epilepsy are noticed at the age of two or three years and constitute the main neurological symptoms, but hemiplegia occasionally occurs, and may be associated with athetosis.

Pick's disease is a rare condition of cerebral atrophy, localized to one or more lobes and usually more or less symmetrical, which comes on after the age of 40 with the production of a presenile dementia and localizing symptoms—agnosia, apraxia, aphasia—which depend on the site of the atrophy. Hemiplegia is rare in this disease, but a pseudo-hemiplegia may be present when apraxia makes the patient disinclined to use the limbs on one side of the body. Air encephalography will show a large pool of air over the area of cortex affected.

Schilder's disease (syn. encephalitis periaxialis diffusa) occurs at any age. There are areas of spreading demyelinization in one or both hemispheres, with or without smaller patches in the brain-stem, pons, and cerebellum. The disease may run its course to a fatal termination in months or years but may also become arrested for many years. The acute cases may be marked by pyrexia and raised intracranial pressure, with headache and papilloedema, but these are absent in subacute and chronic cases. Symptoms depend on the site or sites of the lesions, and hemiplegia may occur by itself, or more often in combination with mental changes, fits, hemianopia, aphasia, apraxia, agnosia, etc. The spinal fluid is usually normal, but excess of protein and a moderate lymphocytic pleocytosis may be found in acute cases.

Hysterical Hemiplegia is limited to the arm and leg; the face escapes. The limbs are usually flaccid, and the reflexes are normal. It is almost always associated with hysterical anaesthesia on the same side of the body. As in all hysterical manifestations, diagnosis depends on four points —absence of objective signs of disease, evidence of psychoneurosis in the past history of the patient, positive signs of psychiatric disturbance, and the removal of the 'paralysis' by suggestion.

Ian Mackenzie.

HICCUP

Hiccup is a very common symptom and is only significant if it persists. It is due to sudden involuntary contraction of the diaphragm checked rapidly by closure of the glottis. Gastric irritation or distension after rapid eating or excessive intake of alcohol are the commonest causes but the following conditions should be considered in persistent cases:

A. **Central:**

  1. Epidemic encephalitis.

  2. Intracranial: Tumour, meningitis, haemorrhage.

  3. Toxic:
  a. Uraemia.
  b. Acute infections and fevers. Pneumonia.

  4. Lesions in the medulla or cord.

  5. Hysteria (rare).

B. **Irritation of the Phrenic Nerve:**

  1. Cervical.

  2. Thoracic.

  3. Diaphragmatic.

C. **Reflex** from stomach, peritoneum, intestines, or other viscera.

Since the reflex stimulus may be trivial, hiccup is often of no clinical significance, e.g., resulting merely from excessive laughter, stimulation of certain reflex spots especially about the chin, tickling, indigestion or wind especially in infants, or occurring spontaneously without obvious cause. The hiccup of *alcoholism* has a character of its own; the circumstances indicate the causation.

Particular types of hiccup that merit attention include:

Peritonitic Hiccup may occur in acute peritonitis, acute haemorrhagic pancreatitis, acute intestinal obstruction, or acute postoperative dilatation of the stomach; its persistence always indicates a grave prognosis.

Hysterical Hiccup. The patient is generally a girl between 15 and 25 years of age, who may hiccup persistently throughout her waking hours for weeks, at the rate of two or three times a minute. The hiccup stops during sleep. The chief difficulty will be to exclude the possibility of epidemic hiccup (*see below*).

Irritation of a Phrenic Nerve by something in the mediastinum may cause recurrent attacks of intractable hiccup. In a child, *tuberculous caseation of bronchial* or *mediastinal lymph-nodes* is now a rarity in most countries. In adults, *malignant* or *lymphomatous deposits* in the mediastinum may be present. There may be symptoms and signs of a primary growth in the bronchus or oeso- phagus. An aortic aneurysm may be present, and rarely a mediastinitis.

The hiccup of pneumonia is due to the accom- panying diaphragmatic pleurisy. Hiccup may occur as a manifestation of pericarditis.

Tabetic crises—*hiccup crises*—are today ex- tremely rare, but may be distressing, prolonged, and intractable.

Epidemic or **Infective Hiccup** was probably a variety of encephalitis lethargica, the inflam- matory process affecting centres in the medulla instead of those in the midbrain; if at the same time there are ocular pareses and other symp- toms of midbrain inflammation the diagnosis is less difficult.

Abdominal Disease. Patients suffering from serious but not urgent abdominal disease occasionally develop distressing hiccup. In some cases the diaphragm is being irritated, for example by a *diaphragmatic hernia*, *subphrenic abscess*, *sub- diaphragmatic peritonitis*, secondary deposits of *carcinoma in the liver*, a *gumma* or *abscess in the liver*, an *infarct in the spleen*, or a *carcinoma of the stomach*; but sometimes the mischief seems far removed from the diaphragm—*a carcinoma of the sigmoid colon*, for instance, or *carcinoma of the uterus*, even when there are no secondary deposits. Hiccup may occur after abdominal or pelvic operations as well as thoracic.

Uraemic Hiccup is rare, but it may be persistent and is always of grave omen. The diagnosis de- pends on the associated evidence of renal disease.

Disorders of the Medullary Centres. Hiccup due to this cause will be associated with other symp- toms of cerebral or spinal disease. Tumours, meningitis, or haemorrhage may be responsible.

F. Dudley Hart.

HIRSUTISM

Introduction. Though the possibility of treatment of idiopathic hirsutism is becoming somewhat more promising than was previously the case, striking results have not been obtained and the possible side-effects of prolonged treatment make one disinclined to embark on it. Small doses of dexamethasone should theoretically suppress excessive production of adrenal androgen but might in time give rise to adrenal atrophy. Fur- thermore, this treatment is often ineffective. Oral contraceptives have also been used to oppose the action of topically produced androgen or to diminish the circulation of free testosterone by means of the oestrogen component. The use of the anti-androgen cyproterone may have undesir- able side-effects and it has not been available sufficiently long, at present, to evaluate its long- term effects.

Furthermore, although high amounts of di- hydrotestosterone and androstenedione have sometimes been found in the skin of the hirsute areas, nevertheless, in many cases the levels of circulating testosterone are normal and it is thought that the hirsutism may be due to in- creased sensitivity to normal concentrations of androgens.

The importance of the differential diagnosis of hirsutism is therefore to decide whether it is a manifestation of some extremely rare and sinister condition such as an adrenal carcinoma or a masculinizing ovarian tumour or whether the condition, though probably incurable, is relatively benign.

Types of Hair Growth

Lanugo: This is the very fine, silky but some- times quite long hair that covers the entire surface of the skin of the developing foetus but which is usually shed in utero during the seventh or eighth month.

Vellus: This is somewhat similar and again may be widely distributed. In most cases it is almost invisible and is certainly never a cause of embarrassment in males. In a female, however, its presence may be suddenly noticed, particularly on the face when she is looking in a mirror with the sun or a light behind her head. She then finds that she has this type of hair over her sternum, on her arms and her legs, and this becomes a case of 'pseudohirsutism'.

Intermediate hair is still soft and silky but tends to grow long and become pigmented. It may become conspicuous and therefore a cause of embarrassment. A combination of vellus and intermediate hair over the face and the shoulders is characteristic of Cushing's syndrome.

Terminal hair is coarse, pigmented, and usually discrete. It is the hair naturally found in the axillae and on the pubis of females, and on the face, chest, and abdomen and limbs of males. When it grows in this distribution in females it constitutes 'hirsutism'.

Degrees of Hair Growth and Distribution. It is important to understand what is meant by 'hirsutism', for many women live miserable lives believing themselves to be disfigured by excessive hair growth whereas the growth of hair is within the normal physiological range—just as there are men who torture themselves by imagining that they have inadequate facial hair growth. 'Hirsutism' applies only to females and means that they are afflicted to some extent with hair growth both facial and on the body which would be regarded as natural for a man but abnormal for a woman. 'Hypertrichosis' should mean literally excessive amount of hair growth but of normal distribution, and could therefore apply also to the male who has a more than average amount of body hair growth. There is, for instance, a condition known as *hypertrichosis lanuginosa* in which the first pelage, the lanugo which is shed in utero in the seventh or eighth month, suddenly regrows and completely covers the face so that the features become unrecognizable. In the *de Lange syndrome* which is associated with short stature (*Amsterdam dwarfism*), the scalp hair reaches down to the bushy and confluent eyebrows and there is also generalized hirsutism of the vellus/ intermediate type. (*Fig.* 418).

The degrees of hair growth may be classified briefly as follows:

In *Alopecia totalis*, all the hair falls out and the patient is left without a hair on his head. He or she loses the eyebrows and eyelashes as well as the axillary and pubic hair and all the body hair.

Non-sexual hair, which is not dependent on sex hormones, constitutes the hair of the scalp, the eyebrows, and the eyelashes. A good example of a

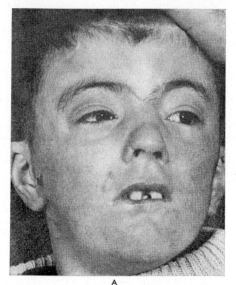

Mediterranean women and many Indian women have a natural tendency to conspicuous growth of vellus hair if not actual terminal hair, whereas Mongolian and Japanese men may not actually need to shave.

The condition of *premature pubarche* (p. 722) is interesting. Pubic hair begins to grow sometimes as early as 2 years of age. No other sign of sexual precocity develops.

Male sexual hair, which is dependent on male levels of sex hormones, is characterized by facial hair which is cultivated extensively and with pride at the moment of writing by the male sex but which is the subject of considerable distress for women. The upper pubic triangle, however, is something that most females nowadays are

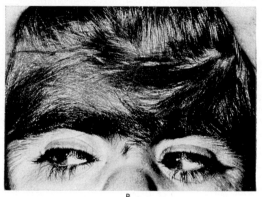

Fig. 418. A, de Lange facies. (*Dr. D. M. MacDonald, Guy's Hospital, London.*) B, Long curly eyelashes, synophrys, and confluent forehead hair. (*Dr. D. M. MacDonald and the British Journal of Dermatology.*)

condition in which only non-sexual hair is found is congenital hypopituitarism, in which the adolescent or young adult is found to have grown no pubic or axillary hair let alone any body hair simply because neither gonadal nor adrenal androgens are being produced. Patients with testicular feminization grow no pubic hair because they cannot respond to the normal amounts of androgen which they are producing.

Ambosexual hair is dependent on female levels of sex hormones and is characterized by axillary hair and the lower triangle of pubic hair, together with a varying degree of intermediate hair on the limbs. It should be pointed out that of 400 consecutive Welsh and English women students at the University of Wales examined 36 were considered to be 'hirsute': 26 per cent of these 400 young women had terminal hair on the face, 17 per cent on the chest or breasts, 35 per cent had abdominal hair mainly concentrated on the linea alba, and 84 per cent had terminal hair on the lower arm and leg and 70 per cent of these had terminal hair on the upper arm and leg. The condition of *pseudohirsutism* must therefore be very common and may sometimes be even more distressing than true hirsutism. One must, of course, take into account under this heading the varying sensitivity of different individuals to the agents which control facial and body hair growth.

determined to demonstrate that they do not possess, or if they do they hasten to rid themselves of it. Hair on the chest, the back, the lumbar region (the satyr's tail), the ears and the tip of the nose are typical male characteristics. Women who share these male hair distributions conspicuously are pathologically hirsute and may also suffer from infrequent periods or amenorrhoea, and seborrhoea and acne—both typical manifestations of male androgens, and it is these women whom one has to examine and investigate carefully before dismissing them with sympathy, reassurance, and advice concerning local depilatory devices.

Hirsutism and Virilism, though not necessarily more sinister than conspicuous hirsutism alone, certainly demand the most careful and intensive investigation. Virilism consists of enlargement of the clitoris, atrophy of the breasts, baldness of the scalp, and increased muscularity. There may even be some deepening of the voice, and amenorrhoea almost invariably accompanies the condition.

Hirsutism (and virilism) may be due to abnormal activity of the adrenal cortex, of the ovary, of the thyroid, or of the growth hormone, or it may be idiopathic.

Adrenal Cortex. *Congenital adrenal hyperplasia* may occur either in the female or the male. In the latter sexual precocity becomes manifest in the first two or three years of life and the condition is known as 'macrogenitosomia precox'. The condition is due to lack of the enzyme system 21-hydroxylase which completes the synthesis of cortisone by the adrenal gland. Androgen, however, which has only 19 carbon atoms, is unaffected by this defect and is released in great quantities, and when it occurs in girls it produces the condition usually referred to as *female pseudohermaphroditism* of which early establishment of hirsutism and virilism is a clinical feature, though probably not the presenting one. Under the stimulus of androgen growth is at first rapid but early closure of the epiphyses results in markedly stunted growth and the child could almost be mistaken for an achondroplastic. The clitoris is enlarged and the internal genitalia consist of normal patent tubes, uterus and cervix, but the lower part of the vagina leads into the posterior portion of the urethra, so that there is only one genito-urinary aperture on to the surface. Breast development does not take place at puberty, but it is to be hoped that the condition will have been recognized before then, for cortisol will lead to complete feminization. High levels of urinary 17-oxosteroids and pregnanetriol confirm the diagnosis.

Adrenogenital Syndrome. The *adrenogenital syndrome*, in contrast to congenital adrenal hyperplasia, is due to postnatal adrenal hyperplasia or to a tumour, adenoma, or carcinoma. Hyperplasia is far more common than tumours, which are rare. The *hyperplasia* may be mild or 'functional' and associated with slight elevation of the urinary 17-oxosteroid output; levels may even be in the upper part of the normal range and the clinical features confined to hirsutism without virilism and oligomenorrhoea or amenorrhoea. It is in these cases that it is claimed that regular ovulatory menstrual cycles may be restored and the hirsutism alleviated by administering doses of corticosteroid sufficient to depress the 17-oxosteroid output. The bilateral hyperplasia, however, may be considerable and even capable of detection by intravenous pyelography and perirenal insufflation, so that the question of surgery rather than medical suppression of adrenal activity has to be considered. *Adrenocortical adenoma* and *carcinoma* are sometimes difficult to distinguish from hyperplasia, though the level of 17-oxosteroids is usually significantly raised and may be very high. Furthermore, the secretory activity of these tumours is autonomous and not affected by corticotrophin. Thus if 2 mg. of dexamethasone are administered daily the urinary 17-oxosteroid output may be appreciably lowered in a case of hyperplasia, but even 8 mg. of dexamethasone daily will not suppress the 17-oxosteroid output in cases of tumour, especially carcinoma. Moreover, increased quantities of dehydroepiandrosterone can be extracted from the urine in tumour cases, which are nearly always accompanied by coarse hirsutism and virilism. Calcification in the tumour can be detected by X-ray in some cases of carcinoma.

Cushing's Syndrome (*see* p. 584) is usually associated with hirsutism, sometimes quite conspicuous in the beard and upper lip areas, but the characteristic feature is a rather widespread vellus hirsutism on the face and over the shoulders. The plethoric moon-shaped face and characteristic distribution of obesity and cutaneous striae make the diagnosis easy in classic cases, and it can be confirmed by finding raised levels of plasma cortisol and urinary 17-oxogenic steroids. If the syndrome is due to bilateral hyperplasia these figures may rise even higher under the stimulus of 'synacthen' 0·25 mg. injected intramuscularly, and will be significantly depressed by dexamethasone, but will remain unaltered if the syndrome is due to a tumour. In the case of a tumour the amount of glucocorticoid being secreted may be sufficient to suppress endogenous corticotrophin and the contralateral adrenal gland may atrophy.

Ovary. *Virilizing tumours of the ovary* are exceedingly rare and indeed many experienced gynaecologists have never seen one. They usually give rise to extreme degrees of virilism because the androgen they produce (testosterone) is biologically very potent though biochemically almost unrecognizable and the urinary 17-oxosteroid levels may be within the normal range. Plasma and urinary estimations of testosterone and epitestosterone will give high levels. Furthermore, injection of chorionic gonadotrophin 2000 I.U. will triple the testosterone output and administration of dexamethasone or oestrogen will lower the plasma testosterone level. In some cases an enlarged ovary may be palpated on pelvic examination. These tumours never develop before puberty.

Polycystic (Stein-Leventhal) ovary syndrome is much more common. The classic clinical picture is one of amenorrhoea, hirsutism, obesity, and palpably enlarged ovaries which on macroscopical examination are large and oyster-shaped with a bluish-white thickened capsule with multiple cystic follicles protruding from the surface. On microscopical examination numerous small follicular cysts are found surrounded by hyperplastic theca interna. Androstenedione has been isolated from the cyst fluid and is the cause of the hirsutism and the 17-oxosteroids may be in the high normal range, though in fact hirsutism occurs only in about 50 per cent of cases. Many cases do not show the classic features. Laparoscopy therefore may be called for to clinch the diagnosis. Clomiphene or bilateral wedge resection leads to reversal of the clinical picture, at any rate temporarily in many cases. The *monocystic ovary syndrome* has recently been described and may behave like the polycystic ovary syndrome and produce hirsutism.

Thyroid. Cases of *congenital cretinism* tend to grow a coat of vellus or intermediate hair to cover the back and extensor surfaces of the skin as though to compensate for the lowered metabolic rate and keep the cold out. This is also seen sometimes in cases of *juvenile myxoedema* and *hypothyroidism*. Isolation studies on the urine have shown proportionately more androsterone than aetiocholanolone.

Acromegaly. Hirsutism is usually found in cases of acromegaly and the urinary 17-oxosteroids may be slightly raised. Occasionally this is associated with concomitant adrenal adenomas.

Iatrogenic. Though there are great individual variations most women are sensitive to administration of androgens therapeutically administered. Some preparations for relief of menopausal symptoms contain both oestrogens and methyltestosterone and frequently give rise to hirsutism, particularly of the upper lip. Preparations given for their protein-anabolic properties are nearly always mildly androgenic and may produce undesirable side-effects.

There is a tendency to develop hirsutism, especially on the arms and legs, in *anorexia nervosa* and many *postmenopausal women* tend to develop facial hirsutism, presumably because of the change of ratio between androgen and oestrogen production.

When all these conditions have been carefully excluded one is justified in making a diagnosis of *idiopathic* or *simple hirsutism*.

P. M. F. Bishop.

HOARSENESS (OR CHANGE IN THE VOICE)

Hoarseness, or a rough, coarse timbre of the voice implies to the laryngologist some abnormality or irregularity of the opposing edges of the vocal cords. It is a symptom which may be the only manifestation, for a long period, of serious disease and it calls for expert attention in order that an accurate diagnosis may be reached.

Hoarseness should be distinguished from *weakness* of the voice which is more liable to be present in neurological lesions of the larynx when the cords are in fact free from disease but their movement is limited.

HOARSENESS IN CHILDREN:

Congenital:
Cysts, malformations
Traumatic:
Foreign body in larynx or upper oesophagus. Scalding of larynx
Infective:
Acute exanthemata, measles, variola, laryngotracheitis, diphtheria
Neoplastic:
Multiple papillomata.

HOARSENESS IN ADULTS:

Traumatic:
Foreign body, injury from intubation. External injury to larynx
Over-use of voice—clergyman's throat, singer's nodes
Abuse of voice—costermonger's shouting
Exposure to irritant gases.

Infective:
Acute:
Acute non-specific laryngitis
Acute infection of pharynx and mouth—quinsy—cervical phlegmon—perichondritis of larynx, producing oedema of larynx
Chronic:
Chronic non-specific laryngitis due to tobacco or alcohol
Keratosis, pachydermia of larynx
Crico-arytenoid joint ankylosis from rheumatoid arthritis or septic infection
Tuberculosis
Syphilis
Leprosy
Reinke's oedema.
Neoplastic:
Cysts, papilloma, fibroma (*Fig.* 419)
Carcinoma (*Fig.* 420).

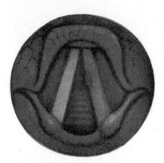

Fig. 419. Papilloma on an inflamed vocal cord. This occurred in a patient over 60, and aroused suspicion of malignancy, but the cord remained mobile, and the growth had not increased markedly three years after first coming under observation.

WEAKNESS OF THE VOICE:

Neurological:
Paralysis of recurrent laryngeal nerve from—
Thyroidectomy
Carcinoma of thyroid gland, of cervical oesophagus, of cervical lymph-nodes
Carcinoma of lung, of mediastinal lymph-nodes (left nerve only)
Aneurysm of subclavian artery
Aneurysm of aorta or mitral stenosis (left nerve only)
Paralysis of vagus nerve at base of skull—pachymeningitis, tuberculosis, syphilis, thrombosis of jugular bulb, cancer of the nasopharynx
Paralysis of the motor centres in the medulla—poliomyelitis, thrombosis of postero-inferior cerebellar artery, bulbar palsy.

WEAKNESS OF THE VOICE UNASSOCIATED WITH TRUE HOARSENESS:
Myasthenia gravis
General debility, convalescence from severe illness
Myxoedema, acromegaly
Functional aphonia.

Many of these diseases are short-lived, and in many the cause is self-evident from the history, so that little trouble will be found in making at least a tentative diagnosis. If the hoarseness should last more than a few days, it calls for examination by a laryngologist skilled in the use of the mirror. Delay may be extremely deleterious to the well-being of the patient.

Three diseases in particular are of serious import, and all may present considerable difficulty in diagnosis—tuberculosis of the larynx, cancer, and neurological disorders.

The characteristic of the tuberculous laryngeal lesion is a hoarse, weak whisper, as distinct from the forceful brassy voice of the syphilitic. Later in tuberculosis, the patient will complain of

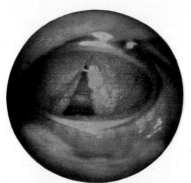

Fig. 420 A. Carcinoma of the vocal cord.

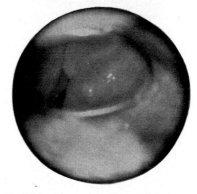

Fig. 420 B. Advanced carcinoma of the larynx.

pain on swallowing, which radiates to the ear. Syphilitic ulcers are grosser than those of tuberculosis, fewer in number, and show fibrotic healing. Tuberculous ulcers are multiple, small, shallow, and they are generally seen along the edge of the epiglottis and on the aryteno-epiglottidean folds as well as on the edges of the vocal cords themselves (mouse nibbled cords). There may be a suggestive pallid oedema of the folds without recognizable ulcers or tubercles. Sputum must be examined for tubercle bacilli, the blood for evidence of syphilis. Radiography of the chest may reveal pre-existing phthisis, or intially the lung fields may seem clear.

The recurrent laryngeal nerves supply all the intrinsic muscles of the larynx except the crico-thyroid. When these nerves, their parent nerve, the vagus, or the motor centre in the medulla are involved in disease or injury, the cord on the affected side will be found to lie immobile near the midline. If both are involved, the adducted position of the two cords narrows the glottis, and stridor will occur on inspiration. Later, the paralysed cords may assume a more lateral position, and breathing will be easier, but the voice will be weaker and 'breathy' in quality. Paralysis of one cord may be completely symptomless.

Hoarseness is a very early sign of cancer of the cord. Preceding keratosis may have given rise to some muffling of the voice and intermittent hoarseness, but once a growth has formed the voice becomes permanently impaired. Cancer of other parts of the larynx, such as the epiglottis and aryteno-epiglottidean folds, may cause a feeling of discomfort on swallowing and slight thickness of the voice, but true hoarseness occurs only later, often after the cervical lymph-nodes have become palpable as a result of cancerous infiltration.

Laryngoscopic biopsy is needed to establish the differential diagnosis between keratosis and cancer, and between the latter and innocent tumours. Naked-eye appearances alone may be misleading; and it is by no means uncommon to confuse tuberculous ulceration and cancer if biopsy is not employed.

The most dangerous diagnoses are hysterical aphonia and 'chronic laryngitis'. Neither should be made unless an adequate examination of the larynx has been carried out.

Miles Foxen.

HYDROGEN ION HOMEOSTASIS (ACID-BASE BALANCE)

Hydrogen ions (H$^+$) generated by metabolic processes may be reutilized or be oxidized to water during oxidative phosphorylation. Since the hydrogen ion concentration of body fluids is critical, any excess must be inactivated as speedily as possible, and ultimately be eliminated from the body.

Because hydrogen ions are the products of metabolism, acidosis is much commoner than alkalosis. For the same reason the term 'hydrogen ion homeostasis' is better than 'acid–base balance'.

BUFFERS

Buffers are the first line of defence in maintaining a constant hydrogen ion concentration in body fluids, and a brief description of the mode of action of buffers is necessary.

An acid is a substance which has the potential to dissociate and release hydrogen ions and so become acidic. If we denote this acid as HB we can see that dissociation also releases B$^-$, the conjugate base of the acid.

$$HB \longrightarrow H^+ + B^-$$

B$^-$ is called a base because it can accept H$^+$ to re-form HB. The proportion of HB dissociated at equilibrium is the dissociation constant

(K) of the acid. Using square brackets to denote concentration, we can express this as:

$$K[HB] = [H^+][B^-] \qquad (1)$$

or

$$[H^+] = K\frac{[HB]}{[B^-]} \quad \text{at equilibrium.} \qquad (2)$$

Acids with high dissociation constants are strong acids, almost all in the form H^+B^- at equilibrium, and therefore being strongly acidic: the conjugate base has a low affinity for H^+. The acids involved in metabolism are *weak* acids, with low dissociation constants which are predominantly in the form HB at equilibrium; their conjugate bases have a high affinity for H^+.

$$H^+ + B^- \longrightarrow HB$$

The weak acid so formed does dissociate a little, providing a 'pool' of hydrogen ion should $[H^+]$ tend to fall. B^- and HB thus form a 'buffer pair', B^- combining with, and therefore inactivating, added H^+, while HB reduces the effect of any tendency to remove H^+ by dissociating. Obviously, if $[B^-]$ and $[HB]$ are equal, buffering against change of $[H^+]$ is maximum. We can see in equations (1) and (2) that these conditions are fulfilled if $K = [H^+]$.

Although some people express hydrogen concentration directly, it is traditional to use pH (log $1/[H^+]$. Taking negative logs throughout equation (2), we get the Henderson-Hasselbalch equation—

$$pH = pK + \log\frac{[B^-]}{[HB]}$$

The most efficient buffer is then one with a pK near the desired pH. The lower the pK of the system, the more acid the solution will tend to be when $[B^-] = [HB]$.

The efficacy of a buffer to keep pH relatively constant depends on:

1. *The pK of the system.* In the extracellular fluid the ideal pK would seem to be near 7·4. As we shall see, bicarbonate is an important special case, since it is converted to CO_2 during buffering, but the concept is of importance in urinary buffering.

2. *The concentration of the buffer.* Buffering capacity for free H^+ must depend on the concentration of the buffer. Even if the pK is ideal, low quantities of B^- can buffer only low quantities of H^+.

Circulating Buffers and the Role of the Lungs. The two important buffers are *bicarbonate* in the extracellular fluid and *haemoglobin* in the erythrocytes. Bicarbonate provides 60 per cent of blood-buffering capacity, and works co-operatively with haemoglobin which is of great importance in respiratory disturbances (*see below*). Plasma proteins and monohydrogen phosphate are of much less importance: the latter, although of suitable pK, circulates at a concentration of only about 1 mmol/l compared with bicarbonate at 25 mmol/l.

The Bicarbonate System. The Henderson-Hasselbalch equation for bicarbonate is often written

$$pH = 6·1 + \log\frac{[HCO_3^-]}{[H_2CO_3]}$$

In fact, carbonic acid dissociates so rapidly to CO_2 and water that it cannot be detected, and the pK of 6·1 is derived from a combined constant of two reactions.

$$H^+ + HCO_3^- \xrightarrow{\hspace{1cm}} H_2CO_3$$
$$\xrightarrow{\hspace{1cm}} CO_2 + H_2O$$

It is usually written as pK'. The denominator in the Henderson-Hasselbalch equation is then the sum of the very small amount of H_2CO_3 and gaseous CO_2 with which it is in equilibrium. In clinical practice the partial pressure of the latter (P_{CO_2}) is measured, and is multiplied by the solubility constant of CO_2 (0·225 if P_{CO_2} is in kPa, or 0·03 if it is in mmHg) to give the denominator.

Although the pK' of 6·1 is apparently far from ideal for buffering extracellular fluid to pH 7·4, the bicarbonate system has a great biological advantage. Since H_2CO_3 dissociates rapidly to CO_2, and since the respiratory rate, and therefore the rate of removal of CO_2, by the *lungs*, is normally finely adjusted to maintain the P_{CO_2} of blood near 5·33 kPa (40 mmHg), the denominator of the Henderson-Hasselbalch equation is accurately controlled.

At such a P_{CO_2} the bicarbonate concentration (the numerator in the equation) is maintained near 25 mmol/l by two important mechanisms, both involving the enzyme carbonate dehydratase (carbonic anhydrase), which catalyses the reaction

$$CO_2 + H_2O \xrightarrow{\hspace{1cm}} H_2CO_3$$

Erythrocytes and renal tubular cells contain the enzyme in high concentration, and CO_2 is rapidly converted to H_2CO_3, the reaction being kept to the right by removal of H^+ as H_2CO_3 is formed and dissociates.

$$H_2CO_3 \xrightarrow{\hspace{1cm}} HCO_3^- + H^+$$

In erythrocytes H^+ is removed by buffering by haemoglobin, while in the kidney it is secreted into the urine, thus removing it from the body. HCO_3^- diffuses into the extracellular fluid from both sites. A change in P_{CO_2} will eventually alter $[HCO_3^-]$ by these two mechanisms, until the ratio between the two, and therefore the pH, returns to normal.

At the ratio determined by the lungs, erythrocytes, and kidneys the pH is about 7·4. In other words, accurate respiratory control removes CO_2 sufficiently fast, compared to generation of bicarbonate by erythrocytes and renal tubular cells, to maintain the pH well above the pK of the system. HCO_3^- and CO_2 are central to buffering in the body, but only work efficiently together with haemoglobin and normal kidneys and lungs.

RENAL CONTROL OF HYDROGEN ION HOMEOSTASIS

In the absence of normal renal function, buffering of added H^+ is limited. As more haemoglobin is converted to the acid form and as the CO_2 resulting from buffering by bicarbonate is lost through the lungs, further addition of hydrogen ions would cause marked pH changes. Only the kidneys can eliminate H^+ from the body and regenerate bicarbonate. Normal urine is usually slightly acid relative to extracellular fluid, reflecting daily production of hydrogen ions in excess of those oxidized.

Hydrogen and potassium ions compete for secretion by renal tubular cells. Renal secretion of hydrogen ions depends, as described above, on the action of carbonate dehydratase. CO_2 released by bicarbonate during buffering or retained by the lungs is reconverted to carbonic acid in the renal tubule, where the H^+ can be secreted in the urine, with regeneration of bicarbonate lost in the original buffering.

Reabsorption of bicarbonate from the glomerular filtrate depends on its conversion to CO_2 by combination with secreted H^+. CO_2 diffuses back into the tubular cell, where it re-forms bicarbonate, the associated hydrogen ion being resecreted. Once bicarbonate has been reabsorbed from the urine the availability of other buffers to keep the urinary free $[H^+]$ low by binding the secreted ions becomes all-important in maintaining secretion. Cation associated with the buffer (mostly Na^+) returns to the bloodstream with HCO_3^- generated during H^+ secretion.

Urinary Buffers. The most important urinary buffer is *monohydrogen phosphate*, which combines with hydrogen ion to form dihydrogen phosphate. Its concentration is very low in the glomerular filtrate (*see above*), but increases as more water than phosphate is reabsorbed during passage down the tubular lumen. Ammonia (NH_3), produced from glutamine in renal tubular cells, can accept H^+ to form ammonium (NH_4^+), and probably has a function in hydrogen ion homeostasis. Minor urinary buffers are urate and creatinine.

MEASUREMENTS TO ASSESS STATE OF HYDROGEN ION HOMEOSTASIS

Assessment of hydrogen ion balance is usually made by measuring the constituents of the bicarbonate buffer pair which is, as we have seen, of central importance. Attempts to correct for haemoglobin concentration and to allow for other buffers are desirable especially in anaemic subjects, but are rarely essential for clinical assessment.

The three measurable components of the bicarbonate system are:

pH—this is measured directly using a glass electrode, on *fresh, heparinized arterial blood withdrawn anaerobically.*

PCO_2—as previously explained, this can be used as a measure of the denominator in the Henderson-Hasselbalch equation. It is either measured directly, using a specific electrode, or derived by measuring the pH of the withdrawn blood after *in vitro* equilibration with gases of known PCO_2. This estimation, like pH, should be performed on *fresh arterial blood, heparinized and withdrawn anaerobically.*

Actual bicarbonate (the circulating bicarbonate concentration) may be derived from the Henderson-Hasselbalch equation, if pH and PCO_2 are known.

It is often more convenient to assess bicarbonate concentration on plasma obtained from venous blood when estimating plasma electrolytes. This is an estimation of the *total CO_2 (TCO_2)* content of the plasma—the sum of $[HCO_3^-]$ $[H_2CO_3]$ and gaseous CO_2. $[HCO_3^-]$ makes, quantitatively, by far the greatest contribution to this, even at the lowest pH found in the body, and TCO_2 is a reasonably valid index of it. If other parameters are not required (usually in metabolic disturbances), TCO_2 estimation, together with clinical assessment, is often adequate.

In addition, further parameters may be derived. We will only consider one, 'Standard Bicarbonate', to show its limitations:

Standard bicarbonate. This is a calculated value, and is an attempt to assess the contribution to a change in actual bicarbonate made by the *respiratory component* of the system, CO_2. If whole blood is equilibrated *in vitro* with gas of known PCO_2, the erythrocyte mechanism described above is brought into play, with a change in $[HCO_3^-]$. Thus the $[HCO_3^-]$ *in vitro* at a normal PCO_2 (5·33 kPa or 40 mmHg) can be derived. Since the renal mechanism *cannot* be reversed *in vitro*, the difference between actual and standard bicarbonate measures the increment of $[HCO_3^-]$ by the erythrocytes alone in response to a raised PCO_2. In practice, more can be learned from pH and PCO_2 readings, especially in chronic respiratory states, in which the renal mechanism contributes to most of the increase in $[HCO_3^-]$.

TERMINOLOGY

Four terms have been used: *acidosis, alkalosis, acidaemia* and *alkalaemia*. The last two are sometimes used to denote actual blood pH changes, 'acidosis' and 'alkalosis' denoting abnormalities which, because of compensatory changes, are associated with a normal blood pH. I prefer to use only the terms 'acidosis' and 'alkalosis', specifying if they are partially or wholly compensated.

CAUSES OF, AND FINDINGS IN, ACIDOSIS

In all forms of acidosis there is a tendency to *hyperkalaemia*, due to replacement of K^+ in cells and urine by H^+.

Metabolic Acidosis. The common finding is a low plasma HCO_3^- (*and therefore TCO_2*), either because it is used up in buffering more rapidly than it can be repleted, or because the cause of the acidosis is loss of bicarbonate. The compensatory response is *hyperpnoea* ('air hunger'), which, by removing at least as much CO_2 as, and often more than, is formed when HCO_3^- buffers H^+, tends to restore the ratio $[HCO_3^-]/P_{CO_2}$ to normal. The P_{CO_2} is therefore *normal or low* depending on the adequacy of the response, and the pH is normal (if fully compensated) or low. In metabolic acidosis the severity can usually adequately be judged by measuring total CO_2 on venous plasma, obviating the necessity for arterial puncture.

CAUSES

1. *Excessive Production or Ingestion of Acid* may 'swamp' normal homeostatic mechanisms.

    a. Ketosis results from impaired carbohydrate metabolism, due to insulin deficiency, with high blood glucose levels (*diabetic ketoacidosis*), or, more rarely, to *starvation* when glucose levels are normal or low. Acetyl CoA metabolism is disturbed, and as it accumulates condensation, followed by reduction, produces aceto-acetic and β-hydroxybutyric acid, respectively.

    Hydrogen ion balance is rapidly restored when the cause is removed, and keto-acidosis rarely merits specific treatment for acidosis.

    b. Lactic acidosis—hypoxia, relative or absolute, impairs carbohydrate metabolism beyond the pyruvate stage. The NAD^+ necessary for glycolysis is reoxidized by reduction of pyruvate to lactate, thus allowing further glycolysis to occur.

$$CH_3COCOO^- + NADH + H^+ \longrightarrow CH_3CHOHCOO^- + NAD^+$$

Pyruvate → Lactate

Lactate accumulates. Because oxidative phosphorylation is also impaired, much of the H^+ produced metabolically by other routes cannot be reutilized or oxidized to water, with resultant acidosis.

Hyperlactaemia with acidosis may be due to:

    i. Relative hypoxia following *severe exercise* ('oxygen debt'). This is rapidly reversed at rest, and is not a clinical problem.

    ii. Tissue anoxia following poor vascular perfusion in *hypotensive states*, such as 'shock', and severe dehydration (including that due to diabetic coma, and other severe illnesses). This is the commonest cause and often occurs in a severe form after *cardiac arrest*, when impaired liver metabolism of lactate contributes to very high plasma levels. Acidosis is severe, and is even out of proportion to the lactate levels.

    iii. Rarely *therapy with biguanides* such as phenformin, which inhibit reconversion of lactate to glucose. It seems that only a few subjects are susceptible to this form, which may therefore be associated with an inborn metabolic error.

    iv. '*Type I*' *glycogen storage disease* (von Gierke's disease). In this condition glycogen conversion to glucose is impaired. Consequent increased metabolism by the glycolytic pathway, especially during fasting, increases pyruvate and lactate production.

    v. Inborn errors of lactate metabolism are very rare. In one, recurrent severe lactic acidosis occurs in infancy.

    Treatment of the cause is often all that is necessary. In severe cases (for instance, after cardiac arrest) bicarbonate should be infused.

    c. Rarely *ingestion of ammonium chloride* causes acidosis. The ammonium forms urea, releasing H^+.

2. *Failure of the Kidneys* to secrete hydrogen ions, with consequent failure to replete bicarbonate.

    a. Inadequate total amount of urinary buffer to accept hydrogen ions and to provide sodium for exchange, when the *glomerular filtration rate is low*. This may be due either to renal circulatory insufficiency in hypotensive states, or to true glomerular disease in acute glomerulonephritis. Most commonly it is associated with tubular dysfunction in generalized renal failure. The plasma urea and creatinine levels will be high.

    b. Non-specific renal tubular damage, impairing, amongst other functions, the ability to secrete H^+, even in the presence of adequate urinary buffer. If the glomeruli are functioning normally there may be hypokalaemia, hypophosphataemia, and hypo-uricaemia, together with other evidence of tubular damage, such as aminoaciduria. This non-specific picture is sometimes called the *Fanconi syndrome*. More often, as stated above, glomerular and tubular failure coexist.

    c. Renal tubular acidosis. This is a group of rare syndromes in which there is isolated deficiency of urinary acidification mechanisms, without other evidence of tubular dysfunction.

3. *Depletion of Bicarbonate*, usually due to prolonged loss of intestinal secretions (for instance, through fistulae). This depletes the numerator in the Henderson-Hasselbalch equation, tending to lower the pH.

$$pK + \log \frac{[HCO_3^-]\downarrow}{P_{CO_2}} = pH\downarrow$$

4. *Surgical Transplantation of the Ureters into the Colon or Ileum* causes intestinal loss of bicarbonate in exchange for urinary chloride and causes hyperchloraemic acidosis.

Respiratory Acidosis. The constant finding is a *high P_{CO_2}. Increases in plasma bicarbonate* are compensatory, and T_{CO_2} cannot be used alone to assess the severity of respiratory acidosis. This assessment can only be made by measuring pH and/or P_{CO_2} on arterial blood, but is only clinically indicated if therapy is likely to be successful.

CAUSES

Any Severe Generalized Lung Disease, such as bronchopneumonia, chronic bronchitis, and emphysema, causes failure of alveolar exchange and retention of CO_2. The denominator in the Henderson-Hasselbalch equation is raised, tending to lower the pH

$$pK + \log \frac{[HCO_3^-]}{[P_{CO_2}\uparrow]} = pH\downarrow$$

The compensatory mechanisms in the erythrocytes and renal tubular cells tend to increase plasma $[HCO_3^-]$ in proportion. The contribution of the erythrocyte mechanism is reflected in the difference between the actual and standard bicarbonate, and is limited by the buffering capacity of haemoglobin. The renal mechanism is unlimited, as hydrogen ions can be lost in the urine, and in chronic disease the standard, as well as the actual, bicarbonate level is elevated; at a steady high P_{CO_2} the renal mechanism will continue to increase plasma $[HCO_3^-]$ until the ratio $[HCO_3^-]/P_{CO_2}$, and therefore the pH, return to normal. Treatment on a respirator is contra-indicated if the pulmonary disease is irreversible, since lowering of P_{CO_2} will be associated with loss of compensation.

Respiratory acidosis does *not* occur in local pulmonary disease, since CO_2 loss can be increased through normal alveoli by hyperventilation. It is also rare in pulmonary oedema, since CO_2 can diffuse through the oedema fluid; hyperventilation in this condition may even cause a *low* P_{CO_2}.

CAUSES OF, AND FINDINGS IN, ALKALOSIS

For the reasons stated in the introduction alkalosis is rare.

In all forms of alkalosis *hypokalaemia* is common, since K^+ replaces the deficient H^+ in cells and urine. In item (3) below, however, the hypokalaemia is primary. Tetany can occur due to reduction in the proportion of the total plasma calcium that is ionized.

Metabolic Alkalosis. The common finding is a high plasma $[HCO_3^-]$ (and therefore total CO_2). P_{CO_2} is rarely altered significantly. If there is no clinically obvious pulmonary dysfunction the commonest cause of a high total CO_2 is potassium depletion.

CAUSES

1. *Excessive Intake of Bicarbonate.* Rarely metabolic alkalosis is due to self-medication with oral bicarbonate for 'indigestion'. More commonly it is iatrogenic, for example due to treatment of cardiac arrest with sodium bicarbonate.

The numerator in the Henderson-Hasselbalch equation is increased, tending to raise the pH.

$$pK + \log \frac{[HCO_3^-]\uparrow}{P_{CO_2}} = pH\uparrow$$

2. *Loss of Unbuffered Hydrogen Ion in Pyloric Stenosis.* This is a rare cause, and is only evident after prolonged vomiting due to pyloric stenosis. Obstruction at the pylorus leads to loss of H^+ with Cl^- in vomitus. Reduction in H^+ causes a rise in pH, and $[HCO_3^-]$ also rises.

$$pH\uparrow = pK + \log \frac{[HCO_3^-]\uparrow}{P_{CO_2}}$$

The P_{CO_2} is usually normal.

Vomiting with a patent pylorus causes loss of bicarbonate as well as HCl, and rarely, if ever, causes alkalosis.

Table I. CAUSES OF ABNORMAL PLASMA BICARBONATE (AND TOTAL CO_2) CONCENTRATION

PLASMA $[HCO_3^-]$ REDUCED	pH	P_{CO_2}	CLINICAL FEATURES	FURTHER RELEVANT CHEMICAL INVESTIGATIONS FOR MAKING DIAGNOSIS
Acidosis, metabolic ($[HCO_3^-]$ affected first) Uncompensated	↓	N	Hyperpnoea. In diabetic ketoacidosis smell of acetone, dehydration	Blood glucose
Fully compensated	N	↓		Plasma urea
Alkalosis, respiratory ($[HCO_3^-]$ change compensatory) Partially compensated	↑	↓	May present with muscle cramps or even tetany	
Fully compensated	N	↓	Hyperpnoea with 'clear' lungs, or with pulmonary oedema	
PLASMA $[HCO_3^-]$ ELEVATED				
Acidosis, respiratory ($[HCO_3^-]$ change compensatory) Partially compensated	↓	↑	Dyspnoea due to severe pulmonary disease	
Fully compensated	N	↑	Cyanosis	
Alkalosis, metabolic ($[HCO_3^-]$ affected early)	↑	N	Look for cause of K^+ loss (diuretics etc.). May be history of ingestion or infusion of sodium bicarbonate. Severe vomiting due to pyloric stenosis	Plasma potassium Plasma chloride

3. *Extracellular Alkalosis in Potassium Depletion.* A deficiency of K^+ results in entry of H^+ into cells and urine. The result is an extracellular alkalosis, although there is intracellular acidosis. The plasma bicarbonate concentration rises as a result of the renal mechanisms associated with H^+ secretion.

Respiratory Alkalosis. The common finding is a *low* P_{CO_2}, with *secondary reduction of* $[HCO_3^-]$ (by the reverse mechanisms of those in respiratory acidosis).

CAUSES. Respiratory alkalosis results from hyperventilation with relatively normal pulmonary function.
1. *Hysterical Overbreathing*, which often presents as tetany, due to reduction in the proportion of calcium ionized (total calcium is normal).
2. *Overtreatment on Respirators.*
3. *Brain Stem Lesions* causing stimulation of the respiratory centre.
4. *Patchy Pulmonary Disease or Pulmonary Oedema*, when the respiratory centre is stimulated by a low P_{O_2} and/or alveolar stretching, with increased loss of CO_2 through normal alveoli or oedema fluid.

Table I summarizes the causes of an abnormal total CO_2.

Joan F. Zilva.

HYPERPYREXIA

The point at which pyrexia becomes hyperpyrexia is arbitrary: by some it is fixed at 105° F., by others at 106° F. (approximately 42° C.). Dangerous and even fatal hyperpyrexia has occurred in perfectly healthy subjects undertaking prolonged violent exercise in circumstances particularly unfavourable to heat loss. It may occur in many different diseases, but is only indirectly of diagnostic significance. The patient will nearly always have exhibited other symptoms or signs pointing to the diagnosis, therefore the following list of maladies in which hyperpyrexia may occur needs little elaboration:

1. Fevers of Microbial, or probably of Microbial, Origin, for example:

Septicaemia
Pyelitis
Malaria
Miliary tuberculosis
Suppurative meningitis
Lymphoma
Thyroid storm
Acute pancreatitis
Malignant endocarditis
Rarely, rheumatic fever.

2. Lesions of the Central Nervous System:

Cerebral haemorrhage, especially pontine, or into an optic thalamus
Head injury
Brain surgery
Cerebral tumour or abscess, especially tumour of the pons Varolii

Fractured spine, especially in the lower cervical or upper dorsal regions.

3. Other Causes:

After burns or scalds
Heat-stroke
Infantile hyperpyrexia
Acute atrophy of the liver.

4. The Taking of Drugs or Poisons, for example:

Dinitrocresol
Dinitrophenol
Picrotoxin
Extracts of poison ivy.

5. Factitious

Extremely high fevers over 106° F. (42° C.) are rare and are usually due to cerebral lesions, as noted above, but may also occur in heat-stroke (heat hyperpyrexia). Hyperpyrexia may sometimes serve as the chief point in distinguishing *pontine haemorrhage* or *heat-stroke* from other forms of coma. It has also been reported, though rarely, in cord lesions involving the intracord portion of the autonomic pathways so that vascular reflexes are affected. This may occur in disseminated sclerosis.

Infantile hyperpyrexia may be caused by high external temperature. Infants, particularly if premature, have difficulty in controlling body temperature, whether due to infection, dehydration, or environmental factors.

Heat hyperpyrexia (heat stroke) is due to exposure to a very high temperature often combined with excessive exercise or lack of circulating air. A systemic febrile disease and/or consumption of excessive alcohol may also be factors. Individuals with ichthyosis or reduced ability to sweat are more at risk than others.

In the past several instances of hyperpyrexia have arisen as the result of the taking of dinitrocresol for the purpose of weight reduction. The drug first raises the metabolic rate and after several days the temperature may rise suddenly to 105° F. (42° C.) or higher. Several drugs may also be responsible for hyperpyrexia usually from an allergic reaction. Large doses of aspirin have rarely been noted as responsible.

Malingerers and hysterics have been known to produce a fictitious rise of temperature, as by compressing the bulb of the thermometer or heating it in a cup of tea or against a hot-water bottle.

F. Dudley Hart.

HYPERSOMNIA

Hypersomnia has to be distinguished from other types of altered consciousness (*see* CONSCIOUSNESS, DISORDERS OF, p. 173) due to a wide variety of conditions. True hypersomnia resembles normal sleep in having a similar electroencephalographic pattern but may differ from normal sleep in its extent and in the fact that it occurs under inappropriate circumstances. A tendency for prolonged sleep by day is often seen among adolescents who may have great difficulty in rising in the morning. Going to bed late may contribute but is not the whole cause. Some patients, again, adolescents in particular, who are emotionally disturbed show a tendency to retreat from their emotional difficulties into sleep. Hypersomnia may also be a feature of a *depressive* illness. Although insomnia together with loss of appetite and weight is very much more common, in a much smaller number who become depressed (about 10 per cent possibly) the reverse occurs; they eat more, are overweight, and sleep unduly.

A rare but striking form of hypersomnia occurs in *narcolepsy*; a condition which, despite statements to the contrary, bears no relation whatsoever to epilepsy, but is one in which a patient may quite suddenly fall asleep at any time of the day, while, for example, holding a conversation or even in the middle of a meal, etc. Narcoleptic sleep, whether by day or night, is light with an EEG pattern resembling normal sleep. The patient is usually easily woken. Left to himself the narcoleptic may pass both the day and night in a series of cat-naps. The conditions under which sleep occurs are also those liable to produce sleep in normal persons although much more profoundly so in narcoleptics: after a meal, when bored or inactive, when travelling by train, when in a hot stuffy room, etc. It is possible that those who are not overtly narcoleptic but who succumb to sleep more readily than others may have a narcoleptic tendency.

Other features of narcolepsy, which are not invariably present, are *cataplexy*: a sudden loss of muscle tone associated with a strong and sudden emotional urge, e.g., laughter, surprise, etc. (this also occurs in normal persons to a lesser degree), and *hypnagogic* or *hypnopompic* hallucinations which usually occur at night, just at the point of falling asleep or waking. As the narcoleptic sleeps lightly by night as well as by day he spends quite a portion of the night hovering half-way between sleep and wakefulness. It is under these circumstances that *hallucinations*, usually visual and auditory, are particularly liable to occur (*see* HALLUCINATIONS, p. 357). Another rarer feature of narcolepsy is *sleep paralysis* in which the subject wakes but is unable, for a short time, to move hand or foot.

In most cases of narcolepsy no obvious cause is demonstrable but the root of the disturbance is considered to lie in the diencephalon. Narcolepsy may also be symptomatic of a variety of neurological disorders and has been recorded as a post-encephalitic phenomenon, in which a reversal of sleep rhythm may occur; following head injury; in association with cerebral tumours, particularly in the region of the midbrain and hypothalamus; with cerebral arteriosclerosis; neurosyphilis; subarachnoid haemorrhage and multiple sclerosis. Hypersomnia verging on stupor may occur also in diabetes, uraemia, and trypanosomiasis.

Periodic attacks of hypersomnia, usually of a few days' duration and recurring every few weeks or months, may be a feature of the very rare *Kleine-Levin syndrome*. The attacks of hypersomnia are associated with excessive hunger, restlessness, irritability, and a degree of mental confusion. The condition occurs chiefly in adolescent or young adult males. Its aetiology is unknown.

W. H. Trethowan.

HYPOCHONDRIASIS

Hypochondriasis is the term used for a variety of states which have as their central theme a morbid concern with bodily function or an unjustified conviction on the part of the patient that he suffers from some or other bodily disease. Hypochondriasis may coexist with a physical illness in the form of anxiety which the illness itself does not warrant, or may be manifested by morbid fears or false beliefs about the body and its organs, or by abnormal bodily sensations or by a combination of these.

Hypochondriasis is a common although not an invariable feature of *anxiety states*. Anxiety or apprehension, of which the cause is unknown to the patient, may attach itself to a physical symptom (*somatization of anxiety*); the physiological concomitants of anxiety may become in this way a subject of undue preoccupation. Palpitations, for example, are often taken to be a sign of heart disease and may form the basis of a cardiac neurosis (*da Costa's* or *effort syndrome*). In *hysterical* patients, a complaint of illness for which there is no organic foundation is frequently part of the clinical picture; many who are chronic invalids suffer in fact more from hypochondriacal symptoms than from physical dysfunction.

The content of an *obsessional state* may be supplied by fears of doubts about disease (*obsessive hypochondriasis*). In depressive disorders the patient's thoughts about his health are coloured by his mood, particularly so in the case of depressions occurring in the involutional period. In severe cases such hypochondriacal beliefs may reach the intensity of delusions; for example, the patient may believe that he is afflicted by cancer or venereal disease, or that his bowels have turned to stone, or even that he is actually dead (*nihilistic delusions*; *Cotard's syndrome*). In younger patients grotesque statements about the body, for instance that the intestines are shrunken, or that the spine has been penetrated by insects, may point to a *schizophrenic* disorder. Sexual hypochondriasis which may find expression in a delusion that the genitals are undergoing atrophy or the patient's sex is changing is not uncommon.

A hypochondriacal attitude towards his disability may be found in a patient with early *cerebral arteriopathy*. The diagnosis in these various disorders must be made on a clinical assessment of the primary condition, of which hypochondriasis is only one component. Hypochondriasis is also frequent after *injury* at *work*, particularly after *head injury* even in the absence of any organic impairment. While compensation may play a part in prolonging this state it is quite clear that with the passage of time, before legal proceedings are completed and as a result of repeated medical examinations and investigations, the injured workman may begin to believe that his condition is much more serious than it really is. Secondary depression may lead to further prolongation.

Where the hypochondriacal complaint is central to the clinical picture, there may be difficulty, firstly, in separating it from the complaint which signifies organic disease and, secondly, in discovering its actual pathogenesis. A morbid body-interest is often betrayed by multiple complaints of pain, numbness, 'creeping', or other unusual sensations, in several regions; the form of the complaint may itself be pathognomonic. Thus, a patient may describe a pain of shooting and burning quality, which begins in the neck and is felt in the back, chest and abdomen, and down both arms and legs. A wide distribution is by no means invariable; a common form of hypochondriacal symptom is a single, persistent localized pain, often in the face. In such cases, which occur without any physical basis, pain is felt constantly, showing little or no fluctuation with time, and little response to analgesics, although, as such patients are often depressed, it may respond to antidepressive medication. A hypochondriacal condition is foreshadowed in earlier life by an immoderate concern with physical health, with the regulation of the bowels and the choice of food, and by the accumulation of patent medicines and 'tonics'. Many people who take pride in physical fitness are apt to be much alarmed by slight signs of ill-health; thus many athletes, and others whose recreation or livelihood depends on bodily skills, are markedly hypochondriacal. The patient's history may show that he comes from a home in which there is, or was, an exaggerated notion about health and ill-health sometimes occasioned by protracted physical illness or hypochondriasis in his relatives.

Where hypochondriasis is a complication of an already-existing illness, suspicion may be aroused by the exaggeration or distortion of symptoms, or the prolongation of illness beyond its usual time. The attitude of the patient towards his condition, where this can be estimated, is an important clue, for the hypochondriac shows an undue concern for his bodily condition.

The significance of hypochondriacal symptoms has, therefore, to be weighed in each case. Mere anxiety about the possibility of some bodily disease may respond to simple reassurance. It may, however, signify a much more profound degree of mental disturbance requiring much fuller exploration. A *hypochondriacal obsession* has to be distinguished from a *hypochondriacal delusion*. The main difference is that in *obsessive* hypochondriasis the patient can never quite convince himself that he has not got the disease he fears he has, although his conviction may wax and wane in intensity, whereas in the case of *delusional* hypochondriasis, nothing will convince him that he has not got the disease he unwaveringly believes he has.

W. H. Trethowan.

HYPOCHONDRIUM (LEFT), PAIN IN

In considering localized abdominal pain it is well to remember the possibility of complete transposition of viscera and to make the appropriate alterations as they are anatomically indicated. Pain in the left hypochondrium may proceed from:

THE STOMACH. Any painful condition of the stomach may cause pain below the left costal margin, particularly a new growth or an ulcer towards the cardiac end. For the differential diagnosis, *see* INDIGESTION, p. 422, *and* EPIGASTRIUM, PAIN IN, p. 254. Flatulent distension of the fundus may also be a cause, diagnosed by the fact that the pain disappears on eructation; it is a familiar consequence of aerophagy.

THE SPLEEN. Some enlargements of the spleen are painful (*see* SPLEEN, ENLARGEMENT OF, p. 746). Pain may be caused by perisplenitis, in which case a friction sound can sometimes be heard on auscultation over the organ. This is probably the cause of pain in many cases of splenic infarction.

THE LEFT KIDNEY. *Pyelitis* and *Stone* in the left kidney may cause pain which has the characters described in the section on pain in the right hypochondrium (*see below*). A mobile left kidney is rarely a cause of pain, but intermittent hydronephrosis from kinking of the ureter may produce it. This can be accurately diagnosed only by pyelography. A perinephric abscess may cause pain in this situation, but more often in the loin where a swelling is evident on bimanual palpation. Infarction is again a possible cause of pain.

THE COLON. A new growth in the splenic flexure of the colon or obstruction of the large bowel lower down may cause pain in the left hypochondrium. In the case of new growth a tumour can usually be felt on bimanual palpation; obstruction will have the usual features. Apart from growth, a mere *accumulation of faeces* in the transverse and descending colon may cause a feeling of pain and weight in the left hypochondrium relieved by the administration of enemata. Swallowed air that is not eructated may cause pain and distension when trapped in the splenic colon, the so-called 'splenic flexure syndrome'.

PLEURISY and HERPES ZOSTER are possible causes. In the first of these a friction-sound will be heard; in the case of herpes, the explanation of pain will be evident on the appearance of the characteristic eruption, but pain may persist long after this has disappeared.

SLIPPING RIB. Abnormal mobility of the lower intercostal joints may cause pain—a condition which is called 'slipping rib'. The pain may be very severe and come on with exertion, especially when this involves stooping and bending: it is at first sharp and stabbing but may be followed by a persistent dull ache. It may simulate the pain of a deep-seated lesion and is apt to be mistaken for gastric ulcer when on the left side, for gall-stones when on the right. The slipping rib may be felt on careful palpation, but in most cases the condition is suggested by the patient's own story of how the pain is brought about. (*See* p. 133.)

SUBDIAPHRAGMATIC ABSCESS. (*See* p. 409.)

Harold Ellis.

HYPOCHONDRIUM (RIGHT), PAIN IN

Pain in the right hypochondrium may proceed from any of the following organs:

Liver and gall-bladder
Duodenum
Head of the pancreas
Right kidney
Appendix vermiformis
Colon
Uterine appendages
Intrathoracic disease
Affections of the spine or chest wall
Subdiaphragmatic abscess
In fascioliasis.

The differential diagnosis is rendered difficult by the circumstance that disease may be simultaneously present in more than one of these situations.

LIVER. Various forms of enlargement of the liver may be attended by pain in the right hypochondrium, e.g., hepatitis, passive congestion, liver fluke infestation, hepatic abscess, carcinoma (*see* LIVER, ENLARGEMENT OF, p. 503).

Diseases of the Gall-bladder are gall-stones, cholecystitis, and carcinoma. In these it will usually be found that there is tenderness on pressure over the gall-bladder, with the characteristic catch in the breath when the patient is asked to take a deep inspiration while the fingers of the observer are pressed in over the organ. In acute cholecystitis there will be pyrexia, and probably rigors; a tender mass may be felt arising in the right subcostal region at the lateral border of the rectus sheath. As the gall-bladder distends it projects thence towards the umbilicus.

The pain of *biliary colic* may be felt chiefly in the right hypochondrium, but tends to radiate through to the back and up towards the right shoulder. It may be closely simulated by both the kinking of a mobile kidney and renal colic. When the attacks occur during the night as well as in the day, biliary colic is more likely. Absence of jaundice does not contra-indicate a diagnosis of gall-bladder disease.

DUODENUM. A *duodenal ulcer* may cause deep-seated pain in the right hypochondrium, usually with the character of hunger-pain (p. 336). Pain due to chronic cholecystitis or appendicitis may also have this character, and an exact differentiation of them may not be possible without X-ray examination or even exploration, not to mention the far from infrequent coexistence of two or even all three of these lesions. The pain in duodenal ulcer occurs in more definite attacks with long intervals of freedom; it is often nocturnal, waking the patient in the small hours of the morning. Typically the patient takes a glass of milk or some alkaline preparation to bed with him as antidote in anticipation of the pain. Biliary colic may also have a nocturnal incidence. Duodenal ulcer is commoner in men, disease of the gall-bladder in women, whilst appendicitis may occur with almost equal frequency in either sex. A history of melaena, or the presence of occult blood in the faeces, would be in favour of ulcer, and support will be afforded by X-ray examination, which in most cases of duodenal ulcer will show typical distortion of the duodenal cap and often demonstrate the ulcer crater itself.

PANCREAS. Malignant disease of the pancreas may cause pain in the right hypochondrium. In this condition a deep-seated tumour may be felt, and there is often jaundice together with a distended gall-bladder. On the other hand, when gall-stones are responsible for jaundice the gall-bladder is usually not distended (*see* p. 444).

RIGHT KIDNEY. A freely *movable right kidney* may, by ureteral kinking, cause sudden attacks of pain in the right hypochondrium—Dietl's crises—which may closely simulate gall-stone colic. Indications of intermittent hydronephrosis should be looked for, e.g., the appearance of a renal tumour and the occasional discharge of large quantities of urine; urinary symptoms may, however, be entirely absent. A certain diagnosis may be impossible without pyelography (p. 479).

Stone in the right kidney may cause chronic pain in the right hypochondrium and back. The kidney may be enlarged and tender on bimanual palpation, the urine may furnish no diagnostic indication although frequently there is slight proteinuria which is often intermittent. There may be macroscopic, or more commonly microscopic, haematuria. X-rays may make the diagnosis clear (*Figs.* 479, 480, p. 473); although some 90 per cent of renal calculi are radiologically opaque, a negative result does not, of course, exclude the possibility of stone. Ureteral catheterization and pyelography may be needed as diagnostic aids.

The pain of *renal colic* may be difficult to distinguish from that of gall-stone colic, lead colic, or appendicitis, but it begins below the lower ribs posteriorly and has a tendency to pass downwards towards the umbilicus and thence into the groin. During or after the attack there may be blood and gravel in the urine.

Pyelonephritis may also be the cause of severe pain. The urine will furnish diagnostic indications (*see* PYURIA, p. 678, and BACTERIURIA, p. 91). The kidney may be recognized as enlarged on bimanual palpation. Even if impalpable, there is usually loin tenderness on deep bimanual palpation. The pain may begin acutely, starting in the loin and right hypochondrium and passing downwards towards the iliac fossa and pelvis. It is specially apt to occur during pregnancy. There are pyuria and rigidity of the muscles both in the loin and in the right side of the abdomen.

A *perinephric abscess* may cause pain in the right hypochondrium and lumbar region. A tender tumour will be felt, the loin may be visibly filled out, and there will be the usual signs of deep-seated suppuration.

APPENDIX. An attack of acute appendicitis may simulate gall-stone colic when the appendix lies in the high retrocolic position. (*See also* EPIGASTRIUM, PAIN IN, p. 254.)

COLON. *New growths* in the neighbourhood of the hepatic flexure may cause pain in the right hypochondrium. A tumour can usually be felt, and signs of chronic intestinal obstruction are present.

UTERINE APPENDAGES. *Salpingitis*, a *twisted ovarian pedicle*, and a *ruptured extra-uterine gestation* may all cause pain in the right side of the abdomen, with its maximum intensity rather below the hypochondriac region. A pelvic examination should establish the diagnosis.

PLEURISY, SLIPPING RIB, and HERPES ZOSTER may be causes of pain in the right hypochondrium as on the left side (p. 407).

SUBDIAPHRAGMATIC ABSCESS. In this condition there will be a history of some responsible antecedent such as acute appendicitis, a perforated gastric or duodenal ulcer, hepatic abscess, or an operation upon the abdomen. The onset of the pain may be sudden or gradual. There may be accompanying referred shoulder-tip pain and occasionally hiccup from diaphragmatic irritation. Pyrexia and leucocytosis point to deep-seated suppuration. The abnormal physical signs are generally few, but those that can be distinguished usually point to trouble at the base of the right lung. The liver is *not*, as a rule, pushed down. The abscess may be located by X-rays, or by the exploring needle, preferably employed when the patient is on the operating-table and one is prepared to open the abscess at once if it is located.

During the autumn of 1958, in the Hampshire market town of Ringwood, several (some 6) patients presented themselves with a mysterious illness characterized by pain in the right hypochondrium and an irregular pyrexia lasting over six weeks. There was high eosinophilia. This was traced by the discovery in the faeces of the ova of the liver fluke *Fasciola hepatica*, due to the habit of eating watercress grown in natural beds. Fresh outbreaks of this condition have been reported from Monmouthshire and Shropshire. Pains in the epigastrium or in the right hypochondrium were almost invariably present.

Harold Ellis.

HYPOTHERMIA

Hypothermia signifies a condition of subnormal temperature and it is generally assumed to refer to the temperatures registered by the thermometer in the mouth. Many cases are missed if clinical thermometers registering only from 35 °C. (95 °F.) are used. A temperature as low as this should be checked with an incubator thermometer or thermocouple. When the body temperature falls below this level physiological changes occur, pulse-rate, blood-pressure, and metabolic rate falling. Shivering begins and as the temperature approaches 30 °C. consciousness becomes impaired: hallucinations may occur. Ventricular fibrillation is the main danger. In the elderly it may occur in subjects living alone in unheated rooms in cold weather. It may complicate or be confused with a cerebrovascular accident. As many as 2000 deaths a year may occur annually in Great Britain from accidental hypothermia in the elderly. The picture may be aggravated by the taking of alcohol or drugs such as chlorpromazine which tend to render the subject poikilothermic. Rapid external rewarming is dangerous as it may cause a sudden loss of peripheral vasoconstriction and circulatory failure. If inadequately protected, immersion in water about 0 °C. will result in the subject losing consciousness within 15 minutes and death within the hour. From a diagnostic point of view hypothermia may be a symptom of importance; for instance, in helping to differentiate the coma due to *opium poisoning* from that due to *pontine haemorrhage*. In both there are bilateral loss of movement, pin-point pupils, and few other signs: in opium poisoning, however, the temperature is usually subnormal while with pontine haemorrhage it tends to rise to the level of hyperpyrexia. The knowledge that hypothermia is common in sufferers from chronic cardiac illness is of significance as indicating the necessity for regarding even slight rises above 37 °C. (98·4 °F.) as possibly being significant. In such patients bacterial endocarditis may be missed.

The chief causes of hypothermia are as follows:

Chronic Debilitating Maladies, such as:

Chronic valvular, and other types of heart disease
Extreme wasting as in malignant disease or starvation
Kwashiorkor
Chronic pancreatitis
Terminal hepatic cirrhosis.

Endocrine Disorders, such as:

Addison's disease
Hypoglycaemic coma and precoma, whatever the cause
Hypopituitarism
Subthyroidism.

Coma due to poisons and drugs through which the power of heat regulation is temporarily lost, particularly:

Opium
Alcohol

Barbiturates
Morphine
The phenothiazines (e.g., chlorpromazine)
Chloral
Anaesthetics.

Cerebral Conditions Rarely in:

Cerebrovascular accidents
Tumours
Abscess.

Shock after **severe injury** or after a serious **operation**, **coronary thrombosis**, or **pulmonary embolus**, or after **overwhelming infections**.

Collapse due to loss of liquid from the tissues from such conditions as:

Severe diarrhoea, choleraic or otherwise
Severe vomiting
Peritonitis
Intestinal obstruction
Haemorrhage.

Exposure to cold, particularly after prolonged immobility in the aged, as after cerebrovascular episodes, or after immersion in cold water.

F. Dudley Hart.

ILIAC FOSSA (LEFT), PAIN IN

As mentioned in the survey of pain in the hypochondrium, in the condition of complete transposition of viscera the substitution of right for left and reversely must automatically follow. Although many of the causes of pain complained of mainly or entirely in the left iliac fossa are the same as those which cause similar pain in the right iliac fossa, there are certain differences, as will be seen on comparing the table on p. 413 with the following:

CAUSES OF PAIN IN THE LEFT ILIAC FOSSA

1. ACUTE PAIN:

Stitch
Acute diverticulitis
Ureteric calculus
Acute pyelonephritis
Salpingitis
Twisted left ovarian cyst pedicle
Oophoritis
Pelvic abscess
Retained left testis
Appendicitis (exceptional cases)
Volvulus of the sigmoid colon
Strangulated retroperitoneal hernia
Local injury.

2. SUBACUTE, CHRONIC, OR RECURRENT PAIN:

Most of the conditions mentioned under Group 1
Carcinoma of the sigmoid colon
Carcinoma of rectum
Impaction of faeces
Colonic diverticular disease
Psoas abscess
Sacro-iliac joint disease
Tuberculous hip
Osteo-arthritis of the spine
Infective arthritis of the lumbar spine
Herpes zoster
Inflamed iliac lymph-nodes

Tuberculous iliac lymph-nodes
Pericolic abscess
Periprostatic abscess
Dysentery
Ulcerative colitis
Aneurysm of the left iliac artery
Sarcoma, osteoma, or other tumour of the left iliac bone
Tuberculous left kidney.

1. Acute Lesions. What is said on pp. 413 et seq., in regard to *ureteral calculus, twisted ovarian cyst pedicle, salpingitis, oophoritis, pelvic abscess, retained testis, periostitis of the ilium, injury,* and *stitch,* applies in the case of the left iliac fossa as it does to the right, so that here we need discuss only *acute diverticulitis, appendicitis, acute pyelonephritis, volvulus of the sigmoid,* and *strangulated retroperitoneal hernia.* Of these, the last two call for immediate operation on account of urgent symptoms of intestinal obstruction, especially persistent constipation and vomiting which becomes faeculent if operative measures are not quickly adopted. The precise nature of the obstruction may not be certain until the abdomen has been opened. Abdominal distension is pronounced although the abdominal wall remains supple unless general peritonitis supervenes. There is visible peristalsis of the oblique or transverse type in the case of strangulated retroperitoneal hernia, a rare condition in which a coil of small intestine becomes herniated through the normally small retrosigmoid pouch of peritoneum. In sigmoid volvulus, distension is at first conspicuous in the left iliac fossa before general colonic dilatation with vertical peristaltic waves develop. Plain X-rays of the abdomen in the erect and supine positions are valuable in demonstrating distorted loops of bowel with fluid levels. The enormously dilated loop of sigmoid in volvulus is characteristic and has been likened to a bent inner tube of a motor-car tyre.

Acute pyelonephritis is a less common cause of pain in the left iliac fossa than of corresponding pain on the right side (p. 414). When it does cause left-sided pain there is nearly always a more severe pain simultaneously on the right side. Acute pyelonephritis affects the right kidney and ureter much more commonly than the left, especially in pregnant women, though why its incidence should be first or solely on the right side is not clear.

Appendicitis is almost the last thing that occurs to one as the cause of acute pain referred entirely to the left iliac fossa, just as it is the first when the pain is on the right side. Apart from transposition of viscera, left-sided pain may occur for two reasons: first, because in some cases the vermiform appendix is so long that the inflammation starting at its tip spreads to the left, the symptoms and swellings being to the left of the middle line instead of as is usual in the right iliac fossa; secondly, because in a few cases pains produced in viscera on one side of the body are referred to the corresponding region on the other side.

Acute diverticulitis has been described as 'left-sided appendicitis', an apt term having regard to its clinical manifestations. It may cause an abscess demanding surgical measures, or an acute attack may resolve without suppuration, as may also happen in appendicitis. The patient is seized with severe pain in the left iliac fossa, and generally vomits. The temperature and pulse-rate rise, the tongue is coated, there is either diarrhoea or constipation or the two may alternate. On abdominal examination acute tenderness is evident, with rigidity of the muscles over the lower left quadrant of the abdomen and fullness or an ill-defined tumour in the same region. On rectal or vaginal examination, tenderness may be elicited when the examining finger is pressed upwards and to the left. Symptoms may abate after a day or two and disappear completely within a fortnight: alternatively they may increase rapidly and call for urgent surgical intervention or they may subside considerably without clearing up altogether, to recur after a few weeks or months. At operation the cause of the persistence of symptoms will be found to be a local thick-walled abscess in the left side of the pelvis, perhaps suggesting a pyosalpinx if the patient is a woman. As in appendicitis, general peritonitis may supervene at any stage. The cause of this common disease is the development of hernial pouches in rows (*Fig.* 185, p. 177) between the longitudinal muscle-bands of the colon. They occur chiefly distal to the splenic flexure. When present but not inflamed they are distinguished by the term *diverticulosis*. The orifice of a diverticulum is usually smaller than the sac and the interior of the intestine looks as if it has been punched with a series of small holes into which the little finger may just pass, each such hole leading into a more or less dilated pouch or sacculus, generally with an appendix epiploica attached to its free end; such a diverticulum is liable to inflammation, resulting in acute diverticulitis. Acute diverticulitis is a disease of the second half of life rather than the first. Either sex may be attacked, females in a majority.

2. Subacute or Chronic Lesions. *Carcinoma* of the *sigmoid colon* or of the *rectum* may cause pain in the colon owing to its distension with accumulated faeces; sometimes this pain is complained of chiefly over the descending colon, and thus in the left iliac fossa. As a rule increasing constipation is a prominent symptom, or a constantly repeated desire to defaecate is experienced without satisfactory relief from the effort. If blood and mucus are passed per rectum, if the patient is over forty, has been free from bowel symptoms until the last two or three months, and has been losing weight, carcinoma is highly probable. A tumour may be felt in the left iliac fossa. Difficulty in diagnosis arises in patients who have long been habitually constipated so that any increase experienced is not conspicuous nor easily assessed. Rectal examination, the sigmoidoscope, X-rays after a barium meal, or after a barium enema, may all be needed to exclude simpler conditions such as *impacted faeces* or *spastic constipation*, which are discussed under CONSTIPATION (p. 173).

Diverticular disease of the left colon may produce signs and symptoms very like those of carcinoma of the pelvic colon.

All the other conditions mentioned in the table above are discussed in the article on ILIAC FOSSA (RIGHT), PAIN IN *below*, and what is said there applies equally to the left iliac fossa.

Harold Ellis.

ILIAC FOSSA (LEFT), SWELLING IN

Normally the left iliac fossa contains iliac and pelvic colon, with a few coils of small intestine and the lower edge of the omentum. A list of swellings is appended, the common ones being marked with a *.

Classification:

SWELLINGS CONNECTED WITH THE NORMAL CONTENTS OF THE LEFT ILIAC FOSSA:
   *Colon spasm
   *Faecal masses
   *Diverticulitis
   *Carcinoma of the colon.

SWELLINGS CONNECTED WITH STRUCTURES NOT USUALLY PRESENT IN THE LEFT ILIAC FOSSA:
   Spleen
   Left kidney
   Metastases in omentum
   *Cysts and tumours of the left ovary
   *Uterine fibroids
   Extension of pelvic peritonitis.

SWELLINGS IN THE POSTERIOR WALL OF THE FOSSA:
   Ilio-psoas abscess
   Tumours of ilium
   Aneurysm of the external iliac artery
   Enlarged glands of the external iliac group.

Colon spasm affects the iliac colon more commonly than any other portion of the large bowel, and is seen typically in thin nervous patients. The spastic colon is felt as a firm, cylindrical, tender swelling lying above and parallel to Poupart's ligament; it varies in size and firmness at different examinations, and will often disappear under the influence of full doses of atropine. *Faecal masses* may be felt in all parts of the colon in the aged, the mentally deficient, or those who habitually neglect themselves; they are recognized by their distribution in the site of the colon, their doughy consistency and pitting on pressure, and their reduction or disappearance after an enema. Masses aggregated in the pelvic colon only, with the transverse colon empty, suggest that a carcinoma lies just below them.

Diverticulitis, a local inflammatory change supervening on diverticulosis, may give rise to a history of gradual obstruction in the colon and a swelling in the left iliac colon that resembles carcinoma very closely. *Carcinoma of the colon* affects the pelvic colon (*Figs.* 421, 422) more often than any other part. If it is of the scirrhous or ring type no lump can be felt, and the condition may not be discovered until intestinal obstruction has supervened. If it infiltrates the bowel wall widely, and especially if it is undergoing colloid degeneration, it forms a swelling that can be felt in the left iliac fossa, and is even more evident on bimanual examination after the bowels have been well cleared by enemata. It is, however, unlikely either in diverticulitis or cancer that the patient has noticed the lump; he comes complaining of

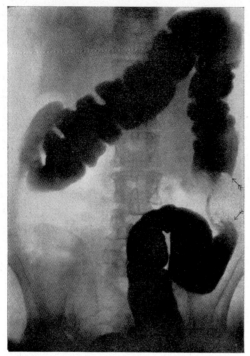

Fig. 421. Radiograph showing the site of a stenosing carcinoma of the lower end of the descending colon. The limits of the carcinoma are indicated by the narrow isthmus of barium shadow between the two arrows. A barium meal had been given, and the barium that had been given by the mouth had reached the upper limit of the cancerous constriction when a barium enema was administered; the latter extended up to the lower limit of the constriction, and the radiograph was then obtained. (Dr. W. H. Coldwell.)

irregularity in the bowels, of increasing constipation, sometimes alternating with diarrhoea, of attacks of distension accompanied by colicky pain in the hypogastrium which are relieved by passing flatus.

When the lesion is in an accessible part of the bowel (within 30 cm. of the anus), passage of the sigmoidoscope and the removal of a piece of tissue for biopsy is an essential part of the examination. Often, however, the lesion will be beyond the reach of the sigmoidoscopic biopsy and laparotomy even may fail to establish the diagnosis, but the presence of diverticula elsewhere, the involvement of several inches of bowel, and wide fixation with no glandular involvement, suggest an inflammatory origin of the swelling. Fibre-optic colonoscopy may be

useful but with good radiography this investigation may delay laparotomy.

Good radiography will usually differentiate between carcinoma and diverticulitis (*Fig.* 423), but laparotomy may be the only course when there is doubt.

Radiographs taken with the so-called 'double-air contrast' technique will sometimes reveal a small lesion which otherwise escapes detection (*Fig.* 424).

Both the *spleen* and the *left kidney* may enter the left iliac fossa, but neither should cause confusion. The left kidney is very rarely displaced. *Metastases in the free margin of the great omentum* are responsible for some of the puzzling swellings in the lower compartments of the abdomen, among them the left iliac fossa: the primary

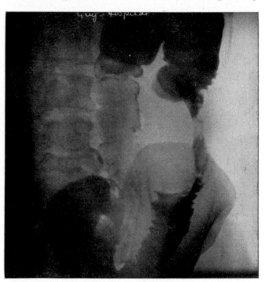

Fig. 422. Filling defect of the colon due to carcinoma. (Dr. T. H. Hills.)

growth is usually in the stomach, and a 'shelf' will usually be felt per rectum in the pouch of Douglas.

Swellings of the uterus and ovary are discussed on page 626. A *pelvic abscess*, such as that arising from inflammation of an appendix lying low in the pelvis, may, as it increases in size, be guided to the left by the pelvic mesocolon so as to present in the left iliac fossa: the swelling is tender, inseparable from the abdominal wall, and occupies the lower part of the fossa. Rectal or vaginal examination will reveal a mass in the pelvis continuous with that in the abdomen. A history of sudden onset with abdominal pain and vomiting can usually be obtained.

An *ilio-psoas abscess* is a fluctuating swelling, placed deeply in the iliac fossa: it is unlikely to attract attention as a swelling, but may be discovered in the examination of a patient with tuberculous disease of the spine, or when the abscess points below Poupart's ligament. *Tumours of the ilium* are rounded and hard, fixed to the bony pelvis, and displacing the colon inwards: a radiograph will confirm the diagnosis.

Aneurysm of the external iliac artery is recognized at once by its expansile pulsation.

Enlarged lymphatic glands. The glands forming a chain round the external iliac vessels may be swollen as the result of pyogenic infection which has spread up through the femoral lymphatics, or from secondary deposit of some malignant growth starting either in the leg, the external genitals, or the pelvis. The largest glandular swellings encountered in this region are those of Hodgkin's disease, which may start in this group.

R. G. Beard.

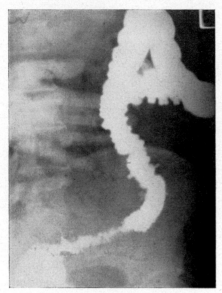

Fig. 423. Diverticulitis of sigmoid colon.

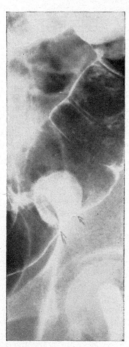

Fig. 424. Malignant polyp of colon shown by 'double-air contrast' barium enema.

ILIAC FOSSA (RIGHT), PAIN IN

A considerable number of conditions may be responsible for pain in this situation. The pains may be acute and severe, or subacute, or chronic with a history of previous similar attacks. These characters do not distinguish any one cause with certainty from the rest, though they may serve as a basis for classification as follows:

CAUSES OF PAIN IN THE RIGHT ILIAC FOSSA

1. ACUTE AND SEVERE PAIN:

Acute appendicitis
Acute salpingitis
Crohn's disease (regional ileitis)
Calculus impacted in right ureter
Acute pyelonephritis
Twisted pedicle of right ovarian cyst
Pelvic abscess
Retained right testis
Suppurative periostitis of the ilium
Stitch
After local injury
Acute inflammation of the iliac or ileocaecal lymph-nodes
Acute destructive myositis of the lower part of the rectus abdominis muscle
Rupture of the lower part of the rectus abdominis muscle
Rupture of the inferior epigastric artery.

2. SUBACUTE, CHRONIC, OR RECURRENT PAIN:

Most of the conditions already enumerated in Group 1
Psoas abscess
Sacro-iliac joint disease
Obturator hernia
Herpes zoster
Osteo-arthritis of the lumbar vertebrae
Infective arthritis of the lumbar vertebrae
Tuberculous hip
Inflamed or tuberculous iliac lymph-nodes
Ileocaecal tuberculosis
Actinomycosis of the caecum
Carcinoma of the caecum
Mobile right kidney
Dysentery
Ulcerative colitis
Typhoid fever
Aneurysm of the right iliac artery
Tuberculous right kidney and ureter
Intestinal obstruction at a distal point in the intestines, due to any cause, such as carcinoma of the sigmoid flexure, etc.
Sarcoma, osteoma, or chondroma of the iliac bone
Lobar pneumonia, pleurisy, other chest conditions, with referred pain.

1. Acute and Severe Pain. In most cases of pain in the right iliac fossa the first diagnosis to be considered is appendicitis. When acute pain is accompanied by an increased pulse-rate, some rise of temperature, vomiting, local rigidity over the right iliac fossa, and perhaps in addition to a sense of resistance, a diffuse palpable fullness, or even a more or less localized tender swelling, together with tenderness of the right side of the rectum on rectal examination, the probability is high that the patient has *acute appendicitis*, and that in most instances surgical measures will be necessary. The temperature subsides on perforation of the appendix or if an abscess forms and is walled off. The pain in cases of acute appendicitis, although frequently experienced at first in the umbilical region, is often associated with a localized acute tenderness referred to McBurney's spot which is situated at the outer point of trisection of a line joining the umbilicus to the right anterior superior iliac spine. More accurately, this exquisite local tenderness is at the site of irritation of the parietal peritoneum by the inflamed appendix; thus it may be far out into the right flank, in the hypochondrium, or only detected on pelvic examination. It has often been noted how unusual is an accompanying headache; in fact its presence suggests some other lesion.

Occasionally, when acute appendicitis has been the apparent diagnosis, some other focal suppuration is found at operation, a *pyosalpinx* or a *suppurating ovarian cyst*, for example, or even *acute suppurative periostitis of the inner surface of the ilium*, a rare condition which may closely simulate acute appendicitis.

Crohn's disease or *regional ileitis* (*Fig.* 425) is a chronic, localized inflammation of the terminal portion of the small intestine giving rise to pain in the right iliac fossa, periodic attacks of diarrhoea, pyrexia, distension, and occasionally vomiting; a palpable lump may be felt, usually in the right side of the abdomen, occult blood may be present in the stool. X-ray examination after an opaque meal may establish a diagnosis by the appearance of the narrow streak of barium (Kantor's string sign) connecting the ileum and caecum.

A *ureteric calculus* generally becomes impacted in the lower end of the ureter close to the bladder. It may produce ureteric colic, the pain being referred to the right iliac fossa so that appendicitis is suspected. There may be local rigidity of the muscles, but no tumour can be felt, and as a rule the patient is much less ill than with appendicitis. The history of recurrent attacks associated perhaps with transient haematuria (macroscopic or microscopic) will help to distinguish the cause, or the diagnosis may be determined only after routine examination, including the use of plain X-rays, pyelography, cystoscopy, and ureteric catheterization. The conditions likely to simulate the X-ray appearance of a stone in the ureter are calcareous iliac lymph-nodes or a phlebolith in a formerly thrombosed iliac vein (*Fig.* 489, p. 478).

It may be possible to distinguish between these three by the relative situations of the shadows, especially if radiographs are taken in different planes with an opaque bougie in the ureter (*Figs.* 479–481, pp. 473–474).

Acute pyelonephritis is a familiar difficulty in the differential diagnosis of appendicitis. Although it is to be expected that the pain should be referred mainly to the kidney, generally the right, it is common for patients suffering from

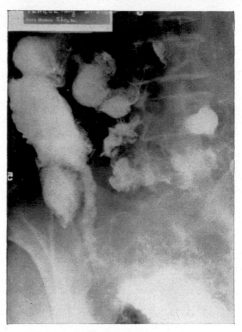

Fig. 425. Crohn's disease, showing irregular and constricted terminal ileum.

this condition to experience pain not in the back or loin but in the front of the lower part of the abdomen, particularly over the right iliac fossa, so simulating appendicitis. Even though the urine be examined and a haze of albumin found together with an excess of leucocytes, the acuteness of the condition may be such that the surgeon may not feel justified in delaying an operation, in waiting for cultures of a catheter specimen of the urine to be made for identification of the *Escherichia coli*. Not a few patients have in such circumstances undergone operation for acute appendicitis when the appendix is found to be perfectly normal.

Twisting of the pedicle of an ovarian cyst upon the right side produces acute abdominal pain, and the diagnosis may be established only when urgent laparotomy is performed. As a rule the pain starts in the lower part of the abdomen before it becomes general, and in the case of a cyst upon the right side it may be referred particularly to the right iliac fossa, so that appendicitis may be simulated, especially as there is tenderness in the right lower quadrant of the abdomen, in which situation a diffuse swelling may be felt, and confirmed on bimanual pelvic examination. Effusion of liquid into the general peritoneal cavity rapidly takes place producing dullness in the flanks; the peritonitis is generally non-suppurative. This emergency calls for urgent laparotomy.

Acute salpingitis or *inflammation of the right ovary* is generally secondary to pelvic inflammation which has been diagnosed on account of other symptoms, such as a vaginal discharge (p. 811), pain in the pelvis (p. 630), or some menstrual irregularity such as menorrhagia (p. 524). The temperature is, as a rule, higher than in appendicitis, and vomiting is usually absent. On vaginal palpation it may be possible to determine the cause, though until laparotomy is performed doubt may exist whether the inflammatory process affects the right uterine appendages or the vermiform appendix. Should the pain in the right iliac fossa be relatively slight in the intermenstrual periods, and severe at the time of the periods themselves, the mischief is more likely to be in the pelvic organs than the appendix. A possible fallacy may result from preceding appendicitis with extensive adhesions which include the uterine appendages, so that the pain, though primarily the result of appendicitis, may be recurrently worse at each monthly period. An important point is that salpingitis and oophoritis, though possibly unilateral, are more commonly bilateral, so that the distribution of the pains is wider in the case of ovarian or Fallopian-tube inflammation than with or after appendicitis.

Acute stitch generally affects the flank in the lower costal region on one side or the other, but the muscles over the right iliac fossa may be involved instead of the abdominal muscles higher up, the acute pain in the right iliac fossa then causing the patient to fear appendicitis. The character of the pain, and the recognition that it is definitely in the abdominal wall, and is unaccompanied by hyperaesthesia or swelling or pyrexia or other evidence of inflammation, should exclude appendicitis, especially since it is transient and related to violent and unaccustomed exertion such as running for a bus.

Retention of the right testis should not be forgotten when a lad at puberty complains of pain in the right iliac fossa suggesting appendicitis. The scrotum should be examined for the identification of both testicles. The testis, if it is in the upper end of the inguinal canal, may cause subacute pain similar to that of mild appendicitis, and at the same time there may be local resistance in the iliac fossa. There is no pyrexia.

Injury to the right iliac fossa may be followed by acute pain. In most instances the history indicates the diagnosis, especially if there is local bruising. Sometimes, however, the patient may have injured himself unknowingly, for instance during times of excitement, or when under the influence of drink, or during a nocturnal attack of epilepsy. The absence of pyrexia and of an increased pulse-rate will be points against acute appendicitis, though there may be local swelling from a deeply situated haematoma and the injured muscles may be rigid.

It is often forgotten that acute, subacute, or chronic *inflammation of the lymph-nodes* in the abdomen may cause pains as severe as those due to similar inflammation elsewhere. The nodes at the ileocaecal junction may become inflamed in children due to virus infection (non-specific mesenteric adenitis), and cause pains referred to McBurney's spot, simulating appendicitis so closely that operation is often performed and a normal appendix removed.

Acute affections of the lower part of the rectus abdominis muscle may not be common, but they should be borne in mind; for when they occur on the right side they may closely simulate appendicitis. The diagnosis is suggested by the contour of the parts locally, the distribution of the pain over a definite entire sector of the muscle, or by local subcutaneous discoloration. Appendicitis may similarly be suggested in rupture of the muscle in this situation when Zenker's degeneration has occurred after such illness as typhoid fever. At operation (for supposed appendicitis) the condition is recognized on incising the muscle. *Rupture of the inferior epigastric artery* with haematoma of the rectus muscle may follow a violent cough or may occur spontaneously in pregnancy. There is local pain followed by the appearance of a lump and later bruising of the overlying skin.

2. Subacute or Chronic Lesions. Passing now to a consideration of the differential diagnosis of conditions which may produce subacute, chronic, or recurrent mild attacks of pain in the right iliac fossa, it is clear that most of the conditions described above will have to be recalled; many additional causes, however, may be confused with subacute or recurrent appendicitis.

Ileocaecal tuberculosis is associated with pulmonary tuberculosis. Although fortunately now rare in Britain, it is still common in other parts of the world. When phthisis is active and extensive the bacilli swallowed are generally so numerous that if ulceration of the bowel occurs the ulcers are diffused widely through the ileum, caecum, and ascending colon. Even in such a case the maximum incidence of the bowel tuberculosis which results from the swallowing of tuberculous sputum is in the region of the ileocaecal valve presumably because the delay in the passage of intestinal contents which occurs in this situation gives the bacilli a better opportunity of attacking the mucous membrane. In less acute cases the tuberculous process is confined entirely to the ileocaecal valve region, involving perhaps the last inch or two of the ileum, the ileocaecal valve itself, the caput caeci, and the first inch or two of the ascending colon. Diarrhoea may result from this chronic ulceration, but this is unusual. Whether or no pyrexia occurs depends upon the degree of activity of the pulmonary lesion. Fullness or even a definitely palpable mass may be felt in the right iliac fossa; carcinoma of the caecum is a condition that naturally calls for differential diagnosis. The presence of tubercle bacilli in the faeces is of crucial significance. A barium follow-through study reveals stricturing in the terminal ileum and caecum; characteristically the latter is elevated higher than usual in the right abdomen by fibrous contracture.

Actinomycosis of the caecum is rare, indeed constant reminder of the possibility is necessary. In some cases the nature of the lesion in the right iliac fossa is suggested by the presence of a chronic inflammatory groin discharge (*Fig.* 692, p. 689), or an ulcerative condition of the jaw or cheek, or of the pleura and chest wall, or of the liver; for these, in addition to the caecum, are the sites most usually affected by actinomycosis. The chronicity of the condition is generally pronounced; the ultimate diagnosis depends upon the discovery of ray fungi from the affected part. Were the caecum involved primarily the symptoms would be more or less like those of either tuberculosis or of carcinoma of the caecum, and laparotomy would probably be resorted to, though large doses of penicillin should be tried in the hope of cure resulting without operation.

Inflamed iliac lymph-nodes may cause pain, tenderness, and obscure swelling in the right iliac fossa, and appendicitis may be closely simulated. There will generally be pyrexia. Spasm of the psoas may cause flexion of the right hip or, failing this, the patient complains of pain on hip extension. If the inflammation in the internal nodes is due to spread from the femoral or inguinal group there will generally be some sore place upon the corresponding area of the skin. But the inflammation of the iliac may occur independently of the inguinal lymph-nodes when the source of the infection is in the pelvis or secondary to periproctic or periprostatic inflammation. Rectal examination may assist the diagnosis.

Tuberculous iliac lymph-nodes generally form part of tabes mesenterica or of tuberculous peritonitis, but the tuberculous deposits may occur mainly, or even entirely, in the nodes in the region of the caecum, in which case it may be difficult without operation to be sure that the patient is not suffering from appendicitis or tuberculous lesions in the caecum itself. When multiple small but firm tender swellings can be felt, as is sometimes possible in a thin person and especially a child, tuberculous adenitis is a reasonable presumption. The X-rays may show multiple shadows in the position which the nodes normally occupy.

Carcinoma of the caecum is generally characterized less by pain in the iliac fossa than by a definite, usually irregular, firm mass, at first movable, later more fixed. The patient is often anaemic, due to persistent loss of blood from the tumour, and, indeed, the mass may be discovered in the investigation of an otherwise symptomless iron-deficiency anaemia. This mass is distinguished from an accumulation of faeces in the caecum by greater firmness, by the fact that it cannot be moulded by the fingers, and that it does not disappear when the bowels are thoroughly evacuated. Carcinoma of the caecum may be simulated by accumulated faeces, the result of obstruction in a distal portion of the bowel; there may for instance be adhesions obstructing the sigmoid colon, or a partial volvulus, or a carcinoma of the rectum, or of the sigmoid colon, leading to partial intestinal obstruction and preventing complete evacuation of the caecum. The pain of which the patient then complains may not be at the site of obstruction but in the right iliac fossa. In such a case, a barium X-ray examination may assist materially in detecting the cause of the symptoms, and examination of the rectum with the finger, or of the sigmoid colon by means of the sigmoidoscope, will be necessary. When there is obstruction to the colon in its distal part it is particularly in the caecum that *stercoral ulcers* are apt to occur, and these may be associated with pain in the right iliac fossa more or less simulating appendicitis.

As a rarity, a *hydatid cyst* may be found in the right iliac fossa, causing pain and a tumour simulating carcinoma even to the extent of producing obstructive symptoms. The diagnosis is seldom possible without laparotomy.

In *dysentery* and *ulcerative colitis* the abdominal pains are usually general, or at least referred now to one, now to another part: occasionally, however, pain may be more pronounced in the right iliac fossa than elsewhere. The diagnosis of a more widespread infection will generally be indicated by the history, especially as of residence in the tropics in the case of dysentery, or of recurrent intractable diarrhoea with passage of blood and mucus in a sufferer from ulcerative colitis. Sigmoidoscopy is invaluable in confirming the diagnosis.

In *typhoid fever* the general symptoms will nearly always be out of all proportion to any pain in the abdomen, but, occasionally, acute pain in the right iliac fossa has been the presenting symptom. Moreover, there is such a thing as typhoidal or paratyphoidal appendicitis, and a perforation low down in the ileum may lead to the formation of a local abscess in the right iliac fossa. The patient, though suffering from typhoid or paratyphoid fever, is likely to be operated upon as a case of appendicitis until the subsequent course of the pyrexia has suggested the possibility of typhoid fever and has demanded appropriate investigation.

Discomfort or actual pain in the right iliac fossa may be the first complaint of patients suffering from a *tumour of the iliac bone*; this tumour may be simple—*osteoma* or *chondroma*, or malignant—*sarcoma*. On palpation the tumour will be felt to be firm or even bony hard, and, unlike other tumours in the iliac fossa, completely fixed to the deep parts.

An *aneurysm of the iliac artery* is very uncommon. It may give rise to considerable pain in the iliac fossa which radiates down the right thigh. The discovery of a tumour with expansile pulsation establishes the diagnosis.

Although both *mobile right kidney* and *other lesions of the right kidney*, especially *tuberculosis*, cause pain in the loin to a more pronounced extent than pain in the right iliac fossa, some patients, especially those suffering from unduly mobile right kidney, complain of more pain in the lower right abdominal quadrant than in the loin, and the difficulty of distinguishing between pain when due to a mobile kidney only and that due to appendicitis occurring in a person who has at the same time a mobile kidney may be considerable. With renal tuberculosis, pus cells and tubercle bacilli may be detected in the urine. With mobile kidney the urine is generally normal, though there may be a little albumin or occasionally a trace of blood: there will be no pyrexia, such as one would expect with coincident appendicitis, and the patient will tell the examiner that she experiences the pain when the kidney is palpated between his two hands and not when he presses into the right iliac fossa without touching the kidney. Cystoscopy, ureteric catheterization, and pyelography in both horizontal and vertical postures may on occasion be necessary before the diagnosis can be made.

Herpes zoster needs bearing in mind when pains are unilateral without objective signs; herpetic pains may be present for 48 hours and perhaps longer before the eruption appears, and also for weeks or months after the eruption has subsided. It is even possible that in some cases there are pains from herpes zoster without any eruption at all. As a rule, with herpes zoster occurring in such a way as to produce pain referred to the right iliac fossa, the pain will not be confined to this situation, but will be referred also to the inner side of the upper part of the thigh and to some point in the right loin, so that renal colic is more likely than appendicitis to be simulated. The characteristic vesicles will be looked for or the slight scabs that may be left for some time after the vesicles have dried up.

The remaining conditions in the list above are those in which pain may be referred to the right iliac fossa from remote lesions. It is well recognized that a patient suffering from *acute pleurisy* at the base of the right lung, or from *pneumonia* in the lower lobe of the right lung, may complain of pain in the lower part of the abdomen rather than in the chest. There are occasions when it is by no means easy to decide whether the patient's lesion is abdominal or thoracic. Even when there are definite lung signs there may be coincident appendicitis. In pulmonary cases there is as a rule neither rigidity nor tenderness in the right iliac fossa when this is a situation of pain.

Chronic pain suggestive of ureteric calculus or of appendicular colic may be complained of when the posterior nerve-roots on the right side are being irritated by bony or other changes in connexion with the lower dorsal or upper lumbar vertebrae, for instance from *spondylitis deformans*

in an early stage, *osteo-arthritis* of the spine, infective changes in the spine of the same nature as *rheumatoid arthritis, spinal caries* with or without *psoas abscess, spinal tumour, prolapse of an intervertebral disk* (p. 86). Although such conditions are chronic, the pains may be acute, and only after much deliberation and repeated examinations will a conclusion be reached that the pains are referred from the spine and not due to primary trouble in the right iliac fossa itself. The X-rays sometimes assist in detecting osteophytic or other bony changes in the vertebrae but absence of radiographic abnormality does not exclude infective spondylitis as the cause, for the inflammatory changes affecting the intercostal nerves as they emerge between the vertebrae may be confined entirely to the soft parts. If the patient's complaints can be analysed successfully it may be found that he has definite localized pain in the back as well as in the iliac fossa.

Harold Ellis.

ILIAC FOSSA (RIGHT), SWELLING IN

A swelling in the right iliac fossa may be noticed accidentally by the patient, or it may be discovered in a routine examination of the abdomen. An attempt should first be made to determine the anatomical site of the swelling, whether it is in the anterior or posterior wall of the fossa; or, if it is in the abdominal cavity, what are its attachments. Its physical characters should then be studied by palpation, percussion, and auscultation: is it an indefinite swelling such as is common in appendicitis, or if well defined what is its shape, and are its outlines smooth or irregular; is it solid or cystic, if solid how hard is it, if cystic does it contain air or fluid; is it tender, does it pulsate, can the sounds of peristalsis be heard around it? By consideration of the site and characters of the swelling, the diagnosis can usually be determined. Distension of the caecum with wind or faeces may cause an obvious swelling in the right iliac fossa; doubt on these points can be cleared up by administering an enema.

The normal contents of the right iliac fossa are the caecum and appendix, with the lower coils of ileum.

Classification:

SWELLINGS CONNECTED WITH THE NORMAL CONTENTS OF THE RIGHT ILIAC FOSSA:

Appendicitis
Carcinoma of the caecum
Regional ileitis
Actinomycosis
Tuberculous mesenteric glands
Intussusception
Ileocaecal tuberculosis
Sarcoma of the intestine
Carcinoma of the appendix.
(These swellings are put down approximately in the order of their frequency.)

SWELLINGS CONNECTED WITH STRUCTURES NOT
USUALLY PRESENT IN THE RIGHT ILIAC FOSSA:
Liver
Gall-bladder
Right kidney
Cysts and tumours of the right ovary
Uterine fibroids.

SWELLINGS IN THE POSTERIOR WALL OF THE FOSSA:
Ilio-psoas abscess
Tumour of ilium
Aneurysm of the external iliac artery
Enlarged glands of the external iliac group.

Appendicitis must be considered first because
it is the commonest lesion in this compartment,
but in appendicitis at the stage when it is usually
encountered, and when it should be diagnosed
and submitted to operation, there is no swelling
that can be seen or felt. The cardinal signs are
pain, first colicky and referred to the umbilicus,
later fixed and felt in the right iliac fossa, vomiting, constipation, with a raised temperature and
pulse-rate; at this stage diminished movement of
the muscles in the right lower quadrant of the
abdomen, with guarding and tenderness over
McBurney's point, will be found, but though the
appendix is probably swollen, it cannot usually
be felt except under anaesthesia. A swelling
indicates a localized peritonitis or an abscess,
and it is commonly met between the second and
tenth days of the attack. Such a swelling is firm,
indefinite in outline, tender, fixed to the posterior
abdominal wall and later to the anterior wall as
well; the muscles are immobile over it, but the
guarding is not widespread and ill defined as in
an early appendicitis: the swelling is first resonant, and becomes dull when it involves the
anterior abdominal wall. The early history is
that outlined above, but by the time a localized
swelling has formed the patient usually feels and
looks better. His temperature and pulse are
moderately raised, and there is a well-marked
leucocytosis. If the abscess is low in the iliac
fossa, micturition may be painful or frequent.
A rectal examination should be made, but in the
localized type of peritonitis characterized by a
swelling in the right iliac fossa, only slight tenderness or none will be found.

Distension of the caecum may be of no importance, but distension of sufficient degree to cause
a visible and palpable swelling, especially when it
occurs in the elderly, is highly suggestive of a
carcinoma in the left half of the colon. A distended caecum causes a marked asymmetry in
the lower half of the abdomen that becomes
obvious as soon as the patient lies down and un-
covers his abdomen. It is rounded, smooth, and
tympanitic. Percussion usually reveals that the
transverse colon is also distended, though it is
rarely visibly so. Thorough investigation to confirm or disprove the suspicion of a colonic cancer
must be undertaken.

Cancer of the caecum, ileocaecal tuberculosis,
and *actinomycosis* must be considered together,
since the distinction between them is often a
matter of considerable difficulty. All three may
be practically symptomless, and the accidental
discovery of a lump in the right iliac fossa may
be the first indication that anything is amiss; in
all three there may have been an attack of
appendicitis shortly before the lump appeared, or
the appendix may have been removed for digestive disturbances accompanied by pain in the
right iliac fossa. Cancer of the caecum is a disease of the old and is uncommon under 50;
there may be diarrhoea or attacks of partial
obstruction, but the typical history is one of
asthenia, anaemia, and loss of weight without
any very obvious bowel symptoms. Tuberculosis,
on the other hand, is commoner in the young, and
usually gives rise to alternating diarrhoea and
constipation, passing later to more obvious
obstruction. The patient often has a history of
previous tuberculosis in some other focus, usually
pulmonary, and may be losing weight and running a temperature in the evenings. Actinomycosis may occur at any age. The patient has
usually been healthy till recently, but a very
common story is that he had an attack of apparently typical appendicitis with a localized abscess,
and that after operation the wound continued to
discharge, and later a lump appeared deep to it.
Where there is no history of appendicitis, there
has been pyrexia and pain in the right iliac fossa
which has led to the discovery of the swelling.
On palpation a carcinoma of the caecum is a
hard, rounded, or knobbly mass in the right iliac
fossa, usually in its upper part, for the caecum is
less commonly involved than the colon opposite
to or just above the ileocaecal junction: the mass
is at first movable. Hyperplastic tuberculosis
usually involves the caecum and the whole ascending colon, rarely the ileum as well: it is therefore
typically longer and more tubular than a carcinoma, and does not feel as hard. An actinomycotic mass may feel exactly like a carcinoma,
but is usually more fixed than one of the same
size; later it softens and discharges pus. This pus
may be charged with yellow granules which under
the microscope are seen to consist of clumps of
a Gram-positive streptothrix. In this event the
diagnosis is confirmed; more usually the granules
are absent and bacteriological examination under
the microscope may fail to reveal the streptothrix
in a number of successive specimens. In these
cases the diagnosis must be made on clinical
grounds depending upon the multiplicity of the
fistulae and the tendency to fibrosis of the surrounding soft tissues. If the bacteriologist fails to
report the streptothrix, he may yet give a lead in
establishing the diagnosis by reporting that the
discharge from the fistula is sterile or near sterile
on culture, that the organisms are few in number,
or that they consist mainly of probable contaminants; for the secretions of *Streptothrix actino-
myces* are distantly allied to streptomycin, and
on occasion inhibit the growth of pyogenic
organisms, a property which as suggested above
may be made use of in making a diagnosis. After
a barium meal a carcinoma shows a filling defect

in the caecal region, a tuberculous lesion a tubular stricture: actinomycosis may give no characteristic picture beyond demonstrating fixity of the whole caecal region. (*Fig.* 426.)

Tuberculous mesenteric glands are common in children up to the age of 8, and those at the termination of the ileocolic artery may form easily palpable swellings. They may cause intermittent

Sarcoma of the intestine is rare, but affects the lower ileum and caecum more commonly than any other part. It is usually found in children, and in its history and the characters of the swelling resembles ileocaecal tuberculosis. *Carcinoma of the appendix* is a tumour of very low malignancy. It usually gives rise to appendicular inflammation and is therefore removed surgically

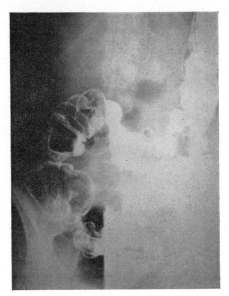

Fig. 426. Tuberculous stricture of ascending colon.

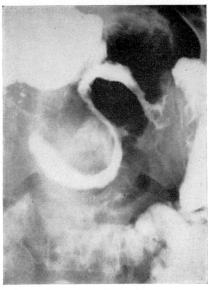

Fig. 427. Ileocaecal Crohn's disease.

colicky pains or a general loss of health, or no symptoms at all. If they become secondarily infected they may resemble an appendix abscess, from which they are distinguished by their more medial position and by the history. A plain radiograph will often demonstrate calcification and thus confirm the diagnosis. *Regional ileitis* or Crohn's disease is a chronic inflammatory process involving the lower ileum, which is then palpable as an indefinite tender mass in the right iliac fossa, resembling an appendix abscess. The disease usually affects young adults between 20 and 40, and the leading symptoms are abdominal pain, loss of weight, pyrexia, diarrhoea, and later chronic intestinal obstruction. The picture thus resembles that of an appendicitis spread over months instead of days. A barium meal will generally demonstrate a long tubular stricture of the lower ileum. (*Fig.* 427.) *Intussusception* usually occurs in healthy male babies round about the end of their first year, and is indicated by vomiting, constipation, the passage of blood and mucus by the rectum, and by bouts of intestinal colic that cause the child to draw up his legs and cry. The intussusception starts in the right fossa and the swelling may be felt here, but usually this compartment is empty and the intussuscepted portion can be felt in the right hypochondrium or above the umbilicus.

while very small, but it is sometimes found as a hard, freely movable tumour the size of a walnut, lying in the right iliac fossa. A lump with these characters, that does not disappear after an enema, should be investigated by laparotomy.

The *liver* if enlarged may reach the right iliac fossa, but should occasion no difficulty in diagnosis: a *Riedel's lobe* or an *enlarged gall-bladder* may, however, be deceptive. Enlargement of the gall-bladder sufficient to give it the appearance of a swelling distinct from the liver is usually the result of a stone blocking the cystic duct, and distension with mucus or mucopus; thus there is no jaundice, and the original obstructive symptoms may have been forgotten. Either swelling is continuous with the liver, and this continuity can be demonstrated by palpation, by the continuity of dullness to percussion from tumour to liver, and by movement on respiration.

The *right kidney* is often sufficiently mobile to reach the right iliac fossa. It is recognized by its shape—which is that of a kidney unless it is considerably enlarged by tumour or hydronephrosis—by its free mobility, which, however, occurs in the radius of the renal pedicle, by a band of resonance over it, and by the way in which it can be returned to the right loin, when it can be felt between the left hand on the loin and the right on the abdomen. Swellings extending into the iliac fossa from the pelvis, and attached to the uterus and its appendages, can usually be felt dipping into the pelvis; they can be displaced downwards but not upwards, and swing about on a 'stalk' that comes from below. Such swellings may be a *cyst* or *tumour of the right ovary*, or a subperitoneal *fibroid of the uterus*. Vaginal and rectal examination will establish the relation of the swelling to the pelvic viscera.

Swellings in the posterior wall of the fossa are discussed in the preceding article on ILIAC FOSSA (LEFT), SWELLING IN (p. 411).

R. G. Beard.

IMPOTENCE

Impotence may be defined as inability to perform the sexual act. It needs to be distinguished from sterility, which is inability to reproduce. Sterility may exist without impotence and an impotent man may be fertile.

Impotence may be complete or partial, temporary or permanent. Sexual power in healthy men varies from time to time and may be temporarily absent or reduced in states of fatigue, anxiety, worry over personal affairs, etc. Temporary impotence of this kind is common during the first weeks of married life, especially if the honeymoon is preceded by a few days or weeks of unusual physical exertion or emotional tension attendant upon the wedding. Likewise the first act of intercourse with a virgin may cause her pain and distress which communicate themselves to her male partner. He may then feel apprehensive of inflicting injury upon her whereupon this reacts upon his capacity for intercourse. Apart from this and in men who marry without prior experience of sexual intercourse, early attempts may be accompanied by considerable apprehension which may have a markedly depressing effect on potency. Failure of these first attempts leads to further anxiety, and so predisposes to unsuccessful repetition. *Premature ejaculation* (*ejaculatio praecox*), the emission of semen before penetration has taken place, is merely a variety of impotence, having the same aetiology.

The causes of impotence may be classified as follows:

1. Impotence Secondary to Physical Abnormality. There are a great many possible causes, most of which are obvious (e.g., congenital or acquired deformation of the penis), or unimportant. Those who are severely or chronically physically ill are likely to be impotent to some degree but are unlikely to complain of it. Those with certain endocrine disorders, e.g., *congenital eunuchoidism, sexual infantilism, Fröhlich's syndrome*, etc., may also be impotent. As they lack sexual desire this, too, is not likely to be a problem. In acquired eunuchoidism, potency may in some cases be retained though the subject is of course sterile. Impotence and lack of sexual desire can also be produced in men who are given natural or synthetic oestrogen compounds and certain other drugs such as chlorotranisene and cyproterone acetate, which may be used in the treatment of certain sexual offenders or for carcinoma of the prostate. Antihypertensive agents such as methyldopa, rauwolfia, and guanethidine also interfere with sexual performance in some male subjects. But despite all these the only really important physical causes of impotence are first and foremost, *diabetes mellitus*, where it may occur as a very early symptom, and spinal cord disorders, e.g., *compression, paraplegia, tabes dorsalis, disseminated sclerosis*, etc. Alcohol, though it increases desire, tends to reduce potency; therefore chronic alcoholism, although psychologically engendered, can be regarded as a physical cause.

In those of advancing years impotence can occur for no very good reason other than as part of the ageing process. Differences in the duration of the persistence of potency into old age are quite probably largely genetically determined.

2. Primary Impotence. Here there is no discoverable organic cause, and impotence is due to abnormal psychological influences. It is much the most common form.

The first factor to be considered is anxiety, for this, especially if chronic, is likely to be inhibitory to erection. Such anxiety may be a symptom of a lifelong neurotic condition; it may be the concomitant of guilt over masturbatory practices in earlier life; or it may be the outcome of a morbid attitude to sex which is the result of faulty sex education. Where masturbation has been continued into adult life and becomes the usual method of sexual outlet, it may establish itself and resist attempts to exchange it for normal sex relations.

Impotence may also be a common early symptom of *depression* occurring as part of a general lowering of vitality. This is of some importance in Asiatics who are more inclined to offer impotence as a primary complaint when depressed than are Europeans, which would seem to reflect among them a greater preoccupancy with the matter. This form of impotence is the easiest of all to treat as it tends to vanish as the depressive state resolves. However, it should be noted that tricyclic antidepressive drugs themselves appear to produce impotence in some patients, and although this may not be permanent their prolonged use may prevent a return of potency when depression has seemingly lifted.

Abnormalities of sexual inclination may be associated with incapacity to perform the sexual act under conventional conditions. In some subjects sexual excitement only occurs in special circumstances, for example, when the limbs are bound, by the use of flagellation, or partial strangulation. In such cases either *suffering* or the *infliction of pain* may be necessary in order to achieve erection. In others sexual intercourse may only be possible with some type of *fetishistic behaviour*, e.g., the partner may have to wear high-heeled shoes during the sexual act. Tight-fitting rubber or leather garments are also a common source of sexual stimulation. In the absence of these special stimuli, as no sex desire is shown in the situations which ought to arouse it, the subject appears impotent. The source of an unusual inclination of this kind is generally to be found in experiences of childhood and adolescence; the subject may go through life unaware of his sexual disposition and unable to achieve a satisfactory sex relationship. The discovery of this disposition may be made only after a lengthy psychiatric inquiry, or it may come to light by chance.

A particular and common instance of this is *homosexuality*, either latent or overt. Potency in heterosexual intercourse is not invariably lost however, although the subject may during a sexual relationship with a female have to resort to homosexual fantasies in order to obtain and maintain erection. Some homosexuals can be classified as *heterophobic* (i.e., they fear women, usually having had highly dominant mothers) rather than being primarily homosexual, although being unable to relate to women they turn to homosexuality as a substitute activity.

Relative impotence is said to exist when the subject cannot effect coitus with one woman but is potent with others; thus, he may be impotent towards his wife, for whom he feels tender affection and respect, but experiences a much stronger sexual desire for women of easy virtue. This condition follows from a separation of the two elements of which feeling for women is compounded—the affectionate and the lustful. It springs from a linking of sex experiences with the furtive and disreputable associations with which they are commonly surrounded at the schoolboy age. If this link survives until the age of marriage, the subject is likely to feel that coitus in some way degrades his wife and should be kept for women of lesser account. It is said that a man who marries a woman who resembles his mother, to whom he is over-attached, is liable to this kind of difficulty.

Failure to complete the sex act can also result from *absence of ejaculation* and no seminal emission. This is sometimes called *coitus reservatus*. This is probably the rarest form of impotence. Its origin is obscure, although it has been suggested that the subjects are either narcissistic, and incapable of 'giving' of themselves, or have only feeble sex desire and do not arrive at a sufficient intensity of excitement to attain ejaculation.

Finally, psychogenic impotence may often profitably be regarded as symptomatic of a *marital disturbance*. While admittedly his potency may not be of the highest order, a wife can, by nagging or some other untoward behaviour, render her husband impotent. Similarly if she fears pregnancy and gives over-ready expression to this he, in his turn, may fear making her pregnant. The implications of this are that treatment is likely to be much more successful if both husband and wife are involved.

W. H. Trethowan.

INDICANURIA

Indican (potassium indoxyl sulphate) is a normal constituent of urine in amounts up to 30 mg. per day. It is formed from indole, which

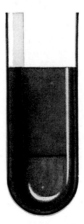

Fig. 428. The calcium hypochlorite and chloroform test for indicanuria.

is derived from the action of intestinal bacteria on tryptophan. It is usually invisible, but urines containing a large excess of indican may darken on exposure to air and very occasionally oxidation to indigo in an alkaline urine may produce a bluish tinge to the phosphate deposit. In such cases typical blue rectangular or needle-like crystals may be seen in the deposit. Tests for indican all depend on the oxidation to indigo blue. The urine is acidified with hydrochloric acid and shaken with chloroform after the addition of a small amount of oxidizing agent such as $FeCl_3$ (Obermayer), or $KClO_3$ (Jaffé), or calcium hypochlorite (*Fig.* 428). The chloroform layer assumes a blue colour when the test is positive.

Excess indican is excreted in the urine if there is malabsorption of tryptophan by the gut, or if the small intestinal fluid contains an abnormally large number of indole-producing bacteria, e.g., *Escherichia coli.* Tryptophan malabsorption occurs in some cases of coeliac disease and especially in the rare hereditary condition known as 'Hartnup disease', in which there is a specific defect of transport of many neutral amino-acids by the gut and by the proximal renal tubular epithelium. A high bacterial content within the small intestine is found in cases of the blind-loop syndrome, including obstructive lesions, small intestinal diverticular disease, and gastrojejuno-colic fistula.

M. D. Milne.

INDIGESTION

When alimentary processes usually unconscious obtrude themselves into the consciousness we speak of 'indigestion', a definition which, if of practical service, is not synonymous with an incapacity to digest food. For gross errors in secretion and even grave visceral disease may be present with presumably some digestive disadvantage but without subjective symptoms of any kind. Alternatively, a patient often complains of indigestion when investigation fails to reveal any abnormality of the digestive tract. Such complaints as pain or discomfort or vaguely unpleasant sensations in the abdomen, vomiting, flatulence, disturbance of appetite, heartburn, acidity, are naturally identified in a patient's mind with the digestive organs, however fallacious as a guide to their aetiology his symptoms may be.

The subject then resolves itself into considering those causes in which the alimentary tract is free from abnormality, those in which the digestive organs are diseased, and those in which they are structurally intact but functionally disturbed.

I. SIMULATION OF SYMPTOMS OF DYSPEPSIA BY OTHER CONDITIONS

The Vomiting of Pregnancy. The possibility of pregnancy should always be present in the mind when one is consulted by a young woman who complains of vomiting and, vaguely, of indigestion. In some instances the patient may herself be unaware of her pregnant state, although pregnancy is in some way responsible.

Cerebral Vomiting. In children particularly, vomiting of cerebral origin may be mistaken for dyspepsia. Incipient meningitis or tumour are the commonest causes of such vomiting. The presence of signs of cerebral irritation (e.g., photophobia, squint, irritability, headache, Kernig's sign, etc.) should make one suspicious of meningitis; paralyses, headache, and optic neuritis point to tumour. Examination of the cerebrospinal fluid obtained by lumbar puncture may be required (p. 123).

Uraemia may masquerade as 'indigestion', characterized by loss of appetite and vomiting (uraemic gastritis), in any form of renal failure but particularly perhaps in cases of enlarged prostate with residual urine with or without pyuria. The 'uraemic odour' in the breath, mental blurring, high arterial tension, and proteinuria should be looked for, and the diagnosis confirmed by estimation of the blood-urea.

Pulmonary Tuberculosis. In cases of early phthisis indigestion may be the chief symptom complained of, commonly associated with loss of appetite, and nausea, with or without vomiting. Careful examination of the chest, both clinically and radiologically, and of the sputum should not be omitted, especially in young subjects complaining of such symptoms.

The Gastric Crises of Tabes are apt to be mistaken for dyspepsia, especially nowadays when neurosyphilis is a clinical rarity. Paroxysmal vomiting of great violence with severe abdominal pain is the usual form they assume and they may simulate gastric ulcer even to the extent of perforation. If the knee-jerks are absent and the pupils immobile to light the diagnosis is easy, but gastric crises may occur early in a case of tabes before any of the usual signs of disease of the cord have manifested themselves. One should inquire in such a case for a history of lightning pains and for any disturbances of micturition. Serological tests of the blood or cerebrospinal fluid may determine the diagnosis. It should be remembered that perforation of an ulcer or the occurrence of other abdominal catastrophe is, of course, possible in a tabetic.

Nervous or **Hysterical Vomiting** is a diagnosis which must be made largely by the method of exclusion. The patient is usually a woman, and other signs of hysteria will almost certainly be present. After the First Great War, a considerable number of cases was seen in soldiers in whom an emotional cause was advanced, e.g., persistence of the memory of the stench of decaying corpses. In general, this symptom has been interpreted as symbolizing disgust through psychological traumata that may be exposed by analysis.

In Chronic Intestinal Obstruction the abdominal pains, and the vomiting which often accompanies them, may be described by a patient as 'indigestion'. In such a case there will be distension of the abdomen often with visible peristalsis, and a history of gradually increasing constipation. A tumour may be felt, or radiographic examination or the sigmoidoscope may establish a diagnosis.

Cholecystitis. In the case of patients, particularly middle-aged or elderly women, who complain of 'wind' and 'spasms' together with nausea, the possibility of gall-stones as the responsible factor should always be considered. A cholecystogram will confirm or refute the clinical diagnosis.

Recurrent Appendicitis may manifest itself chiefly by symptoms which point to the stomach rather than to the vermiform appendix as the seat of the disease. The pain in such a case may have the character of a typical 'hunger-pain', and be relieved by alkalis. The possibility of appendicitis should be specially remembered in the case of children who suffer from irregularly recurring abdominal pains.

Angina Pectoris in one of its forms may be accompanied by much flatulence which leads the patient to consult his doctor for 'indigestion'. The occurrence of the symptoms upon exertion, the tendency of the pain to spread into the left arm, and the frequent presence of a high blood-pressure are all of diagnostic value. (*See* CHEST, PAIN IN, p. 133.) The therapeutic test is of help, the pain being relieved by vasodilators.

Chronic Bronchitis. Patients dyspnoeic from chronic bronchitis and emphysema or from persistent congestive cardiac failure may experience discomfort in the upper abdomen and flatulence, described by them as 'indigestion'.

Migraine. A patient who suffers from this complaint may describe his case as one of 'indigestion' or 'biliousness'. The chief diagnostic point is the occurrence of severe headache and visual disturbances with or preceding the gastric symptoms, and the periodicity of the attacks.

Acute Glaucoma. Vomiting is generally an accompaniment.

Extra-abdominal Causes of Pain are often attributed by patients to indigestion. Examples of these are pleurisy, spinal caries, aortic aneurysm, neoplasm of the spine.

Eructatio Nervosa, due to air-swallowing, or aerophagy, is also usually described as indigestion. (*See* FLATULENCE, p. 303.)

Porphyria may cause acute abdominal pains described by the patient as 'acute indigestion'.

II. FUNCTIONAL VERSUS ORGANIC DYSPEPSIA

If loss of weight or *severe* pain are prominent symptoms the disease is probably *organic*. If these are absent, and the affection has persisted for some time, it is more likely to be a *functional* disorder. Functional pain tends to be present continuously, day in and day out, year after year, compared with the periodicity of organic pain. Finally, the patient with functional symptoms tends to describe these in flowery language and may record his story at length on sheets of paper (Charcot's *le malade avec le petit morceau du papier*).

III. DIFFERENTIAL DIAGNOSIS OF ORGANIC DYSPEPSIAS

The chief organic diseases of the stomach which have to be thought of are: (1) *Carcinoma*; (2) *Ulcer*; (3) *Gastritis*; (4) *Obstructive dilatation*.

1. Carcinoma. A malignant growth in the stomach may be situated either at the *cardiac orifice*, in the *body*, or at the *pylorus*. In the first of these situations it may cause difficulty in swallowing. If at the pylorus it may result in dilatation of the stomach. Growths in the body are those which are most difficult to diagnose. A history of 'indigestion' beginning abruptly in a patient (most often a man) above the age of 40, and not yielding to simple treatment, should arouse suspicion. On the other hand, it must be remembered that in a number of cases the growth starts either in an old ulcer or *de novo* in one who has suffered from chronic gastro-intestinal disturbances, so that a long history of indigestion does not exclude carcinoma. Steady loss of weight and the early appearance of anaemia point to malignant growth; on the other hand, the absence of these signs, and even a temporary gain in weight under treatment, by no means exclude it; but on the whole, loss of weight is always a significant feature. Loss of appetite, and according to some (but not all) observers a special disinclination for meat, are usually early symptoms. Nausea and vomiting supervene later but are rarely absent altogether. Pain in the epigastrium may be present early and is often more or less constant.

It is upon a combination of these symptoms and signs that the clinical diagnosis must be based in the possibly early stage. Later, a tumour may be felt below the left costal margin or in the epigastrium; enlarged lymph-nodes may appear above the left clavicle, and, since Douglas's pouch is frequently implicated, a rectal examination should never be omitted. There may be signs of secondary growths in the liver or at the umbilicus. When ulceration has supervened, blood may be found in the gastric contents—'coffee-grounds' vomit—and occult blood in the stools (p. 73). X-ray examination is of the greatest diagnostic value in all stages. Filling defects and interference with peristalsis are the features to look for. (*Figs.* 356, 357, p. 335.)

In some cases of carcinoma of the body of the stomach, pronounced anaemia is one of the earliest and most striking symptoms. Such cases are frequently confused with Addisonian anaemia. A blood-count will usually suffice to distinguish them, for in gastric carcinoma the red cells are rarely below 2,000,000 per c.mm. whereas in Addisonian anaemia the reduction is greater; in Addisonian anaemia, also, the colour index is about 1 or above it, in carcinoma it is less than 1. Megaloblasts are found in the film in Addisonian anaemia, but not—or only very rarely—in carcinoma. (*See* p. 46.)

Gastroscopy and biopsy of the ulcer are becoming increasingly employed thanks to the development of modern fibre-optic instruments.

In spite of all that has been said above, the early diagnosis of carcinoma of the stomach is a matter of great difficulty, and it may be justifiable to resort to an exploratory operation in a suspicious case which does not clear up after a few weeks' treatment.

2. Ulcer. The characteristic symptom of gastric ulcer is *pain* which comes on after food and is relieved by vomiting. The pain occurs in 'attacks' of a few weeks' duration separated by intervals of freedom. Haematemesis is strongly confirmatory but is absent in the majority. (*See* p. 333.) Duodenal ulcer is also often associated with symptoms that the patient naturally describes vaguely as 'indigestion'; the clinical features are given on p. 336.

An X-ray examination should never be omitted and may reveal an ulcer crater.

3. Gastritis. Chronic 'gastric catarrh' is certainly diagnosed unduly often, the majority of cases so described being really examples of functional dyspepsia. The symptoms are loss of appetite and fullness with a sense of oppressive weight in the epigastrium. Pain is not a feature of gastritis, nausea is common, and vomiting may occur but it is not usually a prominent symptom. There is no characteristic physical sign and a diagnosis cannot be made with certainty without the use of careful X-ray examination, gastroscopy, and gastric biopsy.

4. Dilatation. The presence of dilatation is determined by: (a) Demonstrating that the stomach is enlarged; and (b) Proving the occurrence of stagnation of the contents.

Enlargement of the stomach may be inferred by the presence of a gastric splash 3 or 4 hours after the last meal. Visible peristalsis and even a palpably distended stomach may be present in advanced cases. A history of projectile vomiting, the vomitus containing recognizable undigested food eaten 12 or more hours previously, is all but diagnostic. Examination with X-rays (*Fig. 756, p. 762*) is a more certain method of diagnosing delay in emptying the stomach; normally the meal should have left the stomach in four hours.

Assuming that obstructive dilatation has been diagnosed, one has next to distinguish between *benign* and *malignant obstruction*. A history or signs and symptoms of gastric or duodenal ulcer point to the former; the general symptoms of carcinoma to the latter. A tumour may be felt in either case but is much more common in cancer. Radiography may clinch the diagnosis (*Figs.* 356, 357, p. 335).

One has further to distinguish dilatation from: Hour-glass stomach.

Hour-glass stomach is far commoner in women than in men, and is diagnosed by X-ray examination, which shows the division of the stomach into two pouches (*Fig.* 353, p. 333), though a warning is pertinent not to mistake for organic hour-glass stomach the physiological behaviour of stray peristaltic waves which may produce an hour-glass appearance in a photograph; screen examination shows the constriction to be inconstant in position in the simulated condition, always in the same situation in the true hour-glass stomach.

IV. DIFFERENTIAL DIAGNOSIS OF FUNCTIONAL DYSPEPSIA

Having excluded all the above forms of organic disease, the next task is to determine what particular variety of functional disorder one has to deal with.

Aetiological Classification. Instead of attempting to distinguish different forms of functional dyspepsia on a symptomatic basis, they may be classified according to the particular exciting cause responsible. This method is simple and convenient, and is also useful for purposes of treatment. Adopting it, one may say that functional dyspepsia may be induced by:

a. DIETETIC CAUSES, e.g., unsuitable badly cooked unpalatable food, hasty meals, over-eating, underfeeding, the abuse of alcohol, tea, tobacco, or drugs.

b. PHYSICAL CAUSES, BAD HABITS GENERALLY, e.g., imperfect chewing, defective teeth, oral sepsis, eating when fatigued or cold, deficient exercise, constipation, general and local infective disease, e.g., pulmonary tuberculosis, severe anaemia.

c. MENTAL CAUSES, e.g., over-work, especially extending into the periods of eating and digestion.

d. EMOTIONAL CAUSES, e.g., shock, love-affairs, and in general a faulty mental or nervous adjustment which will include worry and anxiety states, hysteria, and hypochondriasis.

See also STOMACH, TESTS OF FUNCTION OF, p. 762.

Harold Ellis.

INGUINAL SWELLING

Inguinal swellings are properly those in the region of the inguinal canal; that is, related to the inner half of Poupart's ligament and the parts immediately above it. The following are some of the most important: (1) Enlarged glands; (2) Abscess, acute or chronic; (3) Inguinal hernia; (4) Hydrocele of the cord or of a hernial sac; (5) Retained testis; (6) Tumours of the cord and round ligament; (7) Aneurysm.

1. Enlarged Glands. There are three chief groups of glands in the groin. The *inguinal* lie in the subcutaneous tissues about Poupart's ligament and drain the external genitals, the anus, the umbilicus, the lower parts of the abdomen and back, the buttock, and the upper third of the thigh; the *femoral* glands are below the saphenous opening and drain the lower limb below the upper third of the thigh, though the lymphatic drainage is somewhat erratic, so that a sore toe may sometimes induce enlargement of an inguinal gland without enlarging the femoral group at all; the *iliac* glands are deeply placed in the iliac fossa, draining the inguinal and femoral set, and consequently often enlarging secondarily to these, though they also communicate freely with the other abdominal lymphatics and may become infected from them. Enlarged glands in the groin are nearly always multiple, and usually subcutaneous, so that they are easy to recognize as glands. Swellings of the femoral glands are discussed on page 517. The *iliac* glands just above Poupart's ligament are difficult to palpate because they lie deep to the abdominal muscles, but their enlargement is generally secondary to disease of the superficial glands and this often gives the key to the diagnosis of an obscure swelling in the right iliac fossa.

SOME CAUSES OF ENLARGEMENT OF THE GROIN GLANDS. These are: (a) Mechanical or chemical irritation; (b) Septic infection, for instance from genital sores or from sores on the toes or legs; (c) Tubercle; (d) Syphilis; (e) Lymphogranuloma inguinale; (f) Other specific diseases, such as rubella and bubonic plague; (g) Hodgkin's disease (h) Lymphatic leukaemia; (i) Malignant diseases—secondary carcinoma (especially melanotic carcinoma), secondary or primary sarcoma; (j) Filariasis.

a. The glands may become slightly enlarged and tender in young men, particularly in athletes during training, often due to epidermophytosis of the feet. They may also enlarge as a result of the *mechanical irritation* of a truss.

b. Septic infection may follow the *bites of parasites* such as the *Pediculus pubis*, but the glands generally remain movable and rarely suppurate. More commonly a septic sore or recent scar can be discovered upon examination of the area drained by the glands. Septic glands either soon subside, ceasing to be tender after the removal of the source of infection, or enlarge rapidly, become adherent, and suppurate within one to four weeks of their first enlargement.

c. This, and the amount of inflammation of the skin over them, distinguishes septic from *tuberculous* glands, which do not suppurate for some months, and then with but little inflammatory reaction. The source of infection may be a neighbouring tuberculous gland, but is more likely to be a chronic sore on the foot or leg, the tuberculous nature of which has not hitherto been suspected. Epitheliomatous glands may suppurate, and often ulcerate towards the end.

d. The true *syphilitic* gland is hard, movable, painless, and only moderately enlarged, and the existence of the indurated chancre usually makes the diagnosis easy. The *Spirochaeta pallida* may be detected, or Wassermann's serum test may be positive, though a negative reaction is not conclusive. An apparently soft sore (septic) may later become hard and definitely syphilitic; therefore suppuration of a bubo does not disprove syphilitic infection. Instances of mixed infection by sepsis and syphilis are common.

e. Lymphogranuloma inguinale is a venereal infection of the inguinal glands which is met with in coloured patients or in white patients who have lived in close community with coloured people. The glands are swollen and the intervening fibrosis gives to the mass a lobulated, firm feeling. The condition persists for many months with slight tenderness, and eventually the mass may break down and discharging sinuses or ulcers appear on the skin of the groin. In lymphogranuloma inguinale Frei's serological test is positive.

f. In *Hodgkin's disease* the groin glands are rarely affected alone, and the smooth, soft enlargement of many glands without signs of inflammation, associated with increasing anaemia and intermittent pyrexia (*Fig.* 322, p. 298), and possibly enlargement of the spleen suggest the diagnosis. Biopsy may be necessary to clinch the matter, microscopical section in a typical case showing multinucleated 'Hodgkin' cells, increase of reticulum cells, and the presence of large numbers of eosinophils in a gland in which the normal architecture has been destroyed.

g. Blood examination will give pathognomonic results in cases of *lymphatic leukaemia* (*Fig.* 58, p. 56) and filariasis (p. 54).

h. Malignant disease of the groin glands is nearly always epitheliomatous, secondary to a primary epithelioma of the skin or mucous membrane in the area drained by the glands. The primary growth may be small, and the patient may be unaware of its existence; a small growth at the anus, a malignant wart on the scrotum, an epithelioma of the penis still concealed by the prepuce, may be discovered for the first time by a systematic search in suspected areas. The other points in distinguishing epitheliomatous glands are their exceeding hardness, their progressive but slow growth, their early adhesion to the deep fascia and skin, the amount of pain to which they give rise without signs of inflammation. Late in the disease they may suppurate, ulcerate, or slough, with severe haemorrhage. Intraabdominal carcinoma, especially of the ovary or colon, sometimes causes secondary deposits in and consequent enlargement of the inguinal glands.

Melanotic growths of the skin give rise to rapidly growing smooth glands, often cystic; the pigment may be visible through the skin. The primary growth or ulceration in connexion with the skin, particularly of a toe, or a wart, may not show pigmentation, and its serious import may thus be overlooked. Late in the disease, when the tumour is widely disseminated, the urine may give a positive reaction for melanin or melanogen (p. 808).

Sarcoma of the groin glands is rare; it may be primary or secondary. Usually these are not the only glands affected. They grow with rapidity and remain smooth and fairly soft until they attain a great size, when they may fungate through the skin. Biopsy is necessary to distinguish lymphosarcoma from lymphadenoma with certainty. Both conditions may react with amazing rapidity to therapeutic X-rays, a point sometimes of diagnostic value. Lymphosarcoma usually recurs after the preliminary improvement with greater rapidity than lymphadenoma.

i. Filariasis: see (*g*) above.

2. Abscess:

a. Acute abscess in the groin has only one common cause, namely, suppuration of the glands, and a search must always be made for a primary source of infection, especially about the genitals or on the foot or in connexion with a toe. A hernia may occasionally suppurate, and an appendicular abscess may point just above Poupart's ligament; but there is then a history of the characteristic symptoms of appendicitis, and the pus when released has the suggestive smell of the products of the *Esch. coli*. Tuberculous and epitheliomatous glands may suppurate as the result of secondary pyogenic infection.

b. Chronic abscess in the groin may be due to disease of the hip, sacro-iliac joint, or lumbar spine; but such abscesses usually point below Poupart's ligament, the diagnosis should be clear and can be confirmed by radiographic examination. A chronic abscess pointing in the inguinal region is usually due to breaking down tuberculous inguinal glands, or to pus tracking in the extraperitoneal cellular tissues and reaching the inguinal canal along the cord or orund ligament. In the first the history and the observation that the whole abscess is superficial to the external oblique will establish the diagnosis. If the pus is tracking along the inguinal canal, its source may be anywhere in the iliac fossa or pelvis. Actinomycosis of the appendix on the

14*

right side (*Fig.* 692, p. 689), pericolic abscess on the left, and chronic suppuration or tuberculous infection of the uterus and tubes on either side, are among the possible causative conditions.

3. Hernia. In examining swellings in the groin, inguinal hernia must always be considered. An inguinal hernia, unless it is obstructed, gives an impulse on coughing and is reducible. Psoas abscess and saphena varix give these signs, but they are below Poupart's ligament. A femoral hernia may overlap the inguinal region and thus become an inguinal swelling: the points of distinction will be discussed later (*Fig.* 429).

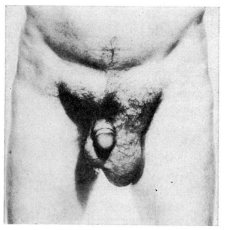

Fig. 429. Right inguinal hernia and left inguinoscrotal hernia. (*Courtesy of the Gordon Museum, Guy's Hospital.*)

The two chief varieties of inguinal hernia, the oblique and the direct, are easily distinguished in their typical forms, but the differentiation is not always possible before operation. An oblique hernia is usually a congenital fault and is therefore the only common type in young people. It descends obliquely from without inwards and downwards when the patient coughs or strains, and disappears obliquely in the opposite direction when it is reduced: it can also be felt to traverse the abdominal wall obliquely, the medial end being superficial and easily felt, the lateral part tailing off into the thickness of the abdominal wall. An oblique sac is tubular, and lies antero-external to the cord. If large, it descends into the scrotum and there lies in front of the testis. Except in old-standing cases, an oblique inguinal hernia, once reduced, does not descend immediately, but needs a cough, strain, or movement to bring it down: once down it is not reduced by simple pressure, but needs a little manipulation in an upward and outward direction. The sac usually contains bowel, and is therefore resonant to percussion and reduces with a gurgle. An inguinal hernia becomes irreducible either because it contains adherent omentum or because it is strangulated. The first is a non-urgent condition. The swelling is usually a typical hernia, and has been reduced previously. It is

dull to percussion and the sac has a coarse granular feel, in which larger knobs of fibrosed omentum can sometimes be felt and moved about. Some gut may also enter the sac, so that it usually gives an impulse on coughing and is partly reducible. An omental hernia may become sealed at its neck by adhesions, and converted into a *hydrocele of a hernial sac*: this is a cystic swelling, distinguished from a bilocular vaginal hydrocele by the history of previous hernia, and by palpating the swelling right up to the inguinal ring. *Strangulated hernia* is an acute surgical emergency: if the hernia contains gut there are the general signs of intestinal obstruction, but if a piece of omentum only is strangulated these signs will be absent and reliance must be placed on the local signs of tenseness: these are tenderness, absence of an impulse on coughing, and dullness to percussion.

A direct hernia is only common after 40, and is seen particularly in men pursuing laborious occupations, and those with poor health and a chronic cough. Both sides are usually affected, not always to the same extent. The swelling is globular rather than tubular, wider, more medial, and higher than an oblique hernia. The cord is not often felt, but it lies in front of the sac. A direct hernia usually appears as soon as the patient stands, coming directly forwards, and reduces on the pressure of a finger, disappearing directly backwards. It very rarely enters the scrotum, becomes obstructed, or strangulates.

A large femoral hernia tends to extend upwards over the inner end of Poupart's ligament, and in fat individuals may resemble an inguinal hernia. It is usually clear, however, that it originates from below Poupart's ligament, whereas an inguinal hernia originates above : the impulse in a femoral hernia comes upwards and the hernia is reduced by pressure downwards and backwards, whereas the inguinal requires pressure upwards and outwards. In a femoral hernia extending upwards, the inguinal part is rounded and movable, and on careful palpation the fixed neck can be traced passing backward to the inner side of the femoral vessels and below Poupart's ligament. In difficult cases it is a good plan to reduce the hernia, then to get the patient to stand up whilst the surgeon makes firm pressure over the internal ring and asks the patient to cough; a femoral hernia may then come down, but not an inguinal. Similarly pressure can be made on the femoral canal; this prevents the descent of a femoral hernia, so that if the swelling now returns it is inguinal. In this connexion it should be noted that femoral hernia is rare in males and in females under maturity. The prevalent belief that femoral hernia is more common than inguinal in grown-up women is wrong, inguinal being more common at all ages and in both sexes.

4. Hydrocele. The neck of an inguinal hernia may become obstructed, usually by omentum, and a hydrocele may develop in the sac. Such a hydrocele extends up to the internal ring. An encysted hydrocele of the cord occupies part of the inguinal canal, and is a rounded oval swelling transilluminated with difficulty; it is rare and seen only in boys. Inguinal hydroceles, being cut off from communication with the abdominal cavity, do not give an expansile impulse on coughing, but they are pushed forwards by the thrust of the abdominal wall.

5. Retained Testicle. The most important points in the diagnosis of this condition are the absence of the organ from its proper place, and the presence of a swelling in the region of the inguinal canal. Occasionally, the testicle may be partially descended and lie within the inguinal canal. More commonly the testicle is ectopic and lies superficial to the inguinal canal. The swelling in the groin may give the characteristic testicular sensation, or the condition may be associated with attacks of pain which have been mistaken for appendicitis or intestinal colic. It is often accompanied by actual or potential inguinal hernia.

6. Tumours of the Cord and Round Ligament. The only common tumours of these structures are (a) Lipoma, (b) Fibromyoma, and (c) Endometrioma of the round ligament. The lipoma is so soft and displaceable that it gives an impulse on coughing and is often mistaken for an omental hernia, especially in stout patients. The fibromyoma is hard and smooth, somewhat simulating the ovary or a thick-walled hydrocele of the canal of Nuck, for either of which it may be mistaken, a certain diagnosis being possible only by exploration. A history of the swelling becoming painful and more swollen at the time of menstruation will suggest endometrioma.

7. Aneurysm and Other Vascular Swellings. Aneurysm of the external iliac artery may be mistaken for a vascular sarcoma arising from the pelvis. It can generally be recognized by the classic signs of aneurysm, such as expansile pulsation, bruit, weakening and delay of the corresponding femoral pulse, and marked reduction of the size of the swelling as a result of pressure on the common iliac artery.

R. G. Beard.

INGUINOSCROTAL SWELLING

Inguinoscrotal swellings almost necessarily arise in the constituents of the spermatic cord or in a persistent funicular process. The following must be considered: (1) *Hernia*, (a) reducible, (b) irreducible, (c) strangulated; (2) *Varicocele*; (3) *Hydrocele*, (a) congenital, (b) of the cord, (c) of a hernial sac; (4) *Traumatic*, inflammatory, or malignant thickening of the cord.

1. Hernia is by far the commonest inguinoscrotal swelling and is the only one that gives an impulse on coughing and that can be reduced into the abdomen. A swelling with this character is therefore an inguinal hernia, almost certainly of the oblique variety (*see* p. 426). The usual hernia containing bowel is resonant to percussion and reduces with a gurgle. One containing omentum has a granular feel, gives a less pronounced impulse on coughing, and requires a little more manipulation to reduce it. An omental hernia may be partly irreducible and may contain knobs of fibrous fat that move about with the sac, but the anatomical relations of the swelling and the impulse on coughing and the partial reduction establish its nature without a doubt. An *irreducible hernia* is usually one containing omentum adherent to the sac. It presents as a tubular swelling along but in front of the cord, going up to the internal ring and extending downwards for a variable distance, but ending below in a rounded fundus. When, as is usually the case, there is a history of a swelling previously reducible there can be no confusion: without such a history exploration is the final appeal. A *strangulated hernia* is also unmistakable in most cases because of the simultaneous onset of symptoms of intestinal obstruction—colicky pain, vomiting, and absolute constipation even to flatus—and of irreducibility in a hernia that was previously reducible. A strangulated hernia containing bowel is at first resonant to percussion, but the accumulation of fluid masks this sign later. The swelling is tense and tender, and the surrounding parts soon become oedematous. Strangulated omentum may cause confusion: there may be some abdominal pain and vomiting at first, but after this the abdominal symptoms subside, but the inguinal swelling remains irreducible and becomes tender. Strangulated omentum may resemble an inflamed hydrocele of the cord, but this last is a very rare condition, and both demand operation. *Torsion of a retained testicle* with strangulation of its vessels may give rise to an inguinal or inguinoscrotal swelling that simulates a strangulated hernia: there may be abdominal pain, vomiting, and local tenderness, and since the funicular process usually extends beyond the testicle into the scrotum and becomes filled with blood, a swelling previously unknown to the patient will appear along the cord. However, vomiting is not so severe as in strangulated hernia and does not persist, and the bowels are not obstructed. In a strangulated Richter's hernia intestinal obstruction is not complete, and this may mislead the diagnostician. Help may be obtained from the history; with a retained testis there will always have been an irreducible swelling, whereas a strangulated hernia is a recent irreducible swelling with or without a previous period when it was reducible; moreover, a retained testis is dull on percussion, and thus distinguished from a strangulated hernia containing bowel, which, in its early stages at any rate, is resonant.

2. A Varicocele is an inguinoscrotal swelling that is chiefly scrotal. It is nearly always on the left side. The distended veins of the pampiniform plexus resemble a 'bag of worms'. With a lax scrotum the blue colour of the veins can be seen. A varicocele is said to give an impulse on coughing, but the sensation is that of a fluid thrill or a small tap on the examining finger rather than an impulse. Squeezing empties the swelling, which refills immediately; recumbency with the scrotum raised also causes it to disappear.

3. Hydrocele. A *congenital hydrocele* is a persistence of the processus funicularis throughout its length, and differs from a congenital hernia in that the communication with the abdomen is shut off, or so nearly shut off that bowel or omentum cannot enter it. The condition is seen most commonly in infants. The swelling fills the tunica vaginalis and obscures the testis, and continues as a tubular prolongation up the inguinal canal. It is elastic or fluctuant, and transilluminates easily. It is distinguished from hernia by the translucency (though in infants a hernia containing bowel may transilluminate to some extent) and by the absence of an impulse on coughing or crying, and of reducibility. Though irreducible, many congenital hydroceles in infants have a small communication with the abdomen, indicated by a reduction in size during the hours of sleep and a tendency to vary in tenseness from time to time. For this reason the sudden appearance of a bilateral congenital hydrocele in a baby is often an index of intraperitoneal mischief, such as tuberculous peritonitis. A completely patent processus funicularis may remain unobserved in infancy, but distend in adult life: in such cases, in place of the usual hydrocele, the patient develops a *bilocular hydrocele*, with the physical characters described above except that it does not vary in size. *Hydrocele of the cord* and *hydrocele of a hernial sac* are described under INGUINAL SWELLINGS (*see* p. 426).

4. Trauma. Since the cord contains vessels and lymphatics enclosed in a tubular fascial sheath, it may become swollen when those structures are injured or inflamed. A *haematoma of the cord* may follow a kick in the groin; following rupture of one of the veins, blood is effused inside the infundibuliform fascia and causes a sausage-shaped swelling extending a variable distance into the scrotum, tender and irreducible. The resemblance to a strangulated hernia is at first considerable, but the history of injury, the absence of abdominal symptoms, and later the appearance of bruising, should make the diagnosis clear. Inflammatory conditions of the testis, particularly acute ones, lead to swelling and tenderness of the cord, and new growths may extend along its lymphatics; the inguinal condition is, however, overshadowed and explained by the scrotal one.

R. G. Beard.

INSOMNIA

Insomnia is clearly a relative term. To one accustomed to seven or eight hours' unbroken sleep, an interval of a minute or two awake may, whatever the reason, seem like half an hour of misery; while an unaccustomed spell of longer duration especially in the small hours, when accompanied by a tossing and turning, may easily convince the sufferer that he has 'barely had a wink of sleep all night'. It has been shown that even depressives who do, for the most part, sleep badly, often sleep better than they think they do, so that their complaints of total insomnia may sometimes have a near, if not actual, delusional basis.

It is difficult to decide what actually is the normal amount of sleep required. Clearly there is much individual variation; other than that determined by age, occupation, and sociocultural circumstances. A 1-month-old infant will sleep for 21 out of 24 hours. At 6 months he may sleep for 18; at 1 year for 15. A 4-year-old child seems to need about 12 hours' sleep while one aged 12 requires about 10. But even within these limits there are wide variations. Insomnia, therefore, is not a disease but a symptom which occurs under very many different circumstances, both physical and mental. Many of these are so obvious as not to require mention in detail, e.g., *pain, itching* or other forms of gross discomfort, such as *respiratory distress*. Environmental discomforts may also contribute, e.g., noise, light, heat, cold, uncomfortable conditions, sleeping in a strange bed, etc.

In infancy sleeplessness is most often due to indigestion, hunger, or other bodily discomforts. Bottle-fed infants may suffer from indigestion and colic; those insufficiently well breast-fed may fail to sleep out of hunger. Other causes are dirty napkins or too many or too few bedclothes leading to overheating or cold. Training plays a part, so that middle-of-the-night insomnia can usually be minimized by gradually extending the period between the late evening and early morning feeds. There are, however, children who appear to be bad sleepers, possibly from constitutional or other causes which are most likely of familial origin, whose insomnia and persistent crying may even contribute to incidents of battering. In older infants, fretfulness due to teething is an obvious cause of misery by day and wakefulness by night. Nocturnal irritation due to threadworms may also be a cause.

While only in a minority of instances is insomnia in childhood due to disease, a few special forms call for passing mention. Sleep disturbance is usual in *chorea* and in *encephalitis* in which latter disorder reversal of rhythm not infrequently occurs with insomnia at night and somnolence by day. In early *hip disease* sleep may be disturbed by starting pains; the child falls asleep, to be awakened by sudden shooting pains in the affected leg or hip. Sudden intense pain due to nocturnal cramp in the calf muscles may also be a source of disturbance.

The more usual causes of insomnia in childhood are psychological. Sleep may be broken by fright in *nightmares* (*see* p. 571) when the child wakes up screaming and frightened but is able to explain that he has had a bad dream, or by *night terrrors*, also known as *pavor nocturnus*, in which the child fully awakes, screaming and frightened but not fully conscious, and unable to recognize those around him. There is no recollection of the fright next day. Some children also cannot sleep except with a nightlight or unless the bedroom door is left ajar. Insomnia in childhood, whether due to bad dreams or not, is usually associated with other neurotic symptoms, e.g., shyness, sleep-walking, nail-biting, thumb-sucking, etc. Some small children sleep better if they are allowed to take a doll, teddy-bear or some other favourite toy or even a piece of rag to bed with them. This, which is called a *transition object*, induces in them a feeling of security under which circumstances they sleep better. In older children worry over matters pertaining to school may be a factor.

Insomnia in Adults may, as in the case of children, be due to faulty *habits*. Some sleep badly because they go to bed too soon after a heavy dinner, a few because they go to bed hungry. Some sleep badly if they drink coffee or tea after dinner, others if they indulge in brainwork after dinner and take their problems to bed with them. While both bodily and mental fatigue promote sleep, some sufferers from insomnia who solicit sleep by pushing fatigue to the point of exhaustion only aggravate this. The observance of fairly regular hours for work, food, and sleep is often neglected by busy men and this neglect frequently results in disturbance of sleep. Sudden changes in the mode or routine of daily life may result in persistent insomnia. In those accustomed to long-distance flights 'jet-lag' and a disturbance of circadian rhythms may interfere with sleep, at least for a few days until there is adjustment to a changed time-cycle. It is to the investigation of these and similar irregularities, trifling as many of them may appear, that one must turn to discover the cause of insomnia in healthy or fairly healthy patients, since treatment rests mainly on their correction. Comparatively trivial disturbances such as abdominal discomfort, cough, frequency of micturition, and irritation of the skin naturally require appropriate attention.

Probably the commonest cause of insomnia in adults is a *depressive illness*. Together with insomnia there is depression of mood, loss of weight and appetite, diminished sexual desire, irritability, lack of concentration, impaired memory, and inability to make decisions. The patient is often able to fall asleep soon after going to bed, may wake in an hour or two and be unable to obtain further rest, except perhaps in short snatches during the remainder of the night. Alternatively, he may sleep for longer but still wake much earlier than he usually does, at 4 or 5 instead of 7 a.m. It is to be noted that even in those who are not depressed a tendency to early waking may occur during late middle age. In *neurotic* states there may be difficulty getting off to sleep or sleep once obtained may be so disturbed by dreams and nightmares that the patient fears trying to go to sleep again. Some *schizophrenic* patients, particularly those in whom the disorder makes its onset insidiously during adolescence and who do little or nothing active by day, become wakeful and restless at night, tramping around the house. In some cases of *dementia*, particularly due to *cerebral arteriopathy*, and in *senile dementia* there may similarly be a reversal of sleep rhythm so that the patient takes frequent naps by day but suffers from restlessness and insomnia by night. In *mania* the press of activity may be so great that the patient simply cannot find time to go to bed. He appears remarkably able to do without sleep at least for a time and until exhaustion sets in.

Alcohol and *drugs* are another important cause. Although the alcoholic having drunk too much often falls readily into an intoxicated slumber, he may wake nonetheless in the small hours, perhaps with a full bladder, but even having relieved this, may be unable to sleep again. Furthermore, someone used to imbibing alcohol in relatively large quantities in the evening may, if deprived of it, be unable to sleep. The same applies to hypnotics, particularly *barbiturate* drugs, but to others also. The danger is that having started to take hypnotics in order to cure a relatively mild insomnia, dependence can occur and insomnia be made worse thereby. Alcohol, barbiturates, and some other hypnotics appear to have a tendency to suppress REM (*rapid eye movement*) sleep, episodes of which occur during normal sleep at intervals during the night on some seven or eight occasions, as can be demonstrated by electroencephalography. After taking hypnotics and some other drugs and then ceasing to use these it may be some weeks before the sleeping EEG pattern returns to normal. Some other drugs such as *amphetamine*, which in themselves may produce wakefulness, may also give rise to a disturbed sleep pattern which may persist for some weeks after the drug is withdrawn.

The onset of an attack of delirium tremens is often marked by nightmares with episodes of wakefulness which may be followed by total insomnia. Patients delirious from other causes may despite some clouding of consciousness be similarly wakeful at night. Sleeplessness is frequent in cirrhosis of the liver, being accompanied also by nocturnal delirium in severer cases; the same may also occur in chronic renal disease with uraemia.

In *heart disease* insomnia is frequently distressing; the patient often has to sleep propped up in bed because of breathlessness whenever the recumbent position is adopted, and when he does fall asleep he is often awakened by palpitation or dyspnoea. The condition is aggravated when compensation fails. Patients with aortic incompetence may be kept awake by the pulsating shock and noise of their own hearts.

Dyspnoea is a common cause of sleeplessness in many *chest 'diseases*. Patients with bronchitis, emphysema, spasmodic asthma, extensive pulmonary adhesions, or pulmonary tuberculosis, and other kindred diseases often pass restless nights because they are awakened by pulmonary dyspnoea soon after falling asleep. With them, as with those suffering from heart disease, the sitting or semi-recumbent position at night is often imperative, the reason being that the amplitude of the diaphragmatic movements is greater when the patient sits than when he lies. Sleeplessness is often a persistent and distressing feature of hypertension. As any treatment that lowers the blood-pressure cures the insomnia, it is possible that high arterial pressure directly prevents sleep. Finally, an important cause of insomnia, particularly in the early hours, is pain and stiffness due to chronic *rheumatic* and other *musculoskeletal disorders.*

W. H. Trethowan.

INTESTINAL PARASITES

Tape-worms. The commonest symptom of the presence of a tape-worm is the passage per rectum of the detached terminal segments in longer or shorter tape-like strips (*Fig.* 430). The only condition for which these might be mistaken is

stage of which is spent in cattle. *T. solium* is derived chiefly from pig-meat, and *Dibothriocephalus latus* occurs mainly in those who live much on freshwater fish. It may be possible to make the diagnosis of *T. saginata* by holding the segments up against a bright light and seeing a median streak of water-channel in addition to one down either edge of each strip, this middle water-channel giving the name to the parasite. The ultimate proof of the nature of a tape-worm, however, is afforded by the characters of the head, that of *T. solium* having four sucking disks, with a rostellum and a double row of 14–20 hooklets (*Fig.* 431). The head of *T. echinococcus*, the short tape-worm of the dog and the source of hydatid cysts in man, also has hooklets, some twenty or more in number in two rows, alternately long and short. The head of *T. saginata* has four circular sucking disks but no rostellum and no hooklets (*Fig.* 432); that of the *Dibothriocephalus latus* has a flattened oval head, with two elongated lateral sucking grooves and, again, neither rostellum nor hooklets (*Fig.* 433). The degree of anaemia, macrocytic in type, is usually greatest with *Dibothriocephalus latus*, least with *T. saginata*, and the same applies to the degree of eosinophilia. The eggs of the tape-worm (*Fig.* 434) are spherical,

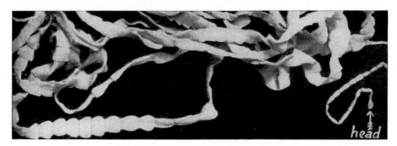

Fig. 430. Part of a tape-worm (*Taenia solium*), a little smaller than actual size.

muco-membranous 'colitis', in which long, narrow, white mucous casts of the bowel may be passed with or independently of the motions. Distinction is afforded by floating the material in water when in the case of a cast of the bowel a central lumen may be found which is not present in the tape-worm. Closer examination will identify the regular segmentation of a tape-worm. If any doubt still remains, examination with a lens will show the glandular structure of the uterus in the tape-worm segments, absent in the strips of mucus in muco-membranous 'colitis'. It is not infrequently stated that picking of the nose and a voracious appetite are symptoms of the presence of some kind of intestinal parasite. This, however, is exceptional; the patient is either symptomless or complains of some abdominal discomfort or diarrhoea. There may be some degree of anaemia and often considerable EOSINOPHILIA (p. 253). The three forms of tape-worm that occur in the human intestine are *Taenia solium*, *T. saginata*, and *Dibothriocephalus latus*, the commonest in Great Britain being the *T. saginata*, the cystic

with a dark-brown central portion and a lighter striated broad capsule.

Microscopical Examination of Faeces. To prepare faeces for microscopical examination for the ova of parasites or for other solid particles, as much as would cover a shilling is placed in a test-tube two-thirds full of normal saline solution. The tube is corked and shaken vigorously in order to break up the faeces as much as possible, then allowed to stand for twenty minutes. The upper part of the fluid remains opaque with fine debris whilst the heavier particles, including the ova of parasites, sink to the bottom. The supernatant opaque fluid is now poured off and the residue again shaken up with normal saline and allowed to stand for another twenty minutes. This process is repeated until the supernatant fluid is clear; and then, when as much of the fluid as possible has been poured away, a drop of the sediment is taken up in a pipette, transferred to a microscope slide, covered, the excess of fluid removed with filter-paper, and the specimen examined either with the $\frac{2}{3}$-in. or $\frac{1}{6}$-in. objective. Vegetable cells, keratin particles, and other debris must be distinguished from the ova of intestinal parasites, but these on the whole are sufficiently characteristic for accurate identification.

Round-worms. The only round-worm that infests man in Great Britain is the *Ascaris lumbricoides.* Ova are ingested in contaminated water or vegetables, hatch in the jejunum and the embryos pass into the portal blood to the heart, thence to the lungs, are coughed up in the sputum, swallowed, and pass once more into the intestine where they mature into adult worms. This

and move about slowly. The only symptoms commonly present are reflex, e.g., in children restlessness and irritability with local results such as frequency of micturition, vaginitis, or pruritus. Thread-worms should be remembered as a possible source of pruritus ani in adults. The **Whip-worm** (*Trichuris trichiura*) inhabits the caecum and large intestine. With its tail it is about 40 mm. (1¼ in.)

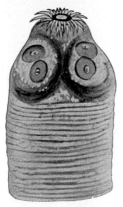

Fig. 431. Head of *Taenia solium* (semidiagrammatic). (×30.) (*From Cammidge's 'Faeces of Children and Adults'.*)

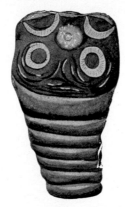

Fig. 432. Head of *Taenia saginata* (semidiagrammatic). (×30.) (*From Cammidge's 'Faeces of Children and Adults'.*)

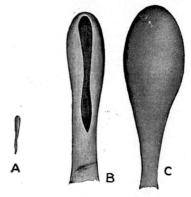

Fig. 433. *Dibothriocephalus latus.* A, Head (natural size). B, Lateral view (×15). C, Dorsal view (×15). (*From Cammidge's 'Faeces of Children and Adults'.*)

Fig. 434. Ovum of *Taenia solium*, semidiagrammatic. (High power.)

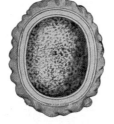

Fig. 435. Ovum of *Ascaris lumbricoides*. (High power.)

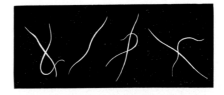

Fig. 436. Thread-worms, magnified about four times.

parasite may give rise to symptoms of intestinal colic or biliary obstruction. The larval form may give rise to pneumonitis during its lung transit, or to urticaria with associated eosinophilia. More often the condition is unsuspected until one of the worms is found in a stool, or in the bed having passed out per anum. If round-worms have been found previously, and if the existence of others is suspected, confirmation may be afforded by discovering the typical ova (*Fig.* 435) in the faeces. These ova are distinguished by their relatively large size, oval shape, and irregular membranous envelope outside the chitinous shell. Eosinophilia is not a feature of infestation by this worm.

Thread-worms. *Oxyuris vermicularis*, if present at all, usually occur in large numbers. They can be detected by naked-eye examination of the faeces. Each parasite is rather less than 3–10 mm. (¼ in.) in length and is colourless (*Fig.* 436); the extremities project like tiny threads from the faecal mass,

in length, and it is often coiled up like a watch-spring; its ovum (*Fig.* 437) has deep-brown central parts and clear terminal knobs. *Whip-worms* are present in some cities to the extent of nearly 10 per cent of all the inhabitants. They

Fig. 437. Ovum of *Trichuris trichiura*. (High power.)

produce no eosinophilia, and symptoms are rare, although appendicitis has been known to be produced by or at least associated with their presence.

The **Hookworm** (*Ancylostoma duodenale*) is not a native parasite in Great Britain, but as the result of introduction from abroad has affected many persons in certain districts, particularly tin-miners in Cornwall. Outbreaks have also occurred in workers in coal-mines in Belgium and in the St. Gotthard tunnel. Ancylostomiasis is prevalent throughout the subtropical world especially in India, Egypt, Brazil, Ceylon, and Jamaica. The infection is carried from faeces to soil; here the ova hatch into larvae which penetrate the skin of the next victim, pass to the lungs, ascend the trachea, are swallowed, and mature into adult worms in the intestine. The symptoms are those of progressive anaemia and asthenia, oedema of the lower extremities, anasarca, shortness of breath, and the occurrence of vesicular and pustular skin eruptions described as 'flowers' of the disease. The appearance of the patient may suggest pernicious anaemia and the blood-count may sometimes seem to confirm this diagnosis, for whereas a great many of the patients have a severe microcytic hypochromic type of anaemia, some have a marked reduction of the red corpuscles and a slightly lower reduction of the haemoglobin so that there is a high colour index. There is generally no leucocytosis, but the differential leucocyte-count nearly always exhibits a high degree of eosinophilia. The administration of anthelmintics such as tetrachlorethylene may lead to the evacuation of the mature worms, which may be recognized in the faeces, each being from 8 to 17 mm. in length. The ova are oval with a clear transparent shell and coiled-up embryo parasite. Melaena may in some cases be consider-able.

The two intestinal parasites which produce the most serious anaemias and other toxic effects in man are *Ancylostoma duodenale* and *Dibothrio-cephalus latus*.

Harold Ellis.

INTRACRANIAL BRUIT

A systolic bruit may be heard over the extra-cranial arteries in the neck, over the orbits, or over the mastoid processes either because there is

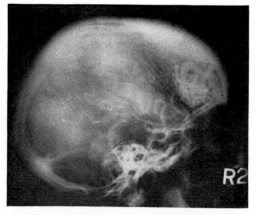

Fig. 438. Carotid angiogram showing cerebral angioma with feeding arteries and a large draining vein.

turbulence due to increased flow in the arteries or because there is turbulence due to stenosis.

A bruit invariably accompanies the pulsating proptosis of a caroticocavernous fistula, usually due to a head injury or to rupture of a carotid

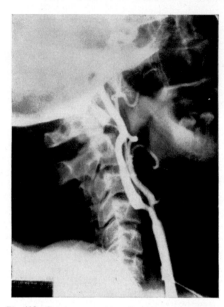

Fig. 439. Common carotid angiogram showing stenosis at the bifurcation over which a bruit was heard.

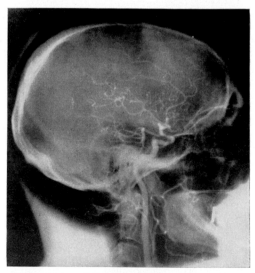

Fig. 440. Right common carotid angiogram showing narrow-ing of the internal carotid in the 'siphon' which was accompanied by a bruit heard over the eyeball.

aneurysm in the cavernous sinus. A bruit may also be heard in the presence of a cerebral angioma (*Fig.* 438), but absence of a murmur does not exclude such a lesion. Increased flow will also occur and a bruit may be heard when one or more extracranial arteries are occluded and also in generalized conditions such as thyrotoxicosis, severe anaemia, and advanced Paget's disease of the skull.

Stenosis of an artery in the neck (*Fig.* 439) can cause a localized bruit and if the narrowing is in the intracranial portion of the carotid artery (*Fig.* 440) a localized bruit may be heard over the orbit.

The systolic bruit of aortic stenosis can be conducted into the neck but it is maximal over the aortic area, unlike the bruit which arises in the carotid itself.

Ian Mackenzie.

JAUNDICE

Jaundice may conveniently be classified according to the predominance of either unconjugated or conjugated bilirubin in the blood (*Fig.* 441).

haemolytic anaemia; 7. Haemolytic disease of the newborn; 8. Micro-angiopathic haemolytic anaemia; 9. Infections; 10. Hypersplenism; 11. Secondary to other conditions.

General. The normal level of serum bilirubin depends upon a balance between red-cell breakdown and liver excretion. Red cells are removed from the circulation by the reticulo-endothelial system and haemoglobin is broken down to form unconjugated bilirubin. An increased rate of red-cell destruction therefore leads to an increase in the serum level of unconjugated bilirubin. Except in the neonate, the liver has an enormous capacity to conjugate and excrete bilirubin; levels of serum bilirubin seldom rise above 85–90 μmol/l (5 mg. per 100 ml.) in haemolytic states and jaundice is usually slight.

Some clinical signs and laboratory findings are common to states of increased haemolysis

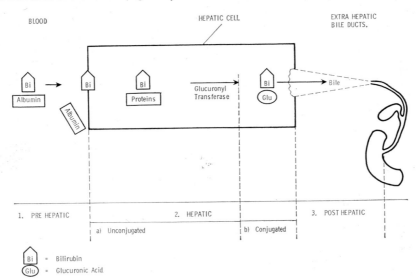

Fig. 441. The classification of jaundice.

GENERAL CLASSIFICATION

UNCONJUGATED HYPERBILIRUBINAEMIA	PREHEPATIC	(Haemolytic anaemia)
	HEPATIC	
CONJUGATED HYPERBILIRUBINAEMIA	HEPATIC	Acute damage Chronic damage Cholestasis
	POSTHEPATIC	

UNCONJUGATED HYPERBILIRUBINAEMIA—PREHEPATIC (HAEMOLYTIC ANAEMIAS)

1. Hereditary spherocytosis; 2. Haemoglobinopathy, Thalassaemia; 3. Paroxysmal nocturnal haemoglobinuria; 4 Congenital non-spherocytic haemolytic anaemias; 5 Drugs and chemicals; 6. Auto-immune

regardless of the cause: the presence of such features in a patient with mild jaundice suggests that increased haemolysis is occurring. Examination reveals the triad of anaemia, jaundice, and splenomegaly. Bilirubin is not found in the urine and stools are of normal colour. There is anaemia and peripheral blood shows reticulocytosis, a sign of increased bone-marrow activity. Examination of the bone-marrow shows hyperplasia of erythropoietic cells. Haemolysis can be confirmed and its extent documented by measurement of red-cell half-life using cells labelled with radioactive chromium.

When haemolysis occurs within the bloodstream, rather than in the reticulo-endothelial system, the plasma haemoglobin level rises from its usual low level. At first haemoglobin is bound to haptoglobins, a protein fraction which forms part of the α_2 globulin band. When haptoglobins are saturated, haemoglobin appears in the plasma bound with albumin as methaemalbumin, and there is haemoglobinuria. In chronic haemolytic states, low levels of haptoglobin are found.

1. Hereditary Spherocytosis. In this congenital condition, inherited as an autosomal dominant, the red-cell membrane 'leaks' sodium and the cell therefore swells, becoming spherical. The increased metabolic activity of the cell required to pump out the extra sodium leads to depletion of membrane phospholipid and the cells become smaller than normal (microspherocytosis). Such cells are prematurely destroyed in the spleen.

The disease is not uncommon in Europeans but is rare in other races. Symptoms usually appear in childhood but the condition has been discovered for the first time in the elderly. Typically, there is a compensated haemolytic state, perhaps with slight anaemia but symptomless. This is interrupted by 'crises' due to increased haemolysis accompanied by anaemia, jaundice, and splenomegaly. Fever is common and pain in the left subchondral area may suggest some abdominal emergency. Spontaneous recovery within a few days is normal. In a few cases there is chronic ulceration of the legs, and children with the disorder may be small and mentally retarded. Pigment gall-stones are not uncommon.

The diagnosis is usually made by examination of a blood-film which shows the characteristic microspherocyte. Because the cells are small and swollen they are more sensitive to disruption in hypotonic saline and this forms the basis of the osmotic fragility curve, which is confirmatory.

Splenectomy is curative and should ideally be carried out after age 5. Transfusion is occasionally required for crises.

2. Sickle-cell Disease. The haemoglobin molecule contains four haem molecules and four polypeptide chains. Substitution of amino-acids in the polypeptide chains leads to the production of various abnormal haemoglobins, the most important of which is haemoglobin S. Cells with this haemoglobin show two abnormalities. In conditions of hypoxia, they form sickle-shaped cells which lead to local thrombosis: these cells also have a short life-span, and there is therefore a chronic haemolytic anaemia.

Haemoglobin S is inherited as an autosomal intermediate character. Homozygotes have sickle-cell disease. Less than half the cells of heterozygotes are abnormal and they are said to have the sickle-cell trait which is not associated with haemolytic anaemia. Sickle-cell disease mainly affects Negroes in Central Africa around the Equator and down to the level of the Zambezi River. It occurs less commonly in countries bordering the Mediterranean, and in the Middle East and India.

The disease usually becomes apparent in early childhood. There is chronic anaemia and mild jaundice interrupted by thrombotic crises which cause polyarthritis, abdominal pain, avascular necrosis of bone, particularly the head of the femur, splenic, pulmonary, and cerebral infarcts, and priapism. These crises are accompanied by fever and leucocytosis. Leg ulcers are common and there is an increased risk of *Salmonella* osteomyelitis. The spleen is palpable in young children but later shrinks because of repeated infarcts. Repeated transfusions are often required and the condition is usually fatal in later childhood.

Diagnosis is confirmed by finding sickle cells in the blood-film and by haemoglobin electrophoresis.

OTHER HAEMOGLOBINOPATHIES. A large number of other abnormal haemoglobins, identifiable by electrophoresis, have now been described. They are usually inherited as autosomal dominant characters and there is a variable degree of haemolysis in homozygotes. An example is haemoglobin-C disease, common in Ghana, in which there is mild anaemia, intermittent jaundice, and splenomegaly.

THALASSAEMIA. In thalassaemia there is suppression of formation of the polypeptide chains of haemoglobin. A normal haemoglobin molecule has two α chains and two β chains and either may be suppressed. The disorder is inherited as an autosomal intermediate, homozygotes having thalassaemia major and heterozygotes thalassaemia minor. α-Thalassaemia major is incompatible with life and α-thalassaemia minor produces no clinical abnormality. β-Thalassaemia major or minor may cause jaundice by increased haemolysis, but anaemia resulting from failure of haemoglobin synthesis dominates the clinical picture.

Thalassaemia is found in countries bordering the Mediterranean and in the Far East. Thalassaemia major is usually apparent in the first year of life, the child being markedly anaemic with splenomegaly. Jaundice is slight or absent. Repeated transfusions are required and death in childhood is usual. The blood-film resembles that of iron deficiency with small pale cells, but the serum iron is normal or raised. These cells are resistant to lysis in hypotonic saline. Haemoglobin electrophoresis reveals raised levels of haemoglobins F and A_2. These haemoglobins, composed of α and γ or δ polypeptide chains, are normally present only in foetal life but production continues as a compensatory phenomenon in thalassaemia.

In thalassaemia minor there is usually a mild anaemia compatible with a normal life. Jaundice does not occur except in a rare type of thalassaemia minor, described in Italy, in which there is a chronic haemolytic state with jaundice. Diagnosis can be difficult but levels of haemoglobin A_2 are again increased.

3. Paroxysmal Nocturnal Haemoglobinuria. Crises in this condition are sometimes accompanied by slight jaundice. There is also anaemia and haemoglobinuria which is usually but not always noticed in the morning, having occurred at night. Patients also have attacks of abdominal pain and venous thrombosis. The spleen is usually enlarged. There are no characteristic features on a blood-film but the diagnosis can be confirmed by Hain's acid haemolysis test. The condition is uncommon with no particular racial incidence and is not hereditary.

4. Congenital Non-spherocytic Haemolytic Anaemia. This is a group of conditions caused by deficiency of enzymes concerned with red-cell glycolysis. The commonest is pyruvate kinase deficiency, which is inherited as an autosomal recessive character. It may also occur as a manifestation of glucose-6-phosphate-dehydrogenase deficiency, particularly in Caucasians. A number of other enzyme deficiencies have been described. Clinical features resemble those of hereditary spherocytosis, a compensated haemolytic state interrupted by crises of increased haemolysis and jaundice often precipitated by infection. Red-cell morphology is normal and the diagnosis is made by measurement of red-cell enzyme levels. Splenectomy has no effect.

5. Haemolytic Anaemia due to Drugs and Chemicals. There are three ways in which drugs and chemicals may cause haemolytic anaemia and jaundice.

A. DIRECT ACTION. Phenylhydrazine, a drug which has been used for the treatment of polycythaemia, causes haemolysis by a direct effect on the red cell. Some organic chemicals such as aniline, benzene, and methyl chloride have a similar effect.

B. GLUCOSE - 6 - PHOSPHATE - DEHYDROGENASE DEFICIENCY. The enzyme glucose-6-phosphate dehydrogenase is required in the red cell for the maintenance of glutathione in the reduced state. Reduced glutathione seems to be required for the integrity of the red-cell membrane. Deficiency of this enzyme therefore leads to an increased susceptibility to haemolysis by oxidant compounds. The deficiency is inherited as a sex-linked intermediate character, affecting mainly males. It is common in Negroes, affecting 10 per cent of Negroes in America, and also in countries bordering the Mediterranean, India, and the Far East.

Acute haemolytic anaemia is mainly associated with the 8-aminoquinoline anti-malarials such as primaquine and pamaquine. Acute haemolysis begins within a day or two of taking the drug in a susceptible subject; there is fever, malaise, and abdominal or loin pain accompanied by pallor, jaundice, and splenomegaly. Haemolysis is predominantly intravascular and haemoglobinuria occurs in severe cases. Even if the drug is continued, recovery follows since only older cells are destroyed. The diagnosis is confirmed by measurement of red-cell glucose-6-phosphate dehydrogenase.

The following drugs have been reported to cause haemolysis in glucose-6-phosphate-dehydrogenase deficient subjects: 8-aminoquinolines, primaquine, and pamaquine; chloroquine; sulphonamides; nitrofurantoin; aspirin in large doses; salts of para-amino salicylic acid (P.A.S.); water-soluble vitamin-K analogues; phenacetin.

Haemolysis may be precipitated by various organic chemicals including naphthalene.

Glucose-6-phosphate-dehydrogenase deficiency is also the underlying defect in favism; in this condition an acute haemolytic episode is precipitated by ingestion of the broad bean, *Vicia faba*, or inhalation of its pollen. Haemolysis begins within hours and jaundice may be striking. The condition is sometimes fatal, but in most cases recovery ensues within a few days. It characteristically occurs in certain families in Italy, Sardinia, Sicily, and Greece, but has been reported in natives of many other countries including Great Britain. Affected subjects are also susceptible to drug-induced haemolysis.

C. IMMUNE MECHANISM. Two types of immune mechanism operate in the production of haemolytic anaemia by drugs:

a. Drug-dependent. In this situation antibodies are formed against red cells in the presence of the drug. Haemolysis is acute, often severe, intravascular, and therefore accompanied by haemoglobinuria in severe cases. Coombs' test is positive. Drugs responsible are: penicillin, salts of para-amino salicylic acid (P.A.S.), quinidine, sulphonamides, stibophen, quinine, and phenacetin.

b. Non-drug Dependent. Twenty per cent of patients taking methyldopa develop a positive Coombs' test and a small proportion of these have a haemolytic anaemia. Antibodies are directed against red cells even in the absence of the drug.

6. Auto-immune Haemolytic Anaemia. Acute or chronic haemolytic anaemias associated with a positive Coombs' test may be classified as follows:

a. Idiopathic, accounting for about 60 per cent of cases.

b. In *malignant disease,* particularly chronic lymphatic leukaemia and reticulum-cell sarcoma.

c. In *infections,* particularly mycoplasma pneumonia.

d. In systemic lupus erythematosus, rheumatoid arthritis, and ulcerative colitis. These conditions occur at any age and are commoner in females; the course is very variable, sometimes acute and self-limiting, sometimes chronic. Jaundice is usual.

e. Paroxysmal cold haemoglobinuria; slight jaundice may occur following attacks of haemoglobinuria.

7. Haemolytic Disease of the Newborn. This condition arises when there is Rhesus incompatibility, a Rhesus-positive foetus immunizing a Rhesus-negative mother. Antibodies reach the foetal circulation and destroy the red cells. A similar condition is rarely produced by ABO incompatibility. The first child is usually unaffected but subsequent children are affected with increasing severity, being jaundiced at birth. The diagnosis is made by detecting antibodies in maternal blood in the later stages of pregnancy. Rhesus incompatibility must be distinguished from other causes of foetal jaundice:

Physiological jaundice due to hepatic immaturity particularly in premature infants.

Glucose-6-phosphate-dehydrogenase deficiency. Neonatal jaundice is not uncommon in susceptible populations, particularly in Mediterranean areas.

Infections, congenital syphilis, rubella, cytomegalic inclusion disease, toxoplasmosis.

Hereditary spherocytosis is a very rare cause.

Overdose with menadiol (Synkavit) especially in premature infants.

8. Micro-angiopathic Haemolytic Anaemia. In this condition, haemolytic anaemia is believed to result from contact of red cells with abnormal vascular endothelium. There are characteristic findings on examination of a blood-film, with distortion and fragmentation of red cells. It occurs in the following:

The haemolytic uraemic syndrome is an acute condition of young children, usually presenting with diarrhoea and vomiting. Subsequently pallor, sometimes jaundice, and oliguria develop. Most patients die of acute renal failure.

Thrombotic thrombocytopenic purpura is a condition of adults, characterized by haemolytic anaemia, purpura, neurological signs, and acute renal failure.

This type of haemolytic anaemia also occurs in malignant hypertension, disseminated malignancy, polyarteritis nodosa, and eclampsia of pregnancy.

9. Infections. Haemolytic anaemia and jaundice may complicate the following infections: septicaemia, particularly *Clostridium welchii*; endocarditis; typhoid; tuberculosis; malaria (blackwater fever); toxoplasmosis; relapsing fever.

Auto-immune haemolytic anaemia may occur, particularly with mycoplasmic pneumonia. Patients with glucose-6-phosphate-dehydrogenase deficiency may have episodes of acute haemolysis precipitated by infection.

10. Hypersplenism may give rise to a chronic haemolytic anaemia with jaundice.

11. Secondary to Other Conditions. A variety of other conditions may give rise to haemolysis and jaundice. In severe cases of *pernicious anaemia*, slight jaundice is common. Haemolysis is sometimes a feature of *acute and chronic leukaemias, lymphomas, Waldenström's macroglobulinaemia, myelosclerosis*, and *carcinomatosis*. Some of these conditions give rise to auto-immune haemolytic anaemia but they may also cause haemolytic anaemia without the presence of detectable antibodies. Haemolysis is also rarely associated with *benign or malignant tumours of the ovary*.

Intravascular haemolysis and jaundice may follow transfusions of mismatched or stale blood, and *cardiac and vascular operations* involving the use of Teflon grafts or artificial valves. Occasionally, large *haematomata* give rise to slight jaundice as the contained blood is reabsorbed. Haemolysis may contribute to jaundice in *liver disease* and occurs in the terminal stages of *renal failure*.

UNCONJUGATED HYPERBILIRUBINAEMIA—HEPATIC

1. FAILURE OF TRANSPORT INTO THE CELL:
   Gilbert's syndrome.
   Male fern extract (flavaspidic acid).

2. IMPAIRED CONJUGATION:
   Absent
     Crigler-Najjar (Type I).
   Low
     Crigler-Najjar (Type II).
     Neonates.
   Inhibited
     3,20-Pregnanediol.
     Lucey-Driscoll syndrome.

Bilirubin is formed from haem and transported in the blood bound to albumin. In this unconjugated, water-insoluble form it reaches the liver cell where it is freed from the albumin and transported across the cell membrane. The membranes of the endoplasm reticulum (microsomes) contain the enzyme glucuronyl transferase and this conjugates bilirubin to a relatively water-soluble glucuronide.

Any condition which interferes with the passage of bilirubin into the hepatic cell, or with the process of conjugation, will result in jaundice. The consequent raised serum level of unconjugated bilirubin may be detected by the diazo reaction of Van de Bergh as the 'indirect' form.

Certain substances, for example phenobarbitone and dicophane, induce the synthesis of many hepatic microsomal enzymes including the specific bilirubin glucuronyl transferase. In situations where it is present in low concentration jaundice may be improved by treatment with an enzyme inducer.

Gilbert's Syndrome. This is the commonest form of familial unconjugated, non-haemolytic hyperbilirubinaemia. The defect lies in the transport of bilirubin from the serum to the liver cell. It is usually diagnosed by chance, particularly in medical students and nurses who are perhaps more likely to notice slight jaundice. It may be discovered routinely following viral hepatitis when the bilirubin fails to return to normal. The jaundice is mild and intermittent but during exacerbations patients often feel vaguely unwell. Mild intercurrent infections may deepen the jaundice. There are no other abnormal physical findings and total serum bilirubin rarely exceeds 50 μmol/l (3 mg. per 100 ml.). All other tests of liver function and red-cell survival are normal.

Occasionally Gilbert's syndrome is associated with an unconjugated bilirubin level of 140–170 μmol/l (8–10 mg. per 100 ml.). In such patients glucuronide conjugation is defective in addition to the transport defect and may be improved by phenobarbitone.

Male Fern Extract (Flavaspidic Acid). Extract of the male fern (*Dryopteris filix mas*) can inhibit the uptake of bilirubin by the hepatic cell. It may act by competing with bilirubin for binding sites on proteins within the cell. It produces a mild, reversible jaundice particularly in patients with Gilbert's disease.

Crigler-Najjar. This condition affects neonates and infants and has been divided into two types, depending on whether glucuronyl transferase is present with reduced activity or is completely absent. Affected infants usually die in the first year of life, although a case has been recorded surviving into adulthood and producing an affected child. Type I patients have severe jaundice (bilirubin above 900 μmol/l (22 mg. per 100 ml.)), some develop kernicterus, and they have no bilirubin in the bile. Type II patients are less severely affected, without kernicterus, and conjugated bilirubin is found in the bile. In Type II patients there is probably a recessive inheritance of a partial enzyme defect. There is no evidence of haemolysis and all other liver-function tests, including bromsulphthalein retention, are normal.

Neonatal Jaundice. The enzyme glucuronyl transferase seems to mature at or shortly after birth, therefore newborn babies, particularly if premature, will possess it in small amounts or in an inactive form. A mild degree of jaundice is common in the neonate and any factor increasing the bilirubin load (for example, haemolysis) will deepen the jaundice and kernicterus may result.

3α-20β-Pregnanediol. Prolonged unconjugated hyperbilirubinaemia in the neonate may be associated with breast-feeding.

It was believed that this was due to inhibition of glucuronyl transferase by 3α-20β-pregnanediol, a steroid secreted in breast-milk. This action has not yet been confirmed.

Lucey-Driscoll Syndrome. This is a more severe and familial form of neonatal jaundice. A substance which inhibits glucuronyl transferase is found in excess in the serum of affected babies and their mothers. The inhibitor has not yet been identified.

CONJUGATED HYPERBILIRUBINAEMIA—HEPATIC

JAUNDICE DUE TO ACUTE HEPATOCELLULAR DAMAGE

This type of jaundice may be caused by infections, poisons, or drugs. The depth of jaundice is variable; serum transaminases are always raised, often to very high levels, while the alkaline phosphatase is usually only moderately raised and may be normal.

INFECTIONS:

Viral hepatitis
Infectious mononucleosis
Yellow fever
Other viral infections
Portal pyaemia
Septicaemia
Leptospirosis
Relapsing fever
Syphilis
Tuberculosis
Other bacterial infections
Protozoan infections.

POISONS:

Carbon tetrachloride
Dicophane (Chlorophenothane, D.D.T.)
Benzene derivatives
Tannic acid
Muscarine

Aflatoxin
4,4-Diaminodiphenylmethane
Phosphorus (yellow form)
Physical agents.

DRUGS:

The hydrazines and related drugs
Halothane
Cytotoxic drugs
The tetracyclines
Paracetamol
Obsolete drugs.

1. Infections

A. VIRAL HEPATITIS. This may be due to the infective hepatitis (I.H.) virus or the serum hepatitis (S.H.) virus. Infective hepatitis has an incubation period of 15–50 days. It occurs most commonly in young adults and an attack confers lifelong immunity. Before jaundice develops there is a period of anorexia for from 3 to 9 days. It is at this time that the urine becomes dark because of bilirubin being excreted. There may be a dull ache in the region of the liver but there is usually no severe pain such as occurs in post-hepatic jaundice. On examination of a peripheral blood-film it is common to find that the white-cell count is depressed. The patient usually feels extremely ill and fever is very common. One in 20 patients develops some kind of urticarial or maculopapular rash. Once jaundice appears it develops rapidly and after 3–10 days the symptoms regress. The liver may be palpable and tender from the pre-icteric stage, but as jaundice appears it becomes non-tender, although it may remain palpable for some months.

Serum hepatitis has a clinical course similar to infective hepatitis but is always preceded by some event which has successfully implanted the virus beneath the surface of the patient's skin. The incubation period is 50–160 days. The amount of infected material required to produce an infection is extremely small. Infections have been caused by tattooing, the shared needles of narcotic addicts, injections of any kind, blood, plasma, fibrinogen, and antihaemophilic globulin transfusions. Outbreaks of serum hepatitis among the staff of renal dialysis units has given especial cause for concern. The discovery of the Australia antigen and of its association with viral hepatitis, particularly serum hepatitis, has proved to be of great importance both in diagnosis and in screening blood donors who might transmit hepatitis.

The progress of the disease usually is to complete resolution in a few weeks with completely normal liver-function tests by 6 months. Occasionally the symptoms and jaundice return in the relapsing form. Fulminant hepatitis results in hepatic cell death and has an inevitably fatal outcome. Subacute hepatitis may smoulder on until liver failure supervenes. In this case the spleen is palpable and there is progressive worsening of the liver-function tests.

B. INFECTIOUS MONONUCLEOSIS. Overt jaundice occurs in 5–10 per cent of cases. This is usually due to hepatocellular damage and raised serum transaminases are found more frequently than jaundice. It should be remembered that haemolysis may also occur in glandular fever. The diagnosis is made by finding atypical lymphocytes in the peripheral blood and a positive test for heterophile antibodies (Paul-Bunnell test). The Epstein-Barr virus, responsible for Burkitt's lymphoma, has recently been shown to be associated with glandular fever also.

C. YELLOW FEVER. This disease is due to the yellow-fever virus transmitted from man and primates by mosquitoes. It occurs in tropical or subtropical climates and is prevalent in West Africa, the West Indies, and Central and South America. The incubation period is 3–4 days and the onset is sudden with rigors, headache, pain in the back and limbs, and constipation. Jaundice is an early symptom but varies in intensity, being much more severe in fatal than in mild cases. The temperature rises to a high level of 102–105° F. (39–41° C.). Albuminuria, vomiting, and haemorrhage from the gums and beneath the skin are conspicuous features.

D. OTHER VIRAL INFECTIONS. Coxsackie B virus and the viruses of cytomegalic inclusion disease, herpes simplex, and rubella are liable to cause jaundice in the neonatal period. The first two of these, plus Q fever, may rarely cause hepatitis in adults.

E. PORTAL PYAEMIA. This condition is due to the spread of infected emboli within the portal system. It is associated with a primary infective focus somewhere within the portal drainage system, e.g., acute appendicitis, and is attended by a very high swinging fever, with rigors and severe prostration. Occasionally the jaundice may be associated with an element of haemolysis compounding that due to the hepatic cellular damage. *Escherichia coli*, *Proteus vulgaris*, *Streptococcus faecalis*, and staphylococci are among the commonest infectious organisms that may be obtained on blood-culture.

F. SEPTICAEMIA. In severe septicaemia there may be considerable hepatic destruction. The patient is desperately ill with hypovolaemic hypotension and tachycardia, a confusing feature of which may be a vasodilated stage—the so-called 'warm shock'. The blood-culture is positive and the spleen palpable.

G. LEPTOSPIROSIS (Weil's Disease). This condition is caused by the *Leptospira icterohaemorrhagiae* which infects the kidney and urine of rats and mice. For this reason the disease is usually found in sewer and agricultural workers. The onset is sudden with pyrexia, pain in the back and limbs, headache, and giddiness, followed in 2–4 days by jaundice, enlargement of the liver and spleen, and nephritis. The jaundice deepens rapidly over a period of 24 hours and the temperature rises to between 103° and 104° F. (40° C.). In an untreated case the pyrexia has two peaks. The initial pyrexia occurs with the onset of the disease and after this has fallen there occurs a secondary rise during the third week. There is generally an associated albuminuria with haematuria and tubular casts in the urine. There may be pulmonary consolidation. Usually there are associated severe haemorrhages, particularly purpura, haemoptysis, haematemesis, epistaxis, and melaena.

The diagnosis is made by finding the *Leptospira* organisms in the patient's blood and later in the urine. The presence of a polymorphonuclear leucocytosis is useful in differentiating Weil's disease from virus hepatitis. Jaundice may occur in *Leptospira canicola* infections also.

H. RELAPSING FEVER. This is due to the motile Gram-negative spiral organism of the *Borrelia* group of which there are seventeen types. Jaundice is a common feature with this contagious fever, which is prevalent in India, occurring in other countries as well in times of famine. There is considerable enlargement of the liver and spleen and a certain amount of abdominal pain and tenderness in most cases. Epistaxis and haematemesis often occur. The most characteristic feature of this disease is the temperature, which rises abruptly to 104° or 105° F. (41° C.) and then remains high for 5–6 days. It then rapidly falls to normal when, after an interval of about a week, it again rises and remains high for 3–4 days (*Fig.* 321, p. 299). During periods of pyrexia the organism may be found in peripheral blood-smears.

I. SYPHILIS. Mild jaundice may be a manifestation of congenital syphilis or rarely of diffuse hepatitis in secondary syphilis. Otherwise jaundice occurring in syphilitic patients has usually been due to syringe-transmitted virus hepatitis.

J. TUBERCULOSIS. Granulomatous hepatitis is the usual lesion in tuberculous infections. Jaundice is unusual but may occur with severe miliary tuberculosis.

K. OTHER BACTERIAL INFECTIONS. Jaundice may occur as part of a severe infection with pneumococci, *Klebsiella pneumoniae*, *Salmonella typhi*, and *Bacteroides*. In such conditions the jaundice is usually caused by cholestasis as well as actual liver-cell damage.

L. PROTOZOAN INFECTIONS. Jaundice in the neonatal period may be caused by congenital toxoplasmosis. Jaundice is unusual in hepatic amoebiasis; indeed, the presence of jaundice with a liver abscess suggests that the abscess is due to a pyogenic organism rather than to *Entamoeba histolytica*.

2. Poisons

A. CARBON TETRACHLORIDE. This substance may be inhaled in the course of a dry-cleaning process or in handling fire extinguishers. Centrizonal hepatic cells show degenerative changes, the extent of which depends upon the amount of carbon tetrachloride taken. Jaundice develops usually within 2 days, the depth being related to the extent of hepatic damage. The liver may be enlarged and tender and hypoprothrombinaemia develops. Serum transaminase values are extremely high. There may be associated acute tubular necrosis with subsequent renal failure.

Similar substances, such as tetrachlorethylene, tetrachlorethane, ethylchloride, and methyl chloride, will also produce hepatic necrosis.

B. DICOPHANE (CHLOROPHENOTHANE, D.D.T.). This substance is used as an insecticide and in very large doses it is toxic to the liver. It is possible for it to cause fatty change and hepato-cellular necrosis.

C. BENZENE DERIVATIVES. This is a rare cause of hepatotoxicity and the substances included in this group are trinitrotoluene, dinitrophenol, and toluene.

D. TANNIC ACID. The toxic nature of this substance became important following the application of tannic acid to burned areas of skin. In addition, tannic acid has been added to barium sulphate to improve the definition of barium enema. Unfortunately it is absorbed from the colon and several deaths from hepatic necrosis have been reported following this procedure.

E. MUSCARINE. Poisoning with this substance follows the ingestion of *Amanita* mushrooms, including the three varieties *A. phalloides*, *A. muscaria*, and *A. verna*. The mushrooms have the appearance of edible mushrooms and grow under oak trees. There is nausea, abdominal pain, and diarrhoea 8–12 hours after ingestion. This lasts for 3–4 days. It is then followed by a period of comparative improvement, the illusion being rapidly shattered by massive cell destruction in the liver, kidney, and central nervous system.

F. AFLATOXIN. This substance is derived from *Aspergillus flavus* and may be ingested following the fungal contamination of ground-nuts.

G. 4,4-DIAMINODIPHENYLMETHANE. This substance is interesting because it was spilt on the floor of a van subsequently used to transport wholemeal flour to a bakery. It contaminated the flour, was made into loaves, and resulted in the acute onset of severe, intermittent, right upper-quadrant pain lasting for $1–1\frac{1}{2}$ days, followed by fever, malaise, and jaundice.

H. PHOSPHORUS (YELLOW FORM). This may be taken by accident or with suicidal intent. It causes jaundice and often death in a few days.

I. PHYSICAL AGENTS. Hyperpyrexia, severe burns, and irradiation of the liver can all cause jaundice by hepatocellular damage.

3. Drugs

A. THE HYDRAZINES AND RELATED DRUGS. This group of drugs includes the monoamine oxidase inhibitors: iproniazid, phenelzine, pheniprazine, isocarboxazid, phenoxypropazine, and tranylcypromine; and the antituberculous drugs: isoniazid, ethionamide, and pyrazinamide.

These drugs all cause an illness that is difficult to distinguish from acute viral hepatitis. It is unrelated to the dose or duration of the drug therapy and may occur up to 3 weeks after stopping treatment. The mortality is high and those who survive the initial illness may show progression to cirrhosis of the liver. Recurrence follows further treatment with the original drug or another member of the group.

B. HALOTHANE. Fever and jaundice may rarely follow the administration of this widely used anaesthetic agent. If a second anaesthetic with the same agent is then used a severe, even fatal, hepatitis-like illness may follow. Although this is extremely rare, authorities feel that repeated halothane administrations within 6 months of each other are unwise.

C. CYTOTOXIC DRUGS. Many of the cytotoxic drugs currently in use as a means of therapy for carcinoma will produce hepatic damage. For example, jaundice may occur after treatment with 6-mercaptopurine or methotrexate.

D. THE TETRACYCLINES. Usually innocuous, this group of drugs may affect the liver, particularly if used in high intravenous dosage in late pregnancy or in the malnourished.

E. PARACETAMOL. Jaundice is associated only with overdosage of this drug.

F. OBSOLETE DRUGS. For completeness drugs now withdrawn must be mentioned. These include: Cincophen, zoxazolamine, and ibufenac

JAUNDICE DUE TO CHRONIC HEPATOCELLULAR DAMAGE

CIRRHOSIS:

> Cryptogenic
> Viral
> Alcoholic
> Cardiac failure
> Hepatic venous obstruction
> Chronic active hepatitis
> Prolonged cholestasis and biliary cirrhosis
> Hepatolenticular degeneration
> Haemochromatosis
> Fibrocystic disease
> Galactosaemia
> Congenital syphilis
> Schistosomiasis
> Glycogen-storage diseases.

AMYLOIDOSIS.

TUMOURS:

> Primary carcinoma of liver
> Secondary tumours
> Reticulo-endothelial disease and the liver.

Chronic Hepatocellular Damage. The liver may be affected by many forms of chronic disease and hepatocellular failure may result whether the liver-cell damage is due to infection, degeneration, infiltration, or malignancy. In all cases jaundice can occur due to the failure of the liver cells to metabolize bilirubin. The level of jaundice is roughly correlated with the degree of liver-cell failure and other features of failure, such as foetor, 'flap', neurological changes, and ascites, should be sought.

1. Cirrhosis. The diagnosis of cirrhosis may be suspected clinically but it can only be confirmed by histological examination of a piece of liver. There are five essential features that must be present before a diagnosis of cirrhosis can be made: changes must be generalized throughout the liver, there must be destruction of cells with fibrosis and nodule formation, the lobular architecture is disturbed, there is regeneration of parenchymal cells, and there must be no actual cellular necrosis. Subclassifications may be made based on the size of the regenerating nodules. Thus cirrhosis may be referred to as macronodular, micronodular, or mixed. Jaundice implies that liver-cell destruction is greater than cell regeneration and is always serious. Biochemical tests of liver function may be normal in the early stages of the disease but will be abnormal when jaundice is present. Bromsulphthalein retention and prothrombin time are the most sensitive tests of cellular function, the transaminases will be abnormal with cellular failure but the alkaline phosphatase is often normal. Signs of cirrhosis must be distinguished from those of liver-cell failure.

The diagnosis of cirrhosis must be suspected if the patient has a firm, enlarged liver, spider naevi, palmar erythema, or white nails. Splenomegaly indicates the presence of portal hypertension and possibly varices. Hepatocellular failure may produce testicular atrophy, gynaecomastia, sweet-smelling breath (foetor hepaticus), mental deterioration and coma, ascites and oedema, bruising, and cyanosis. There are many causes of cirrhosis and in all types liver-cell failure may occur with subsequent production of jaundice.

A. CRYPTOGENIC. Most cirrhosis in Great Britain is of unknown aetiology and is therefore referred to as 'cryptogenic'. It is slightly more common in males than in females. Diagnosis is by exclusion and the absence of past or family history of any known cause of cirrhosis. Portal hypertension and splenomegaly commonly develop and patients may present with haematemesis. Needle-aspiration biopsy of the liver will show macronodular cirrhosis.

B. VIRAL. Since viral hepatitis is a common and often subclinical disease it is difficult to be certain of its exact relationship to cirrhosis. In Britain about a third of patients give a history of previous jaundice but only a few patients have had serial liver biopsies showing the progression from acute hepatitis to macronodular cirrhosis. Studies of Australia antigen have so far failed to show any significant correlation with cirrhosis. The role of the virus must therefore remain doubtful and clinically this form of cirrhosis is indistinguishable from the cryptogenic form.

C. ALCOHOLIC. There is no doubt about the aetiological role of alcohol in the production of cirrhosis. In Western countries its incidence can be directly related to the quantity of alcohol consumed. The incidence is larger in the United States and France than it is in Britain but even in this country it is on the increase. The incidence of cirrhosis amongst severe alcoholics is 1 in 12 but the type of alcohol indulged in does not seem to matter. Either micronodular or macronodular cirrhosis may develop. The diagnosis is made mainly on the history although many alcoholics are evasive and many deny that they drink heavily. There are often clinical clues as to the aetiology. There may, for example, be signs of malnutrition such as sore tongue, peripheral neuropathy, anaemia, scurvy, and beriberi. In addition about 25 per cent of patients will have Dupuytren's contractures and painless parotid enlargement. Peptic ulcer is also common in this form of cirrhosis.

Jaundice in an alcoholic may also be due to acute alcoholic hepatitis and the differential diagnosis may be made by liver biopsy.

D. CARDIAC FAILURE. Long-standing congestive cardiac failure may result in irreversible changes in the liver with the eventual production of centrilobular cirrhosis. This is particularly common in patients with mitral stenosis and tricuspid incompetence. It is not sufficient to make a diagnosis of cardiac cirrhosis just on the presence of prolonged cardiac failure and jaundice since patients in cardiac failure may become jaundiced without the presence of cirrhosis. Features of portal hypertension are usually absent except in very severe cardiac cirrhosis associated with constrictive pericarditis. As with other types of cirrhosis the definitive diagnosis must be made by biopsy.

E. HEPATIC VENOUS OBSTRUCTION (Budd-Chiari Syndrome). This is a rare condition in which the hepatic veins are obstructed by tumour or thrombosis. There may also be a congenital form due to maldevelopment of the veins. Although the underlying cause is usually unknown it has been reported as a complication of the use of oral contraceptives and it may sometimes be due to clotting disorders such as polycythaemia rubra vera. The resultant venous congestion is considerable and may result in secondary cirrhosis. The patient may have signs of malignant disease or some other underlying disorder and pressure over the liver will fail to fill the jugular veins. Liver biopsy will show centrizonal venous congestion as in cardiac cirrhosis, and hepatic venography may be impossible or show narrow, occluded hepatic veins. Superior venocavography shows the patency of the superior vena cava, and selective coeliac axis arteriography shows a small hepatic artery with branches of fine calibre.

F. CHRONIC ACTIVE HEPATITIS. This condition has been variously described as 'lupoid hepatitis', 'plasma-cell hepatitis', and 'chronic liver disease in young women'. Classification is still disputed but at present it is usually described in histological terms depending on the findings of liver biopsy. It is said to be 'aggressive' when there is destruction of the limiting plate of parenchymal cells around portal tracts, necrosis of groups of cells, and fibrous septa in the parenchyma. It is 'persistent' when these changes are absent and this latter condition proceeds to cirrhosis less often than the 'aggressive' type.

A proportion of patients give a history of acute viral hepatitis at the start of their illness. Studies of Australia antigen show no consistent relationship with this form of chronic hepatitis but it remains possible that there is an aetiological association with infective, as opposed to serum, hepatitis. There are certainly other aetiological factors involved and there is considerable disturbance of immunity.

It is usually a disease of young people, over half the patients presenting between the ages of 10 and 20, and 75 per cent of them are female. The onset is usually insidious with vague, non-specific symptoms followed by the development of jaundice which does not remit. Attacks of pyrexia are common and spider naevi are nearly always present. Some young patients have cutaneous striae, females have amenorrhea, but malaise and jaundice increase if a period does occur. The spleen is usually enlarged relatively more than the liver and in the young acne is a common finding. About half the patients also have symptoms suggesting that this is a systemic disorder rather than a primary liver disease. Such symptoms are: arthralgia, purpura, erythema, vasculitis, ulcerative colitis, pulmonary fibrosis, hypertension, and the nephrotic syndrome. Differentiation must obviously be made from disseminated lupus erythematosus which can produce any of these findings. As the name 'lupoid hepatitis' suggests, it was originally thought that the liver disease was part of the syndrome of disseminated lupus, but it does appear to be a separate entity.

The definitive diagnosis is by liver biopsy, but the combination of the clinical picture with biochemical and serological findings will usually give the diagnosis. The biochemical picture is of very active hepatocellular disease with very high transaminases but only moderately raised alkaline phosphatase. These values will fluctuate in the course of the disease. Serum γ-globulin levels particularly IgG are very high but albumin is normal until the terminal changes of liver failure. Immunofluorescent tests for antibodies show 50 per cent positive for smooth muscle, 50 per cent positive for renal glomeruli, and about 30 per cent positive for mitochondrial antibodies. LE cells may be found in 15 per cent of patients—usually those with fever and arthralgia—but antinuclear factor may be positive in as many as 50 per cent of patients, with tests for rheumatoid factor positive in 20 per cent.

G. PROLONGED CHOLESTASIS AND BILIARY CIRRHOSIS. Prolonged cholestasis, whether of intrahepatic or extrahepatic origin, can result in cirrhosis. This is known as biliary cirrhosis and may be secondary to any of the causes of cholestasis or may be primary. Of the secondary causes it is more likely to occur with partial biliary obstruction than with gall-stones and it has never been described following carcinoma of the head of the pancreas, possibly because patients die before cirrhosis can develop. The histological changes of fibrosis and nodule formation are present but regeneration is less than in other forms of cirrhosis.

Primary Biliary Cirrhosis. In this condition there is no known cause for the cholestasis, but an accurate pathological description is 'chronic, non-suppurative, destructive cholangitis'. It is predominantly a disease of women in the age-group 35–70 years, and clinical evidence of disease may be present for some years before the histological criteria for cirrhosis are fulfilled. Itching is usually the presenting symptom and the patients are often covered with scratch-marks even if their jaundice is not very deep. The other features of cholestatic jaundice will be present so that urine will be dark and stools pale. The liver will be enlarged, smooth, and firm and the spleen is often palpable. Xanthomata are frequently present in the skin and tendons and the serum cholesterol will be raised. Other serological findings are a greatly raised alkaline phosphatase (about 50 K.A. units) and only moderately raised transaminases. Primary biliary cirrhosis is a disorder of immune mechanisms and the diagnosis may be made on the combination of clinical and biochemical findings with serological tests. Mitochondrial antibodies are present in over 90 per cent of patients, and there is nearly always a raised level of IgM immunoglobulin. Other tests such as antinuclear factor and smooth muscle antibodies may be positive but are less specific.

H. HEPATOLENTICULAR DEGENERATION (Wilson's Disease). This is a rare, familial disorder of copper metabolism mainly affecting young people. Increased amounts of copper are deposited in the tissues, the most characteristic sites being the basal ganglia of the brain, producing extra-pyramidal signs, the liver, producing cirrhosis, and the cornea, producing the characteristic greenish-brown Kayser-Fleischer rings. Differential diagnosis from other forms of cirrhosis is made on family history, the eye signs, and the reduced level of serum caeruloplasmin.

I. HAEMOCHROMATOSIS. All types of iron-storage disease whether due to overload, as in haemosiderosis, or to abnormal metabolism, as in haemochromatosis, may lead to cirrhosis.

Idiopathic haemochromatosis is an inborn error of metabolism in which, over many years, iron accumulates in various tissues and organs. The liver and the pancreas are particularly involved producing the typical picture of 'bronzed diabetes'. The heart and kidneys may also be involved. Ninety-five per cent of the patients are male and important clinical features are the deeply pigmented skin (which may obscure jaundice), hepatomegaly, cardiomyopathy, diabetes, diminished sexual activity, and loss of body hair due to testicular involvement. The grey-slaty pigmentation is not due to the deposition of iron in the skin but to increased melanin deposits in combination with a thin epidermis; pigmentation can also occur in the mouth. The diagnosis may be confirmed by liver biopsy which will show iron deposits at the periphery of the nodules, but care must be taken to distinguish it from alcoholic cirrhosis with secondary deposition of iron. In addition, serum iron is raised to about 220 μg. per 100 ml. with about 90 per cent saturation of binding proteins.

J. FIBROCYSTIC DISEASE (Mucoviscidosis). This is a congenital abnormality of mucous secretion and the commonest hepatic abnormality is fatty change. On rare occasions cirrhosis may develop with portal hypertension. The familiar pulmonary and pancreatic features will always be predominant.

K. GALACTOSAEMIA. This inborn error of carbohydrate metabolism is due to lack of galactose-1-phosphate uridyl transferase in liver and red blood-cells. It is an autosomal recessive condition presenting in infants as feeding difficulties, diarrhoea, and jaundice due to fatty change which progresses to cirrhosis. Unless recognized and treated early it is usually fatal, but survivors become mentally retarded and develop cataracts. In a few rare cases the disease is mild and has, on one occasion, been diagnosed in a patient aged 63.

L. CONGENITAL SYPHILIS. Acquired syphilis does not produce cirrhosis but in the, fortunately now rare, cases of congenital syphilis the liver is invaded by spirochaetes and the resultant fibrous reaction leads to a true pericellular cirrhosis. If the infant survives the other stigmata of congenital syphilis will be present and the Wassermann reaction will be positive.

M. SCHISTOSOMIASIS. Infestation with schistosomiasis is said to produce periportal fibrosis and 'pipe-stem' cirrhosis. It is now thought that the association with cirrhosis in countries where the parasite is endemic may be due to other aetiological factors.

N. GLYCOGEN-STORAGE DISEASES. These are a complex series of hereditary disorders of carbohydrate metabolism which result in retention of glycogen in the tissues. The types that may involve the liver are Von Gierke's (type I), Pompe's (type II), Cori's (type III), Anderson's (type IV), and Hers's (type VI). Of these only type IV progresses to cirrhosis, hepatocellular failure, and jaundice and it is extremely rare. In this condition death from liver failure is in early childhood. Type VI exclusively involves the liver but only very rarely proceeds to liver-cell failure and jaundice.

2. Amyloidosis. The liver may be involved by infiltration with amyloid both in the primary disease and where it is secondary to any cause such as chronic infection, myelomatosis, or rheumatoid arthritis. Amyloid is a mucopolysaccharide which stains metachromatically with crystal violet and shows birefringence with Congo-red staining. The liver is enlarged and rubbery and the patient may show other features of amyloidosis such as the nephrotic syndrome, cardiac failure, or malabsorption. Hepatocellular failure and hence jaundice are rare in this condition and the diagnosis is made by liver biopsy or rectal biopsy.

3. Tumours. The liver may be affected by both benign and malignant tumours but only the latter will cause jaundice. Of malignant tumours, secondary deposits are twenty-five times more common than are primary malignant growths.

A. PRIMARY CARCINOMA OF LIVER (Hepatoma). There is a definite relationship between cirrhosis of the liver and the development of hepatoma. The incidence of carcinoma in cirrhosis varies in different series between 15 per cent and 60 per cent. It is less common in alcoholics and there is a definite geographical variation, with a particularly high incidence in South and South-east Africa.

Although many toxins have been shown to produce primary liver tumours in animals there is no definite evidence that they are significant in man with the possible exception of thorotrast. This radioactive dye was previously used as a contrast medium in radiology and 24 cases of carcinoma have been reported following its intravenous administration. Hepatocellular carcinoma has a latent period of 20 years following administration of thorotrast.

The tumours may occur at any age and are more common in males with a ratio of about 5 : 1. Primary liver carcinoma should be suspected in any patient with cirrhosis who deteriorates or in whom a lump is felt in the liver. Jaundice is usually a terminal feature, is not always present, and is never deep, the depth of jaundice bearing no relation to the extent of hepatic involvement. A rub is occasionally heard over the tumour and arterial murmurs may be present. Diagnosis is by liver biopsy and liver scan and a clue may be obtained by measuring the α-foeto-proteins. These are raised in a high proportion of African cases, but only in about 15 per cent of Caucasians with liver carcinoma.

Primary Sarcoma of the Liver and Malignant Haemangio-endothelioma. These extremely rare tumours may cause jaundice in their terminal stages. Malignant haemangio-endothelioma may follow 15 years after injections of thorotrast.

B. SECONDARY TUMOURS. The liver is the most frequent site of blood-borne metastatic tumours, whether drained by systemic or portal veins. It is involved in about a third of all cancers including half of those in stomach, gut, breast, and lung. The liver may be normal in size or grossly enlarged with palpable hard deposits. Jaundice may be absent and it is usually mild. Serum bilirubin values greater than 35 μmol/l (2 mg. per 100 ml.) imply invasion of major bile-ducts.

C. RETICULO-ENDOTHELIAL DISEASE AND THE LIVER. The reticulo-endothelial cells of the liver may be involved by any malignant disease involving this system. However, jaundice is mild and usually related to increased haemolysis. In Hodgkin's disease deep jaundice may be related to intrahepatic deposits and is terminal. Very occasionally an obscure form of intrahepatic cholestasis may be seen in Hodgkin's disease; its aetiology is unknown.

INTRAHEPATIC CHOLESTASIS

Drug-induced cholestasis
Primary biliary cirrhosis
Pregnancy
Haemolytic disease of the newborn
Congenital biliary atresia
Virus hepatitis
Other types of cirrhosis
Sclerosing cholangitis
Carcinoma of the intrahepatic bile-ducts
Dubin-Johnson and Rotor syndromes.

General. The characteristics of obstructive jaundice, itching, pale stools, and dark urine, a predominance of conjugated bilirubin, and a serum alkaline phosphatase level greater than 30 K.A. units per 100 ml., are found in a group of conditions in which cholestasis occurs within the liver. It is important to distinguish this situation from extrahepatic obstruction to avoid unnecessary and possibly dangerous surgical exploration. A history of drug-ingestion should be sought. The liver is often enlarged but pain and fever are normally absent. Liver biopsy, percutaneous cholangiography, and response to prednisone may provide further information. In extrahepatic obstruction, percutaneous cholangiography reveals dilated bile-ducts within the liver and a block below. In intrahepatic cholestasis the bile-ducts are not dilated and no obstruction is seen.

A. DRUG-INDUCED CHOLESTASIS. There are two groups of drugs which cause intrahepatic cholestasis. The first, or sensitivity type, is commonest with chlorpromazine but occurs with other phenothiazines and also with para-aminosalicylic acid, chlorpropamide, thiazides, erythromycin, and nitrofurantoin. The second, or non-sensitivity type, was first described with methyltestosterone but occurs with all C17-α-alkyl-substituted testosterones such as norethis-terone and norethandrolone, and also with sulphadiazine. With drugs of the chlorpromazine type, jaundice may occur with a single dose, while with the non-sensitivity type this complication is dose-related and normally occurs after several months of treatment. Jaundice may develop up to 6 weeks after ingestion of chlorpromazine.

Jaundice is insidious in onset and is associated with itching, malaise, pale stools, and dark urine. An eosinophilia is sometimes present in the sensitivity type and there are characteristic histological changes. Spontaneous recovery occurs in a few weeks, or occasionally months, and steroids have no effect.

B. PRIMARY BILIARY CIRRHOSIS. *See above*, p. 441.

C. PREGNANCY. Some women develop intra-hepatic cholestasis in the last trimester of pregnancy. The condition appears to be due to a genetically determined sensitivity to the effects of sex hormones and affected women also develop jaundice on the contraceptive pill.

D. HAEMOLYTIC DISEASE OF THE NEWBORN. Occasionally infants with severe haemolysis develop a cholestatic picture, probably caused by liver-cell damage. This has also been called the 'inspissated bile syndrome'.

E. CONGENITAL BILIARY ATRESIA causes jaundice apparent a few days after birth.

F. VIRUS HEPATITIS may present with a cholestatic picture. The diagnosis is often suggested by the history but in difficult cases relief of jaundice with a course of prednisolone distinguishes the condition from extrahepatic obstruction.

G. OTHER TYPES OF CIRRHOSIS. Alcoholic and postnecrotic cirrhosis are occasionally complicated by transient cholestasis.

H. SCLEROSING CHOLANGITIS.
Primary Sclerosing Cholangitis. In this condition there is progressive fibrosis of the intra- and extrahepatic bile-ducts which appear narrow and irregular on cholangiography. Aetiology is unknown but there is an association with ulcerative colitis in many cases.
Secondary Sclerosing Cholangitis. In the presence of prolonged extrahepatic biliary obstruction, possibly associated with biliary infection, a similar sclerosing cholangitis may develop. This most commonly follows postoperative strictures of the bile-duct but is occasionally associated with stones or tumours.

I. CARCINOMA OF THE INTRAHEPATIC BILE-DUCT is a rare but confusing cause of intrahepatic cholestasis. Tumours are usually slow-growing and cause insidious jaundice. Diagnosis may be suspected on cholangiography but exploration is usually necessary to confirm.

J. DUBIN-JOHNSON AND ROTOR SYNDROMES. These are rare, chronic, benign, intermittent conditions producing jaundice with conjugated hyperbilirubinaemia. In the Dubin-Johnson type the liver is greenish-black and contains a brown pigment believed to be melanin. Jaundice is rarely deep and the alkaline phosphatase remains normal. Diagnosis may be made by a brom-sulphthalein retention test in which, after an initial fall, the serum level of BSP increases after 2 hours and remains detectable for 48 hours. This is believed to be due to poor transport into the biliary canaliculi.

Rotor type resembles Dubin-Johnson clinically and biochemically, the main difference being the absence of brown pigment in the liver. Both types of jaundice have an excellent prognosis.

CONJUGATED HYPERBILIRUBINAEMIA —POSTHEPATIC

CAUSES WITHIN THE LUMEN OF THE COMMON BILE-DUCT:

Gall-stones
Parasites.

CAUSES AFFECTING THE WALL OF THE DUCT:

Accidental division
Acute pancreatitis
Chronic pancreatitis
Carcinoma of the bile-duct
Congenital obliteration of the bile-duct.

CAUSES COMPRESSING THE BILE-DUCT OR INVADING IT FROM THE OUTSIDE:

Peritoneal adhesions
Enlarged portal lymph-nodes
Tumours
Aneurysm of the hepatic artery
Hydatid cyst
Retroperitoneal cyst
Duodenal diverticulum.

General. This is the extrahepatic form of cholestasis and is associated with failure of conjugated bile to reach the intestine. The major and minor bile-ducts become dilated and bile-plugs may be seen in the bile canaliculae on light microscopy. Electron microscopy shows the microvilli of the hepatic biliary canaliculae to be blunted and abnormal. The architecture of the liver is usually normal although long-standing obstruction may result in some hepatic enlargement and the development of biliary cirrhosis. Infective episodes of cholangitis, accompanied by fever often associated with rigors, result in an acceleration of hepatic damage.

The serum bilirubin rises and may reach very high levels, most of it being conjugated. The patient appears to be yellow, later a deep orange-yellow occasionally tinged with green as the condition progresses. Since bilirubin is bound to albumin, superficial parts of the body of high protein content appear to be more yellow than other parts. The urine is dark, containing an excess of bilirubin, and gives a positive reaction using a Bili-Labstix.

If the obstruction is complete the faeces are pale and clay-coloured, and, since bile-salts are

CAUSES WITHIN THE LUMEN OF THE COMMON BILE-DUCT:

A. GALL-STONES. This constitutes the most common cause of extrahepatic cholestasis. Gall-stones are usually associated with a long history of flatulent dyspepsia possibly interspersed with episodes of cholecystitis. On examination there may be few abdominal physical signs apart from slight tenderness in the region of the gall-bladder. The liver is usually enlarged and tender, the spleen cannot be felt. Jaundice due to stone may fluctuate. Testing of the faeces for occult blood is usually negative. Plain X-ray of the abdomen is ineffective for diagnosis in 60 per cent of cases because of the lack of radiotranslucency of cholesterol stones. Apart from cholesterol stones, pigment stones may produce obstruction in cases of acholuric jaundice. When infection has occurred the stones may be coated with calcium and phosphate salts and produce the characteristic ring shadows (*Fig.* 442). Gall-stones when in the gall-bladder are most satisfactorily demonstrated by cholecystogram in the

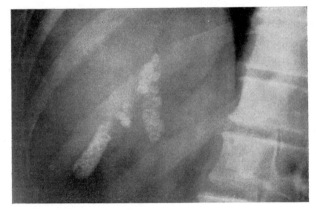

Fig. 442. Multiple gall-stones situated in the gall-bladder and common bile-duct. Patient presented with obstructive jaundice.

essential for normal fat absorption, bulky by virtue of increased fat. One consequence of reduced fat absorption is failure to absorb vitamin K. This in turn results in hypoprothrombinaemia and a prolonged prothrombin time. In addition, calcium forms insoluble calcium soaps with intestinal fat and is not available for absorption. The urine in complete obstruction contains no urobilinogen. Serum alkaline phosphatase rises and is usually above 30 K.A. units. Also 5-nucleatidase is usually raised. In long-standing obstructive jaundice the serum lipids are raised. One-quarter of these is represented by cholesterol and this explains the development of xanthomata. Serum albumin is generally normal until liver damage later supervenes. This will be indicated by raised transaminases. With changes in the albumin there may be a slight relative increase in the α_2 and β-globulins.

majority of cases. If this is not possible because of failure to concentrate the dye, an intravenous cholangiogram or 'drip' cholangiogram with tomography will usually be successful not only in demonstrating the gall-bladder but also the major bile-ducts. But, when there is significant obstructive jaundice with a total bilirubin above approximately 50 μmol/l (3 mg. per 100 ml.), cholangiography is not only ineffective but also dangerous since renal damage may occur. The level of the obstruction can be demonstrated in this case, providing bleeding time and clotting time are normal, by percutaneous cholangiography (*Fig.* 443); this should be reserved as a preoperative investigation, however, because of the dangers of haemorrhage and biliary peritonitis. Cannulation of the ampulla of Vater followed by injection of radio-opaque dye is now possible by means of an endoscopic technique (ERCP, Endoscopic

Retrograde Cholangio-Pancreatography). This has the great advantage of being iron-invasive, allowing inspection of the duodenal mucosa and of demonstrating the level of obstruction in the bile-duct. Occasionally the only way in which it is possible to make the diagnosis is by laparotomy, operative cholangiography via the cystic duct (*Fig.* 444), and exploration of the common bile-duct.

either at operation or soon after by the development of jaundice or a persistent biliary fistula. One circumstance that has resulted in damage to the common bile-duct is the practice of cholecystectomy during an acute attack of cholecystitis, often a technically difficult procedure. Although possible, division by external trauma is rare.

B. ACUTE PANCREATITIS. Jaundice in this condition is quite common but is usually of a minor

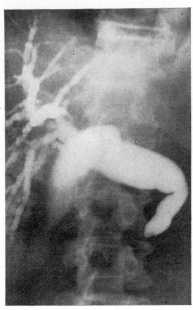

Fig. 443. Percutaneous transhepatic cholangiogram. The lower end of the common bile-duct is obstructed by a carcinoma of the pancreas. (*By courtesy of Dr. J. Gleeson.*)

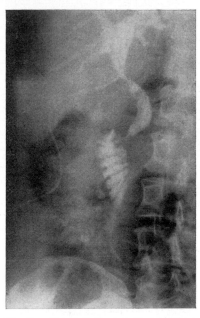

Fig. 444. Operative cholangiogram via a T tube in the common bile-duct. Multiple stones in the common bile-duct. Note the gall-stones that have passed on into the intestine.

B. PARASITES:

Distomata. These include *Opisthorus tenuicollis*, *Clonorchis sinensis*, and *Paragonimus westermani*. Infestation results from eating inadequately cooked fish or, in the third case, crabs and crayfish. *Ascarides. Ascaris lumbricoides*, the adult worm resembling in size and shape the common earthworm, occurs most commonly in the tropics. The ingested mature ova hatch in the duodenum and the larvae penetrate the intestinal wall entering the portal circulation. They then enter the liver and pass to the heart and lungs. From here they burrow through the pulmonary vessels and enter the bronchi. They migrate to the pharynx and are then swallowed. Haemoptysis, bronchitis, and pneumonia may occur and be associated with eosinophilia. Occasionally the adult worm blocks the bile-ducts and they have even caused intestinal obstruction. Diagnosis is by recognition of a worm or ova in the faeces.

CAUSES AFFECTING THE WALL OF THE DUCT:

A. ACCIDENTAL DIVISION. This is fortunately rare. When it occurs it is usually recognized

nature compared with the primary disease. The patient generally has an acute attack of abdominal pain, radiating through to the back. There may be associated hypovolaemia depending on the severity of the attack. The serum amylase may be above 1000 Somogyi units; the calcium is often depressed, particularly in severe attacks, and the blood-glucose elevated with associated glycosuria. Plain X-ray of the abdomen may reveal a localized area of ileus producing the characteristic 'sentinel loop' of intestine.

C. CHRONIC PANCREATITIS. In this case the obstruction is produced by cicatricial contraction of the terminal duct system. The diagnosis may be suggested by pancreatic calcification seen on X-ray and confirmed by the secretin test. Rarely, recurrent jaundice has been reported in chronic relapsing pancreatitis.

D. CARCINOMA OF THE BILE-DUCT. Epithelial tumours of these ducts are probably as common as carcinoma of the head of the pancreas. Occurring slightly more often in men than in women, they arise in the age-range 50–70. The most frequent site is the common bile-duct where the incidence is three times that of the ampulla of Vater. Diagnosis depends on demonstration of typical posthepatic conjugated jaundice and often is only made at laparotomy.

E. Congenital Obliteration of the Bile-duct. Over 75 per cent of infants with this condition have no major hepatic bile-ducts. In only just over 10 per cent are the major hepatic ducts present with atresia of the *extra*-hepatic ducts, but in both cases the effect initially is the same, jaundice usually appearing within 2–3 days of birth. The jaundice deepens and the infant dies, unless the atresia is relieved, with liver failure at 3–6 months.

The condition has to be distinguished from the physiological neonatal jaundice, Rh-incompatibility, congenital spherocytosis, congenital syphilis, and the rarer forms of glucuronyl transferase defects such as occur in Crigler-Najjar, Lucey-Driscoll syndromes and depression by 3α-20β-pregnanediol. In obliteration of the bile-duct the faeces are white from birth, although when the bilirubin rises to very high levels they become tinged with yellow.

CAUSES COMPRESSING THE BILE-DUCT OR INVADING IT FROM THE OUTSIDE:

A. Peritoneal Adhesions. As a cause of ductal obstruction these are rare, since the only portion of the common hepatic and common bile-duct in the peritoneal cavity is the supraduodenal portion. The most common type of adhesions are those caused by a localized collection of bile resulting from a leak following exploration of the common bile-duct. In this case there will obviously be a history of a recent operation and the biochemical picture typical of obstruction at this level.

B. Enlarged Portal Lymph-nodes. Again, this is an extremely rare cause of obstructive jaundice. Usually there is some indication of the primary cause for involvement of the nodes. A possible exception is in the case of secondary syphilis, a condition which, according to many venereologists, is becoming more common in men who indulge in homosexual practices. In this case there may be very little indication of the syphilis except that serological tests are positive and penicillin produces a rapid cure.

C. Tumours. Malignant tumours of the liver, whether primary or secondary, may invade the bile-duct by virtue of their proximity. Similarly the liver may be so involved as to be largely destroyed, the result being a mixture of hepatic cell destruction and intrahepatic conjugated jaundice.

Carcinoma of the head of the pancreas quite commonly presents with obstructive jaundice. The jaundice is progressive, often painless, and may be associated with enlargement of the gall-bladder. Courvoisier's law states that in the jaundiced patient a palpable gall-bladder indicates that the jaundice is not due to stone (*Fig.* 445). The reason for this is that if gall-stones are present they will have produced such an inflammatory reaction in the wall of the gall-bladder that it cannot distend by virtue of back-pressure. It must be emphasized that this law can only be

interpreted as it is stated and the converse in the jaundiced patient is by no means always true. Islet-cell carcinomas, whether carcinoid, β-cell, or non-β-cell, may also produce the picture of obstructive jaundice.

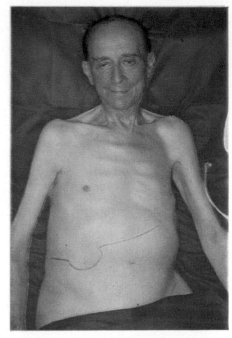

Fig. 446. Jaundiced patient with enlarged gall-bladder. Jaundice due to a carcinoma of the pancreas.

Carcinoma of the ampulla of Vater is associated with fluctuating jaundice and, since it is an ulcerative lesion projecting into the duodenum, a positive occult blood. In this condition the absence of bile from the faeces together with intestinal bleeding combines to give rise to the 'silver stool'. The biochemical picture is that previously described for posthepatic jaundice. Endoscopic visualization of the duodenum in the region of the ampulla of Vater is an essential investigation in cases of obstructive jaundice, so that carcinoma of the ampulla can be diagnosed with certainty before operation. In both this condition and carcinoma of the head of the pancreas barium-meal examination is often helpful. In the latter case an 'inverted 3' sign is occasionally present on the medial wall of the duodenal loop. Hypotonic duodenography provides greater detail of the mucosal appearances of the duodenal wall. Carcinoma of the duodenum occurs but is excessively rare. It may invade and block the common bile-duct, either when it lies behind the duodenum or more often at the ampulla. A barium meal is usually diagnostic.

Jaundice due to carcinoma of the stomach is generally due to hepatic metastases but occasionally a juxta-pyloric carcinoma may infiltrate the common bile-duct. A barium meal provides the diagnosis.

The hepatic flexure of the colon is related to the front of the right kidney and is lateral to the right side of the common bile-duct. Because of this relationship a carcinoma arising in this portion of the colon may obstruct it. This usually betokens an advanced stage in this condition and some bowel symptoms, such as a change in bowel habit with frank bleeding per rectum or a positive occult blood, will generally be present. A barium enema provides a diagnostic picture.

As with the above condition, malignant renal tumours on the right may extend to involve the bile-ducts. Intravenous pyelography will generally serve to make the diagnosis. Occasionally right renal arteriography is required to differentiate some benign renal swellings, e.g., cysts, from malignant ones.

Tumours of the suprarenal are rare but when they do occur may obstruct the bile-duct.

Tumours of the female genital tract, if giving rise to jaundice, usually do so by virtue of secondary deposits within the liver. However, occasionally secondary disease occurs so as to obstruct specifically the bile-duct. One such case of a patient with a carcinoma of the cervix diagnosed and treated 5 years previously presented and was treated as though she had a carcinoma of the head of the pancreas. It was only on histological examination of the removed head of the pancreas that it was found that she had a solitary secondary deposit from the carcinoma of the cervix.

Tumours of the omentum are generally secondary in nature, although non-epithelial sarcomas may arise in this situation. If associated with jaundice, it is usually by virtue of generalized disease but may be by bile-duct obstruction. In such cases laparoscopy may be a diagnostic technique, particularly since biopsies may be taken by this route.

D. ANEURYSM OF THE HEPATIC ARTERY. Aneurysm of the hepatic artery is rare. Diagnosis may only be made by either arteriography or laparotomy.

E. HYDATID CYSTS. These result when man acts as the intermediate host of the cestode, *Taenia echinococcus*. The definitive host is the dog, human infection occurring when ova from infected canine faeces are ingested. Hydatid cysts may occur anywhere in the body and commonly appear within the liver substance. They have also been found in the free edge of the gastrohepatic omentum producing stretching and obliteration of the common bile-duct. They are rare in Great Britain and awareness of the condition is therefore necessary together with the finding of a palpable abdominal mass before the correct diagnosis is made. The Casoni skin test is usually positive but is less reliable than the complement-fixation test.

F. RETROPERITONEAL CYSTS. A retroperitoneal cyst is a rare condition of unknown aetiology which occasionally may obstruct the bile-duct.

G. DUODENAL DIVERTICULUM. True duodenal diverticulae are common, occurring in the second, third, fourth, and first parts of the duodenum in that order of frequency. Those in the second part of the duodenum arise from the medial side just above the point of entry of the common bile-duct. A case has been reported in which one of these diverticulae has resulted in obstruction of the lower end of the common bile-duct. The diagnosis was provided in this case by barium meal with associated oral cholecystography.

C. Wastell.

JAW, LOWER, PAIN IN

Pain in the lower jaw—unaccompanied by any swelling (*see* JAW, LOWER, SWELLING OF, *below*) —is generally due to *dental caries*, i.e., toothache. The decayed tooth may be obvious at once, or it may be so hidden as to call for the services of a skilled dentist, assisted by radiographs of the jaw. Occasionally an unerupted molar may be the cause of the pain.

Trigeminal Neuralgia. Here pain is the only primary symptom. In solitary isolation and with crushing severity it comprises the whole clinical picture, and consideration of its character and distribution provides the diagnosis. Unilateral, and limited in the first place to one division of the 5th nerve, the pain may remain confined to that division for many years, but sooner or later spreads to include another. Should it be bilateral or should more than one division be involved from the beginning, a diagnosis of trigeminal neuralgia is likely to be incorrect. The pain most commonly begins in the second division and is felt in the upper jaw and teeth, upper lip, molar region, and lower eyelid, the earliest stabs often being noticed at the junction of the side of the nose with the upper lip. Less commonly does it begin in the third division, when the lower jaw, teeth and lip, the oral part of the tongue, and the external auditory meatus are affected. Only rarely is the first division attacked. This rigid anatomical distribution serves to distinguish it from complaints such as dental neuralgia and sinus infection where the area of pain is determined by the area of local disease. In character the pain is periodic, but an attack may last for several days or even weeks. Remissions are complete but get progressively shorter. During an attack there is a continuous dull ache to which the slightest stimulus, such as a draught or light touch, may act as a detonator releasing a violent explosion of pain, which may last for a few minutes or an hour or more. It is likened to rapidly repeated stabs of a red-hot needle and is accompanied by unilateral flushing of the face, running of the eye, and distortion of the features by involuntary muscular contractions. Physical examination reveals the skin over the affected area to be hyperaesthetic, but there is complete absence of other sensory or motor changes, a most important diagnostic point.

Diagnosis of local neoplasms is usually arrived at on grounds other than pain. Involvement of the fifth nerve in an intracranial neoplasm is distinguishable from trigeminal neuralgia by its unremitting character, the involvement of other nerves, and the presence of sensory and motor changes.

Herpes zoster is painful both before and at the time of the skin eruption, when the diagnosis should not be difficult, and later when in the form of post-herpetic neuralgia it may cause agony equal to that experienced in the idiopathic form. As distinct from the latter it commonly occurs in the ophthalmic division of the nerve, but it may involve the third division of the 5th nerve, and therefore the region of the lower jaw; even when the eruption has died away, a history of its existence should be obtainable.

R. G. Beard.

JAW, LOWER, SWELLING OF

Swelling of the lower jaw may sometimes be mistaken for, or masked by, swelling of the cellular tissues in front of it. The real site of the swelling is first to be ascertained by opening the mouth and running the finger along the outer and inner borders of the mandible and comparing the two sides.

The causes of enlargement may be subdivided as follows:

(1) *Injury*. (2) *Inflammatory affections*. (3) *Tumours*: Innocent—fibroma, osteoma, giant-cell tumour, odontoma; Malignant—sarcoma, epithelioma. (4) *Acromegaly*. (5) *Leontiasis ossea*. (6) *Paget's disease*. (7) *Generalized osteitis fibrosa*.

1. Injury. A *haematoma* or traumatic *periostitis* may follow a blow. If the injury has caused a *fracture*, the abnormal mobility of the fragments, the irregularity of the line of the teeth and arch of the jaw, the laceration of the gums, serve to indicate the injury. The nearer the line of fracture is to the symphysis the more marked is the mobility, and diagnosis is only difficult when the fracture is of the ascending ramus and underneath the masseter muscle. A radiograph may then be needed. Fracture of the mandible is commonly compound, and therefore is often complicated by septic infection. Later, *callus* will form a tumour which might be mistaken for one of some other kind unless the course of the case has been watched.

2. Inflammatory Affections. *Alveolar Abscess* is a common swelling, associated with toothache. An ordinary gumboil forms on the outer side of the gum, and is quite superficial. A more troublesome form of abscess is that which develops at the root of a tooth, which, generally carious, may yet appear healthy on the surface. Pus usually points between the gum and the cheek, but it may travel a long way between the bone and the mucous membrane, and point on the cheek, in the submaxillary region, or on the chin. As in the case of injury, periostitis extending up under the muscle may be difficult to diagnose, and it is sometimes mistaken for parotitis. In the early

stages the only sign is toothache, but as suppuration becomes established there are also pain, swelling of the gums, furred tongue, trismus, enlargement of the upper cervical lymphatic glands, and raised temperature. The presence of a septic tooth indicates the diagnosis. Chronic periostitis with new bone formation may be difficult to distinguish clinically from a tumour.

NECROSIS OF THE JAW, often preceded by an acute periosteal abscess, may follow injury, alveolar abscess, syphilis, or mercurial or phosphorus poisoning, and in rare cases one of the acute exanthemata or typhoid fever. In many cases it may be impossible to say whether the bone is necrosed or not, for the signs are much the same as in suppuration in connexion with alveolar abscess. It can only be diagnosed for certain if a piece of loose bone can be felt with a probe or be seen by the aid of a radiograph. Its presence may be inferred by the profuseness and long continuance of the discharge.

SYPHILITIC DISEASE of the lower jaw in the form of osteoperiostitis or gumma is rare; if there is doubt, a serological reaction will be of service.

ACTINOMYCOSIS. A long-standing and obstinate suppuration about the lower jaw with indurated cellulitis of the neck and formation of sinuses in the skin (*Fig.* 446) should lead to the suspicion of the nature of the trouble. In the beginning it gives rise to inflammatory changes which simulate alveolar abscess, and the similarity is increased by the presence of carious teeth, through which the fungus may gain access to the jaw; in the pus, the small yellow granules are to be sought for, and the Gram-staining mycelium on microscopical examination.

3. Tumours. In many cases there is no difficulty in deciding whether a swelling is inflammatory or a new growth; in the early stages, however—and an early diagnosis in the case of malignant disease is of extreme importance—there may be grave doubt; therefore inflammatory mischief should be excluded by a careful, thorough examination of the mouth and teeth for any source of infection, and it is frequently advisable to invite the co-operation of a dentist. If malignancy is a possibility the condition should be regarded as such until proved otherwise, and a radiographic examination should never be omitted.

Under 'tumours of the jaw' must be considered a group of conditions known as *epulides*. This term, meaning 'on the gums', refers in its widest sense to a variety of lesions including angiomata, granulomata, adenomata of salivary type, and even malignant neoplasms. The name is better restricted to two pathological types: one, where fibrous tissue predominates, the fibroid epulis; and the other, the so-called 'myeloid epulis', where large numbers of giant cells dominate the histological picture, which resembles that of the benign giant-cell tumour of long bones. The epulides are marginal tumours commonly occurring in the region of the bicuspid and canine teeth on upper and lower jaws. The only symptom is the swelling, small when presented for advice; the fibroid variety tends to be smooth, pink, or grey, and sometimes pedunculated, the giant-cell type dark red, sessile, and lobulated, with somewhat overhanging edges. Although these tumours may grow to a large size and may recur locally, they do not metastasize and they do not invade bone, being therefore radiologically negative. (*Fig.* 447.)

is elicited; pulsation is an occasional feature. Radiographs confirm the thinning of the cortex which is perforated early, and show trabeculae traversing the tumour; and there is no osteogenic or periosteal reaction, while the edges are sharply defined—all features distinguishing the condition from a bone sarcoma. (*Fig.* 448.)

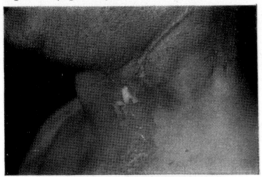

Fig. 446. Actinomycosis.

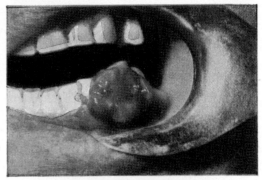

Fig. 447. Giant-cell (myeloid) epulis.

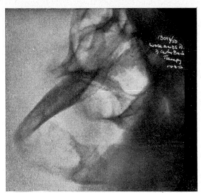

Fig. 448. Gaint-cell tumour of the mandible, showing trabeculation. (*Dr. T. H. Hills.*)

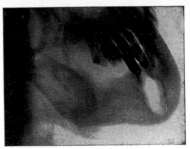

Fig. 449. Radiograph showing a dental cyst of the right mandible, connected with a crowned second bicuspid tooth. (*Dr. J. H. Mather.*)

Another marginal benign tumour of the jaw is the *osteoma*. This is also a symptomless swelling, but in contradistinction to the epulis it is bony, hard, and frequently occurs in the region of the permanent molars, a rare site for the epulis. A radiograph shows a dome-shaped mass of dense bone with clear-cut margins.

Central tumours eventually expand the jaw on all aspects, but in the early stages the expansion is often asymmetrical, the outer surface being commonly more affected than the inner. Very careful running of the finger along the apparently unaffected surface may, however, reveal slight deviation from the normal. Central tumours include the benign giant-cell tumour and the tumours of dental origin. Pain is not a prominent symptom; most of these lesions are noticed on account of deformity. The *giant-cell tumour* occurs most frequently near the symphysis, and presents the same character as elsewhere. The expansion is considerable and the bone is greatly thinned until in some cases 'egg-shell crackling'

No comprehensive classification of tumours of dental origin, or *odontomes*, will be given as none has received general acceptance. The pathology is difficult and the clinical picture varied. The tooth is developed from epithelial and mesodermal tissues; tumours of either element or both (composite odontome) are therefore possible. Seen in a radiograph these lesions appear as central swellings which may be monocystic, polycystic, or solid. The commonest monocystic swelling is the dental cyst, a condition developing in relation to the root of a tooth, especially the canines and incisors of the upper jaw. Less common is the dentigerous cyst (follicular odontome) which develops around an unerupted tooth so that the crown and not the root is intracystic. The tooth may be one of the permanent set, in which case it will be noted as absent from its normal place, or there may be a supernumerary in the cyst, or even several undeveloped denticles. Radiographs will show the relation of dental elements to the cyst and, by the sharpness of the margins, will distinguish a dental cyst from the ill-defined root granuloma. (*Figs.* 449, 450.) Both these cysts belong to the epithelial group, being lined by squamous epithelium. A third variety of this group used to be known as an epithelial odontome, and later as multiloculated cystic disease of the jaw. Clinically this is yet another form of painless expansion of the jaw which may attain a great size if untreated. 'Egg-shell crackling' may be obtained, and radiologically the tumour may closely resemble a giant-cell tumour, although trabeculation is usually greater, pulsation

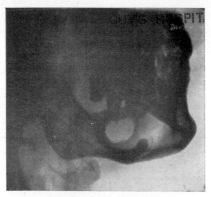

Fig. 450. Dentigerous cyst showing unerupted tooth.
(*Dr. T. H. Hills.*)

most unlikely, and frequently some teeth are missing. Histologically the majority of these polycystic tumours have recently been recognized as originating in the enamel organ; the picture is varied and complicated, but the presence of enameloblasts has warranted the name *adamantinoma*, which is now the accepted term. A point to remember is that an adamantinoma may be monocystic or solid, when only microscopy can give the diagnosis in the first case from the closely related condition of dentigerous cyst, and in the second, from a solid odontome. Similarly only microscopy will distinguish between a polycystic adamantinoma and localized osteitis fibrosa, cases of which have been reported in the jaw, although in the latter condition there should be no missing or abnormal teeth. Mesodermal and composite odontomes form well-defined solid central tumours usually associated with missing teeth.

Malignant tumours of the mandible have the same significance as elsewhere. Osteogenic sarcoma, chondrosarcoma, and fibrosarcoma are found. Growth of these tumours is not necessarily rapid, although rapidity of growth raises suspicion. Involvement of soft tissues is to be regarded with the greatest gravity; this never occurs in benign neoplasms, although it may with inflammatory conditions. Short of microscopy, radiographic diagnosis offers the most help. Periosteal reaction with new bone formation, and osteolysis with ill-defined edges and irregular erosion, are all characteristics of malignancy. Metastasis has occasionally been reported in cases of adamantinoma, which must therefore be regarded as potentially malignant, although the majority are locally invasive only.

Epithelioma—better termed 'squamous-celled carcinoma'—is a very insidious and dangerous form of growth, and in its early stages very apt to be overlooked. It may start as a small ulceration of the gum about a decayed tooth, and so be mistaken for a simple ulcer, and it may not be until a large tumour has formed that the condition is recognized, when most valuable time will have been lost from the point of view of treatment. The diagnosis will be made by careful examination, and noting that the ulcerated gum is hard and indurated and does not heal when the decayed tooth is removed. The name 'boring epithelioma' has been well applied to this condition. To make the diagnosis sure a piece from the edge of the ulcer should be removed for histological examination at the earliest moment that suspicion is aroused as to its malignancy. An epithelioma may also spread from the tongue or floor of the mouth and cause a swelling involving the jaw. The diagnosis here is obvious.

Four diseases in which the mandible becomes enlarged, but in which the swelling is not confined to the one bone, and is only one of the manifestations of the complaint, remain to be mentioned:

4. Acromegaly. The lower jaw is often conspicuously enlarged in this disease, becoming prominent and massive (*Fig.* 295A, p. 277). There is hypertrophy of the whole bone rather than a swelling in it. The other bones of the face are enlarged, the superciliary ridges are exaggerated, and the general effect of the disease is to give the patient a dull, coarse-featured appearance. In addition, the bones of the hands and feet become much enlarged; also, in the late stages of this very chronic illness, headache and muscular debility become prominent symptoms, and, owing to swelling of the pituitary body (*see Fig.* 411, p. 390), bilateral temporal hemianopia is to be expected (*Fig.* 409, p. 389).

5. Leontiasis Ossea is the name given to a rare disease in which great overgrowth of the facial and cranial bones is the distinguishing feature. It usually begins in childhood and is not likely to be confounded with any of the above-mentioned swellings, except perhaps acromegaly, from which it is distinguished by the absence of changes in the hands and feet, and absence of hypertrophy of the soft tissues of the lips.

6. Paget's Disease (*see also* p. 109) occurs in elderly patients and is characterized by preliminary softening and bending of the bones, followed by recalcification. During the course of the disease the bones become enormously thickened, and cases are recorded where the thickening has first been noticed in the jaws.

7. Generalized Osteitis Fibrosa (*see also* p. 108) is a disease due to parathyroid overactivity. There is widespread decalcification and fibrosis, with the formation of giant-cell tumours. Occasionally attention may first be drawn to the condition by a lesion in the jaw.

R. G. Beard.

JAW, UPPER, PAIN IN

Pain in the upper jaw, as in the lower, may be due to dental infections, trigeminal neuralgia, odontoma, myeloma, and other new growth; but an additional source of pain here arises from lesions of the maxillary antrum. Involvement of the temporomandibular joint in infective, tempo-ritic, or traumatic lesions may be associated with spasm of the masseter muscle.

Affections of the Maxillary Antrum. Infective conditions of the antrum vary from mucosal congestion to a true empyema. Pain is greatest in the acute case when the ostium is blocked and no outlet is available for the inflammatory exudate; in a chronic case with a patent ostium there may be little more than a dull ache. The boundaries of antral pain are the floor of the orbit, the outer wall of the nose, and the roof of the mouth, in any of which pain, tenderness, and inflammatory reaction may be experienced. A septic tooth may be present at the same time as an antral infection—may indeed be responsible for the infection. The possibility of a dual condition should not be overlooked although the tooth alone may be the cause of the patient's trouble. Pus seen on examination of the middle meatus indicates the presence of disease in one of the anterior group of sinuses—frontal, maxillary, or anterior ethmoidal; valuable aid in distinguishing between these is available in transillumination. With a completely translucent antrum there are, in addition to the clear red glow of the cheek, a crescent of light below the eye and a glowing pupil. Such an appearance means the absence of disease. Partial translucency, if symmetrical, may not be proof of disease but inequality of translucency on the two sides rouses a strong suspicion that the dimmer of the two is pathological. A radiograph adds further information; more detail of the depth of the obscurity is obtained, a fluid level or the outline of a polyp may be visible, or the usually sharp margins of the cavity may be blurred by thickened mucosa. A growth starting in the antrum but not big enough to cause a swelling may be mistaken for purely inflammatory trouble; superadded infection may indeed be the dominant feature. However, it is seldom that one is consulted for a neoplasm of the antrum until it has made its presence felt by the swelling of one or more of the antral walls. It should be observed that inflammatory disease of the antrum virtually never causes expansion of the bony wall, and that such a finding is therefore strong evidence of neoplastic disease. The oedema of the soft tissue over the antrum in inflammatory lesions may, however, make this a difficult point to determine, and particular attention should be paid to any evidence of blunting of the normally sharp infra-orbital margin. A blood-stained discharge from one nostril, in the absence of a bleeding point in the nose itself, should rouse suspicion. An antrum the subject of a neoplasm is dull to transillumination, and casts an abnormal shadow on the radiograph. Antrum puncture,

which is performed through the inferior meatus, will give conclusive evidence of the presence or absence of pus, and is therefore a very important diagnostic procedure, but it does not necessarily reveal the presence of a small growth.

R. G. Beard.

JAW, UPPER, SWELLING OF

The remarks made in the article on JAW, LOWER, SWELLING OF (p. 448), apply equally to swellings in the upper jaw; dental cysts, for example, are perhaps rather more common in the upper jaw, and giant-cell tumours are not infrequent. Tumours arising in the maxillary antrum merit special mention, however, for many cause no pain or discomfort until the late stages. Benign osteomata occasionally give rise to swelling of the antrum. Malignant tumours are more common and are usually carcinomata or endotheliomata arising in the mucous membrane; sarcomata are rare (*Fig.* 451). Rapid growth,

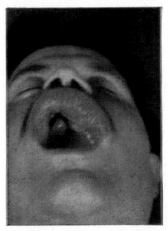

Fig. 451.   Sarcoma of the maxilla protruding into the palate.

bulging into and invasion of surrounding fossae, pain, discharge of blood and pus from one nostril, and invasion of the overlying skin, are momentous indications of malignant disease. The first evidence of bulging into the orbital fossa may be blockage of the tear duct or unilateral proptosis, and of bulging into the nasal cavity blockage of the airway on one side. On the facial and palatal aspects the swelling is visually obvious. In the case, though, of slow-growing tumours, and in the early stages, differentiation between innocent growths and suppuration is extremely difficult. It should be noted that inflammatory swellings virtually never deform the bony wall of the maxilla, and are confined, for the most part, to the soft tissues around. Clinical or radiological evidence of bony distortion is therefore very much in favour of a neoplastic lesion. Often the first sign of bony expansion is the blunting of the normally sharp infra-orbital margin. Transillumination is to be employed, also puncture of the antrum, and if necessary exploration and histological examination of the parts removed.

R. G. Beard.

JOINTS, AFFECTIONS OF

A List of the Arthropathies:

1. CONGENITAL:

Achondroplasia
Angiokeratoma corporis diffusum (Fabry's disease)
Arthrogryposis multiplex congenita
Camptodactyly
Congenital indifference to pain
Dysplasia epiphysalis multiplex
Ehlers-Danlos syndrome
Familial dysautonomia (Riley-Day syndrome)
Hurler's syndrome (gargoylism)
Hypermobility syndrome
Marfan's syndrome
Morquio-Brailsford osteochondrodystrophy
Osteodysplasty
Osteogenesis imperfecta.

2. DEGENERATIVE, TRAUMATIC, AND OCCUPATIONAL:

Ankylosing vertebral hyperostosis
Osteoarthrosis
Occupational syndromes, e.g., porter's neck, wicket-keeper's fingers.
Mseleni joint disease
Traumatic syndromes, e.g., traumatic haemarthrosis.

3. DIETETIC:

Kashin-Beck disease
Rickets
Scurvy.

4. ENDOCRINE:

Acromegaly
Cretinous and myxoedematous arthropathy
Hyperparathyroidism
Idiopathic hypoparathyroidism
Thyroid acropachy.

5. HAEMATOLOGICAL:

Agammaglobulinaemia
Anticoagulant therapy
Haemophilia and allied disorders
Leukaemia
Sickle-cell disease.

6. IDIOPATHIC:

Ankylosing spondylitis
Caplan's syndrome
Crohn's disease
Dermatomyositis and polymyositis
Erythema multiforme (Stevens-Johnson syndrome)
Familial Mediterranean fever and other periodic disorders
Felty's syndrome
Intermittent hydrarthrosis
Osteochondritis dissecans
Osteochondrosis

Palindromic rheumatism
Pigmented villonodular synovitis
Psoriatic arthropathy
Relapsing polychondritis
Rheumatoid arthritis
Sarcoidosis
Schönlein-Henoch (anaphylactoid) purpura
Scleroderma
Sjögren's syndrome
Still's disease
Systemic lupus erythematosus
Ulcerative colitis
Whipple's disease (intestinal lipodystrophy).

7. INFECTIVE:

Infections due to Bacteria, Spirochaetes, and Mycoplasma:
Anthrax
Brucella abortus and melitensis arthritis
Cat-scratch fever
Clutton's joints
Diphtheria
Erysipelas
Glanders
Gonococcal arthritis
Haverhillia
Kala-azar
Leprosy
Meningococcal fever
Mycoplasma pneumoniae (Eaton's agent)
Pneumococcal
Pseudomonas pseudomallei
Rat-bite fever
Secondary syphilis
Subacute and acute bacterial endocarditis
Tuberculosis
Typhoid and paratyphoid fever
Weil's disease (*Leptospirosis ictero-haemorrhagica*)
Yaws.

Infections due to Viruses:
Behçet's disease
Chikungunya
Echo virus infection
Epidemic Australian arthritis
Glandular fever (infectious mononucleosis)
Infective and serum hepatitis
Influenza
Lymphogranuloma venerans
Measles
Mumps
O'Nyong-Nyong fever
Poliomyelitis
Psittacosis
Rubella
Smallpox.

Infections due to Fungi:
Actinomycosis
Aspergillosis
Blastomycosis
Coccidioidomycosis
Cryptococcosis (torulosis)
Histoplasmosis
Madeira foot (mycetoma pedis)
Sporotrichosis.

Infections due to Protozoa:
Amoebiasis.

Infections due to Worms:
Chylous arthritis
Dracunculosis (Guinea-worm arthritis)
Filariasis
Trichiniasis.

8. Post-infective and Post-inflammatory:

Jaccoud's arthritis
Osteitis pubis (post-prostatectomy syndrome)
Post-coronary thrombosis (Dressler's) syndrome
Post-dysenteric
Post-scarlatinal
Reiter's (Brodie's) syndrome
Rheumatic fever
Subacute pancreatitis.

9. Metabolic:

Amyloidosis
Biliary and alcoholic cirrhosis
Calcinosis circumscripta (pyrophosphate arthro-pathy)
Calcinosis uraemica
Chondrocalcinosis articularis
Disseminated lipogranulomatosis (Farber's disease)
Familial hypercholesterolaemia
Familial lipochrome pigmentary arthritis
Gaucher's disease
Gout
Haemochromatosis
Multicentric reticulohistocytosis (lipoid dermato-arthritis)
Myositis ossificans
Ochronosis
Osteomalacia
Osteoporosis
Renal transplant and haemodialysis syndrome
Wilson's disease.

10. Vascular:

Avascular necrosis (fat, caisson, etc.)
Polyarteritis nodosa
Polymyalgia arteritica (giant-cell arteritis and polymyalgia rheumatica)
Takayasu's (pulseless) disease
Wegener's granulomatosis.

11. Neoplastic: Arthropathies associated with benign and malignant tumours:

Chondrosarcoma
Haemangioma
Left atrial myxoma
Lymphoma
Metastatic malignant disease
Multiple myelomatosis
Osteoid osteoma
Paget sarcoma
Pseudohypertrophic pulmonary osteo-arthropathy
Synovioma.

12. Neuropathic:

Carpal tunnel median nerve compression
Charcot's joints, tabetic or syringomyelic
Diabetic arthropathy (neuropathic and infective)
Osborne's syndrome (ulnar nerve compression) and other compression neuropathies
Paraplegia syndrome
Shoulder–hand syndrome
Ulcero-osteolytic neuropathy.

13. Therapeutic:

Alcoholism
Anticoagulants
Barbiturates
Corticosteroid arthropathy
Hydrallazine syndrome (procaine amide, oral contraceptives, etc.)
Isoniazid shoulder–hand syndrome
Serum sickness.

14. Miscellaneous:

Acro-osteolysis syndrome
Degos' syndrome
Dupuytren's contracture
Knuckle pads (Hale-White)
Paget's disease of bone
Periostitis deformans (Soriano)
Septic focus syndrome
Xyphoid syndrome.

As a glance at the list will show, joints are affected in a large number of conditions in medicine (*see also Figs.* 452–455). The affection may be acute, as in rheumatic fever, gout, or traumatic hydrarthrosis; acute relapsing becoming chronic, as in rheumatoid arthritis or Reiter's disease; chronic with acute onset, as in some cases of generalized osteo-arthrosis; or insidious and

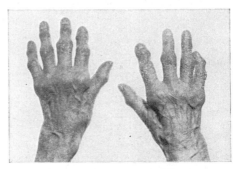

Fig. 452. Typical osteo-arthrotic (Granny's) hands. The bony enlargement and distortion is essentially bony secondary to degenerative changes in the cartilages.

chronic as in most cases of osteo-arthrosis. The affection may be of one joint, a monarthritis, as may be seen in tuberculous arthritis; or it may be the starting point of a polyarthritis, as is seen not infrequently in psoriatic arthropathy, in which a number of joints are eventually affected. The pattern of joint involvement may be important: rheumatoid arthritis affecting initially and chiefly peripheral joints; ankylosing spondylitis affecting the sacro-iliacs and spine; polymyalgia rheumatica affecting the girdle joints, pelvis, and shoulders. The terminal interphalangeal joints are affected commonly in osteo-arthrosis (Heberden's nodes) and psoriatic arthropathy, occasionally in adolescent rheumatoid arthritis, and less commonly in adult rheumatoid arthritis. Interphalangeal involvement of the toes is rare in rheumatoid arthritis but more common in the arthritis associated with ulcerative colitis or Reiter's disease. Joint involvement may be in the form of a flitting and transient polyarthritis, as in rheumatic fever, some cases of systemic lupus erythematosus, and a number of other conditions, or in a recurring or palindromic pattern subsiding completely between inflammatory episodes, as in some cases of rheumatoid arthritis.

Joints may be swollen because of:

1. Bony enlargement, as in osteo-arthrosis or Charcot's joints in tabes dorsalis or syringomyelia.

2. New periosteal bone deposition, as in pseudo-hypertrophic pulmonary osteo-arthropathy or thyroid acropachy.

3. Increase in normal joint fluid, as in traumatic synovitis.

4. Inflammatory sterile fluid, as in rheumatoid arthritis.

5. Blood-stained fluid, as in traumatic haemarthrosis and haemophilia.

pain, stiffness, tenderness, and weakness. These five factors in variable combinations cause the dysfunction typical of the particular arthritic disease in question. In scleroderma (progressive systemic sclerosis) stiffness is the dominant component; in gout swelling, tenderness, and pain. The joints in rheumatoid arthritis vary and differ depending on acuity and stage of the disease process: stiffness in early rheumatoid disease is largely due to joint-swelling, in advanced disease

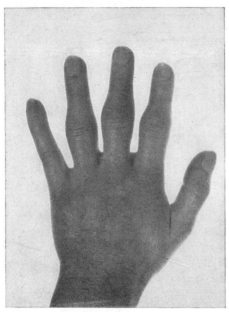

Fig. 453. Typical spindling of proximal interphalangeal joints in rheumatoid arthritis. The swelling is due to inflammatory changes and increased fluid in these joints.

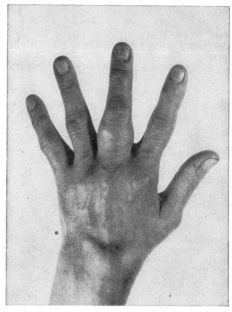

Fig. 454. Swelling in a rheumatoid hand due to inflammatory changes in extensor tendon sheaths.

6. Purulent infected fluid, as in gonococcal arthritis or staphylococcal pyarthrosis.

7. Synovial proliferation, as in rheumatoid arthritis.

8. Fluid containing crystals, as in gout or chondrocalcinosis articularis.

9. Rarely because of malignant changes, as in sarcoma and secondary carcinoma.

Not infrequently joints are swollen from a combination of two or more of these factors. Swelling of synovial tendon sheaths or bursae alongside joints may also contribute greatly to the clinical picture, symmetrical involvement of extensor sheaths on the dorsum of the wrists being very typical of rheumatoid arthritis. Subacromial and semimembranosus bursal involvement may contribute much swelling when shoulders or knees are affected by an inflammatory arthritis. If there is doubt regarding the presence of infecting organisms aspiration should be performed. This will often contribute useful information in other non-infective conditions such as gout, chondrocalcinosis, or haemarthrosis if diagnosis is in doubt.

Joints affected by any disease process may show a variable blend of five factors: swelling,

to irreversible change, even in some patients to the point of bony or fibrous ankylosis. In other cases destruction of joint tissue in rheumatoid arthritis causes hypermobility, the so-called 'lorgnette' or 'telescope fingers' being examples of this.

Two of the cardinal signs of inflammation, heat and redness, are often absent in inflammatory arthritis, while in acute pyarthrosis the joint is hot and in gout hot and red. In most cases of rheumatoid arthritis the joints tend to be cold and moist without erythema, though swollen, painful, and tender. The so-called 'liver palm' is common in rheumatoid arthritis and in systemic lupus erythematosus, palms and finger-tips being often a bright pink, but the joints themselves of normal colour though swollen, the superficial capillaries not being dilated. Inflammatory arthropathies usually cause most discomfort in the early morning, the tissues becoming 'gelled' with disuse in the night. This early morning increase in pain and stiffness of fingers, wrists, and shoulders in particular is characteristic of rheumatoid and similar arthropathies; in ankylosing spondylitis a similar increase in stiffness and pain is seen in spine, hips, and shoulders. Painful morning stiffness is also seen characteristically in polymyalgia rheumatica in shoulders and hips. Characteristic of median nerve carpal tunnel compression are the unpleasant paraesthesiae, variously described by the patient as 'pins and needles', electric shocks, hot tinglings, and so on, worse at night and preventing sleep.

There are very many possible causes of joint involvement in systemic disease. These are listed

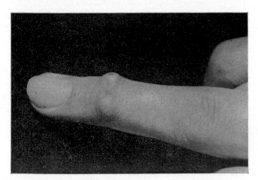

Fig. 455. Rheumatoid nodules masquerading as Heberden's nodes. Note the necrotic (arteritic) centre in the upper one.

in the accompanying table. Not all can be discussed and described; the following account merely deals with the more common and distinctive of them.

1. Congenital Arthropathies. *Arthrogryposis multiplex congenita* is a rare congenital condition characterized by joint contractions, usually symmetrical and multiple, affecting lower limbs rather than upper and distal joints more than proximal ones. The subcutaneous tissues may be thick, doughy, or gelatinous. While usually apparent at birth and readily recognized, if the patient is not seen until adult life the condition may be confused with advanced rheumatoid arthritis with joint contractions of fingers, knees, elbows, and wrists. It is usually, but not always, painless, though secondary degenerative changes may occur later and cause considerable discomfort, particularly in the hips which may become dislocated. Other congenital abnormalities may be present, such as small or absent patellae, high palate, hypospadias, micrognathia, mental deficiency, and cardiovascular abnormalities.

Camptodactyly is an innocent congenital condition where the little fingers are flexed with thickening of the proximal interphalangeal joints. It is a relatively common condition and important only in that it may cause confusion with osteoarthrosis. Other fingers are less often affected.

In *congenital indifference to pain* the patient traumatizes the joints and other tissues repeatedly and may develop secondary traumatic osteoarthrosis or even Charcot's joints. Such patients are usually mentally normal but are constantly suffering the effects of injury, fractures, bruises, dislocations, cuts, and scratches, as they do not experience pain as do normal subjects. It is a rare condition.

Dysplasia epiphysalis multiplex is inherited as an autosomal dominant trait. The epiphyses of the long bones become deformed, the hips most commonly. Any or all of the epiphyses of the long bones may be affected, with resultant osteoarthrosis, particularly of hips and knees, beginning in early life. The sufferers are often of short stature with short, squat digits.

The *Ehlers-Danlos syndrome* is a rare genetically determined disorder of connective tissue, characterized by hypermobile joints and hyperextensible skin which tends to split if mildly injured with resulting gaping scars. There are probably five separate entities included in this title, in one of which sudden death is common. Joint subluxations and dislocations occur if the joints are unnaturally mobile and effusions into knees are common. Dislocations of clavicle, patellae, shoulders, radii, and hips may occur and recur several times. Other developmental abnormalities are common, such as kyphoscoliosis, anterior wedging of vertebrae, spina bifida occulta, club-foot, and genu recurvatum. Bleeding may occur in superficial tissues, or from vagina, rectum, or mouth, and haemarthrosis may occur. Children may be backward in walking and develop a tabetic-like gait. In the sixth to ninth months of pregnancy joints may become more lax and subluxable than previously.

Familial dysautonomia (Riley-Day syndrome) is a congenital disorder almost completely confined to Ashkenazic Jews, transmitted as an autosomal recessive gene. Among many manifestations relative insensitivity to pain may lead to Charcot's joints in early adolescence in knee or shoulder.

Hurler's syndrome (gargoylism). In the classic syndrome, though the onset is from 6 months to 2 years of age, the typical picture of gargoylism does not appear until 4–5 years later, the child showing coarse features with thick lips, large bulging head, and flattened nose. (*Fig.* 236, p. 221.) The cervical spine is short with kyphosis of upper lumbar and lower dorsal spines. Acetabula are shallow, epiphyses flattened, irregular, and retarded in development. Limitation of joint movement is common, particularly abduction of shoulders and hips and extension of fingers, and contractions may occur of hips and elbows, the hands becoming clawed. The children are often intellectually impaired and rarely live beyond 20 years of age.

In the *hypermobility syndrome* generalized joint laxity occurs as an isolated finding, giving rise to recurrent joint pains and effusions, particularly after vigorous exercise. Symptoms, more common in females than males, usually start before the age of 15. Knees are most commonly affected. Degenerative changes may begin early in the fourth decade. These children, who often consider themselves to be 'double-jointed', often suffer quite severe cramp-like pains in the legs after sporting activities.

The picture of *Marfan's syndrome* is of a tall, thin, loose-jointed, youth or girl with long extremities, especially the fingers (arachnodactyly), dislocated lenses, tremulous irides, and cardiovascular abnormalities, particularly dilatation of ascending aorta and aortic incompetence. Fifty per cent of these patients present with backache, pains in joints, and/or effusions. Joints may dislocate readily, hips or shoulders most commonly. Many other abnormalities may be present, pigeon chest and pectus excavatum particularly. Sexes are affected equally. In these

sternum and prominent chin appearing a year later. Growth usually ceases at 10 years, the child showing a short trunk with kyphosis, knock knees, flat feet, waddling gait, muscle weakness, and increased laxity of joints. Mentally they are normal. A number of varieties of this disorder exist and it may well consist of a number of different entities.

Osteodysplasty (Melnick and Needles syndrome) is another inherited skeletal dysplasia, probably a congenital disorder of skeletal growth which leads to early degenerative changes in the large

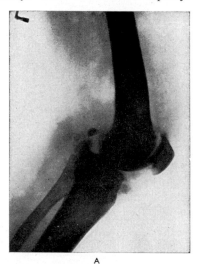 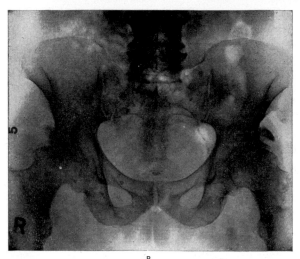

Fig. 456. A, Osteo-arthrosis of the knee-joint; B, Osteo-arthrosis of the hip-joints. (*Dr. T. A. Hills.*)

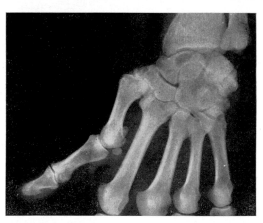

Fig. 457. Severe osteo-arthrosis of the carpometacarpal joint of the thumb. (*Dr. Keith Jefferson.*)

thin, tall, gangling subjects the distance from pubis to sole exceeds that of pubis to vertex, and arm span is greater than height. Distal bones are longer than proximal. Subcutaneous fat is sparse.

In the *Morquio-Brailsford osteochondrodystrophy* the children appear normal until 1–2 years of age when kyphosis is seen with protrusion of

weight-bearing joints, including the spine. X-rays show curvature of the long bones of the limbs with irregular cortex and widening and thinning of the metaphyses. These changes may roughly resemble those of rickets, but ribs, clavicles, and scapulae are also deformed.

The outstanding abnormality in *osteogenesis imperfecta* is the ease with which bones may be fractured. In addition joints are unduly mobile, thinness of the sclerotics give the eyes the typical pale-blue appearance, and there is atrophy of the skin with a tendency to subcutaneous haemorrhage. Joints dislocate readily and growth may be arrested by multiple small fractures in epiphyses. Spine and chest deformities may occur and deafness is not unusual. Ligaments are weakened and tendon ruptures may occur.

This list of congenital non-infective arthropathies is not complete and the different causes are not yet clear enough to classify them all accurately. Undue laxity, with recurrent subluxations or increased friability or fragility of tissues, leads to premature degenerative changes in the joints affected. Other coexistent congenital abnormalities are common.

2. Degenerative. By *osteo-arthrosis* is meant the various painful syndromes arising primarily from degenerative changes in the joints (*Figs.* 456, 457). Age brings degenerative changes, but the pains experienced vary greatly depending on personality, degree of change, and joints affected. Such changes are more likely to occur in any joint previously injured by fracture or dislocation or even mild subluxation, or in any joint which is congenitally abnormal or, because of mechanical factors, working abnormally in the face of abnormal stresses. Repeated small 'micro-traumata' may also predispose to degenerative changes. Endocrine factors may play a part in some cases as in the so-called *generalized osteoarthrosis* which usually affects women 1–5 years or more before or after the menopause. Most commonly affected joints are the terminal interphalangeal joints of the fingers (Heberden's nodes), the thumb bases (carpometacarpal and metacarpophalangeal joints of the thumbs), cervical and lumbar spines, knees and hips, and acromioclavicular joints. Less commonly affected

above 30 mm. per hour (Westergren) in osteoarthrosis and are usually normal, as are haemoglobin and plasma proteins. Tests for rheumatoid factors are negative. In the cervical spine degenerative changes centre essentially around the lower 5th, 6th, and 7th intervertebral disks, the pain often fanning up into the occiput, over the head, and into the shoulders, neck movements being restricted and painful. In rheumatoid disease, particularly in childhood, involvement is more diffuse throughout the cervical spine though pains may also be referred in a similar manner. Subluxation of the 1st on the 2nd cervical vertebrae, which occurs in rheumatoid arthritis and ankylosing spondylitis, is not seen in osteo-arthrosis. A lateral X-ray of the cervical spine will readily distinguish the rough irregularity of disk degeneration from the straight, even intervertebral bridging of ankylosing spondylitis. The

DIFFERENTIAL DIAGNOSIS OF OSTEO-ARTHRITIC AND RHEUMATOID JOINTS

OSTEO-ARTHROSIS	RHEUMATOID ARTHRITIS
Gnarled, knobbly and bony	Spindle soft-tissue swellings of joints
Terminal interphalangeal joint involvement common (Heberden's nodes)	Terminal interphalangeal joint less commonly involved
Metacarpophalangeal and proximal interphalangeal joints less commonly involved	Metacarpophalangeal and proximal interphalangeal joints commonly involved
Wrists rarely affected	Wrists very commonly affected
Tendon sheaths not involved	Swelling of tendon sheaths common
Affected joints not usually tender	Affected joints usually tender
Terminal phalanges tend to deviate towards middle line	Metacarpophalangeal ulnar deviation common
No bony rarefaction in X-rays	Periarthrodal bony rarefaction in X-rays the rule
Bony surface erosions rare in X-rays	Bony surface erosions common in X-rays
No excess fluid in joints unless recently traumatized	Increased fluid in joints often palpable

are proximal interphalangeal and metacarpophalangeal joints. Although essentially degenerative, the Heberden's node may in some cases be tender, red, and inflamed in its early stages. Most serious in terms of crippling is hip involvement, the knee coming next. Finger and thumb joints, though a painful nuisance, are less likely to cause major disablement. The hand in generalized osteoarthrosis differs from that in rheumatoid arthritis as shown in the table above.

In the knee effusions may occur as a result of traumatic aggravation and there may be considerable synovial proliferation also. It is not, therefore, always easy to distinguish an osteoarthritic knee from a rheumatoid one, but the pattern of the disease elsewhere in the body and the absence of systemic features in osteo-arthrosis usually suffices to distinguish the two. In any joint, the absence of inflammatory swelling, nodules, and of enlarged lymph-nodes favours osteo-arthrosis rather than inflammatory arthritis. Sedimentation-rates are rarely elevated

condition known as 'ankylosing hyperostosis' of the spine is a degenerative one occurring not infrequently in diabetics (*see* BACK, PAIN IN, p. 86), usually in the lower dorsal area.

3. Dietetic. *Kashin-Beck's disease* is a condition apparently based on fusarial infection of flour. In the valleys in Siberia where it occurs degenerative changes in joints and spine appear in relatively young people as a result of cartilage destruction. It has not been seen in Great Britain. *Rickets* is much less common than it was and for this reason may be more readily missed. Presenting symptoms may be pains and tenderness over bones, particularly back, hips, thighs, and legs generally. The pains are usually aggravated by rising from resting positions and by exercise. The dangers of missed diagnosis lie in permanent bony deformities in the pelvis and lower extremities and in the thorax. Pelvic deformities, the most serious in the female child, usually occur in the first year of life. In *scurvy* the child is listless and apathetic with poor appetite. Bones may be painful and tender from subperiosteal haemorrhages and tender swellings may be palpated. The disease is seldom seen in adults; when it occurs dietetic deficiencies are usually due to neglect, alcoholism, or obsessional food fads, sometimes medically induced.

4. Endocrine. In *acromegaly* recurrent pains in spine and limb joints may be mistaken for those occurring in osteo- or rheumatoid arthritis. Effusions may occur in knees and carpal tunnel compression is not uncommon. The joints may be hypermobile in the early stages due to enlargement of the cartilages, and subluxations and

the early stages of the disease before the more classic symptoms of myxoedema occur (*Fig.* 458). Carpal tunnel compression occurs not infrequently and arthralgia is a common complaint. Signs of inflammation are absent but synovial thickening and, occasionally, effusions may occur, knees and hands being most commonly affected. Traumatic lesions are not uncommon and hip pain may be due to a slipped femoral epiphysis.

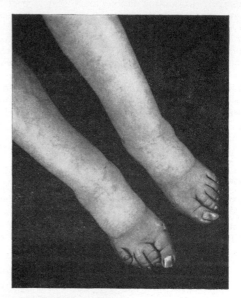

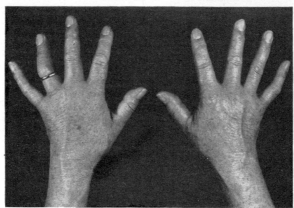

Fig. 458.   Typical facies and swelling of hands, feet, and ankles in myxoedema.

traumatic effusions may occur as in the other hypermobility syndromes. Later bony overgrowth limits and restricts movement, so that the picture resembles more that of osteo-arthrosis or, because of the fixed bent spine, advanced ankylosing spondylitis.

In the original description of *myxoedema* in 1873 by Sir William Gull muscular stiffness, joint swelling, and broad spade-like hands were noted. The hands in this condition may be mistaken for those of early rheumatoid arthritis in

In *hyperparathyroidism*, as in some cases of osteomalacia, crush lesions may occur in juxta-articular bone with a traumatic type of synovitis, with effusions and impaired function of the affected joints. Calcification is as common in synovial membrane and cartilage in these cases as it is rare in rheumatoid arthritis, a point of distinction between the two conditions. In idiopathic hypoparathyroidism back pain and stiffness may cause a clinical picture similar to that of ankylosing spondylitis, but though ligamentous calcification is present sacro-iliac joints are normal. It is associated with hypocalcaemia, cataracts, fits, tetany, and rashes. In *thyroid acropachy* subperiosteal thickening is seen in metacarpal and phalangeal bones of the hand in patients with hyperthyroidism who have in many cases been treated and rendered euthyroid. Exophthalmos is common and the so-called 'pretibial myxoedema' may be present. The somewhat thickened hand resembles that seen in pseudohypertrophic pulmonary osteo-arthropathy, but the condition is milder and less extensive, being usually confined to the hands.

5. Haematological. It is wise to perform a full blood-count, sedimentation-rate, and examination of plasma proteins in obscure cases of arthritis. Approximately 25 per cent of patients with *agammaglobulinaemia*, congenital or acquired, develop a non-suppurative arthritis not unlike rheumatoid arthritis, the joints showing effusions, pain, tenderness, and stiffness. The condition is usually asymmetrical, is unaccompanied by radiological changes, and may be transient, subsiding in a few weeks without sequelae, or may persist for years but with little residual change. Biopsy of synovial tissue does not distinguish between the two conditions. The sedimentation-rate is usually normal and tests for rheumatoid factor are negative. Recurrent infection with the usual pyogenic organisms is common.

Haemarthrosis may occur in *haemophilia* (factor VIII deficiency) and allied disorders, such as *Christmas disease* (factor IX deficiency), and in patients on anticoagulant therapy, but is rare in von Willebrand's disease. In *leukaemia* haemorrhages are common and flitting pains resembling rheumatic fever are not uncommon in acute leukaemia, which, taken in conjunction with a systolic apical cardiac murmur, may cause diagnostic confusion particularly in acute aleukaemic leukaemia. Pains in bones and joints occur not infrequently in acute leukaemia in childhood and in chronic leukaemia in adults, both myeloid and lymphatic. In children Still's disease is often misdiagnosed. In *sickle-cell anaemia* painful crises occur which are characteristic of the disorder, and these may not only be felt in the abdomen but in bones and joints in children or adults. Although the most common symptoms are those of anaemia, some patients have no complaints except during crises. Aseptic necrosis of bone may occur, particularly in the head of the humerus or femur, X-rays showing subsequently areas of increased density and areas of necrosis. The course of the disease is that of a chronic haemolytic process punctuated by periodic painful crises. Chronic ulceration of the lower legs is relatively common and scars are commonly to be seen around the malleoli.

6. Idiopathic. The classic picture of *ankylosing spondylitis* is that of a young male adult with stiff back and chest and often of neck and hips also. The sedimentation-rate is elevated, anterior uveitis is present in 25 per cent of cases at some stage in the disease course, and X-rays show typical changes in sacro-iliac joints and usually in the dorsolumbar spine. Peripheral joint involvement may occur but is usually, though not always, transient. Knee effusions are not uncommon. The pattern of the disorder is essentially central, spine and girdle joints being predominantly affected, peripheral small joints rarely and transiently. This is the opposite of rheumatoid arthritis. Nodules do not occur and rheumatoid factor is absent in the serum. The tissue antigen HLA-B 27 is found in over 90 per cent of patients. *Caplan's syndrome* is the association of rheumatoid arthritis and coarse lung opacities in X-rays of miners with progressive fibrosis of the lungs. In *Crohn's disease*, arthralgia or arthritis may occur in spine or peripheral joints, as it may in *ulcerative colitis* and less commonly in *Whipple's disease* (intestinal lipodystrophy). In all of these, rheumatoid factor is absent from the blood and rheumatoid nodules are not seen. In the arthropathy of ulcerative colitis, the best documented of these three disorders, onset is usually between the ages of 15 and 45 years. It is usually symmetrical and often monarticular with short exacerbations and usually complete recovery, joint erosions being rare and minor in character. It affects both sexes equally and usually begins acutely, affecting one knee or ankle primarily, subsequent attacks being of similar pattern. The arthritis commences usually long after the colitis and may coincide with an exacerbation of the disease. In all three conditions, ulcerative colitis, Crohn's disease, and Whipple's disease, a picture similar to that of ankylosing spondylitis may eventually appear after some years. In *polymyositis* and *dermatomyositis* minimal or moderate transitory arthralgia or arthritis occurs in about one-third of cases. Effusions are less common but may occur. Fingers and knees are most commonly affected. The skin and muscle manifestations point to the true diagnosis, muscles of the pelvic girdle and thighs and shoulder-girdle becoming weak. The association with malignant disease in adult cases should be kept in mind. The diagnosis *erythema multiforme* probably covers several different entities, some mild, some severe, the so-called Stevens-Johnson syndrome being a severe variant. Arthritis or arthralgia may occur along with other inflammatory reactions in skin, eye, mouth, and elsewhere. *Familial Mediterranean fever* is an ill-understood disorder characterized by recurrent and sometimes periodic attacks of arthralgia or arthritis. It occurs predominantly in people of Mediterranean origins, Armenians, Arabs, and Jews. Onset is in childhood or adolescence, episodes of fever recurring with polyserositis, abdominal pain, urticaria and other rashes, arthralgia and arthritis, and later amyloid nephrosis. Joint manifestations occur in one-third to one-half of the cases, usually arthralgia but sometimes mono- or polyarthritis. The acute episodes last only a few days, most cases showing no permanent sequelae.

In *Felty's syndrome* splenomegaly, enlargement of lymph-nodes, neutropenia, and sometimes pigmentation of the skin are superimposed on the usual picture of rheumatoid arthritis. The only reason for maintaining the title in what is merely a variant of rheumatoid arthritis is to emphasize the importance of the neutropenia, for intercurrent infections are the rule and splenectomy may be necessary. Leg ulcers are relatively common, the usual site being the lower shin anteriorly. (*Fig.* 459.)

Intermittent hydrarthrosis, or recurring effusions, usually into the knee, may occur in a variety of arthropathies; in rheumatoid arthritis or ankylosing spondylitis, for instance, it may be the initial presenting symptom. Hydrarthrosis

and early adult life, possibly ischaemic in origin. Early X-rays show dense fragments in the epiphysis and a broadening of the epiphysial line with, later, areas of rarefaction and condensation so that a core of dense bone is seen in a porotic matrix. The epiphyses are affected during the periods of their greatest activity, for instance the femoral head from 4 to 12 years (Legg-Calve-Perthes disease), the tibial tubercle from 10 to 16 years (Osgood-Schlatter disease). *Palindromic*

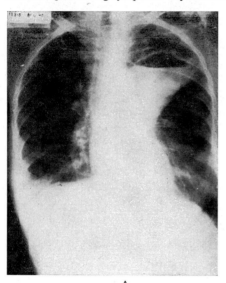

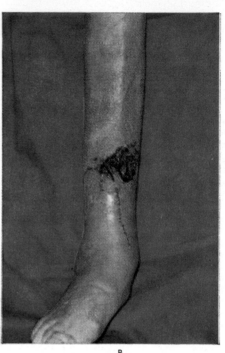

A   B

Fig. 459. A, Lung abscess in neutropenic Felty's syndrome. B, Leg ulcer in Felty's syndrome.

may, however, be a manifestation of infective systemic disease such as syphilis or brucellosis. There is usually complete or almost complete remission between attacks. Repeated trauma may cause the condition in osteo-arthrosis and it may be a sign of osteochrondritis dissecans; in other words, it is a physical sign and not a diagnosis. Some patients recover without showing signs of any other disorder.

In *osteochondritis dissecans* flakes of articular cartilage, sometimes with a portion of the underlying bone, become detached for no apparent reason, the condition manifesting itself as recurring attacks of arthritis, the commonest site (85 per cent) being the knee. The radial head is the next most common site, hip and ankles being rarely involved. The condition may be bilateral. X-rays are usually diagnostic. It occurs most commonly in adolescents and young adults. In *osteochondrosis* the diagnosis is also essentially a radiological one. It is essentially a disturbance of epiphysial ossification seen in early childhood

rheumatism is a name given to recurring episodic arthritis due to many causes, the most common probably being rheumatoid arthritis in an early phase. *Pigmented villonodular synovitis* presents as a persistent relatively painless but sometimes painful synovial proliferation with blood-stained joint fluid. The synovial proliferation forms brown nodular masses, possibly due to haemangiomata, in the synovia, which become traumatized, inflamed, and hyperplastic, the hyperplastic synovial cells containing haemosiderin. The condition is usually monarticular, commonly of the knee, and occurs in young adults, males rather than females. The joints may lock repeatedly. The aspirated joint fluid is characteristically blood-stained or dark brown in colour.

In *psoriatic arthropathy* (*Fig.* 461) the arthritis usually but not invariably follows the skin disorder by several years. The seronegative, nonnodular polyarthritis tends to be more patchy and less evenly symmetrical than rheumatoid arthritis, and the terminal interphalangeal joints of the fingers are frequently affected, particularly if the nails are affected by the pitting, ridging, and separation of psoriasis. When all these joints of the fingers are affected by inflammatory arthritis the digit resembles a hot sausage, as was noted many years ago by French rheumatologists. In some cases the sacro-iliac joints of the spine

occasionally death. *Rheumatoid arthritis (Figs.* 460, 463) is sufficiently well known as to need no description. It is as well to remember that tendons and tendon sheaths and bursae are commonly involved by the inflammatory process and these add to the clinical picture. *Still's disease*, chronic polyarthritis in childhood or early adolescence, differs only in that splenomegaly and lymphadenopathy

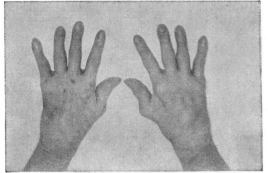

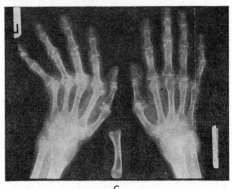

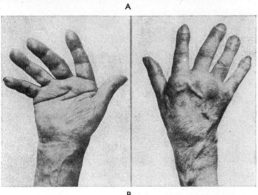

Fig. 460. A, Hands in rheumatoid arthritis. In addition to arthritic changes extensor tendon sheaths are involved. Rheumatoid nodules and vasculitic lesions are present. B, Rheumatoid arthritis with ulnar deviation and palmar contraction (pseudo-Dupuytren). C, Unusual unilateral ulnar deviation with gross bilateral carpal rheumatoid changes. Changes in metacarpophalangeal joints are more marked in the left than in the right hand.

are more common, tests for rheumatoid factor usually negative, involvement of terminal interphalangeal joints of fingers and cervical spine more common (*Fig.* 462), and skin rashes of maculopapular type more common. In the eye iritis with band opacity in the cornea occurs, sometimes with secondary cataract formation; these are not seen in rheumatoid arthritis in adults. Growth in general may be arrested if the disease is severe and premature fusing may occur in epiphyses adjacent to involved joints. Pericarditis is more common in Still's disease than in adult rhematoid arthritis.

Sarcoidosis. The arthropathy associated with this disorder is often accompanied by erythema nodosum; a weak or negative tuberculin reaction

are involved, the clinical picture being that of an ankylosing spondylitis. *Relapsing (or atrophic) polychondritis* is an unpleasant and rare disorder where the cartilages of joint, ear, nose, and trachea soften and collapse, leading to arthritic changes, facial changes, dyspnoea or stridor, and

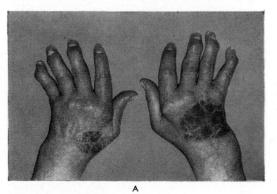

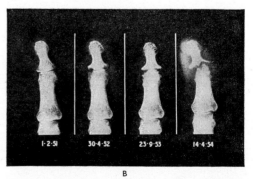

Fig. 461. A, Psoriatic arthropathy, showing involvement of terminal interphalangeal joints. B, Advance of destructive changes in psoriatic arthropathy.

is usual and the Kveim test may be positive. The arthropathy may be no more than a migratory arthralgia or it may be a true polyarthritis with pain, fever, systemic upset, and swelling of several joints, usually the larger ones. The majority of cases are less widely distributed than in most

the outstanding symptom is a maculo-petechial and sometimes papular rash over buttocks and extensor surfaces of the lower limbs particularly. Urticaria and purpura may occur. Pain, swelling, and stiffness of joints, most commonly ankles and knees, is usually transient and lasts only a few

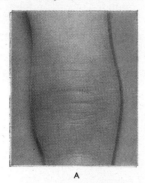
A

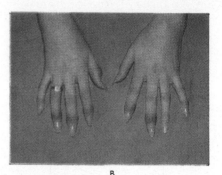
B

Fig. 462. Involvement of terminal interphalangeal joints in juvenile chronic polyarthritis.

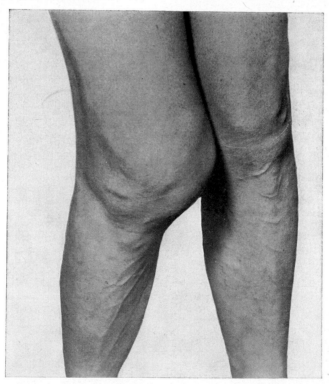

Fig. 463. Disorganization of the right knee-joint in chronic rheumatoid arthritis. (Dr. P. H. Kendall.)

polyarthropathies and most subside in a few weeks. Hilar node enlargement is common in chest X-rays, and glands may be palpable in the neck and axilla in some cases. Splenomegaly may be present.

Schönlein-Henoch (*anaphylactoid*) *purpura.* Commonest in children under 12 years of age,

days. About 10 per cent of cases develop chronic nephritis.

In *Scleroderma* (progressive systemic sclerosis) the skin is stretched tight over the underlying tissues (*Fig.* 464), the joints being intact, though initially they may show changes resembling rheumatoid arthritis.

In *systemic lupus erythematosus* any or all systems of the body may be involved in addition to the joints, which are not invariably involved, though arthralgia is usually present at some stage in the course of the disease. The patient, usually a female, is more ill than arthritic in most cases, though joint involvement is present in about two-thirds of patients. The finding of numerous antibodies, including anti-nuclear factor, in high titre and DNA-antibody and LE cells in the blood is strong confirmatory diagnostic evidence. The pattern of joint involvement may be flitting,

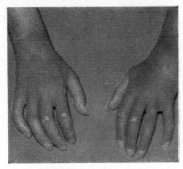

Fig. 464. Scleroderma (progressive systemic sclerosis).

resembling rheumatic fever, or more constant, resembling rheumatoid arthritis. The coexistence of skin lesions and visceral manifestations suggests the correct diagnosis, the typical lupus butterfly rash over nose and cheeks being particularly characteristic. Neutropenia and anaemia are common, thrombocytopenia not uncommon. Asthma, proteinuria, neurological signs, splenomegaly, retinal exudates, and a number of other coexistent findings in any arthritic should make one think of this disorder. Epileptiform fits occur in about 10 per cent of cases. Patients with neurological and renal involvement fare worst.

7. Infective Arthropathies. In the infective arthropathies the infecting organism is present in locomotor tissues: in gonococcal arthritis, for instance, gonococci are isolated from the infected joints or joint, and the condition responds to appropriate antibodies. Once a not uncommon arthropathy, the advent of antibiotics which rapidly cured the acute gonococcal infection rendered it very rare in Britain—until recently. Now it is again increasing in frequency, possibly related to homosexual practices in men and the use of oral contraceptives in women. Any of the infections due to bacteria, spirochaetes, or mycoplasma may, if there is destruction of tissue, lead to chronic changes in bones and joints, but often they leave little or no residual disability. In these days of holidays abroad on the Mediterranean conditions such as Kala-azar, previously unknown in residents of this country, can occur with resultant arthralgia, fever, and splenomegaly.

Viral arthropathies are uncommon in Great Britain, with the exception of *rubella arthritis*.

This mild and transient condition closely resembles rheumatoid arthritis but in a few days or weeks resolves completely. It is the best example in Britain today of an acute infective arthropathy, due to an infectious disease, which affects the same joints in the same manner as rheumatoid arthritis, but resolves rapidly without sequelae within a few days or weeks. Joint symptoms usually appear within 1–3 days of the onset of the disorder, usually just after the appearance of the rash. Arthritis may also follow prophylactic rubella vaccination. Joint symptoms may also occur, though less commonly, in *infective mononucleosis*. In Africa cases of an infective viral arthropathy have been reported, variously called *O'Nyong-Nyong fever* or *Chikungunya* (*breakbone fever*) according to the geographical area in which they occur. Although the conditions listed do not frequently give rise to arthropathies it is as well to remember that they can do so; certain of them, e.g., filariasis, probably do so more commonly than is generally thought.

8. Post-infective and Post-inflammatory Arthropathies. The commonest example of this syndrome, now that rheumatic fever is less often seen, is *Reiter's* (*Brodie's*) *disease*, which may follow dysentery or venereal infection, either gonococcal or non-specific urethritis. Of the three components, arthritis, urethritis, and conjunctivitis, the last is often transient or absent and the second may not be mentioned by the patient; the history, therefore, has to be taken not only carefully but diplomatically. Incomplete forms of the triad are frequent. The infective agent remains unknown, arthritic symptoms appearing a few days or up to 3 weeks after the initial symptoms of the causative infection. Lesions of buccal mucosa, of the glans penis or prepuce (balanitis circinata), or of skin (keratoderma blenorrhagia) often suggest the correct diagnosis, as does the distribution of affected joints; ankles, heels, and knees are relatively more often affected and joints of the upper extremity less, the disease joint pattern being otherwise similar to that of rheumatoid arthritis but less widespread. Later, sacro-iliac changes may occur and sometimes a clinical picture similar to that seen in ankylosing spondylitis. In such cases, as in other examples of ankylosing spondylitis associated with other disorders, the tissue antigen HLA-B 27 is usually present. Rheumatoid factor is absent in the blood; nodules do not occur. When skin manifestations are present the condition may closely resemble that of psoriatic arthropathy. The interphalangeal joints of the toes, rarely involved in rheumatoid arthritis, may be affected in Reiter's disease. Iridocyclitis and iritis, rare in rheumatoid arthritis, are not uncommon in Reiter's disease. *Rheumatic fever* is seen much less often today than previously. It is as well to remember that many other arthropathies may present in similar form, joints being successively affected and remitting rapidly, the so-called 'flitting pains' rippling round the locomotor system. Not only may rheumatoid arthritis present in this way, but also systemic lupus erythematosus, ankylosing spondylitis, Hodgkin's disease, leukaemia, undulant fever, and a number of other disorders. The heart is relatively rarely seriously involved if the condition first occurs over the age of 17 years.

with fever, arthralgia, and sometimes arthritis. The arthropathy occurring after *prostatectomy*, and sometimes after gynaecological operations, affects hips particularly, the patient lying in great pain with hips partly flexed. On rising from his bed he may have to walk backwards as forward

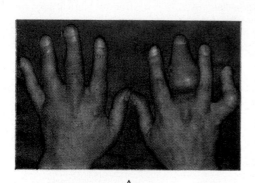 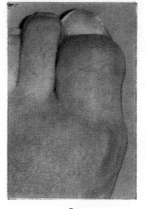 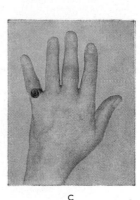

A   B   C

Fig. 465. A, Severe tophaceous gout. B, Acute gout in big toe. C, Acute gout in middle and little finger.

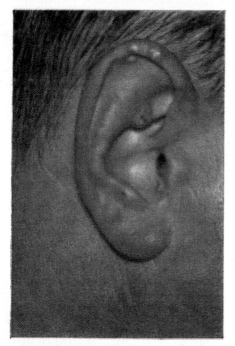

Fig. 466. Typical tophi in ear. They are opaque to trans-illumination.

Jaccoud's arthritis is an extremely rare disorder following repeated attacks of rheumatic fever, characterized by ulnar deviation of the fingers and hyperextension of the proximal interphalangeal joints without bone destruction. The syndrome following *coronary thrombosis* occurs around 2–3 weeks or more after the acute episode,

progression is too painful. The disorder is usually rapidly relieved by draining a pocket of fluid or infective material from behind the symphysis pubis, though only occasionally is true osteitis pubis present.

9. Metabolic Disorders. The commonest of these is gout. This disorder is characterized by the sudden agonizing nature of the acute attack which is often so severe as to make the patient, almost always an adult male, feel he must have broken a bone in his foot, but for the fact that the disorder frequently starts in bed in the early morning about 5–6 a.m. There are usually clear signs of inflammation, the skin being tense, shiny, hot, and red over the big toe, metatarsophalangeal joint, ankle, or hand, the first named being the commonest site. Acute attacks may also occur in the knee. (*Figs.* 465–467.)

Although hyperuricaemia is usually present it is not invariably so, and an elevated plasma uric acid level occurs in many other disorders and is not in itself diagnostic. The presence of tophi in ears or elsewhere suggests the diagnosis although the symptoms and signs are usually pathognomonic. The only absolute proof is the identification of urate crystals from the affected joint under the polarizing microscope. In some cases these turn out to be not urate but calcium pyrophosphate, the condition being 'calcium gout' or *chondrocalcinosis articularis*. This condition affects knees most commonly but other joints are also affected, often in symmetrical fashion, with the appearance of calcification in the joint cartilages. Acute inflammatory episodes occur also with deposition of calcium salts in uraemia in the soft tissues alongside, rather than in the joints. This is seen in chronic uraemia and in patients following *renal transplantations* from cadavers or living donors other than identical twins. Polyarthritis with effusions, often in the knees, may occur in these renal-grafted patients who may, though not rheumatoid, have a positive rheumatoid factor sheep-cell agglutination (Rose-Waaler) test in the blood.

In *calcinosis circumscripta* calcium salts (carbonate and phosphate) may be deposited under the skin but they are again para-articular rather than in the joint tissues, which appear normal. *Amyloidosis* may be secondary to rheumatoid arthritis, ankylosing spondylitis, and (more rarely) Reiter's disease, but it also may occur in primary form associated with pains and swellings in joints, and, occurring with multiple myelomatosis, may

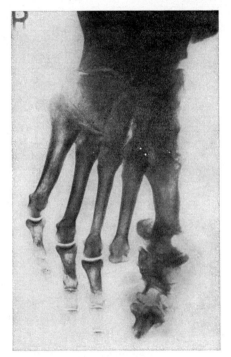

Fig. 467. Severe destructive tophaceous gout. The second toe was even more severely affected and was removed.

cause the median nerve carpal tunnel compression syndrome. Joint symptoms and backache in particular occur in *ochronosis*. Here the diagnosis is made by examination of the urine for homogentisic acid and the cartilage of the ears for pigmentation. X-rays of the spine are typical, heavy calcification occurring in the intervertebral cartilages.

Reticulohistiocytosis (*lipoid dermato-arthritis*) may be mistaken for rheumatoid arthritis in adults as changes in fingers and tenosynovitis occur, but the presence of yellow nodules on ears, forehead, neck, forearms, and elsewhere, with groups of purple papules, suggests the true diagnosis which is confirmed by biopsy. In advanced cases erosion of phalanges leads to shortening of the fingers.

In *Wilson's disease*, characterized by accumulation of copper in the tissues, arthritic changes, commonest in hands, wrists, and knees, may start about the age of 30. Associated features are hepatic cirrhosis, neuropsychiatric disease, and the Kayser-Fleischer green-brown ring around the cornea.

10. Vascular. *Avascular necrosis* occurs in Caisson disease (nitrogen or air embolism), from fat embolism, and occasionally in chronic alcoholism. The hips are often bilaterally involved with destruction of parts of the heads of the femora but shoulders may also be affected. One or both knees may be affected. *Giant-cell* (*cranial*) *arteritis* and polymyalgia rheumatica are probably two facets of the same condition, best termed 'polymyalgia arteritica', as on existing evidence both conditions are due to an arteritis in the

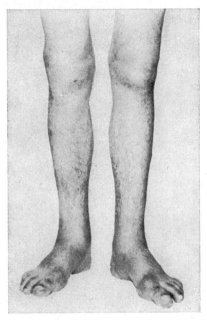

Fig. 468. Hydrarthrosis of knees and swelling of ankles and feet due to bronchial carcinoma, causing pseudo-hypertrophic pulmonary osteo-arthropathy.

elderly of those vessels having an internal elastic lamina. Renal and cerebral vessels are therefore spared. The patients, usually over the age of 60, are of either sex, have marked morning stiffness, sedimentation-rates around 60–100 mm. in 1 hour (Westergren), and pains and stiffness of shoulder and hip girdles. When temporal vessels are involved a splitting headache is often present, and the main danger is to vision if the central artery of the retina becomes affected. Pulses may disappear and haemic murmurs be apparent at the points of arterial narrowing. Sternoclavicular joints may be affected, but the disorder as far as the girdle joints in general are concerned is one of pain and stiffness in hips and shoulders without progressive clinical or radiological change and eventually with full recovery. Diagnosis is confirmed by arterial biopsy. In *polyarteritis nodosa* arthralgia is much more common than actual arthritis, but any joint may be affected in any pattern, local or general, severe or mild, flitting or constant. The appearance of nodules clinches the diagnosis but occurs in only a minority of cases and many biopsies may have to be done before the diagnosis is confirmed. Eosinophilia occurs in only about 15 per cent of cases. Bronchial spasm is among the more common manifestations elsewhere but all

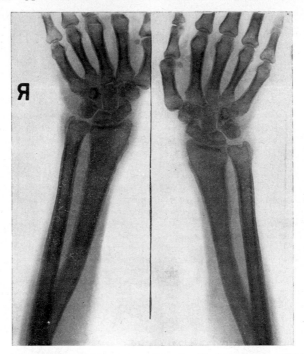

Fig. 469. Pseudo-hypertrophic pulmonary osteo-arthropathy of the radius and ulna. (*Dr. T. H. Hills.*)

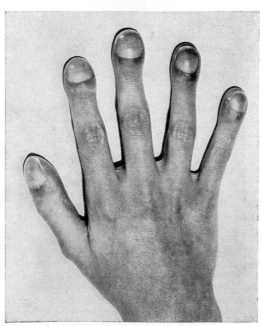
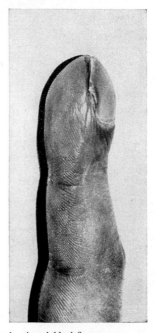

Fig. 470. Pseudo-hypertrophic pulmonary osteo-arthropathy, showing clubbed fingers.

symptoms may be involved: it is this multi-system distribution of symptoms which may suggest the diagnosis.

11. Neoplastic. *Metastatic malignant disease* or *multiple myelomatosis* usually causes bony rather than joint changes. The serum alkaline phosphatase, often elevated in the former, is usually normal in the latter as there is no osteoblastic activity in myelomatosis. Joint changes do occur, however, in *pseudohypertrophic pulmonary osteoarthropathy* (*Figs.* 468, 470), a condition mostly associated with a bronchial carcinoma, usually a peripheral one. Removal of the primary lesion leads to rapid resolution of the effusions and arthritic changes in the more commonly affected joints, the knees and ankles. Fingers and toes are clubbed and the extremities show a thickening based on new subperiosteal bone deposition which can be seen in X-rays (*Fig.* 469).

Osteoid osteoma. Although not a disease of joints this benign disorder should be mentioned because of the pain it causes and the difficulties in differential diagnosis. Initially an intermittent painful condition, the pain becomes more

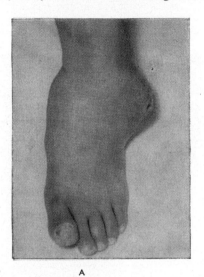

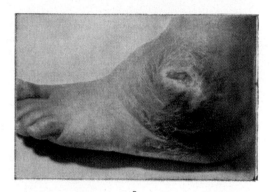

Fig. 471. Charcot's disease of ankle showing, A, disorganization of the joint, and, B, gummatous ulcer. (*Mr. R. G. Beard.*)

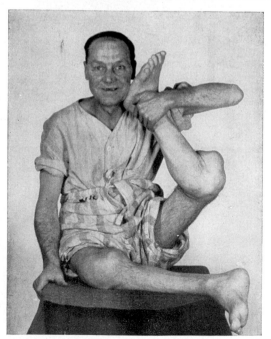

Fig. 472. Charcot's disease of the knee-joints showing the extraordinary mobility arising from joint destruction. The absence of pain is evident from the facies. (*Dr. Ralph Kauntze.*)

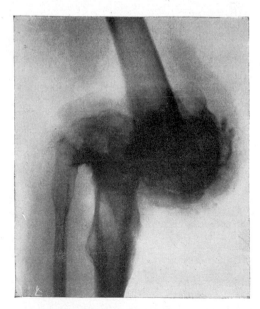

Fig. 473. Charcot's disease of the knee-joint with pathological dislocation. (*Dr. Cochrane Shanks.*)

persistent and severe, often aggravated by movement. There are no physical signs. It affects young adults and adolescents, and although any bone except the skull may be affected, the commonest to be involved are femur and tibia, which account for half the cases. X-rays show a characteristic central opacity surrounded by a trans-

of bone islands surround a grossly deformed or disorganized joint, the X-ray appearances resembling an ossified map of Greece. *Syringomyelia* affects chiefly shoulder and elbow; knee, ankle, hip, and spine are more common in tabes dorsalis (*Figs*. 471, 474). Diabetic arthropathy is different in that clinical and radiological signs of infection are often present along with poor vascularization and signs of peripheral neuropathy: the condition is usually confined to the feet and toes. *Osborne's syndrome* is due to ulnar nerve compression beneath the arcuate ligament just below

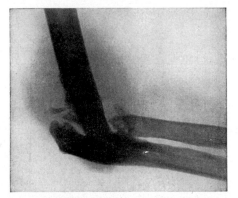

Fig. 474 Charcot's disease of the elbow-joint with pathological dislocation. (*Dr. T. H. Hills.*)

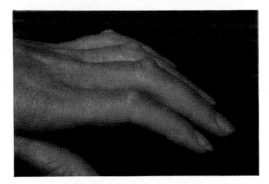

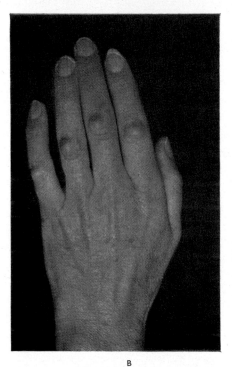

A   B

Fig. 475. Extra-articular knuckle-pads (Knobbly Knuckles, K.K. syndrome, Garrod's fatty or Hale-White's painful pads). They are fibrous, are not painful, and are only important in differential diagnosis from rheumatoid and osteo-arthritic nodes.

lucent zone, surrounded in turn by a zone of sclerosis. It may affect the bones of the spine, where it is often very difficult to diagnose and is usually unsuspected. Back pains are sometimes worse in the night than in the day.

12. Neuropathic. Although the *median nerve carpal tunnel compression syndrome* is not strictly a joint affection, it is so often a manifestation of rheumatoid arthritis that it should be mentioned. It is not infrequently the first sign of this disorder. Other causes are pregnancy, acromegaly, myxoedema, multiple myelomatosis, and amyloidosis. There is also an idiopathic variety with no apparent cause. Characteristic symptoms are tinglings and hot and cold electrical sensations up the arms interfering with sleep. *Charcot's joints* are characterized by their gross deformity, painlessness, and florid X-rays, where numbers

the elbow. In the *shoulder–hand syndrome*, a reflex dystrophy, trophic changes often follow soon after injury to the shoulder or weeks or months after coronary thrombosis, but a similar syndrome has been reported in patients on antituberculous therapy and in other pathological conditions. The shoulder is stiff and painful, the skin of the hand shiny and smooth and sometimes hyperaesthetic, the muscles atrophic. There is no joint swelling, though initially there may be considerable swelling of the whole hand and fingers. X-rays show initially osteoporosis of humeral head and wrist, later a more diffuse ground-glass picture. In many cases there is no apparent cause for the condition.

Ulcero-osteolytic neuropathy, a condition described in the Bantu in South Africa, occurs primarily in the feet.

13. Therapeutic. *Alcoholics* are more likely to sustain fractures than normal people; often an anicteric cirrhosis of the liver is present also. They are also more prone to septic arthritis and avascular necrosis of bone than normal people. Prolonged *corticosteroid therapy* may also be associated with septic arthritis, osteoporosis and fractures, and in some cases with gross changes in rheumatoid joints used too much under cover of the drug given locally or systemically. Crush fractures of lumbar or dorsal vertebrae are not uncommon. A condition very similar to systemic lupus erythematosus with LE cells present in the blood can be due to a large range of drugs, the commonest being procaine amide. This is the so-called *hydrallazine syndrome.* Symptoms disappear on stopping the drug. It has also been reported with oral contraceptives, though such cases are very rare.

14. Miscellaneous. The *knuckle pads* seen not infrequently on the dorsal aspects of the proximal interphalangeal joints of the fingers (*Fig.* 475) are usually not accompanied by any symptoms and are best disregarded. They are due to fibrous thickenings the size of small orange-pips and are not part of the clinical picture of osteo-arthrosis or of any other form of arthritis. They are not associated with any bony changes, though in some cases they occur with *Dupuytren's contraction* which, in turn, is occasionally associated with Peyronie's disease (induratio penis plastica). The palmar contractions occurring in rheumatoid arthritis may on occasion closely resemble Dupuytren's contraction. The *septic focus syndrome* is a rare disorder where diffuse aches and pains in and around joints are rapidly relieved by removal of a septic focus or drainage of an abscess. No residual changes are left in the tissues. Lastly, the *xiphoid syndrome* refers to pains which stem from a displaced or mobile xiphisternum, often the result of trauma. This simple condition is only noteworthy in that it may be mistaken for more serious disorders of stomach, duodenum, gall-bladder, or heart.

F. Dudley Hart.

KELOID

A keloid (*Fig.* 476) is a new growth of dense fibrous tissue and is the final result of hypertrophy of scar tissue. The cause of this hypertrophy is obscure, but certain individuals, especially Negroes, appear to be particularly prone to keloid formation, and this tendency is made use of in Africa for tribal markings. It most commonly occurs after severe scalds and is not rare in burns generally and vaccination scars. There is no evidence that keloids arise spontaneously although some appear to do so. The first sign is a pinkish thickening of the apparently normal scar tissue; this may extend beyond the area of the original scar in claw-like processes and the overlying epidermis is thin, smooth, and glossy, and may be a little tender. Rarely telangiectases occur on the surface. Later the lesions become white and very dense in texture. They are occasionally painful. Spontaneous improvement occurs in many cases.

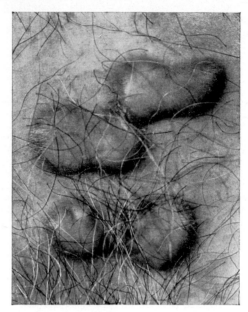

Fig. 476. Keloid on the chest, following trivial injury.

Acne keloid or *nuchae*—dermatitis papillaris capillitii—is not a true keloid. It is the result of a chronic staphylococcal infection of the nuchal area, and consists of numerous pustules each of which is surrounded by dense fibrous tissue. The infection is usually secondary to ingrowing hairs in the area.

P. D. Samman.

KETO-ACIDOSIS

If carbohydrate metabolism is reduced most of the body's energy requirements come from fat breakdown. Under these circumstances acetyl coenzyme A metabolism by the tricarboxylic acid cycle does not keep pace with its production. Condensation of acetyl CoA is catalysed enzymatically in liver and kidney to form aceto-acetate.

$$2CH_3COSCoA + H_2O \longrightarrow CH_3COCH_2COO^- + H^+ + 2CoASH$$

Acetyl CoA   Aceto-acetate

Reduced NAD reacts with aceto-acetate to form β-hydroxybutyrate, regenerating the NAD^+ required for further fat breakdown, in the same way as does lactate production from pyruvate in anaerobic carbohydrate metabolism (*see* p. 403).

$$CH_3COCH_2COO^- + NADH + H^+ \longrightarrow CH_3CHOHCH_2COO^- + NAD^+$$

β-Hydroxybutyrate

Since formation of aceto-acetate liberates hydrogen ion, effectively aceto-acetic and β-hydroxybutyric *acids* are formed, accounting for the acidosis in ketosis. Some acetone (which is *not* acidic) is formed spontaneously from aceto-acetic acid, causing the characteristic smell on the breath of severely ketotic patients.

$$CH_3COCH_2COO^- + H^+ \longrightarrow CH_3COCH_3 + CO_2$$
$$\text{Acetone}$$

Aceto-acetic acid, β-hydroxybutyric acid, and acetone are sometimes called 'ketone bodies', and overproduction is known as 'ketosis' or 'keto-acidosis'. Accumulation in the plasma causes *ketonaemia*, and appearance in the urine, due to glomerular 'overflow', is called *ketonuria*.

Significant ketosis is always associated with acidosis, with a reduced plasma bicarbonate level (*see* p. 402). It is the acidosis, not the ketosis itself, that is harmful.

Tests for ketosis. The usual tests detect predominantly aceto-acetate. β-Hydroxybutyrate does not react.

Urinary Ketones. All tests should be carried out on fresh urine, since aceto-acetate decomposes and acetone is volatile. If urine *must* be kept it should be refrigerated, to slow these reactions.

Rothera's test. This is the basis of the reaction given by 'Ketostix' and 'Ketotest' (strips and tablets made by Ames). Aceto-acetate, and to a lesser extent acetone, react with sodium nitroprusside in alkaline solution to give a purple colour. In the original test about 3 ml of urine is saturated with solid ammonium sulphate, and a crystal of sodium nitroprusside and a few drops of concentrated ammonia are added.

The *advantage* of the test is its almost complete specificity for aceto-acetate. Bromsulphthalein (BSP), phenosulphthalein (PSP), and phenolphthalein (a constituent of some purgatives) are all purple in alkaline solution; if the urine is purple on addition of sodium hydroxide *without* nitroprusside the cause will be evident.

A *disadvantage* is that sensitivity is such that even clinically insignificant concentrations are detected. The original test detects 0·5 mmol/l or more, and the commercial tests more than 1–2 mmol/l.

Ferric chloride (Gerhardt's) test. Ferric chloride solution (10 per cent) is added drop by drop to a few millilitres of urine, with shaking, until it clears. A reddish purple colour develops in the presence of aceto-acetate.

The *advantage* of the test is that the sensitivity is such that it detects only clinically significant levels of aceto-acetate (2·5–5 mmol/l).

The *disadvantage* is its non-specificity. A large number of compounds, of which the most important is salicylates, react to give a purple colour (many others give other colours). Since heat accelerates the decomposition of aceto-acetate, retesting a further specimen after boiling for a few minutes gives a negative result with ketones, but a positive one with other substances.

It should be remembered that *both* ketones and salicylates may be present in the same specimen, and a persisting positive reaction does not exclude ketonuria unless Rothera's test is negative.

Plasma ketones. Plasma aceto-acetate concentration can be estimated roughly using 'Ketostix'. This may be useful to confirm the diagnosis of ketosis if urine cannot be obtained. The actual level is of less importance for two reasons:

1. 'Ketones' are only harmful because of the associated acidosis. The severity of the acidosis is best judged as described on p. 403.

2. The degree of acidosis cannot be equated directly with the level of ketones as estimated by 'Ketostix', since the test does not detect β-hydroxybutyrate (associated with hydrogen ion production) but does to some extent react with acetone (which is not acidic).

Causes of ketosis

1. *Diabetic keto-acidosis* is due to failure to metabolize glucose in the absence of insulin, or in the presence of insulin antagonists. This is the most severe form of keto-acidosis and is associated with *hyperglycaemia*. The patient is usually dehydrated and may be overbreathing due to acidosis. In severe cases the odour of acetone may be detectable on the breath. Treatment with fluid and insulin is required urgently.

2. *Glucose deficiency.* Carbohydrate metabolism is reduced after even a short period of fasting, and mild ketosis may be detectable after as short a period as 24 hours. This is of no pathological significance, and is not severe enough to cause significant acidosis. It will disappear when food is taken. The blood glucose is a normal fasting level.

More marked ketosis occurs after prolonged fasting, whether due to unavailability of food in starvation, or due to rigid reducing diets or anorexia nervosa. Food intake may be hindered by vomiting or oesophageal obstruction. These cases may be associated with a significant degree of acidosis, and the *blood-glucose concentration may be low* in the late stages. Intravenous administration of glucose may be indicated. Ketotic hypoglycaemia, similar to that due to starvation, occurs in some young children after febrile illnesses or short periods of fasting.

Joan F. Zilva.

KIDNEY, ENLARGEMENT OF

A renal swelling may be so slight that it is only found upon clinical examination, or it may be large enough to attract the patient's attention. Hydronephrosis, pyonephrosis, renal tuberculosis or abscess, new growth, or cysts (single or multiple) in the kidney have to be diagnosed not only from one another but also from other tumours simulating a renal swelling. The characteristic points of a renal tumour are:

1. *The large intestine is in front of the tumour.* When either kidney is merely slightly enlarged, both large and small intestine will be in front of

it; but when the organ is so enlarged as to reach the anterior abdominal wall the coils of small intestine are pushed aside. The anatomical relation of the large intestine to the kidney, and the absence of a mesentery, do not allow of the same mobility of the colon, which usually retains its position in front of the kidney, although it is sometimes pushed downwards by a tumour projecting forwards from the lower pole. Hence an area of resonance can usually be obtained in front of a renal swelling; if the colon is empty it can sometimes be felt in a thin subject and rolled by the fingers on the surface of the tumour. Bowel is never placed in front of a splenic tumour, and only rarely in front of a hepatic tumour.

2. The *area of dullness to percussion* is continuous from the lateral aspect of the swelling to the midline posteriorly—that is, there is no area of resonance between the mass and the vertebral spines, as with a splenic or ovarian tumour.

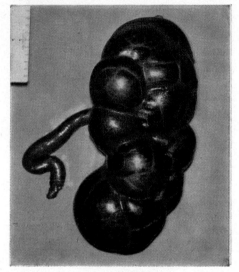

Fig. 477. Enormous hydronephrosis due to a small stone impacted in the distal ureter. The kidney was so large that it could readily be felt on rectal as well as abdominal examination yet it has retained its reniform shape.

3. A renal tumour usually *retains the shape of the kidney*; it is rounded at its borders and poles, and does not possess any edge or sharp margin, as do splenic or hepatic swellings (*Fig.* 477). The surface of the tumour may present rounded, smooth, raised bosses in cases of renal growths or in polycystic disease.

4. A *renal tumour* in the process of enlargement *projects forwards and downwards*. It may fill up the natural hollow of the loin, but seldom causes any prominence posteriorly. A perinephric abscess, which often simulates a renal swelling, may cause a distinct prominence in the loin.

5. A renal tumour may be movable downwards or inwards, unless it is fixed in the loin by preceding inflammation, or by the spread of carcinoma into the perirenal tissues; an enlarged

kidney can be felt bimanually, and if grasped between the two hands *can be pushed into the loin*. A renal tumour rarely descends into the iliac fossa but it may be present there in congenital ectopia or in cases of excessive mobility.

6. When a renal tumour is large enough to reach the anterior abdominal wall it commonly comes in contact with it at the level of the umbilicus, at the same time bulging out the iliocostal space. There is usually a line of resonance between the upper margin of the tumour and the hepatic dullness.

7. A *varicocele* may be developed on the same side as the renal tumour. This is especially significant on the right side although it is a rare finding.

8. With a renal tumour there may be *changes in the urine* pointing to renal disease; but on the other hand, the urine at any one time may be normal, free from blood or pus, from the fact that the ureter of the diseased side is blocked, or that the disease does not involve the renal pelvis.

9. In exceptional cases, a tumour of the right kidney may extend upwards towards the dome of the diaphragm, rotating the liver so that the anterior margin of the latter descends below the costal margin, and prevents satisfactory palpation of the renal areas.

Although, from the above physical characters, it would seem that a renal tumour should present little difficulty in diagnosis, yet it is by no means infrequent to find that a tumour possessing several of these characters may give rise to considerable doubt in the determination of the organ from which it arises. The following points will assist in the diagnosis of renal swellings from other tumours with which they are likely to be confused.

1. Tumours of the Gall-bladder are placed immediately below the costal margin, so that no interval exists between the tumour and the lower margin of the liver. They are usually oval in outline, with the long axis in the line between the 9th right costal cartilage and the umbilicus; are freely movable with the respiratory movements, and movable from side to side about an axis at the costal margin. There is dullness on percussion over them, and they cannot be felt in the loin or be grasped bimanually. With a tumour of the gall-bladder there may be attacks of colic, with or without jaundice. A good radiograph may show the outline of a distended gall-bladder distinct from the shadow of the kidney, and gallstones may sometimes be seen, while a cholecystographic examination will show that no contrast medium enters the gall-bladder.

2. Enlargements of the Liver pass downwards from beneath the costal margin so that there is no line of resonance, or area in which the hand can be depressed, between the tumour and the costal margin. Hepatic tumours do not impair the normal resonance in the loin in the same manner as a renal tumour does. A tongue-shaped lobe of the liver (Riedel's lobe) may cause difficulty in diagnosis; but here the lower margin is seldom so rounded as is that of a renal tumour, nor will the mass be felt in the loin on bimanual examination. A tumour or cyst in the concave aspect, or of the left lobe, of the liver is especially liable to cause error in diagnosis, whereas, on the other hand, a tumour of the right kidney which projects upwards behind the liver may so rotate the latter that its anterior margin descends below the costal margin and completely obscures the kidney. In a case of a large carcinoma of the right kidney, the liver may in this way be so depressed as to render palpation of the kidney impossible. A pyelographic examination may reveal a normal renal picture or on the other hand may indicate a hydronephrosis or renal growth.

3. Enlargements of the Spleen descend from beneath the left costal margin, and have no bowel in front of them. The edge of a splenic tumour is usually well defined and often notched, and there is resonance between the posterior aspect of the tumour and the spinal column. A splenic tumour is more movable than is a left renal tumour. A blood-count may help in deciding in favour of a splenic enlargement, and a pyelogram may show a normal kidney.

4. Perinephric Effusions, whether of blood, pus, or urine, may form a tumour in the loin which upon physical examination may be mistaken for a renal swelling. A perinephric effusion may arise from some suppurative condition of the kidney, so that the previous history and examination of the urine will not assist in differentiation; or it may be due to conditions entirely distinct from renal disease. An effusion of blood around the kidney is, in nearly all cases, caused by an injury to the loin, and will be accompanied by other signs of injury. It may, however, occur from the spontaneous growth and rupture of a renal neoplasm. A perinephric abscess forms a less well-defined tumour than that caused by a renal swelling, is more acute in its general symptoms, such as pain and temperature, and fills up the iliocostal space. The skin over it may be thickened or oedematous, and fluctuation may be felt to be more superficial than in a renal swelling. A perinephric abscess may result from suppuration about a carcinoma or diverticulum of the large bowel, from appendiceal inflammation, or from suppuration in a perinephric haematoma due to injury; it may be a sequel to a specific blow, or be due to a haematogenous infection. Bilateral palpation and comparison of the loins may detect perinephric swelling by the way the loin is filled out and becomes even convex on the affected side. This is best seen by laying the patient prone and carefully inspecting both sides. A high leucocyte count in the blood with increased percentage of polymorphonuclear cells would be in favour of perinephric inflammation.

5. Tumours arising from the Pelvic Organs, from the ovary or uterus, may in some cases simulate renal tumours. An ovarian cyst with a long pedicle occupying the loin may be mistaken for an enlarged or movable kidney, and any sudden attacks of pain occurring from torsion of the

pedicle may be looked upon as due to renal colic. The usual ovarian cyst or uterine fibroid will seldom be confused with a renal swelling, for it is placed in the mid-line of the body, can be felt to come up from the pelvis, and can be felt on bimanual vaginal examination to be attached to the uterus or its appendages. These tumours give rise to dullness anteriorly, and do not alter the normal resonance in the loin. In cases of malignant ovarian tumours associated with ascites the lumbar resonance may be lost, but on turning the patient over on one side the previously dull note becomes replaced by resonance in the uppermost loin. In the case of an ovarian cyst with a long pedicle, or of a uterine fibroid of pedunculated, subserous form, the position in

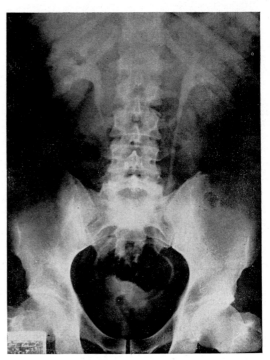

Fig. 478. Normal excretion urogram, 30-min. film after removal of compression. The calices are cupped, the left ureter is filled completely and the right partially.

the loin may sometimes suggest a renal tumour; it will be found, however, to occupy a more anterior position in the abdomen than a renal tumour, and to possess a much greater range of movement, and it does not slip back into the loin under the costal margin in the same manner as an enlarged kidney does; there is resonance posteriorly, the kidney may be actually palpated as well as the abdominal tumour, while a distinct connexion with the pelvic organs can sometimes be traced from the tumour when the latter is drawn up.

In contradistinction to the above a very large cystic renal swelling may be mistaken for an ovarian cyst. It may occupy the greater part of the abdomen, and even be felt per vaginam to be encroaching upon the pelvis; but on careful examination of a renal tumour of this form there will be no line of resonance between the mass and the vertebral column posteriorly, the natural hollow of the loin will be filled up, and there is frequently a distinct bulging in the lower thoracic wall, together with an increased length of the iliocostal space on the affected side. Some assistance may be obtained from the history; a hydronephrosis may have been first noticed as a tumour starting under the costal margin and gradually increasing downwards towards the iliac fossa and inwards across the median line, whereas an ovarian tumour may have been noticed to increase upwards from the pelvis. With an ovarian or pelvic tumour, a pyelogram will show a normal renal pelvis.

may not complain of constipation, but may in fact have a small daily evacuation from the overloaded bowel.

8. Inflammatory Thickenings about the Appendix will be diagnosed from renal tumours by the situation of the pain and by the swelling being in the iliac fossa rather than in the loin. In some cases, however, the pain may be referred to the lumbar region, or an appendiceal inflammatory mass may spread upwards. This is especially so when the appendix is retrocaecal in position. The onset of the trouble, the acute symptoms, and the febrile disturbance will usually distinguish these cases from renal lesions.

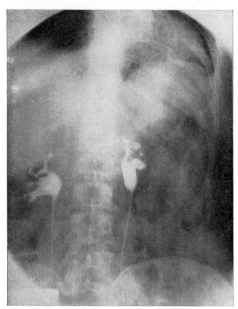

Fig. 479. Retrograde pyelogram. The right kidney is normal. On the left the calices are clubbed and the pelvis dilated from the presence of a calculus which is hidden by the contrast medium.

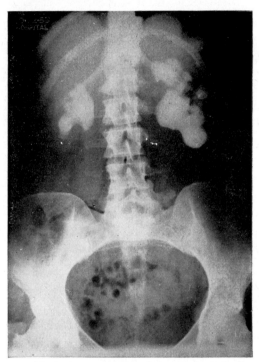

Fig. 480. Radiograph showing bilateral renal calculi. On the left the dendritic stone forms a cast of the renal pelvis and calices.

6. Suprarenal Tumours may occasionally be of sufficient size to form an abdominal tumour, presenting a rounded, movable swelling in the hypochondrium. It is sometimes possible to distinguish them from renal tumours by radiography after presacral insufflation of oxygen into the retroperitoneal tissue (*see* p. 479), or, more certainly, by aortography.

7. Faecal Accumulations in the Colon, Caecum, or Sigmoid Flexure may give rise to a tumour and pain of a colicky nature in the loin; the tumour can sometimes be indented by the examining fingers. They will be distinguished from renal swellings by the general intestinal symptoms, flatulence, and the changes in form consequent on the administration of large enemata. A patient with a collection of faeces in the colon

9. Malignant Growth of the Large Intestine, especially of the ascending or descending colon, may form a tumour in the loin which closely resembles a renal swelling. The mass formed by the growth may be grasped bimanually, is movable in the same directions as a renal tumour, and comes forward under the costal margin. The percussion note over the front of the lump is resonant, and there is usually an aching pain in the loin. If the growth has infiltrated through the wall of the bowel uncovered by peritoneum, the perirenal tissues may be thickened, or albuminuria may be produced by direct invasion of the kidney, when the case will even more resemble a renal lesion. Carcinoma of the large intestine should be suspected if there is any irregularity in the action of the bowels, mucus or blood in the motions, or any symptom of incipient obstruction in the intestine. The tumour may be irregular and nodular, whereas a renal tumour presents rounded margins. The occurrence of a tumour in either side, associated with discomfort or palpable distension of the caecum from the accumulation of faeces, would render a growth in the colon the more suspicious. The appearances seen with the X-rays at a suitable interval after a barium meal or enema (*Fig.* 184, p. 177) may assist in arriving at the diagnosis by showing organic intestinal stenosis. Pyelography will show a shadow of a normal renal pelvis (*see Fig.* 478).

10. Tumours of the Omentum, Mesentery, or Pancreas, either cystic or malignant, are more median in position, do not project into the loin, and seldom resemble a renal tumour. Retroperitoneal and perirenal tumours may closely simulate renal tumours but can be distinguished on pyelography; they displace the ureter medially or laterally.

In many cases in which difficulty arises in the diagnosis of a swelling in the loin great help may be obtained by excretion urography (p. 481) or by retrograde pyelography by the injection into the renal pelvis and calices of a medium opaque to X-rays, through a ureteric catheter. By these means the renal pelvis and calices may be outlined clearly in their normal position, and any change in position or shape may indicate that the swelling is of renal origin.

THE DIFFERENTIAL DIAGNOSIS OF RADIOGRAPHIC SHADOWS IN THE ABDOMEN AND THE PELVIS

It is necessary for the true interpretation of radiographs that a clear conception should be held of the various conditions which may cast a shadow on an X-ray negative. In the diagnosis of cases of urinary disease much information may be gained by the use of X-rays, and not merely in the confirmation of the presence of calculi in some part of the urinary tract; in a good negative the outline and the size of the kidney can be seen, while, by means of excretion urography or by the direct injection of the ureter and the pelvis of the kidney with a radio-opaque solution, the size, position, and shape of either may be outlined accurately and compared with the normal (*Figs.* 478, 479). Whereas formerly only the presence of a distinct shadow was of value, the recent advances in radiology render a negative report, except in the few instances of a calculus of pure uric acid, almost of equal value. In a good negative after efficient alimentary preparation the outline of a normal kidney should be visible, lying opposite the bodies of the 1st, 2nd, and 3rd lumbar vertebrae (*Fig.* 478), and having an excursion of from 4 to 5 cm. in forced inspiration and expiration. A *renal calculus* (*Figs.* 479, 480) in a radiograph casts a shadow superimposed upon the renal shadow. If it is of triangular or branched outline,

it is almost certainly a renal calculus; but others may give a shadow of even, uniform density, of sharp outline, yet clearly renal as shown by the manner in which the opacity moves equally with the renal shadow in respiratory movements. In a negative taken laterally through the transverse axis of the patient, a renal calculus should make a shadow superimposed upon the bodies of the upper lumbar vertebrae, usually the second, unless the kidney is enlarged, when the shadow of a calculus may be displaced in front of the vertebral bodies. A stone composed of pure uric acid may give no shadow on a radiograph; one of calcium oxalate gives the most dense shadow; next in order of density is the phosphatic; those of urates, cystine, and xanthine give a less definite shadow. A radiolucent stone may,

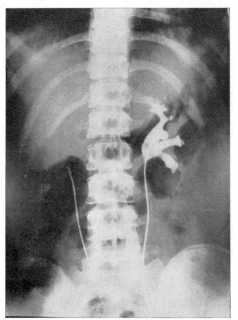

Fig. 481. Pyelogram outlining a pure uric acid stone in the left kidney. It gave no shadow on the plain film.

however, be shown as a negative shadow in an excretion or retrograde pyelogram; it must be distinguished from a tumour of the renal pelvis, an air bubble, or blood-clot. In the case of a stone the contrast medium is more likely to surround the shadow completely (*Fig.* 481) whilst a tumour will be attached at some point (*Fig.* 482). Blood-clot is irregular and an air bubble can be displaced in a second radiograph.

The shape of a shadow in the renal area will often indicate its position in the kidney and an excretion pyelogram will confirm it (*Fig.* 483). There are, however, several other conditions which may cast a shadow in the renal area, and it is necessary to differentiate these from the shadow of a renal calculus. The following are the most frequent:

1. Intestinal contents
2. Calcification of mesenteric lymph-nodes
3. Gall-stones, on the right side
4. Calcification of the costal cartilages
5. Caseous masses in a tuberculous kidney
6. Areas of calcification in a renal growth
7. Foreign bodies.

1. INTESTINAL CONTENTS may cast a shadow in the renal area owing to inefficient preparation of the patient or to the fact that he has recently taken as medicine bismuth, magnesium salts, etc. If any doubt exists a second examination should be made after further purgation. There may be some residue in the intestine from a recent barium-meal examination.

2. CALCIFICATION OF THE ABDOMINAL OR MESEN-TERIC LYMPH-NODES may cause a shadow in any part of the abdominal cavity. Though they are most frequently seen near the lower lumbar verte-brae or about the sacro-iliac joint, and therefore external to the renal shadow, they may be super-imposed upon the latter and cause difficulty in diagnosis. The shadow of a calcified node is usually mottled in appearance, small areas in the shadow showing increased density owing to the irregular deposition of lime salts; calcareous nodes are frequently multiple, but their chief characteristic is their range of mobility. Thus if more than one negative is taken with varying degrees of compression the shadows of calcareous nodes may show a varying position with regard to the renal shadow, whilst in a lateral view a glandular shadow is usually in front of the bodies of the vertebrae and not superimposed upon them. A calcified node may be placed im-mediately in front of the kidney and move equally with it, causing great difficulty in diag-nosis; or there may be a calculus in one kidney and calcareous nodes imitating calculi on the other side.

A pyelogram will show the relation of a calculus to the renal pelvis (*Fig.* 483).

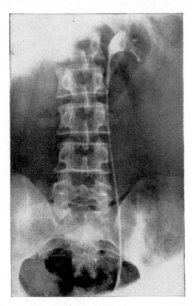

Fig. 482. Pyelogram showing a benign tumour in the left renal pelvis.

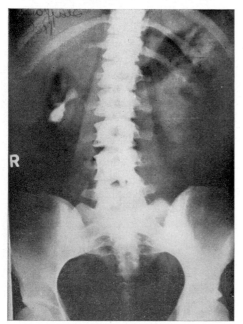

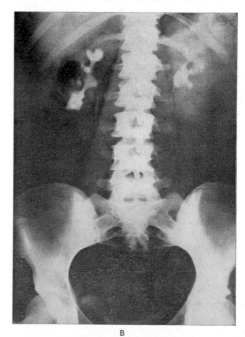

A   B

Fig. 483. A, Radiograph showing a dumb-bell shadow in the right renal area. B, The excretion urogram shows that the shadow is a stone occupying the lowest calix and pelvis of the right kidney. Treated by partial nephrectomy.

3. GALL-STONES may give a shadow in the renal area on the right side. They are frequently multiple, and may be seen to be faceted in a fusiform collection presenting the shape of the distended gall-bladder (*Fig.* 484). A single gall-stone

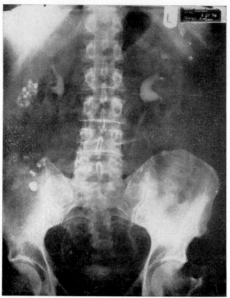

Fig. 484. Intravenous pyelogram showing also a collection of faceted stones in the gall-bladder, calcified mesenteric glands in the right iliac fossa, and phleboliths in the pelvis.

superimposed on the renal shadow may cause difficulty; the shadow of a gall-stone is less dense than is that of a renal stone, and it is frequently more dense in the central than in the peripheral part. In a lateral view a stone in the gall-bladder will occupy an anterior position in the abdomen, though one impacted in the common bile-duct may be seen opposite the body of the 1st or 2nd lumbar vertebra; in this case there will probably be jaundice. In a cholecystographic examination a gall-stone may cause a filling defect (negative shadow) in the area of the gall-bladder occupied by the dye. The distribution of stones in a horseshoe kidney may cause confusion until a pyelogram is done (*Fig.* 485).

4. CALCIFICATION OF THE COSTAL CARTILAGES may give a shadow in the renal area in an antero-posterior negative. The shadows are not dense, are hazy in outline, and tend to assume a horizontal or oblique axis. In a lateral view they will be placed immediately under the anterior abdominal wall.

5. CASEOUS MASSES IN A TUBERCULOUS KIDNEY. The shadow in this condition is rarely so defined as is that of a calculus, is of moderate density with blurred and indistinct margins, appearing as one or more blotches in the renal area; but occasionally, from the deposition of lime salts, it may be very like the radiograph of a calculus. (*Fig.* 361, p. 343.)

6. CALCAREOUS AREAS IN A RENAL CARCINOMA. Rarely faint ill-defined areas may be present in a renal carcinoma. There will, however, be symptoms of growth, such as haematuria and renal tumour, whilst a pyelographic examination will show deformity of the pelvis and renal calices.

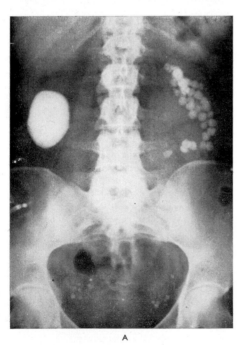

A

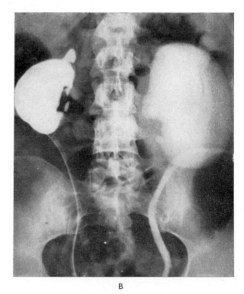

B

Fig. 485. A, Large single dense shadow on the right and multiple small ones on the left. B, Pyelography shows that the shadows are enclosed in the dilated pelves of a horse-shoe kidney. Note the inwardly pointing calices and the flower-vase pattern of the ureters.

7. A FOREIGN BODY, such as a shrapnel bullet, lying in front of or behind the kidney may mimic a calculus (*see Fig.* 486).

The line of the *normal ureter* lies anatomically along or just internal to the tips of the transverse processes of the 2nd to the 5th lumbar vertebrae, passes with a slight curve outwards in front of the sacro-iliac articulation, and then with a marked curve forwards and inwards to the base of the bladder. A shadow in this line may be due to a calculus in the ureter, but it must be differentiated carefully from other conditions. A calculus is usually small, rounded, or oval, with a long axis in the line of the ureter (*Fig.* 487). It may be found in any part of the course

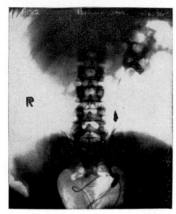

Fig. 486. Piece of shrapnel in the line of the left ureter. There is no dilatation of the ureter above the shadow. (Retrograde pyelogram.)

of the ureter, but it is seen most frequently in the lower end just before it enters the bladder. The conditions which may give a shadow that is likely to be mistaken for a ureteric calculus are:

1. A calcified lymphatic node
2. A concretion in the appendix or the intestinal contents
3. Phleboliths in the pelvis
4. A foreign body.

1. CALCIFIED LYMPH-NODES in the line of the ureter are placed most frequently in the angle between the last lumbar vertebra and the ala of the sacrum. They are usually multiple, forming a group in this situation in triangular form rather than in the longitudinal axis of the ureter; they are mottled in appearance, of irregular density, and are so movable that their position varies in successive radiographs. Should difficulty arise, the examination should be repeated after a radio-opaque catheter has been passed into the ureter by means of a cystoscope. In many cases a stereoscopic examination of the area with a catheter in the ureter or an X-ray by the 'double-shift' technique in which two exposures are made on the same film, the tube being moved laterally before the second exposure is made,

will show that the suspicious shadow is some distance from the ureter. A catheter may often be passed up the ureter alongside and past a calculus in the duct, but a stereoscopic examination will show that the two are actually in contact with each other.

2. A CONCRETION IN THE APPENDIX may occasionally give rise to a shadow in the line of the right ureter, suggesting a calculus with very similar clinical symptoms. Further examination with a radio-opaque catheter in the ureter will show that the shadow is extra-ureteric.

3. PHLEBOLITHS IN THE PELVIS are liable to be mistaken for ureteric calculi, but they often have a characteristic ring-like appearance. They are usually multiple and are placed towards the peripheral areas of the pelvis, often about the level of the ischial spine. A stereoscopic examination with an opaque catheter in the ureter will differentiate them from calculi, though it may not be possible to distinguish them from calcareous glands. It must not be forgotten that a calculus may be present in the ureter in addition to phleboliths, but the distinction can be made by excretion pyelography or radiography after the passage of a ureteric catheter (*see Fig.* 63, p. 64). *Figs.* 487, 488 show that the shadow of the ureter does not impinge on any of the numerous phleboliths present in the pelvis.

4. FOREIGN BODIES, especially after periods of war, may occasionally lie near the line of the ureter. They are usually more dense than calculi. (*Fig.* 486.)

A shadow may be present in a pelvic radiograph which must be differentiated from that of a vesical calculus. The latter is usually rounded or oval, occupies a fairly central position in the pelvis, and may show rings of varying density owing to the deposition of layers of urinary salts of different composition (*Fig.* 371, p. 347). Occasionally one or more vesical calculi may form a shadow in a more lateral position in successive negatives, when a suspicion of their presence in a diverticulum in the bladder will arise. The diagnosis of this condition is discussed below. The following conditions may give rise to radiographic shadows in the pelvis:

1. Prostatic calculi
2. Calcification of a uterine fibroid
3. Opaque masses in a dermoid cyst of the ovary
4. Phosphatic encrustation upon a vesical growth
5. Foreign bodies in the bladder
6. Urethral calculi.

1. PROSTATIC CALCULI may be single or multiple, but in the radiograph they occupy a position very low in the pelvis, often behind the shadow of the pubes (*Fig.* 489). They would not be seen by a cystoscope, but might be felt during the passage of any instrument through the prostatic urethra when the latter is ulcerated by the stone. They are palpable in the gland per rectum, either as a hard, inelastic nodule embedded in the prostate, or by the grating of multiple calculi on each other on pressure.

2. CALCIFICATION OF A FIBROID TUMOUR OF THE UTERUS gives a large, irregular shadow of varying degree of density (*Fig.* 490). Bimanual palpation of a tumour moving with the uterus would point to the diagnosis.

3. OVARIAN DERMOIDS may give rise to irregular shadows in the pelvis due to the formation

foreign bodies have been found in the bladder, either introduced by intent or by the accidental breaking off of a piece of catheter or the like. In some cases the shadow will show a central area of different density or even a metallic nucleus.

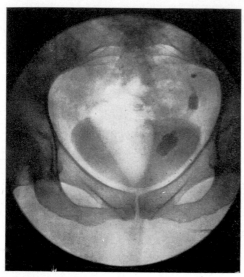

Fig. 487 Radiograph of three stones in the pelvic ureter: excretion urography, 30-min. film. (*Dr. Norman Henderson.*)

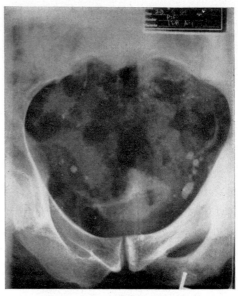

Fig. 488. Excretion pyelogram showing numerous phleboliths in the pelvis; the left ureter is seen passing between them. Note the 'bite' defect in the bladder caused by a solid carcinoma.

of bone or teeth in the cyst. They may be present in young adult life, and a tumour would be palpated on abdominal or pelvic examination.

4. PHOSPHATIC ENCRUSTATION UPON A VESICAL TUMOUR may occur in a case of growth in the presence of cystitis and give rise to faint ill-defined shadows in the pelvic radiograph. A cystoscopic examination will reveal the true nature of the lesion.

5. FOREIGN BODIES in the bladder may become so encrusted with urinary salts that a shadow like that of a calculus may be present. A variety of

6. URETHRAL CALCULI may be retained in the canal behind a stricture and enlarge in situ. They form a shadow in a radiograph above or below the pubic arch (*Fig.* 491).

Much assistance in the diagnosis of urinary disease apart from the presence of calculi may

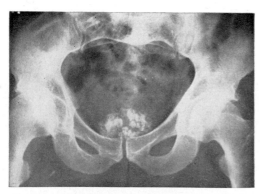

Fig. 489. Radiograph showing shadows in the pelvis due to multiple prostatic calculi.

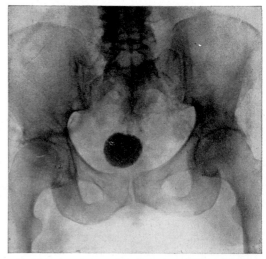

Fig. 490. Calcified fibroid simulating vesical calculus.

be afforded by means of radiography supplemented by methods used by the urologist. A good negative taken in a thin subject may show the outline and size of the kidneys so plainly that one of them may be demonstrated to be enlarged, or the irregularity of outline may give rise to a suspicion of malignant growth. Methods have been devised by which more information may be gained—for example, by the injection of gas into the presacral tissues or by direct

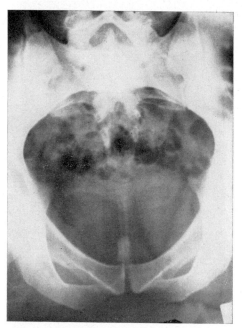

Fig. 491. Radiograph showing a shadow due to a cystine calculus in the prostatic urethra.

introduction into the renal pelvis, calices, and ureter of radio-opaque solutions, or by the injection into the circulation of radio-opaque dye which is excreted by the kidneys, or by the injection of such substances into the aorta.

Presacral gas insufflation consists in distending the fatty tissue around the kidney with oxygen, CO_2, or air; by this method a more distinct outline of the kidney is obtained. The injection is made into the retroperitoneal tissues in the presacral hollow. The needle is inserted beside the coccyx and is guided by a finger in the rectum; 800 ml. of filtered oxygen or air are *slowly* injected, the patient being turned to the opposite side after half the amount has passed in. He should then walk about for 15 minutes before films are taken in the anteroposterior and oblique positions, and tomographs if thought necessary. The outline of the kidneys can usually be clearly demonstrated and sometimes that of the liver and spleen. The method is harmless and usually painless (*Fig.* 492). Nowadays it is usually reserved for outlining suprarenal rather than renal masses.

The injection of radio-opaque solutions into the renal pelvis and ureter, combined with radiography (*retrograde pyelography* and *ureterography*), has a wide application and renders more precise information than can be obtained by the perirenal insufflation method; the two investigations can be successfully combined. A dilute solution of 25 per cent sodium diatrizoate ('Hypaque') or 35 per cent meglumine iothalamate, the drug used for excretion urography, is used. For this method of pyelography (the 'ascending') a ureteric catheter is passed by means of the cystoscope to the renal pelvis; the solution is injected very slowly by means of a small syringe or allowed to run in by gravitation until the patient begins to feel discomfort in the loin, an accurate measure of the amount of fluid injected

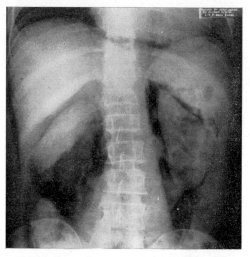

Fig. 492. Presacral oxygen combined with intravenous pyelography, showing normal kidneys.

being recorded. The pelvis of the normal kidney will hold an average of 6 ml. before pain is produced. A radiograph is taken immediately, when an exact outline of the renal pelvis and calices is displayed as a dense shadow (*see Fig.* 479, p. 473, and *Fig.* 494). In cases of renal distension a much larger amount can be injected before pain is produced. In these cases it is better in practice to take a succession of radiographs with the increasing amounts of fluid injected rather than to await the onset of pain. Thus if on examination it is found that the patient feels no discomfort after the injection of about 10 ml., the injection should be stopped and a radiograph taken; further injection is then made and a second or even a third negative exposed. In renal distension the first radiograph may show only a blurred shadow from the dilution of the solution with the fluid in the renal pelvis, but the subsequent negatives will show the extent of the distension and whether the stress is thrown on the renal tissue or on the pelvis. In cases of suspected hydronephrosis it is advisable to draw off the urine in the distended kidney by the catheter before the injection is begun (*Figs.* 493–496).

This examination can be conducted under a local anaesthetic so that the patient can indicate when the discomfort due to the distension of the renal pelvis begins. Frequently the patient is able to affirm that the pain produced by the injection is exactly similar to that experienced during his previous clinical attacks—often a valuable point in diagnosis. The examination can be conducted under low spinal anaesthesia or a caudal block, but many patients prefer a general anaesthetic and this is quite safe if the

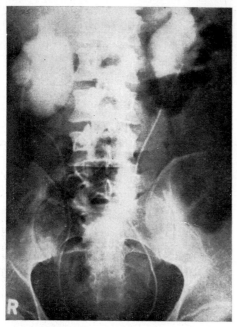

Fig. 493. Retrograde pyelograms in a case of bilateral hydronephrosis associated with pelvi-ureteric obstruction.

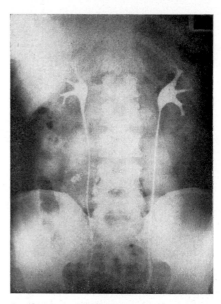

Fig. 494. A normal bilateral retrograde pyelogram.

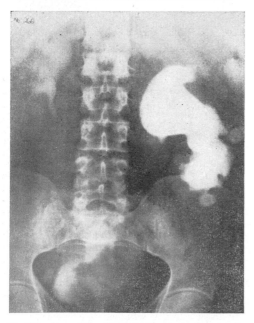

Fig. 495. An excretion pyelogram showing a giant calculus in the left kidney. Note the filling defect in the bladder caused by a large papillary tumour.

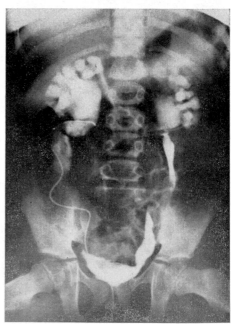

Fig. 496. Retrograde pyelogram showing bilateral congenital hydro-ureter and hydronephrosis in a girl.

injection is made slowly. Occasionally a calculus which has only yielded a faint shadow in a radiograph is shown much more distinctly after an injection of contrast medium around it. Incipient dilatation of the renal pelvis, changes in the normal outline of the pelvis or calices, or kinking of the upper ureter can be identified readily.

The determination of a normal renal pelvis by radiography has also aided the diagnosis in many cases of doubtful abdominal tumours in which the clinical data have raised a suspicion of renal disease. There may be doubt as to whether a tumour palpable in the abdomen and causing pain in the loin is a renal tumour or whether it originates in the colon, gall-bladder, pancreas, or suprarenal gland. Examination by pyelography may demonstrate a normal renal pelvis which would in many cases exclude any disease of the kidney. In one case a patient, aged 47, complained of pain in her left loin, where a rounded tumour presenting the characters of a renal swelling was felt. She gave a history of slight haematuria and the urine contained a small amount of albumin and pus. On cystoscopic examination there was subacute cystitis; the ureteric orifices appeared to be normal, and the urinary efflux from each was stained a deep blue colour within five minutes of an intravenous injection of indigocarmine. A pyelographic examination of the left kidney showed that the renal pelvis and calices were small and normal, so that the diagnosis of renal disease was negatived. Abdominal exploration revealed a carcinoma of the colon near the splenic flexure, for which resection was performed. Thus pyelography may be used not only in the diagnosis of a renal lesion, but also as a means of excluding renal disease in cases in which the diagnosis may be difficult.

To obtain a radiograph of the ureter it is advisable to pass a ureteric catheter with an acorn tip only a short distance into the ureter before making the injection; in this way any dilatation or deviation from the normal line of the ureter is demonstrated, whereas the passage of the catheter along the whole length of the canal might straighten out the latter. In some cases the passage of the catheter may be obstructed in the ureter; in these the injection should be made with the catheter in situ, when the fluid may find its way past the obstruction and radiography may show a dilated or tortuous ureter (*Fig.* 496) with dilatation of the pelvis of the kidney.

Occasionally a radiographic picture of the bladder is required to determine the size of a diverticulum, the vesical opening of which has been found on cystoscopy. For this purpose the same type and concentration of dye is used as in retrograde pyelography. Radiographs are then taken in both the anteroposterior and the oblique planes; it is also of advantage to repeat the exposures after the patient has voluntarily voided the vesical contents, when the diverticulum

may be seen to remain filled with the solution. (*See Fig.* 691, p. 688.)

Excretion urography is a method of pyelography consisting of the *intravenous injection* of non-toxic fluids of high iodine content and depends upon the excretion of the radio-opaque solution by the kidney. For this purpose 40–60 ml. of 45 per cent sodium diatrizoate ('Hypaque') or meglumine iothalamate 60 per cent is injected into a vein after the patient has abstained from drinking any liquid for at least six hours. Radiographs are then taken at intervals of 1, 5, 15, and 30 minutes after the injection. In cases in which the kidneys are of normal efficiency, a distinct shadow should be obtained of the renal pelvis and calices of each side in the first picture, increasing in definition in the second (*see Fig.* 478, p. 472). The outlines of the ureters may be seen and in the later pictures the bladder is outlined in the pelvis. This test differs from the ascending method in being dependent upon the functional efficiency of the kidney; if this is impaired the test may fail to show any shadow owing to lack of excretion of the fluid, and therefore it may be used as a test of function as well as a radiographic test. The simplicity of the method has much to recommend it, but it must be said that the outlines of the renal pelvis and calices may be indistinct, and insufficient to rely upon for accurate diagnosis, in which case it has to be sometimes supplemented by the ascending method. In cases in which there is obstruction to the ureter, dilatation of the latter and of the renal pelvis may be distinctly seen. In cases of vesical tumour a distinct filling defect may be seen in the bladder in the later negatives (*see Fig.* 488, p. 478). It is often advisable to carry out the examination while the patient is maintained in a modified Trendelenburg position, by which means increased definition of the renal pelvis and calices may be obtained. Compression of the lower ends of the ureters by a pneumatic belt and pads suitably placed after the first pictures have been taken improves the definition and filling even more. The interpretation of the films is not easy, and requires a good deal of experience.

By cine-radiography and the use of an image-intensifier during pyelography it is possible to see the contractions of the renal pelvis and ureter and the site of an obstruction. The emptying contraction of the bladder can be watched and any diverticulum be seen to fill up during the act of micturition.

Aortography is done by the translumbar route or by catheterization of the femoral artery (Seldinger's method). In the translumbar method 20–30 ml. of 60 per cent meglumine iothalamate are injected directly into the upper part of the abdominal aorta in order to outline the renal vascular system. It is carried out under general or local anaesthesia with the patient in the prone position; a long needle, up to 10 in. in length, is introduced from the left side of the body of the 1st lumbar vertebra below the last rib and passed forwards, inwards, and upwards to enter the aorta above the origin of the renal arteries; 30 ml of solution are injected quickly and films are taken as soon as the injection starts and as rapidly as possible whilst it continues. The early ones show the arterial system and the later ones show the nephrographic phase when the whole of the renal substance is opacified; they may also show the veins and sometimes some filling of the pelvis. (*Fig.* 497.)

to be functionless and shrunken, when it cannot be felt; but the remaining organ may be enlarged in a compensatory degree and may be distinctly palpable. One must remember the danger of regarding an enlarged kidney as the diseased organ when it may in reality be the only functioning one. The kidney of normal size and position is not palpable from the abdomen, or on bimanual examination with one hand on the loin; but, in a thin subject, the lower pole may be felt

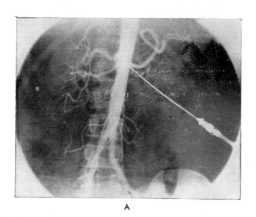

A

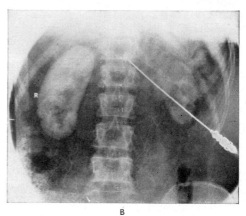

B

Fig. 497. A, Aortogram done by the translumbar method; arterial phase. The right renal artery, seen below the hepatic, is of normal size. The left, seen below the splenic, is small. B, Nephrographic phase in the same case. The left kidney is small and less densely opacified than the right; it contained a papillary carcinoma in the upper calix.

In the femoral approach by the Seldinger technique (now by far the more commonly used) a fine catheter is passed into the femoral artery and up the aorta as far as the renal vessels where the contrast medium is injected. A method of selective renal angiography has been developed in which the tip of the catheter can be turned to enter one or other renal artery; this gives the best demonstration of the renal vessels but it requires the use of an image intensifier with a television monitor.

The investigation is of value in demonstrating new growths of the kidney, where pooling of the contrast occurs in the growth, and in detecting congenital abnormalities. It has been of use in verifying the existence of a solitary kidney. It can also differentiate tumours from cysts, which may also be aspirated under radiological control.

Nephrotomography. In this investigation 45 per cent sodium diatrizoate or 60 per cent meglumine iothalamate is injected rapidly into an antecubital vein, and a series of tomograms is taken at 1-cm. levels through the whole thickness of the kidney. This investigation has its greatest value in distinguishing a renal tumour from a cyst; the tumour is irregularly and densely opacified; the cyst contains no vessels and remains radiolucent. (*Figs.* 498, 499.)

A kidney may be enlarged and yet not palpable from the fact that it is either wholly above the costal margin or obscured by the liver or the thick abdominal walls of the patient. On the other hand a kidney may be so diseased as

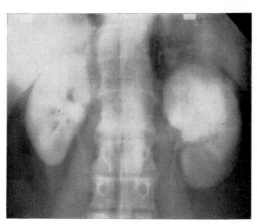

Fig. 498. Nephrotomogram showing a solid tumour (carcinoma) in the upper pole of the left kidney. (*Figs.* 498, 499 *reproduced by courtesy of Dr. John L. Emmett.*)

to descend between the hands on the patient's taking a full inspiration; if, therefore, a kidney can be felt easily on bimanual examination, it is either unduly mobile or enlarged. If is often difficult to say if a kidney that is movable is also enlarged to a slight degree; and a kidney which was thought clinically to be enlarged has often been found to be of normal size when exposed; this is in part due to the thick coverings of the abdominal wall, or to the amount of fatty tissue surrounding the organ.

If the kidney is definitely enlarged, it remains to determine the nature of the enlargement; in this one is guided, not only by the physical characters of the tumour present, but also by other symptoms that are associated with it, more especially, perhaps, by the altered characters of the urine. The kidney may be enlarged only slightly, as in tuberculosis, pyelonephritis, incipient hydronephrosis, or carcinoma; or may be enlarged to a considerable degree in polycystic disease, hydro- or pyonephrosis, and in some forms of malignant growth. From the physical examination of the enlarged organ it is often possible to say that the swelling is fluid or solid in nature, but it is seldom that a true diagnosis of the lesion can be made from palpation of the kidney alone. In the following diseases, in which renal enlargement is usually present, the diagnosis must be arrived at by the consideration of associated symptoms.

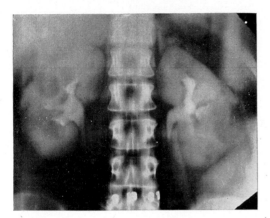

Fig. 499. Nephrotomogram showing multiple circular radiolucent areas in both kidneys indicating multiple bilateral renal cysts.

In *renal tuberculosis* the disease occurs in a miliary or in a caseous form. Miliary tuberculosis occurs as a part of a general tuberculosis, usually in children, is bilateral, and causes no tumour. The caseous variety occurs most frequently in young adults who have had tuberculosis elsewhere in the body, as a disease in one kidney, in which one or several foci may be present. These enlarge and soften to form a tuberculous abscess, which invades the medullary tissues, to open eventually and discharge its contents into the renal pelvis. (*Fig.* 362, p. 343.) The kidney is slightly enlarged and tender, and there are persistent pyuria and haematuria in small amounts. The epithelial lining of the ureter is quickly invaded by the tuberculous process, becoming thickened and infiltrated, and at the same time shortened, so that cystoscopically the ureteric orifice is seen to be drawn upwards (*Fig.* 684, p. 680). An early symptom of renal tuberculosis is increased frequency of micturition, even before the bladder has become infected in the downward progress of the disease. The

ureter may be felt to be thickened per rectum or per vaginam, or other tuberculous foci may be found in the prostate, vesiculae seminales, or epididymes in the male. A thorough search should be made for tubercle bacilli in the urine by microscopy, specific culture, and guinea-pig inoculation. In cases in which caseous areas are present in the kidney, a radiograph may show blurred, indistinct shadows in the renal area, and a pyelographic examination will show a lack of definition of one or more renal calices (*Fig.* 500) and occasionally cavitation of the kidney.

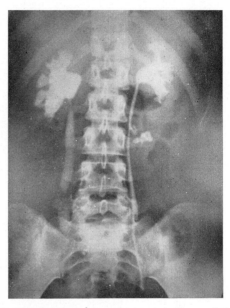

Fig. 500. Pyelogram showing tuberculous disease of the right kidney and ureter. The pelvis is dilated and the lower calices are clubbed. The ureter is narrowed at its upper end but dilated below. The left kidney is normal. Note the calcified tuberculous mesenteric lymph-nodes to the left of L3.

Intravenous pyelography may fail to show a shadow on the affected side owing to inefficient function of the kidney in the excretion of the dye.

In *pyelonephritis* the kidney may be slightly enlarged, together with renal pain, pyuria, and general malaise. Pyelonephritis is usually bilateral, and due to some infective or obstructive lesion in the lower urinary tract, symptoms of which are usually obvious (*see* PYURIA, p. 678). Bacteriological examination by culture of a catheter specimen of urine is essential to the diagnosis.

Malignant tumours of the kidney give rise either to an irregular nodular enlargement of the kidney, or to a general, uniform, solid tumour. There is usually aching pain in the loin, with intermittent attacks of profuse haematuria that occur when the growth has infiltrated the renal pelvis or sometimes sooner. The bleeding may be so profuse that clots are formed in the renal calices, pyramidal in shape, which in their passage down the ureter give rise to typical colic. Long worm-shaped clots from formation in the ureter may also be present. The malignant tumours found in the kidney are of several varieties, and their origin and exact pathological nature have given rise to much discussion in recent years. The true sarcoma exists, but is rare, forming but a small percentage of the malignant renal tumours. It gives rise to renal enlargement and intermittent haematuria, is usually extremely malignant, and is accompanied by early metastases. The more common type of renal tumour in the parenchyma of the kidney, the adenocarcinoma, arises in the renal tubular epithelium. It was formerly supposed to arise in small aberrant areas of suprarenal tissue which

symptoms are slight. Haematuria occurs without any apparent exciting cause, and there may be renal colic from the passage of clots down the ureter; the tumour may be of fair size before any haematuria is noticed. Metastases to lungs, brain, liver, and bones (skull, vertebrae, pelvis, ribs, upper humerus, and upper femur) are common and, indeed, these manifestations may be the first evidence of the presence of the renal primary.

Another form of malignant tumour that occurs in the kidney is that which arises from embryonic tissues, and to which the name of nephroblastoma (Wilms's tumour) has been applied. These tumours are formed of mixed tissues, such as striated and non-striated muscle, cartilage or

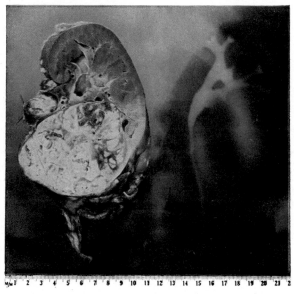

Fig. 501. Pyelogram showing a filling defect in the lower pole with elongation and displacement of the lowest calix. The superimposed kidney contains an adenocarcinoma in the lower pole which produced the defect. (*Middlesex Hospital Photographic Department.*)

may be found in this situation and was known as a hypernephroma (Grawitz tumour). The tumours described by Grawitz, however, the 'so-called lipomata', were small, multiple, and often benign. The malignant tumours arise in any part of the kidney, are often fairly well defined from the renal tissues, and are seen on macroscopical section to contain areas of yellow colour and areas of organizing blood-clot from former interstitial haemorrhage (*Fig.* 501). Microscopically, they show large polyhedral cells, with clear cytoplasm, arranged in an alveolar, tubular, or papillary formation somewhat resembling the suprarenal cortical tissue; in some specimens granular cells predominate. They are now classified under the term 'adenocarcinoma'. Their rate of growth varies enormously, but the main symptoms are fairly constant. There is aching in the loin, and enlargement of the kidney may be found on examination, but at first the

bone, and epithelial structures in tubular or glandular form. They grow in the renal tissues, expanding these to form a spurious capsule. They occur most frequently in children, and haematuria is infrequent. These tumours are of rapid growth, are exceedingly malignant, and the existence of a large tumour in the loin may be the earliest symptom.

Thus, the occurrence of a renal tumour, accompanied by intermittent attacks of haematuria, especially if profuse, should always give suspicion of renal growth in an adult. Renal tuberculosis and calculus both may give rise to renal enlargement, but the haematuria is seldom profuse; with calculus, the haematuria is often brought on or increased by exertion, whereas with growth it may come on at any time, even during rest. At the same time it should be remembered that both profuse haematuria and renal enlargement may arise from a vesical tumour which obstructs the normal flow of urine from the ureteric orifice; in all cases, therefore, a full urological examination should be made before any operative measure is carried out. The rapid development of a *varicocele*, especially on the right side, is rare but is a point significant of renal growth. The pyelographic picture of a renal growth is usually distinctive. There is displacement or destruction of one or more calices

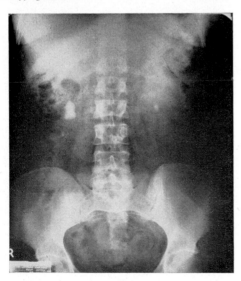

Fig. 502. Pyelogram in a case of carcinoma of the right kidney. The crescentic filling defect is characteristic of a space-occupying lesion.

and deformity of the renal pelvis, with frequently a filling defect in the latter (*Fig.* 502). A filling defect in the pelvis alone, perhaps with dilatation of the calices, is more suggestive of a pelvic new growth of the papillary type.

Hydronephrosis and *pyonephrosis* form definite enlargements of the kidney, which may attain a large size. The tumour is oval or rounded, smooth, and gives a sense of tenseness or elasticity, while occasionally distinct fluctuation may be obtained. Pyelography assists the diagnosis very materially (pp. 479 et seq. and *Fig.* 502). A hydronephrosis occurs when there is a partial ureteric obstruction, or in cases of repeated attacks of temporarily complete obstruction to the ureter. Bilateral hydronephrosis may also arise from the back-pressure due to any obstruction of the normal passage of urine from the bladder. Hydronephrosis is often accompanied by renal pain, sometimes by renal colic, and occasionally by haematuria. The tumour may show marked changes in size, from the varying character of the lesion producing the obstruction; thus, if the ureter is wholly blocked, the tumour will increase in size and become more tense, whilst if the obstruction is partially relieved the tumour will diminish, synchronously with the passage of a larger quantity of urine of low specific gravity. The presence of any obstruction to the normal flow of urine from the kidney predisposes to the onset of infection of the kidney by micro-organisms, so that a hydronephrosis may become converted into a pyonephrosis, or the latter may arise from the obstruction to the ureter of a kidney alread they seat of pyelitis. The physical examination of a kidney distended with urine or with pus shows practically no difference between them, but with pyonephrosis

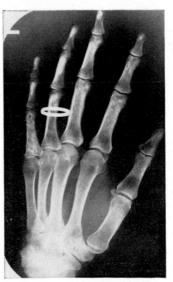

A   B

Fig. 503. A, Recurrent bilateral calculi of the kidneys in a woman with a parathyroid adenoma. (Plain X-ray of abdomen.) B, The left hand of the same patient showing cystic changes in the 5th proximal phalanx.

other indications are usually present to assist the diagnosis. Examination of the urine will reveal the presence of pus at some time, although, if the ureter is wholly obstructed at the time of examination, pus may be absent if the other kidney and the bladder are normal. If, however, the pyonephrosis is renal calculus, so that a careful inquiry into the history of the case for symptoms of calculus may give important indications, and X-ray examination may be of service (pp. 474 et seq.) unless the stone has been passed. Very occasionally palpation of a kidney enlarged from

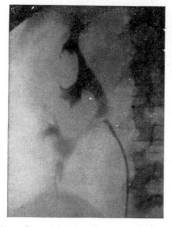
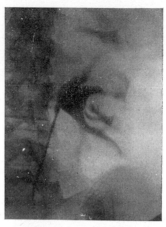

Fig. 504. Ascending pyelograms in a case of bilateral polycystic disease of the kidneys, after injection of sodium iodide. Note the elongation of the calices on each side. (*Professor J. M. W. Morison.*)

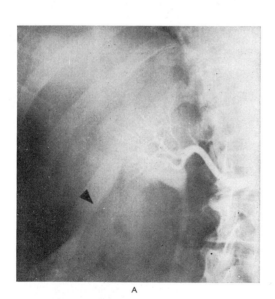
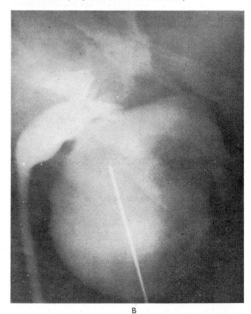

A   B

Fig. 505. Arteriogram demonstrating a renal cyst. A, Demonstrates (anterior view) the avascular filling defect. B, Demonstrates the cyst after aspiration and confirmation of the diagnosis by injection of contrast medium (posterior view). (*F. Starer.*)

ureter is blocked only partially, pus will be found in the urine; in the intermittent form, pus may be present in large quantities at intervals coinciding with the decrease in the size of the renal tumour. With pyonephrosis, also, there will be the general evidence of suppuration, namely, raised temperature, sweating, pallor, and often diarrhoea. The most frequent causation of calculous disease will give rise to distinct crepitation from the friction of one stone upon another. *Fig.* 503 illustrates recurrent bilateral calculi of the kidneys in a woman with raised serum calcium and lowered serum phosphate. After removal of the parathyroid tumour and pyelolithotomy there has been no more stone formation and the case also demonstrates the relationship between urinary calculi and the parathyroid glands, because of the influence of the latter upon the calcium metabolism of the body.

Hydatid cyst of the kidney may give rise to a tumour in the loin exactly resembling a hydronephrosis, and would usually be diagnosed as such. The discovery of hooklets (*Fig.* 74, p. 79) or hydatid elements in the urine, or in the fluid aspirated from a renal cyst, will point to the nature of the disease.

Polycystic disease of the kidney may occur in children or in adults, and forms a tumour which is commonly lateral, though that of one side may be larger than the other. In adults the disease causes practically no trouble, except the presence of the tumour, in the early stages, but later, symptoms of renal insufficiency develop, with thirst, drowsiness, and vomiting. The tumour gives the usual physical signs of a renal enlargement, and may attain a great size on both sides. In thin subjects rounded prominences may be felt on the surface of the tumour. There may be aching pain in the loins, and, occasionally, marked haematuria. The urine is of low specific gravity, is increased in amount, and in the absence of blood often contains a small amount of protein. The disease is usually accompanied by arteriosclerosis and raised blood-pressure. Indeed, death may result from hypertensive cardiac failure or a cerebrovascular accident. The character of the urine and the bilateral renal tumour are usually sufficient data upon which to form a diagnosis, but with a unilateral tumour, such as occasionally occurs, the diagnosis is very difficult. A hydronephrotic or pyonephrotic kidney may give evidence of fluctuation which will not be obtained with a polycystic kidney. The pyelographic picture of polycystic disease (*Fig.* 504) shows the calices to be considerably lengthened and drawn out by the disease, but shows no cavitation and rarely any pelvic dilatation as in a hydronephrosis (*Fig.* 493, p. 479).

A large *solitary cyst* of the kidney may produce a renal tumour and may cause aching in one loin. A pyelographic examination shows the calices to be displaced by the enlarging cyst, and in spite of the absence of haematuria, a diagnosis of renal growth is usually made and the true cause of the disease is only found by aortography; the renal cyst is avascular in contrast to the marked tumour circulation seen in a renal carcinoma. The cyst can then be confirmed by aspiration under X-ray control. (*Fig.* 505.)

Harold Ellis.

KIDNEY, TESTS OF FUNCTION OF

The kidney is an important organ for maintaining the chemical composition of the body within narrow limits. The glomerulus is a passive filter, allowing fluid of the same composition as extracellular fluid to pass into the tubular lumen: thus the filtrate contains very little protein, but is otherwise almost identical with plasma. The tubules actively adjust the composition of this filtrate by reabsorption from and secretion into it, and the difference in composition between plasma and urine reflects tubular function.

Renal disease usually affects both tubules and glomeruli. However, sometimes damage to one is so predominant that the effects appear to be purely tubular or purely glomerular. Glomerular dysfunction, without renal disease, can be the consequence of reduced blood flow, and therefore of reduced filtration.

GLOMERULAR FUNCTION

No test of glomerular function can distinguish between true renal disease and dysfunction due to reduced renal blood flow. However, the presence of cells, protein, and casts in the urine suggests renal pathology.

If glomerular function is grossly reduced, the most obvious clinical sign is *oliguria* (less than 400 ml. of urine in 24 hours), or even complete anuria. Substances depending mainly on passive filtration for their excretion accumulate in the extracellular fluid. Amongst other constituents, the concentrations of plasma *urea* and *creatinine* rise. Urea originates from breakdown of dietary and tissue protein, and levels are more affected than those of creatinine by changes in protein intake, tissue damage, or gastro-intestinal haemorrhage. However, it is most unlikely that plasma urea concentration will much exceed the 'normal range' if renal function is absolutely normal, even if the diet is grossly abnormal or if there has been massive trauma; certainly urea levels over about 16 mmol/l (100 mg./dl.) signify renal dysfunction. For this reason, and because precision of urea estimation is better than that of creatinine at near normal limits, I feel that plasma urea is often more sensitive as an index of renal dysfunction; however, many workers prefer creatinine estimation. If the concentration of either is significantly elevated, the glomerular filtration rate is reduced, and no further tests of renal function are necessary.

The kidneys have a large reserve capacity, and normal levels of urea and creatinine do not exclude glomerular dysfunction, minor degrees of which may be detectable using clearance tests. In clinical practice urea and creatinine clearances are most commonly used. The theoretical concept of clearance is the volume of blood which could be completely cleared of the substance in unit time. This may be calculated by measuring the amount excreted in an *accurately* timed specimen (concentration in that specimen (U) times volume (V)), dividing by the time of collection (T) to give the amount in unit time, and dividing by the concentration in the plasma (P):

$$\text{Clearance} = \frac{U \cdot V}{T \cdot P}$$

The units of concentration must be the same for U and P. It should be noted that the biggest difficulty of the test is ensuring an accurate and complete collection of the timed specimen. The longer the period of collection, the lower the percentage error is likely to be.

If the clearance is to be a true measure of glomerular function, the substance to be measured should neither be reabsorbed nor secreted by tubular cells. Only inulin is thought to fulfil these criteria. It is not suitable for routine clinical use, since constant infusion is needed to maintain a steady blood-level of a substance foreign to the body. Urea diffuses out of the tubular lumen and creatinine is secreted into it by about the same small amount, and urea clearance is slightly lower and creatinine clearance slightly higher than inulin clearance. However, either parallels inulin clearance accurately enough for clinical use. The clearance of urea is not affected by diet. Infected or stale urine should not be used since both urea and creatinine may be destroyed by bacterial action. Urea is more likely to be significantly affected than creatinine, although this action may be partially inhibited by using mercurial salts as preservative.

TUBULAR FUNCTION

The renal tubules alter the composition of the glomerular filtrate by reabsorption and secretion of different constituents. The degree of reabsorption is often hormonally controlled. For instance, reabsorption of water is increased by antidiuretic hormone, and of sodium by aldosterone; both of these hormones circulate in high levels if the subject is water depleted, and both disappear on water loading.

Chronic Tubular Disease. Tests of tubular function may be necessary if a relatively 'pure' tubular lesion is suspected (for instance, in the presence of hypercalcaemia). If such a lesion is present, the patient will be polyuric, due to failure to reabsorb water normally. Plasma potassium, urate, and phosphate levels may be low (in the presence of glomerular dysfunction they are high), also due to failure of normal reabsorption, and bicarbonate concentration is often reduced because of failure of the mechanisms of hydrogen ion secretion (*see* HYDROGEN ION HOMEOSTASIS, p. 402). If glomerular function is near normal, levels of urea and creatinine (excretion of which are not significantly affected by tubular action) are not raised in the plasma, although, if water loss causes glomerular insufficiency, they may rise slightly. Amino-acids, normally reabsorbed in the proximal tubule, may be present in abnormal amounts in the urine. Such tubular lesions are sometimes known as the 'Fanconi syndrome'.

Water Concentration Test. This is the simplest test for suspected tubular disease. It depends on the fact that water restriction leads to antidiuretic hormone (ADH) secretion. If distal tubular function is normal this, in turn, causes reabsorption of water from the tubular lumen. As water is reabsorbed, urinary solute concentration rises, until urinary osmolality and specific gravity are well above those of plasma.

Procedure. Food and water are withheld after 18.00 hours. At 07.00 hours on the following day the bladder is emptied and the specimen discarded. At 08.00 hours the bladder is again emptied, and if the osmolality of this specimen is 850 mmol/kg (specific gravity 1·022) or above the test may be terminated. If it is below this figure the measurement should be repeated on a specimen passed at 09.00 hours. Plasma osmolality may be estimated, and the plasma-to-urine ratio should be above 3. Failure to concentrate indicates either impaired tubular response to ADH or lack of the hormone. If the latter diagnosis (diabetes insipidus) is suspected, the test should be repeated after injection of 5 units of the oily suspension of pitressin tannate at 19.00 hours. If the result is now normal diabetes insipidus is the likely diagnosis, if it is still abnormal tubular damage is likely.

Osmolality will be affected by glycosuria, 150 mmol/l (2·7 g./dl.) contributing 150 mmol/kg to the osmolality reading. The same concentration adds 0·001 to the specific gravity, which also gives falsely high readings in the presence of proteinuria and contrast media used in intravenous pyelography. In these circumstances high readings do not indicate normal tubular function. Specific gravity readings should be made with care. Hydrometers are usually calibrated at 15° C., and measurements should not be made on freshly passed urine; 0·001 should be added to the reading for every 3° C. above 15° C. The hydrometer should be floating freely; if it touches the wall of the container false readings will be obtained.

Acute Renal Failure. In suspected acute renal failure the tests of tubular function fulfil a different purpose. An acute 'shock' episode produces hypotension, and a consequently reduced glomerular filtration rate, even without renal damage. Neither plasma urea and creatinine levels, nor their clearances, can distinguish the 'prerenal' phase from the phase when reduced blood flow has caused renal damage. Since, in renal damage of this kind, both glomeruli and tubules are affected, evidence of tubular insufficiency will indicate renal pathology. In the presence of both tubular and glomerular lesions the plasma findings will reflect the reduced GFR, but analysis of the urine may detect tubular dysfunction.

If the patient is still collapsed or dehydrated the conditions are similar to those of the water deprivation test, and in the presence of normal renal function osmolality (and specific gravity) will be high. Urinary sodium concentration will be negligible due to maximum aldosterone secretion. If, however, the tubules are unable to respond to the hormones because of renal disease, any urine passed will be inappropriately dilute and have a sodium concentration over 30 mmol/l. It must be stressed that once the patient has been rehydrated the *appropriate* response is to pass a dilute urine of high sodium concentration, and these tests cannot be used to determine if renal disease is present, since stringent fluid restriction is not justified. The presence of protein and casts in the urine and continuing oliguria are then in favour of renal damage.

Joan F. Zilva.

LASSITUDE OR WEARINESS

This is a feature of many, many diseases. It is a symptom of many, many patients, with and without disease. It is so non-specific as to have little value in differential diagnosis. Patients with heart disease, infectious, inflammatory, and many other conditions will often add lassitude to the end of a long list of complaints. But one of the most difficult problems in clinical medicine is the patient who just does not feel well but who has no symptoms to suggest disease of a particular site or system. The following conditions are those which deserve consideration in such a case.
MALIGNANT DISEASE. Lassitude may be the only symptom of patients with malignant disease, sometimes even with widely disseminated disease. Certain tumours which are notorious for the silence of their primaries and which may therefore present in this way include carcinoma of the caecum and large bowel, carcinoma of the ovary, and carcinoma of the bronchus.

Lymphomas also have this habit and lassitude is an important symptom in young adults with conditions like Hodgkin's disease. The peripheral blood is often normal though the E.S.R. may be raised. Bone-marrow may be helpful but in the absence of lymphadenopathy, lymphangiography is a particularly useful investigation.
ANAEMIA. Lassitude is a characteristic symptom of anaemia, whatever the cause. An insidious onset of anaemia, presenting only with lassitude, is most likely in iron deficiency, pernicious anaemia, dietary disorders, malabsorption, and chronic renal failure. Inspection of the mucous membranes followed by estimation of haemoglobin level and examination of a blood-film is essential.
OTHER BLOOD DISEASES. Patients with polycythaemia rubra vera, like those with anaemia, complain of being easily tired. This diagnosis is often suggested by the patient's appearance and hepatosplenomegaly is a usual finding. In chronic leukaemias and myelofibrosis there is often a period of several years of lassitude and other minor symptoms before the diagnosis becomes apparent. Again there is hepatosplenomegaly with characteristic changes in peripheral blood and bone-marrow.
INFECTIONS. Tuberculosis is a typical example of an infection which may present with mild constitutional symptoms such as lassitude. This may be accompanied by fever and night sweats but not necessarily by cough or haemoptysis. Chest X-ray is therefore an essential investigation. Tuberculosis of the gut and tuberculous disease elsewhere may present similarly. In patients with rheumatic heart disease, lassitude may be the main symptom of infective endocarditis, almost always accompanied by fever. Surface signs such as splinter haemorrhages, clubbing, and Osler's nodes are unusual and culture should be carried out if there is even a suspicion and repeated for as long as the suspicion remains.

Lassitude is a prominent feature of infectious mononucleosis which should be considered particularly in older children and young adults. Lymphadenopathy is usual and there may be splenomegaly. The diagnosis is made by examination of peripheral blood which shows increased and atypical mononuclear cells. The Paul-Bunnell test is useful confirmation. Lassitude may persist for many months. Many other infections begin with lassitude and it is only when more characteristic features develop that a diagnosis can be made.
CONNECTIVE TISSUE DISORDERS. Lassitude is seldom the major feature of connective tissue disorders though it may be prominent in systemic lupus erythematosus and occasionally in temporal arteritis. Examination of the temporal arteries is essential in elderly patients with lassitude or fever, who may not have headaches. A high E.S.R. is a useful clue to the presence of these disorders.
ENDOCRINE DISORDERS. Lassitude may be a striking feature of hypothyroidism and it is easy to overlook other diagnostic symptoms and signs, especially in an early case.
PSYCHIATRIC DISORDERS. Weariness and lack of desire to do anything are features of depression and are common complaints in patients in problem situations, whether financial, domestic, or marital. Inquiry should be made for other symptoms of depression such as sleep disturbance.
GASTRO-INTESTINAL DISORDERS. It is characteristic of coeliac disease that the symptoms are insidious and may not be obviously related to the gastro-intestinal tract: lassitude is common. Careful inquiry about bowel habits should be made. Clues will usually be found in the blood (megaloblastic anaemia) but it may be necessary to proceed to faecal fat estimation and small-bowel biopsy. Crohn's disease may present similarly with little or no abdominal pain or bowel disturbance.
DRUGS. Some people feel weary because they are taking (often unnecessarily) drugs like tranquillizers.
NORMALITY. Many normal people complain of lassitude. Whether due to the stresses and cares of life, extremes of weather or unaccustomed exertion, it leads to fear of disease and medical consultation.

E. C. Huskisson.

LEG, ULCERATION OF

Ulceration of the leg may be classified under four headings: (1) *Non-infective ulcers*; these include those that are not due to any specific

16*

infection, but which are caused by various factors that interfere with the vitality of the part by injury, poor circulation, or deficient innervation of the tissue. (2) *Infective ulcers* resulting from the direct action of a definite specific infection, e.g., tuberculosis or syphilis. (3) *Ulcerating tumours*; these are malignant tumours, which have originated in or invaded the skin. (4) Ulcers associated with leukaemic states and other blood disorders.

Non-infective Ulcers. There are usually several aetiological factors at work, of which circulatory disturbance is the most frequent and the most important, and may alone be sufficient cause. With trauma and mild non-specific infection added, the situation is ripe for the development

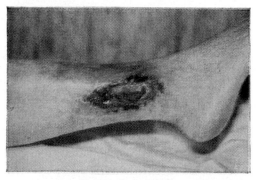

Fig. 506. Varicose ulcer.

of an indolent ulcer. These conditions obtain in the following varieties:

1. NUTRITIONAL ULCER. Following childbirth or surgical operations, or during the course of recumbency from any disease, especially in patients over the age of 40, there is a liability to thrombosis of the small veins of the calf. This is manifested by a slight pyrexia, a glossiness, indicative of early oedema, over one ankle-joint, an area of tenderness in one calf not present on the opposite side, and pain in one calf on strongly dorsiflexing the foot with the knee straight. The condition may spread into one of the main veins of the leg, and considerable oedema of the limb follows. Such cases, if followed up for a number of years, almost invariably develop a chronic oedema, with ulceration subsequently. The ulceration is usually determined by trauma; and some slight knock causing an abrasion which would normally heal is the starting-point of a chronic ulcer.

2. An almost precisely similar condition is caused by *varicose veins* and for the same reason— namely, deficient venous return leading to oedema and circulatory insufficiency (*Fig.* 506). Not infrequently both factors operate together, and in such cases treatment of the varicose veins is essential and may be sufficient to lead to healing of the ulcer.

In cases of extreme chronicity the serological tests for syphilis should be made, as this may be a factor, and a biopsy is taken from the edge of the ulcer to preclude carcinoma.

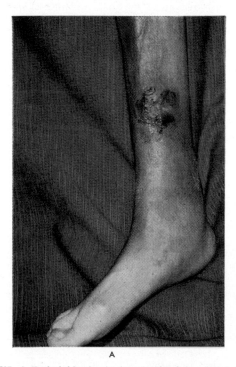

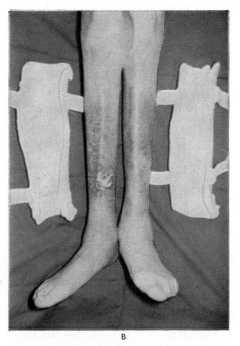

Fig. 507. A, Typical shin ulcer in rheumatoid arthritis. This lady with Felty's syndrome had recurrent shin ulcers due to trivial injuries (or traumas). She wore these shin pads (B) to prevent their recurrence. (*Dr. F. Dudley Hart.*)

3. ULCERATION DUE TO ARTERIAL DISEASE. Atheroma, arteriosclerosis, thrombo-angiitis obliterans, all lead to poor circulation and so to loss of nutrition. Ulcerative conditions are common in such cases and even gangrene may result. Such ulceration can start as a result of tissue infarction in large or small blood vessels (arteries or arterioles) due to many causes, thrombotic or embolic. Ulcers over the shin are not uncommon in advanced rheumatoid arthritis, particularly in Felty's syndrome (rheumatoid arthritis with splenomegaly and neutropenia and a tendency to sepsis). (*See* p. 460.) (*Fig.* 507.) They also occur in polyarteritis nodosa, scleroderma, systemic lupus erythematosus, and allergic vasculitis.

4. LYMPHATIC OBSTRUCTION also leads to loss of nutrition, and ulceration may result. The best instance is seen in elephantiasis due to *Filaria sanguinis hominis*. In this country elephantiasis is rare. Other instances that may be cited are swellings of the leg following a badly united fracture and the cicatricial contractions of extensive burns.

5. DEFICIENT INNERVATION leads to loss of nutrition. Examples are seen in infantile palsy; rubbing of the boot or pressure of an instrument is liable to be followed by an obstinate ulcer. In cases of hemiplegia, even when the patient is lying on a water-bed, ulceration in the form of bed-sores will occur much more rapidly on the paralysed side than on the other. Perforating ulcer of the foot is a well-known sequel of *tabes dorsalis* and *diabetes mellitus*.

6. TRAUMA, unless it is continuous, is not alone sufficient to cause an ulcer in healthy people, in whom any abrasion usually heals without trouble. Infection with pyogenic organisms may lead to chronicity, not forgetting the rare cases where the diphtheria organism is the agent. Interference with the normal contraction of scar tissue may also retard healing, as when the lesion is situated over and adherent to a bone.

7. PHYSICAL AGENTS. Burns due to heat or to radium need no elaboration, nor do the ulcers which result from the inadvertent permeation of the subcutaneous tissues by the sclerosing fluids used for the injection of varicose veins. Cold is a factor in the production of ulcerating chilblains, but here once again deficiencies of circulation play a part.

8. DIABETES MELLITUS needs special mention. In this disease ulceration and gangrene (p. 313) are prone to occur because the resistance of the sugar-laden tissues to infection is lowered, because the arteries are the subject of endarteritis and the nerves of peripheral neuritis.

9. Varicose or syphilitic ulceration of the leg may be simulated by a *malingerer* who wishes to escape conscription or for some other reason desires to make out that he is ill; nitric acid or other corrosive may have been rubbed into the leg, and the diagnosis may be obscure unless the circumstances of the case are well known. Sometimes the diagnosis is suggested by the rectangular or other definite shape of the ulcer itself.

BLOOD DYSCRASIAS. Ulcers of the leg may also occur in sickle-cell anaemia, thalassaemia, polycythaemia rubra vera, thrombotic thrombocytopenic purpura, and hereditary spherocytosis, all of which should be considered where the aetiology is not evident. Ulceration of the leg, particularly on the lateral aspect, may occur in leukaemia.

Infective Ulcers. The legs may be attacked by any form of acute infective ulcer such as *anthrax* or *glanders*, but such an event is rare. The chief ulcers that belong to this group are chronic, and due to syphilis or tuberculosis.

SYPHILITIC ULCERS are the result of gummata which have formed in the subcutaneous tissues. These ulcerated gummata tend to occur in the upper part of the leg, and if in the lower part, on the outer aspect; they are almost always circular, and present a punched-out appearance; they are generally multiple and tend to run into each other (*Figs.* 508, 509), so that the ulcer has a

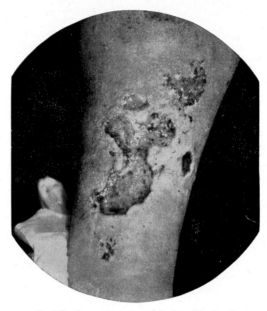

Fig. 508. Gummatous ulcer of the leg. (*Dr. Dore.*)

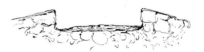

Fig. 509. Diagram of a gummatous ulcer. Cleanly punched out. Slough on base.

serpiginous outline. They are today rarely seen. Diagnosis can in most cases be made on the distribution and shape of the ulcer; on the presence of other signs of syphilis; and by finding a positive serological reaction.

There are rare cases of subacute or chronic sores and ulcers of the leg, as of other parts of the body, which have been shown microscopically to arise from various skin fungi. *Blastomycosis*, *sporotrichosis*, and *actinomycosis* of the skin are examples of this group. They are granulomatous eruptions sometimes associated with subcutaneous abscesses and multiple sinuses, sometimes simulating tertiary syphilitic lesions; their exact nature is determined by means of the microscope. Another fungus infection, one occurring in a tropical climate, is *Madura foot*, where the whole foot may become broadened, swollen, and distorted by the formation of suppurating granulomatous tissue.

TUBERCULOUS ULCERS usually follow the formation and bursting of tuberculous abscesses, starting either in the subcutaneous tissue or in a bone, and the history may help materially in diagnosis. The ulcer is very chronic, and is characterized by undermining of the skin for a considerable distance from the edge (*Fig.* 510). Lupus vulgaris,

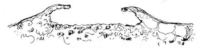

Fig. 510. Diagram of a tuberculous ulcer. Undermined edges.

a form of primary tuberculosis of the skin, is not often found on the leg, though it may occur there as in any cutaneous area. A useful guiding rule is that lupus never starts later than the age of 20 and lasts for years, whereas a gumma starts at a later period and tends to heal spontaneously. In lupus the chief characteristic is the presence of minute, semi-transparent nodules at the margin of the ulcer and in the skin around, resembling apple jelly. A particular variety of tuberculous ulcer of the legs is described on page 576 under the heading of erythema induratum scrofulosorum, or Bazin's disease.

Leg ulcers may also be seen in amoebiasis, chancroid, diphtheria, leprosy, yaws, tularaemia, osteomyelitis, kala-azar, and granuloma inguinale, all of which should be considered particularly in recent immigrants. The so-called 'phagedenic ulcer' of feet or legs is a chronic lesion caused by mixed bacterial infection that occurs in persons suffering from neglect or starvation.

DYSPROTEINAEMIAS. Leg ulcers may be seen in association with cryoglobulinaemia and macroglobulinaemia.

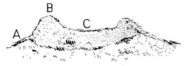

Fig. 511. Diagram of an epitheliomatous ulcer. Growth in excess of destruction. A. Normal skin; B, Heaped-up edges; C, Ulcerated portion.

Ulcerating Tumours

EPITHELIOMA may develop in a simple varicose ulcer that has existed for many years (Marjolin's ulcer). The change may be very slow, or rapid. The ulcer spreads, the edges become heaped-up, everted, and indurated (*Figs.* 511, 514). The femoral lymphatic glands become enlarged, and if

the disease is allowed to progress, the bone is attacked. If any doubt arises as to a change in the character of an ulcer, a piece from the edge should be removed for histological examination. The appearance of bare bone at the base of a

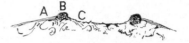

Fig. 512. Diagram of a rodent ulcer. A, Normal skin; B, Smooth, wire-like edges; C, Shallow cavity. (*From Rutherford Morison's 'Introduction to Surgery'*.)

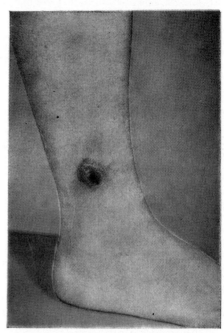

Fig. 513. Malignant melanoma.

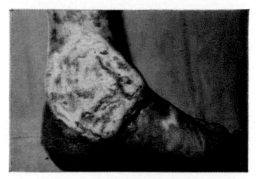

Fig. 514. Marjolin's ulcer. (*Mr. Nils Eckhoff.*)

varicose ulcer should always arouse the gravest suspicion that malignant change has taken place. RODENT ULCER (*Fig.* 512) (*see also Fig.* 285, p. 271) usually attacks the face, though it may be found on any part of the body.

MALIGNANT MELANOMA may ulcerate and bleed. It should not be biopsied but excised widely. (*See Fig.* 513.)

SARCOMA, starting in the deeper tissues, may fungate through the skin and give rise to an irregular breaking-down mass, which is obviously malignant, but may be mistaken for epithelioma unless there is previous knowledge of a malignant bony tumour or unless histological examination is made. Hodgkin's disease and mycosis fungoides may also be associated with ulcers of the leg.

Pyoderma gangrenosum. In this condition, often associated with ulcerative colitis or regional ileitis, the ulcers may be multiple and cover large areas of the leg. The ulcers tend to have ragged blue-red overhanging edges and necrotic bases. They often start as pustules or tender red nodules, often from minor trauma.

R. G. Beard.

LEUCOCYTOSIS

Leucocytosis denotes an increase above the normal in the number of leucocytes per c.mm. of blood. The normal figures range between 5000 and 10,000 per c.mm.: but the figure not only varies greatly from one individual to another, but also in the same individual from day to day and at different times of the day. A physiological leucocytosis may occur after muscular exercise and exposure to sunlight and during digestion; while independently of other effects the leucocyte count tends to alter during the day, reaching a maximum in the early morning and early afternoon, and falling to a minimum in the late morning and during the night. A leucocytosis is normal during the first week of life and often occurs during pregnancy and parturition and at the time of menstruation. Most commonly a leucocytosis is due to an increase in the number of the polymorphonuclear neutrophil cells (*neutrophilia*); but in a few conditions the leucocytosis is due to an increase in lymphocytes (*lymphocytosis*). An increase in eosinophils (*see* EOSINOPHILIA, p. 253) or in monocytes (*monocytosis*) is seldom great enough to affect appreciably the height of the total white-cell count: in certain cases of acute leukaemia, however, monocytic cells may constitute as much as 90 per cent of a total count of several hundred thousand per c.mm. A gross increase in the basophil cells (*basophilia*) is extremely rare except in chronic myelogenous leukaemia, when they sometimes rise to 20 or 30 per cent of the total count.

Although a leucocyte count near the upper limit of normal, or slightly above it, cannot by itself be regarded as significant, it will immediately become so if it is found that the differential count is abnormal. Thus a count of 10,000 per c.mm. would be regarded as a definite leucocytosis if the polymorphonuclear cells were over 70 per cent, and as a definite lymphocytosis if the lymphocytes constituted 40 per cent to 50 per cent of the cells.

It is, however, important to think of these changes in the individual types of cells in absolute numbers rather than in percentages. An immediate increase in the neutrophil count is usually a result of the mobilization of leucocyte stores which are distributed along the margins of small blood-vessels in the visceral tissues and especially in the bone-marrow. The polymorphs liberated are all mature and well lobed. A continual demand for leucocytes results in an increase in bone-marrow activity producing more cells, and those that are released into the peripheral blood then often show certain immature characteristics; many of them are metamyelocytes and occasionally some are myelocytes. This appearance of immature forms of neutrophils is known as 'a shift to the left'.

There are two main groups of conditions in which the examination of the leucocytes is of special importance in diagnosis, namely: (1) in diseases of the blood, especially cases of leukaemia, the differential diagnosis of which is discussed under ANAEMIA (p. 25); and (2) in infective conditions. However, important changes occur in the total and differential white-cell counts in many other conditions, more particularly after severe haemorrhage, in trauma, malignant disease, cachexia, toxaemias, and poisoning with drugs. In severe infections the neutrophils may show toxic changes which consist of an exaggeration in the staining of their granules.

NEUTROPHILIA. The commonest form of leucocytosis is a *neutrophil leucocytosis*, and though it tends to be most marked in infections, it may occur in a number of other conditions:

1. *Haemorrhage.* Following the sudden loss of a large amount of blood, as after a large haematemesis or postpartum haemorrhage, there may be a big increase in neutrophils, bringing the total count up to 20,000 or more per c.mm.

2. *Metabolic conditions.* A neutrophil leucocytosis may be associated with the intoxication of an acute attack of gout, uraemia, or diabetic coma.

3. *Malignancy.* It frequently occurs in persons suffering from malignant disease, especially of the alimentary tract with metastases in the liver. Retroperitoneal sarcoma may present with pyrexia (39·5° C.), tachycardia, and a white-cell count of 16,000–20,000 with 80–90 per cent neutrophils, as may Hodgkin's disease.

4. *Poisons.* Leucocytosis sometimes results from certain drugs and poisons, including, among many others, ether, chloroform, carbon monoxide, lead, turpentine, castor oil.

5. *Tissue damage.* A neutrophil leucocytosis may be produced by tissue damage; or it may arise in conditions such as intestinal obstruction, infarction in different parts of the body, and gangrene, especially of the lung, in which one or more factors may play a part.

6. *Infections.* The highest neutrophil leucocytoses, apart from those found in chronic myelogenous leukaemia, are most frequently seen in infections, particularly those which tend to be

associated with the formation of pus and in which the responsible organism is the staphylococcus, pneumococcus, streptococcus, meningococcus, gonococcus, or *Escherichia coli*. Nevertheless a neutrophil leucocytosis of greater or less degree usually occurs in all of the following infective conditions: rheumatic fever, erysipelas, tonsillitis, diphtheria, scarlet fever, cholera, anthrax, in the early stages of smallpox and chicken-pox, in lobar pneumonia, bronchopneumonia, empyema, in the acute form of pulmonary tuberculosis and in phthisis with secondary infected cavities, in meningitis, peritonitis, appendicitis, cholecystitis, salpingitis, osteomyelitis, otitis, pyelitis, pyonephrosis, pyelonephritis, urethritis, pyaemia, and septicaemia. The outpouring of polymorphonuclear cells is liable to be specially abundant in septicaemias, provided the patient is not completely overwhelmed by the severity of the infection, and also in suppurative conditions, particularly if the pus is confined under pressure. In the infective conditions enumerated above, a more or less well-developed neutrophil leucocytosis is the general rule: on the other hand, there are a limited number of infective conditions which usually do not produce a neutrophil leucocytosis, and while some of these give rise to a lymphocytosis others depress the number of neutrophil leucocytes and cause a LEUCOPENIA (*see* p. 455).

LYMPHOCYTOSIS. A *lymphocytosis*, by which is meant an increase in the number in excess of 1500 per c.mm., and not merely in the percentage, of lymphocytes, occurs most markedly, apart from chronic lymphatic leukaemia, in whooping-cough and glandular fever. In whooping-cough the total white-cell count may reach 50,000 or more per c.mm., of which over 80 per cent may be lymphocytes. In glandular fever the total count seldom greatly exceeds 30,000 per c.mm. with lymphocytes up to about 80 per cent; but among the lymphocytes there are numerous abnormal forms, often resembling lymphoblasts or unusual monocytes. In German measles there usually occurs, about the third or fourth day of the disease, a moderate lymphocytosis which may include a number of plasma cells. A mild lymphocytosis is occasionally seen in influenza, measles, mumps, malaria, Malta fever, abortus fever, in syphilis, particularly congenital syphilis, and in chronic tuberculous disease which is not secondarily infected. A lymphocytosis is the rule in the later stages of smallpox and chicken-pox, and in the convalescent phase of any infection which produces a neutrophil leucocytosis in its active stages. It must also be realized that a lymphocytosis is normal in early infancy and may persist, though in lessening degree, even beyond the age of puberty, especially in girls.

Although the causes of a leucocytosis are so numerous and varied, the discovery that there is or is not a leucocytosis, and if there is, whether it is a neutrophil leucocytosis or a lymphocytosis, is frequently of great value in diagnosis. A definite neutrophil leucocytosis may be the deciding factor which leads to an operation in a doubtful case of appendicitis. In the absence of clinical indications of lobar pneumonia or some septicaemic condition, a leucocytosis of 30,000 or more per c.mm. is strongly suggestive of suppuration somewhere in the body. A secondary rise in the neutrophil count following its fall after the crisis of a lobar pneumonia is usually an indication of the development of an empyema. Again, when an abscess has been drained and the neutrophil count has been decreased as a result, a subsequent increase in the count will suggest the collection of a further pocket of pus. When the physical signs show that there is fluid in the chest, it may be helpful to know that a serous effusion produces only a slight leucocytosis, whereas an empyema usually gives rise to a high polymorphonuclear leucocytosis. The presence of a neutrophil leucocytosis may help to distinguish a coronary thrombosis from a simple anginal attack, or may suggest that in a case of valvular disease of the heart an infective endocarditis has supervened. Examples of this sort may be multiplied without limit, and there can be no doubt that with increasing experience the examination of the white cells may be helpful in differential diagnosis.

Information regarding the severity, prognosis, and progress of an infection may be obtained from a consideration of the degree to which the nuclei of the polymorphonuclear cells are lobulated. There is no doubt that cells with single unlobulated nuclei are less mature than those with multilobed nuclei; and the relative proportions of these cells and of still more primitive forms have an important bearing on the severity of the infection. The following classification is convenient: myelocytes have round or oval nuclei; metamyelocytes have indented or kidney-shaped nuclei; 'juvenile' forms have fat, sausage-shaped nuclei; in single-lobed forms the nuclei are narrow and compact, but still unlobulated; finally the multilobed forms are placed in classes 2, 3, 4, and 5, according to the number of their lobes, class 5 containing those in which there are five or more lobes. Lobes are not regarded as separate unless the connexion between them is reduced to a single fine chromatin filament. In the Arneth, Cooke, and Schilling counts these classes are combined or subdivided in various groups, and the percentage of cells in each group is determined. Since there are several ways of selecting the groups and since the criteria for deciding to which group a given cell belongs are difficult to define precisely, the results depend very much on individual judgement. In normal blood there are no myelocytes or metamyelocytes and only a very occasional juvenile form. Depending on individual methods of counting, the single-lobed forms constitute 10–20 per cent of the polymorphonuclear cells, two-lobed forms 25–35 per cent, three-lobed forms 35–45 per cent, four-lobed forms about 15 per cent, and forms with five or more lobes about 2 per cent. In an acute infection the relative proportions will be shifted in the direction of diminishing maturity, a so-called 'shift to the left'.

For a given type of infection the height of the polymorphonuclear leucocytosis is dependent in the first place on the severity of the infection, and in the scond place on the ability of the patient to react to it. The severer the infection the higher the leucocytosis, but if the infection is overwhelming the marrow response may begin to fail and the leucocytosis diminish. On the other hand, the amount of the left shift seems to run parallel to the strain put upon the bone-marrow by the infection. The greater the shift the more seriously is the patient affected: but while a considerable shift in association with a high leucocytosis is not necessarily of bad import, an extreme shift with a feeble polynucleosis, or a leucopenia, is of grave significance. A shift to the right is commonly found in pernicious anaemia and occasionally in the leucocytosis associated with malignant disease.

The condition known as *toxic granulation* consists in an exaggeration of the number, size, and depth of staining of the granules in the neutrophil leucocytes. It is most marked in severe, *long-standing* infections. It may be seen with very high or very low total white-cell counts, and when the left shift is negligible or extreme. It does not occur in all *acute* infections, however severe.

A further test of value on granulocytes is the estimation of their content of the enzyme alkaline phosphatase (NAP). This may be done by suitable staining procedures on a blood smear and the enzyme concentration assessed visually. NAP is increased in reactive leucocytosis, in polycythaemia and leukaemoid states, but it is usually low in acute and chronic myeloid leukaemia.

LEUKAEMOID REACTION. This name is given to conditions in which in one way or another the blood-picture may be suggestive of leukaemia. Perhaps the commonest of these is glandular fever, in which the lymphocytes may constitute 90 per cent of a total count of over 30,000 per c.mm. Many cells, closely resembling lymphoblasts, may be present and suggest the diagnosis of acute leukaemia. In whooping-cough the high lymphocytosis may simulate that of chronic lymphatic leukaemia. A high lymphocytosis superficially resembling that of leukaemia is seen occasionally in children with congenital syphilis, rickets, and tuberculosis. Very high polymorphonuclear leucocyte counts are liable to occur in chronic suppuration, but it is excessively rare for the left shift to be so extreme as that which is characteristic of chronic myelogenous leukaemia. A much closer resemblance to chronic myelogenous leukaemia is found in certain cases of malignant disease with metastases in the bones and in miliary tuberculosis. There may then arise the picture of leuco-erythroblastic anaemia with large numbers of primitive white cells and nucleated red cells (*see* p. 54).

T. A. J. Prankerd.

LEUCOPENIA

Leucopenia denotes a reduction below the lower limits of normal in the number of leucocytes per c.mm. of the blood. If the number is appreciably less than 4000 per c.mm. one can say that there is a leucopenia, but one not infrequently finds counts between 4000 and 5000 which have little significance. A leucopenia is almost always due to a diminution in the number of neutrophil granulocytes, or occasionally lymphocytes; it is therefore more rational to assess the severity of a leucopenia by the reduction of the affected cells rather than by the reduction in the total white-count. In fact there are certain conditions in which a gross depression of granulocytes may be associated with a normal or even high total white-cell count. Since a leucopenia is generally due to a diminution of the neutrophil granulocytes and does not often involve a reduction in the number of lymphocytes, it follows that a leucopenia is usually associated with an increase in the *percentage* of lymphocytes, a so-called *relative lymphocytosis*. This is of course of no significance in itself, but it must be carefully distinguished from an absolute lymphocytosis, which may be of great diagnostic importance. When there is an almost total reduction in the number of circulating granulocytes, the condition is known as 'agranulocytosis'.

Neutrophils are an important component of the body's defences against infection by virtue of their phagocytic and intracellular bacterial-killing activities. When the neutrophil count is less than 700 per c.mm. these defences become impaired and the risks of infection become appreciable. In some conditions neutrophils may be present in normal numbers but are defective in function, thus rendering the body equally susceptible to infection.

Neutropenia occurs in the following conditions:

1. Infections:

a. BACTERIA: Typhoid, paratyphoid, and brucellosis.

b. VIRUSES: Influenza, measles, rubella, dengue, sand-fly fever, and rickettsia.

c. PROTOZOA: Malaria, kala-azar, and relapsing fever.

d. Any type of overwhelmingly severe bacterial infection; miliary tuberculosis.

2. Haemopoietic Diseases. Aplastic anaemia, acute leukaemia, agranulocytosis (*see under* POISONING, *below*), megaloblastic anaemia, iron-deficiency anaemia, hypersplenism, and bone-marrow infiltration.

3. Poisoning with various chemical and physical agents, particularly: Benzene, amidopyrine, sulphonamides, thiouracil, arsenic, gold, the nitrogen mustards, chloramphenicol, and streptomycin. Also after exposure to X-rays and radioactive substances.

4. In cachectic and debilitated states and in chronic toxic conditions.

5. In anaphylactic shock and in the early stage of reaction to the injection of foreign protein.

6. Miscellaneous conditions; disseminated lupus erythematosus, myxoedema, hypopituitarism, and cirrhosis of the liver.

Of the infections producing leucopenia, typhoid is the most important. Here the leucopenia is practically constant and present from the onset of the disease, persisting unless perforation, or other complication leading to pus formation, supervenes. It is thus a valuable point in distinguishing typhoid from suppurative lesions or from the majority of acute infections which produce a leucocytosis. The other infections listed produce a less regular leucopenia. *Brucellosis* may start with a slight leucocytosis, but as the disease progresses anaemia and leucopenia develop. Blood-cultures and the agglutination test are the chief aids to its diagnosis. In *influenza* the leucopenia follows an initial leucocytosis which may reappear if complications arise. In *measles*, and particularly in *rubella*, the leucopenia may be associated with the presence of plasma cells. *Dengue* produces a moderate but fairly regular leucopenia appearing as early as the first or second day. *Malaria* generally produces a moderate leucopenia which is very frequently associated with an increase in the monocytes of the blood. In *kala-azar* leucopenia is accompanied by anaemia; the diagnosis is established by finding Leishman-Donovan bodies after splenic or sternal puncture. In any *overwhelming infection*, when the prognosis is usually hopeless from the start, there may be a severe leucopenia, while the granulocytes which remain give an Arneth count with a gross left-shift.

Leucopenia due to disease of the haemopoietic system, whether primary, or secondary to some known poison, has already been dealt with under ANAEMIA (*see* pp. 25 et seq.). It must be noted here, however, that the most extreme forms of leucopenia are usually of this type. In many of the cases the association with a severe anaemia or some other obvious abnormality of the blood will lead directly to the proper diagnosis, but this is not always the case. Thus the presence of anaemia, leucopenia, and thrombocytopenia strongly suggests the diagnosis of bone-marrow failure, infiltration, or hypersplenism. Acute leukaemia is more often associated with a leucopenia than a leucocytosis. In elucidating a haematological cause for leucopenia, bone-marrow aspiration or biopsy are important diagnostic procedures. The latter particularly is important in making the diagnosis of aplastic anaemia, as the mere failure to aspirate bone-marrow is not a sufficient diagnostic finding.

In pure agranulocytosis anaemia is either negligible or absent. But here the diagnosis may be difficult unless a careful inquiry is made into the administration of drugs such as amidopyrine, sulphonamides, or thiouracil, or the exposure to any poisons. In drug-induced agranulocytosis the patient may be very ill with high fever and there may be a gangrenous ulceration of gums, tonsils, soft palate, and pharynx. The surrounding tissues show little or no reaction; and an examination of a blood-film shows the complete, or almost complete, absence of granulocytes. Death usually occurs within a few days.

This condition may be fatal but in some instances, after stopping the offending drug and with the administration of adrenocortical steroids, the agranulocytosis may disappear and normal cells reappear in the peripheral blood. Monitoring of the blood-count of a patient on potentially toxic drugs may serve to prevent this condition developing if the drug is stopped when leucopenia first begins to appear. However, in some instances the fall in white-cell count may be acute and without warning.

The chemicals listed above under poisons most commonly affect the white cells alone, but also occasionally affect the red cells and platelets. With benzene, and the derivatives of benzene, all three elements are equally liable to be affected, consequently with benzene poisoning the leucopenia is generally but one manifestation of an aplastic anaemia. X-rays and radioactive substances, though affecting the white cells first, finally produce a picture of aplastic anaemia. Chloramphenicol (chloromycetin) and gold have been the cause of a number of fatal cases of leucopenia, sometimes as a part of a general marrow aplasia. The complication has generally arisen after prolonged treatment; but sometimes when a first course has been given without ill effect it has developed rapidly during a second course, suggesting a sensitization phenomenon, particularly Felty's syndrome.

In cachectic and certain toxic conditions a moderate leucopenia is common, for example in cirrhosis of the liver and in long-standing chronic rheumatoid arthritis, particularly Felty's syndrome.

Functional Leucocyte Defects

1. Bactericidal—Phagocytic / bacterial - killing deficiencies:
   Chronic granulomatous disease.
   Chediak-Higashi syndrome.
   Myeloperoxidase deficiency.
   Glucose-6-phosphate dehydrogenase deficiency (leucocyte type)
   Certain drugs.
2. Migratory and chemotactic deficiencies:
   Not yet well defined.

T. A. J. Prankerd.

LIMBS, LOWER, PAIN IN

Limitation of space precludes a comprehensive discussion of all surgical and medical causes of pain in the leg, and the present section will be confined to pain referred to the lower limb from elsewhere, together with a brief reference to vascular disorders and some comments on pain in the foot.

SCIATICA

The term 'sciatica' is applied to pain radiating from the buttock, down the back of the thigh, and along the posterior or lateral aspect of the calf to the foot; it may be used for pain distributed through any considerable part of this territory, but should not be applied to pain limited to the buttock or other small area.

THE CAUSES OF SCIATIC PAIN

A. Affections of the Nerve-roots, Lumbo-sacral Plexus, and Sciatic Nerve

1. Cauda equina: Neurofibroma or other tumour; backward protrusion of intervertebral disk; irritation of meninges by haemorrhage, infection, and intrathecal injections; hydatid cyst; post-herpetic neuralgia.
2. Lumbar vertebrae: Disk lesions; spondylosis; Pott's disease; osteomyelitis; tumours; fracture-dislocations; spondylolisthesis.
3. Lumbosacral plexus: Cysts and tumours of pelvic adnexa and rectum; the uterus during labour; pelvic inflammation (very rare).
4. Sciatic nerve: Neurofibroma; penetrating injuries.

B. Extraneural Disease

1. Sacro-iliac joints: Subluxation, tuberculous and non-tubercular arthritis; ankylosing spondylitis and other spondylarthropathies.
2. Sacrum and pelvic bones: Primary and secondary neoplasm.
3. Soft tissues: gluteal bursitis.

The causes of sciatica are many, but the vast majority of all cases is due to lesions of the lumbar intervertebral disks, spondylosis, or sacro-iliac disease. A list of the aetiological possibilities is given above, but it is important to distinguish between sciatica due to implication of the nerve or its roots on the one hand, and sciatic pain referred from extraneural lesions on the other. Complaints of paraesthesiae, in the shape of tingling, numbness, or 'pins and needles', always indicate that sensory pathways are directly involved, but paraesthesia may be absent. They never occur in 'referred' pain. Aggravation of pain or paraesthesiae by flexion of the hip (which stretches the cauda equina) is a reliable indication of a root lesion. Flexion of the neck can cause a surge of paraesthesiae down the trunk into the limbs—hermitte's or the 'barber's chair' sign—in disseminated sclerosis, subacute combined degeneration of the cord, and cervical spondylosis or tumour. Pain down the leg on coughing occurs in root lesions and in acute extraneural disease of the spine, pelvis, and sacro-iliac joints; its value is therefore slight. Of the objective signs, pain induced by straight-leg raising (Lasègue's sign) is more likely to be present in neural lesions than in the others, but it is unreliable. Muscular weakness, sensory loss, and depression or loss of the ankle-jerk indicate a neural lesion. Wasting of muscles usually has the same significance, but may occur from disuse or pain from extraneural disease. On the other hand, radicular pain of recent onset may be unassociated with objective neurological signs, and the ankle-jerks (S.1) will remain normal in sciatica due to an irritative lesion of the 5th lumbar root. Neurological signs may be present at a higher level, e.g., loss of the knee-jerk, wasting of the quadriceps, in sciatica due to a lesion affecting the cauda equina.

Lesions of the cauda equina are uncommon. *Tumours*, notably slowly growing neurofibromata, may cause intermittent sciatic pain for months or even years before the diagnosis is established; neurological signs may be relatively late in appearing, but lumbar puncture will usually reveal a raised protein in the spinal fluid and there may be a partial or complete block. Backward protrusion of the lower intervertebral lumbar disks or of the lumbo-sacral disk may compress the cauda equina, with unilateral or bilateral sciatica; if the second or third disk is involved, there may be pain in the front of the thigh and objective changes in the distribution of the third and fourth lumbar roots in addition to those within the sciatic distribution. The spinal fluid may or may not show evidence of block and the protein may be raised above normal. Meningeal irritation from local meningitis, haemorrhage, or intrathecal injections can give rise to severe bilateral sciatica, usually of short duration and obvious origin.

Posterolateral herniation of the nucleus pulposus of the intervertebral disks at the L.4/5 and L.5/S.1 spaces is the common cause of acute sciatica. There is usually a history of acute lumbago of sudden onset, either immediately preceding the sciatica or at a more remote date. Trauma—amounting to little more than a slight strain—is present in more than half of all cases. But both trauma and lumbago may be absent. The sciatica is usually unilateral, occasionally bilateral, and rarely alternating. Paraesthesiae are often felt in the big toe and lateral aspect of the foot (L.5) or on the sole of the foot and back of ankle (S.1). The lumbar spine is stiff and tender, and there may be a reduction of the normal lumbar lordosis, with or without scoliosis. Tenderness of the lumbar muscles, the glutei, hamstrings, and calf is common, and deep pressure may cause an exacerbation of the sciatic pain, while infiltration of these 'trigger' points with procaine may provide considerable relief. Weakness is usually slight, and is best seen in the extensor hallucis longus (L.5); wasting of the calf is sometimes seen in S.1 root lesions. Hypalgesia and hypaesthesia are found in a limited portion of the periphery of the affected root area; deeper and more extensive sensory loss is exceptional. The ankle-jerk is depressed or lost when the first sacral root is involved. The spinal fluid is often normal; in other cases there is a rise of the protein content. Radiographs of the lumbar spine may or may not show significant narrowing of the affected disk space. Contrast myelography may demonstrate the herniation, but this method is not used unless there is reason to suspect some other lesion such as a tumour of the cauda equina, or unless there is difficulty in localizing the lesion, if operative treatment is contemplated.

Spondylosis is not uncommon as a cause of root pains in the neck, upper limb, and leg. The symptoms and signs are not unlike those of a disk herniation; indeed protrusion of the annulus fibrosus is an integral part of spinal osteo-arthritis and plays a part in the production of root pain. There is usually a history of chronic, intermittent pains in the lower back, recurrent attacks of sciatica, and evidence of osteo-arthritis elsewhere in the spine and in the larger joints of the limbs. More than one root may be involved, either simultaneously or at different times, but objective neurological changes are rather less prominent than in disk herniations in younger subjects. Radiographs of the spine will eventually show narrowing of the disks, with lipping, and, at a later stage, irregularity of the intervertebral facets. It is essential to remember, however, that the spondylosis seen on radiography may not be the cause of the pain in the leg. *Pott's disease* occasionally involves the lower lumbar vertebrae, with local pain and stiffness and sciatic radiation. The latter may be due to involvement of the dural sheaths of the lumbosacral roots or to collapse of the vertebrae with root pressure; pain extending to the buttock and back of thigh, without neurological signs, may be in the nature of a referred pain from the diseased vertebra itself, without implication of the nerve-roots. Radiographs of the spine will ultimately show rarefaction and collapse, and it is wise to radiograph the chest as well in any suspicious case of sciatica, for the presence of pulmonary tuberculosis may provide an early clue as to the nature of the process in the vertebrae. *Osteomyelitis of the lumbar vertebrae* is a rare cause of sciatica. Fracture-dislocations are clinically obvious, but *spondylolisthesis* (forward or backward displacement of the 5th lumbar vertebrae upon the sacrum) requires radiography for diagnosis; the presence of this deformity does not prove that it is the cause of sciatic pain, since it can be present without discomfort. When sciatica is so caused, however, it is usually bilateral, and neurological signs—motor, sensory, and reflex—are usually severe. *Pelvic disease* is a rare cause of sciatica, and when it does produce it the symptoms in the leg are usually overshadowed by the clinically obvious pelvic condition. Exception to this rule will not be missed if rectal or vaginal examination is done in every case of sciatica for which there is no obvious cause. In such cases the pain is usually intense and may have a burning (causalgic) quality, while wasting is rapid, sensory loss profound, and loss of the ankle-jerks invariable. These symptoms and signs may be unilateral or bilateral. Acute sciatic pain occurring during *parturition* is usually a transient event due to pressure of the foetal head upon the lumbosacral trunk as it crosses the pelvic rim. Permanent paralysis of the muscles below the nerve has occurred after prolonged dystocia. Persistent sciatica following parturition is occasionally due to herniation of a lumbar disk. *Tumours of the sciatic nerve* are exceedingly rare; the presence of other evidence of von Recklinghausen's disease (neurofibromatosis) is suggestive, and the signs—motor, sensory, and reflex—of a lesion of the nerve itself are well marked.

Extraneural disease may give rise to referred sciatic pain, without paraesthesiae and without objective neurological signs. An outstanding example is disease of the sacro-iliac joint. *Subluxation* may occur during pregnancy or after pregnancy, but subluxation also happens in males as a result of severe injuries. Pain is felt over the joint and buttock, and may radiate down the back of the thigh to behind the knee, but no farther. It is aggravated by walking and by torsion movements of the trunk, and sometimes by coughing. If uncorrected, it leads to faulty posture and a resultant ache in the lower back. Subluxation is apt to make the patient feel uncertain of his legs, which may be described as 'useless' immediately after the dislocation has taken place. Pain is induced by forced abduction or adduction of the flexed thigh, and by extension of the thigh. Compression of the iliac crests is an unreliable method of inducing pain, and a poor test. *Arthritis of the joint* may be tuberculous, pyogenic, osteo-arthritic, or part of ankylosing spondylitis. The signs and symptoms have a general similarity to those described in subluxation, but the manipulative tests are less likely to induce pain and may remain negative throughout the course of the disease. In tuberculous sacro-iliac disease, X-ray signs are late in appearing, but pulmonary tuberculosis is often present, the sedimentation-rate is raised, and a cold abscess may point over the joint or in the gluteal fold. Acute suppurative arthritis is a rare condition complicating septicaemia or pyaemia. Chronic infective arthritis of a single sacro-iliac joint in otherwise healthy persons is very like tuberculous arthritis. Sciatic pain is rare in ankylosing spondylitis, but when the sacro-iliac joints are involved early, pain in the buttock and upper part of the thighs is due to the sacro-iliac lesion. Tumours of the iliac bones and sacrum are an occasional cause of pain down the back of the thigh. Their recognition depends on radiography.

Opinion is today in general against 'muscular rheumatism', or 'fibrositis' as permissible diagnosis. Some authorities believe that fibrositic nodules in the muscles, fascia, and aponeurosis of the lower back and buttock give rise to referred pain down the leg. It is more likely that fibrositis represents muscle spasms due to root involvement which is also causing the pain. *Fat herniation*, wherein lobules of deep fat herniate through the deep fascia and become strangulated, has been recorded as an occasional cause of referred sciatica.

PAIN IN THE FRONT OF THE THIGH

Pain down the front of the thigh to the knee may be referred from the hip, as in tuberculosis and osteo-arthrosis of that joint, from the upper part of the iliac bone, or from the 2nd or 3rd lumbar vertebra. In such cases there may be wasting of the quadriceps, but there is no weakness, sensory loss, or interference with the patellar reflex. The presence of these neurological signs means that the pain is due to a lesion implicating the 2nd or 3rd lumbar roots or the femoral nerve itself. There is no evidence that interstitial neuritis of the nerve ever occurs, although this was the popular explanation of femoral pain with abnormal neurological signs in former years. Most cases are due to spondylosis of the upper lumbar vertebrae with protrusion of the upper lumbar disks. Some are due to diabetes and a very small number are due to Pott's disease, or disease of the meninges and cauda equina. As in sciatica, X-ray examination and lumbar puncture are desirable in every case.

Pain sometimes occurs not only down the front of the thigh, but extends down the front of the shin to the inner aspect of the foot. This distribution indicates a lesion of the 4th lumbar root, and the aetiological possibilities are the same as for

The pain and numbness tend to develop in men in middle life, sometimes as a result of weight increase, but it has also been described as a local manifestation of systemic disease, e.g., typhoid or malaria.

On examination sensory loss may be demonstrated over a somewhat variable area on the lateral aspect of the thigh corresponding to the whole or part of the distribution of the lateral cutaneous nerve.

Dieting may be sufficient to relieve the symptoms but an operation to decompress the nerve may be necessary if the pain is severe. The sensory loss is of no consequence.

PAIN IN THE FOOT

Pain in the foot is usually due to local disease or abnormality and seldom occurs as a referred pain from elsewhere, radicular or non-radicular.

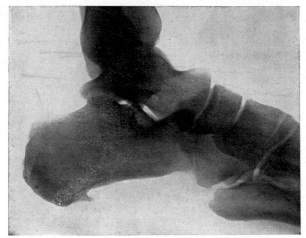

Fig. 515. Radiograph of a 'spur' on the under-surface of the os calcis causing painful heel. (*Dr. Lindsay Locke.*

lesions of the 5th lumbar and 1st sacral roots, as detailed in the section on sciatica. The knee-jerk is occasionally depressed or lost in such cases.

Obturator pain, down the inner aspect of the thigh, is commonly due to disease of the hip-joint, rarely to obturator hernia or gross neoplastic or inflammatory disease within the pelvis.

Meralgia Paraesthetica. The lateral cutaneous nerve of the thigh is sometimes compressed as it passes from the pelvis under the lateral aspect of the inguinal ligament where it may become involved in the insertion of the sartorius muscle. This compression may give rise to numbness over the lateral aspect of the thigh and to pain. Hence the name meralgia paraesthetica. The pain develops typically on exertion and may be severe enough to halt the patient so that this is one of the causes of intermittent claudication (intermittent limping) and thus resembles the symptoms caused by ischaemia in the leg. The pain is relieved by rest but may return with further exertion.

Cases are occasionally encountered in which a sharp pain in the side of the foot, the big toe, the lateral border of the foot, or the lateral border of the ankle, has been the first manifestation of a root pain, but root pains usually spare the foot and favour the upper part of the limb. It is therefore profitable to pay particular attention to the foot itself when it is painful. Gout, rheumatoid arthritis, tuberculosis, bunions, plantar warts, calcanodynia from Reiter's disease or from a calcanean spur (*Fig.* 515), flat-foot, metatarsalgia, and march fracture (*pied forcé*) are to be remembered. Raynaud's disease may cause severe pain in the toes before and after the phase of local asphyxia; it is usually present in the fingers as well, and the relationship of symptoms to cold will make diagnosis easy. *Erythromelalgia* is a less common abnormality of the superficial vessels of the foot; it, too, may occur in the hands or elsewhere. It sometimes occurs in otherwise normal subjects, but is also found in the early stages of chronic arsenical poisoning, polycythaemia, and syringomyelia. Pain is the first symptom. It is burning in quality, and may be severe. It may be continuous or remittent, and is aggravated by heat, dependency, and walking. Hyperidrosis of the foot is common. The pain is soon followed by the appearance of cutaneous flushing, going on to cyanosis, and there is increased pulsation of the vessels. Tenderness is extreme, and in long-standing cases there is some oedema of the affected part. Painful feet are a feature of the *polyneuritis* caused by alcohol and arsenic, and are a conspicuous symptom in the neuropathy which occurs in starvation. Many cases of this occurred in the prison camps of the Far East during the Second World War and were attributed with doubtful accuracy to vitamin-B deficiency. Objective neurological signs—weakness, wasting, sensory loss, and depression of the ankle-jerk and knee-jerk—were present in all but the milder cases.

TABES DORSALIS

The lightning pains of tabes are more often complained of in the legs than in any other part of the body. Unlike the neuralgias, they are usually bilateral and not referred to the distribution of any particular peripheral nerve. The 'lightning' pains are so characteristic that they can hardly be compared with pains of any other origin. Whether trivial and 'niggling', or so intense as to draw sweat and cries from the most heroic of sufferers, they are always short and lightning-like in duration, often rapidly repeated in the paroxysms, irregularly periodic in their attacks, and variable in their localization. Some patients describe their lightning pains as sharp stabs, or as if the flesh had been raised and pinched between two fingers and then let go. The area in which a paroxysm of pain occurs is never much larger than the palm of a hand, and it often remains hypersensitive for hours after the paroxysm has passed. Many patients, when asked if they suffer from pains, emphatically deny it, but readily admit to 'rheumatics', and then describe in a graphic manner the lightning pains of tabes. In addition to lightning pains, sufferers from tabes often complain of dull aching or boring pains, which are more continuous and less intermittent than those just described. Tabetic pains may precede all other signs and symptoms of the disease, in which case their diagnosis may be difficult. The following points should be investigated carefully when pains answering to the description given above are complained of:

(*a*) A history of syphilis;
(*b*) Pupils not reacting to light but reacting on convergence;
(*c*) Absent knee- and ankle-jerks;
(*d*) Loss of sensation to pain below the knees, and over the trunk and inner arms;
(*e*) Lymphocytosis in the cerebrospinal fluid;
(*f*) Positive TPI and VDRL tests in the blood and cerebrospinal fluid (though they may be negative).

A particularly valuable sign of tabes is the impaired pain sensibility in the calf and other muscles when they are squeezed. Lightning pains may also occur in diabetes mellitus.

PAIN IN CONNEXION WITH DISTURBANCES OF THE CIRCULATION

INTERMITTENT CLAUDICATION. This term is applied to a condition which depends on an insufficient blood-supply to the muscles of the lower extremities when they are called into activity during locomotion. It occurs in atheroma, with or without thrombosis, and in embolism, Buerger's disease, and, rarely, syphilitic endarteritis; it is aggravated by anaemia.

The patient complains of pain in one or both legs, generally in the calf muscles, coming on after walking a certain distance, and disappearing with rest. The pain becomes so intolerable that he is obliged to stand or sit still until it passes off. As time goes on, the distance he can walk in comfort becomes progressively shorter. Examination of the affected limbs reveals nothing obvious; they are well nourished, powerful, and normal in regard to sensation and reflexes. Probably, however, the arteries at the ankle will be pulseless, and the popliteal pulsation behind the knee-joint may not be felt. The femoral artery can usually be felt to pulsate in a normal manner. After the exertion of walking the foot may appear unduly pale; with rest, the returning flush of normal colour spreads gradually over its surface. Sometimes ischaemia affects the cauda equina (intermittent claudication of the cauda equina) when the peripheral pulses are found to be normal. However, if he continues to walk pain will develop in the legs and paraesthesiae may develop in the feet. The ankle-jerks may disappear. The condition is not uncommon, and its diagnosis is not difficult if the characteristic history of pain coming on during the act of walking is borne in mind and leads to the search for the signs referred to above. The importance of its recognition needs no emphasis in view of its tendency to go on to gangrene.

REFERRED PAIN IN VISCERAL DISEASE

On theoretical grounds pain in the sole of the foot and back of the leg (S.1, S.2) might be expected as a referred phenomenon in pelvic disease, but in practice this is exceedingly rare, and when pain does occur in this situation it is usually the result of pressure upon or infiltration of the sciatic plexus in the pelvis; vaginal or rectal examination will demonstrate a pelvic mass.

Ian Mackenzie.

LIMBS, UPPER, PAIN IN

This section will not deal with the diagnosis of gross lesions such as arthritis, bone tumours, or the results of injuries and strains, but with the more complex forms of brachial pains which are referred to the limb from the lower cervical area and the region of the brachial plexus.

Lesions in the Cervical Spine and Cord:

Disk lesions	Tumours of the spine
Spondylosis	Paralytic radiculitis
Syringomyelia	Pachymeningitis
Fracture-dislocations	cervicalis
Tumours of the spinal	Pott's disease
cord	Tumours of the menin-
Post-herpetic neuralgia	ges and roots

Lesions of the Brachial Plexus:

Cervical ribs	Pressure of subclavian
Malignant and inflam-	aneurysm
matory infiltration	Scalenus anterior syn-
from apex of lung	drome
Costoclavicular com-	
pression	

Pain referred from Viscera:

Angina pectoris and	Syphilitic aortitis
coronary thrombosis	

Pain referred from Extraneural Lesions:

Periarthritis of the	Tendonitis of supra-
shoulder-joint	spinatus tendon
Tendonitis of long head	
of biceps	

LESIONS IN THE CERVICAL SPINE AND CERVICAL CORD. Herniation of the disks at the C.5/6 and C.6/7 intervertebral spaces is an exceedingly common cause of pain in the upper limb. There may or may not be a history of recurrent stiff neck. Pain gradually spreads from the back of the neck, across the back of the shoulder, down the arm and forearm to the wrist. The pain may be aggravated by movements of the neck, by downward pressure on the head, and by movement of the limb itself. Pain may also be felt deep to the scapula and, in the pectoralis major, below the clavicle, i.e., in muscles supplied by the affected root. Paraesthesiae in the thumb and index finger and depression of the supinator jerk indicate a lesion of the 6th cervical root, and paraesthesiae in the index and middle fingers with loss of the triceps reflex are usually found in lesions involving the 7th cervical root. Weakness in the appropriate muscles may be found but sensory loss is rare. The spinal fluid is normal except in the case of the larger herniations, when the protein content may be raised. Especially is this so when the spinal cord itself is compressed, but paraesthesiae and evidence of pyramidal damage will then be present in the legs. Narrowing of the L5/6 or L6/7 disk spaces, with lipping of the adjacent margins of the vertebral bodies, may be present, but it is so common a finding in otherwise normal persons over the age of 40 that it is not necessarily significant. Contrast myelography will usually demonstrate the protrusion of the disk, either by a niche in the column of opaque substance or as an obliteration of the dural sheath of the affected root, but it will not necessarily disclose the presence of a protrusion situated in the intervertebral foramen.

Spondylosis of the cervical spine can produce three sets of symptoms which may occur alone or in combination. First, pain and stiffness of the neck, usually recurrent and commonly called 'rheumatism' or 'fibrositis'. Secondly, pain down one or both arms, radiating in radicular fashion and associated with the same type of motor, and reflex changes as occur in prolapsed disks. Thirdly, compression of the cervical cord and anterior spinal artery giving: (1) weakness, wasting, and fibrillation in the upper limbs, with reduction or loss of the tendon reflexes at the level of the compression; (2) paraesthesiae in arms and legs, with or without some slight impairment of sensibility in the hands and feet; (3) evidence of pyramidal involvement, weakness, spasticity, increased tendon reflexes, and extensor plantars in the legs. The combination of atrophic weakness in the arms and spastic weakness in the legs has a superficial resemblance to amyotrophic lateral sclerosis, from which spondylosis may as a rule be distinguished by a history of paraesthesiae, the presence of sensory impairment, and myelographic evidence of compression. There may or may not be stiffness of the neck and pain down the arms in spondylosis. After the age of 40, radiographic evidence of spondylosis does not necessarily mean that the patient's symptoms are due to it.

The other spinal conditions which have been listed as causes of brachial pain are far less common than either of the foregoing. *Pott's disease, fracture-dislocations,* and primary or secondary *neoplasms* of the vertebral bodies may give rise to root pain, with or without motor, sensory, and reflex changes. Diagnosis is confirmed by X-ray examination. *Tumours of the meninges and roots* usually cause symptoms in the legs, from compression of the pyramidal and sensory tracts, as well as pain in the arm. A raised protein in the spinal fluid will indicate the need for confirmation by contrast myelography, the contrast medium being introduced by lumbar and/or cisternal puncture. *Syringomyelia* occasionally causes pain in the arm, but it is a late symptom and by the time it appears there will be the characteristic dissociated sensory loss, atrophy of the muscles, and loss of reflexes in the arms, with pyramidal signs below the level of the lesion. *Pachymeningitis cervicalis hypertrophica* is a rare condition, sometimes syphilitic in origin, which causes diffuse pain in both arms, together with paraesthesiae, widespread atrophy, loss of reflexes, and variable sensory loss; more than one root is implicated. The spinal fluid contains an excess of lymphocytes and protein, and serological tests are positive in the fluid and in the blood in syphilitic cases. This is a rare condition, and pain in the arm should not be attributed to it on the sole evidence of a positive serological test. *Herpes zoster* may give rise to persistent pains in the arm, especially in elderly subjects. The history of an eruption and residual pigmented scars, will indicate the correct diagnosis; paralysis of one or more muscles of the limb, and cutaneous hypalgesia or hyperaesthesia in the affected area, are present in a minority of cases. *Paralytic brachial radiculitis* (syn. infective radiculitis, neuralgic amyotrophy) is a cause of acute and severe pain in the shoulder and upper arm; the pain lasts several days, and the muscles in which it is felt become paralysed and wasted; the pain does not persist, and if there is any considerable degree of paralysis, the weakened limb is apt to ache after it has been used.

THE BRACHIAL PLEXUS is liable to irritation by a cervical rib, over which the lower cord is angulated as it passes into the axilla. Pain is felt

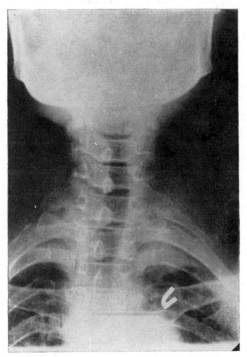

Fig. 516. Radiograph of cervical ribs in an adult. These are bilateral but more fully developed on the left.

behind the clavicle and down the inner aspect of the arm; atrophy of the hypothenar eminence and of the interossei, paraesthesiae and hypaesthesia of L8 and T1, and Raynaud's phenomena in the fingers are common findings. Palpation of the neck may disclose the accessory rib, and radiographs will confirm this finding unless it takes the form of a fibrous band (*Fig.* 516). The irritation of the plexus sometimes leads to reactionary fibrosis around it, and in such cases pain is intense. The subclavian artery is displaced upwards by the accessory rib or band, and in this situation it is liable to compression between the rib and the clavicle during movements of the arm; aneurysmal dilatation of the artery may occur, and emboli arising therefrom may lead to gangrene of the finger-tips.

Similar symptoms are sometimes seen in the absence of a cervical rib. In such cases, it appears

that the descent of the shoulder which occurs in middle life causes an angulation of the plexus and of the artery over a normal first rib; this may cause no symptoms at all, or the only complaint may be of pins and needles in the finger-tips (from subclavian compression), or the full-blown picture of a cervical rib may result. In such cases passive manipulation of the affected arm will usually disclose a position in which the symptoms are aggravated and the pulse disappears at the wrist. Highly characteristic of these cases is the patient's complaint of waking up in the night with 'pins and needles' in the fingers, for recumbency favours such compression. The paraesthesiae are usually felt in the little and ring fingers, but if the subclavian artery itself is compressed the whole hand and the distal half of the forearm may feel numb on waking. In the carpal tunnel syndrome, on the other hand, the little finger may be free from paraesthesiae, which never extend higher than the wrist. Nevertheless, pains and various unpleasant sensations in the arm or arms, particularly at night, may be due to median nerve compression at the wrist, and are relieved by division of the transverse carpal ligament. Aggravation of symptoms by the carrying of heavy weights is also noted by some patients, but it is inconstant and also occurs in brachial pain from other causes. In some subjects symptoms are relieved by freeing the scalenus anterior from its attachment to the front rib; the muscle retracts, and so provides more room for the artery and plexus. This has given rise to the idea that the muscle actually compresses the neurovascular bundle, whence the name 'scalenus syndrome'. A disturbance of the normal anatomical relationships between the plexus, the artery, the clavicle, and the uppermost rib is common to all these conditions; combinations and permutations of the various factors involved provide a wide range of clinical pictures. Pain in the arm is occasionally due to pressure on or infiltration of the brachial plexus by *enlarged glands* (carcinoma, lympho-sarcoma, Hodgkin's disease), but palpation of the axilla and of the posterior triangle of the neck will eventually reveal these conditions. Less obvious are the cases in which the plexus is involved by upward spread of a *bronchogenic carcinoma* situated in the superior pulmonary sulcus (Pancoast's tumour) or by apical inflammatory disease, but radiographs of the lung apex will make the diagnosis clear. In all these conditions, pain is very severe, and there is often a curious absence of weakness, sensory loss, or reflex changes in the early stages, but once the plexus is actually infiltrated, there is rapid onset of paralysis and comparatively little sensory loss.

Reference of pain to the arm (usually the left) is a common and easily recognized feature of *angina pectoris, coronary thrombosis,* and *syphilitic aortitis.* The majority of cases, in the past diagnosed as 'fibrositis', are today susceptible of other explanations. Pain over the deltoid and down the outer surface of the arm, aggravated by abduction of the limb, is a fairly common result of degenerative lesions in the region of the shoulder-joint—a *periarthritis*. Degeneration, with or without calcification, in the tendon of the supraspinatus or in the long head of the biceps are variants of this condition. Painful limitation of movement, of abduction in particular, affords a ready means of recognizing the condition.

Ian Mackenzie.

LINEAE ALBICANTES

Lineae albicantes or striae atrophicae are scars of the skin due to loss of elasticity of the skin after undue stretching. Commonly occurring on the abdomen, they are a sign of past pregnancy or obesity; they also occur on the breasts or thighs and buttocks. They may appear on the knees after typhoid fever. Curiously they do not often occur after swelling of a limb due to thrombosis or oedema. Occasionally they occur spontaneously. At first they are of a purplish colour, but later turn white and they are, of course, permanent. The appearance of purplish striae over the lower abdomen and thighs is a typical feature of Cushing's syndrome. They often appear following treatment with corticosteroids systemically and may also arise from the use of steroids topically especially if used under occlusion.

P. D. Samman.

LIPS, AFFECTIONS OF

Inflammation of the lips is known as *cheilitis* and this is usually followed by peeling of the mucous membrane. This is seen in its simplest form from exposure to severe weather. It may also be due to hypersensitivity to substances such as lipstick, when it is usually the colouring matter that causes the trouble, and toothpastes. Occasionally there may be a reaction to nail varnish. This occurs with the habit of resting the chin in the palm of the hand with the nails touching the lips.

Cheilitis exfoliativa is an intractable disease of the lips, the cause of which is unknown. The lips become inflamed and peel incessantly for months or even years. They ultimately get well spontaneously. Chronic dental sepsis may be responsible for some cases of cheilitis, as may riboflavin deficiency. In all cases of cheilitis there is a sensation of heat and discomfort and there may be difficulty in eating.

Fordyce's disease affects the lips and buccal mucous membrane. Numerous yellow or white milium-like bodies form under the mucous membrane. These are due to sebaceous glands and are therefore physiological. They may, however, cause stiffening of the lips with a good deal of discomfort.

Herpes simplex may affect the lips, either in an occasional attack or in a recurrent form, and it may be associated with pyrexial diseases, notably typhoid fever and pneumonia, and is frequently precipitated by sunlight. Some unfortunate patients have recurrences with every trivial upper-respiratory infection, the commonest being simple coryza.

A *primary syphilitic chancre* may occur on the lip, where it is characterized by its extreme induration and painlessness and shotty enlargement of the lymph-nodes under the chin. The mucous patches of secondary syphilis occur on the inner sides of the lips.

The lips may be the seat of a patch of *leucoplakia* and *epithelioma* also occurs there. The latter may start as a very small crack or papule. The lips are affected in a number of skin diseases such as dermatitis affecting the face, and seborrhoeic dermatitis. In lupus erythematosus (discoid type) and lichen planus the lips may be involved, and in urticaria there may be swelling of the lips. Giant urticaria commonly picks out the lips for recurrent attacks.

Perlèche is a low-grade inflammation of the lips usually affecting children. It starts at the angles of the mouth, with whitening and maceration of the mucosa; later there is inflammation and desquamation. Possibly lip-sucking is a cause of the disease. In adults it is often due to maceration from saliva resulting from over closure of the mouth due to ill-fitting dentures. Very rarely *impetigo contagiosa* and *erythema multiforme* affect the lips. In infants a monilia infection of the lips and tongue occurs and is known as *thrush*. It consists of a white deposit on the mucous membrane.

P. D. Samman.

LIVER, ENLARGEMENT OF

In adults the liver is about $\frac{1}{36}$, but at birth it is $\frac{1}{24}$ to $\frac{1}{18}$, of the whole body-weight, so that in infants and young children it is relatively larger than in adults. For this reason the normal liver in a child may be thought to be enlarged. In thin people whose abdominal muscles are lax, the lower edge of the normal liver can on deep inspiration in the supine position be felt to descend to touch the fingers if they are thrust up under the ribs outside the right rectus; in the upright position it may descend half an inch lower than this. In the epigastric angle a small portion of the liver is in contact with the anterior abdominal wall, but this cannot as a rule be felt through the recti abdominales muscles.

On percussion, the hepatic dullness to the left of the sternum cannot be distinguished from that due to the heart. On the right it begins at the middle of the xiphoid process of the sternum; in the right nipple line it reaches the upper part of the fifth intercostal space; in the mid-axillary line, the seventh; in the line of the angle of the scapula, the ninth. In health the edge of the liver is firm and uniform and the surface feels smooth. If the liver is transposed, the right lobe is small and the left large. Occasionally either lobe is dwarfed by disease, e.g., cirrhosis. A tongue-like projection of the right lobe may protrude from its lower right-hand part, generally in the nipple line, or to the right of this. This projection, known as *Riedel's lobe*, is commoner in women than in men. It may give rise to difficulties of diagnosis: if the connexion between it and the liver is only peritoneum it may be mistaken for a mobile kidney, especially as in such a case there may be a band of resonance between it and the liver. The lobe may be confused with a large gall-bladder or any tumour to be found on the right side of the abdomen.

Many conditions quite unconnected with the liver cause an apparent alteration in its size.

Alterations in the chest may lead to displacement of the liver giving a fictitious impression of enlargement. Deformities of the chest due to rickets or curvature of the spine may lead to great depression of the liver. A pericardial effusion may, if extremely large, depress the liver. A subdiaphragmatic abscess is rarely responsible, as the adhesions in connexion with such an abscess generally prevent any movement of the liver, but it can occur.

It is unusual for enlargement of the liver to lead to upward extension of the hepatic dullness; the weight of the enlarged liver leads to its descent. Elevation of the upper limit of hepatic dullness is best observed when some local disease of the liver directly implicates the diaphragm. Thus, an amoebic abscess of the liver may elevate the diaphragm; a hydatid cyst will have a similar action. When there is extension upwards of the upper hepatic dullness it is a local extension forming a dome-shaped addition to the hepatic dullness. Very large collections of ascitic fluid or very large abdominal tumours may push the liver up, but displacement in such circumstances is rare, for such conditions will more readily compress the intestines and bulge the abdominal walls. A subdiaphragmatic abscess may cause extension of liver dullness upwards. The hepatic dullness may be altered by gas, and may also be almost obliterated by the descent of an emphysematous lung; lowering of the upper margin of the hepatic dullness from this cause is common. In emphysema, too, the lower ribs stand so far forwards in a position of partial inspiration that it may be impossible to feel the lower edge of the liver. Free gas in the peritoneal cavity may diminish the hepatic dullness as in perforative peritonitis and therapeutic pneumoperitoneum. On the other hand, partial obliteration of the hepatic dullness may be due to gaseous distension of the colon. A large collection of ascitic fluid often makes estimation of the size of the liver impossible.

Hepatoptosis and *wandering liver* are terms applied to a liver which leaves its normal situation. A liver which is only displaced may erroneously be thought to be enlarged. It only rarely occurs and may be best seen after a therapeutic pneumoperitoneum when air separates the liver from the dome of the diaphragm. A displaced liver may form a protrusion of the abdominal walls, especially when the musculature is lax. It is easily palpable, moves up and down with respiration, and can usually be pushed or may even fall back into its normal position when the patient lies down. It is movable laterally and can be rotated with the hands about a horizontal axis. There may be no symptoms, but the patient usually complains of a dragging pain and a heaviness in the hepatic region which is much worse in the erect posture.

The main pathological enlargements of the liver, and the chief points to be utilized in the diagnosis of each are as follows.

Acute Infections. In a number of acute infections ranging from infective hepatitis and infectious mononucleosis to malaria hepatic enlargement with variable tenderness may occur.

Venous Congestion of the Liver, or Nutmeg Liver. This results from chronic congestive heart failure, whatever the cause. The enlargement of the liver is uniform, it may reach to the umbilicus or lower, its edge is firm, its surface smooth. When the heart failure is acute, pain and tenderness are common from rapid stretching of the hepatic capsule; but when hepatic enlargement has persisted for weeks the liver is no longer painful or tender. In severe cases there is usually a slight degree of jaundice. Dyspeptic symptoms are frequent. Ascites may be present, generally accompanied by oedema of the feet and legs.

In a severe degree of nutmeg liver the organ may pulsate. In such a case the tricuspid orifice must be incompetent and the right ventricle must be beating strongly, sending into the vena cava and hepatic veins a strong pulse wave, causing the whole organ to expand synchronously with each contraction of the right side of the heart. Such incompetence of the tricuspid orifice is nearly always secondary to rheumatic mitral disease; tricuspid disease alone is never present. Care must be taken to avoid mistaking for hepatic pulsation a thrust downwards of the liver by the contraction of a hypertrophied heart, or the thrust forwards by a pulsating aorta. The distinguishing feature of true from transmitted pulsation is that, when one hand is placed on the front and the other on the back of the abdomen over the enlarged, congested liver, the two hands can be felt to be separated at each heart beat. Pulsation of the veins of the neck is generally evident in subjects in whom the liver can be felt to pulsate.

Obstruction to the Common Bile-duct, whatever the cause, is associated with uniform enlargement of the liver since the bile is dammed back into it, with, in consequence, swelling. Jaundice will always be present, and the differential diagnosis is discussed under JAUNDICE, p. 433.

Suppuration within the Liver. Multiple pyaemic abscesses within the liver, which constitute part of the condition known as *portal pyaemia*, do not as a rule produce as much enlargement of the liver as one might expect, nor do multiple abscesses connected with the bile-ducts—*suppurative cholangitis*—unless there is sufficient obstruction to cause jaundice. Rigors, pyrexia, and tenderness of the liver are prominent features in the majority of cases. Enlargement of the liver is more often present with a *large single abscess*. There is usually a history of dysentery, for amoebic infection is the commonest cause of a large single ('tropical') abscess. On rare occasions, a single abscess may be secondary to non-dysenteric intestinal ulceration or to other specific fevers; it may be due to a suppuration around a gall-stone; it may spread from some neighbouring suppuration, e.g., a perinephric abscess; or again, it may be caused by suppuration of a hydatid cyst or of a hepatic haematoma caused by injury. The presence of any of these may help the diagnosis; but in many cases, even when the abscess is due to the amoebiasis, the antecedent history may be unhelpful or misleading, since the dysenteric ulcers of the intestine may have healed years before the symptoms of hepatic abscess appear. Tropical abscess occurs most commonly in men between the ages of twenty-five and forty-five: it is more frequent in Europeans than natives. Eighty per cent are in the right lobe, usually in its upper part. The colour of the pus depends upon the amount of broken-down hepatic tissue present: if there is none, it is yellow; if there is much, it resembles anchovy paste, an appearance regarded as characteristic. Amoebae may be identified in the pus, or more often in the granulation tissue forming the wall of the abscess. Bacteria may be present, but in a long-standing abscess the pus is often sterile. The symptoms and physical signs to which attention must be directed are as follows: GENERAL. The most important is pyrexia. The rise of temperature is at first slight and irregular; gradually it becomes hectic, with a wide daily excursion, say from 37° C. in the morning to 39·5° or 40° C. in the evening. The patient is thought to have malaria, but examination of the blood shows no malarial organisms, and there is leucocytosis, in contrast to malaria in which leucopenia is more usual. Intermissions may occur with the temperature normal for weeks, followed by a week or so of pyrexia. In Great Britain mistakes in diagnosis are only too likely. A man afflicted with tropical abscess, perhaps acquired in India, may return to England and suffer attacks of pyrexia separated by such long intervals of normal temperature that he may be thought to have recurrent influenza. Severe rigors with profuse sweats provide a strong resemblance to malaria. In mild cases the rigor is reduced to a mere feeling of chilliness. The pulse is rapid in proportion to the temperature. Jaundice may be present, but is not usual. In severe cases the patient is exceedingly ill and weak, anaemic, and wasted to a skeleton, but if there are long intervals of apyrexia the general health is not greatly impaired.

LOCAL. The abscess is most often at the upper part of the right lobe, grows upwards between the layers of the coronary ligament thus forming an extraperitoneal subphrenic swelling which softens the diaphragm and pushes it up, giving a dome-shaped area of dullness varying in size from one to several inches across, added to the top of the normal line of the hepatic dullness. It may be visible in a radiograph as an upward bulge of the right cupola of the diaphragm. It is usually posterior to the mid-axillary line. In some instances the abscess is so situated that a rounded swelling may be felt, or even seen, on the liver when the patient draws a deep breath. The measurement round the lower part of the chest may be greater on the affected side, the intercostal spaces may be obliterated, and if the abscess is very large, the lower ribs may bulge. Not uncommonly the abscess is much smaller and in a position that demands the greatest skill for its detection. The whole of the hepatic area should be pressed carefully by one finger, for local tenderness is often a diagnostic aid. If the abscess presents in the abdomen the rectus muscle over it may be rigid. Pain is variable; it may be produced by coughing, drawing a deep breath, or by shaking the patient. In about one-sixth of the cases pain is referred to the right shoulder; if the abscess is in the left lobe, there may be pain in the left shoulder. If the abscess comes close to the skin there may be oedema and redness over it, and, in rare cases, fluctuation. The liver is often enlarged generally as well as locally. A large abscess may be seen in the X-rays. A lateral radiograph is particularly useful. A filling defect will be demonstrated if a liver scan is performed. If it implicates the diaphragm, infection may spread through it and cause pleurisy, empyema, pneumonitis, or gangrene of the lung, but this is not nearly so common as with other subphrenic abscesses. Hepatic pus, sometimes of an almost diagnostic anchovy-sauce colour and consistence, may be coughed up when the abscess has ruptured into the lung, may be vomited when it has ruptured into the stomach, or passed by the bowel when it has ruptured into the intestine. Needling the suspected area is a useful diagnostic procedure.

Cirrhosis of the Liver. Cirrhosis is defined as widespread hepatic fibrosis with nodular regeneration of hepatic parenchyma. Here we have to consider only the stage at which the liver is enlarged. It has been known to weigh as much as 200 oz., although anything over 100 oz. is exceptional. In the early stages the liver is not altered in shape, and the surface and edge are smooth; later, as the fibrous tissue contracts, the surface becomes finely uneven; this unevenness with progressive hardness increases, until the irregularities (compared to hobnails) can be felt through the abdominal wall. At this stage the edge of the liver is irregular and very firm. In distinction from cancer, no irregularity from cirrhosis ever exceeds the size of a small cherry, nor is it ever umbilicated or ever enlarged suddenly, whereas a cancerous nodule may be umbilicated and may enlarge suddenly from haemorrhage into it. A cirrhotic liver is usually not painful, unless there is local perihepatitis. In cirrhosis the spleen is often enlarged, sometimes to a considerable extent. Associated portal hypertension may lead to the development of varices in the oesophagus and proximal stomach. These may give rise to haematemesis, which may be accompanied at some period by melaena. Occasionally, dilatation of the veins around the umbilicus is conspicuous. Rarely a venous hum, continuous, loud, high-pitched, with increase in intensity on inspiration, may be heard immediately over, or below, the xiphoid process. It may occur also in syphilitic cirrhosis, Hanot's cirrhosis, and Banti's syndrome (chronic congestive splenomegaly). Cirrhosis is commoner in men than in women in the proportion of three to one, and patients are usually over thirty. There may be much impairment of strength, wasting, a sallow pigmented facies, dilated venules on the cheek, a red nose, a furred tongue which is often tremulous, foetor hepaticus, and a dry, harsh skin. Spider naevi in the upper part of the body appear, as in any condition of gross hepatic dysfunction. Both sexes tend to lose axillary and pubic hair and men need to shave less; they may also develop gynaecomastia, lose their libido, and develop testicular atrophy. The pulse becomes weaker as the disease progresses, and the end is usually by cardiac failure. In about one-third of the advanced cases the evening temperature will be found to be a little raised. Jaundice occurs at some stage in about one-third of the cases; it rarely if ever becomes as deep as that seen in cancer of the liver. Ascites occurs in 50 per cent of all cases of cirrhosis, but generally in the latest stages only. If ascites is abundant the enlarged liver can be felt only by dipping, i.e., pressing the hand down suddenly on the liver, so dispersing the fluid which is over it. Tympanites, not uncommon in severe cases of cirrhosis, may make it difficult to feel the liver. The urine is usually scanty, of high specific gravity, very acid, high-coloured, and full of urates; it generally contains urobilin and sometimes bile. Sufferers from cirrhosis may have delirium tremens, and apart from this cirrhosis towards the end is often accompanied by nervous symptoms, especially mental obfuscation, delusions, and coma, even in those who have not recently taken alcohol and are not jaundiced. There may be a typical 'flapping tremor' of the outstretched hands. In severe cases the ankles swell. Cirrhosis may, however, exist without symptoms; in between a third and a half of all cases of cirrhosis in the post-mortem room death is attributable to some other lesion, and in many of these no symptoms of cirrhosis have been observed during life.

The difficulties of diagnosis fall into one of two classes: the cause of ASCITES (p. 75), and the cause of the enlargement of the liver. If it is clear that the liver is undoubtedly enlarged, it is often difficult to decide between cancer and cirrhosis. Moreover cancer and cirrhosis may co-exist; a large percentage of hepatomas and a rather smaller number of cholangiomas arise in cirrhotic livers. Their presence should be suspected if pain occurs in the upper abdomen or the right side of the chest, on the appearance of a new mass in the liver, particularly if tender, of a bruit or friction rub over the liver, or the sudden appearance or sudden deepening of jaundice. This last is characteristic of cholangiomas. Syphilis of the liver does not cause much difficulty in differentiation; the irregularities of the surface are much larger than the hobnails of cirrhosis, the patient is rarely jaundiced, and hardly ever has ascites. The manifestations of a syphilitic liver are nearly always entirely local; only rarely is it associated with general symptoms. It is now extremely rarely seen. Obstruction of the common bile-duct leads to a large smooth liver. When due to a gall-stone there is usually deeper jaundice than in cirrhosis, but no ascites; the stools are pallid, which is unusual in cirrhosis, and there is commonly a history of gall-stone colic. So-called malarial cirrhosis occurs only in those who have drunk to excess, and is then to be ascribed to alcohol.

Hanot's Cirrhosis—often called 'primary biliary cirrhosis'—is rare. It usually occurs in middle-aged or elderly women; the reason for this is unknown. The onset is gradual; pain is absent but pruritus may be marked. The liver is firm, enlarged, and smooth, long-standing jaundice is present, the spleen is enlarged. Jaundice is an early and fluctuating symptom and persists till the end, very slowly becoming darker with the passage of time. Ascites is rare and its development means that the end is near. The fingers may become clubbed. In the later stages there may be purpura and gastro-intestinal haemorrhage.

Chronic Active Hepatitis (*see* p. 440), formerly called *lupoid hepatitis*, resembles primary biliary cirrhosis in many ways but usually occurs in younger patients, female rather than male.

'**Veno-occlusive disease**' of the liver has recently been recognized as a distinct entity. Usually, but not entirely, in children, there is sudden development of hepatomegaly and ascites and this cannot always be distinguished from cirrhosis. There is direct mechanical obstruction to hepatic venous outflow and destruction of liver cells. In infants under twelve months the mortality is high. It is seen particularly in Jamaica and the probable cause is the action of certain plant toxins, especially 'bush tea'. It is concluded that many cases of the Budd-Chiari syndrome are examples of veno-occlusive disease.

In *polycythaemia vera*, occlusion of the hepatic veins by thrombosis leads to hepatosplenomegaly. But hepatosplenomegaly may occur as part of the uncomplicated disease process, congestion and extramedullary haematopoietic foci occurring not infrequently and sometimes cirrhosis of the liver. In *chronic haemolytic* disorders hepatomegaly may occur. In addition to polycythaemia vera, other supposed causes of such thrombosis are trauma, pregnancy, peritonitis, carcinoma of the gall-bladder, malignant growth in the inferior vena cava, hepatoma, hepatic abscess, sickle-cell anaemia. The number of correct ante-mortem diagnoses is very small and, until comparatively recent advance in surgical therapy, no practical significance was accorded to its recognition.

Haemochromatosis. In this disorder, also known as bronzed diabetes, the liver is enlarged, hard, and cirrhotic, exactly like that of an ordinary cirrhosis. As a consequence of metabolic disturbances, ferritin and haemosiderin (from iron) is deposited in the tissues, especially the liver; to a lesser extent in the pancreas, spleen, heart, and salivary glands. The face has usually a blue-grey or leaden colour, the rest of the body has a bronzed (brown-black) coloration. The mucous membranes are affected in about 16 per cent of cases. There are in addition endocrine changes in the pituitary and adrenal cortex. The hair of the axillae and chest disappears, pubic hair has the feminine distribution (the great majority of sufferers are males), the testes become small and atrophic, the hair of the head and face becomes soft and silky so that shaving and hair cutting are unnecessary. Cardiac failure is a usual cause of death. Pigmentation of the skin, the nature of which may be revealed in a biopsy, the absence of jaundice, and the presence of sugar in the urine sufficiently distinguish the disease. In less characteristic cases, the diagnosis may be in doubt until a post-mortem examination is made; the cirrhotic liver, which is generally of considerable size, is then found to give a typical Perl's prussian-blue reaction similar to that seen in Addisonian anaemia, which is not the case in ordinary cirrhotic livers.

Syphilis of the Liver. Syphilis when it affects the liver may in the secondary stage cause temporary enlargement. Later, it produces in it gummata and gross bands of fibrous tissue traversing the liver irregularly and leaving large areas of healthy substance. The presence of recent gummata, gummata that have begun to shrink, bands of contracting fibrous tissue, and pieces of normal liver, all combine to make a syphilitic liver very lumpy and irregular. It may be enlarged but not to the size of a large cirrhotic liver, unless amyloid disease is present. It is much more irregular, and indeed usually resembles a cancerous rather than a cirrhotic liver, but it seldom produces clinical symptoms; if detected during life the discovery is generally accidental. It occurs at a younger age than cancer; there are none of the other signs of cancer, but there may be some of syphilis, and serological tests will be positive; ascites and jaundice do not occur as features of this disease unless an enlarged lymph-node presses on the portal vein. It is today a rarity in Great Britain.

In children, congenital syphilis may produce in the liver precisely the same effects as those of the acquired disease in adults, but it may alternatively cause a generalized smooth, hard enlargement due to pericellular cirrhosis. The hardness of the smooth big liver in a child suggests the diagnosis and positive serological tests clinch it.

Secondary Carcinoma of the Liver is the commonest tumour of the liver (*Fig.* 517). Symptoms may be present of the primary malignant disease, which include those arising from the portal territory as a whole (stomach, pancreas, large bowel, etc.), as well as breast, bronchus, kidney, and many other less common sites. Carcinoid tumours have a particular proclivity to metastasize to the liver. Not infrequently the features of hepatic carcinoma are the first indication of any illness. On the other hand, in about half the cases of hepatic carcinoma no symptoms of it are present, and it remains unrecognized until post-mortem examination, the primary disease killing while the hepatic disease is still at an early stage. Seventy-five per cent of all the patients are between 40 and 70 years old, and hepatic carcinoma is all but unknown under the age of 20. If the disease gives rise to symptoms, enlargement of the liver can usually be defined both by percussion and palpation. There is no other disease in which such a huge liver may be found, weights up to 15 kg. ($33\frac{1}{2}$ lb.) have been recorded. The increase in the weight of the liver may be so great that the patient actually gains a little in spite of the general wasting caused by the cancer. The organ may be felt well below the ribs, even far below the umbilicus. It may be so big as to be visible through the abdominal wall, moving with respiration. Upward increase of the hepatic dullness may occur. The edge is hard, and often irregular; when the secondary nodules are numerous the whole organ is uneven, knobbly, and hard to the touch, and the lumps on it can sometimes be felt to be umbilicated, a feature absolutely diagnostic of cancer. If much softening has occurred a faint sense of fluctuation may be detected; in a few instances local peritonitis causes a rub. Occasionally the cancer grows so rapidly that the liver increases obviously in size in a week; very rarely a nodule may enlarge suddenly from haemorrhage into it. Either of these points is almost proof that the enlargement is due to carcinoma and in both cases there is usually marked local pain and tenderness. It must not be forgotten, however, that not all livers enlarged from malignant disease have palpable nodules, for these may be in such a situation that they cannot be felt, they may be too small to be felt, or the growth may be diffused through the whole liver. About half the sufferers have pain in the hepatic region; pain may also be experienced near the right shoulder and down the right arm. If the liver is very large there is a sense of dragging and fullness in the right hypochondrium. Jaundice occurs in perhaps 50 per cent of cases. The most frequent cause of long-standing jaundice is cancer of the liver, which produces a deeper yellow discoloration of the skin than any other disease; in course of time this colour changes to deep olive-green. Deep jaundice implies invasion and obstruction of the major intrahepatic bile-ducts. The wasting becomes extreme, the skin dry and shrivelled, the patient weaker and weaker, his pulse feebler, his respiration shallow, and finally he dies comatose. ASCITES (p. 75) occurs in late cases or in those associated with carcinomatosis peritonei. The urine usually contains bile. Rapidly growing carcinoma of the liver is often associated with an evening rise of temperature.

Some recapitulation of features in differential diagnosis may be added. The cirrhotic liver is uniformly enlarged, and the palpable nodules are small, they are never umbilicated, and never increase rapidly in size. If jaundice is present and

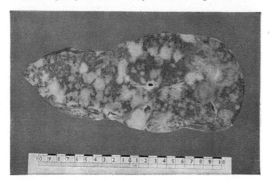

Fig. 517. Liver almost replaced by secondary deposits. The primary site was a carcinoma of the breast.

the patient has a large cirrhotic liver the jaundice is never very deep, and remains yellow, never acquiring the dark olive-green colour seen in biliary obstruction. In cirrhosis, clay-coloured motions or dilatation of the gall-bladder are not found, but a large spleen is not unusual. Extreme wasting and dryness of the skin are more common in cancer. A moderate leucocytosis is often found in both diseases in the late stages. The discovery of cancer elsewhere is of course all but conclusive. Syphilis of the liver has already been described sufficiently to indicate the points of difference. Difficulty of diagnosis may be experienced in cases in which owing to non-malignant obstruction of the bile-duct, usually by a gall-stone, there are enlargement of the liver and jaundice. These patients, however, rarely have the extreme wasted look with dry shrivelled skin so frequently seen in cancer; the hepatic enlargement is uniform and never so great as it may be in cancer; the jaundice seldom becomes green. If it disappears for a time, it means that the gall-stone has shifted; that the jaundice due to secondary deposits should disappear even temporarily is almost unknown. Rigors are common in cases of gall-stones. The age, history, and detection of growth elsewhere will be of help. When we are in doubt as to whether a patient has an impacted gall-stone or a malignant growth, exploration, sadly, almost always reveals a growth. Hydatid tumours of the liver are seldom confused with cancer, for the liver is smooth and regular and is not tender. The hydatid tumour causes neither pain, jaundice, ascites, nor general emaciation. There is no leucocytosis, but eosinophilia is usual. The Casoni test is helpful.

Primary Carcinoma of the Liver is comparatively rare in Britain, although common in the Far East and in East Africa, and is usually secondary to cirrhosis; the liver has the same character as in the secondary form, but there are no symptoms of a primary growth elsewhere. It is almost always a disease of adult life. It usually progresses more rapidly than secondary cancer; most of the patients are dead within three months from the onset of symptoms so that the jaundice has not time to become dark green. Wasting, and other general signs, including slight pyrexia, are present. During life, primary can hardly ever be diagnosed from secondary cancer of the liver, for even when the liver appears clinically to be the only organ affected, it often transpires that there has been primary disease elsewhere, relatively inconspicuous, giving no symptoms, and not detected till after death.

Secondary Melanoma of the Liver may reach a considerable size; a primary lesion in the choroid is notorious in this respect; 'beware of the man with a glass eye and an enlarged liver' is a well-known medical aphorism.

Primary Sarcoma of the Liver is very rare, and during life cannot be distinguished from carcinoma.

Adenomata of the Liver are also very rare; they are single and hardly ever of sufficient size to be detected during life.

Hodgkin's Disease of the Liver. New formations consisting of lymphoid tissue, generally diffused through the whole liver but sometimes occurring in nodules, may be seen in those dying from Hodgkin's disease or from lymphatic leukaemia. The nodules cannot be detected during life, but in a few cases the diffuse variety makes the liver uniformly enlarged; it is smooth, its surface and edge are firm, it is painless, not tender, never of great size, and there is no jaundice. Leukaemic cases will be identified by the blood-count.

Angiomata. It is not uncommon to find small angiomata in the liver in the post-mortem room, but they are rarely large enough to give symptoms to suggest the diagnosis. Larger angiomata may be mistaken for secondary deposits either on liver scan or at laparotomy; it is as well to remember that not all multiple tumours of the liver are necessarily malignant. Sometimes when a large tumour of the liver has been thought to be a carcinoma, and yet the patient has seemed well enough to justify operation, the growth has turned out to be a cavernous angioma and amenable to excision. In other, less happy, cases the tumour is a malignant haemangioblastoma.

Fatty Liver. This is very common, but the enlargement of a fatty liver is usually not sufficient to be detected during life, particularly because the subjects are so obese that palpation of the liver is difficult or impossible. A fatty liver, if palpable, is uniformly enlarged, has a rounded edge, feels a little softer than natural, with a smooth surface; there is neither pain nor tenderness, jaundice does not occur. Alcoholic excess is the commonest cause of fatty liver in Britain today, but protein malnutrition, as in kwashiorkor, is not uncommon in Africa and elsewhere. Fatty livers also occur in adult patients with diabetes mellitus, the grossly obese, and in some chronic wasting disorders, such as chronic tuberculosis and ulcerative colitis. Phosphorus poisoning is responsible for the largest examples, when a weight of 4·5 or 6·5 kg. has been recorded.

Amyloid Liver. The liver is uniformly enlarged; the increase in size may be considerable—up to as much as 6 kg. Indeed, next to cancer, amyloid disease causes the largest livers that we meet. It is smooth, firm, with a sharp and hard edge; it causes no pain, and is not tender. The spleen may also be enlarged considerably and uniformly, there may be albuminuria from amyloid disease of the kidneys, or diarrhoea from amyloid disease of the intestine. The condition may be primary, occurring without pre-existing disease, or may follow long-continued suppuration, e.g., psoas abscess, bronchiectasis, chronic phthisis with cavitation, chronic hip-joint disease with sinuses, chronic osteomyelitis, ulcerative colitis, and long-standing syphilis, even if this has not caused any suppuration. It may also complicate myeloma, advanced rheumatoid arthritis, and ankylosing spondylitis. Diagnosis has been made on the affinity of amyloid for Congo red. Rectal biopsy and liver biopsy reveal amyloid infiltration; the former is a far safer procedure than the latter.

Tuberculosis of the Liver. It is exceedingly rare for a tuberculous deposit in the liver to form a mass sufficiently large to be detected clinically.

Sarcoidosis. Hepatomegaly occurs in a minority of cases, around 20 per cent or less. It may be the only sign of the liver being involved, jaundice and signs of hepatic dysfunction being very rare.

Gaucher's Disease. Accumulations of Gaucher cells, large reticulo-endothelial cells containing glucocerebrosides, in liver and spleen account for the splenohepatomegaly in this disorder. Diagnosis is by liver biopsy. Other lipoid storage diseases in which liver enlargement is present include *Niemann-Pick* disease, a rare inherited condition, in which hepatomegaly and retarded development are noted in infancy.

Actinomycosis of the liver could hardly be diagnosed without laparotomy unless the patient were known to have actinomycosis elsewhere. It is very rare, and has seldom been recognized in the liver until after the patient's death, even when the illness has been long-drawn-out with ample opportunity for repeated clinical and laboratory investigations. The illness it causes was serious and as a rule fatal, but modern antibiotic therapy has justified a more hopeful prognosis. There may be intervals of improvement, but in the main the course is progressively downhill, simulating carcinoma in some respects, severe internal infection in others, yet without distinctive characters which enable any certain diagnosis to be made. If detected during life, there would be a local enlargement of the liver with pus in an irregular cavity with shaggy walls and trabeculae, in which the characteristic little sulphur-coloured granules would be identified with the naked eye, and the ray fungus on microscopical examination.

Hydatid Disease of the Liver can hardly be recognized unless the cyst causes a discoverable tumour of the liver which may on occasion be huge. Hydatid cysts of the liver may contain 30 pints or more. If the tumour can be felt, it is rounded, smooth, localized, and regular, features that distinguish it from cancerous or syphilitic livers in which the tumours are irregular and rough. The patient's country of origin is a useful clue to diagnosis; hydatid disease is particularly common in Australia, Iceland, Cyprus, Greece, the Middle East, and South America. It is rare in Great Britain apart from some areas in Wales. A hydatid tumour is neither tender nor painful, thus differing from an abscess. If the tumour projects from the lower part of the liver it may simulate a gall-bladder. A large hydatid cyst of the lower part of the right lobe of the liver causes considerable intra-abdominal enlargement of that lobe; on the other hand if, as is frequently the case, it grows between the layers of the coronary ligament, it pushes up the diaphragm. In hydatid cysts calcification may develop in their walls rendering them visible in X-rays. If a hydatid tumour is deep within the liver the swelling feels hard, if it comes to the surface the tumour feels tense—often too tense for fluctuation. The so-called 'hydatid thrill', perceptible in the finger lying on the tumour when it is struck by a finger of the other hand, is not often felt; it may be obtained over any tense collection of fluid, but if it is present in this situation it is of considerable diagnostic value, for other tense cysts are very unusual in the liver. Occasionally two or even three hydatid cysts are present in the liver; each then has the characteristics of a single cyst, but the diagnosis of these cases may give much difficulty. It is excessively rare for hydatids to cause pressure symptoms; if jaundice occurs it is probably caused by rupture of the cyst into the bile-passages. A huge cyst may displace the heart. EOSINOPHILIA (p. 253), sometimes considerable, is found when the cyst is still living, but not when it is obsolete. If the hydatid fluid becomes absorbed the patient may have urticaria. Hydatid liquid does not, as in the case of an ordinary pleuritic effusion, give an albuminous precipitate when heated. Hooklets (*see Fig.* 74, p. 79) may be found in centrifugalized hydatid fluid. Hydatid cysts sometimes suppurate, in which event they can hardly be distinguished from other forms of single solitary abscess.

The Casoni intradermal test and the complement-fixation test are positive in about three-quarters of cases; of various serological tests, the indirect haemagglutination test appears to be the most sensitive. Aspiration of cysts for diagnostic purposes is dangerous as it may disseminate the infection or cause an anaphylactic reaction.

Schistosomiasis (Bilharziasis) Mansoni and **S. japonica** may both cause hepatic enlargement, diagnosis being made on finding ova in stool or rectal mucosal biopsy. Intradermal and complement-fixation tests are also useful. In areas where intestinal (Mansoni) bilharziasis is endemic the presence of ova in the stools does not prove the diagnosis. Portal hypertension may develop as a late complication.

Kala-azar. Although splenomegaly may dominate the clinical scene, hepatomegaly and lymphadenopathy also occur, often later after the splenic enlargement has been present for many months. The liver is rarely tender.

Liver Biopsy. In the few cases in which diagnosis cannot be achieved on clinical grounds, microscopical examination of a portion of liver removed by a special cannula may be of great value. The right 8th intercostal space in the mid-axillary line is the usual point of entry. After a preliminary i.m. injection of 10 mg. vitamin K the area is anaesthetized in depth and the cannula, attached to a special syringe and stylet, is rapidly plunged into the liver and withdrawn while the patient holds his breath in full expiration. In skilled hands the danger of bleeding in non-jaundiced patients is slight.

Liver biopsy is also of great value in determining the nature of some rare forms of jaundice in which the liver may be normal in size. Thus intermittent jaundice may occur in *congenital hyperbilirubinaemia*, the common form being Gilbert's disease. Apart from the jaundice it is symptomless and is harmless. If haemolytic and hepatic diseases be excluded it may be diagnosed, especially if there is a family history of the complaint. The serum bilirubin is raised to levels of 2–3 mg. per 100 ml. There is no bile in the urine. Bouts of jaundice date from childhood. At times the discoloration deepens in association with malaise, nausea, and discomfort in the liver area. The fault lies in a hereditary defect in the uptake of bilirubin by the liver cells. Liver biopsy is normal.

The Dubin-Johnson type of chronic benign intermittent jaundice differs in that the circulating pigment is conjugated and thus bilirubin appears in the urine. Furthermore, microscopically the liver cells are seen to be greenish-black (black-liver jaundice) due to a brown pigment containing neither iron nor bile. The bromsulphthalein (BSP) excretion test is diagnostic. After an initial fall of serum BSP there follows a rise, so that the value at 210 minutes exceeds that at 45 minutes.

(*See also* LIVER, TESTS OF FUNCTION OF.)

Harold Ellis.

LIVER, TESTS OF FUNCTION OF

Although the term 'liver function tests' is hallowed by tradition, very few of the investigations now included in this blanket description really do test function. Some detect hepatic cell damage which, if minor, is not necessarily associated with demonstrable loss of function of the organ as a whole; others may suggest the aetiology of the disease.

Apart from the hepatic parenchymal cells, which carry out most of the 'liver functions', other types of cell line the biliary tract. The liver also contains cells of the reticulo-endothelial system. Different disease processes involve these cells in different proportions. Jaundice can accompany any of these syndromes and will be discussed first.

Jaundice. Jaundice, once the only available index of liver disease, is evidence of a raised circulating bilirubin concentration: levels greater than about 34 mmol/l (2 mg/dl) are usually clinically detectable. Bilirubin is a product of haemoglobin breakdown, which occurs mainly in the spleen. It is carried to the liver bound to albumin (as unconjugated bilirubin). After splitting off from protein, it is transported by an active process into the liver cells where it is conjugated with glucuronic acid. Unconjugated bilirubin accumulates in the plasma in haemolytic anaemia, when its production exceeds the liver's capacity to excrete it. In the absence of haemolysis jaundice indicates liver or biliary disease. Impaired transport into hepatic cells, or impaired conjugation within them, causes *unconjugated hyperbilirubinaemia*, which is therefore an accompaniment of extensive *hepatocellular* damage. The conjugated bilirubin is secreted into the bile, and accumulates in the plasma if this secretion is impaired, or if there is obstruction of biliary flow (cholestasis). Some rise in both conjugated and unconjugated fractions usually accompanies liver cell damage, although occasionally the conjugated fraction is predominantly and markedly increased. The highest levels of *conjugated bilirubin* result from extensive *biliary obstruction*.

Inborn errors may affect different stages in hepatic transport of bilirubin. *Gilbert's disease* is the commonest manifestation and is probably associated with a transport defect into the cell; there is therefore a slight rise in unconjugated bilirubin. The *Dubin-Johnson syndrome*, in which there is a slightly raised conjugated bilirubin, is due to defective secretion of bilirubin out of the cell and into the bile. Both these conditions are harmless. By contrast, the *Crigler-Najjar syndrome*, probably due to a deficiency of the conjugating enzyme, is associated with very high levels of unconjugated bilirubin, and may cause kernicterus and death in infancy.

Only conjugated bilirubin (non-protein bound) can pass the renal glomerulus, and bilirubinuria indicates conjugated hyperbilirubinaemia. It is suggested by the passage of dark-orange urine, especially if, after shaking, the froth is orange (if the dark colour is due to a concentrated urine the froth is white). More minor degrees may be detected with 'Ictotest'—a strip test manufactured by Ames. Urobilinogen is the colourless product of bacterial action on conjugated bilirubin reaching the intestinal lumen via the bile. After reabsorption it is excreted in the bile, any excess over liver excretory capacity appearing in the urine. Although urinary excretion is sometimes slightly increased in hepatocellular damage, many other factors, such as urinary pH, affect it, and its detection is of doubtful value as a liver function test; complete absence is compatible with failure of bile to reach the intestinal lumen due to total biliary obstruction.

Tests of Hepatic Parenchymal Cells. The hepatic parenchymal cells are predominantly affected in *hepatitis* of any aetiology—whether acute or chronic—and by *infiltration* of the liver, as with secondary malignant deposits. They are involved, together with reticulo-endothelial cells, in *cirrhosis*. They may be secondarily involved in obstructive biliary conditions, due to regurgitation of bile; in this case evidence of biliary involvement is predominant.

Tests of Hepatic Cell Damage. These tests may be the only abnormal ones when mild, or patchy, cell damage spares enough relatively normal cells to maintain apparently normal function. They are often the only abnormal findings in acute conditions, before tests of synthetic function, such as serum albumin concentration, become abnormal. Their sensitivity is such that they may be slightly affected in many intercurrent illnesses not primarily involving the liver; in these conditions this abnormality is not necessarily of clinical significance, and they are likely to return to normal with recovery from the primary illness. It is important to take the full clinical picture into account before embarking on extensive, and sometimes potentially dangerous, investigations (such as liver biopsy).

The tests depend on detection of intracellular constituents in abnormal amounts in the plasma. *Enzymes* can be detected in very low concentrations because their catalytic activity can be measured. Like all such tests, results should be interpreted with the following points in mind.

1. If excretion and breakdown are steady, *levels* of circulating enzymes depend on:

   a. The rate of release from cells (*rate of damage*).

   b. The *extent of damage.*

Rapid damage of relatively few cells (for instance, in acute hepatitis) may cause higher levels than more extensive but slowly progressing damage (as in cirrhosis). The rate of fall towards normal may be rapid in the first case, but levels may be steady, or rise slowly, in the second. Moreover, very extensive damage, as in acute liver atrophy, may leave so few cells to undergo further damage that falling levels, far from indicating recovery, are terminal. Neither single nor serial estimations are therefore necessarily of prognostic value.

2. The use of plasma enzymes to *localize* cell damage to a particular organ depends on the fact that different tissues contain enzymes in different proportions. For instance, liver parenchymal cells contain high concentrations of aspartate and alanine transaminases (AST and ALT), and of lactate dehydrogenase (LD). Most enzymes are present to some extent in nearly all cells, and no enzyme (or even pattern of enzymes) is truly specific to one tissue. For instance, extensive trauma and circulatory failure cause leakage of many types of enzyme from all cells, and the pattern is then of no diagnostic value, while malignant tissue may elaborate enzymes (such as LD) usually thought to be 'specific' to a few tissues. Haemolysis (*in vitro* and *in vivo*) and other blood diseases such as leukaemias and megaloblastic anaemias can also cause elevation of LD and AST.

If these points are borne in mind, the tests can often be useful.

Patterns in Liver Disease. These tests are the best ones for detecting acute hepatocellular disease. Probably the most useful enzymes for detecting liver cell damage are the transaminases (AST and ALT). Many other enzymes including isocitrate dehydrogenase and lactate dehydrogenase are also elevated when there is hepatocellular damage, but their estimation offers no great advantage for this purpose. γ-Glutamyl-transpeptidase activity is a very sensitive index, and may either be used as a primary test or, in suspected liver disease, if other enzymes are normal.

AST occurs in both the mitochondria and the cytoplasm of liver cells, while ALT is found in cytoplasms only. In *acute hepatocellular damage* (viral or toxic) both reach very high levels, and, although ALT is higher than AST, either may be used as an index of liver disease. In chronic hepatitis (either chronic aggressive or chronic persistent) rises are less marked, and ALT is more sensitive than AST measurement. Deposits or infiltration of the liver (as by secondary malignant deposits) cause a more marked rise of AST than ALT, and a similar pattern is found in *cirrhosis*. Hepatocellular damage can occur with biliary obstruction.

It is important to note that the sensitivity of transaminase estimation is such that all other tests of 'liver function' (including plasma bilirubin and alkaline phosphatase concentration) are often normal when transaminase levels are raised.

Tests of Hepatic Cell Function. These tests are most affected in chronic liver disease, especially in cirrhosis. The liver, like other organs, has a large reserve capacity, and impaired function is only demonstrable when much of the liver parenchyma has been damaged.

Albumin is synthesized in the liver. Hypo-albuminaemia is a relatively common non-specific finding. It may occur in extensive chronic liver disease, when it is accompanied by the other protein findings discussed below; these protein abnormalities may be the only findings in cirrhosis.

Many coagulation factors also depend on hepatic synthesis. A prolonged prothrombin time, not reversed by parenteral administration of vitamin K, may be demonstrable. In advanced cases haemorrhages may occur.

Jaundice due to impaired bilirubin metabolism by liver cells may accompany extensive disease.

Typically, both conjugated and unconjugated fractions are elevated.

If other tests are normal, a *bromosulphthalein* (BSP) *retention test* may help to indicate liver dysfunction; it is unnecessary if other evidence is present. BSP is conjugated and secreted by normal liver cells. Significant retention in the bloodstream (in the absence of obstructive jaundice) indicates impaired hepatic function. The test is very sensitive, and may be slightly impaired in many illnesses, including those associated with pyrexia, and in congestive cardiac failure.

Tests of Biliary Tract Involvement. These are the tests most affected in obstructive disease of the biliary tract, or in cholangitis.

Biliary Tract Enzymes. The cells lining the biliary tracts (intra- and extrahepatic) contain high concentrations of *alkaline phosphatase, 5'-nucleotidase* and γ-*glutamyl-transpeptidase.* Any disease

conjugated fraction is predominant. In cholangitis, when large space-occupying lesions spare areas of normal liver, bilirubin levels may be normal, or only slightly raised.

Other Tests. The *prothrombin time* may be prolonged due to malabsorption of the fat-soluble vitamin K when bile salts cannot enter the intestine. Unlike the prolonged prothrombin time due to hepatocellular damage, it can be corrected by parenteral administration of vitamin K. As mentioned above, the bromosulphthalein retention test cannot distinguish between hepatocellular and biliary jaundice. In primary biliary cirrhosis *plasma cholesterol* levels may be markedly elevated.

Tests indicating Involvement of the Reticulo-endothelial System. The reticulo-endothelial cells manufacture immunoglobulins, and abnormal immunoglobin levels are found in many liver

Table I. RESULTS OF LABORATORY TESTS IN LIVER DISEASE

	TRANSAMINASES	ALKALINE PHOSPHATASE	ALBUMIN	γ-GLOBULINS AND IMMUNO-GLOBULINS	BILIRUBIN	OTHER LABORATORY FINDINGS
Acute hepatitis	Both very high, ALT more than AST	N or slightly ↑	Usually N	Usually N (IgM may be slightly raised in viral)	Variable	
Chronic hepatitis	ALT more than AST (AST may be normal)	N or slightly ↑	N or slightly ↓	Diffuse ↑ (IgG)	Variable often N	
Cirrhosis	AST more than ALT (both may be normal)	N or slightly ↑	Usually ↓	Diffuse ↑ (IgA)	Often N	PT may be prolonged. *Not* reversed by i.m. vitamin K
Complete biliary obstruction	Variable	↑ ↑	Usually N	Usually N	C↑ ↑	PT may be prolonged but reversed by i.m. vitamin K
Biliary cirrhosis	Variable	↑ ↑	N or slightly ↓	IgM↑	C↑	Cholesterol↑ ↑

N = normal; C = conjugated bilirubin; ALT = alanine transaminase; AST = aspartate transaminase; PT = prothrombin time.

primarily affecting the biliary tree causes raised plasma levels of these enzymes, which may be due either to damage to, or proliferation of, the cells. Unless liver cells are also damaged, transaminases are little affected. A similar pattern may be due to large space-occupying lesions in the liver (such as a hydatid cyst or primary hepatoma). Alkaline phosphatase activity is usually adequate as a test of biliary tract involvement if there is other evidence of liver disease, such as abnormal transaminase or bilirubin levels. However, circulating alkaline phosphatase also originates from bone. γ-Glutamyl-transpeptidase and 5'-nucleotidase are not raised in bony disease, and either estimation may help to elucidate the rare cases where the origin of a raised plasma alkaline phosphatase is obscure; they cannot be used to assess whether, in the presence of liver disease, bone is also involved.

Bilirubin. The highest plasma bilirubin levels are found in obstructive biliary disease. The

diseases. Overactivity of the reticulo-endothelial system is reflected in the diffusely raised γ-globulin of many chronic liver diseases. IgA and IgG overlap β- and γ-globulin on the routine electrophoretic strip; IgA is predominantly elevated in *cirrhosis* and IgG in *chronic active hepatitis* which may, therefore, be associated with β–γ fusion. IgM is the predominant fraction in primary biliary cirrhosis, in which the β and γ fractions remain separated.

Tests indicating the Aetiology of the Disease.

Hepatitis Associated Antigen (*HAA*; *Australian Antigen*) usually indicates a viral origin for hepatitis. *Circulating antibodies* to mitochondria, smooth muscle, and nuclei (antinuclear factor) occur in chronic active hepatitis, cryptogenic cirrhosis, and primary biliary cirrhosis.

α-*Fetoprotein* (AFP) may be detectable in the blood of some patients with primary hepatoma.

Joan F. Zilva.

LYMPH-NODE (LYMPHATIC GLAND) ENLARGEMENT

1. GENERALIZED ENLARGEMENT

In certain diseases many of the lymph-nodes in the body are enlarged—generalized nodular enlargement, as distinct from enlargement of local groups of nodes only. This distinction is not absolute, however, for in some patients suffering from a malady which usually causes general lymphatic nodular enlargement the changes may be confined to local groups.

The following disorders should be considered:

α. **Primary Disorders of Lymph-nodes and Blood-forming Organs:**

    Acute lymphatic and myelocytic leukaemia
    Chronic lymphatic leukaemia (early)
    Chronic myeloid leukaemia (late)
    Polycythaemia rubra vera (late)
    Lymphoma (Hodgkin's disease, lymphosarcoma, and reticulum-cell sarcoma).

2. **Infections:**

    Diffuse skin infection or inflammation
    Infectious mononucleosis
    Secondary syphilis
    Toxoplasmosis
    Dengue
    Tuberculosis (rarely)
    Listerosis
    Filariasis
    Leishmaniasis
    Scrub typhus.

3. **Hypersensitivity Reactions and Connective-tissue Disorders:**

    Serum sickness
    Systemic lupus erythematosus
    Rheumatoid arthritis
    Still's disease
    Drug reactions.

4. **Miscellaneous:**

    Sarcoidosis

General nodular enlargement usually implies simultaneous affection of the cervical, axillary, epitrochlear, and inguinal nodes; those in the popliteal space or above the internal condyle of the humerus are less often affected. The various groups within the abdomen can seldom be palpated, whilst enlargement of the mediastinal and bronchial groups may only be demonstrated by X-rays or lymphangiograms.

When a case of generalized lymphatic nodular enlargement presents itself, the first investigation should be a blood-count; chronic lymphatic leukaemia may at once be identified (p. 56). *Chronic myeloid leukaemia* in its late stages may be accompanied by generalized lymph-node enlargement. At this stage anaemia is usually marked, as it is also in advanced chronic lymphatic leukaemia. *Polycythaemia rubra vera* in its late stages may present not only with marked splenomegaly but with diffuse lymph-node enlargement and often anaemia. (*See* p. 749.)

HODGKIN'S DISEASE nearly always starts with swelling of one group of nodes, especially those in the neck. There is usually moderate enlargement of the spleen, and in the course of weeks or months swelling of other groups of lymphatic nodes occurs, especially those in the axillae and in the thorax, the resultant masses being sometimes of considerable size (*see Figs.* 53, 54, p. 44), though the individual nodes remain distinct from one another, do not tend to break down and suppurate, and do not become fixed either to the skin or to the deeper parts as usually happens if they are tuberculous, inflammatory, or due to secondary deposits of malignant disease. The occurrence of pyrexia especially of a peculiar relapsing type (Pel-Ebstein) may assist in diagnosis, reduction of fever by radiotherapy being another diagnostic feature. Ingestion of alcohol may cause pain at the site of the lesion, thus assisting in differential diagnosis. The blood changes in Hodgkin's disease are variable; the majority of cases exhibit a leucocytosis and eosinophilia, in some instances of high degree. Biopsy of a suitable and characteristic lymph-node will clinch the diagnosis.

The diagnosis of *lymphosarcoma* and reticulum-cell sarcoma is by biopsy, clinical manifestations being very similar. Lymphosarcoma is particularly prone to affect the mediastinal or bronchial nodes, and a fair number of mediastinal new growths is due to lymphosarcoma of the mediastinal nodes. Pruritis occurs but less commonly than in Hodgkin's disease.

DENGUE, an arbovirus infection, is associated, unlike most, with a diffuse lymphadenopathy.

SYPHILITIC NODES seldom attain any considerable degree of enlargement. The first to be involved are those in the neighbourhood of the chancre, and therefore most often those in the groin, spreading later to all the nodes in the body, including those in the occipital region which are not as a rule affected except by syphilis, pediculosis capitis with sores, impetigo capitis, suppurating ring-worm (kerion), lymphatic leukaemia, and rubella. The epitrochlear nodes also are usually palpable. Syphilitic nodes are almond-shaped and firm, painless, or at most slightly tender, and they do not become adherent to the skin or to the deeper parts. They may remain palpable for months after the other signs of secondary syphilis have disappeared. The difficulty in their diagnosis does not arise when chancre or roseola is present, but later their nature may not be obvious unless there is a clear history of syphilis, or serum tests are positive.

In INFECTIOUS MONONUCLEOSIS, although the cervical nodes in particular are conspicuous, generalized enlargement may occur. There may be a high degree of lymphocytosis so that a provisional erroneous diagnosis of lymphatic leukaemia may be made or neutropenia may be present, suggesting a drug reaction. In some cases a positive Wassermann reaction has led to confusion with syphilis. Splenomegaly occurs in 50 per cent of cases, maximal in the second and third weeks of the illness. A grey membrane resembling a diphtheritic lesion but confined to the tonsils is relatively common. As an early diagnostic sign a petechial eruption has been pointed out at the junction of the soft and hard palate, appearing on the fourth day of the illness and persisting for three or four days.

In RHEUMATOID ARTHRITIS, while generalized lymph-node enlargement is occasionally present

splenomegaly is more common than in the adult.

DRUGS: A large number of drugs may cause generalized lymph-node enlargement, anti-leprosy,

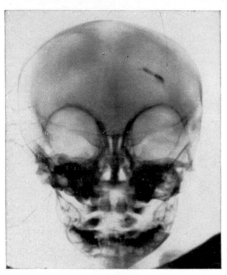

Fig. 518. Intracerebral calcification in a child with toxoplasmosis.

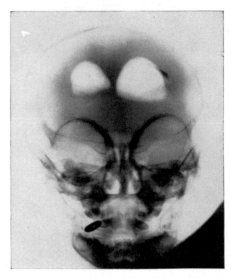

Fig. 519. The same as in *Fig.* 469 with the addition of a ventriculogram. Note the dilatation of the left lateral ventricle.

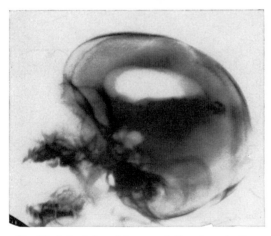

Fig. 520. Lateral view of the same skull as shown in *Figs.* 518, 519. (*By kind permission of Dr. Noel Olivier Richards. Radiograph by Dr. John Rae.*)

in most cases it is confined to those nodes draining actively inflamed joints—axillary, inguinal, and epitrochlear. Supraclavicular node enlargement is rare and when it occurs some other pathology, such as lymphoma, infectious mononucleosis, or lymphatic leukaemia, should be suspected. Splenomegaly is rare (around 3–5 per cent) in adults, though it is part of Felty's syndrome (rheumatoid arthritis with neutropenia and lymph-node enlargement).

In STILL'S DISEASE (*chronic polyarthritis* in childhood) lymph-node enlargement with

anti-thyroid, isoniazid, hydantoin derivatives, and a number of others, particularly if they cause a diffuse rash.

TUBERCULOSIS of lymph-nodes is more often local than general; occasionally, however, one meets with a case in which the inguinal and axillary as well as the cervical and internal nodes are all enlarged as the result of tuberculous infection. This then closely simulates Hodgkin's disease, and to establish the diagnosis it may be necessary to excise one of the affected nodes and examine it histologically and bacteriologically. The occurrence of caseation is confirmatory of tuberculosis. It should be realized that tuberculosis may occur in lymph-nodes affected by Hodgkin's disease or carcinoma.

In SARCOIDOSIS any of the lymph-nodes may be affected throughout the body. In other reticuloses, Gaucher's, Hans-Christian-Schüller, Niemann-Pick, Tay-Sachs diseases, there may also be corresponding lymphadenopathies.

TOXOPLASMOSIS. This is a congenital condition acquired in utero, from an infected but symptomless mother, in which there is extensive damage to the developing brain tissue with multiple intracerebral calcifications (*see* Figs. 518–520) and chronic retinitis. But there is also an acquired form in adults in which lymphadenopathy is common and so prominent as to suggest primary lymphatic disease. It takes the form of an illness with abrupt onset, high fever, acute pneumonitis, myocarditis, and general enlargement of lymph-nodes. In this variety there is no intracranial calcification or chronic retinitis. Maculopapular rashes often appear early in the illness and tend to disappear in a few days.

II. LOCALIZED LYMPH-NODE ENLARGEMENT

In all the above diseases in which enlargement of the lymphatic glands may be general a localized distribution may be encountered, either permanently or in an early stage. In addition the following must be included:

Local sepsis in skin or mucous membranes from which the lymphatics drain into the particular nodes that are involved
Tuberculous disease
Secondary malignant disease
Mycosis fungoides
Acute infections such as cat-scratch fever, brucellosis, rubella, plague, blastomycosis, syphilis, kala-azar, glanders, lymphogranuloma venereum, arbovirus infections, melioidosis, trypanosomiasis, tularaemia, and coccidioidomycosis.

Occipital Nodes. These may be enlarged as the result of leukaemia, Hodgkin's disease, rubella, syphilis, or tuberculosis, often with simultaneous enlargement of other nodes. When enlargement is restricted to the occipital nodes, by far the likeliest cause is rubella or septic absorption from the posterior region of the scalp, particularly from *impetigo, seborrhoeic dermatitis, suppurating ringworm* (*kerion*), *suppurating wen or sebaceous cyst, suppurating scalp wound,* or *pediculosis capitis*. Nits should be looked for in the hair. These may be found in the most unexpected circumstances: irritation of the skin at the back of the neck may have been speciously attributed to the rubbing of a collar.

Pre-auricular Nodes. The common cause for enlargement of the pre-auricular nodes is *septic infection* of the skin of the cheek, eyelid, ear, or temporal region of the scalp. Rarer causes are *epithelioma, rodent ulcer, lupus vulgaris*. The nodes may also be the site of *melanotic sarcoma*, the primary growth being in the eye or from a pigmented mole elsewhere in the body.

Acute Infections

Cat-scratch Fever. This is most commonly seen in children. After an incubation period of 7–10 days an inflamed papule appears at the site of the injury and enlarged nodes which suppurate appear in various situations apart from anatomical relationship to the lesion. The illness persists for about 3 weeks.

In *undulant fever* (*brucellosis*) lymph-nodes are affected in about 50 per cent of cases, cervical nodes most commonly. In *filariasis*, lymphadenitis almost always accompanies lymphangitis, the inguinal femoral and epitrochlear nodes being most commonly involved. *Melioidosis* can present as an acute, subacute, or chronic inflammatory condition, with or without suppuration anywhere in or on the surface of the body with appropriate lymphadenitis. In *African trypanosomiasis* tender lymphadenopathy is almost invariably present, the nodes becoming gradually indurated. Those of the posterior cervical triangles are typically involved (Winterbottom's sign). It has been said that irregular fever, lymphadenopathy, and circinate erythema in a European resident in Africa less than 7 years should arouse suspicion of the diagnosis. In *tularaemia*, although generalized lymphadenopathy may occur, regional enlargement in relation to local infection is the rule. It is often very marked, more so than in most infections. Coccidioidomycosis may be benign or disseminated and severe. Lung lesions and hilar and mediastinal adenitis are common. In *plague*, pain and tenderness are present in the infected regional lymph-nodes (buboes), 70 per cent of which are in the inguinal or femoral areas. *Blastomycosis*, a fungus infection of the skin and viscera, may, in both North and South American varieties spread to involve the lymph-nodes.

Submaxillary Nodes. The commonest cause for enlargement of these is oral infection. Tonsillitis and inflammation of the fauces are responsible for most cases in which a firm node becomes palpable just beneath and behind the angle of the jaw; the enlargement is generally greater upon one side than upon the other. The nodes are painful in the acute stages and in a few cases the infection is so severe that suppurative adenitis with an abscess results. All kinds of inflammation of the throat may cause this nodular enlargement—follicular tonsillitis, quinsy, diphtheria, scarlet fever, Vincent's angina, secondary syphilis. Infectious mononucleosis should always be kept in mind. The nature of the infecting organism is ascertained by bacteriological culture of swabbings from the tonsils or fauces, but the organisms obtained may sometimes be superimposed on another condition, such as infectious mononucleosis or secondary syphilis, and lead to a wrong diagnosis. Vincent's angina produces nodular enlargement less frequently than do other severe forms of sore throat.

The enlargement may be due to tuberculosis even when the swollen node is solitary, unilateral, and confined to the region of the angle of the jaw where a tonsillar inflammatory cause might seem more probable. Persistence of the swollen node, its gradual adherence to the skin, or the development of other nodes farther down the neck and a lilac-red discoloration of the skin encourage a revision from an initial diagnosis of inflammatory node to that of tubercle, especially if the patient is a child.

Inflammatory changes in nodes farther forward beneath the jaws are often secondary to caries of a tooth or to some variety of stomatitis. Less acute enlargement, going on to much greater size than is usual with inflammatory adenitis, may result from secondary deposits of *malignant disease* in the submaxillary nodes when there is squamous-celled carcinoma (epithelioma) of the tongue, lip, gum, cheek, nose, palate, fauces, tonsil, pharynx, or larynx. The diagnosis in these cases depends upon the presence of an obvious primary epithelioma: for confirmation, biopsy is performed.

Cervical Nodes. Enlargement of the nodes in the neck may be either unilateral or bilateral. If unilateral, if only a few nodes are involved, and if the history is short, the cause is probably *inflammatory*, particularly if there has been any sore place on the skin of the neck, the buccal mucosa, or in the throat, or if the patient has otitis media. Acute cervical adenitis often with sore throat is one of the chief features of infectious mononucleosis (*see* p. 785). *Pediculosis capitis* is a not uncommon cause of enlarged cervical nodes in children. It is sometimes difficult, however, to decide when the enlargement is merely inflammatory and when it is due to some more serious lesion, particularly *tuberculosis* or *sarcoidosis* on the one hand or *Hodgkin's disease* or *lymphosarcoma* on the other. The longer the glandular swellings persist, the less likely are they to be of purely inflammatory origin. The younger the patient the more likely are they to be tuberculous or due to sarcoidosis. If they are present on both sides of the neck, tend to become adherent to one another and to the skin, and are tender notwithstanding their having been present for some time, they are probably tuberculous. Spontaneous breaking down of the nodes with a red indolent condition of the skin around a discharging sinus and very slow healing, are developments to be forestalled whenever possible. Such conditions are almost certainly tuberculous when there is no question of a late stage of malignant disease. There may be confirmatory evidence in the shape of tuberculous lesions elsewhere, especially in a joint, the spine, or the peritoneum. Patients with tuberculosis of the lymph-nodes are unlikely to develop ordinary phthisis, so that the absence of lung signs is no indication that the nodes are not tuberculous. Hodgkin's disease is sometimes so restricted in its earlier lesions as to affect the cervical lymphatic nodes long before other groups are involved. On biopsy Hodgkin's disease is readily distinguishable from the giant-cell changes of tuberculosis in most cases, and bacteriological cultures are negative.

Secondary carcinoma of the nodes in the neck is suggested when the past or present existence of a primary growth is known, generally a squamous-celled carcinoma (epithelioma) of the tongue, lip, gum, cheek, face, palate, pharynx, larynx, or oesophagus. In some cases of oesophageal carcinoma, metastatic nodes may precede the occurrence of symptoms of stenosis.

Sarcomatous nodes in the neck are rare; the chief variety is lymphosarcoma.

Supraclavicular Nodes. When the nodes immediately above the clavicle, especially those on the left side in the region of the attachment of the sternomastoid muscle, are enlarged without affection of other lymphatic nodes in the neck, they suggest a *primary new growth in the chest or abdomen*, with secondary deposits ascending along the course of the thoracic duct to affect the nodes close to the entry of the duct at the junction of the left jugular and left subclavian veins. Although usually absent, the value of the sign (*Troisier's*) when present is considerable. The primary carcinoma may be the stomach, bronchus, gall-bladder, pancreas, colon, rectum, ovary, testicle, prostate, kidney, or suprarenal; excision and microscopical examination of the left supraclavicular node may indicate the site of the primary growth. The right supraclavicular node may be enlarged in a similar way, but less often—and generally not as the result of intra-abdominal but of *intrathoracic new growth*, particularly bronchial carcinoma or squamous-cell carcinoma of the oesophagus. Apart from new growth, supraclavicular lymph-adenitis may occur in septic or infective conditions of the skin of the neck and upper extremity, the pharynx, larynx, oesophagus or thyroid.

Axillary Nodes. The three main causes for localized enlargement of the nodes in one axilla are: *Septic absorption* from sore places upon the fingers, arm, breast, shoulder, or upper part of the back; *secondary deposits* of carcinoma from the breast; and *Hodgkin's disease*. Tuberculous axillary nodes without obvious affection of those in the neck are uncommon, although tuberculosis of the breast might be responsible. The source of sepsis may be slight, perhaps no more than inflammation around or under a finger-nail. Inflammatory nodes are generally painful, and associated with pyrexia. Lymphatic leukaemia will be excluded by the absence of pathognomonic blood changes; the breasts should be palpated carefully lest an unsuspected carcinoma be present. Axillary nodes are enlarged in most active cases of rheumatoid and similar inflammatory arthropathies; Hodgkin's disease will suggest itself only if other more likely causes are excluded, but biopsy will clinch the diagnosis. If diagnosis is delayed in Hodgkin's disease other lymphatic nodes will in due course become enlarged (*see* Figs. 53, 54, p. 44): concomitant enlargement of the spleen is usually present.

Epitrochlear Nodes. The most common cause of enlargement of the epitrochlear gland is infection of the fingers, hand, or forearm. The site of primary infection is generally in the skin—a whitlow, wound, or sore—but it may be more deep-seated, as in cases of infective synovitis, arthritis, or periarthritis. They are relatively common in rheumatoid arthritis where the hand and wrist on that side are actively involved. The finding of these nodes is a good point in differential diagnosis from generalized osteoarthrosis.

Mediastinal and Bronchial Nodes. Their enlargement is surmised when there are signs of bronchial obstruction, laryngeal paralysis, or stenosis of either the innominate vein or the superior or inferior vena cava. The commonest cause by far is a primary bronchial carcinoma. Hiccup may be produced. Radiographs and bronchoscopy confirm the diagnosis; tomographs are often helpful. Inflammatory or caseous bronchial or mediastinal nodes seldom if ever obstruct a bronchus to the extent that malignant nodes often do. When, as happens in rare cases, a caseous node does obstruct a bronchus, it will usually be on the right side as a form of early post-primary tuberculous disease in a child or young adult. In pulmonary sarcoidosis (*see* DYSPNOEA) great non-obstructive enlargement of the hilar nodes is usually unaccompanied by lymphadenopathy elsewhere. Erythema nodosum is often present.

Mesenteric Nodes. Any *inflammatory* condition of the bowel may lead to their enlargement, particularly if there is ulceration of the mucous membrane, as in cases of *ulcerative colitis, dysentery, tuberculosis of the bowel, typhoid fever,* or *undulant* (*brucellar*) *fever*. Non-specific mesenteric adenitis in children accepted as of viral origin may be one aspect of 'the periodic syndrome'. In cases of *tuberculous peritonitis*, the masses that are felt in the abdomen are hardly ever the nodes themselves, but extensive inflammatory and caseous mattings of which nodes may form the nucleus.

Malignant new growth, such as primary carcinoma of the stomach or colon, ovary, uterus, or testis, may cause extensive secondary deposits in the mesenteric and retroperitoneal lymphatic nodes, usually most marked in the immediate neighbourhood of the primary growth but extending thence in the direction of the liver until the portal nodes are involved.

Iliac and Pelvic Nodes. What has been said in regard to mesenteric nodes applies here also, but in this situation the affected nodes are more easily palpated. In cases of suspected *malignant disease*, nodules of secondary deposits in lymphatic nodes may sometimes be felt on careful palpation of the iliac fossa or upon making a rectal or vaginal examination.

Inguinal and Femoral Lymphatic Nodes. The commonest cause of localized enlargement of the inguinal lymphatic nodes is infection in the area of lymphatic distribution. Search should be made for sources of infection between the toes, upon the feet, legs, thighs, buttocks, lower part of the back, scrotum, penis, perineal and vulval regions. A urethral discharge, gonorrhoeal or otherwise, may be responsible. Most of these cases are associated with constitutional symptoms, especially pyrexia, and with local pain and reddening. The nodes may break down into abscesses—buboes. The venereal disease, lymphogranuloma venereum, is a venereally transmitted infection caused by a small intracellular bacterium, the chlamydia.

Another, but less common, cause for localized enlargement of the inguinal nodes is *carcinoma* —secondary to squamous-celled carcinoma (epithelioma) of the scrotum, prepuce, penis, perineal region, anus, clitoris, labium majus, labium minus, vagina, leg, or foot.

Melanotic sarcoma is a rare cause of enlargement of the inguinal lymphatic nodes to a degree out of all proportion to the size of the primary growth. The nature of this enlargement may be quite obscure unless the dark tinge of the growth can be seen through the skin, or there is melanuria (*see* p. 808), or a careful examination reveals a small primary new growth of the skin.

Popliteal Nodes are seldom palpable, and are discovered as a rule rather because there are enlarged lymphatic nodes elsewhere than from any symptoms which attract attention to the popliteal space itself. Almost the only cause for their enlargement is infection either from joints or from the skin of the toes, feet, or legs, comparable to the conditions which produce enlargement of the epitrochlear nodes in the arm.

F. Dudley Hart.

MACULES

Macule is the term applied to any change in a limited area of the skin without elevation or depression. Such lesions may be permanent or temporary, inflammatory or neoplastic. The term is often restricted to lesions of small size

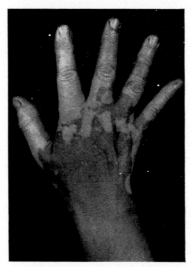

Fig. 521. Leucoderma.

up to 1–2 cm. across, larger lesions being referred to as 'patches' or 'areas'. The distinction is, however, unimportant so that lesions of any size or shape may be included. The origin of macules is varied. Thus purpura is due to the passage of blood into the skin; erythema to hyperaemia, and here we have the classic macules of measles and rubella; telangiectasia is permanent capillary dilatation of the skin, and when combined with patches of pigmentation and atrophy is an important feature of an X-ray or radium scar (*see Fig.* 14, p. 19); capillary or spider naevus is a benign vascular neoplasm; a freckle or lentigo is a macular area of increased pigmentation of the skin and many moles and naevi are macular in character; *leucoderma* or *vitiligo* (*Fig.* 521) is complete absence of pigmentation in areas of skin of varying size—this disease is more apparent after exposure to sunlight, when it is shown up by the surrounding zones of increased pigmentation. Brown macules may be the final stage in any inflammatory disorder of the skin, but they are particularly well marked after varicose dermatitis and lichen planus.

The *macular syphilide* is one of the most characteristic lesions of secondary syphilis. The eruption (*Fig.* 522), erythematous in character and named 'syphilitic roseola', begins as a macular mottling, resembling measles but rather

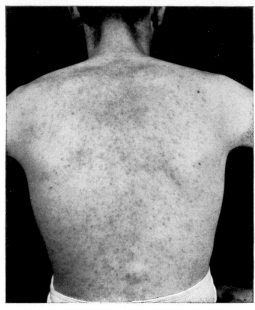

Fig. 522. Macular syphilide.

more dusky, distributed over the chest and abdomen. Generally after about a fortnight from its appearance the rash begins to fade, giving place to a papular or follicular eruption on trunk, limbs, face, and neck. An important diagnostic feature is the complete absence of itching in all eruptions due to syphilis and the presence in nearly every case of signs of a primary sore. In every case of secondary syphilis the Wassermann reaction or some other suitable test will prove positive.

The macular syphilide is distinguished from *Tinea versicolor* (*see* p. 727) by the ease with which the scaly patches can be demonstrated by scratching and by the detection of the fungus microscopically in the latter condition; from the erythematous drug rashes by their more vivid redness and the presence of itching and burning; from seborrhoeic dermatitis by the pinkish-yellow colour of the latter disease and by its scaliness; from measles by the crescentic character of the eruption, the coryza, cough, and the different distribution; and from pityriasis rosea (*see* p. 704) by the history of the herald patch, the distribution, the face and extremities usually being free, the pinkish-fawn colour, and the characteristic scaliness.

In the earliest stage of *leprosy*, erythematous macules appear on the face, limbs, or trunk, varying in colour according to the natural pigmentation of the skin, but in white races usually of a light red. The colour is brightest at the edge; the centre may become white and atrophic. In coloured races there is a loss of pigment. The macules vary in size; they are smooth and shining with a well-defined outline. Some infiltration is usually present. After a time the macules and the neighbouring areas of apparently normal skin become more or less anaesthetic. Depigmented areas must be distinguished from vitiligo and the pale areas which often accompany pityriasis versicolor, and less often eczema such as pityriasis alba on the face of boys in the summer months. The presence of anaesthesia is of great importance in the differential diagnosis of leprosy, as it is almost invariably present, if not in the lesions themselves, then in some neighbouring area of the skin. Its commonest sites are towards the centre of the macule, and in the hands and feet. Enlargement of superficial nerves can often be detected.

The lepra bacillus (*Mycobacterium leprae*) should be looked for in biopsy preparations of the lesions or in the nasal secretion.

P. D. Samman.

MALLET FINGER

Mallet finger is a condition in which a terminal phalanx is maintained in a position of acute flexion; it is diagnosable at sight. It is usually

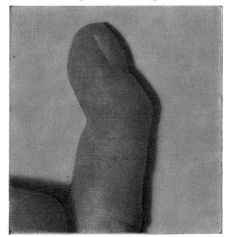

Fig. 523. Mallet finger. (*Courtesy of the Gordon Museum, Guy's Hospital.*)

the result of injury, and the deformity is due either to detachment of the insertion of the extensor aponeurosis into the base of the dorsal aspect of the terminal phalanx, a fracture of the base of the phalanx, or to stretching and attenuation of the aponeurosis, so that the flexor tendon attached anteriorly to the base of the terminal phalanx draws the latter into the position of acute flexion (*Fig.* 523). *R. G. Beard.*

MAMMARY SWELLING

Method of Examination. The patient should stand stripped to the waist, so that a clear view of both breasts, the thorax, axillae, and supra-clavicular fossae may be obtained. The surgeon should sit with his eyes level with the nipples. Both breasts should first be looked at as a whole, to see whether they are symmetrical in size, contour, and level, and whether the two nipples are in the same site and of the same circumference, prominence, and inclination. One breast may always have been smaller or one nipple depressed, but any recent change is highly significant. The patient should then lie on a couch and the breasts be studied in detail for evidence of local enlargement or shrinking, and for abnormalities such as redness of the skin, dilatation of veins, tumour, or ulcer. If no difference is at first noticed, the patient should be asked to raise both arms slowly above the head and bring them down again to the side, since differences previously invisible, particularly dimpling of the skin from attachment of a lump, may come into view as the breast glides over the chest wall. Next the breasts are felt, using first the flat of the hand, passing systematically over all parts, examining comparable sectors on the two sides simultaneously; afterwards the fingers are used for more detailed examination of any irregularity that may have been discovered or suspected. The axillae should also be palpated carefully for enlarged glands, particular attention being paid to the inner wall along the pectoralis minor and to the apex. In cases of suspected cancer the supra- and infra-clavicular fossae should also be examined for fullness or enlarged glands, and the chest and liver should be investigated for signs of secondary growth. Examination from behind with the patient sitting may be used to check any abnormalities seen, felt, or suspected in the lying position.

Transillumination may be applied to any localized swelling; it will identify a cyst containing clear fluid, but it is valueless as a means of distinction between solid tumours. X-ray mammography may be helpful in some cases.

Classification:

SWELLINGS OF THE WHOLE BREAST:
Bilateral:
 Pregnancy
 Lactation
 Hypertrophy
 In males from stilboestrol administration
Unilateral:
 Fibro-adenosis of the newborn
 Fibro-adenosis (usually bilateral)
 Puberty
 Unilateral hypertrophy.

LOCAL SWELLINGS IN THE BREAST:
 Acute mastitis
 Tuberculous abscess
 Fat necrosis
 Single cysts:
  Galactocele
  Single cysts in fibro-adenosis

Innocent tumours:
 Hard fibro-adenoma
 Soft fibro-adenoma
 Duct papilloma
 Lipoma
Malignant:
 Carcinoma
 Sarcoma.

MULTIPLE SWELLINGS, USUALLY INVOLVING BOTH BREASTS:
 Fibro-adenosis
 Multiple cysts.

SWELLINGS THAT ARE NOT OF THE BREAST:
 Retromammary abscess:
  From disease of rib
  Chronic empyema
 Chondroma of chest wall
 Deformities of the ribs.

Swelling in Pregnancy and Lactation is normal, and only liable to cause confusion when the patient is unaware of her condition. Both breasts are enlarged equally and feel tense and nodular. The superficial veins are usually prominent, and on gentle squeezing a few drops of milk are discharged from the nipple. Montgomery's tubercles will be evident.

True Hypertrophy is rare. The enlargement is of two types; the commoner where multiple fibro-adenomata cause a bilateral enlargement of varying consistency, and the less common consisting in a diffuse lipomatosis of both breasts sometimes attaining prodigious proportions. The condition is usually bilateral, but may be one-sided, in which case it is very disfiguring.

Unilateral Enlargements are usually found in the undeveloped breast. In the *newborn* one breast is often enlarged to the limits of its infantile size, and may discharge a little serous fluid from the nipple. The enlargement used to be attributed to the manipulation of midwives, but it is more probably due to an endocrine imbalance consequent on the withdrawal of the maternal endocrines in the foetal circulation, and subsides rapidly unless perpetuated by meddlesome applications. In girls at *puberty* one breast may enlarge several months before the other, and may distress a solicitous mother; unless there are obvious signs of an inflammatory change, no notice need be taken of unilateral enlargement of the breast in girls from 10 to 13. Uniform enlargement of one breast also occurs in *men* usually after the age of 40, and nodular plaques may appear in both sexes at puberty as a result of endocrine disturbance.

Acute Mastitis usually occurs during lactation, occasionally during pregnancy, and is most often due to infection with pyogenic organisms which have gained entrance through cracks in the nipple At the beginning of the illness there is shivering, followed by fever and a feeling of weight and pain in the breast; the pain soon becomes very acute. In the early stages the swelling is limited to one part of the breast, which feels more resistant than normal; the skin is not reddened at first, nor are the lymphatic glands enlarged. Pressure over the swelling may cause extrusion of a drop of pus from the nipple, and this is distinguished from milk by its viscidity and yellow colour. Later, fluctuation may become evident, and, as the inflammation approaches the skin, this becomes red and oedematous, and ultimately an abscess may point and burst through it; at the same time other foci of suppuration form, until the breast may be a bag of pus. The presence of fever and the intense tenderness of one portion of the breast are sufficient to distinguish acute mastitis from physiological engorgement.

It is not uncommon to find a small *alveolar abscess*, the size of a hazel nut, in virgins.

Tuberculous Abscess is not so uncommon as might be supposed, and a certain number of cases of chronic mastitis and chronic abscess are really tuberculous. The disease is insidious, starting as a painless irregular swelling, the periphery of which is hard and the centre soft. Later, the skin becomes reddened, and an abscess forms which may burst and leave a sinus. It differs from an acute abscess in that the duration is much longer, there is little or no pain or fever, and the pus, if examined, reveals no organisms on culture unless there has been secondary infection; direct examination of stained films of the pus may show tubercle bacilli. The facts that the history is a long one, that the swelling or the edges of it are hard, and that the axillary glands may be enlarged, render this condition liable to be confounded with carcinoma of the ordinary form, or one in which suppuration has occurred.

Local Fat Necrosis following a blow on the breast, or even a saline infusion, may give rise to a tumour almost indistinguishable from cancer. It is hard, irregular in outline, and fixed to the skin. Points of distinction are the previous history of severe injury at the exact spot where the swelling lies, the impression given on palpation that the lump is *on* rather than *of* the breast, and the absence of hard glands in the axilla. Sometimes a period of two or three weeks' observation is justifiable, in which time a traumatic swelling should decrease in size, but if there is any real doubt about its nature it should be excised with a wide ellipse of surrounding breast tissue, and submitted to section.

Galactocele, a cyst containing milk, is formed by dilatation of one of the larger ducts owing to obstruction. Galactoceles occur only during lactation and very rarely in the later months of pregnancy; they form oval fluctuating swellings lying in the central zone of the breast just outside the areola, and on pressure milk can sometimes be squeezed out of the nipple.

Single Cysts in Fibro-adenosis usually lie on the deep surface of the breast, so that their outline is obscured and they bear a considerable resemblance to carcinoma. The absence of skin dimpling and of any alteration in the size or shape of the breast as a whole or in the appearance of the nipple, and a sensation of elasticity when the swelling is pressed firmly, suggest the diagnosis. These cysts are discussed further on page 521.

Innocent Tumours. A fibro-adenoma is the only common innocent tumour of the breast, and the *hard fibro-adenoma* is far commoner than the soft variety. The hard fibro-adenoma is an encapsulated tumour, generally single, but sometimes multiple, and varying in size. It is firm, with the consistency of hard rubber, rounded, or with irregular rounded projections, and clearly outlined. Most characteristic is the ease with which it can be moved under the skin and in the substance of the breast, to neither of which does it appear to have any attachment. These tumours generally occur between the ages of 18 and 30, and though they are quite painless, they are so firm that they are usually discovered by the patient. The *soft fibro-adenoma* sometimes occurs in older women, being found between the ages of 40 and 45, although exceptions to this rule may be found in both directions, that is a hard fibro-adenoma may arise in the fourth decade and a soft fibro-adenoma in the third. Generally the tumour has elements of both types when examined under the microscope, but the predominance of one type gives it the overall characteristics detected on clinical examination. Soft fibro-adenoma has the rounded outline, the absence of fixation to skin or fascia, and the remarkably free mobility of a hard fibro-adenoma, but it is usually larger when first noticed, it is softer and almost elastic in consistency, and it grows fairly rapidly. Owing to its size it can usually be seen as well as felt. It may undergo cystic degeneration, and then enlarge fairly rapidly giving a sense of fluctuation. A hard fibro-adenoma can usually be recognized without difficulty but if it is placed so deeply that its outline is obscured, it may resemble a carcinoma. Points of distinction are the free mobility, the normal shape and consistency of the breast, the absence of enlarged glands, and the age. A carcinoma may occur under 30, but it is usually diffuse and rapidly growing, and not a small, hard, mobile lump. A soft fibro-adenoma is clearly a rounded tumour separate from the breast and pushing it aside. It can be mistaken only for a sarcoma or a lipoma; but a sarcoma, though it appears separate from the breast, has not the free mobility of a fibro-adenoma; further it is excessively rare. A *lipoma* may occur in the breast as elsewhere, and has the same characters.

A *duct papilloma* is a small rounded tumour near the nipple; when it is handled a serous or blood-stained discharge may appear at the nipple. There is no means of distinguishing a duct papilloma from an early intraduct carcinoma, and the part should always be removed for diagnosis.

Malignant Tumours of the breast are nearly always primary. Sarcoma is very rare, but *carcinoma* is common and the most important tumour that affects the breast. It is essentially a disease of the female breast, only about 1 per cent of the cases occurring in males. It is common in both married and unmarried women, and may occur at any age after puberty, though the majority are in women between 35 and 60. In advanced cases the disease is obvious; the tumour is large and hard, attached to and ultimately, if not removed, fungating through the skin and becoming fixed to the chest wall; the axillary glands are enlarged and hard and the patient is often cachectic. Such cases are beyond any but palliative treatment, and the importance of diagnosis lies in the recognition of the early case, where the only sign is a small lump which the patient has probably discovered accidentally. Usually there is no pain and the patient looks and feels perfectly well. The lump may lie in any part of the breast, but typically is intermediate between the nipple and the periphery, and is more commonly in the upper and outer quadrant than in the other three. It can usually be felt with the flat of the hand. These lumps may be stony hard, but any consistency may be met with. Its outline is usually not sharply defined. In the early stage it is freely movable over the pectoral muscles and under the skin, but it is not so movable in the breast substance as is a fibro-adenoma. Very soon bands of fibrous tissue that connect the breast with the skin become involved, and by their contraction prevent free movement of the skin over the swelling, and cause, first dimpling when the tumour is displaced, later puckering visible all the time. If the tumour is anywhere near the centre of the breast, the nipple becomes retracted; a nipple may have been always depressed, but if one previously well formed becomes retracted the sign is of serious import. Fixation to the deep fascia, which usually comes later, can be demonstrated by making the patient press her hands on the iliac crests to fix the pectoralis major, when the involved breast will be found to move less on the muscle than the normal one. Many cancerous tumours, even when extensive infiltration has occurred, cause shrinkage, so that the affected breast may appear smaller than the healthy one, and in the atrophic form the gland may almost disappear. In the ordinary form it will be rare to find any discharge from the nipple; a blood-stained discharge often indicates an intraduct carcinoma (*see* NIPPLE, DISCHARGE FROM, p. 572). After a while the axillary glands become enlarged and hard. Too much attention should not be given to the absence of palpable glands; in a fat patient they may be enlarged but impalpable, and in any case it is hoped to recognize cancer before the glands are involved.

This tumour, if fully intraduct, cannot be felt, and announces its presence only by a blood-stained discharge from the nipple.

Sarcoma of the breast is rare. It generally occurs in women under the age of 40. In the early stages it is not easily distinguishable from a fibro-adenoma, particularly one which is enlarging rapidly on account of a cyst or intracystic growth. It is soft, vascular, grows quickly, at first seems to push the breast aside, but later infiltrates its tissues and eventually fungates through the skin.

Fibro-adenosis (syn. Chronic Mastitis) is a diffuse induration of the breast lobules. It may affect one segment of the breast only, or the whole organ. It takes the form of hardening of part of the breast, usually the upper and outer quadrant or the axillary tail, without alteration of its shape as a whole. The swelling is firmer than the normal breast, but is not easily felt with the flat of the hand. It is often tender, and inclined to ache just before the periods. The generalized form affects the whole breast, and usually both sides. It is seen most commonly in thin women between 35 and 50, and is characterized by a general lumpiness of the whole breast. The lumps may not be felt with the flat of the hand, but when the breast is picked up between the fingers they appear as irregularly rounded swellings of rubbery consistency, on the whole arranged radially, but not clearly defined, each lump fading off into others of the same nature. The axillary glands may be palpable, but they are not hard and are often tender. A cyst in fibro-adenosis gives rise to a lump more easily palpable than the rest, and often resembling carcinoma. If the cyst is lax and superficial it can be recognized by its fluctuation and translucency, but if it is deeply placed and tense its nature is less obvious.

Multiple Cystic Disease of the breast is usually regarded as a variety of fibro-adenosis. One breast, sometimes both, becomes filled with cysts, some microscopic, others as large as walnuts, with all intermediate sizes, so that the organ has a bossy appearance. The diagnosis is usually simple. No accurate figures are available as to the 'precancerous tendency' of fibro-adenosis with or without cysts, and, since the disease fibro-adenosis is one which merges imperceptibly with the normal, no hard-and-fast line can be drawn, either clinically or histologically, between what is physiological and what is pathological. Nevertheless, statistics lend colour to the impression that carcinoma is more common in women who have previously complained of nodularity of the breasts than in those who have not. In women with large cysts, however, malignant change is exceptionally rare. In any event the malignant tendency of such lesions is not sufficiently great to warrant mastectomy as a precautionary measure. Periodic examination is a better procedure and far from alarming the patient usually produces a sense of security and a feeling that the worry and responsibility are being taken off her own shoulders.

The diagnosis of a single lump in the breast, where cancer must be taken into consideration, may cause considerable difficulty. A lump definite enough to be felt with the flat of the hand and hard enough to resemble cancer is either a hard fibro-adenoma, a tense cyst in fibro-adenosis, a localized lump of fibro-adenosis, or a carcinoma. A fibro-adenoma is usually found in women under 30, is less hard than a carcinoma, and is of rounded outline, but its contour may be obscured by surrounding fibro-adenosis. A cyst in fibro-adenosis is usually round and elastic, but if it is deep its outline is obscured, and if it is tense it may feel hard. A carcinoma is undoubtedly solid, and has an ill-defined outline; where these characters are present or where there is the slightest suggestion of skin dimpling, local flattening of the breast, or alteration in the nipple, cancer must be diagnosed.

The diagnosis of cancer at this early stage is intensely important, for only then is the prospect of cure high, but not one to be made lightly since it implies removal of the whole breast with the pectoral muscles and axillary contents. Local resection of a doubtful lump is imperative. It is important that this procedure should be carried out in an institution where, should the lump turn out to be a cancer, there will not be delay of more than a day or two before definitive treatment is carried out.

The proper course is to proceed as follows. First, consent must be obtained for a radical operation if need be, and, as the first step, the tumour is excised locally and examined by the naked eye, or with frozen section. The cut surface of a tumour is usually characteristic: a cancer cuts with a grating feel like an unripe pear, its cut surface is concave, and is a dirty white with specks of grey or brown that turn deep orange when nitric acid is applied to them; a fibro-adenoma is pearly white, with a sharp outline and a convex cut surface; a cyst contains fluid, and the fibro-adenosis around it is white and smooth with irregular margins which may include fat islets. The subsequent procedure then depends upon the condition diagnosed, and radical mastectomy is proceeded with forthwith if there is no doubt that the lump is a cancer.

Swellings Pushing the Breast Forward are often mistaken by the patient for breast tumours. A *retromammary abscess* is most commonly tuberculous, arising in an underlying rib or in a mediastinal abscess that has tracked along a branch of the internal mammary artery. Sometimes an empyema points beneath the breast, usually in the 5th or 6th intercostal space in the midclavicular line. A *chondroma* is a hard nodular swelling springing from one of the ribs and tilting the breast or pushing it aside. *Deformities of the ribs* may also cause confusion; the commonest is a prominence of the costochondral junction of the third rib, which may be forked and join two cartilages. The condition is often bilateral, and may be associated with other abnormalities of the ribs or vertebrae.

R. G. Beard.

MARASMUS

Translated literally marasmus is a 'withering' or 'growing lean', so that no more specific application is justifiable beyond that which is WEIGHT, LOSS OF (*see* p. 837). But in common usage the term is applied to progressive emaciation in infants and young children. The alternative description is *infantile atrophy*. Marasmus, then, is the name applied to extreme chronic malnutrition for which numerous causes may be responsible. Actual loss of weight is usually the outstanding criterion; the point at which an infant becomes marasmic is indeterminate, but as a reasonable if arbitrary estimate it may be so described when one-fifth to one-third of its body-weight has been lost. The condition presents an unmistakable appearance. The face, which is pinched and grey, has a curiously senile expression. The eyes and the fontanelles are sunken, the skin is tightly stretched over the bones of the skull, whereas on the limbs and body generally the skin is thin and inelastic through dehydration and loss of subcutaneous fat so that it hangs in festoons on the stick-like arms and legs. The thorax is particularly wasted and the ribs are unduly prominent. The bony fingers are often stuffed into the mouth as if to obtain nourishment. If protein depletion is a marked feature the belly may be swollen with ascites and the legs with oedema ('starvation oedema'), giving a peculiarly disproportionate appearance between the wasted and swollen parts of the anatomy. In the absence of any acute infection the temperature is subnormal and the child is usually apathetic.

Among the very many conditions which may produce this condition are included the following: starvation (either from neglect, extreme poverty, or the breakdown of normal civilized behaviour as usually occurs in modern warfare); persistent vomiting (for example, hiatus hernia) or diarrhoea; chronic infections (the urinary tract, tuberculosis, congenital syphilis, and parasitic infestations); malabsorption—of fat in coeliac disease and fibrocystic disease of the pancreas, of sugar in carbohydrate intolerance, or of protein in protein-losing enteropathy; Hirschsprung's disease; a group of conditions associated with polyuria, that is to say diabetes mellitus, diabetes insipidus, hypercalcaemia, renal acidosis, and renal failure; and, rarely in children, thyrotoxicosis, Addison's disease, and malignant disease. Severe cyanotic congenital heart disease which is not corrected may be associated with marked failure to thrive.

Starvation comprehends a variety of causes. Because of social and political circumstances the child may simply not receive enough calories. Because of ignorance, feeding may be imperfect both as regards quantity and quality. (*See* KWASHIORKOR *below*.) Because of structural imperfections, such as hare-lip, cleft palate, or feebleness from prematurity the infant may be unable to suck. Because of an oesophageal stricture dysphagia may prevent adequate intake of food and persistent vomiting will have a similar disastrous effect.

Chronic infections include serious involvement of the upper renal tract, in which circumstances associated uraemia, for example in advanced bilateral congenital hydronephrosis, may be an aggravating factor. Congenital syphilis was once a potent cause of marasmus although its classic features of snuffles, skin lesions, Parrot's nodes, condylomata, and enlargement of the liver and spleen are now rarely seen. Advanced miliary tuberculosis is now fortunately rare in Great Britain, as is neglected tuberculous disease of bone with its associated discharging sinuses leading to secondarily infected abscess cavities.

Malabsorption is a potent cause of weight-loss in children. Fibrocystic disease of the pancreas and coeliac disease are associated with gross steatorrhoea. Disaccharidase deficiency may result in the infant being unable to split disaccharides into absorbable monosaccharides. Lactase deficiency is the commonest example but the enzymes responsible for splitting sucrose and maltose may be affected. Not only is the child prevented from absorbing sugar, but this remains in the small intestine to aggravate the condition by causing diarrhoea by osmosis. Protein-losing enteropathy due to a variety of small intestinal diseases, including Crohn's disease, may result in protein loss into the bowel lumen.

Diabetes mellitus may have a relatively acute onset in children, with thirst, polyuria, and severe loss of weight.

Kwashiorkor is a condition seen chiefly in Central Africa but it has been widely described in other tropical and subtropical parts of the world and even in Europe. It is a state produced by gross protein deficiency and is usually due to incorrect feeding. The majority of sufferers are infants under the age of 2 years who, when breast-feeding is discontinued, are placed on a diet mainly of cereals with little if any animal protein; this may be because of shortage of suitable foods or deeply ingrained superstitions. In addition to the failure of growth, there is oedema of the legs, a distended abdomen, and very typical depigmentation of the skin and hair which produces a reddish hue in Negro babies. In the world today it is probably the commonest cause of marasmus.

Harold Ellis.

MELAENA

Melaena (*see also* ANUS, BLOOD PASSED THROUGH, p. 67) is the term applied to the black motion resulting from haemorrhage that has occurred in the alimentary canal at a high enough level for chemical alteration to have taken place, or after the swallowing of blood derived from haemoptysis (p. 352) or epistaxis (p. 256). The appearance has led to the familiar term 'tarry stool', a useful appellation, since it well describes its black, treacly appearance and its sticky nature, which renders it difficult to flush down the toilet. By feeding volunteer healthy medical students with increasing aliquots of their own blood it has been shown that between 50 and 80 ml. were sufficient to have this effect.

Melaena may be simulated by other conditions which render the stools dark or black, notably after taking iron by mouth in large quantities (the iron being converted into the sulphide), or following the ingestion of charcoal biscuits or much red wine. Certain foods such as bilberries or the black cherries in Switzerland may impart an intense dark colour to the motions and the same appearance is possible through the excretion of large amounts of bile pigments. Where there is occasion for doubt the diagnosis can be confirmed by laboratory investigation of the stool.

Usually melaena is due to bleeding from the oesophagus, stomach, or duodenum, and under these circumstances there will often have been *haematemesis* (p. 329) before the melaena is apparent. If melaena occurs alone from these sources it usually indicates that the rate of bleeding is relatively slow; rapid haemorrhage would almost certainly be accompanied by the vomiting of blood. However, it is not an uncommon experience for a patient to collapse from faintness in the absence of any other symptoms where an explanation is forthcoming subsequently by the passage of a tarry stool as evidence of internal bleeding.

The vast majority of patients with melaena will be found to have bled from lesions situated at or above the duodenum. The commonest, amounting to perhaps 85 per cent of patients, will be from peptic ulceration which includes duodenal and gastric ulcers, acute gastric erosions, and peptic oesophagitis. Increasing numbers are due to the erosions associated with the ingestion of aspirin in its various forms, phenylbutazone, indomethacin, or other antirheumatic agents.

Lesions lower down the bowel from the duodenum, as a rule, give rise to dark- or bright-red blood in the stools rather than melaena, but melaena may occur in the relatively uncommon group of causes of small intestinal bleeding which include haemorrhage in *typhoid fever* from an ulcerated Peyer's patch in the upper ileum or from an ulcer in the jejunum, from a *leiomyoma* or *haemangioma* of the upper jejunum, in *mesenteric thrombosis* or *embolism*, following direct injury to the abdomen by a blow or crush resulting in *contusion of the bowel*, and, particularly in children, from a peptic ulcer in a *Meckel's diverticulum*. Any of the *blood dyscrasias* may result in oozing from the mucosa in the alimentary canal and the commonest cause of this today is anticoagulant therapy. However, sharp haemorrhage from the small bowel usually results in unchanged blood, rather than tarry stools, being passed per rectum.

It is not uncommon for a patient with a chronic peptic ulcer to give a history of having passed a melaena stool on one or more occasions during the history of his disease. It is impossible to judge the severity of such bleeds from the patient's description of the stools so more emphasis should be laid on whether or not such episodes were accompanied by collapse, faintness, and sweating; whether or not the patient required admission to hospital; and whether or not the clinician dealing with the problem at that time deemed the situation serious enough to require blood transfusion. All of these would indicate the loss of a minimum of 600 ml., or probably more, of blood.

Harold Ellis.

MENORRHAGIA

Menorrhagia signifies excessive menstrual flow, or undue prolongation of the time during which it takes place. The patient is free from bleeding during the intermenstrual periods, the term METRORRHAGIA or IRREGULAR UTERINE BLEEDING (p. 531) being reserved for bleeding which occurs between the periods. Careful distinction between these symptoms often serves to distinguish very important conditions, and they should not be confounded with one another. Pure menorrhagia is an important symptom of many well-defined conditions which do not, as a rule, give rise to irregular bleeding. Both these terms must be limited carefully to patients who menstruate, and must not be used for bleeding after the menopause.

The diagnosis of menorrhagia may be difficult because of the absence of anaemia or other signs of severe menstrual blood-loss. The diagnosis has to be accepted when the patient complains of having to use more than a dozen and a half pads per menstrual period or when she loses clots or has flooding. Experiments using radioactive chromium to label red cells show that some women may suffer excessive menstrual loss without becoming anaemic, while others may show all the signs of a severe iron-deficiency anaemia due to chronic blood-loss.

Diagnoses such as *chronic metritis* and *sub-involution* are no longer made as causes of menorrhagia, for the excess of menstrual loss in women without abnormal physical signs is believed to be endocrine in origin. Acute endometritis of gonococcal or pyogenic origin tends to cure itself owing to the shedding of the endometrium during menstruation. *Tuberculous endometritis* is found in 2–5 per cent of those seeking advice for infertility. It is due to spread from the Fallopian tubes and is therefore associated with menorrhagia due to the tuberculous salpingo-oophoritis. If a tuberculous infection is suspected the uterine curettings should be examined for the typical tubercles and the organism isolated by culture or guinea-pig inoculation.

1. Endocrine System.

Menorrhagia of puberty is mainly due to hypofunction of the anterior pituitary body, with consequent failure of ovulation and want of a corpus luteum. The ovaries contain unruptured Graafian follicles, there is increased oestrogen formation, and a lack of the luteal hormone progesterone. These cases often right themselves as the pituitary gradually assumes its normal cyclic activities.

Menorrhagia of mature women without obvious lesions of the generative or other systems is thought to be due to an imbalance between the secretion by the ovary of oestrogen and progesterone, with an increase in oestrogen and a complete lack of or a deficiency of progesterone. When there is a complete absence of progesterone in the second half of the menstrual cycle the cycle is referred to as *anovular*, drawing attention to failure of ovulation and formation of a corpus luteum. The condition may be diagnosed by a study of basal temperature charts, there being no post-ovulatory rise in basal temperature, or by examination of endometrial curettings, which show evidence only of oestrogenic hypertrophy. Sometimes the ovaries become cystic and the endometrium undergoes polypoidal thickening with a characteristic microscopic appearance known as 'Swiss cheese' endometrium or 'cystic glandular hyperplasia'. This condition is known as *metropathia haemorrhagica*. Bouts of amenorrhoea of some weeks are followed by prolonged irregular bleeding, a symptom-complex which does not properly come under the heading 'Menorrhagia'.

Menorrhagia in relation to the menopause and in the years preceding is the result of increasing failure of the ovarian functions and consequent upset in balance between the secretion of oestrogen and progesterone.

Polymenorrhoea is the name given to a form of irregular and excessive menstruation in which the cycle is shortened from the usual 28 days to 21 days or even less; this is due to disturbed balance of internal secretions, causing ovulation to occur too early in the cycle; in some cases two corpora lutea have been found at the same stage of development; in many cases fibroids are present.

2. Generative System.

In considering this, some diseases will be easy to discover, others will require some special method of examination. For instance, of all the causes of pure menorrhagia, *fibromyoma* (fibroids) of the uterus stands out as the only important growth associated with this symptom, and a simple bimanual examination, as a rule, suffices to show that such a tumour exists. The chief characteristics of a fibromyoma of the uterus are these: the uterus itself is enlarged and in almost every instance the enlargement is asymmetrical, the typical shape of the organ being altered according to the number and size of the fibroids it contains; as there may be more than one tumour in the uterus, its shape may be exceedingly irregular; the consistence of the tumour is hard and unyielding as a rule, but pathological changes in these tumours are common, some of them leading to softening, others to cystic changes. The tumour and cervix always move together if the organ can be moved at all. The only difficulty in diagnosis, as a rule, lies in distinguishing a fibromyoma of the uterus from an ovarian cyst, and sometimes this is difficult, for it is not always possible to say that a given tumour is actually the enlarged uterus. It must be remembered, however, that the symptom under discussion is menorrhagia, and ovarian tumours almost never give rise to it. Ovarian tumours usually cause no disturbance of menstruation at all, unless they are double and destroy both ovaries completely, in which case they cause amenorrhoea. If the tumour cannot be diagnosed by simple examination, the uterine sound should be used if no possibility of pregnancy exists—and with pure menorrhagia pregnancy *is* impossible. In most cases of fibromyoma the sound passes beyond the normal 6 cm., and it may pass as much as 11 cm.; in cases of subperitoneal fibroids the uterus may not be much enlarged, but in such cases menorrhagia is not usually present. With ovarian tumours the length of the uterine cavity is not increased. In general, however, it is unnecessary to use the sound for the diagnosis of a fibromyoma. Adenomyoma of the uterus produces symmetrical enlargement as a rule, but cannot be distinguished from fibromyoma until after removal.

Chronic salpingo-oophoritis (in the form of a pyosalpinx, a hydrosalpinx, a tubo-ovarian abscess, or chronic interstitial salpingitis) and *ovarian endometriosis* both give rise to menorrhagia due to pelvic congestion, but dysmenorrhoea, pelvic pain, dyspareunia, and backache are usually more prominent symptoms. In either

3. Circulatory System. Any lesion of the heart, liver, or lungs which leads to back-pressure in the venous system may in theory cause hyperaemia of the pelvic organs and consequent excessive menstrual losses. It does not follow, however, that this will be the case, because the sufferers from these diseases are sometimes anaemic as far as the *quality* of the blood goes, and consequently may lack the stimulus to menstruate at all. However, it happens very occasionally that menorrhagia is caused by uncompensated valvular lesions of the heart, cirrhosis of the liver, or emphysema of the lungs.

Anaemia. The quality of the blood itself may be a cause of menorrhagia if it is deficient in calcium salts or other factors, leading to retardation of the coagulation-time. Modern methods of estimating coagulation-time enable us to distinguish these cases with some certainty, and thus

CAUSES OF MENORRHAGIA

1. OF ENDOCRINE ORIGIN	2. IN THE GENERATIVE SYSTEM	3. IN THE CIRCULATORY SYSTEM	4. IN THE NERVOUS SYSTEM
At puberty	Fibromyomata	Uncompensated valvular disease of the heart	Excessive coitus
At maturity without obvious lesions	Salpingo-oophoritis (chronic)	Cirrhosis of the liver	Prevention of conception
In relation to the menopause, and in the years preceding	Endometriosis	Emphysema of the lungs	
	Adenomyoma	Hyperthyroidism	*A Single Excessive Period*
	Tuberculous endometritis	Hypothyroidism	Fright
	Intra-uterine contraceptive device	Chronic alcoholism	Violent emotion
			Sudden changes of temperature
	Acute Infectious Diseases	*The Blood Itself*	Cold bath
	Influenza	Deficient coagulability	Dancing
	Enteric	Scorbutus	Hunting
	Cholera	Purpura	Gymnastics
	Scarlatina	Haemophilia	Bicycling, etc.
	Variola	Lymphatic leukaemia	
	Malaria	Splenomedullary leukaemia	
	Diphtheria		
	Measles	*High Blood-pressure*	
		Arteriosclerosis	

case a firm tender swelling in the pouch of Douglas is felt on bimanual palpation. It is often not possible to differentiate between these two conditions until a laparotomy is performed. Examination of the uterine curettings will reveal a tuberculous origin of the pelvic inflammation.

Retroversion and retroflexion of the uterus may be associated with menorrhagia, but, in the absence of other causes, an endocrine imbalance is the reason for the excess menstrual loss, the abnormal position of the uterus merely being coincidental.

Intra-uterine contraceptive device. There is almost always some increase of the menstrual blood loss with the use of these devices, and in some cases the loss amounts to menorrhagia.

Exanthemata. The various exanthems are likely to cause menorrhagia except in those instances where they give rise to anaemia, but the symptom only occurs during the acute phase of the disease, the periods becoming normal again with improvement in the general condition.

point out a line of treatment. Often, however, there is an underlying cause, such as an endocrine imbalance, which is responsible for both the menorrhagia and the anaemia. Removal of the cause then cures the anaemia.

Thrombocytopaenia. Severe menorrhagia may complicate this condition. As soon as it is cured the period loss becomes normal.

High blood-pressure must be reckoned as a cause of menorrhagia at any period of life, but particularly when nearing the onset of the menopause. Menopausal menorrhagia much more often depends upon one of the well-defined lesions of the uterus described above than on high blood-pressure, but cases occur in which the blood-pressure seems alone responsible. The high blood-pressure in some such cases may eventually prove to be connected with the internal secretion of the ductless glands; and in many women who have raised blood-pressure about the time of the menopause the blood-pressure readings become normal again spontaneously a year or two later. Normal menstruation depends in part at least on the normal balance being preserved between the various internal secretions, the ovarian and thyroid on the one hand being balanced by the suprarenal and pituitary on the other, and any disturbance of this balance may result in oligomenorrhoea or amenorrhoea, as occurs in hyperthyroidism, or in menorrhagia as occurs in myxoedema.

4. The Nervous System alone is never a cause of menorrhagia. Emotional upsets such as are liable to occur at the time of the menopause may be connected with an endocrine cause of menorrhagia but usually are probably coincidental.

T. L. T. Lewis.

MENTAL SUBNORMALITY

Whereas up until relatively recently mental subnormality was defined in terms of IQ (*Intelligence Quotient*) and, according to degree of severity, mental defectives were classified as 'idiots', 'imbeciles', 'feeble-minded' ('morons'), etc., in the United Kingdom the Mental Health Act of 1959 swept away these somewhat pejorative terms and, disregarding intelligence as such, placed all mentally subnormal persons in two categories only: designated as *subnormal* and *severely subnormal*. Those in the latter category are by definition regarded as being incapable of independent existence and in need of continuous care and protection; while the merely, as opposed to the severely, subnormal are those who may be expected to benefit from special education or training to the point where it may be anticipated that they will be capable of functioning independently. It should be noted that this new simplified classification which has not met with universal approval, breaks away from tradition by being based on social rather than upon medico-psychological criteria, the primary concern being with how a mentally subnormal person functions within his own particular environment, rather than with any theoretical speculations about how the level of his intelligence may affect performance. In practice, however, it may be suggested that a subnormal individual is likely to be one whose intelligence is below two standard deviations of the mean (IQ about 70) whereas one who is severely subnormal will probably have an IQ of 50 or less.

Mental subnormality may first suggest itself because of an apparent deficiency of reasoning power or because of abnormalities of behaviour often resembling those of mental illness. In infancy and childhood suspicion may be aroused if the rate of development as shown by the attainment of landmarks such as walking and talking is delayed, or if a child at school cannot, by reason of an apparent intellectual deficit, keep up with others of comparable age. In adults, absence of foresight or everyday prudence may point to the diagnosis. Thus, mental subnormality may come to light for the very first time following a criminal charge, the court having called for an examination of the offender's mental state.

As there is a very large number of disorders which give rise to varying degrees of mental subnormality, only the commoner and more important varieties will be considered and passing mention made of some others. Several types of aetiological classification are possible though none is entirely satisfactory. The one followed here is a division into categories based on whether *primary* or *intrinsic* factors are the most important; these are usually of genetic origin—or *secondary* or *extrinsic* factors—in which the disorder is not inherent but acquired during gestation, perinatally, or postnatally. In other cases both instrinsic and extrinsic factors are mixed and cannot be satisfactorily separated.

Mainly Primary

1. SIMPLE AMENTIA. In a majority of cases without obvious physical abnormality or disease, mental subnormality may be regarded as a biological variant of simple genetic origin. Thus dull children tend to be born of dull parents, although it should be noted, other things being equal, that successive generations may demonstrate a *regression towards the mean*, which partly explains why their numbers do not increase. Also, although certainly in large part genetically determined, *simple* or *subcultural amentia* is now regarded partly as a product of environment. Whereas inheritance probably largely determines potential, whether this potential is realized is most likely to be due to the environment in which the child is reared. By the same token, just as dull parents give birth to dull children, by virtue of their own dullness they tend to raise their children in a dull, unstimulating environment.

2. CHROMOSOMAL ABERRATIONS. By far the most important of these is *Mongolism* (*Down's syndrome*) which is currently estimated to occur in about 1 in 550 live births. The most usual form is associated with *trisomy* of chromosome 21. As these are children born of mothers of advancing age, the risk of recurrence is neligible. However, in the much smaller proportion of mongols born to younger parents in which a *translocation defect* or *mosaicism* is present (i.e., about 6 per cent), there is a hereditary factor operative which may give as high as a 1 in 3 risk of a further mongol birth. Luckily it is now possible, as in the case of a number of other disorders, to detect the condition antenatally by amniocentesis, thus indicating the advisability of a therapeutic abortion. Mongolism is characterized by certain easily recognized physical peculiarities. The skull is small and brachycephalic. The face is expressionless; the palpebral fissures are usually narrow sloping downwards and inwards; epicanthic folds are often present. Convergent squint is common, and there is a special liability to infection of the conjunctivae and eyelids. The tongue is fissured and the hair dry and scanty. The hands and feet are broad and clumsy, and

height below average. The voice is harsh, circulation is usually poor, and congenital heart disease is common. Mongols also have a special liability to respiratory disorders and leukaemia. There is always some retardation of mental development—mostly fairly severe.

There are a number of other conditions characterized by chromosomal abnormalities in which mental subnormality may be a feature. One of the more important of these is *Klinefelter's syndrome*, a condition occurring in males and characterized by gynaecomastia, aspermatogenesis, hypospadias, and other physical defects. The patients usually have an XXY chromosome complement. In these intelligence may be only slightly reduced although in other cases in which

inheritance. Sporadic cases also occur. The principal features are mental subnormality (not invariably present), epileptic fits, and a variety of skin lesions. The most important of these is *adenoma sebaceum* which takes the form of a butterfly rash on the face, due to an overgrowth of sebaceous glands and capillaries which lead finally to the formation of nodules. These are not present at birth but appear at about 5–7 years of age. A similar rash can occur in relatives without other manifestations of the disorder. *Café-au-lait spots* and *shagreen patches* are also common. Other of the numerous features include *retinal phakomata, neuroglial nodules*, and *tumours* in the brain, a *candle-guttering* appearance within the lateral ventricles and intracranial calcification,

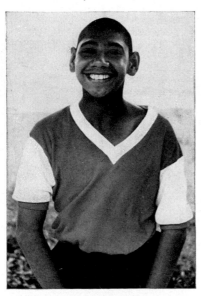

Fig. 524. Microcephaly.

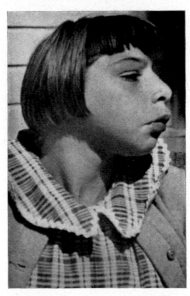

Fig. 525. Microcephaly. Side-view showing bird-like profile.

the number of X's is increased (XXXY, XXXXY), intelligence tends to be progressively impaired. Whereas in *Turner's syndrome* (XO) which is to some extent the female equivalent of Klinefelter's syndrome, the association with mental defect is less common. This may be very much more marked in *Triple-X* females (so-called '*superfemales*'), in which the majority show some degree of mental retardation, often severe. Finally, in this section some consideration may be given to the male *XYY syndrome*. Those with this constitution are said to be characterized by undue tallness, a degree of mental subnormality and a tendency to antisocial behaviour, though these last two characteristics have recently been called into question.

3. HEREDITARY DISORDERS. By far the most important of these is *tuberous sclerosis (epiloia)*, a development disturbance related to *neurofibromatosis (Von Recklinghausen's syndrome)*, which is usually due to an irregular type of dominant

and a variety of tumours affecting other organs (e.g., *hypernephroma, rhabdomyoma*, etc.).

4. OTHER DEVELOPMENTAL ANOMALIES. There are a large number of these, some of which may be partly genetically determined. The first to be considered is *microcephaly*, a term used in two ways: to denote an abnormally *small cranium* which may occur in a variety of disorders causing mental subnormality, some of which are due to adverse influences during early gestation, or to denote a specific and genetically determined (recessive) condition which has other features also. In addition to a small skull which slopes sharply backward, the occiput is flattened. This, with a chin which recedes gives the head a bird-like appearance. The scalp is often corrugated causing the top of the head to be longitudinally grooved. Microcephalic patients are short in stature, usually under 5 ft.; some also suffer from spastic paraplegia or quadriplegia. Most are severely subnormal (*Figs.* 524, 525).

Other developmental anomalies particularly affecting the head include *acrocephaly (oxycephaly)* in which there is an overgrowth of the vertex, *exophthalmos*, a *divergent squint*, and *optic atrophy*. This may be associated with *syndactyly* of the hand or foot ('lobster claw'). *Hypertelorism* is caused by abnormal growth of the sphenoid bones giving rise to eyes which are unusually widely spaced (*Fig.* 526). The degree of subnormality may not be severe.

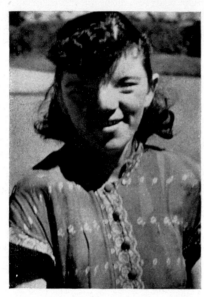

Fig. 526. Hypertelorism.

A more important series of developmental errors may be those generally included in the *craniorachischisis* series which includes *congenital hydrocephalus* and *spina bifida*, which latter anomaly ranges from an asymptomatic form, usually affecting the lower lumbar spine or sacrum only and discovered as a rule accidentally by X-ray (*spina bifida occulta*), and via the several varieties of *spina bifida cystica* in which a *meningocele* or *meningomyelocele* may be present, at the other extreme *anencephaly* which is not compatible with life. Spina bifida may also be associated with the *Arnold-Chiari malformation*, characterized by downward herniation of parts of the medulla and cerebellum through the foramen magnum. There has been a regrettable tendency in recent years to perform repair operations on moderately severe spina bifida cases; for although life may be prolonged thereby, most of the patients grow up to be severely mentally handicapped. More recently it has been shown that severe cases with herniation or imperfect closure of the foetal spinal canal can be detected by amniocentesis, which may reveal the presence of α-fetoprotein. Thus, as in the case of mongolism, a rational approach to prevention by therapeutic abortion becomes feasible; especially in view of the fact that a mother who has

previously borne an anencephalic child or one with spina bifida may well bear another; although the nature of the underlying reasons for this are not yet understood.

Other developmental anomalies include the *Sturge-Kalischer-Weber syndrome (naevoid amentia)* in which the most striking feature is the presence of extensive *facial angiomata* usually associated with *meningeal angiomata*, giving rise to epilepsy, mental subnormality, and occasionally to limb pareses (*Fig.* 527). Yet another example is the *Laurence-Moon-Biedl syndrome*, which is probably the result of an incompletely recessive gene and consists, when fully developed, of four main features: *retinitis pigmentosa, polydactyly, mental subnormality*, and *pituitary dystrophy* which in turn gives rise to *obesity, hypogonadism*, and *depressed sexual function*. Partial forms occur.

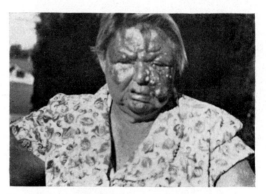

Fig. 527. Sturge-Kalischer-Weber syndrome (naevoid amentia).

Primary and Secondary

These comprise a variety of conditions, some of which are due to disturbances of protein, carbohydrate, and lipid metabolism.

1. DISTURBANCE OF PROTEIN METABOLISM. In *phenylketonuria (phenylpyruvic oligophrenia)* the basic disturbance is a blockage in the conversion of phenylalanine to tyrosine as a result of which phenylpyruvic acid is excreted in the urine giving a positive ferric chloride response. Abnormally increased amounts of phenylpyruvic acid may also be detected in capillary blood. The condition is inherited as an autosomal recessive. If untreated, physical development may be normal but some dwarfing of stature and a degree of microcephaly may occur. There is a tendency to reduced pigmentation in the skin and hair although this is not invariable. Some degree of mental subnormality is usual but can be prevented if a phenylalanine-free diet is administered early enough. Diagnosis in infancy is therefore essential and screening of neonates by either blood- or urine-testing may identify cases which otherwise might pass undetected. Other disturbances of protein metabolism include *Hartnup disease* in which a number of abnormal amino-acids appear in the urine. The disorder may give rise to cerebellar ataxia and a scaly skin

rash which appears on exposed body surfaces. Mental subnormality is usually moderate in degree and other psychiatric symptoms may be present. In *maple-syrup urine disease (leucinosis)* large amounts of valine, leucine, and isoleucine are excreted in the urine. There is also a high concentration in other body fluids. The principal clinical features are failure to thrive, epileptic convulsions, and increasing spastic paralysis leading to opisthotonos. Inheritance is probably due to a recessive gene.

2. DISTURBANCES OF CARBOHYDRATE METABOLISM. These include *galactosaemia* due to the absence of glycolytic enzyme. The condition is characterized by hepatosplenomegaly, jaundice, cataracts, progressive mental retardation, and death in untreated cases. Prevention may be achieved by giving a lactose-free diet. *Hypoglycaemia* may be *familial* giving rise to cerebral damage with attendant subnormality or *acquired* as a result of insulin overdosage in the treatment of juvenile diabetes.

3. DISTURBANCES OF LIPID METABOLISM. *Cerebromacular degeneration (Tay-Sachs's disease; amaurotic family idiocy)* is most commonly found among Jews. Its most characteristic feature is a cherry-red spot on the macula, which appears at about 3 months of age. Optic atrophy and blindness follow. Muscular rigidity, spasm, and an exaggerated startle reaction to a loud noise may be present. Death invariably occurs within 2 years. Other disorders of lipid metabolism which also have a predilection for children of Jewish descent are *Gaucher's* and *Niemann-Pick's diseases* in which there is an abnormal accumulation of lipids in the reticulo-endothelial system, in neurons and in the liver, spleen, and bones. In *gargoylism (Hurler's disease)* dwarfism and dorsolumbar kyphosis occur together with an abnormally large skull, a depressed nasal bridge, and prominent supra-orbital ridges. Corneal opacities and hepatosplenomegaly are usually present. The degree of mental subnormality tends to be severe.

Cretinism, while endemic in iodine-poor soil areas, is more often sporadic and due either to congenital thyroid aplasia or to some kind of biochemical failure of thyroid function. There may be some apparent resemblance between *cretins* and *mongols*. But the signs of cretinism do not usually appear for a few months while those of mongolism are present at birth. In cretinism there is puffiness of the eyes and lips and an enlarged tongue. The skin is coarse, dry, and icteric; the abdomen swollen often with an umbilical hernia. None of these is characteristic of mongolism. Cretins tend to be irritable or apathetic; whilst mongols are often lively, good-humoured, and tractable.

Mainly Secondary

1. DEVELOPMENTAL AND TRAUMATIC. Mental subnormality in this group is usually caused either by *brain injury* at birth or *Rhesus incompatibility*. The extent of subnormality and the degree of physical disability vary from mild to severe. *Spastic paralysis* results from damage to the pyramidal system while extrapyramidal involvement may give rise to *choreoathetosis*. Epileptiform attacks are common. Apart from these there are probably other, at present more obscure, causes of spastic diplegia. Not all are mentally subnormal.

2. INFECTIVE. Mental subnormality may follow meningitis in childhood which may be either of *meningococcal* or *tuberculous* origin. *Congenital syphilis* is now a fairly rare cause. It may be recognized by the presence of the characteristic stigmata. While *encephalitis* may give rise to mental subnormality, disturbance of behaviour is particularly prominent. Post-encephalitics tend to be highly distractible and difficult to manage. Distractibility and failure to concentrate or persevere may lead to an inability to learn and in consequence to mental subnormality.

3. EPILEPSY. The common association between mental subnormality and epilepsy is usually due to some kind of underlying brain disease which gives rise to both. However, epilepsy itself can give rise to subnormality—*epileptic amentia*—this being more likely in those children who have very frequent fits. Sometimes a fairly severe degree of mental subnormality may follow a bout of *status epilepticus* in a child of reasonably normal mentality. This is probably the result of *cerebral anoxia* sustained during repeated seizures.

W. H. Trethowan.

MERYCISM (RUMINATION)

Merycism means cud-chewing or rumination, a rare symptom in man with usually no evidence of disease. In typical cases there is no difficulty in identifying the condition, for the act is voluntary; more or less unchanged food returns to the mouth. It may occur in several members of the same family, either as a congenital peculiarity or as the result of imitation. It is generally only a habit, especially in highly strung subjects by whom it is even regarded as a sort of accomplishment.

It may occur in infants and lead to considerable loss of weight. Unless the child is observed closely the condition may be overlooked. In the act of regurgitation some food may spill from the mouth, leading to increasing loss of weight and often to incorrect diagnosis and unnecessary investigation.

Harold Ellis.

METEORISM

Meteorism, or tympanites, is the term used to denote distension of the abdomen with gas within the alimentary canal. The term is also used for gas free in the peritoneal cavity either from a perforation in the alimentary tract or from laparotomy. It is seldom itself of diagnostic importance, the nature of the case being determined on other grounds. It is of grave omen in cases of *general peritonitis*, appendicitis, or typhoid fever. The usual accompanying features are persistent vomiting, dry furred tongue, abdominal rigidity and the absence of intestinal movements, rising pulse-rate, the facies Hippocratica, and impairment of note in the flanks.

Intestinal obstruction, whether acute, subacute, or chronic, and whether due to strangulated hernia, peritoneal band, volvulus, new growth, intussusception, or other cause, often leads to extreme meteorism, with visible peristalsis, the passage of neither faeces nor flatus, and persistent vomiting which becomes faeculent. Peritonitis ultimately supervenes with the features already mentioned.

Acute pancreatitis, whether haemorrhagic or not, may cause meteorism. The symptoms are variable, but they nearly always suggest an acute abdominal condition. The onset with very acute pain in the epigastrium may at first suggest perforated gastric ulcer, but the abdomen remains supple as in obstruction, more often than rigid as in peritonitis. Diagnosis includes estimation of serum amylase and other special tests. (*See* STEATORRHOEA.)

Meteorism in cases of *lobar pneumonia, typhoid fever, dysentery*, and other severe illnesses in which the bowel is affected is chiefly of importance in that it may lead to an erroneous suspicion of general peritonitis. The diagnosis is often difficult, and there may be grave anxiety and doubt whether the abdomen should be opened or not. One important point in typhoid fever is that perforation is generally accompanied by a sudden drop in the temperature and an equally sudden rise in the pulse-rate.

When the vessels in the mesentery are affected by *thrombosis* or *embolism*, acute meteorism results, with all the signs of intestinal obstruction. In milder cases recovery may ensue spontaneously after days of anxious watching; in severer cases peritonitis develops and the nature of the condition may be quite obscure until laparotomy is performed. Aneurysm of the abdominal aorta in elderly people sometimes leads to bouts of subacute or even quite acute abdominal symptoms, during which meteorism, vomiting, and severe and recurrent colic-like pains may produce a clinical picture closely resembling acute obstruction. The diagnosis can be made by detecting a pulsatile swelling, feeble or absent pulses in the legs, and by X-ray if the vessel wall is calcified.

Interference with the *mesenteric plexuses of nerves* has sometimes led to severe meteorism after abdominal *injury*, for instance after a motor-car smash, or in cases of *tabes mesenterica*, or infiltrating intra-abdominal *new growth*. Gross distension may be seen in *paralytic ileus* which follows any abdominal operation, whether involving intraperitoneal or retroperitoneal structures and which may sometimes be prolonged and severe. A similar picture is seen

in advanced untreated myxoedema, and rarely after acute coronary occlusion or retroperitoneal haemorrhage, as in patients on anticoagulant therapy.

Paralysis of the bowel and tympanites may result from affections of the *spinal cord*, notably from transverse myelitis, whether due to primary softening of the cord from syphilitic or other spinal arterial thromboses, from compression by spinal caries, new growth, or aneurysm, or from destruction of the dorsal region of the cord by a crushing, a stab, or a bullet wound. There will generally be PARAPLEGIA (p. 618).

Diabetes mellitus often indicates its impending termination in coma by the onset of abdominal pains, with more or less meteorism. Meteorism often occurs in the late stages of *cirrhosis of the liver*.

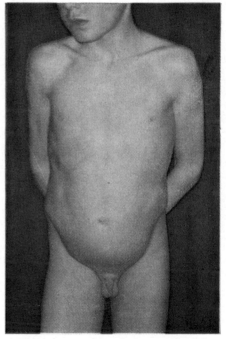

Fig. 528. Hirschsprung's disease in a child of 10; note the distended abdomen, the lack of development, and the wide sub-costal angle.

Particular mention may be made of *Hirschsprung's disease* (megacolon)—idiopathic distension of the rectum and sigmoid colon and sometimes the whole of the large intestine in children and young people (*Fig.* 528). Careful examination indicates that the enormous gaseous distension of the abdomen is not due to general tympanites, but to ballooning of what may seem at first to be stomach, but which is proved otherwise by the swelling appearing to arise from the left iliac fossa and by the X-ray shadows after a barium meal or enema. Obstinate constipation, or symptoms of recurrent intestinal obstruction, are usual in these cases which are due to a disturbance of the normal balance between the sympathetic and parasympathetic nerve supply to the anus, rectum, or lower colon.

Hysteria. Meteorism may occur as a hysterical manifestation. The essentials of diagnosis are recognition that the condition is in fact meteorism, and not pregnancy, ascites, ovarian cyst or other tumour—phantom tumours are difficult to diagnose without examination under an anaesthetic.

Harold Ellis.

METRORRHAGIA

Metrorrhagia means loss of blood from the uterus between the menstrual periods, and the term should be applied strictly only to irregular haemorrhages during menstrual life. It may be used for losses of actual blood or for blood-stained discharges in which mucus is mixed with blood. There has been a tendency of late to refer only to *Menorrhagia* (p. 524) and to *Metrorrhagia*, including all types of irregular vaginal bleeding, whether they occur during menstrual life, before puberty, after the menopause, or during pregnancy. For the purposes of discussion irregular vaginal bleeding will be considered here under three headings: (*A*) Irregular bleeding during menstrual life; (*B*) Irregular bleeding before puberty and after the menopause; (*C*) Irregular bleeding during pregnancy.

A. IRREGULAR BLEEDING DURING MENSTRUAL LIFE

1. The Lesions of the Generative Organs which give rise to metrorrhagia are well defined as a rule, as in the case of carcinoma of the cervix uteri, when the cervix is replaced by a mass of friable growth which bleeds readily on being probed or touched with the finger. A growth of the body of the uterus is more difficult to diagnose and in all instances microscopical examination of material removed by curettage is required; in fact, with the exception of obvious mucous polypi, fibroid polypi, and advanced growths of the cervix, all the growths of the uterus require a preliminary histological examination for their exact diagnosis.

It is not out of place here to suggest the best way to make histological preparations from curetted material, a matter of great importance to the patient, because it is often difficult to distinguish between cancer and thickened endometrium unless the very best microscope sections can be secured. The curetted material must be obtained after dilatation, with a sharp curette, and the larger the fragments removed the more easy will be the histologist's work. Anaesthesia is frequently given except in the case of cervical growths. A Danish suction machine (the Vabra) can be used safely on patients in the out-patient department for diagnostic purposes. The curettings obtained are quite satisfactory for histology. In doubtful cervical growths a rectangular-shaped biopsy should be cut out, including some normal tissue if possible. If malignant cells have been seen in a vaginal or cervical smear and the cervix looks grossly normal, intra-epithelial carcinoma of the cervix (carcinoma-in-situ) will be suspected. A large cone-shaped biopsy of the cervix should be removed with the scalpel so that many sections can be microscopically examined, placing them immediately in an efficient fixing fluid, the best being formalin 10 ml., 0·75 per cent salt solution 90 ml. Twenty-four hours in this fluid gives good fixation, after which the tissues can be dehydrated in successive strengths of alcohol, cleared in xylol, and finally embedded and infiltrated with paraffin wax. Sections cut from these paraffin blocks are the best obtainable, far superior to any freezing method or celloidin infiltration. If the stained sections are submitted to a histologist who has experience of uterine growths, there should be no doubtful specimens. If, however, the tissues are fixed improperly, or thick sections cut, the most skilled histologist will be unable to give a definite and reliable diagnosis.

Carcinoma of the body of the uterus, carcinoma of the cervical canal, early carcinoma of the cervix, sarcoma of the uterus, chorionic carcinoma, some sloughing fibroids, tuberculous endometritis, can be distinguished from one another only by investigations carried out on these lines. The fact that all these lesions produce metrorrhagia, and may give rise to haemorrhage on coitus, walking, straining at stool, or bimanual manipulation of the uterus, makes it imperative that we should have histological confirmation of the nature of the lesion before making an exact diagnosis.

The relation of *fibromyoma* to metrorrhagia as opposed to pure menorrhagia, which is the rule with these tumours, is interesting. Fibroids only produce irregular bleeding when they are submucous and in process of extrusion, when they are infected and sloughing, or when they are actually polypoid. The reason for this is that in these conditions the tumours are always partly strangulated by uterine contractions, and therefore in a state of gross venous congestion; hence they bleed more or less constantly, without provocation. The occurrence of irregular bleeding in a person who is known to have fibroids almost always means one of these conditions, and, commonly, extrusion of the tumour from the uterus. On the other hand, it must not be overlooked that carcinoma may develop in the endometrium with a fibroid also present, or that a fibroid may become sarcomatous, or that a sarcoma may arise *de novo* in the uterus and attack a pre-existing fibroid. Rapid enlargement of a uterus, with irregular haemorrhage, is very suspicious of a *sarcoma*, but as it is not uncommon for several fibroids to be present in the same uterus, it is also common for rapid enlargement to occur as a result of cystic changes in one of them, whilst haemorrhage may take place due to extrusion of another.

Pure *carcinoma of the body of the uterus* rarely produces much enlargement of the organ, and any increase in size is not very rapid. It must be remembered that normally the postmenopausal uterus shrinks considerably in size; thus a uterus of a size which would be regarded as normal in a younger woman indicates abnormal enlargement in a woman past the menopause.

Chorionic carcinoma, fortunately a very rare condition, follows hydatidiform mole in about 50 per cent of the recorded cases, and it always follows pregnancy, never having been seen in the uterus in a case where pregnancy could be

The differential diagnosis of bleeding due to *carcinoma, erosion,* and *tuberculosis of the cervix* is often difficult in the early stages. Erosions of the cervix do not as a rule cause bleeding; if there has been irregular bleeding or the cervix bleeds during examination malignancy should be suspected and arrangements made to obtain a biopsy. In advanced cancer the friable hardness of the growth distinguishes it at once from the tough leathery hardness present in erosions. In the former, the growth can be broken down with the finger; in the latter, the soft velvety erosion can be scraped off the tough leathery and fibrous cervix beneath. Nothing, however, but sections

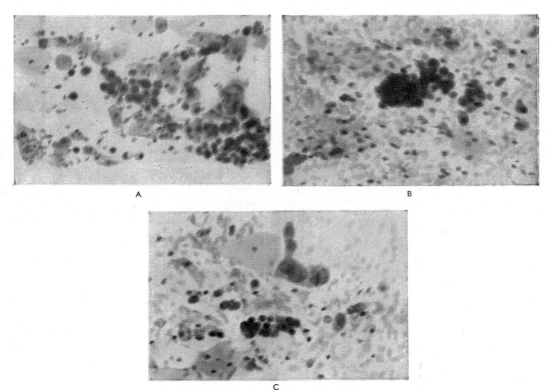

Fig. 529. Abnormal cervical smear from carcinoma in situ. (*Dr. J. Vale.*)

excluded, although the pregnancy may have occurred some years before. It is associated with profuse bleeding and the rapid development of a foetid discharge due to decomposition of blood and necrosing tissues in utero. Carcinoma of the body of the uterus rarely produces foul discharges until the condition is advanced. Secondary deposits of chorionic carcinoma appear as small plum-coloured ulcerating nodules in the vagina or in the lungs, causing haemoptysis. The patient rapidly becomes ill with pyrexia and profound anaemia. A high titre of chorionic gonadotrophin is found in the urine. The diagnosis depends upon the finding of masses of trophoblastic cells in uterine curettings without any evidence of villous formation.

made from biopsies of the cervix enables us to distinguish carcinoma or erosion from tuberculosis in the early stages. Tuberculosis of the cervix is usually mistaken for carcinoma, but the difference is clear enough in microscope sections. On occasions sectional biopsy of the cervix reveals a 'carcinoma in situ' or pre-invasive carcinoma. In this condition the epithelial cells throughout the whole depth of the cervical mucosa have the typical appearance of cancer cells but no invasion of the deeper tissues of the cervix has taken place. This condition has been known to become a true cancer, although many years may elapse before this takes place. Only a small proportion of the cases of carcinoma in situ of the cervix becomes invasive cancer even if left untreated. The small possibility of true cancer supervening, however, makes treatment desirable in most cases. They are usually found in the first place by routine cervical smears. (*Fig.* 529.)

Mucous polypi and *fibroid polypi* are common causes of intermenstrual bleeding, and are usually quite definite growths. The mucous polypus is soft, strawberry-red in colour, pedunculated, and contains cystic spaces filled with glairy mucus. It rarely gives rise to a malignant growth. The fibroid polypus is hard, and shows the glistening whorled appearance so well known in fibromyomata on section. These growths are liable to infection and sloughing, and are then apt to be mistaken for carcinoma or sarcoma. The microscope alone will enable the difference to be made out.

2. Dysfunctional Uterine Bleeding. Until it becomes possible to obtain accurate estimations of the various sex hormones in the blood and

ovary. This state of excess oestrogen secretion affecting the endometrium leads to marked endometrial hyperplasia (Schröder's disease or metropathia haemorrhagica (*see* p. 524). In other cases, however, there is no endometrial hyperplasia present; indeed, the endometrium may be atrophic; again in others the endometrium may be in the secretory phase so that we know ovulation has taken place. In such cases a quantitative imbalance of the sex hormones is assumed, although the cause may lie in the uterine musculature or its autonomic nerve-supply. It may be that the closer relationship between the pituitary and ovarian functions is disturbed, leading to a temporarily excessive drop in the oestrogen level in the blood because of the inhibition or excessive action of the pituitary gonadotrophins. In other cases it is thought that the endometrium is unable to respond to the stimulation of the ovarian or pituitary hormone in a normal

CAUSES OF IRREGULAR BLEEDING DURING MENSTRUAL LIFE

1. GENERATIVE SYSTEM	2. ENDOCRINE
Malignant Growths: Carcinoma of cervix Carcinoma of body of uterus Sarcoma Chorionic carcinoma Carcinoma of Fallopian tube Carcinoma of the ovary *Benign Growths*: Submucous fibroid Fibroid polypus Mucous polypus Endometrial polypus *Inflammatory Lesions*: Erosion of cervix Endometriosis Tuberculosis of uterus	Dysfunctional uterine bleeding Metropathia haemorrhagica Irregular shedding of the endometrium Oestrogen withdrawal bleeding Granulosa-cell tumour

urine during the various phases of the menstrual cycle, not only will a full knowledge of the mechanism of normal menstruation remain unknown, but more so, that of dysfunctional bleeding. At present these estimations are difficult and not very accurate.

Dysfunctional bleeding may occur at any age between puberty and the menopause, but 50 per cent occur between the ages of 40 and 50, about 10 per cent at puberty, and the remainder between these ages. Then bleeding is more commonly a menorrhagia, although the interval between the bleedings may be shortened. Particularly is this the case in this type of bleeding occurring about puberty and the menopause. The bleeding may be profuse or only slightly in excess of normal. In other cases intermenstrual bleeding occurs, continuing for some weeks. It is usually preceded by amenorrhoea for some weeks. In a large proportion of these cases ovulation fails to occur. Schröder was able to demonstrate the absence of corpora lutea and the persistence of unruptured follicles in the

manner (those cases with atrophic endometrium). In other cases irregular shedding of the endometrium takes place leading to prolongation of the desquamative phase of the menstrual cycle. In these cases menstruation is very prolonged, and a late curetting in the bleeding phase reveals islands of secretory endometrium, when normal regenerated endometrium should be found.

There are no gross abnormal physical signs to be found on pelvic examination in cases of dysfunction bleeding. The diagnosis largely depends on curettage. Amenorrhoea followed by prolonged irregular bleeding (the usual pattern) may be caused by pregnancy and abortion (threatened or incomplete), or by the menopause followed by carcinoma of the body of the uterus. In the absence of symptoms and signs of pregnancy curetting the uterus is essential to exclude malignancy in the uterus or retained products of gestation.

Oestrogen withdrawal bleeding. Women commonly take oestrogen preparations to control menopausal symptoms or to prevent conception. Irregular uterine bleeding may occur while the drugs are being taken or following their withdrawal. It is impossible in such cases to exclude malignant growths inside the uterus without uterine curettage which should always be done.

Bleeding associated with ovulation. It is not uncommon for women to bleed very slightly about midway between the periods at the time of ovulation. When this is accompanied by lower abdominal pain (*Mittelschmerz*) the diagnosis is easy, but in some patients curettage will be necessary to be certain.

Bleeding due to granulosa-cell tumour. When irregular bleeding occurs in the presence of an ovarian swelling the possibility of a granulosa-cell tumour arises. Removal of the tumour and histology reveal its nature. The presence of an intra-uterine lesion and a non-secreting ovarian tumour must not be overlooked.

B. IRREGULAR BLEEDING BEFORE PUBERTY AND AFTER THE MENOPAUSE

The bleeding which occurs from the vagina occasionally in newborn infants is usually thought to depend upon a temporary high concentration of oestrogen in the foetal circulation. It is usually trivial, but a fatal case has been reported.

After the menopause the differentiation of *malignant growths, polypi,* and *senile endometritis* can only be established in the same way as in cases

adherent, and the separation brought about by the examining finger may cause bleeding. *Pyometra,* or distension of the uterus with pus, may cause haemorrhage, with a foul discharge; although it is almost always due to malignant growth, it may be only the result of infection. The only growth of the ovary which produces uterine haemorrhage is the granulosa-cell tumour. This may occur at almost any age after puberty. (*See* PELVIC SWELLING, p. 626.)

C. IRREGULAR BLEEDING DURING PREGNANCY

In relation to a recent pregnancy, haemorrhage may result from simple subinvolution, from retained products of conception, or from chorionic carcinoma. The differentiation of these conditions can be established only by exploration of the uterine cavity, with, if necessary, the assistance of the microscope. Such conditions may be termed 'secondary postpartum haemorrhage' in cases occurring within a few days of delivery.

Haemorrhage from the pregnant uterus almost always means separation of the placenta or of the embryo from its attachments, but malignant growth of the cervix, erosions, and polypi may have to be considered. Haemorrhage from a pregnant uterus is never due to malignant growth of the body of the organ, because pregnancy is impossible with this lesion. There are, however, two great difficulties in connexion with pregnancy haemorrhages; these are to differentiate:

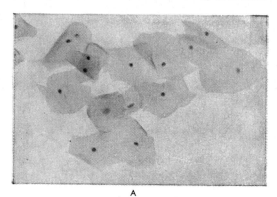
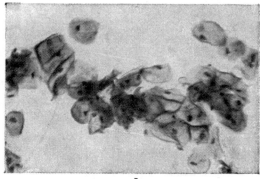

Fig. 530. A, Normal non-pregnant vaginal smear. B, Normal pregnant smear showing good progesterone response. (*Dr. J. Vale.*)

occurring during menstrual life, that is by uterine curettage. At the present day owing to the frequent and often unnecessary use of oestrogen preparations, particularly at the menopause, it is probable that oestrogen withdrawal bleeding is one of the commonest causes of postmenopausal bleeding. In any doubtful case routine dilatation and curettage of the uterus must never be omitted. *Senile adhesive vaginitis* must not be overlooked as a possible cause; the vaginal walls at the fornices become inflamed and form granulation tissue which may bleed if the surfaces rub together; the surfaces may be partly

(1) The uterine haemorrhage which occurs along with *extra-uterine gestation* from that due to *threatened abortion*; and (2) The bleeding of *placenta praevia* from that due to the *separation of a normally situated placenta.*

In the first case, arising very early in pregnancy, generally when only one menstrual period has been missed, or is overdue, the external haemorrhage occurs when the extra-uterine gestation is separated from its tubal or other attachments and is converted into a tubal mole, when it becomes extruded from the fimbriated extremity of the tube, or when the tube ruptures, events which cause acute pain in the lower part of the abdomen, faintness, and possibly collapse from internal haemorrhage. Along with these the uterus will be found not obviously enlarged, whilst there is some sort of swelling in one or the other posterior quarter of the pelvis. Even if no actual swelling can be defined, bimanual palpation will elicit very marked tenderness, which may be excruciating, due to the presence of blood clot in the peritoneal cavity. In the case of ectopic gestation the abdominal pain is severe. It is often referred to the shoulder. It is much more severe than that experienced in an intra-uterine abortion and it almost always precedes the onset of vaginal bleeding; on the other hand the vaginal blood-loss in an inevitable abortion is much more than that in ectopic gestation, which is usually scanty.

products of conception have been passed and recognized. Retained products of gestation can be diagnosed by means of ultrasound scanning.

If repeated small haemorrhages occur into the chorio-decidual space in early pregnancy a carneous mole results. This is often retained in the uterus for several months and then spontaneously expelled (missed abortion). A brown blood-stained vaginal discharge is present and the uterus ceases to enlarge. On examination the uterus is found smaller than it should be for the estimated duration of pregnancy. A pregnancy test may be negative but it is not always so.

A hydatidiform mole should be suspected when rapid increase in size of the uterus occurs during the early months of pregnancy, associated

CAUSES OF IRREGULAR BLEEDING

BEFORE PUBERTY AND AFTER MENOPAUSE	DURING PREGNANCY
Uterine bleeding in the newborn	Threatened, inevitable, or incomplete abortion
Malignant growth of the uterus	Carneous mole
Polypi	Hydatidiform mole
Senile endometritis	Antepartum haemorrhage
Senile granular vaginitis	Secondary postpartum haemorrhage
Pyometra	Subinvolution
Granulosa-cell tumour of ovary	Chorionic carcinoma
Oestrogen withdrawal bleeding	Extra-uterine gestation
	Malignant growth of cervix or vagina
	Erosion
	Polypi

Haemorrhage due to threatened abortion cannot be diagnosed unless the presence of an intra-uterine pregnancy can be established; therefore we must look for the definite signs of a normal pregnancy, which in the early months will be: amenorrhoea, morning sickness, breast swelling, darkening of the nipple, dark secondary areola around the nipple, enlargement of the uterus, Hegar's sign, Braun's sign, and blue discoloration of the cervix and vaginal walls. Hegar's sign consists in extreme softening of the upper part of the cervix and lower part of the uterine body associated with the as yet unsoftened vaginal portion and globular tense fundus; it is found from the 6th to the 8th week. Braun's sign consists in the irregular shape of the uterus from the 8th to the 12th week; one side is larger than the other, and an ill-defined groove is found between them. Ultrasound scanning can be very useful because the pregnancy sac can be visualized in the uterus and the size of the embryo measured to make sure of the duration of the pregnancy. Absence of a pregnancy sac in the uterus with a mass outside of the uterus (sometimes seen to contain a pregnancy sac) makes the diagnosis of ectopic pregnancy a certainty. The diagnosis of inevitable abortion depends upon finding some part of the uterine contents presenting through the dilating cervix. Incomplete abortion is difficult to diagnose, unless some definite

with uterine bleeding. The uterus may be the size of that of a six months' pregnancy, when the estimated duration of pregnancy is only two months. In such a case the pregnancy test would be positive in dilutions of 1 : 100 or thereabouts, while in a normal pregnancy it is positive only in a dilution of 1 : 20. The appearance shown by ultra-sound on a diasonograph is characteristic, and is a great step forward in the means of diagnosis.

In a case of chorionic carcinoma the pregnancy test will usually be found positive in dilutions of 1 : 100 and upwards. This disease should always be suspected on recurrence of bleeding after curettage following a miscarriage or the passage of a hydatidiform mole. A careful microscopical examination of all curettings is therefore essential.

Although when irregular bleeding has occurred during pregnancy there may not be time to wait for laboratory reports upon the tests for pregnancy, these may be mentioned here, for they may afford strongly positive, even if not entirely infallible, evidence of the existence of pregnancy in doubtful cases. Each depends upon the fact that the urine of a pregnant woman contains gonadotrophins, which are proof positive of the presence of live chorionic villi in the uterus, tubes, or ovaries. The urine of the pregnant woman injected into virgin mice in the Zondek and

Aschheim tests, or into the virgin rabbit in the Friedman test, causes one or both ovaries of the injected animal to develop haemorrhagic follicles or corpora lutea. In the case of mice 0·4 ml. of the patient's fresh detoxicated urine is injected intramuscularly twice daily for six doses and the animal's ovaries are inspected 100 hours after the first injection. In the case of the rabbit 5–10 ml. of urine is injected intravenously and the ovaries examined 24–48 hours later. Two rabbits are usually used. In Hogben's test 2 ml. of concentrate obtained from 40 ml. of urine are injected into the dorsal lymph-sac of the clawed toad (*Xenopus laevis*). The test is positive when the toad spawns, and 50–200 ova are discharged from the oviduct between 6 and 15 hours after injection. In Franks's test 2 ml. of urine are injected subcutaneously into a standard immature rat which is killed 24 hours later. A positive test is shown by a diffuse pink or red flush of the ovaries. In a negative test they are pale yellowish-white in colour. Recently immunological tests for pregnancy have been introduced. They depend upon the fact that antibodies can be produced in an animal by injecting human chorionic gonadotrophin into it. Serum (0·5 ml.) containing these antibodies is mixed with 0·5 ml. urine to be tested and incubated at 37° C. for one hour. Latex particles or sheep's blood-cells coated with chorionic gonadotrophin are then added to the mixture. If agglutination takes place the test is negative; if no agglutination takes place the test is positive. These tests are of great value in the diagnosis of pregnancy and have an accuracy of at least 98 per cent. Vaginal smears are helpful in diagnosis (*Fig.* 530).

Bleeding due to *placenta praevia* generally occurs after the 6th month of pregnancy. The only definite sign is the feeling of the placenta through the cervix when it will admit of this method of investigation. The suggestive signs are those due to the filling up of the lower uterine segment by the placenta. The presenting part remains high up and movable, not engaged in the brim, and cannot be made to do so. There is a sensation of increased thickness between the vaginal fornices and the presenting part; a straight X-ray examination may show the placenta in the upper uterine segment of the uterus, thus excluding its presence in the lower segment. Lateral and anteroposterior radiographs may show abnormal displacement of the foetal head forwards, backwards, or to one or other side of the pelvic brim, thus indicating the position of the placenta in the lower uterine segment. The placenta can be easily localized by ultrasound using a diasonograph and the severity of a placenta praevia accurately determined. Where repeated haemorrhages occur, examination under anaesthesia in the operating theatre will reveal the presence of the placenta in the lower segment. Before this examination the patient must be all prepared for an immediate Caesarean section to be undertaken should this be considered necessary at the time of examination. In those cases in which placenta praevia can be excluded a diagnosis of accidental haemorrhage (bleeding from a normally situated placental site) can be made.

T. L. T. Lewis.

MICTURITION, ABNORMALITIES OF

A person in health micturates about five times during the twenty-four hours, the total amount of urine passed being about 1500 ml., or 50 oz. This varies according to the amount of liquid taken, the amount lost by perspiration and by respiration, vomiting, diarrhoea, etc. The act of micturition is controlled by a nervous mechanism, a stretch reflex from the bladder starting an impulse which causes contraction of the main detrusor muscle; its fibres are continued down to the floor of the posterior urethra and their contraction serves also to open the internal urethral orifice. The special centre controlling the motor functions of the bladder is in the spinal cord at the level of the conus medullaris, whilst the brain can inhibit this centre in response to impulses received. The abnormalities of micturition which are met with in practice depend partly upon lesions of some portion of the urinary apparatus, and partly upon some change in the nervous mechanism controlling the act, and will be discussed from these points of view, and under ENURESIS (p. 253).

Increased Frequency of Micturition. A large number of diseases of the genito-urinary tract are accompanied by increased frequency of micturition. The symptom may be due to *polyuria*, there being an increased amount of urine to be passed, or to *vesical irritability*, or to *diminution of the bladder capacity* below the normal 10–15 oz. Thus in *diabetes mellitus, diabetes insipidus*, and *chronic nephritis* the increased amount of urine will cause an increased frequency of desire to micturate, provided the capacity of the bladder is unaltered. Polyuria is also produced by *excessive drinking*, especially of tea or coffee, which contain diuretics; in *hysteria* there is also polyuria, an exaggeration of the reflex nervous polyuria also present in states of mental anxiety or fear, exemplified in student days by 'examination frequency'. The rate of filling also influences the frequency, rapid filling provoking the stretch reflex earlier than slow filling, when the bladder may distend considerably before the stretch reflex is provoked. If the total amount of urine remains normal increased frequency of micturition may be due to some lesion of the genito-urinary apparatus, and consideration of the other symptoms of a case will often point to a definite diagnosis. Increased frequency does not necessarily imply that the bladder is the seat of the disease, as the symptom is present with any form of pyelitis or with prostatic enlargement.

It is important to ascertain the relationship between micturition during the day and during the night. Normally, a healthy person should not wake during the night to pass urine, unless an excess of fluid has been taken before retiring, but if any inflammatory condition is present in the bladder, micturition will be present during the night, as well as increased in frequency during the day. Any form of *cystitis*, or acute inflammatory conditions of the *prostate* or neighbouring organs, will cause increased frequency by both day and night.

With *vesical calculus* there is increased frequency during the day, but often no urination is necessary during the night. The frequency during the day is increased with activity or exercise, or by the jolting movements of travelling, but is absent during a period of rest, particularly because, in the supine position, the calculus rolls away from the sensitive internal urethral orifice area to the posterior part of the bladder. If the presence of a calculus has excited cystitis, increased frequency of micturition will be present by both day and night.

With *prostatic enlargement*, whether simple or carcinomatous, the increased frequency is most marked at night, and is commonly the first symptom of the disease noticed by the patient, generally a man of about sixty. The bladder is not emptied completely, so that the addition of a relatively small amount of urine from the kidneys soon fills up the incompletely emptied viscus and sets up afresh the desire to micturate.

Vesical carcinoma causes increased frequency of micturition by both day and night, as the infiltration of the vesical wall prevents the bladder from being distended without pain, and it is frequently associated with cystitis.

In *renal colic* caused by *calculus* or *blood-clot* there may be increased desire to micturate, and the symptom may result from *pyelitis*, inflammatory diseases of the pelvic organs, such as *salpingitis*, *pyosalpinx*, or a low-placed *appendicitis*, or infiltration of the bladder by *carcinoma* of the *uterus*, *rectum*, or *colon*, or by the extension of inflammation to the bladder from *diverticulitis of the colon*.

In *renal tuberculosis* increased frequency of micturition is often present before any infection of the bladder or change in the ureteric orifice can be detected by the cystoscope.

Increased frequency of micturition may be produced by mechanical obstruction to the normal vesical distension by a tumour occupying the pelvis, and is seen commonly with *ovarian cyst*, *uterine fibroid*, or a *gravid uterus*, particularly in the early months of pregnancy if the uterus is retroverted; these tumours will be found upon vaginal examination.

In children, increased frequency of micturition may be due to *balanitis*, a *small urinary meatus*, *worms*, or *calculus*. With urine of *high acidity*, with *oxaluria* (p. 610), with *phosphaturia*, with *bacteriuria* (p. 91), and after alcohol increased frequency may be present without other symptoms.

Diminution of the bladder capacity may be due to a large stone or new growth occupying some of the available space, or to the presence of a large amount of residual urine, as in chronic prostatic obstruction. Reduction in size can also be caused by fibrosis of the bladder wall. Fibrosis is seen in the absence of urinary infection in chronic interstitial cystitis (Hunner's ulcer). It is present in its most advanced degree in the 'thimble bladder' of the late stage of vesical tuberculosis.

Changes in the Stream of Urine. An abnormality of the stream of urine may be due to a congenital deficiency of the terminal urethra, as in *hypospadias* or *epispadias*, or to some lesion mechanically obstructing the stream. Most commonly this is due to a *stricture* of the urethra. If the stricture is situated in the penile portion, the stream of urine is of small calibre but of fair force, while if the stricture is in the bulbous urethra the mechanical effect upon the stream of urine passing through the stricture into the urethra of wider calibre beyond the stricture is that the force is diminished, whilst the actual stream as it leaves the meatus is not thinned. A stricture at or near the urethral meatus forms a thin but forcible stream; the stream may be twisted or forked because it has insufficient force to expand the lips of the meatus (*Fig. 531*). A patient the subject of urethral stricture commonly complains

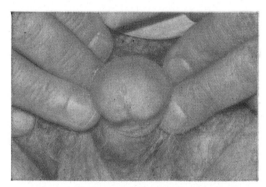

Fig. 531. Pinhole external urethral meatus.

that he cannot expel the last few drops of urine, but that some dribbling of urine occurs from the meatus when he thinks he has completely emptied the bladder. This terminal dribbling is due to the emptying of the dilated portion of the urethra behind the stricture. Similar dribbling may result from the bladder musculature losing its contractile force, or from disease of the nervous system affecting the motor paths to the bladder.

Obstruction to micturition by an *enlarged prostate* causes the stream of urine to be slow and forceless, so that it may fall vertically from the meatus instead of in the usual arched manner.

In any case presenting an abnormality in the stream of urine careful inquiry should be made to ascertain if the stream has become gradually and progressively narrowed, as in stricture, or if the alteration in the force of the stream is accompanied by increased frequency of urination, as in prostatic hypertrophy in an elderly patient, or by urethral discharge in a case suggestive of acute prostatitis. A stricture may be diagnosed with certainty by careful urethroscopic examination under air or water distension, or, failing this, by the obstruction offered to the passage of a catheter or bougie. Prostatic enlargement or inflammation will be suggested by the history of the case, and confirmed by a digital examination of the gland per rectum. Occasionally symptoms are produced by an enlarged median prostatic lobe with normal lateral lobes so that rectal examination of the gland is surprisingly normal (*prostatisme sans prostate*); in such cases the diagnosis is made by intravenous pyelography, which demonstrates the prostate bulging up into the bladder, and is confirmed by cystoscopy. In the absence of a mechanical obstruction in the urethra examination should be conducted for disease of the spinal cord by full neurological examination, and by a complete examination of the cerebrospinal fluid withdrawn by lumbar puncture (p. 123).

Sudden stoppage of the flow of urine during micturition may be caused by a small, movable *vesical calculus*, if the latter happens to engage in the internal urethral orifice or becomes impacted in the urethra. The same sudden cessation of the flow is caused occasionally by a tuft of a vesical *papillomatous tumour* blocking the urethral opening during micturition. Usually the flow will be resumed after a few seconds unless the calculus has passed into the urethra, when it may be passed naturally or require to be removed by surgical means. If the symptom recurs, a cystoscopic examination of the bladder will distinguish readily between the two conditions.

The same sudden cessation of the stream may occur without any intravesical lesion as the result of *spasmodic contraction of the bladder*. Patients subject to this trouble (so-called *stammering bladder*) can at times pass urine quite normally, but at others the stream is interrupted frequently, or they may be unable to pass urine at all, especially in the presence of a second person.

Difficulty of Micturition. Frequently associated with some change in the character of the stream of urine, a patient may complain of difficulty in micturition, either as a hesitation in commencing the flow or a need to strain to maintain it. This, again, is most common with *urethral stricture* or *prostatic enlargement*; in the latter case the difficulty is greater when the bladder is over-full, the stretched detrusor acting at a mechanical disadvantage. It may be due to impaction of a *calculus* in the urethra or to the formation of *blood-clot* in the bladder. A calculus may be passed into the urethra and become arrested in the canal, without wholly obstructing the passage of urine. It is not uncommon for a calculus to occupy the dilated portion of the urethra behind a stricture, or occasionally a *prostatic calculus*

projects from the gland into the lumen of the posterior urethra. A calculus so placed may increase in size by the further deposition of urinary salts whilst in the urethra, and cause difficulty in micturition; it may be felt in the canal from the outside, upon rectal examination, or upon passing a soft bougie into the urethra. Even if placed behind a stricture it may be felt by a fine guide or bougie passed to dilate the stricture. In an X-ray film of the pelvis, prostatic calculi are seen as increased densities behind the symphysis pubis, whilst a calculus impacted in the urethra casts a shadow in the angle of the pubic arch (*Fig.* 372, p. 348). Difficulty in micturition may also arise from *prostatic inflammation* or from *tuberculous disease of the prostate.*

Difficulty in micturition due to the presence of *blood-clot in the bladder* will usually be indicated by the previous passage of blood-stained urine and by the constant efforts to micturate. Difficulty in micturition may be due to tight phimosis or to a pin-hole meatus.

Difficulty in micturition in the female may be caused by a *pelvic tumour* by the drag or direct pressure on the urethra or vesical neck. This may occur with a *uterine fibroid* or a *pregnant retroverted uterus*. Occasionally, difficulty is produced by the direct infiltration of the urethra by a *carcinoma* of the vaginal wall or vulva, or by a primary carcinoma of the urethra. Stricture of the urethra also occurs occasionally in women and there is sometimes no obvious cause for this.

Difficulty in micturition is not uncommon in *disease of the nervous system*, causing paralysis or paresis of the detrusor muscle of the bladder. This may be due to *trauma* producing spinal cord transection or contusion, or to *myelitis, tabes, multiple sclerosis, tumour of the spinal meninges or cord, secondary deposits in the vertebrae*, or *syringomyelia*. It must be remembered that it is not uncommon for the early cord-changes of tabes to affect the urinary organs, and that difficulty in passing urine may be complained of when the urethra and bladder are normal. Difficulty, usually preceded by increased frequency and sometimes followed by retention of urine, can occur in *herpes zoster* affecting the lower sacral segments (*see also* p. 540).

Atony of the bladder wall without any affection of the nervous mechanism, from recurring overdistension of the bladder, may cause difficulty in micturition; it sometimes persists after prostatectomy when there has been prolonged chronic retention of urine before operation.

Retention of Urine—by which is implied the acute or gradual accumulation of urine in the bladder, with inability to pass any per urethram—may arise from *mechanical causes* obstructing the urethra, or from *derangement of the nervous system*. Retention of urine must be distinguished from ANURIA (p. 63), or failure of the kidneys to secrete urine, for in retention the kidneys are still functioning, and the urine is collecting in the distended bladder. Retention of urine occurring suddenly produces severe pain and strangury (except in cases of neurological origin, e.g., spinal transection), but in cases of old-standing obstruction the bladder may be distended enormously without pain. If the retention remains unrelieved urine may continually dribble away per urethram, when a condition resembling incontinence of urine is produced; this condition has to be distinguished from *true incontinence* of urine due to injury or paralysis of the vesical sphincter muscle. In true incontinence the bladder remains empty, urine flows away as soon as it passes down into the bladder, and there is no obstruction in the urethra; whereas in the condition of involuntary passage of urine from an unrelieved distended bladder—*incontinence from overflow*, or *false incontinence*—the bladder may be felt distended in the suprapubic region, and there exists some nerve disease or some mechanical obstruction in the urethra or at the internal urethral orifice. (*Fig.* 532.)

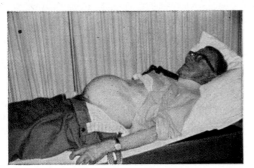

Fig. 532. Swelling in the lower abdomen caused by retention of urine due to enlarged prostate.

The common causes of retention of urine are *urethral stricture* and *prostatic enlargement*. In stricture it does not necessarily follow that the urethra is occluded entirely by the fibrosis, but rather that some spasm or congestion is present at the stricture, from exposure to cold or indulgence in alcohol, when a small catheter may be passed. In elderly men with *prostatic hypertrophy*, acute retention may occur early in the disease from a congested condition of the enlarged gland, or in the later stages be due to actual obstruction of the urethra by a localized enlargement of the gland. It is more likely to occur if the call to micturate has not been obeyed and the bladder has become distended. A catheter can usually be passed readily, but in cases of chronic retention, especially in those of old-standing obstruction in which the kidneys are probably affected by the backward pressure, *the urine must be drawn off very slowly* and must not be allowed to reaccumulate; particular care must be devoted to *asepsis*, otherwise fatal anuria may be induced.

A case of acute retention of urine from *stricture of the urethra* will generally be that of a comparatively young patient, who will give a history of former gonorrhoea or urethral injury, gradually increasing difficulty in micturition, narrowing of the stream, and inability to finish the flow completely without some dribbling of urine. Examination of the urethra by an endoscope, or by the passage of olivary-pointed flexible bougies, will reveal the presence of a stricture.

In *prostatic enlargement* the patient is usually above the age of 55 years, has been troubled with increasing frequency in micturition, especially at night, with straining and loss of force in the stream of urine. Per rectum, the prostate may be found to be enlarged both from above downwards and laterally; it may be smooth, uniform in consistence, elastic, and movable in the pelvic space in the case of adenomatous enlargement, or nodular, hard, irregular, and fixed in the case of carcinoma; the subjective symptoms of both are very similar. In some cases the prostate may not appear to be much enlarged upon rectal examination, though it is causing an intravesical tumour which obstructs urination, or a firm fibrous collar around the internal urethral orifice which gives rise to marked prostatic symptoms. In prostatic cases, even a large catheter of bicoudé form can usually be passed into the bladder readily. Retention of urine may also be present in cases of *acute prostatitis* or of *prostatic abscess*, when a history of recent urethral discharge will be obtained. It should be remembered that the onset of acute prostatitis in the course of an acute urethral infection may coincide with a considerable decrease or even absence of urethral discharge.

Acute retention of urine may be produced by other causes than the above. A *small calculus* may be passed into the urethra and totally obstruct the passage of urine. This may occur at any age, and the calculus become arrested at some narrow portion of the canal—usually at the meatus or at the membranous urethra. The urethra may lodge a calculus for some time with comparatively little pain; but more often the stone passes into the canal during micturition, causing a sudden pain, with cessation of the flow of urine and dribbling of a few drops of blood. The calculus may be palpated if it lies in the penile urethra or in the perineum, or will be felt on passing an instrument into the urethra.

Retention may be caused by the blockage of the internal urethral orifice by the free portion of a *pedunculated vesical tumour*. On any attempt at micturition the growth is forced into the orifice and obstructs it. These cases are rare, but can be detected on cystoscopy.

Retention of urine may occur with *traumatic rupture of the urethra*, often associated with fracture of the pelvis. The history of injury and the appearance of blood at the external urethral orifice and a haematoma in the perineum will point to the diagnosis (*Fig.* 533).

Retention of urine may also occur with *paralysis* of the *motor nerves* of the detrusor muscle of the bladder, or interference with the spinal centres by compression paraplegia, tabes dorsalis, or myelitis, each being diagnosed on examination of the nervous system; *prolapse of an intervertebral disk* will sometimes cause it from direct pressure on the emerging nerve roots. When retention occurs in *herpes zoster* there is a herpetic rash on the buttock or over the sacrum and a patch of acute oedematous congestion on the corresponding side of the bladder on cystoscopy. After operations upon the rectum or neighbouring organs retention may occur from reflex spasm.

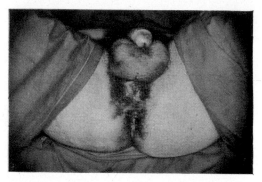

Fig. 533. Traumatic rupture of the urethra showing blood from meatus and perineal haematoma limited by attachment of Colles' fascia.

In other cases, retention of urine is present in association with other symptoms of *hysteria*; but care must be taken not to give a diagnosis of hysteria until all other causes of retention are excluded. These cases usually occur in children or in young women.

Retention of urine occurring after operations about the anal or rectal areas or for hernia, etc., will be diagnosed readily, but it must be remembered that the appearance of piles or a hernia in an elderly man may be due to the straining on micturition caused by moderate prostatic enlargement. In such cases it is better to remove the prostate and deal with the hernia at the same operation, and to leave any operation for piles until after prostatectomy.

Incontinence of Urine. The normal ability of the bladder to remain continent depends on the preservation of the balance between the tone of the detrusor muscle and that of the external sphincter of the urethra. When the sphincter is incompetent the condition of *true incontinence* results; when the detrusor is at fault the bladder fills until urine overflows through the urethra and *false incontinence* ensues. There are also various conditions of *partial*, intermittent, or temporary incontinence due to different causes. In *true incontinence* urine flows out continuously as it enters the bladder. Damage to the sphincter by mechanical causes or interference with its nerve-supply will produce this condition.

Mechanical damage is occasionally caused by injury to the sphincter during prostatectomy. If the mucosa of the membranous urethra is avulsed during enucleation of the prostate incontinence is likely to follow; subsequent fibrous contraction may restore continence at the expense of the formation of a stricture and if this is kept moderately dilated a reasonable degree of continence may be obtained. Injury to the sphincter is not common but is more frequent after transurethral resection than after open prostatectomy. It can follow total prostatectomy for carcinoma of the prostrate (now seldom performed), or be due to the downward extension of the malignant process itself to involve the membranous urethra.

Injury to the external sphincter by gunshot wounds or accidental trauma is more often followed by stricture than by incontinence, but this depends on the extent of the injury.

Neurogenic causes of incontinence may be due to *upper motor neuron lesions, lower motor neuron lesions*, or *lesions of the spinal tracts*. A complete transverse division of the cord above the lumbar enlargement produces an *upper motor neuron lesion*. It is followed by retention of urine until overflow incontinence occurs. The reflex centre in the cord is intact. If the bladder can be kept free from infection the final result may be one of automatic micturition; in this condition urine is passed forcibly, at intervals, with no voluntary control and little or no residual urine after each act of voiding. If sepsis, bed-sores, or other complications occur, as happens too often, a small contracted bladder is likely to ensue from which urine dribbles continuously. Similar effects can follow transverse myelitis or tumours of the spinal cord.

Injuries involving both a transverse lesion of the cord *and* the lumbar enlargement are inevitably associated with continuous incontinence.

In *lower motor neuron* lesions affecting the sacral part of the cord or the cauda equina the bladder is cut off from its reflex centre but the detrusor muscle has some inherent reflex activity. The bladder distends at first and overflows, but can in some cases be induced to contract by external pressure or other forms of stimulation so that a degree of continence is retained; if infection can be avoided it will be more efficient.

Peripheral neuritis (e.g., diabetic or tabetic) can produce similar effects. Damage to the autonomic supply to the detrusor may result from pelvic surgery and, in particular, may follow abdomino-perineal excision of the rectum.

Lesions of the spinal tracts interfere with the cerebral inhibitory impulses to the micturition centre in the conus medullaris. They occur in some cases of partial traumatic transection of the cord and in such diseases as disseminated sclerosis and syringomyelia. In disseminated sclerosis there may be sudden contractions of the detrusor muscle which cause precipitant micturition without warning. As the disease advances the detrusor may become paralysed so that the bladder distends and overflow incontinence occurs.

In *false incontinence* the bladder remains distended; the detrusor muscle is overstretched or may be paralysed but the condition is generally due to unrelieved urethral obstruction from an enlarged prostate or a stricture. Urine dribbles away by overflow and at night the bed is often wet.

Partial or transient incontinence occurs in some patients after prostatectomy but clears up as the prostatic cavity heals and sepsis is eradicated. It is more persistent in aged or debilitated patients.

Stress incontinence in women sometimes follows the trauma of childbirth and is due to overstretching of the connective-tissue supports of the bladder neck. Any sudden increase of intra-abdominal pressure as in sneezing, coughing, or stooping is liable to cause a leak of urine. The vaginal vault is lax and there may be a cystocele or a rectocele. Pressure by one finger on the urethra will generally control the leak on coughing and this test is used as an indication for the type of surgical treatment to be employed.

Certain *congenital anomalies* will also cause continuous true incontinence until corrected surgically. In congenital *ectopia vesicae* (exstrophy of the bladder) there is a failure in the development of the abdominal wall and the anterior wall of the bladder; there is a wide gap in the front of the bony pelvis. The mucous membrane of the bladder is exposed and the

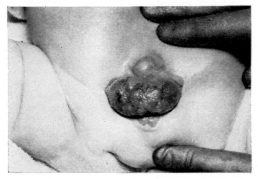

Fig. 534. Ectopia vesicae in a boy of 6 months. The bladder mucosa protrudes and urine drips constantly from the ureters.

two ureteric orifices can be seen with urine dripping from them (*Fig.* 534).

An *ectopic ureter* may open into the vagina or urethra in the female, in which case there is a continuous leak of urine. This ureter as a rule drains a duplex kidney and when a pyelogram shows this condition in a case of apparent incontinence search must be made for the ectopic orifice. The intravenous injection of indigocarmine (4 ml. of 0·4 per cent solution) will facilitate its finding (*Fig.* 535).

Incontinence from a fistula. In some cases of vesico-vaginal or utero-vesical fistula when the opening is large there may be continuous incontinence. In uretero-vaginal fistula the leak may appear to be intermittent.

Pain during Micturition. Pain may be present *during* or *immediately after* micturition, and it is important to ascertain not only the period at which it is present, but also the actual *location* of the pain. If pain is present in the urethra during

micturition it usually indicates that a stricture or some inflammatory process is present, the latter being evidenced by a urethral discharge (*see* URETHRAL DISCHARGE, p. 805). If pain is experienced *immediately after* micturition, and felt as a tingling or pricking sensation in the glans penis, there is some inflammatory or irritant process at the trigonal region of the bladder. Formerly this symptom was looked upon as diagnostic of vesical calculus, and though it is almost a constant symptom of the latter, provided the calculus is not trapped in a post-prostatic pouch, it is also present in cystitis, tuberculous or otherwise, in

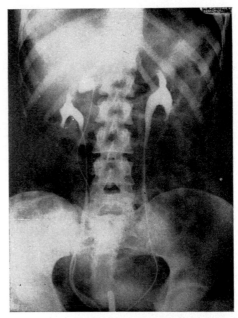

Fig. 535. Pyelogram in a case of incontinence of urine in a woman. There is a duplex kidney on the right; the ureter from its upper segment drained into the vestibule.

vesical carcinoma which is infiltrating the bladder base, and in acute or subacute prostatic infections. Prostatic infection can be diagnosed by the history of the case, usually following an acute urethritis, and by a rectal examination and examination of a smear after prostatic massage. Tuberculous cystitis usually occurs in young adults, and frequently other tuberculous lesions are present in the genito-urinary organs, such as the epididymis, vas deferens, seminal vesicles, or prostate, as well as the kidney, whilst the urine contains not only blood and pus but tubercle bacilli. Cystitis from other causes and vesical growth or calculus can be ascertained upon cystoscopic examination.

In male children *meatal ulcer*, usually consequent upon ammoniacal dermatitis in a circumcised infant, is a cause of pain and screaming on micturition.

Pain may be felt in the *perineum* during and after micturition in cases of prostatic disease, especially if much straining occurs during micturition, or may be felt in both the perineum and the anal area in cases of vesical carcinoma.

In the female, pain is felt at the urethral orifice and in the vulva after micturition in cases of cystitis or vesical carcinoma, and in some cases of urethral caruncle.

It should be noted that in either sex severe pain may be present at the termination of the urethra after micturition when a *calculus* is impacted in the *vesical end of the ureter* (*Fig.* 487, p. 477), especially if the latter is partially prolapsed into the bladder. The patient may hold her urine for hours rather than pass it, owing to the pain that follows micturition.

Micturition through Fistulae. Urine may pass, either wholly or in part, through a fistulous track communicating with the urinary organs, such opening being the result of preceding disease or injury. Occasionally, owing to congenital malformation of the urethra or bladder, urine passes by an opening in the perineum, pubes, or into the vagina. Urinary fistulae in connexion with the urethra are most common as the result of periurethral abscess, stricture, or of some operation; and in the case in which a penile fistula is present it is necessary to ascertain if the calibre of the urethra is in any way narrowed by cicatricial inflammation. A fistula may open in the perineum as the result of inflammation and extravasation behind a stricture following an operation upon the lower urinary organs, or in the female into the vagina from damage during parturition or some vaginal operation. In cases in which a fistula opens into the vaginal fornix the urine may leak from the bladder or from the lower end of the ureter. The opening is usually small and embedded in an area of cicatricial tissue, so that it is very difficult to pass a probe along the track. In these cases, evidence of the nature of the fistula may be obtained by filling the bladder with some sterile coloured solution, such as weak methylene blue; if the opening is in communication with the bladder, coloured solution will appear on a swab placed in the vagina, but if the urine comes from the ureter no stain will be found. In the latter case an intravenous injection of indigocarmine (4 ml. of 0·4 per cent) will cause a blue coloration in the vagina within a few minutes. Evidence may also be obtained by means of the cystoscope, when a cicatricial area may be found in the bladder surrounding a retracted fistulous opening, or the ureteric orifice of one side may be found displaced from its normal situation by the scar contraction when the ureter is at fault. A ureter is occasionally accidentally injured or divided during an abdominal operation on the uterus or the pelvic colon, followed by the formation of a urinary fistula. It may be difficult to tell which ureter is injured until an intravenous injection of indigocarmine is given and the coloured urine is seen to come down the uninjured side on cystoscopic examination. In these cases of ureteric injury it may be impossible to pass a bougie into the

ureter more than a very short distance, the tip being arrested by the scar tissue. At Caesarean section performed by the modern lower segment operation a utero-vesical fistula sometimes occurs, either by direct injury to the bladder or by the formation of a haematoma between the two organs which becomes infected. Urine may leak intermittently from the vagina or there may be continuous incontinence in some cases.

A urinary fistula may be present in the suprapubic area in connexion with the bladder, or in the lumbar area communicating with the kidney, as the result of operations on these two organs. A fistula has been seen in the iliac fossa as the result of an operation on the ureter, or after the opening of an abscess formed around the ureter from the ulceration caused by a ureteric calculus; in one case a urinary fistula containing calculi opened above the pubes—the result of an extensive gunshot wound of the pubes and bladder.

Disorders of Micturition from Diseases of the Nervous System. In most of the foregoing paragraphs symptoms referable to the urinary organs have been stated to be due in some cases to disease of the nervous system, such as myelitis, multiple sclerosis, tabes dorsalis, or paraplegia; in spite of repetition it is advisable to gather these under one heading. The control of the act of micturition depends upon the integrity of the nervous system; for although special centres exist in the lower segments of the spinal area presiding over the motor functions of the bladder, the impulse controlling centres is supplied by the brain after a stimulus has been conveyed to the latter by the sensory nerve-fibres from the bladder. Reflex contraction of the detrusor with reciprocal opening of the bladder neck is dependent on the integrity of the spinal centre; the nerves subserving emptying are of the parasympathetic system which carries both impulses of stretch and those producing contraction. Some afferent impulses are carried by the sympathetic, but its main function is concerned with the control of blood-vessels and of the sexual function. In the diagnosis of all neurological disturbances of the bladder it is most important to exclude all lesions of the urinary apparatus, and not to overlook the fact that vesical symptoms are often produced by some lesion in the kidney when the bladder on careful examination appears quite normal.

IRRITABILITY OF THE SENSORY NERVES OF THE BLADDER. Some patients experience an urgent and frequent desire to pass urine, often every half-hour, though no objective symptoms of disease can be found and all inflammatory lesions can be excluded; there is no pain and no increased frequency of micturition during the night. The cases have received the name of *cystalgia, hyperaesthesia vesicae,* and *irritable bladder.*

IRRITABILITY OF THE MOTOR NERVES OF THE BLADDER. In this condition there is a spasmodic contraction of the sphincter muscle of the bladder, with resulting retention of urine or great difficulty in micturition. There is no stricture or urethral obstruction, as shown by the ease with which a catheter is passed, nor is there any prostatic enlargement. The neurosis is not confined to the male sex, and is seen in hysteria as well as in those nervous affections which affect the spinal centres, such as myelitis, lateral sclerosis, and tabes dorsalis.

PARALYSIS OF THE MOTOR NERVES OF THE BLADDER may affect the peripheral nerves or spinal elements, but the results as regards the bladder are the same. If the nerves supplying the detrusor muscle or its spinal centre are paralysed, retention of urine occurs, and the patient can expel urine only by muscular effort of or pressure upon the abdominal wall. In many cases only part of the motor tract is affected, so that the power of the bladder is not abolished but merely diminished, and a portion of the urine is retained in the bladder after micturition. The bladder may be affected thus in compression of the spinal cord by fracture, or haemorrhage into the membranes, in myelitis, tumour, paraplegia, and tabes dorsalis, or prolapsed intervertebral disk.

DESTRUCTION OF THE SPINAL CENTRES FOR MICTURITION, by injury, softening, or compression, gives rise to incontinence without distension of the bladder. The urine dribbles from the urethra as fast as it enters the bladder.

DRUG-INDUCED DISORDERS OF MICTURITION. Drugs must always be considered when there is unexplained dysfunction in any system of the body, and the urinary tract is no exception. Oral diuretics are taken today by many patients and cause polyuria, frequency, and sometimes incontinence. Some antidepressants, such as amitriptyline, may cause dysuria and urinary retention with dribbling not only in men but also in women. Complete urinary retention may also occur with this drug, though more rarely urinary retention has also been reported with ganglion-blocking agents, imipramine, the antihistaminics, the monoamineoxidase inhibitors, propranolol, and several other drugs. With any unexplained disturbance of micturition the question of its being induced by drug therapy should always be considered.

Harold Ellis.

MOUTH, PIGMENTATION OF

Pigmentation of the mouth generally consists of flecks, streaks, or spots of brown or grey discoloration of the mucosa, especially upon the inner aspect of the cheeks along a line roughly corresponding to the level of the closed teeth. Other sites for their distribution are the mucous surface of the lips, seen best when these are everted in a good light; the roof of the mouth, generally upon the soft palate or upon the posterior part of the hard palate rather than more anteriorly; occasionally upon the gums; and sometimes upon the sides of the tongue. Such pigmentation of the buccal mucosa immediately suggests *Addison's disease* (*Fig.* 536), especially if there is at the same time generalized brown pigmentation of the skin with asthenia and low

blood-pressure. Buccal pigmentation is also a frequent feature in persons who have *Negro blood* in their ancestry, but may occur idiopathically with no obvious associated disorder and without Negro ancestry.

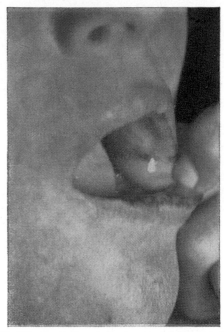

Fig. 536. Buccal pigmentation in untreated Addison's disease. Under treatment with cortisone all pigmentation disappeared within a few weeks.

Arsenic, whether used medicinally, administered surreptitiously, or absorbed in the course of occupation, may lead to marked pigmentation of the skin, and Addison's disease may be simulated, especially as pigmentation may also occur on the mucous membranes particularly of the lips and cheeks, as well as upon the skin. In arsenical cases there may be evidence of peripheral neuritis and of hyperkeratosis of the soles and palms; an abnormally high percentage of arsenic can be extracted from the hair.

Bismuth may also produce a somewhat similar pigmentation in the mouth; it is, however, grey rather than brown. *Silver*, at one time used fairly freely medicinally, may be another cause. Argyrism at the present day is very rare although it occasionally occurs in certain occupations and also through the absorption of silver salts from nasal or vesical irrigation. The 'blue line' of *lead* is usually too characteristic for misinterpretation to occur. Mercury, lead, or bismuth poisoning may show as a dark line along the gingival margins, particularly when oral hygiene is poor.

Pigmentation of the buccal mucosa suggesting Addison's disease is occasionally seen in *chronic cachectic conditions*, such as pulmonary tuberculosis or carcinomatosis, in which the suprarenal glands have at autopsy appeared to be healthy.

In familial intestinal polyposis (Peutz-Jegher syndrome) pigmentation of the face and mouth in the form of melanin spots is seen, as it may also with metastatic malignant melanoma and, rarely, intermittent acute porphyria and acanthosis nigricans.

F. Dudley Hart.

MOVEMENTS, INVOLUNTARY

These fall into seven groups: (1) *Tremor*, a rhythmical to-and-fro movement, fast or slow, which may involve the head, tongue, limbs, or portions of limbs. (2) *Athetosis* (mobile spasm), a sinuous writhing movement usually seen in the upper limb and lower limb, and sometimes in the face. (3) *Choreiform* movements, brief twitches which are unsustained, irregular in time and situation, and pleomorphic. (4) *Clonic spasm* (myoclonus), shock-like contractions of a muscle or a portion of a muscle, which may or may not cause displacement of the part, and which are usually repetitive for several seconds. (5) *Tonic spasm*, a sustained tetanus of a group of muscles. (6) *Fibrillation* (fasciculation), a fine flickering contraction of bundles of muscle-fibres, visible in superficial muscles as an intermittent shimmering of the skin. (7) *Habit spasms or tics*—a co-ordinated movement of some part of the body, often repeated, and purposeless.

1. TREMOR

Tremor is said to be present when the normally smooth and continuous contraction of a muscle at work, or the uniform tone of the muscle at rest, are interrupted by a rhythmic succession of perceptible contractions of opposing muscle groups which cause an oscillation of the affected part. Tremors are of various amplitudes, periods, and distributions in different diseases, in different cases of the same disease, and at different times in a single case; it is therefore seldom possible to make a diagnosis on the nature of the tremor alone, without a consideration of other symptoms and signs. The distinction commonly drawn between tremors which occur at rest and those which are prominent during activity (action or intention tremor) is not absolute. For instance, the tremor of disseminated sclerosis is seen on exertion, and that of Parkinsonism occurs at 'rest', but both are abolished by complete rest (i.e., sleep). Moreover, it is customary to regard action tremor as a movement elicited by and accompanying voluntary action, yet the tremor of the fingers which is seen when the hands are held out horizontally is not called an action tremor, but it is important to understand that this tremor of a part *unsupported* although not strictly in action can be interpreted in exactly the same way. To avoid the ambiguity which arises from symptomatic classification, the present account will be based on aetiological groups rather than on the nature of the tremor.

1. Physiological Tremor is seen after exposure to cold, in fatigue, and during convalescence after exhausting illness.

2 Congenital Tremor is often familial. It is seen in childhood and usually passes off in adult life, but may return in periods of emotional stress or physical illness. It affects the upper limb, and occasionally the head, and is brought out by voluntary movement and by emotion. It is not accompanied by other signs of disease. Sometimes it appears for the first time in adult life and may then become progressively worse.

3. Senile Tremor takes the form of a moderately fine rhythmic oscillation of the fingers, and often affects the head and lower jaw. It is not associated with rigidity or with other abnormal physical signs, and it gives rise to no difficulties in diagnosis.

4. Toxic Tremor is best illustrated by the fine tremor of chronic alcoholism. It is rapid and somewhat irregular, and is most marked during activity, especially early in the morning before the first drink of the day. In some cases it becomes very coarse, and has the features of an action tremor. It may be difficult to elicit a history of alcoholism, or to ascertain how much is being taken, but the presence of nausea, morning vomiting of mucus, paraesthesiae in the extremities, tenderness of the calves, and depression of the tendon reflexes will afford diagnostic assistance. While it is true that a fine tremor of the fingers is a feature of *nicotine poisoning*, it is doubtful whether excessive smoking is a common cause of tremor; heavy smoking is often a symptom of an anxiety state, itself a cause of tremor. Toxic tremor is seen in overdosage with *sodium diphenyl-hydantoinate*; it may be associated with ataxia, slurring speech, mental aberration, spongy gums, skin rashes, drug fever, and leucopenia. The *barbiturates* can cause similar tremor and ataxia, but the gums are unaffected and they have a greater sedative effect, which ranges from confusion to coma. Poisoning by *heavy metals* (mercury, lead, antimony, manganese, gold, and bismuth) may cause a fine tremor of the fingers. Addicts to *cocaine* and *opium* or its derivatives develop a tremor of the hands, lips, and tongue when deprived of their drugs. *Uraemia* and *cholaemia* are responsible for a rather coarse tremor of the hands, lips, and tongue, which appears during movement, but this symptom is overshadowed by other and more serious features of these diseases and has no diagnostic value.

5. Tremor in Metabolic Diseases. Tremor is an important feature of thyrotoxicosis and hypoglycaemia. In *hyperthyroidism* there is a fine, rapid, regular tremor of the outstretched fingers; in severe cases it may spread to the legs, and there may be sporadic attacks of trembling which affect the entire body. The tremor is aggravated by emotion and exertion, and is accompanied by exophthalmos, lid-lag, thyroid enlargement, loss of weight, tachycardia, nervousness, and a raised basal metabolic rate. Difficulty may arise in distinguishing this tremor from the similar tremor of an anxiety state, in which condition there is often a comparable loss of weight, sweating, tachycardia, and nervousness. The tremor of *hypoglycaemia* is seen in minor degrees in otherwise normal persons after strenuous exertion on an empty stomach; it is quickly relieved by eating sweets or a carbohydrate meal. Overdosage with insulin gives rise to a similar fine tremor associated with a sense of weakness and with sweating, and similar symptoms occur in the presence of a tumour of the islets of Langerhans. In chronic liver disease there may be a picture of an organic psychosis which may be accompanied by a 'flapping' tremor. This tremor is coarse, irregular, and bilateral and is characterized by flexion–extension movements of the wrists. This tremor may precede or follow the period of mental confusion. It is convenient to include in this metabolic group two curious conditions found in rickety children, *head nodding* and *spasmus nutans*. The former occurs in infants under two years of age; the head is rolled from side to side when the child is lying down, but ceases when he sits up. The incessant friction of the head on the pillow rubs the hair off the back of the scalp. Spasmus nutans is a rotatory movement of the head associated with a fine nystagmus, and it occurs in rickety infants who have been kept in poorly lighted rooms; it passes off in the summer but may recur in the winter until the child is of age to get out of the house in the colder weather.

6. Tremor in Disease of the Nervous System. Tremor occurs in disease of the frontal lobe, the corpus striatum, the red nucleus, the cerebellum and its pontine connexions, and the olive. In the majority of cases diagnosis depends less upon the characteristics of the tremor than upon satellite signs, but if it is the initial symptom its features require close study.

Frontal lesions—new growths, focal injury, abscess—can cause a rapid fine tremor of the contralateral arm and leg. Disease of the corpus striatum, in particular of the lenticular nucleus, is accompanied by a highly characteristic to-and-fro tremor of the contralateral limbs, which may also affect the lower jaw and head when the disease is bilateral. The face is always spared. It is best seen in *paralysis agitans* (Parkinson's disease), after middle age, but also occurs as a result of encephalitis lethargica, and in hepatolenticular degeneration (Wilson's disease), neoplastic disease and vascular lesions of the lenticular nucleus, severe head injuries, carbon-monoxide poisoning, and manganese poisoning, and with phenothiazine drugs such as chlorpromazine. It is usually a rather coarse to-and-fro movement at the rate of from four to eight oscillations per second. It produces the alternating movements of the thumb and finger known as 'pill-rolling', often combined with alternating pronation and supination of the forearm, and flexion-extension movements of the wrist. In mild cases it is temporarily inhibited by voluntary movements, and it ceases during sleep. It is associated sooner or later

with muscular rigidity, a monotonous voice, a bent and rigid carriage, a shuffling gait, and a notable absence of the 'fidgets' of normal persons. In advanced cases the gait is festinant: the patient starts to walk with difficulty, but accelerates as he goes along as if chasing his own centre of gravity. If given a slight push, he has difficulty in stopping himself (propulsion and retropulsion). Movement is interfered with by rigidity and tremor, but muscular weakness is absent until the terminal stages of the disease, except in the small hand muscles, in which weakness as well as rigidity may be responsible for some of the early disability. Mental capacity, ocular movements, and the superficial reflexes remain normal, and the tendon reflexes remain brisk until they are abolished by the rigidity of the muscles. *Post-encephalitic Parkinsonism* presents a similar picture in so far as tremor and rigidity are concerned, but it occurs in younger persons, there is often a history of a febrile illness with cerebral symptoms months or years before, and there are often, but not invariably, other features not seen in paralysis agitans—mental and moral deterioration, ocular palsies, oculogyric crises (p. 550), ptyalism, inversion of the sleep rhythm, obesity, etc. Although the tremor and rigidity are presumably due to smouldering activity of the virus, the spinal fluid is normal in this 'chronic' stage.

The *encephalomyelitis* which occurs after the specific fevers of childhood occasionally manifests itself as a slow rhythmic tremor of the head and extremities, with or without rigidity, but the condition clears up entirely within a few weeks. Parkinsonian tremor and rigidity occasionally appear during convalescence from *severe head injuries*; it does not progress, but is usually associated with intellectual loss, change of personality for the worse, and, in many cases, with signs of injury to the cranial nerves and long tracts. Paralysis agitans (*Fig.* 537) developing many years after a head injury should not be attributed to the injury. *Hepatolenticular degeneration* (Wilson's disease) is a rare familial condition characterized by excessive copper storage and marked by Parkinsonian tremor, rigidity, emotional over-action, and hepatic cirrhosis, coming on in young persons, and associated in some instances with the presence of a ring of golden-yellow pigment in the cornea near the limbus—the Kayser-Fleischer ring. *Carbonmonoxide poisoning* is a rare cause of Parkinsonian tremor; the anoxia to which the brain is subjected at the time of exposure is often the cause of immediate death, but amongst those that survive there may be evidence of permanent damage—intellectual loss, childishness, Parkinsonian tremor with or without rigidity, and signs of pyramidal lesions.

Manganese poisoning, now rare, affects workmen in certain industries (steel, paint, linoleum, etc.); lethargy, depression, Parkinsonian tremor, and rigidity are present. *Vascular accidents* are rarely a cause of this type of tremor, but both

18

tremor and rigidity sometimes occur as a result of progressive generalized cerebral arteriosclerosis. Unlike paralysis agitans, such cases often suffer from supranuclear paralysis of conjugate ocular movement, bulbar palsy, and mental deterioration. *Neoplastic infiltration* of the basal ganglia is a very rare cause of unilateral Parkinsonism; the presence of headache, papilloedema, and symptoms indicating involvement of the internal capsule serve to indicate the correct diagnosis.

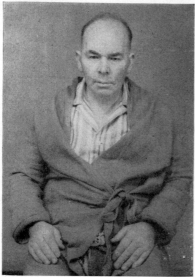

Fig. 537. Paralysis agitans showing expressionless gaze and typical rigid immobility. (*Dr. R. G. Ollerenshaw, Manchester Royal Infirmary.*)

General paralysis of the insane is often, but by no means invariably, marked by a fine irregular tremor of the tongue, lips, and outstretched fingers. At first it appears only when the affected parts are in use, as in lighting a cigarette, exposing the teeth, or protruding the tongue, but if the condition is allowed to progress it becomes coarse and may impart a tremulous element to speech. Mental deterioration, euphoria, or depression, and early signs of pyramidal degeneration make their appearance, and there is always a positive Wassermann reaction in the spinal fluid. Argyll Robertson pupils are present in a minority of cases; optic atrophy and loss of the tendon reflexes indicate that tabes dorsalis is also present (tabo-paresis).

Lesions of the red nucleus give rise to a slow rhythmic tremor of the contralateral hand and foot; it is increased by excitement and voluntary movement and ceases during sleep. A lesion in this region is likely to cause additional symptoms, such as nuclear paralysis of the third nerve on the side of the lesion, or a crossed hemiplegia or hemianaesthesia. When a unilateral lesion of the midbrain involves the third nerve as it passes through the red nucleus and thus causes an ipsilateral third nerve palsy with contralateral tremor, this is called Benedikt's syndrome.

The tremor which occurs in some cases of disease affecting the cerebellum or its connexions in the peduncles and pons is a coarse irregular jerking, absent at rest and brought out by movement, i.e., an action tremor, sometimes called 'intention tremor' (*Fig.* 538). It is due to lack of postural control, which normally imparts smoothness to voluntary movements. Action tremor is common in disseminated sclerosis, and also occurs in neoplastic, traumatic, vascular, and inflammatory conditions of the cerebellum, in alcoholism, in the heredofamilial ataxias (e.g., Friedreich's ataxia), and in olivo-ponto-cerebellar

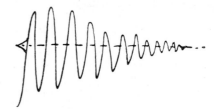

Fig. 538. Movements in intention tremor.

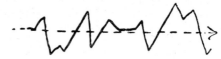

Fig. 539. Movements in ataxy. The dotted lines show the direction of the movement attempted.

atrophy (*Fig.* 539). It may occur when the cerebellum is compressed by a neurofibroma growing from the 8th nerve, and has been recorded in gliomata involving the superior cerebellar peduncle and pons. It is usually associated with other cerebellar signs, such as nystagmus and inco-ordination, but these may be overshadowed by the tremor.

There is a rare form of tremor which may be confined to the soft palate, or may involve the palate, pharynx, larynx, face, platysma, and diaphragm—all on the affected side. The tremor is fast and regular, and is associated with degeneration of the olive in elderly persons; it is sometimes referred to as 'palatal nystagmus' or 'myoclonus'.

Tremor is a common phenomenon in *anxiety states*; it is seen in the fingers when the hands are held out, and may involve the tongue and corners of the mouth when the patient is asked to show the teeth and protrude the tongue. It is fine and rapid and is associated with other somatic manifestations of anxiety—tachycardia, sweating, stabbing left inframammary pain, spastic colon, functional dyspepsia, or other visceral neurosis. Psychiatric investigation will reveal the source of the anxiety, thereby making a positive diagnosis, for the fact that a patient has a cause for anxiety, and manifests a tremor, does not mean that the two are interrelated or that organic disease is necessarily absent. Any form of tremor may be encountered in *hysteria,* and here again it is necessary to exclude organic disease, to identify the psychological factor as a positive illness, and finally to prove the point by showing that the tremor can be influenced by suggestion. It must be remembered that tremor, in common with other involuntary movements, is usually aggravated by emotion such as anxiety or fear. Cynical comments to the effect that a patient is malingering because the movement is only present 'when you watch him' are singularly naïve.

2. ATHETOSIS

The involuntary movements of athetosis, sometimes called mobile spasm, are usually confined to the upper limb, occasionally involve the feet, and may implicate the face. (*Fig.* 540.) In the upper limb the movements are most marked

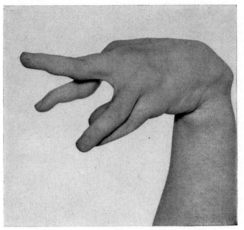

Fig. 540. The hand in athetosis.

in the fingers and wrist, but in severe cases they spread to the forearm and shoulder. They consist of smooth, sinuous, writhing movements; in a typical case the fingers slowly flex, then extend, one by one, and spread widely, while the thumb alternately adducts and abducts and the wrist flexes and extends. The movements are aggravated by emotion, by attempted use of the affected limb, and by voluntary movement of the opposite limb. Athetosis may occur in limbs which possess normal power, or some degree of muscular weakness, but it disappears if paralysis occurs. Furthermore, it is associated with hemiparesis in children, and especially young children, rather than in adults. *Congenital double athetosis* makes its appearance in the first year of life. The arms and face are involved, speech is distorted by movements of the lips and tongue, and swallowing may be affected. In severe cases, the lips may exhibit the movements. The child is late in reaching the milestones of development and some degree of mental deficiency is common. The movements cease during sleep. The condition is sometimes due to a lesion of the corpus striatum, which is broken up into cellular masses separated by a

network of fine nerve-fibres (the 'status marmoratus' of Vogt). Athetosis is a frequent accompaniment of *infantile hemiplegia, double hemiplegia,* and *cerebral diplegia,* conditions which represent symptomatic variants of a common pathology. Each of these may be due to maldevelopment of the brain in utero, to atrophic lobar sclerosis (a degenerative condition of the foetal brain), to birth injury, or to infantile encephalitis of as yet unspecified type. It is often impossible to decide which of these four possibilities is operative in a given case. Prognosis depends more upon the severity of the disability than on the aetiology. The paralysis and athetosis are often associated with mental defect, epilepsy, and a general constitutional delicacy which manifests itself as a failure to thrive and a poor resistance to infections and operative procedures. When there is sufficient mental capacity to make the child teachable, re-educational exercises carried out continuously from the age of three years sometimes prove effective in reducing athetosis. It is important, therefore, to exercise care in assessing the intelligence of these children, and to remember that athetosis, grimacing, and dysarthria may give too pessimistic an impression of the child's capabilities. A rare cause of double athetosis appearing within a few weeks of birth is *icterus gravis neonatorum.* The condition is due to *Rhesus* incompatibility in the parents. At autopsy there is found an intense bile-staining of certain nuclear masses of the brain—notably the lenticular and caudate nuclei. Jaundice is noted within three days of birth, and is intense. Tonic and clonic convulsions may occur, and between the spasms there is often intense rigidity of the musculature, with opisthotonos, trismus, and spasm of the bulbar muscles. At other times the muscles may be flaccid. Athetosis develops within a few weeks, and an intense erythroblastic anaemia is present. In those who survive there is mental deficiency, emotional instability, athetosis, striatal rigidity, and occasionally hemiparesis with an extensor plantar response. Epilepsy may occur, and bulbar palsies may persist. Athetoid movements of the trunk and proximal muscles of the limbs occur as a part of the syndrome known as *torsion spasm* (syn. dystonia musculorum deformans). This is an extrapyramidal syndrome which occurs in a variety of states, notably as a sequel to epidemic encephalitis, and as an expression of hepatolenticular degeneration. The neck, trunk, and pelvic girdles are seized by mobile spasm, which induces a variety of contortions, e.g., the arms are rotated internally and carried behind the back, the head is pulled back or to one side, the trunk is powerfully flexed, is extended or carried to one side, and the legs are extended, with the feet in equinovarus. But many variations are seen. Spasms come on abruptly, waxing and waning during a bout, and they disappear during repose or sleep and are greatly aggravated by voluntary movements and by emotion. They interfere greatly with movement and with gait. Even between the spasms there is an underlying basis of fluctuating hypertonia which has gained the name 'dystonia', but this periodic accession of tone is probably merely a larval attack of mobile spasm. Persistent extrapyramidal rigidity has been described, and contracture of the feet and tendo Achillis is not infrequent. Epilepsy, and other focal symptoms dependent on the nature and site of the causal lesions, may also be present. Diagnosis in the majority of cases lies between hepatolenticular degeneration, with its hepatic cirrhosis, Parkinsonism, rigidity and tremor, emotional over-action, and corneal pigmentation, and encephalitis lethargica. In the last-named, the torsion spasm is often confined to one limb or one side, and there may be a history of the acute phase of the disease together with changes of personality, seborrhoea, sialorrhoea, oculogyric crises, or other suggestive features. A few cases are due to other degenerative processes of the corpus striatum, the nature of which is not understood.

3. CHOREA

Chorea is characterized by involuntary movements which are jerky, irregular, sudden, and pleomorphic, in contrast to the slow, writhing, and repetitive spasms of athetosis. Choreiform movements, in pure form, are best seen in *Sydenham's chorea*. The movements involve the face, tongue, extremities, and muscles of respiration. They are absent when the patient is relaxed, except in the most severe cases, but any attempt at voluntary movement, and any excitement, provoke the movements at once. Natural gestures and the movements of facial expression are exaggerated, and voluntary movements of the limbs are distorted and embarrassed by sharp and irregular involuntary movements of brief duration. These movements, and the hypotonia which is also present, combine to produce a wild inco-ordination of the upper limbs and of gait. Even when gross movements are not visible, there is a characteristic irregular fluctuation in the strength of the grip. Articulation is distorted by movements of the lips, tongue, pharynx, and muscles of respiration. Swallowing may be disturbed. On taking a rapid deep breath incoordination may be seen clinically and radiographically between intercostal and diaphragmatic components (Czerny's sign). The symptoms are usually bilateral, but they may predominate or be confined to one side (hemichorea). The tendon reflexes are diminished in quiet phases, but involuntary movements which occur simultaneously with percussion of the tendons may produce an unduly prolonged contraction. Pendular knee-jerks are also seen. Muscle power is usually somewhat reduced, and fatiguability is extreme. Sensation, sphincter control, and the superficial reflexes are unaffected, but emotional instability and insomnia are common, and delirium is not unknown. Sydenham's chorea occurs typically in children between the ages of six years and puberty, but it may occur in association with pregnancy, in the second and third decades;

this form (chorea gravidarum) ceases shortly after the termination of the pregnancy. It tends to occur in those who previously suffered from rheumatic chorea in childhood. Chorea is regarded as rheumatic because other manifestations of acute rheumatism—carditis or polyarthritis—precede or follow some 75 per cent of all cases.

Senile chorea is an entirely different disease; it occurs in the sixth or later decades and lasts indefinitely. The movements are typically choreiform, are comparatively mild in degree, and are unassociated with hypotonia or inco-ordination. They are often confined to the legs. *Huntington's chorea* is a rare hereditary disease coming on as a rule at about the age of 40 years, and characterized by involuntary movements almost identical with those of Sydenham's chorea but accompanied by progressive mental failure with delusions. The choreiform movements are seldom severe, but inco-ordination may be well marked. Facial grimaces, dysarthria, jerks of the head, and abrupt movements of the trunk and limbs impart an easily recognizable clinical impression. The condition is due to a slow degeneration of the cells of the cerebral cortex and of the corpus striatum, with neuroglial increase and meningeal thickening—a marked contrast to the scarcely discernible histological changes in the cortex and basal ganglia of patients with Sydenham's chorea. Choreiform movements occasionally occur in the acute phase of *encephalitis lethargica*; the association with stupor, pyrexia, ocular palsies, and pleocytosis in the cerebrospinal fluid will make the diagnosis clear. *Congenital chorea* is sometimes seen as an association of *congenital hemiplegia and diplegia*, but it is less common than athetosis; movements of a transitional type, which are more athetotic than choreiform, are not uncommon in these conditions. They are referred to as choreo-athetosis. One interesting but rare variety is the *Lesch Nyhan* syndrome in childhood, where choreo-athetosis is associated as a familial defect with spasticity, mental deficiency, aggressive behaviour directed to others as well as themselves, and hyperuricaemia. In other cases congenital chorea or choreo-athetosis occurs without evidence of pyramidal disease; the movements are associated with a marked hypotonia. Disturbance of speech, difficulty in swallowing, and facial grimaces are present, and mental development is retarded. The term *hemiballismus* is applied to cases in which there are violent choreiform movements of large amplitude limited to one side of the body. It is due to disease (usually vascular) of the sub-thalamic nucleus of Luys. Co-ordination and power may be normal, but excitement and emotional disturbances result in a wild thrashing about of the affected arm and leg, with a risk of severe injury to both the patient and the bystander. In one case, the patient, an inmate of an institution for mental defectives, could not constrain the flail-like movements of the right arm and leg when he was excited; at the weekly cinema show he was unable to remain in a chair but sat on the floor at a safe distance from his fellow patients so that he could safely indulge his somewhat unusual physical response to the events portrayed on the screen.

In *hysteria* choreiform movements are rare except in the case of young adults who have had Sydenham's chorea in earlier years; in such cases the pattern of the hysterical illness is provided by the original disease. It is easy to confuse psychogenic tics with chorea, but the former are repetitive and stereotyped, unlike the constantly changing movements of the latter.

4. MYOCLONUS

The term 'myoclonus' refers to a shock-like contraction of a group of muscles, a single muscle, or a portion of a muscle. Whether the affected part is displaced or not depends on the severity and situation of the myoclonus. The best and most common example is seen in the clonic phase of a major *epileptic fit*. In *Jacksonian epilepsy*, on the other hand, clonic movements limited to a limb, or to the face, or to one side of the body may constitute the entire fit. The episodic incidence and brief duration of the attack distinguish epileptic myoclonus from other varieties of myoclonus, but there is a rare variant, *epilepsia partialis continuans*, in which almost continuous twitching occurs in one segment of the body, usually the hand. This localized myoclonus may spread at times to initiate a major convulsion. Where this condition is a manifestation of idiopathic epilepsy, it may occur periodically over many years, but it also occurs over a period of days or weeks in irritative lesions of the motor cortex, as in thrombophlebitis of cortical veins, abscesses in or immediately beneath the cortex, and cerebral tumours. Another variant is *myoclonic epilepsy*, which takes the form of occasional irregular twitches of some part of the body. These movements—colloquially known as 'the jumps' —are quite common in epileptic subjects, occurring between the major attacks, but they sometimes occur as the sole manifestation of epilepsy. The movements are abrupt and constant. One patient's wife complained that he often kicked her violently in bed; a child was penalized by her parents for 'clumsiness'; she often knocked things over when the arm was suddenly displaced by a myoclonic jerk. The combination of these sporadic myoclonic movements with attacks of major epilepsy is sometimes seen as a familial condition—Unverricht's *familial myoclonic epilepsy*. These manifestations and accompaniment of epilepsy must not be confused with the momentary twitching of a limb which happens to normal persons when falling asleep; such movements are particularly prominent in conditions of fatigue and anxiety, and may even prevent sleep.

The paramyoclonus of Friedreich is a rare disease of adult life characterized by sudden involuntary twitches of the muscles of the limbs, limb girdles, and face. The clonic twitches are sometimes symmetrical, and involve different muscles at different times; they continue throughout the day and may be at their worst when the patient is at rest in bed. They are usually averted by voluntary movement. The twitches do not as a rule displace the limbs, but in exceptional cases they give rise to violent movements which may throw the patient to the floor or out of bed. The nervous system is otherwise normal. *Encephalitis lethargica* occasionally causes powerful myoclonic jerks of the face, neck, shoulders, diaphragm, abdomen, arms, or legs, which prevent sleep and cause tachycardia and profuse sweating. These symptoms occur in the acute phase and they eventually give place to the more familiar sequelae of the disease, but chronic encephalitic myoclonus has also been described as a sequel of the acute disease. Diffuse myoclonic movements are a prominent feature of *subacute inclusion encephalitis*, a rare but fatal disease of childhood marked by slowly increasing intellectual deterioration, bodily wasting, myoclonus, a characteristic electro-encephalographic picture, and death in from one to three years. *Epidemic hiccup*, an affection which lasts for days or weeks, is generally regarded as an abortive form of encephalitis lethargica; the muscles of the abdominal wall are often involved as well as the diaphragm; the more familiar post-prandial hiccup is a myoclonus of the diaphragm due to irritation by a distended stomach, and a similar affection may result from any local irritant above or below the diaphragm. The hiccup of uraemia, usually thought to be due to 'metabolic intoxication', is often relieved by getting rid of abdominal distension. *Hyperpnoeic myoclonus* may be artificially produced in the muscles of the limb or limbs below a compression lesion of the spinal cord. The myoclonus is limited to the large proximal muscles of the limbs, and it ceases when the hyperventilation is stopped.

Clonic facial spasm is characterized by clonic contraction of one or more muscles of the face and may extend to the platysma on the affected side. Twitches succeed each other at inconstant intervals and may be confined to one muscle or appear in different muscles successively. Aetiology is complicated. It may be the sole manifestation of Jacksonian epilepsy, in which case it occurs in well-defined incidents with intervals of normality. It can be caused by irritation of the facial nerve, by pontine lesions, gummatous meningitis, acoustic neuroma, disease of the petrous temporal bone and of the middle ear, or by affection of the facial nerve outside the skull. In such cases motor and sensory signs of organic disease may be present. But in a larger group no physical explanation is to be found, and the condition is known as *facial hemispasm*.

5. TONIC SPASM

'Tonic spasm' is a clinician's term for what physiologists call a tetanus—a sustained contraction of a muscle or group of muscles. Tonic spasm displaces the affected part and maintains the altered position until the spasm ceases, in contrast to the intermittent shock-like contracture of myoclonus. Tonic spasm is seen in the tonic phase of a *major epileptic seizure*, in *decerebrate rigidity*, in *tetanus* and *tetany*, in the *flexor and extensor spasms of paraplegia*, and in postencephalitic *oculogyric crises*.

In *epilepsy* all the voluntary muscles, including those of respiration, become rigid for a few seconds. The jaws are clenched, the neck and trunk are stiff, and the limbs are rigid. This is usually followed by the clonic phase, but cases are not rare in which no clonic contractions occur. Tonic fits are usually a manifestation of epilepsy, but they occasionally occur in the advanced stages of cerebellar tumour. The onset of such a *cerebellar* fit is sudden, with unconsciousness, cyanosis, and dilatation of the pupils. There is tonic head retraction, opisthotonos, tonic extension of the elbow with supination of the forearm, flexion of the wrist and fingers, and extension of the hips, knees, and ankles—a condition of decerebrate rigidity. In unilateral cerebellar fits the tonic spasm is more marked in the ipsilateral limbs than on the other side, and there is a spiral rotation of the limbs, head, and trunk towards the healthy side, so that the patient comes to lie prone with the face corresponding to the side of the lesion pressing in the pillow. It may be remarked in passing that cerebellar tumours occasionally give rise to a typical epileptic fit with tonic and clonic stages. Persistent decerebrate rigidity is occasionally seen in gross lesions of the brain-stem between the vestibular nucleus below and the superior colliculus above.

Tonic spasm is the central feature of infection by the *Clostridium tetani*. In generalized tetanus all the muscles become affected, but spasm appears first in muscles with short motor nerves —the jaw, face, and neck, with progressive spread to the spinal and abdominal muscles and finally to the limbs. The tonic spasm varies from time to time; paroxysms of intense spasm, induced by excitement, noise, or handling the limbs, throws the musculature into excruciatingly painful contractions, with opisthotonos, head retraction, trismus, risus sardonicus, and rigid extension of the legs; or the body may be bent forward (emprosthotonos) and the limbs flexed if the spasm occurs in the flexor groups. These acute painful paroxysms last for a few seconds, and recur at intervals; they may cause death by asphyxia or heart failure. In mild or chronic cases of tetanus the symptoms will be less severe and less generalized—recurrent risus sardonicus, slight stiffness of the neck, and difficulty in opening the mouth. Another important variant is *local tetanus*, in which the bacillus secretes its exotoxin in quantities sufficient to cause local tonic spasm but insufficient to cause generalized spasm. This is particularly likely to occur when partial immunity has been induced by passive immunization. The affected part is rigid, and the stiffness persists during sleep and under spinal anaesthesia. It is often painless, and the periodic

exacerbation which characterizes generalized tetanus may be completely absent. This condition, like all forms of tetanus, is most common in field warfare, and there is a real danger of mistaking it for *hysteria*, or for *reflex spasms* following a painful wound to the affected part. Persistence of the rigidity during sleep will readily indicate the true diagnosis. *Strychnine poisoning* gives rise to recurrent tonic spasms, but trismus is absent or appears late, the extremities are first and most severely affected, the muscles are completely relaxed between spasms, and the symptoms develop within an hour or two of the administration of the poison. During an attack of *tetany* there are paroxysmal tonic spasms of the hands and the feet. The hand assumes a conical attitude, the fingers being extended at the interphalangeal joints, adducted, and slightly flexed at the metacarpophalangeal joints; the thumb is adducted and the palm hollowed (*main d'accoucheur*). The toes are flexed towards the sole, the ankle plantar flexed, and the foot inverted. The spasm may last from a few minutes to two hours or more, and is often painful. It may persist during sleep. Even in the absence of spontaneous spasm, an attack can be induced by arresting the circulation in a limb for 3–4 minutes (Trousseau's sign). Percussion of superficial motor nerves (e.g., the facial) will reproduce the spasm (Chvostek's sign).

In *paraplegia* attacks of tonic spasm occur below the level of the lesion. In incomplete lesions of the spinal cord, the legs are maintained in a position of extension; intermittent exacerbations of the rigidity occur in response to peripheral stimuli, giving rise to tonic extensor spasms. In complete transection of the cord there is paraplegia in flexion, and troublesome flexor spasms occur from time to time. These may be associated with reflex evacuation of the bladder and rectum and with sweating. This mass reflex occurs both as a result of peripheral stimulation and spontaneously. *Oculogyric crises* constitute an unusual form of tonic spasm, the result of epidemic encephalitis lethargica, and now also known to be provoked by drugs of the phenothiazine group. These consist of attacks of involuntary upward movement of the eyes. At times there may be deviation to one or other side or even downwards. The attacks may be brief or last some hours and nothing that the patient may do appears to influence them. A similar tonic spasm of the *masticatory muscles* is also encountered as a sequel of encephalitis, occurring during meals; the patient suddenly becomes unable to open or close his mouth until the spasm passes off.

6. FIBRILLATION AND FASCICULATION

The term 'fibrillation' is used for irregular flickering contractions of small groups of muscle-fibres, visible as a brief shimmering movement under the skin. No displacement of the affected part occurs. It is aggravated by cold, fatigue, and mechanical stimulation. Persistent fibrillation of a rather coarser character, involving a larger collection of muscle-fibres, is called 'fasciculation'.

Fibrillation and fasciculation are occasionally seen as a generalized affection of otherwise normal young adults. This condition, known as 'benign' fasciculation, spares the face but occurs in the muscles of the limbs and trunk. It is unassociated with other signs of disease and the prognosis is good. Of greater importance is the fibrillation and fasciculation which occur in disease of the lower motor neurons, e.g., *motor neuron disease* in which wasting is present or is about to commence, the recovery phase of *acute anterior poliomyelitis, Werdnig-Hoffman progressive muscular atrophy* of infants, *peroneal muscular atrophy, syringomyelia, compression of the cauda equina,* and occasionally in *polyneuritis* and *partial section of large nerves* such as the sciatic and the median. Fibrillation is not always visible in peripheral nerve lesions or in poliomyelitis, but the fine action potentials which mark its presence are always present in the electromyogram. *Fibrillation and fasciculation are conspicuous by their absence in all muscular dystrophies, including dystrophia myotonica.*

7. HABIT SPASMS AND TICS

There must be few involuntary movements of organic origin that have not been reproduced in hysteria at some time or another. Such incidents are usually brief, lasting days or weeks, and the movements are usually cured by psychotherapy. There is, however, a more important and more intractable group of psychogenic involuntary movements, called *tics* or *habit spasms*, which are a manifestation of the obsessional-compulsive neurosis. These differ from hysterically-determined movements in character, duration, and intractability. They are characterized by sudden, rapid, co-ordinated movements, always of the same nature and in the same region, occurring intermittently, aggravated by emotion and ceasing in sleep. They often appear to afford relief to a feeling of emotional tension. They are sometimes associated with compulsive ideas or utterances, and the personality is marked by obsessional traits. They may last for years, or throughout life, and, in common with the other features of obsessional neurosis, they are singularly resistant to psychotherapy. It is convenient to divide the tic into four clinical groups; combinations are not uncommon:

1. Simple Tic consists in a sudden twitch-like movement in which a purposive element may be discerned, such as a movement of the shoulder and neck intended to adjust an uncomfortable collar, a sniff to clear the nose, blinking the eyes persisting after conjunctivitis or exposure to strong light, and so on. Simple tics are common in children and on the whole they run a favourable course, ceasing either spontaneously or as a result of psychiatric treatment. Others persist into adult life.

2. Generalized Convulsive Tic (Gilles de la Tourette's disease) is a more serious affection which usually appears about the age of puberty and is characterized by complicated and widespread tics, associated in many cases with explosive utterances, echolalia, coprolalia (repetition of blasphemous or obscene words), and obvious mental aberration. The movements are polymorphic, numerous, and violent; as in other forms of tic, the nervous system is otherwise normal and there is at present no pathological evidence in support of an organic aetiology. Such cases are singularly resistant to treatment.

3. Co-ordinated Tics are rare. Under a condition of emotional stress, the patient carries out some complicated and co-ordinated act, thereby relieving mental tension. This emotional relief is a characteristic feature of all tics: the patient feels that he must 'twitch or burst', as one described it. It is clear that the involuntary movement or activity has a profound emotional significance for the sufferer, founded doubtless on some past experience and occurring thereafter as a conditioned expression of a subconscious compulsion.

4. Psychical Tics take the form of imperative ideas, or explosive utterances. These features may occur alone, or in association with convulsive tic. Although the patient is much distressed by these phenomena, and desires above all things to avoid them, they keep on breaking through in an embarrassing manner at inappropriate times. Explosive utterances may be meaningless sounds, or words, or sentences—often obscene and out of character. Psychical tics, no less than the motor variants, are often associated with other obsessive–compulsive features such as agaraphobia, claustrophobia, and so on.

SPASMODIC TORTICOLLIS

There is some doubt whether spasmodic torticollis is a psychogenic tic, or is the result of some as yet unspecified organic disease of the nervous system although current opinion tends towards the latter. Nevertheless, emphasis is still concentrated on psychogenic factors and, for the time being, it is classified as a tic. It is a disease of adult life and is twice as common in women as in men. The majority of cases are marked by neuropathic heredity and are themselves highly strung, obsessional, or unstable. In such cases, the onset may be traced to a simple tic, which, in turn, started as a voluntary movement to adjust an uncomfortable collar, or as an occupational habit. A small boy, unhappy at his first public school, found his Eton collar uncomfortable; he eased it by inclining his head to his shoulder, and from this there developed a severe torticollis—which was later cured by a dramatic manipulation of his neck. A pianist was in the habit of jerking his head to the left when striking a chord with the left hand; after his wife committed suicide this movement became an involuntary spasmodic torticollis, and it is pertinent to record that while she was still with him he always sought relief from the annoyance she caused him by resort to the piano. Torticollis has been known to follow epidemic encephalitis, but there is no justification for assuming that the movements were directly caused by a focal lesion since the change of personality which is so frequent after this disease might serve as the basis for a psychogenic tic.

The spasm may be tonic, or clonic, or both. The head is retracted and turned to the side, while the shoulder is raised; in severe cases the face, scaleni, and upper extremity may all be involved. In other cases the head is drawn backwards (retrocolic spasm) and this is usually accompanied by overaction of the frontalis, the skin of the forehead being wrinkled. The movements are intermittent, being increased in severity and amplitude by emotion, and by fatigue; they cease during sleep. When persistent, fatigue of the affected muscles gives rise to an unpleasant dull ache. The disease fluctuates, remissions and exacerbations occurring throughout life, and psychiatric treatment is seldom effective.

Ian Mackenzie.

MUSCULAR ATROPHY

Atrophy of muscles will be considered under the following headings: (1) Atrophy as part of general bodily wasting; (2) Atrophy due to disuse of a limb; (3) Atrophy due to vascular disease in a limb; (4) Atrophy due to injury and disease of the anterior horn cells and peripheral nerves; (5) Atrophy due to disease of muscles.

1. GENERAL BODILY WASTING

Muscular atrophy is often seen in general wasting of the tissues due to chronic and subacute disease such as tuberculosis, malignant disease, neglected or undiagnosed diabetes mellitus, hyperthyroidism, malaria, hookworm infestation, conditions associated with chronic diarrhoea, and anorexia nervosa. It is also seen in old age.

2. DISUSE

Disuse of a limb gives rise to extreme degrees of wasting. The best example is provided by the results of prolonged immobilization in fractures of the long bones. It also occurs in muscles acting upon a painful or ankylosed joint, and in rheumatoid arthritis. Hysterical paralysis gives rise to wasting only when maintained for years, and this is unusual. Voluntary disuse, practised by some votaries of Eastern cults, can lead to extreme 'withering' of the entire limb, e.g., when penance demands that the arm be held above the head in perpetuity.

3. VASCULAR DISEASE

Arterial occlusion is variable in its effects. In tourniquet paralysis, surgical ligation of a major vessel, thrombosis, and embolism of the great vessels, the degree of wasting depends on the efficiency of the collateral circulation. In many instances the muscles become fibrosed and hard rather than wasted and flabby. In other cases, there is a true atrophy of muscles due to ischaemia

of the motor nerves, as in some cases of Buerger's disease (p. 315), and in polyarteritis nodosa (pp. 466, 556). A special variety of ischaemic palsy, known as Volkmann's contracture, is the result of fractures in the region of the elbow: oedema and haemorrhage into the soft tissues interfere with the circulation distal to the elbow and cause fibrosis of the flexors of the wrist and fingers, and of the intrinsic muscles of the hand. The affected muscles are hard in consistency, and wasting is comparatively slight owing to replacement with fibrous tissue.

4. LESIONS OF THE LOWER MOTOR NEURON

Lesions of the lower motor neuron are responsible for the majority of all cases of muscular atrophy encountered in clinical practice. The muscles are weak, flaccid, and wasted. Fibrillation is seen. Electromyography shows fibrillation potentials on mechanical stimulation by the exploring needle and spontaneous fibrillation and fasciculation potentials at rest. The tendon reflexes are depressed or abolished in the affected part unless, as in motor neuron disease, there is a coincident pyramidal lesion, in which case they usually remain brisk as long as there is any power of contraction left in the muscles concerned. It is convenient to classify the causes of this form of atrophy according to whether the lesion is in the spinal cord, the motor roots, or the peripheral nerves.

The Spinal Cord. Destruction of anterior horn cells may occur at the site of *fracture-dislocation* of the spine, or as a result of backward protrusion of an *intervertebral disk* in the cervical and thoracic regions. Primary and secondary *tumours* have a similar effect. In these instances, atrophy is confined to the muscles which are innervated by the affected portion of the cord, any paralysis which may appear below the level of the lesion being of an upper-motor neuron type, with spasticity and weakness but no atrophy. On the other hand, these same conditions cause atrophic paralysis below the level of the lesion when the cauda equina is affected. *Acute anterior poliomyelitis* is the most common cause of atrophy of spinal origin, and although the maximum incidence may be upon one or more contiguous segments of the cord, scattered paralyses elsewhere, and sparing of muscles within the zone most affected, lend a highly characteristic touch to the total picture (*Fig.* 541). *Syringomyelia, haematomyelia,* and *intramedullary tumour* give rise to atrophy of more or less segmental distribution, but sensory loss and the evidence of pressure upon the long tracts of the spinal cord serve to establish the diagnosis. *Motor neuron disease* is a common cause of atrophy in adult life; in the form of progressive muscular atrophy (Aran-Duchenne) the wasting usually starts in the upper limbs (*Fig.* 542), but the first sign may be on the trunk or in the legs; in amyotrophic lateral sclerosis atrophy in the upper limbs is associated with spastic weakness in the legs; in the bulbar form wasting is seen in the tongue (*Fig.* 543); sensation and the sphincters are normal. The rare *syphilitic amyotrophy* may mimic motor neuron disease, but the tendon reflexes are depressed and the Wassermann reaction is positive. The symmetrical atrophy of the distal portion of the leg which characterizes *peroneal muscular atrophy* (Charcot-Marie-Tooth, *Fig.* 544) is readily distinguished from all other forms of progressive

atrophy by its distribution, the disproportion between gross atrophy and slight weakness, the depression of the ankle-jerk, and slight sensory loss in the feet. Later the small hand muscles become involved (*Fig.* 545). Atrophic paralysis of one or more muscles occasionally occurs in *herpes zoster*; the rash, pain, and lymphocytosis in the spinal fluid in the acute phase confirm the diagnosis. Sudden paralysis of a muscle group in a limb may be caused by thrombosis of a branch of the anterior spinal artery. If the main vessel itself is occluded there is softening of the anterior half of the cord on both sides over one or two segments, causing a lower-motor

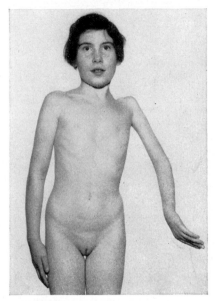

Fig. 541. Atrophy of the muscles of the left shoulder and upper arm, the result of former acute anterior poliomyelitis—infantile paralysis. (*Dr. R. G. Ollerenshaw, Manchester Royal Infirmary.*)

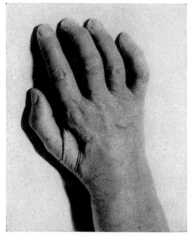

Fig. 542. The dorsum of the right hand, showing atrophy of all the interossei muscles, in a case of early progressive muscular atrophy. The wasting of the abductor indicis is particularly marked. The ring and little fingers are beginning to become contracted into 'main-en-griffe' attitude.

neuron paralysis at the level of the lesion and spastic weakness or paralysis below it—one form of transverse myelitis. Thrombosis of the vessel or its branches occurs in atheroma,

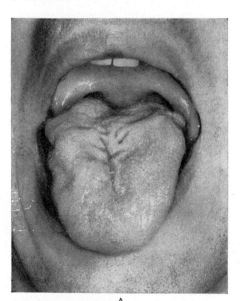

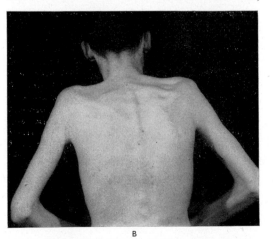

A   B

Fig. 543. Progressive muscular atrophy (motor neuron disease of bulbar type, showing (A) wasting of tongue and (B) muscles of shoulder-girdle. (*Dr. R. G. Ollerenshaw, Manchester Royal Infirmary.*)

meningovascular syphilis, and tumours of the cord.

The Spinal Roots. A lesion of a single root seldom causes much atrophy, since most muscles are supplied by several roots; an exception is the first thoracic root, which supplies the small muscles

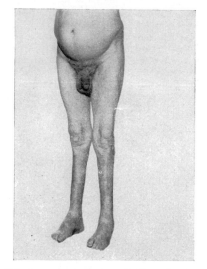

Fig. 544. Peroneal muscular atrophy illustrating characteristic distal wasting. (*Dr. M. J. McArdle.*)

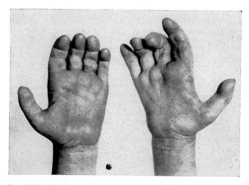

Fig. 545. Peroneal muscular atrophy illustrating wasting of small muscles of the hand. (*Dr. M. J. McArdle.*)

of the hand; the motor cranial nerves—the motor fifth, the facial, and the hypoglossal nerves—are the same in this respect. Spinal-root lesions are seen in *fracture-dislocation*, in *spondylolisthesis*, posterolateral herniation of the *intervertebral disks*, *osteo-arthritis* of the spine, *extramedullary tumours*, *meningeal fibrosis* after meningitis, *meningitis serosa circumscripta*, and *infective radiculitis*.

The Peripheral Nerves. Injuries, pressure lesions, and a large number of toxic and infective neuropathies commonly referred to as 'polyneuritis' constitute the three major subdivisions of this group.

Injuries from stab wounds, gunshot wounds, fractures, and dislocations in the vicinity of motor nerves, and from traction on the arm during delivery, form a large and diagnostically simple group. (*Fig. 546.*)

Pressure on motor nerves causes a 'pressure neuritis'; the radial nerve is easily compressed against the shaft of the humerus; the lower cord of the brachial plexus is liable to pressure and friction in the presence of a cervical rib; the ulnar nerve is liable to repeated injury if the groove in which it lies behind the elbow is unduly shallow, especially in association with cubitus valgus; the median nerve is sometimes compressed within its tunnel under the transverse carpal ligament; the lumbosacral cord may be compressed against the sacrum by the foetal head in difficult labour, with consequent paralysis and atrophy of the muscles below the knee; the external popliteal (common) nerve is exposed to pressure where it

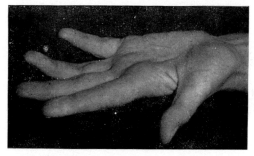

Fig. 546. The hand in a case of ulnar paralysis, showing the 'main-en-griffe' attitude of the little and ring fingers. (*Dr. R. A. Henson.*)

winds around the neck of the fibula. Pressure lesions of mixed motor and sensory nerves are remarkable for the fact that sensory loss is usually slight, whereas atrophy and paralysis are marked.

Peripheral neuritis and *polyneuritis* are omnibus terms for a wide variety of conditions, diverse as to aetiology and pathology but having a certain clinical similarity in that multiple nerves are affected and the signs are most marked peripherally. Thus atrophy and weakness are greater in the hand than in the arm, and in the foot than in the thigh. The disability may affect both the upper and lower limbs, or it may spread to the trunk and face, but whatever its extent it is usually more or less symmetrically disposed on the two sides of the body. Sensory loss is greatest at the periphery of the limbs, shading off proximally, but may spread to the trunk and face. It may be superficial, or both superficial and deep, or there may be no loss at all. Sphincter disturbances are uncommon. Tendon reflexes are reduced or absent in the affected limbs. These clinical features are found in varying combinations in different forms of polyneuritis, but to this basic pattern there are added special features, either in the history or in the results of physical examination, which enable us to establish the aetiology in some instances.

THE CAUSES OF PERIPHERAL NEURITIS OR POLY-NEURITIS

1. *Infections*: 'Infective' polyneuritis (Guillain-Barré) is quite common. It is febrile at the onset, with a rapidly advancing motor and sensory polyneuritis which may also involve the seventh cranial nerve, and is characterized by the presence in the spinal fluid of a normal cell-count but a high protein (e.g., from 70 to 300 mg. per c.mm.). It must be remembered, however, that the protein may be raised in any severe form of polyneuritis. Respiratory paralysis may cause death within a day or two of the onset. This form of polyneuritis constitutes one variety of Landry's paralysis (*see below*). *Diphtheritic polyneuritis* is due to the action of the diphtherial exotoxin on the peripheral nerves; when the infection is in the upper respiratory tract or fauces, palatal and ocular symptoms usually precede the weakness and sensory loss in the limbs by days or even weeks. Cutaneous diphtheria (due to diphtheritic infection of open wounds, veld sores, balanitis) is particularly liable to cause polyneuritis because of failure to recognize that the wound is infected by the Klebs-Loeffler bacillus; consequently antitoxin is not given until paralysis appears, by which time it is too late to arrest it. In cutaneous diphtheria sensory loss and paralysis appear first in the immediate vicinity of the lesion. In the past peripheral neuritis has been listed as a common complication of many *infections and specific fevers* such as typhoid, dysentery, etc., but surveys of large numbers of cases in the First World War by Walshe in the Middle East, and in the Second World War by Elliott in India, failed to confirm this belief. When polyneuritis is reported, it usually turns out to be due to vitamin-B deficiency. There have, however, been reports of wasting, weakness, loss of tendon reflexes, and deep hypalgesia, of symmetrical distribution, in severe generalized tuberculous adenitis. *Leprosy* is a true infective polyneuritis; its distribution is seldom symmetrical, and the diagnosis is made on the thickening of the nerve-trunks and the presence of the typical cutaneous lesions.

2. *Polyneuritis due to Drugs, Industrial Poisons, and Physical Agents*: The list of substances which are known to be capable of causing a toxic polyneuritis is extensive, but Public Health legislation has enforced prophylaxis to such good effect that these intoxications are becoming rare in civilized communities. The general features of this group are those of a polyneuritis—i.e., a symmetrical and atrophic palsy of the limbs, maximal peripherally, associated with loss of tendon reflexes and a variable degree of sensory change. The pathology is that of a degenerative process of the nerves rather than an inflammatory condition: toxic polyneuropathy would be a more accurate designation, but the term polyneuritis has the sanction of tradition. The most important agents are: *alcohol, antimony, arsenic, benzene* and its derivatives, *carbon monoxide* and *carbon tetrachloride, emetine, lead, mercury, petrol containing tetra-ethyl lead, phosphorus, sulphonal, sulphonamides, thallium, trilene, trional,* and *triorthocresyl phosphate* and '*apiol*'. Diagnosis depends primarily on establishing that there has been exposure to the noxious agent. (*Fig. 547.*)

3. *Polyneuritis due to Metabolic Factors: Diabetic polyneuritis* is often latent—wasting and tenderness of the calf muscles, and absence of the ankle-jerks being found in the absence of symptoms. In more severe cases there is pain, weakness,

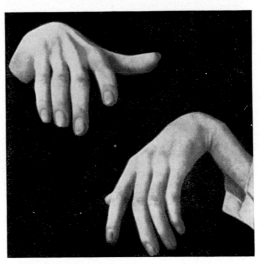

Fig. 547. Wrist-drop after diphtheria, similar to that of plumbism.

wasting, peripheral sensory loss, and absence of the tendon reflexes. These symptoms and signs are usually confined to the lower limbs, and the combination of 'shooting' pains, absent reflexes, and ataxia due to loss of postural sensibility may lead to an erroneous diagnosis of tabes. Rarely, acute severe diabetes is responsible for a more severe polyneuritis, with atrophy, weakness, reflex changes, and sensory loss in all four limbs.

Polyneuritis in acute porphyria is a rare condition in which there are one or more attacks characterized by gastro-intestinal colic, the passage of urine containing porphyrins, which becomes burgundy coloured on exposure to light, and severe polyneuritis which is often fatal owing to respiratory paralysis. It occurs both idiopathically and as a result of poisoning by drugs, especially barbiturates. This condition must not be confused with congenital porphyrinuria, in which polyneuritis does not occur but which may be associated with hydroa vacciniforme. In *congenital alkaptonuria* the urine turns black after it has been passed; it is associated with ochronosis but is not a cause of polyneuritis.

4. *Polyneuritis in Deficiency Diseases*: In beriberi, due to deficiency of vitamin B_1, there is weakness and wasting of peripheral distribution, with loss of tendon reflexes and a variable, but usually slight, degree of peripheral sensory loss. It may

be associated with nutritional oedema and—in acute forms—cardiac dilatation and weakness. Muscular wasting and weakness are greater in the legs than in the upper limbs, and the high-steppage gait associated with foot-drop from any cause is usually seen in severe cases. A related condition, known as the *captivity syndrome* because of its appearance amongst prisoners of war who have been starved for prolonged periods, is characterized by polyneuritis, proprioceptive sensory loss from degeneration of the posterior columns of the spinal cord, and loss of central vision due to a retrobulbar neuritis. A painful glossitis and cheilitis, due to vitamin-B_2 deficiency, is a common concomitant of both beriberi and the captivity syndrome. *Subacute combined degeneration of the cord* presents a combination of pyramidal, posterior column, and peripheral neuritic features in variable combination, associated with pernicious anaemia, a histamine-fast achlorhydria, and absence of Castle's intrinsic factor in the stomach. Rarely, cases occur without either pernicious anaemia or achlorhydria, but which respond promptly to treatment with vitamin B_{12}. Polyneuritis is manifested by tingling in the hands and feet, pain, cramps, moderate atrophy and flaccid weakness, peripheral sensory loss, and ultimate loss of the tendon reflexes. This picture is often obscured by the early appearance of pyramidal signs—spasticity, increased reflexes, and extensor plantar responses, and by ataxia due to degeneration of the posterior columns which convey postural sensibility. Loss of central vision due to a retrobulbar neuritis is a rare finding; it may precede the anaemia and the other neurological symptoms. *Pellagra*, due to vitamin-B_2 deficiency, is characterized by a painful glossitis, flatulent dyspepsia, skin lesions which are symmetrically disposed in the parts of the body exposed to sunlight and friction, mental symptoms varying between simple depression and irritability to a frank organic psychosis, and a neurological picture similar to subacute combined degeneration of the cord—a polyneuritis combined with the features of pyramidal and posterior column degeneration.

The *polyneuritis of pregnancy*, often regarded as of metabolic origin, is probably due to deficiency of the vitamin B complex, for it is seen in the later months, when the body requirements for vitamin B are said to be increased sixfold, and it is especially frequent in pregnancy complicated by hyperemesis gravidarum. The occasional occurrence of retrobulbar neuritis in pregnancy is obviously of interest in this connexion, occurring as it does in other conditions of vitamin-B deficiency. *Visceral carcinoma* is occasionally responsible for a polyneuritis with atrophic weakness, peripheral sensory loss, and reduced and absent reflexes. Cases are also described in which deep sensory loss was present in both the limbs and trunk, without specific weakness or wasting, associated with a small carcinoma of the stomach; post-mortem examination showed degeneration of sensory ganglia and peripheral

sensory nerves without any significant degree of degeneration in the motor fibres. Polyneuritis may also occur in Hodgkin's disease.

5. *Hyperpyrexia*: Polyneuritis is a rare sequel of hyperpyrexia.

6. *Miscellaneous Causes of Polyneuritis*: There remains a small heterogeneous group of diseases, the causation of which is obscure.

Uveoparotic polyneuritis is a rare manifestation of sarcoidosis. As a rule the onset is marked by a short febrile illness, followed by bilateral nonsuppurative parotitis, iritis, cyclitis, and a polyneuritis involving the facial nerves, less often the other cranial nerves, and occasionally the peripheral nerves with weakness, atrophy, and loss of tendon reflexes. A rash resembling erythema nodosum sometimes occurs. The course of the disease is prolonged, extending over many months, and there is a marked tendency to relapses, but recovery usually occurs.

Chronic polyneuritis of unknown origin has been described, with marked wasting, weakness, and loss of tendon reflexes, but without sensory loss; it lasts for months, or even years; recovery is usual, but death sometimes occurs, and postmortems have revealed chromatolysis of anterior horn cells and degeneration of the efferent motor fibres. A similar 'motor' polyneuritis has been seen as a recurrent condition, three or more attacks being experienced during the first twenty years of life.

Pink disease (syn. acrodynia, erythroedema), an acute affection of infants, seems to have been due to mercury administered in teething powders or ointments and since the withdrawal of these products and calomel from the market pink disease has disappeared. *Familial hypertrophic polyneuritis* is a rare heredo-familial disease in which there is hypertrophy of the sheath of Schwann, increase of interstitial tissue, degeneration of the nerve-fibres, and degenerative changes in the posterior column. There is a slowly progressive atrophic palsy and sensory loss, both peripheral in distribution, and both occurring in the lower limbs long before the upper limbs are affected. Proprioceptive sensory loss leads to an ataxia. There is a pathognomonic thickening of the peripheral nerves, which are easily felt under the skin. *Polyneuritis cranialis* is a rare condition of adult life characterized by palsies of cranial nerves, coming on consecutively and usually over one side only, and unassociated with gross disease of the meninges or the bones of the skull. The onset is acute and full recovery is uncommon. *Polyarteritis nodosa*, a disease characterized by inflammation and thrombosis of the smaller arteries, includes polyneuritis amongst its protean manifestation. Superimposed upon a background of remittent pyrexia, wasting, leucocytosis, and eosinophilia, are symptoms referable to tissues or organs which are involved, singly or together, by the arterial lesions. Palsies of one or more peripheral nerves are more common than a general polyneuritis, but the latter does occur. Atrophy, weakness, loss of tendon reflexes, and peripheral sensory loss appropriate to the nerve or nerves involved, are seen. Muscular atrophy is intensified by the presence of arterial lesions in the muscles themselves.

Finally, reference must be made to the vexed question of *Landry's acute ascending paralysis.* Landry originally described a condition in which paralysis spread rapidly from the legs to the trunk, arms, and bulbar nuclei, without sphincter disturbances and with very slight sensory loss in the hands and feet, ending fatally from respiratory paralysis and showing no pathological changes at post mortem. This last point is of little importance inasmuch as the histological techniques available in 1859 were limited. It is uncertain whether Landry's paralysis is a disease or a syndrome; acute febrile polyneuritis (Guillain-Barré type), polyneuritis due to known toxins, and the polyneuritis of acute porphyria may present similar features. If we exclude the very slight sensory changes described by Landry, an acute ascending paralysis is seen in *poliomyelitis, paralytic rabies, poisoning from the bite of the wood tick (Fig. 548), and potassium intoxication.* The last-named is a rare condition, but it is important in that early recognition and prompt treatment

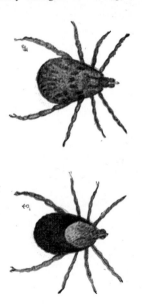

Fig. 548. *Dermacentor venustus* (wood tick), male (top) and female. (×4.) (*Surgeon-General Sir W. P. MacArthur.*)

may save life. When the blood-potassium is unduly high, as in some cases of chronic nephritis, neuromuscular transmission of impulses is impeded and paralysis of the legs rapidly develops; the arms and bulbar muscles may also be affected. The blood-pressure falls and the electrocardiogram shows an abnormally high T wave in all leads. The condition rapidly responds to intravenous saline. A similar clinical condition has been seen when the potassium is very low, as a result of a

too enthusiastic administration of desoxycorticosterone in Addison's disease, in primary aldosteronism, and in chronic nephritis with potassium depletion, but in these cases the electrocardiogram has a low T wave and may show atrio-ventricular block; the paralysis passes off after the administration of large doses of potassium chloride. Sudden death may occur in both high-and low-potassium forms of this condition.

5. DISEASE OF MUSCLES

Diseases of muscles are an infrequent cause of muscular atrophy. *Congenital absence* of a muscle or portion of muscle should not lead to confusion. The sternocostal portion of the pectoralis major is most often involved, but absence of the trapezius, quadriceps, serratus magnus, semi-membranosus, sternomastoids, deltoid, rhomboids, or biceps is sometimes noted. Other skeletal abnormalities are often found in such cases. *Rupture of a muscle* or its tendon leads to atrophy. *Inflammatory diseases* — suppurative myositis, trichiniasis, cysticercosis—do not lead to significant atrophy. *Dermatomyositis* causes fibrosis of muscles, with moderate atrophy and gross incapacity from fibrosis and consequent contracture. More common than the foregoing are the *heredofamilial myopathies* (syn. muscular dystrophies). Males are more often affected than females and the onset is usually in childhood. The essential clinical feature of all types is progressive and symmetrical wasting and weakness of the muscles of the limb girdles and the proximal segments of the limbs, early depression or loss of tendon reflexes, absence of fibrillation, and normal sensation. There may be characteristic electromyographic changes. In the pseudohypertrophic form, which is confined to males, wasting of some muscles is accompanied by enlargement of others, especially the glutei, the calves, spinati, and deltoids, but even the hypertrophied muscles are weak (*Fig.* 549). In the facio-scapulo-humeral and scapulo-humeral types, the disease appears just before puberty, or even in early adult life, and progress is slower. The distribution of wasting is much the same as in the pseudohypertrophic variety, but hypertrophy does not occur.

Amyotonia congenita (Oppenheim's disease) is a familial condition characterized pathologically by abnormalities in both the muscles and in the anterior horn cells, and clinically by profound muscular weakness and atonia with absence of tendon-reflexes. A universal atonia is noticed soon after birth, but atrophy is obscured by the normal subcutaneous fat and does not become obvious until the child grows up. The disease is rare, and many of the cases die in infancy.

Dystrophia myotonica is a heredofamilial disease which appears in the third or fourth decade and is characterized by wasting of the distal muscles of the limbs, of the sternomastoids, and of the facial muscles, together with delayed relaxation of voluntary muscles, and the appearance of premature baldness, cataract, mental deterioration, and testicular atrophy in the patient and in other members of the family. Percussion of the affected muscles gives rise to a persistent local spasm, visible and palpable as a distinct lump. The myotonia is not necessarily confined to the muscles which are atrophied, and it varies in intensity from day to day. Atrophy is occasionally found in long-standing cases of *myasthenia gravis*; the characteristic fatigability of the

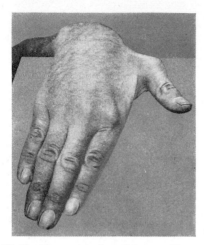

Fig. 549. Hand from a case of pseudohypertrophic muscular paralysis, showing the marked wasting of the abductor indicis.

muscles and the response to prostigmin afford a reliable guide to diagnosis. In thyrotoxicosis there is a generalized loss of weight with some wasting of muscles, but *thyrotoxic myopathy* is a different matter. Weakness and wasting of the pelvic and shoulder girdles develop, with impairment or loss of the related tendon-reflexes, in association with a mild degree of thyrotoxicosis. It is important to identify this condition because partial thyroidectomy is curative if it is carried out in the early stages of the condition. The resemblance to a non-familial muscular dystrophy can be very close in chronic cases.

Ian Mackenzie.

NAILS, AFFECTIONS OF

The nails become involved in many cutaneous affections, commonly dermatitis, psoriasis, epidermolysis bullosa, pemphigus, exfoliative dermatitis, and rarely in lichen planus, Darier's disease, and alopecia areata. In *dermatitis* (*Fig.* 558), when the terminal phalanges of the fingers are affected, there is roughening and ridging of the nail plate, and successive exacerbations of the disease may be recorded by the indentations of the plate so formed. There may also be pitting coarser than that seen in psoriasis (*Figs.* 551–553). In *ringworm of the nails* (*Fig.* 550) caused by *T. mentagrophytes* (*gypseum*) or *T. rubrum* (*purpureum*) one or more of the nails may be involved. The disease affects the plate itself, which first loses its

lustre, then becomes discoloured, and finally friable. Often there is heaping up of tissue under the plate. The diagnosis may be confirmed by finding the causal fungus in scrapings of nail material. It is sometimes difficult to differentiate this condition from psoriasis of the nails, especially when, as not infrequently occurs, the nails only are involved. In *psoriasis* one of the most constant features is pitting of the nails (*Fig.* 551), which may take place before any other sign of the disease appears. Other nail changes in psoriasis are discoloration (*Fig.* 552) and onycholysis (*Fig.* 553) or separation

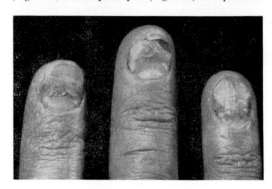

Fig. 550. Ringworm of the nails. (*Dr. Peter Hansell.*)

of the nail from its bed; these may be accompanied by or followed by the formation of a granular mass under the nail; in the final stage the nail becomes 'worm-eaten', cracked and split, friable, and disintegrated. It is worth bearing in mind that psoriasis of the nails is much more common than ringworm of the nails. In chronic paronychia (*Fig.* 554), which is due to combined monilial and bacterial infection, pockets form under the posterior nail folds, which will admit the top of a probe up to an eighth of an inch. Very occasionally pus may be expressed from these pockets, from which cultures of the yeast may be made. In profile the raised nail folds over the pockets have a characteristic bolster-like appearance. The changes in the nail plate are secondary. This disease occurs in those who are obliged to keep their hands wet for long periods, notably housewives, charwomen, barmen, and fishmongers. It is much commoner in women than in men.

In *epidermolysis bullosa* the repeated blister formation at the finger-ends causes atrophy of the skin and loss of nails. The naked-eye appearances of the nail change may indicate the diagnosis at once, or lesions elsewhere may help one in forming an opinion. In *pachyonychia congenita* the nail plates are thick, hard, and firmly attached to the nail beds. It may be associated with follicular, keratotic grey-coloured papules on the extensor surfaces. Blistering and maceration with secondary infection may take place around and between the toes and leucokeratosis of the tongue may be present. In congenital ectodermal defect the nails may be absent; more often they are short and fail to reach the free edge of the digit.

Trophic changes in the nails are not at all uncommon, and while they sometimes occur in general illness more often they are of unknown aetiology. Transverse furrows (*Beau's lines*) usually follow acute illnesses. They are formed at the time of the illness but will not appear on

Longitudinal ridging more often has no apparent cause. Brittleness (*onychorrhexis*) or softness of the nails with splitting or terracing of the free edge is more common in women than in men. The cause is unknown but repeated wetting and drying may be a factor of importance. It has been thought to be aggravated by the use of nail varnish and varnish removers, but many cases occur in women who do not use nail polish.

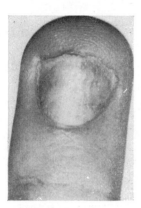

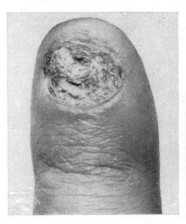

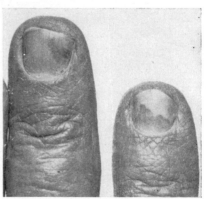

Fig. 551. Nail psoriasis: pitting. (*Dr. Peter Hansell.*)

Fig. 552. Nail psoriasis: discoloration, distortion, and thickening of nail plate. (*Dr. Peter Hansell.*)

Fig. 553. Nail psoriasis: onycholysis. (*Dr. Peter Hansell.*)

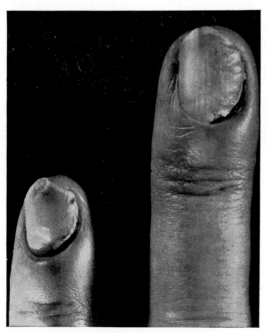

Fig. 554. Monilia of the nail fold.

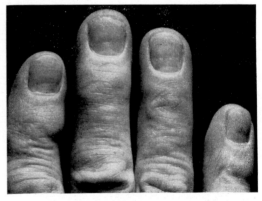

Fig. 555. Nails: Beau's lines. (*Dr. Peter Hansell.*)

Spoon nails (*koilonychia*) occur in anaemia due to iron deficiency and are part of the Plummer-Vinson syndrome. In hypo-albuminaemia the appearance of paired narrow white bands running transversely across the nail plate has been described. The nails may appear white in some cases of hepatic cirrhosis; all degrees of whiteness may be found in chronic congestive heart failure, pulmonary tuberculosis, diabetes, rheumatoid arthritis, and some forms of carcinoma. Red half-moons are seen in some cases of cardiac failure. Hypertrophy of the nails (*onychauxis*) occurs more often on the toes and may lead to onychogryphosis.

the nail plate for about 6–8 weeks and then move steadily forward with the growth of the nail, finally being lost at 5–6 months (*Figs.* 555, 556).

Leuconychia totalis (*Fig.* 557) is a rare congenital anomaly in which the whole nail plate is white. Leuconychia striata and punctata (white lines or dots) are much more common but are of no significance. In leuconychia the changes are in the nail plate itself. Whitening from other causes is due to changes in the nail bed.

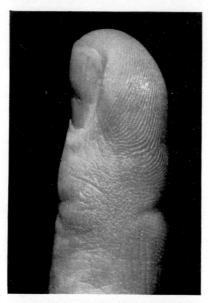

Fig. 556. Nail: Beau's line, side view.
(*Dr. Peter Hansell.*)

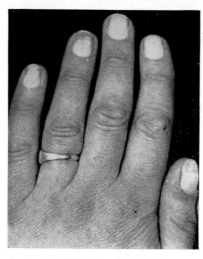

Fig. 557. Leuconychia totalis.
(*St. John's Hospital.*)

The nails may be shed in many acute skin diseases that involve the fingers, notably in exfoliative dermatitis, and this also occurs occasionally in severe secondary syphilis. In X-ray burns affecting the fingers the nails may be destroyed.

Onychia, or inflammation of the nail, is usually septic in origin, but it may be the result of trauma or contact with irritants at work; rarely it is syphilitic or tuberculous in origin. It usually terminates in shedding of the affected nail. *Paraonychia*, or whitlow, is usually obvious, but a primary chancre of the finger may sometimes imitate it.

Trauma is responsible for many nail deformities. Single injuries produce haematomata which may lead to temporary nail loss or to permanent splits if the nail matrix is injured. Repeated minor traumata may be inflicted in several ways. Probably the commonest is nail biting where the usual deformity produced is a short ragged nail and is often complicated by the appearance of peri-ungual warts (*Fig.* 559). Hang nails are spicules of hard material from the edges of the nail folds and are often due to nail biting and may give rise to minor local sepsis. Excess manicuring, especially pushing back the cuticle, may lead to cross ridging of some nails and a similar appearance is produced by a habit tic of playing with the nails (*Fig.* 560). Ill-fitting footwear is responsible for ingrowing toe-nails and probably for most cases of onychogryphosis; it may also lead to repeated shedding of selected nails, usually the great toe nails.

Impaired peripheral circulation is also responsible for numerous cases of nail dystrophy. The most characteristic is due to symptoms of Raynaud's phenomenon of many years' duration and consists of thin nails, ridged longitudinally and in places showing partial onycholysis. There are

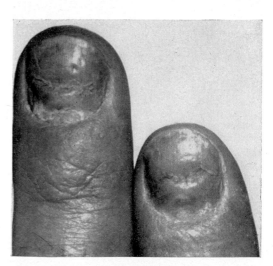

Fig. 558. Nails in dermatitis: coarse pitting and cross ridging. (*Dr. Peter Hansell.*)

variations in colour on the nail surfaces, some areas being redder than normal and others paler. The thin ridged nail is brittle and is therefore usually kept cut short by the patient (*Fig.* 561).

In the *yellow nail syndrome* all nails take on a pale yellow or greenish-yellow colour. The nails grow very slowly. The cuticles are deficient and the nail plate is overcurved in its long axis. The nails may come loose from their beds and be shed but are slowly replaced. The condition is often accompanied by lymphoedema and various chest abnormalities may be present including

and which often starts with pitting of the nail plate. Nearly always there are signs of psoriasis elsewhere on the body. Secondary changes in the nail plate, the result of inflammation of the nail fold, such as that caused by monilia (*Fig.* 554, p. 559), or of inflammation around the nail fold

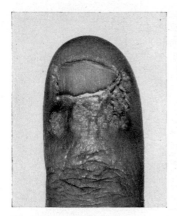 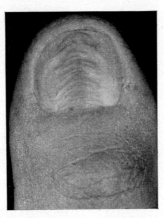 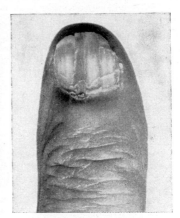

Fig. 559. Nail biting and peri-ungual warts. (*Dr. Peter Hansell.*)

Fig. 560. Traumatic nail dystrophy: habit tic of playing with the nail. (*St. John's Hospital.*)

Fig. 561. Nail dystrophy due to impaired peripheral circulation: Raynaud's disease. (*Dr. Peter Hansell.*)

chronic bronchitis, bronchiectasis, or pleural effusion.

Haemorrhages below the nail are common. They may be the result of trauma or disease and may be petechial (splinter) or more extensive. Haemorrhages are common in fungus infections of the nail plate, psoriasis, and dermatitis. Splinter haemorrhages are terminal arterial emboli in the nail bed and consist of a homogeneous mass of blood embedded in a layer of squamous cells adherent to the undersurface of the nail bed. They occur in trichinosis (in 60–70 per cent of cases), subacute bacterial endocarditis, a few cases of uninfected mitral stenosis, and rarely in peptic ulcer, hypertension, and malignant neoplasms. They may, however, occur with jarring trauma as in hockey players, and at times for no apparent cause in healthy persons.

P. D. Samman.

NAILS, FUNGOUS AFFECTIONS OF

Ringworm of the nails (*see also Fig.* 550, p. 558) is common. It may affect any or all of the nails, and may be confined to the nails alone or may be associated on the feet with interdigital ringworm of the toes.

At first there is a greyness and dullness of the nail plate, which soon becomes spongy or brittle. Later, disintegration of nail tissue occurs. In the friable diseased nail substance the fungus, either *Trychophyton mentagrophytes* or *T. rubrum*, can usually be found. Clinically the condition is most difficult to distinguish from psoriasis of the nail (*Fig.* 551–553, p. 559), which is more common

as in dermatitis, are of the nature of ridging and there is no friability of nail tissue (*Fig.* 558, p. 560).

P. D. Samman.

NAPKIN-REGION ERUPTIONS

In infants the commonest napkin-area eruption is *Jacquet's erythema*. It occurs in the following forms: (1) erythematous, (2) erythematovesicular, (3) papular, and (4) ulcerating. These may develop consecutively or coincidently. The commonest are the erythematous and the papular. It is caused by the irritation set up by moist or soiled napkins, sometimes by the ammonia from decomposed urine, and in this connexion it must be remembered that certain soaps and washing powders left in the napkins may act as skin irritants. The chief sites of the eruption are the buttocks, and scrotum or vulva. In the simple erythema the rash may be limited to the genitalia, the inner sides of the thighs, and the perineum, but it may spread to the lumbar region, the lower abdomen, and down the legs. In the erythemato-vesicular form there appear on the affected areas small bright-red erosions which may become confluent; these erosions are the result of ruptured vesicles, of which a few may be found at the edge of the reddened area. Occasionally papules appear, giving rise to the so-called erythemato-papular type of the disease. In the fourth form of the eruption the erosions ulcerate.

A scaly erythema of the napkin area may be due to infection with *monilia*. Small, thin-walled pustules are usually present at the edges of the lesion. Occasionally the skin lesions of *congenital syphilis*, which approximate to those of the secondary stage of the disease in adults, are confined to the napkin area. Moist condylomata around the anus and vulva are not uncommon in this disease. Other signs of syphilis are usually with a small triangular area of papules on the lower part of each buttock, is absolutely diagnostic of the disease. In *psoriasis* (*Fig.* 562) the eruption is sometimes severe in this area, while on the usual sites—the knees and elbows—the lesions may be quite insignificant. *Intertrigo*

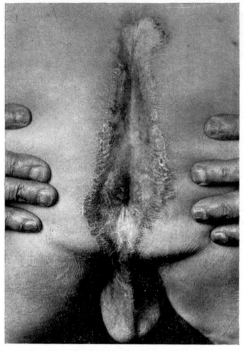

Fig. 562. Psoriasis of the gluteal fold and nails. No other parts were involved and until the nails were examined the diagnosis was obscure. (*Dr. Peter Hansell.*)

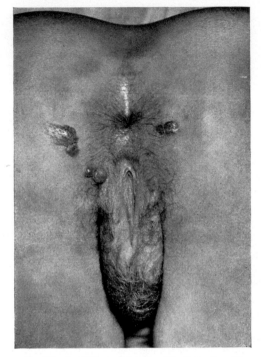

Fig. 563. Syphilitic condylomata. (*Dr. Peter Hansell.*)

present, so that diagnosis should be simple. In *bullous impetigo of the newborn*, badly named 'pemphigus neonatorum', the lesions may be restricted to the buttocks and thighs, but more usually other areas are involved. The disease is due either to a streptococcus or to a staphylococcus and is the infantile form of impetigo contagiosum of older children and adults. Atopic eczema may involve the napkin area as well as other areas. Psoriasis occasionally involves the napkin area in infancy.

In adults the same region may be involved in a number of affections. In *tinea cruris* (ringworm of the groin or dhobie itch) and *erythrasma* the eruption is confined to this region; the differential diagnosis of these affections is given under RINGWORM (p. 726). In *pediculosis pubis* (crab-louse or crabs) the pubic hair alone is usually affected, but the parasite may wander to the hair on any part of the body, including the beard, the eyelashes, and eyebrows, though never the scalp. The diagnosis of this condition is generally obvious. In scabies, when the lesions on the hands and wrists are slight, a solitary papule on the penis (glans or shaft), together commonly affects the folds between the buttocks and between the thighs. Other conditions occurring in this area are *pruritus ani* and *vulvae* (p. 660). In *syphilis* the commonest site for the moist papule is around the anus and genitalia (*Fig.* 563).

P. D. Samman.

NASAL DISCHARGE

A discharge from the nose may be unilateral or bilateral and consist of clear watery fluid, of clear mucoid fluid, of varying degrees of tenacity, or purulent, or again mucopurulent. It may be evil-smelling or free from odour or it may be blood-stained. Frank bleeding from the nose or epistaxis is dealt with under another section (*see* p. 256).

Clear Watery Nasal Discharge. *Cerebrospinal rhinorrhoea* may occur following fractures of the base of the skull in the anterior fossae, as a complication of transphenoidal hypophysectomy or, very rarely, in the case of a ruptured *meningocele* in this region. In order to confirm the presence of C.S.F. the patient is positioned with the head tilted slightly forwards. Clear fluid, in every way resembling water, drips from the nose and is collected in a test-tube. The presence of sugar in this fluid confirms that it is C.S.F.

Clear Mucoid Nasal Discharge. Copious clear mucoid nasal discharge almost as freely flowing as water is present in *nasal allergy* and may be accompanied by excoriation of the skin of the nasal vestibule and upper lip. A relatively physiologically inert foreign body such as a glass bead or small stone may be present for weeks or even months before symptoms become apparent. Conversely cotton-wool, paper, or such substances as rubber will set up symptoms within hours.

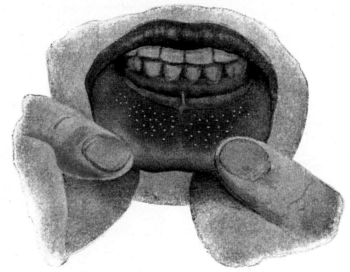

Fig. 564. Koplik's spots.

associated with violent attacks of sneezing, lacrimation, and conjunctival injection. The diagnosis is confirmed by the history and by skin sensitivity tests. Nasal allergy is liable to be confused with *non-specific vasomotor rhinitis*, which is very common. Numerous factors are present in the aetiology of this troublesome condition and these include changes of environmental temperature and humidity, mechanical irritation from dusts and vapours, psychological factors, pregnancy, and drug reactions. Ophthalmic symptoms do not occur as in some cases of nasal allergy but the rhinorrhoea may persist for hours or days on end and the patient with vasomotor instability not infrequently carries a box of paper tissues under the arm or in the handbag. The diagnosis is reached after excluding nasal allergy.

Slightly more 'mucoid' but still perfectly clear nasal discharge occurs in the coryzal phase of the *common cold*, *influenza*, and the *acute exanthemata*. The coryza of measles is likely to be profuse and associated with conjunctival injection and sometimes with Koplik's spots (*Fig.* 564), which may be present for as long as two days before the skin eruption appears. The white spots are the size of a pin's head on the inner aspect of the cheeks and lips, and on the gums.

Purulent Nasal Discharge. A unilateral offensive nasal discharge in a child is almost pathognomonic of a *nasal foreign body*, and is often

Chronic sinus infection produces a unilateral or bilateral mucopurulent discharge which is unlikely to be offensive except in some cases which occur as a result of dental infection. The paranasal sinuses most likely to be infected are the maxillary antra, and, on examination, discharge is seen in the floor and middle meatus of the nasal cavity and also in the corresponding side of the nasopharynx. The diagnosis is sometimes aided by sinus radiography which demonstrates opacity or fluid levels in the sinuses, but sinus X-rays are frequently misinterpreted and absolute confirmation of infection can only be made by antral proof—puncture and lavage (*Fig.* 565).

In childhood sinus infection is predisposed to by *enlarged adenoids* and not infrequently follows measles. Some children, through *neglect of hygiene* and proper attention, are never instructed in nose-blowing and tend to have a perpetual mucoid nasal discharge, at times purulent.

Rhinitis caseosa is an uncommon condition associated with the formation of offensive cheesy material in the nose and a purulent nasal discharge. Microscopical examination of the caseous debris shows numerous organisms and sometimes cholesterin crystals.

Bloodstained Nasal Discharge. *Malignant growths* of the nasal cavities, the paranasal air-sinuses, and the nasopharynx cause a bloodstained nasal discharge. A friable mass in the nasal cavity or an ulcer in the nasopharynx is the usual finding and the diagnosis is confirmed histologically. *Rodent ulcer* may occur in the nasal vestibule. *Non-healing granuloma* of the Wegener or Stewart type is almost invariably associated with a blood-stained nasal discharge and neoplasm must be carefully excluded by biopsy.

In *diphtheritic rhinitis* there is liable to be excoriation of the skin of the nasal vestibules,

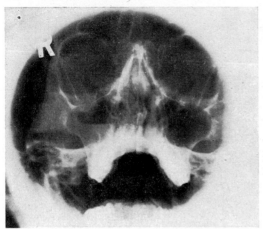

Fig. 565. Radiograph showing fluid-level in the right maxillary antrum and reported as 'sinus infection'. Sinus radiography is very misleading and in this case clear sterile fluid in the antrum had resulted from an allergic attack.

the nasal mucosa is congested, and a greyish adherent membrane may be present. Bacteriological examination of nasal swabs and scrapings is confirmatory.

Lupus of the nose is uncommon, but may cause slight bloodstaining and foetor, the early lesion being a reddish firm nodule at the mucocutaneous junction of the columellar skin and the nasal septum. Biopsy will show the typical histological picture. Other infections associated with a bloodstained discharge are *membranous rhinitis* which can occur as a result of pneumococcal and streptococcal infections, *gumma* of the nasal septum, *atrophic rhinitis* with crusting, and *leprosy*. Very rarely yaws (framboesia) is seen in the nose and resembles syphilis as an ulcerative lesion of the nasal septum causing ulceration and finally extensive destruction.

Of the diseases caused by pathogenic fungi and yeasts which infect the nose *rhinosporidiosis* is probably the most common and usually affects males in Ceylon and India. The characteristic lesion is a friable bleeding polypus which contains the spores of *Rhinosporidium seeberi*. Allied but less common conditions which may be responsible for a bloodstained discharge are *rhynophycomycosis, mucormycosis, aspergillosis*, and *actinomycosis*. Finally, may be mentioned the loathsome condition of *myiasis* which is not uncommon in some tropical countries, particularly India. The nasal cavities are infested by the larvae of certain flies and in advanced cases

cartilage and bone are destroyed and the paranasal sinuses may become filled with crawling maggots.

Miles Foxen.

NASAL OBSTRUCTION

All the conditions mentioned in the section on nasal discharge are likely to cause nasal obstruction owing to the associated inflammation and oedema of the mucous membrane. There are, however, some disorders which simply cause a blockage of one or both nasal passages and are less commonly associated with discharge. These are as follows.

Deflection of the nasal septum is probably the most common condition causing nasal obstruction and may arise from a variety of causes. It may be familial or originate as a result of pressure

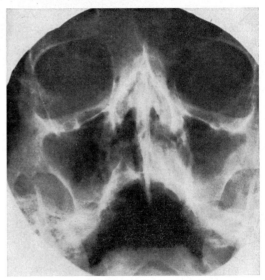

Fig. 566. Thickened lining mucosa in the maxillary antra in a case of vasomotor rhinitis. (*Dr. Lorna Davison.*)

during parturition, but more commonly it follows trauma incurred in early childhood or in sporting activities, personal assault, or accident. The obstruction may be unilateral or affect both nasal passages and over the course of years may gradually worsen. Commonly, the obstruction is found to be due to more than one factor, e.g., a deflected nasal septum associated with hypertrophy of the turbinates.

The diagnosis of deflected nasal septum is made without difficulty using a nasal speculum and head-mirror or lamp, but it must be remembered that other pathology may be obscured by the obstruction.

Vasomotor rhinitis (*Fig.* 566) has been mentioned in the section dealing with nasal discharge, but it commonly occurs without discharge, causing the so-called 'stuffy-nose'. Not infrequently patients notice that at one time one nasal passage is more obstructed and within hours the problem is worse on the other side. This alternating obstruction is merely the result of the normal nasal cycle which passes unnoticed in those with clear noses but becomes obvious in the partially obstructed. On examination, the inferior turbinates may be enormous and in chronic cases present a morulated appearance. They vary in colour from very pale to bright red and some of the worst cases occur in those addicted to vasoconstrictor drops and sprays—*vasomotor rhinitis medicamentosa.*

Nasal polypi are commonly associated with asthma or nasal allergy though the allergic diathesis is not always present. They are smooth insensitive swellings, often oyster-coloured, and usually originate in the middle nasal meatus though in advanced cases the entire nasal cavity becomes filled with them, precluding adequate

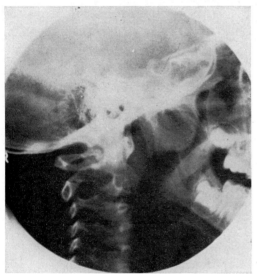

Fig. 567. Enlarged adenoids. (*Dr. Lorna Davison.*)

views of the septum and turbinates and causing total nasal obstruction—and, often, anosmia. An unusual variety is the *antrochoanal polypus* which passes posteriorly from the antrum and may be seen hanging in the nasopharynx. It poses a diagnostic trap for although the patient may complain of very severe nasal obstruction anterior rhinoscopy sometimes reveals no abnormality and the polyp is only seen with the post-nasal mirror.

Haematoma of the septum occasionally follows trauma and causes severe obstruction. It is seen as a fluctuant tense reddish swelling of the septum filling both sides of the nose. If the haematoma is left untreated an *abscess of the septum* may form and this is associated with acute tenderness and redness of the nose, and with pyrexia.

In newborn infants *bilateral imperforate choanae* will cause choking and asphyxia when they attempt to suck. The diagnosis, which is a matter of urgency, is confirmed by the failure to pass soft rubber catheters from nose to nasopharynx and by radiography using opaque media.

In young children *adenoidal enlargement (Fig. 567)* is always to be suspected when nasal obstruction is present. It is, of course, associated with mouth-breathing and snoring, but some care is needed in establishing the fact that the child's nasal airways are genuinely obstructed and that it is not mouth-breathing through habit. A lateral radiograph of the nasopharynx is of some value in this respect but a careful clinical examination, and if necessary examination under an anaesthetic, may be required.

Miles Foxen.

NAUSEA

Nausea is so frequently the precursor of vomiting that the combination term 'nausea and vomiting' is almost automatically employed as if it were invariable. But there are instances of vomiting without accompaniment of nausea and many of nausea that is not followed by vomiting, so that it deserves some discussion as an isolated symptom.

There must be very few who have not at some time experienced nausea which may be described by the familiar expression 'feeling sick' with the certainty that everybody will understand what is meant. An ill-defined sensation is felt at the back of the throat and in the pit of the stomach. Vasomotor disturbances are frequent accompaniments—dizziness, headache, sweating, as well as a feeling of weakness and of malaise.

It seems that the stimulus causing nausea is the same as that causing visceral pain but of lower intensity. The stomach is in a state of hypotonus, hypo-secretion, hypomotility, absence of peristalsis, and, as a consequence, there is stasis of contents. In general, nausea is combated by things that engender appetite and induced by those that destroy appetite. Acute peripheral pain, certain emotions, and suggestion by hypnosis are similarly effective. X-ray examination during an episode of nausea has shown that the lower border of the stomach descends two or three inches (evidently as the result of sudden relaxation of the abdominal muscles) so stretching the oesophagus and gastric walls and thus exerting tension on nerve-endings. The tension may be relieved by the passage of a peristaltic wave, and sufferers are accustomed to swallow repeatedly, a process that may re-establish normal peristaltic rhythm and terminate the backflow of gastric contents—so-called 'reverse peristalsis'.

Reference to vomiting (p. 829) will obviate enumeration of the majority of causes of nausea. Conditions in which nausea without vomiting is not infrequent are: jaundice, cholecystitis, chronic gastritis, carcinoma of the stomach (in which it may be the sole symptom), the early stages of cardiac failure, of pulmonary tuberculosis and of chronic renal disease; and pregnancy (especially in the early morning), labyrinthine disease, and anxiety. Some of these are explainable as the result of the stomach losing its normal functional efficiency through sharing the general consequences of illness. In others, the stomach expresses by nausea the disturbances illustrated in the case of the vasomotor system by pallor and collapse.

Nausea may be the result of drug administration (e.g., digitalis or aspirin), and the patient complaining of nausea should always be asked what medicines, if any, he is taking.

C. Wastell.

NECK, STIFF

This occurs in a number of diseases entirely different in character, and its significance may be either grave or trivial. Stiffness is rarely the only symptom, but it may be the first thing complained of, or it may be a complication arising in the course of a disease. It is not right to assume that the trouble is trivial, or vaguely to designate it as 'rheumatic', without a thorough investigation. It is necessary first to inquire into the history, when it may become obvious that it follows, say, an injury, or has arisen during the course of some disease, and is not primary. Next examine the patient with the head, thorax, and shoulders bared, and see whether there is any swelling or abnormality present, also the extent of possible movement, and whether or not it is the movement that causes pain; if possible, locate the seat of the pain. A complete clinical examination should be made, not only of the nose and throat but of the entire patient, particularly the locomotor and nervous systems. X-rays may reveal unsuspected disease or injury, but before relating the symptom to degenerative changes one should remember that some narrowing of the lower cervical disk spaces is almost invariably present after middle age.

The important causes of stiff neck may be classified as follows:

CONGENITAL:
  Congenital torticollis or wry-neck.
  Congenital deformities, e.g., Klippel-Feil.
ACQUIRED
  Acute:
    Infective:
      Reflex spasm due to adenitis from otitis media, tonsillitis, etc.
      Infective inflammatory bone lesions.
      Epidemic cervical myalgia.
    Traumatic:
      Fractures ⎫
      Dislocations ⎬ of cervical spine.
      Subluxations ⎪
      Strains ⎭
      Lesions of an intervertebral disk.
      Injuries to soft parts, haematoma in muscle, etc.

Degenerative:
  Cervical spondylosis.
Chronic:
  Arthritic:
    Still's disease
    Rheumatoid arthritis
    Ankylosing spondylitis
    Other spondylarthropathies
  Infective:
    Infective arthritis
    Tuberculous disease of spine
  Post-traumatic:
    Untreated acute traumatic lesions
    Contractures following burns, nerve injuries, etc.
  Neoplastic.
  Acute systemic infections:
    Meningitis
    Typhus
    Leptospirosis
    Brain abscess
    Poliomyelitis
    Psittacosis
    Subdural empyema
    Arbovirus infections
    Crimean haemorrhagic fever
    Tetanus, etc.

With the exception of congenital torticollis, contractures, gummata, and possibly some late cases of untreated injury and a few cases of arthritis, all these conditions are more or less painful.

CONGENITAL TORTICOLLIS or WRY-NECK is due to a contraction of the sternomastoid muscle on one side, generally considered to be the result of an injury during labour, possibly ischaemic in nature. The muscle stands out as a tight band in the neck, and its contraction leads to a characteristic deformity. The head is pulled down towards the affected side, and the face and chin are tilted towards the opposite shoulder. The movements of the head are necessarily restricted owing to the shortening of the one muscle, and in long-standing cases this leads to a marked asymmetry of the face. The consequences are not limited to the head and neck, for the spine shares in the general obliquity, and shows marked lateral curvature in old cases.

EXPOSURE TO COLD or SLEEPING IN A CRAMPED POSITION may give rise to a transient stiff neck associated with no other symptoms. There is generally a distinct history of the patient waking up in the morning with a stiff neck, and the diagnosis is made by exclusion.

EPIDEMIC CERVICAL MYALGIA. An epidemic form of stiff painful neck has been described, abating in a few days with symptomatic treatment only, but confirmation of its infective nature has yet to be obtained.

INFLAMMATION OF THE LYMPHATIC GLANDS and the cellular tissues of the neck may cause local stiffness, whether the infecting focus be a boil or carbuncle, or a carious tooth, an inflamed tonsil, pediculosis capitis, or other similar cause. In a mild case the neck can be moved, but movement is painful and therefore it is held stiffly. With a more severe reaction reflex muscle spasm is present. The diagnosis is as a rule easy.

SPONTANEOUS SUBLUXATION OF THE ATLAS occasionally occurs as a result of hyperaemic decalcification due to local inflammatory lesions such as acute tonsillitis. Atlanto-axial subluxation is seen not infrequently in advanced cases of rheumatoid arthritis and in patients with ankylosing spondylitis.

INJURIES TO THE NECK. These vary from soft-tissue injuries and strains to fractures and dislocations. Although some are fatal early there is a most important and not infrequent type of case where there is a subluxation without cord involvement, the only symptoms being stiffness and pain.

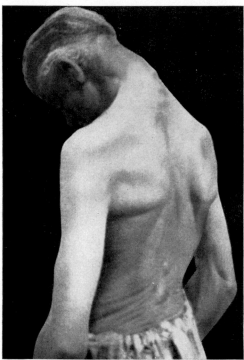

Fig. 568. Ankylosing spondylitis—'poker-back'. The patient was unable to raise his head, though he could just nod and shake it slightly. Except for the atlas and axis, the whole vertebral column was fixed.

These are easy to miss; and as a permanent disability may result if the condition is not treated it is essential to make a correct diagnosis. This can only be made with certainty by good radiographs, the lateral view of which will show slight anterior displacement of the upper vertebra or tilting and asymmetry of the articular processes between the two vertebrae involved. The deformity is rendered more obvious when the spine is X-rayed in the flexed position, and may be missed in extension.

DEGENERATIVE. The commonest cause of stiffness of the neck is degenerative disease of bone, joint, and cartilage, i.e., osteoarthrosis. This is a common disorder of the group of patients over 60

years of age. Pains are commonly referred from the painful stiff neck into the occiput and out towards the shoulders.

SPASMODIC TORTICOLLIS is an unusual form due to spasms of the sternomastoid and other muscles of the neck. The spasms are intermittent, coming on suddenly, sometimes with great pain, the affected muscles relaxing after a variable time, and during sleep. Tics and hysterical symptoms may occur in a similar manner.

INFECTIVE ARTHRITIS OF THE CERVICAL VERTEBRAE. Following infective diseases such as scarlet fever, typhoid fever, paratyphoid fever, diphtheria, and tonsillitis, especially in children, there may ensue a very chronic form of infective arthritis affecting one of several of the cervical vertebrae, and sometimes proceeding to complete bony ankylosis.

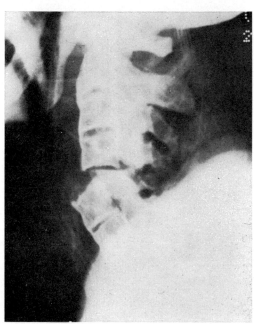

Fig. 569. A broken neck in ankylosing spondylitis. Such rigid necks are more prone to such traumatic lesions than are normal supple ones. (Courtesy of the Gordon Photographic Museum, Guy's Hospital.)

ARTHRITIS. Stiffness of the neck is less common in rheumatoid arthritis of adult life than in childhood (Still's disease). It is more common, however, in cases of ankylosing spondylitis, where the neck and head may be held in a completely fixed position (see Figs. 568, 569). A similar picture may more rarely be seen in the spondyl-arthritic varieties of psoriatic arthropathy, Reiter's disease, and the arthropathy associated with ulcerative colitis and Crohn's disease.

CERVICAL CARIES. (Fig. 570.) The greatest care must be taken not to overlook tuberculous disease of the cervical vertebrae as a cause of reflex muscular rigidity of the neck. Pain and rigidity are among the earliest signs; the pain is increased by the least movement, and the child—for it is generally a child that is affected—takes the greatest precaution to avoid any movement, even holding the head between the two hands. The position of the head varies; it is most often held very stiff and straight, the natural backward curve of the neck being lost. In the late stages there may be an angular or lateral curve.

BURNS. A self-evident cause of stiffness is the cicatricial contraction following a burn on the neck.

NEW GROWTH in one of the cervical vertebrae may cause progressive stiff neck, and generally much local pain on movement; the diagnosis may suggest itself when the patient is known to have had a new growth elsewhere, specially a carcinoma of the breast or of the thyroid gland; cases of primary new growth of the vertebra are fortunately rare.

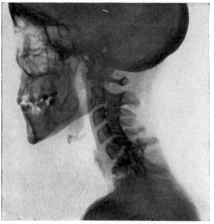

Fig. 570. Cervical caries showing collapse of bodies of 6th and 7th cervical vertebrae. (*Dr. T. H. Hills.*)

ACUTE SYSTEMIC INFECTIONS. Many acute infections are accompanied by a stiff neck (meningism), particularly in children; pneumonia, once a common cause in childhood, is now much less so. Fever is almost always present. Meningitis from any cause almost always causes some neck rigidity. Neck stiffness may be an early prodromal sign in paralytic or non-paralytic poliomyelitis and changes in the cerebrospinal fluid are found. Phlebotomus (sandfly) fever, an arbovirus acute infection, presents as fever, malaise, myalgia, and sometimes headache, in some cases with findings of an aseptic meningitis. Stiffness of the neck may be an early sign of tetanus, but other signs, such as trismus (inability to open the mouth due to tonic contraction of the jaw muscles) rapidly appear (*see* p. 802). *F. Dudley Hart.*

NECK, SWELLING OF

Anatomy. The neck on either side is divided into anterior and posterior triangles by the sternomastoid muscle arising from the sternum, sternoclavicular junction and medial third of the clavicle below and being inserted into the mastoid process of the temporal bone above. At the upper end of the anterior triangle the digastric muscle defines the lower borders of a subsidiary space known as the digastric triangle, and at the lower end of the posterior triangle the posterior belly of the omohyoid muscle defines the upper border of a subsidiary space known as the supraclavicular fossa.

The sternomastoid muscles are enclosed within the deep cervical fascia which splits to embrace them. If even a part of a mass in the neck overlaps either border of the sternomastoid muscle then, by putting one or other of these muscles into contraction, the relation of the mass to the sternomastoid muscle and so to the deep fascia can readily be determined. This method is applicable to practically all masses in the neck except the majority of those situated in the midline. The right sternomastoid muscle is put into contraction by rotating the head to the left while resistance is applied to the chin and vice versa; both sternomastoids are made to contract when the forehead is pressed forwards against resistance.

Lumps in the neck arising from structures superficial to the deep cervical fascia are not specific to the neck. Thus, sebaceous cysts, lipomata, carbuncles, and so on, are common, particularly in or deep to the skin at the back of the neck. It is the masses deep to the deep cervical fascia which have particular relevance in regard to the neck and it is the differential diagnosis of these that must be considered.

It is conventional to divide swellings in the neck into midline swellings and lateral swellings, but this is a little misleading as nearly all so-called 'midline swellings' deviate slightly to one side or the other. They can, however, be divided appropriately into masses arising from unpaired midline structures and masses arising from paired lateral structures.

1. Masses arising from Unpaired Midline Structures

a. THYROGLOSSAL CYST. The thyroid gland is developed from an epithelial-lined duct which grows downwards from the region of the foramen caecum of the tongue, passing close in front of and then behind the hyoid bone, and so towards the site of the adult isthmus from which the lateral lobes expand. A cyst may form in any part of this track by failure of obliteration of the duct, but the most common site is at the lower border of the hyoid bone, anterior to the thyrohyoid membrane. These cysts usually appear at about puberty and enlarge to a variable size slightly to one or other side of the midline. They are fluctuant, globular masses which, if superficial, may transilluminate. If the jaw is held open and the tongue steadily protruded, the swelling will rise in the neck demonstrating its attachment to the hyoid bone. These cysts occasionally become infected and may rupture, leading to a fistula. (*Fig.* 571.)

b. SWELLINGS ARISING FROM THE ISTHMUS OF THE THYROID GLAND. All those pathological conditions described on page 788 and giving rise to

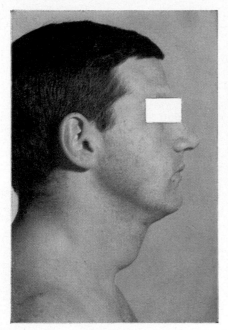
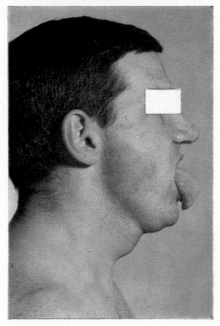

Fig. 571.   Thyroglossal cyst showing elevation on protruding tongue.

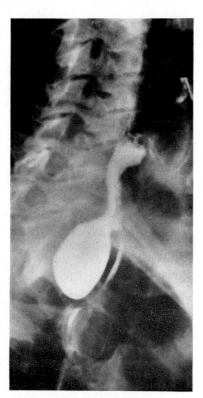

Fig. 572. Pharyngeal pouch filled with barium.
(*Dr. Keith Jefferson.*)

swellings of the thyroid gland can arise in the isthmus. It should be repeated once more that practically all thyroid swellings move up and down on deglutition owing to their intimate relation to the larynx and upper part of the trachea the movements of which they follow during this act.

c. PHARYNGEAL POUCH (*Fig.* 572). At the back of the inferior constrictor muscle of the pharynx there is a triangular area, between the upper border of the transversely running fibres of the crico-pharyngeus below and the lower border of the obliquely running fibres of the thyro-pharyngeus above, where the wall is deficient in muscle. Through this defect, a pouch of mucosa, covered only by the substantia propria of the pharynx, may protrude. This pouch gradually enlarges usually towards the left side of the neck and tends to fill up when food or fluid is swallowed. At first this is just a nuisance and gives rise to an uncomfortable feeling on swallowing together with a rapidly developing swelling which may be emptied by pressing on the mass. Later, the mass becomes sufficiently large to press upon the oesophagus, against which it lies, to produce severe dysphagia with inanition.

Food is apt to stagnate within the pouch and this leads to diverticulitis which may spread giving rise to pharyngitis or oesophagitis, and so adding to the burden of dysphagia. This condition may appear at any age, but usually arises during the third and fourth decades. Treatment, after attention to the nutritional needs of the patient, is by surgical excision.

d. Rare Cases of Swelling arising in Midline Structures

i. Subhyoid bursa, a cystic swelling arising behind the hyoid bone and indistinguishable clinically from a thyroglossal cyst.

ii. Perichondritis of the thyroid cartilage.

iii. A carcinoma of the larynx, trachea, or oesophagus penetrating the walls of these viscera and protruding to one or other side.

iv. The so-called 'Delphic lymph-gland', which lies in the midline on the thyro-hyoid membrane, may enlarge in carcinoma of the thyroid gland and may be the first evidence of this disease.

v. Laryngocele (*Figs.* 573, 574).

In addition to the horizontal system, there is a vertical system ranged along the internal jugular vein. At the upper end there is the upper deep cervical group, common to both systems, and at the lower end the lower deep cervical group with subsidiary groups in between. The lower deep cervical group of lymph-glands is in relation to the internal jugular vein where it is crossed by the posterior belly of the omohyoid, and one large gland of this group—the jugulo-omohyoid gland—is again of significance in relation to pathological processes in the tongue receiving lymphatics from this organ without the interposition of any intervening lymphatic glands; so

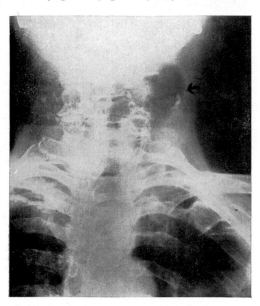

Fig. 573. Radiograph of left-sided laryngocele.

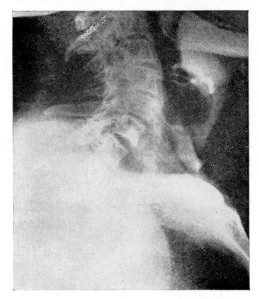

Fig. 574 The same as *Fig.* 573, lateral view.

2. Masses arising from Paired Lateral Structures

a. Lymph-glands. The commonest swellings in the neck are undoubtedly due to pathological processes arising in the lymphatic glands, usually secondary to some inflammatory or neoplastic process in one of the organs which they drain, but sometimes, as in lymphosarcoma, appearing to arise primarily within these glands.

The distribution of the lymphatic glands in the neck is variable, but the general disposition is as follows. In the upper part of the neck there is a horizontally disposed system consisting of the submental, suprahyoid, submaxillary, and upper deep cervical groups. The names of these groups indicate sufficiently their situation except for the upper deep cervical group which is situated in relation to the internal jugular vein where it is crossed by the posterior belly of the digastric muscle. One important gland of this group—the jugulo-digastric gland—is particularly significant in relation to pathological conditions of the tongue. These glands all drain from before backwards.

that, for instance, a carcinoma of the side of the tongue can give rise to secondary deposits in the supraclavicular fossa, where this gland is situated, without the enlargement of any of the systems in the upper part of the neck. It remains to mention the Delphic gland on the thyro-hyoid membrane already referred to. The differential diagnosis of the various types of enlarged lymph-glands is described on page 513.

b. Thyroid Swellings. These, which are the second commonest cause of swellings situated laterally in the neck, are fully described on page 788. Nearly all these swellings move up and down with deglutition, by which property they may be recognized. There are, however, some exceptions to this rule. If the mass is very large and fills one or both anterior triangles and perhaps the midline as well, there may not be room for the thyroid to move on deglutition. Again, in certain types of carcinoma with infiltration of the pretracheal muscles the growth may not move on deglutition. This is because the larynx, which causes the thyroid to move, cannot itself do so as there is no elasticity left in the infiltrated pretracheal muscles. Indeed it is this tethering of the larynx by infiltration of the surrounding structures which leads to dysphagia in carcinoma of the thyroid, as can readily be appreciated by anyone who attempts to swallow while holding down his thyroid cartilage by placing a finger on its upper border. Sometimes in a nodular goitre the excursion of the mass on swallowing or on coughing may be so considerable that it rises up from and 'plunges down' into the superior mediastinum or retroclavicular spaces during these movements. This so-called 'plunging goitre' is only a type of retrosternal or retroclavicular goitre with an abnormally free range of movement. Its very mobility argues that it will probably be a simple matter to deal with surgically.

c. More Rare Cases of Swelling laterally placed in the Neck

i. *Branchial cyst*: This is a congenital condition arising in the remains of a branchial cleft and giving rise to a cystic swelling in the lateral part of the neck. The condition may arise at any age, but usually occurs in young people and is rare after the age of 40. The swelling, which varies in size, usually protrudes into the anterior triangle from the deep surface of the upper part of the sternomastoid muscle. It is usually rather soft and fluctuates readily, but it is generally too deeply situated to demonstrate translucency. Occasionally these cysts become infected, when the differential diagnosis from breaking-down tuberculous glands may be difficult.

Ordinarily the sternomastoid muscle tends to spread over and be attached to a mass of breaking-down tuberculous glands, whereas it is inclined to go into spasm and retreat from an inflamed branchial cyst. However, the diagnosis can usually be determined by aspiration, which will yield either tuberculous pus or, on the other hand, purulent fluid containing numerous cholesterol crystals which is typical of an inflamed branchial cyst.

Although not strictly a swelling in the neck, it should be mentioned here that the unobliterated branchial cleft, instead of forming a cyst, may communicate with the exterior, usually just medial to the sternal head of the sternomastoid muscle below and into the pharynx in the supratonsillar fossa above, forming a branchial fistula.

ii. *'Sternomastoid tumour'*: As a result of birth or intra-uterine injury, some fibres of the sternomastoid muscle may be torn and a haematoma appears in this muscle. This gives rise to a lump which may persist and prevent the proper development of the muscle, leading to wry neck.

iii. *Cervical rib*: Another congenital abnormality which may give rise to a swelling in the supraclavicular fossa is cervical rib. The swelling may be due to the rib itself or there may be a pulsatile swelling due to a 'post-stenotic' dilatation of the subclavian artery. This condition is dealt with on page 502.

iv. A rare congenital abnormality is *cystic hygroma*, a lymphangiomatous condition arising usually in the supraclavicular fossa of infants. It forms a soft, fluctuating, translucent, and painless swelling which may grow rapidly. These masses are liable to attacks of infection.

v. *Aneurysm and arteriovenous fistula*: The large vessels of the neck are liable to the same pathological changes as vessels elsewhere. Aneurysms may occur in the cervical part of the subclavian artery, or the carotid arteries. A penetrating injury of the neck, as by a metallic fragment, may damage both the carotid artery and the internal jugular vein, leading to an arteriovenous fistula.

vi. *Carotid body tumour*: This is a rare lesion arising in the chromaffin tissue situated behind the bifurcation of the common carotid artery. It appears at any time after infancy as a very firm 'potato-like' tumour in close association with the carotid sheath so that pulsation is usually, but not invariably, transmitted to it. Its steady growth over a period of years serves to distinguish it from tuberculous cervical adenitis with which it may readily be confused. Occasionally there is stimulation of the cervical sympathetic which serves to confirm the diagnosis.

vii. *Swellings of the submaxillary salivary gland* arise in the digastric triangle and are described on page 697. Ludwig's angina is an acute inflammatory process of the cellular tissue around the submaxillary gland, usually arising from the floor of the mouth or the teeth. The physical signs extend into the floor of the mouth and give rise to considerable oedema which, without treatment, may spread to the glottis and demand tracheotomy.

viii. *Actinomycosis* is a chronic inflammatory swelling of the cellular tissue about the angle of the mandible. The diffuse induration with the eventual development of multiple sinuses and the accompanying trismus should make the diagnosis obvious. Late in the disease, 'sulphur granules' containing the streptothrix may be discharged, but the diagnosis should not await bacteriological confirmation which may be equivocal in the early stages.

ix. *Spinal abscess*: In certain cases of tuberculosis of the cervical spine, the abscess may track from the retropharyngeal region laterally, and present as a fluctuant mass in the upper part of the posterior triangle and deep to the insertion of the sternomastoid muscle. The accompanying stiffness of the neck together with the general evidence of a chronic infection should alert the examiner to this possibility. If untreated, the abscess breaks down, discharges and forms multiple sinuses in the apex of the posterior triangle.

R. G. Beard.

NIGHTMARES

A nightmare is the term generally applied to a dream accompanied by a particularly unpleasant and vivid emotion, such as fear, horror, or desperation. A closely related phenomenon which occurs during childhood is given the name 'night terror' (*pavor nocturnus*). A distinction is sometimes drawn between the nightmare and night terror on the ground that in the latter there is a more obvious expression of fear, the child may act out his dream experience, and cry or scream, and may later have no recollection of what has happened. Although a physical abnormality, most commonly a febrile state due to measles or some other infection, is a common cause, repeated nightmares or night terrors in a physically healthy child should as a rule be taken as a sign of an emotional disturbance, and an inquiry made for other symptoms. Frequent nightmares are more likely to occur in children of neurotic parents; the liability to attacks being increased by an unhappy or unsettled home atmosphere and by sources of particular stress, such as rivalry between children in the family, or injurious experiences at school. Sometimes no cause can be found, but it cannot be inferred from this that the attacks have a physical precipitant, for the psychological factors responsible for them may only be uncovered by special methods of examination—for example, the analysis of play activities.

Nightmares in adults may also be due to toxic or infective causes although in the latter case not so commonly as in children. The onset of *delirium tremens* may be marked initially by the occurrence of terrifying dreams which are shortly transferred into equally terrifying hallucinations. Physical causes apart, nightmares may also signify internal unrest. An overwhelming experience, which has not been assimilated by the mind, may recur in the form of a terrifying dream. This was a common occurrence in the traumatic neuroses of war, when a soldier who broke down in battle sometimes became the victim of nightmares in which he re-experienced the critical factors leading to breakdown. Surgical operations and accidents may also act as precipitants of nightmares if the individual is, for some psychological reason, especially vulnerable to experiences of this kind. Bad dreams, however, need not follow on any special event; they can also be a sign of excitation of tension in the mind which rises to the surface when conscious control of mental processes is abrogated during sleep. Dreams can often offer an important clue to the content of a neurotic illness; for example, the woman whose mind is occupied by conflict of feelings towards her children may dream that one of them has been cut by a knife: the dream here represents a fear that injury will overtake the child, and may also indicate an unconscious fear of doing the child harm. An overconscientious man who believes he is failing in his task may dream that he is being pursued by a threatening figure, a symbol of his own conscience. Continued anxiety from any cause can manifest itself in disturbed sleep and anxiety dreams. The presence of nightmares therefore should suggest a need to review a patient's present state and life situation so that the source of tension can be traced.

A condition which may be confused with the simple nightmare is *epilepsy* in which attacks occur at night. A history of seizures or of tongue-biting or bed-wetting during the attack may point to the diagnosis. An electro-encephalogram may supply confirmatory evidence.

W. H. Trethowan.

NIPPLE, DISCHARGE FROM

Discharge from the nipple may be divided into three classes:

1. Normal Discharges. A discharge of milk from the breast during pregnancy is not uncommon especially in multiparae; both then and during lactation it is usually of small amount except when the child is put to the breast, but occasionally the flow at other times may be sufficient to be distressing.

2. Normal Discharges at Abnormal Times. A secretion similar to colostrum sometimes occurs from the breasts of both sexes in the newly born and again at puberty; it is due to endocrine stimulation but it may predispose to a true infective mastitis, when the breast, already tender and swollen, becomes hot and red, and the discharge may change from being clear to purulent.

Occasionally the normal secretion of milk during lactation is prolonged for many months or years after the stimulus of suckling has been removed. This is probably due to some endocrine abnormality and, apart from being a serious nuisance and sometimes a source of anxiety to the patient, has no sinister significance. It usually resolves spontaneously and unpredictably after a varying period with or without the aid of endocrine therapy.

3. Abnormal Discharges:
a. SEROUS FLUID. A discharge of serous fluid from the nipple is a common accompaniment of fibro-adenosis, particularly when the epithelial changes of the disease affect the ducts near the nipple. This additional symptom of fibro-adenosis does not usually signify a more treacherous change in the breast tissue, although a simple serous discharge may accompany innocent papillomata of the duct.

b. PIGMENTED FLUIDS:
i. *Green Fluid.* When the colour is due to melanin or pigments other than derivatives of haemoglobin, its admixture with yellow serum gives to the resultant discharges a green colour of varying shades. If the discharge is very dark, dilution with water will disclose the green colour. In cases of real difficulty the discharge may be submitted to spectroscopic or chemical assay for haemoglobin. Such discharges have precisely the same significance as the non-pigmented serous discharges discussed above.
ii. *Haemorrhagic.* Blood-stained discharges can usually be recognized on sight; the colour is red to black, and again if there is real doubt the final arbiters are the spectroscope and the chemical test. Blood-stained discharges are indicative of

duct papilloma, fibro-adenosis with excessive epithelial proliferation, and intra-duct carcinoma, in that order of frequency.

The nipple should be examined through a magnifying glass and a bead of blood or a speck of clot may reveal from which of the twenty or so ducts the bleeding is arising. Such evidence is important in determining from which section of the breast the bleeding is originating. Having examined the nipple thus, it should be wiped clean and (with the breast rendered moderately tense by an assistant if available) the tip of the finger is pressed on to the breast at successive sites, working spirally from the nipple, and paying particular attention to the subareolar region, where the source of the bleeding lies in the majority of cases. By this means it will be found possible to cause blood to issue from the nipple on pressure over quite a restricted area, whereas pressure elsewhere has no effect. If the affected duct has been previously identified the significant area will be found to lie in the segment of the breast drained by that duct, and the pathological region is confirmed. The segment of the breast affected should be removed by local operation, and the pathological condition causing the bleeding determined by naked-eye inspection and histological study. Further treatment depends upon the nature of the lesion so determined. Solitary papillomata adjacent to the nipple are the commonest cause of this symptom, and if removed in this way bleeding seldom recurs.

Should it be impossible to localize the origin of the bleeding, and with care and practice this is most unusual, the diagnosis depends on an assessment of probabilities. The younger the patient the more likely is the cause to be benign; the older the patient the more likely to be malignant. In bleeding from an unidentifiable source, a patient under 35 years of age should be observed for some months, when the bleeding may cease spontaneously. In a patient over 40 years of age only a short period of observation is wise. In either case persistence of the symptoms is an indication for operation, and total, though not radical, operation should be advised.

4. Grumous Material. The discharge of 'cheese-like' material or material having the consistency of tooth-paste or putty, grey or green in colour, indicates the condition known as 'comedo-mastitis'. This condition, unlike the usual varieties of fibro-adenosis, is more common in multiparae, but is probably closely allied to fibro-adenosis. It has the same significance in regard to precancerous tendencies as fibro-adenosis, that is, the tendency is so slight that it may be ignored, and it demands the same watchful and symptomatic treatment.

5. Pus, or pus mixed with milk, generally indicates acute suppurative mastitis; the other signs of inflammation or abscess are well marked as a rule, so that there is no difficulty in arriving at a diagnosis. A *tuberculous lesion* also causes a discharge of pus, and it may simulate carcinoma; the discharge may contain demonstrable tubercle

bacilli, but guinea-pig inoculation or a radiograph of the chest will very likely be required before a positive answer on the nature of the infection can be given.

R. G. Beard.

NODULES

Nodules are solid elevations of the skin, larger than papules and smaller than tumours, and thus may be a stage in the growth of tumours; they may be neoplastic, hypertrophic, or inflammatory.

Rodent ulcer (basal-cell carcinoma) usually starts as a small hard nodule on the face; as a rule it is single, but when more than one are present there may be a great number. The latter tend to occur in blonde or red-headed individuals who have spent a long time exposed to strong sunlight (tropics, Australia). The lesion is hard and pearly and may not ulcerate for a long time. It is of a low grade of malignancy, spreading only locally and slowly without healing. It must be distinguished from a wart, mole, fibroma, or papilloma.

Granuloma pyogenicum (botryomycoma) (*Fig.* 575) is a small, firm, cherry-red nodular excrescence which sometimes arises on an area of sepsis, such as an infected abrasion. It consists of hypertrophic granulation tissue and bleeds easily on slight trauma.

Molluscum sebaceum (kerato-acanthoma) (*Fig.* 576) is a small hard warty nodule affecting the face. It has an histology very similar to squamous-cell carcinoma but is in fact benign with little tendency to spread or ulcerate, nor does it metastasize. If left untreated it may disappear in 5–6 months. It must be distinguished from a simple wart, being harder in consistency and less hyperkeratotic, and also from squamous-cell carcinoma.

The nodules of *lupus vulgaris* (*Fig.* 577) are soft, brownish-red, and translucent, and on pressure with a piece of glass (diascopy) resemble 'apple jelly'. They arise in the corium and at first appear as minute papules, which grow in size and extend upwards. Later a patch of nodules is formed which may be covered with scales. The process is usually a slow one and there may be ulceration. Usually, however, the centre of the lesion undergoes involution with scarring, while fresh nodules appear at the periphery. When ulceration occurs there may be secondary infection, causing pain, which is otherwise absent. On the nose and pinnae ulceration of the cartilage takes place. The commonest site to be affected is the face, especially the nose, but it may occur on the limbs and buttocks. It begins in childhood and is a direct tuberculous infection. It is mainly a disease of the poorer sections of the community. Typical cases are easily identified by the history and the presence of the apple-jelly nodules, but it may have to be distinguished from lupus erythematosus, rodent ulcer, epithelioma, scrofuloderma, and syphilis. It is worth noting that syphilis will cause in a matter of weeks the amount of ulceration that is produced by lupus in years. When lupus vulgaris has been treated with X-rays, sooner or later

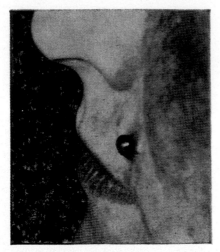

Fig. 575. Pyogenic granuloma. (*Dr. Peter Hansell.*)

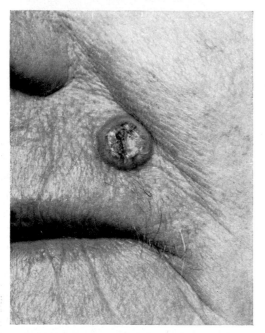

Fig. 576. Molluscum sebaceum. (*Dr. Peter Hansell.*)

an epithelioma (squamous-cell) will appear on the site. This complication is now happily a rarity.

Small isolated nodules are a feature of the 'swimming-pool granuloma', which is due to direct inoculation of *Mycobacterium balnei*.

Similar lesions may be caused by other mycobacteria, e.g., *M. ulcerans* or by leishmaniasis (*see under* FACE, ULCERATIONS OF, p. 272).

Lupus erythematosus is seldom nodular (*Fig.* 578) but in the fixed type a small nodule may form in the spreading edge.

There is a nodular or hypertrophic form of *lichen planus*, in which a few giant lesions occur, usually on the extensor surfaces of the knees and elbows. It must be distinguished from nodular prurigo (Hebra's prurigo).

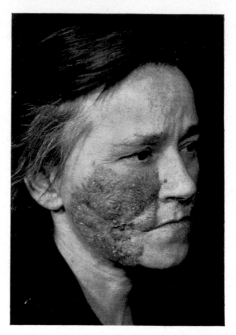

Fig. 577. Lupus vulgaris.

In *scrofuloderma*, which is tuberculous ulceration of the skin over caseating tuberculous glands or tuberculosis of bones or joints usually in connexion with a sinus, there may be nodule formation.

Late *syphilitic lesions* (*Fig.* 579) of the skin are sometimes nodular, and the nodules soon break down to form gummatous ulcers; the process is a rapid one and there is a tendency for them to spread. When healing occurs a characteristic tissue-paper scar is left. Syphilitic nodules are often a deep red or purple colour and free from pain or itching. The Wassermann reaction is always positive.

Yaws (framboesia) is an endemic tropical spirochaetal disease in which nodules are an important symptom. After an incubation period of several weeks a group of papules appears at the site of inoculation, usually the face or extremities. These become crusted and ulcerate; this stage is usually accompanied by mild constitutional symptoms. This is the primary stage and after a few months it heals spontaneously. Some months later the secondary yaws appear; these consist of numerous amber-coloured nodules present all over the body and are soft, crusted, granulomatous lesions. This stage lasts up to about six months and heals spontaneously, leaving no mark. As a rule this is the termination of the disease, but occasionally there is a tertiary stage with gummatous ulceration. Rarely this is associated with periostitis, chronic synovitis, and juxta-articular nodes. The diagnosis as a rule presents no difficulty as it is endemic in certain countries.

with primary tuberculosis, early sarcoidosis, streptococcal infections, and occasionally as a drug eruption. In sarcoidosis it is accompanied by bilateral hilar-gland enlargement, oedema of

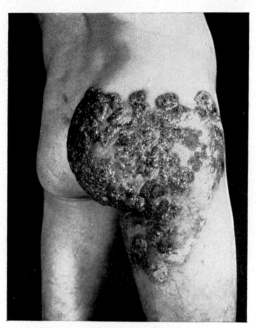

Fig. 579. Nodular late syphilide. Note tissue-paper scars already appearing at the bottom of the patch.

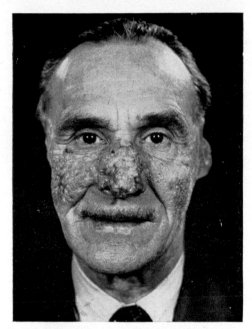

Fig. 578. Very rare nodular type of lupus erythematosus.

Nodules (*Fig.* 580) are a feature of the lepromatous type of *leprosy* in which the skin and subcutaneous tissues are particularly involved. The nodules (leproma) may appear at varying periods after the macules (p. 517), with or without fever or other constitutional disturbance. They appear anywhere on the body, but often on the face, scalp, and ears, and are at first ill defined. Later they become brown or yellowish-brown firm lumps. The development is slow and the so-called 'leonine' facies is a characteristic symptom of the disease. Later ulceration and mutilation occur, especially on the extremities.

There is a nodular form of *verruca peruana* (Peruvian wart, Oroya fever) when nodules appear on the limbs, particularly around the joints. These are painful and may break down to form fungating masses.

In *erythema nodosum* painful red or purplish nodules appear on the fronts of both legs below the knees. Occasionally they occur on the arms, thighs, or calves of the legs. The disease affects mainly children and young adults. It is an important sign of underlying disease. It may occur

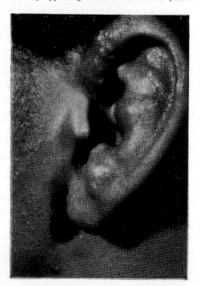

Fig. 580. Lepromatous nodules on ear. (*Dr. Peter Hansell.*)

the ankles, and often infiltration into pre-existing scars. A transient arthritis may occur. In some countries it is a manifestation of deep fungous infections. A rather special form, *erythema nodosum leprosum*, is a frequent accompaniment of treatment of nodular leprosy. The lesions never ulcerate, but slowly subside, leaving bruises. Diagnosis should be simple, the age-group affected and the colour of the lesions distinguishing it from nodular phlebitis, which affects the middle aged and elderly.

The bases of them are inclined to be foul and the surrounding tissues heaped-up and purple in colour. They affect young adults, a fact which serves to differentiate the ulcers from gummata as also does their multiplicity and bilateral

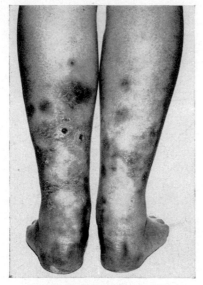

Fig. 581. Erythema induratum (Bazin).
(*Dr. Peter Hansell.*)

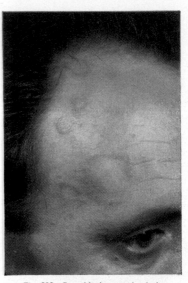

Fig. 582. Sarcoidosis: annular lesions.
(*Dr. Peter Hansell.*)

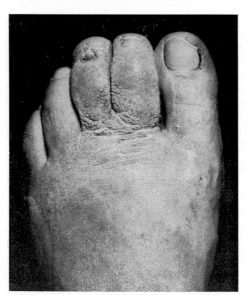

Fig. 583. Sarcoidosis: skin and bone involvement of foot.
(*Dr. Peter Hansell.*)

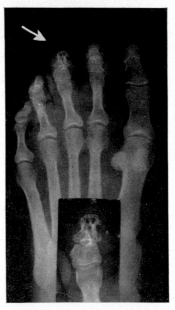

Fig. 584. Sarcoidosis: X-ray of foot. Same patient as *Fig.* 526. (*Dr. Peter Hansell.*)

Erythema induratum scrofulosorum (Bazin's disease) (*Fig.* 581), which is a tuberculous ulceration, starts as nodules in the calves of the legs. These are definitely subcutaneous and soon break down to form indurated irregular ulcers.

arrangement. Erythema nodosum occurs with primary tuberculosis, while erythema induratum occurs in the later stages of the disease. The *subcutaneous sarcoid of Darier-Roussy*, which affects the limbs, resembles Bazin's disease closely.

In *Boeck's sarcoid* sharply defined, elastic, brown, intracutaneous and subcutaneous papules or nodules occur, usually symmetrically distributed over the face and extremities. After reaching

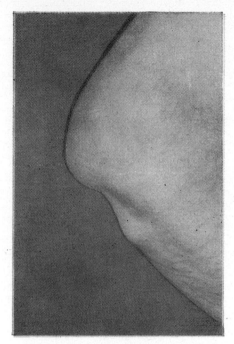

Fig. 585. Typical rheumatoid nodule just below elbow.

In *neurofibromatosis* (von Recklinghausen's disease) multiple nodules, up to thousands, occur in the skin. Although the majority of the little tumours are neurofibromatous in origin, lipomata

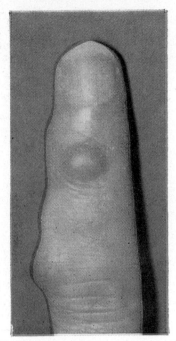

Fig. 586. Rheumatoid nodules over finger in active sero-positive disease.

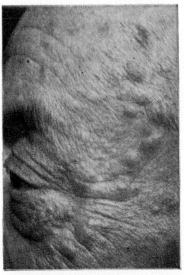

Fig. 587. Nodular leukaemic infiltrations. (*Dr. Peter Hansell.*)

a certain age the lesions remain stationary for months or years and then undergo spontaneous regression. Ulceration never occurs. Other skin lesions also occur in sarcoidosis. These include infiltrations into pre-existing scars, annular lesions (*Fig.* 582) especially on the face, and the condition known as *lupus pernio* in which infiltrations occur on exposed areas, nose, ears, and digits. When the digits are involved the underlying bone is often involved (*Figs.* 583, 584). Lupus pernio is not uncommon in Europe but seldom seen in the U.S.A., whilst papular and nodular lesions are very common in the American Negro.

Subcutaneous nodules sometimes appear in the course of a severe attack of *rheumatic fever*. About the size of a pea, they occur over any of the bones which lie close under the skin. Much more common are the nodules of rheumatoid arthritis, which occur over bony prominences under the skin at points of pressure, the commonest site being over the ulna just below the elbow joint (*Figs.* 585, 586). They are painless, only rarely ulcerate, and vary in size from a pin-head to 1–2 cm. in diameter. Larger ones may be seen over the sacrum. When they occur rheumatoid factor is usually present in high titre (Rose-Waaler or Latex test) in the serum.

Heberden's nodes are small bony swellings on the terminal interphalangeal joints; they are commoner in women and are a sign of *osteo-arthrosis*.

and simple fibromata occur as well. All forms of lesions may later become pedunculated. There are always also present *café au lait* patches and some of the subcutaneous nodules cause a

19

wrinkling and blueness of the overlying skin. Sometimes the lesions are associated with great pain and occasionally mental changes are also present.

In all forms of leukaemia there may occasionally be nodular deposits in the skin (*Fig.* 587). These vary in colour from skin-colour to plum or purple. The diagnosis is as a rule already obvious before the lesions form.

Histiocytoma is a localized form of cutaneous reticulo-endotheliosis. The lesion is a small, solitary, round or oval nodule, grey to violet in colour, with a slightly scaly surface. The exact diagnosis depends upon a histological examination.

The very rare *multiple idiopathic haemorrhagic sarcoma* (Kaposi) is not a sarcoma in the accepted sense of the word, and is characterized by the slow appearance of purple-coloured nodules around the ankles and on the feet. These may ulcerate and eventually heal or they may disappear spontaneously. Some cases are, however, progressive and truly neoplastic. The neoplastic variant is relatively common in parts of Africa. It is a disorder of middle age and affects men more than women. The diagnosis must be made by biopsy, when the histology will show dilatation of capillaries and proliferation of interstitial connective tissue slightly resembling sarcoma in appearance. In older cases there will be fibrosis as well.

P. D. Samman.

NOSE, REGURGITATION OF FOOD THROUGH

Regurgitation of food through the nose may be only a temporary accident, the result of an unsuccessful attempt to stave off a sneeze, a cough, or a burst of laughter when the mouth is full of food or fluid; or it may result from an explosive return of gas from the stomach or oesophagus, particularly after drinking gassy fluids. Pathological regurgitation of food through the nose results from two main groups of causes, namely:

1. Structural Imperfections of the Palate:

Congenital: cleft palate
Acquired perforation: (*a*) traumatic oro-antral fistula after extraction of upper molar teeth, (*b*) syphilitic, (*c*) malignant, (*d*) tuberculous, (*e*) actinomycotic.

2. Paresis or Paralysis of the Soft Palate or of the Pharynx:

Post-diphtheritic
The result of bulbar paralysis
Postoperative
The result of pseudo-bulbar paralysis.

Simple inspection of the roof of the mouth is generally sufficient to decide whether the cause belongs to group 1 or to group 2. The median and symmetrical imperfection of a congenital cleft palate is obvious, and there is the history of the trouble dating from birth.

There may be a hare-lip or other congenital abnormality at the same time. When an ulcerative process is still in progress there may for a time be some doubt as to whether it is syphilitic, malignant, tuberculous, or actinomycotic. The history may help, or the healing of the ulcer under antisyphilitic treatment, or the result of serological tests. If it is important to arrive at the correct diagnosis as early as possible a small portion of the pathological tissue may be excised and examined microscopically, or scrapings from the ulcer examined directly for the *Spirochaeta pallida*, for tubercle bacilli, or for ray fungi. Tuberculous ulceration of the palate is rare, and is generally associated with definite phthisis. Lupus occasionally occurs. A new growth of the palate may be epithelioma, endothelioma, or sarcoma, the distinction between these depending mainly on the microscope.

Diphtheria. If there is no structural defect of the palate, the regurgitation of food through the nose is due to paralysis, possible causes being acute poliomyelitis or diphtheria. The occurrence of diphtheria may have been recognized at the time, but the attack may have been so slight as either to have caused no definite illness, or else to have been regarded as simple sore throat. The palate alone may be paralysed, generally the whole soft palate but occasionally one side only, giving rise to a nasal character of voice as well as to the regurgitation; or there may also be paresis of the ciliary eye muscles, causing difficulty in reading; or general peripheral neuritis affecting the limbs and heart. The trouble may not come on for three or four weeks after the diphtheritic attack, and therefore it may no longer be possible to detect Klebs-Löffler bacilli in swabbings from the tonsils or fauces; but it is important to look for them, both directly and by means of cultures. The paresis recovers in time, sometimes quickly, but often not until three months or more have elapsed.

Postoperative Cases. Very occasionally, surgical removal of tonsils or adenoids is followed by a temporary weakness of the soft palate.

Bulbar Paralysis. When this affects the palate and causes regurgitation of food through the nose there have generally been other symptoms for some time. The malady is slowly progressive, and starts with paresis of the lips and tongue; swallowing is difficult, not so much because of the regurgitation as because the tongue is unable to thrust the bolus back between the fauces. The constant dribbling of saliva from the angles of the mouth is characteristic. The title 'labio-glosso-pharyngo-laryngeal paralysis' indicates the usual sequence of events. Unilateral palato-pharyngo-laryngeal paralysis is due to involvement of the nucleus ambiguus, from such conditions as haemorrhage, thrombosis, embolism, or disseminated sclerosis. Unilateral paresis of palate and pharynx may also occur when the vagus and spinal accessory nerves are attacked in the jugular foramen, usually by a cancer of the nasopharynx.

Bulbar paralysis may be associated with progressive muscular atrophy, and it may be distinguished from pseudo-bulbar paralysis by the atrophy of the tongue, which occurs in the former but not in the latter. Bulbar paralysis is due to a lesion in the medulla oblongata, whereas pseudo-bulbar paralysis, with similar symptoms but no wasting of the tongue, is due to bilateral cortical softening. In either case the patients are generally elderly.

Miles Foxen.

NYSTAGMUS

Nystagmus is a rapid and oscillatory movement of the eyes, independent of the normal movements, which are not affected. In nystagmus of ocular cause the movements are usually pendular, whereas in disease of the central nervous system there is a rapid component and a slow component. Several varieties of associated tremor of the two eyes are comprised under the term 'nystagmus'. These are: (1) Searching movements; (2) Pseudo-nystagmus; and (3) Nystagmus proper.

1. Wide purposeful and slow movements of the eyes in all directions are usually seen in people who are born blind or have lost the power of fixation as the result of some lesion of the retina or choroid at the macula. The eyes appear to be seeking for something but never rest on any definite object.

2. 'Pseudo-nystagmus' is the term applied to rapid jerking movements of the eyes when they are carried to the extreme positions. About one in five normal individuals will show this type of nystagmus expecially when aggravated by fatigue.

3. Nystagmus proper is the term applied to the condition in which the eyes make rapid regular oscillations about a fixed point, not only at the extremity of an excursion but when the eyes are otherwise at rest and looking directly forward. The oscillations may be in the vertical or in the horizontal meridian, or may exhibit a rotatory or circular movement. The condition is usually bilateral, though it may affect only one eye, and rarely the character of the nystagmus may differ in the two eyes. An interesting form is latent nystagmus, in which steady fixation is dependent upon the binocular reflexes. On covering one eye nystagmoid movements are immediately set up in the other.

Nystagmus commonly occurs as a congenital anomaly. Otherwise it is caused by:

a. Conditions causing defective vision in the early months of life. As a result of such affections, the macular region is not differentiated in function from the surrounding portions of the retina as is the usual course in the early months of infant life, and power of fixation is never acquired. Conditions which may thus cause nystagmus are *ophthalmia neonatorum*, *congenital cataract*, *albinism*, and certain cases in which there is an unusual distribution of the retinal pigment.

In the form called 'spasmus nutans' the nystagmus is associated with nodding movements of the head. It occurs in the first year of life, and disappears spontaneously.

b. Conditions developing in later life, as for example *miner's nystagmus*, in which it is caused by continued work in a dim light, where the central vision necessary for steady fixation is comparatively ineffective. Although there is usually a large functional factor in its development, it improves on return to work in good illumination (aided by an anticipated financial compensation).

c. Some general nervous diseases. Such are *disseminated sclerosis* (p. 622), *syringomyelia* (p. 623), and *Friedreich's ataxia* (p. 623); and in *lesions of the cerebellum*, whether inflammatory or neoplastic, nystagmus is usually a marked feature. When there are irritative lesions coarse movement occurs when the eyes are directed towards the side of the lesion and fine movement towards the opposite side.

Nystagmus has been reported in *peripheral neuritis* and *myasthenia gravis*. A form called *myoclonic nystagmus* is associated with spasmodic movements of the head and body, and increased knee-jerks.

d. Disease of the internal ear involving the semicircular canals not amounting to bilateral destruction; this *labyrinthine nystagmus* can be reproduced by syringeing the ear with hot or cold water, rotation, or the passage of a galvanic current.

e. Certain poisons, notably *manganese*; it is met with amongst those who work at manganese-ore mines; it may also result from *plumbism*.

P. Trevor-Roper.

OBESITY

Careful observations have failed to demonstrate metabolic abnormalities such as increased alimentary absorptinn, diminished basal metabolic rate, reduced specific dynamic action, lowered respiratory quotient, fluid retention, or expenditure of energy, sufficient to account for obesity. On the contrary, a study of predicted and actual weight-loss in fat subjects on low-calorie diets shows such close correlation that physiologists interested in metabolism maintain that 'fat comes only from food, and obesity results only from eating more than is needed to meet the energy requirements of the body'.

If this is so there is no need to consider the 'differential diagnosis' of obesity. If the patient is over-weight the diagnosis is 'obesity due to excessive food consumption in relation to energy requirements'.

It is difficult, however, for the clinician to agree always with this uncompromising attitude. He encounters patients who, in his opinion, are genuinely anxious to lose weight and do not appear to him to be consuming excessive quantities of food—patients who tell him that they literally cannot eat as much food as they did before they became obese because they feel bloated whenever they begin to eat; patients who put on an alarming amount of weight during pregnancy, or immediately afterwards, and have the greatest difficulty in losing it subsequently; patients who do not begin to lose their excessive weight on a 1250-calorie diet, though they do so satisfactorily on a 750-calorie diet; patients who put on some pounds in weight during the premenstrual week, presumably as the result of water retention and do not lose all of it during the rest of the cycle so that they steadily increase in weight; and unfortunate children who struggle with a diet while their brothers and sisters eat heartily and remain slender. No wonder the clinician is apt to invoke such factors as fluid retention, abnormal metabolic reactions, or disturbances of endocrine function, though it must at once be admitted that he has produced singularly little evidence, apart from that usually erroneous abstract, his 'clinical impression', to support the existence of these factors.

Nevertheless, it may be helpful to try to define 'obesity'. In the first place 'over-weight' is not necessarily synonymous with adiposity. A professional weight-lifter may be over-weight because he has over-developed his muscles. Those who study body-composition and obesity have abandoned the weighing-machine as a yard-stick in favour of caliper-measurements of skin-folds. These provide the most accurate simple method of estimating fat in the human subject. The so-called Harpenden skin-fold caliper used over the mid-point of the biceps gives a measurement which represents limb fat and used under the angle of the scapula a measurement representing trunk fat. Somatotyping classifies human physique into three groups: 'endomorphs' with substantial abdominal, hip, thigh, and upper arm measurements; 'mesomorphs' with massive chest measurements and a slender waist; and 'ectomorphs' who are thin, long, and lanky. Clearly an extreme endomorph is likely to be above the standard weight and would therefore be considered obese, whereas an extreme mesomorph is conspicuously muscular and may therefore also be overweight. The ectomorph is the fortunate person in terms of this problem who is unlikely to become overweight however many dietary indiscretions he commits and however much physical training he undergoes. Clearly some people just get fat and others do not.

Then there are studies which show that in the third decade, 10 per cent of the body-weight consists of fat, whereas in the fifth decade more than 20 per cent consists of fat, though the total bodyweight remains within the normal standard limits. In other words, one of the features of the ageing processes is to replace body protein by fat. This may well be an important factor in the genesis of the 'middle-age spread'. Furthermore, in cases of obesity, the fat cells are both larger and more numerous than normal fat-containing cells.

The Influence of the Hypothalamus. It has been established that bilateral destruction of the paired paraventricular nuclei gives rise, in experimental animals, to obesity as the result of the development of a voracious appetite, and it has been shown by the use of pair-fed control animals that this disorder of appetite is the only cause of the obesity in these cases. Numerous clinical conditions in which there is evidence of hypothalamic involvement are commonly associated with obesity. They are as follows:

GENETIC DISORDERS WITH HYPOTHALAMIC INVOLVEMENT:

Laurence-Moon-Biedl syndrome (obesity, retarded sexual development, retinitis pigmentosa, polydactyly, and mental deficiency)
Morgagni-Stewart-Morel syndrome (obesity, hyperostosis frontalis interna, virilism).

TRAUMA:

Injuries to the base of the skull, e.g., fractures or gunshot wounds, followed by obesity.

INFLAMMATION:

Meningitis—followed by obesity
Encephalitis
Post-encephalitic obesity
Encephalitis associated with exanthemata and virus diseases: e.g., measles, scarlet fever, and mumps, followed by obesity.

TUMOURS IN THE REGION OF THE MIDBRAIN:

Pineal tumours
Third ventricle tumours
Xanthomata—Hand-Schüller-Christian syndrome (xanthomatous deposits in the skin, hypercholesterolaemia, defects of membranous bone radiologically evident in the skull, diabetes insipidus, exophthalmos, adiposogenital dystrophy, and dwarfism)
Chromophobe adenomata of the pituitary
Cranio-pharyngiomata.

There are certain other classic symptoms which may result from lesions in the midbrain. They are:
1. HYPOGENITALISM. This is seen especially in cases in which the lesion has developed before puberty. The most classic example is true *Fröhlich's syndrome* in which a lesion, demonstrable by X-rays or other means, is found in the region of the hypothalamus, and is accompanied by inadequate or retarded development of the genitalia—so-called *dystrophia adiposogenitalis*. It is a rare condition, too commonly diagnosed. In most fat boys before puberty the scrotum is ill-defined and the pea-sized testicles may readily retract from it and become impalpable in the pubic 'sporran', in which the shaft and indeed the whole structure of the penis may be enveloped. To push back the 'sporran' is to convince oneself of the normal development of the genitalia. (*Fig.* 588.)
2. STUNTING OF GROWTH. This completes the classic triad of Fröhlich's disease, and is found

also in other hypothalamic disorders, such as the Laurence-Moon-Biedl syndrome (*Fig.* 589). Most fat children, however, are above the average height for their age, for overeating seems to increase stature as well as girth.

is Dickens's Fat Boy, concerning whom Mr. Wardle was constantly exclaiming, 'Damn that boy; he's gone to sleep again.' Indeed, the *Pickwick syndrome* is the title applied to the clinical triad of obesity, cyanosis, and somnolence, and

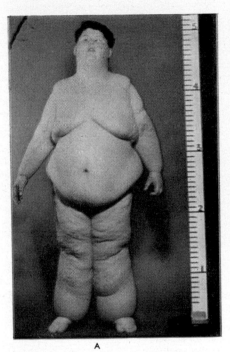
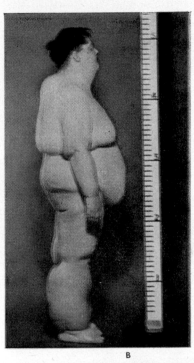

A   B

Fig. 588. True Fröhlich's syndrome. Note obesity and short stature. (*Courtesy of the Gordon Photographic Museum, Guy's Hospital.*)

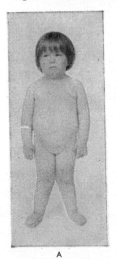
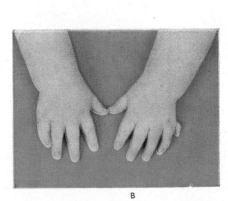
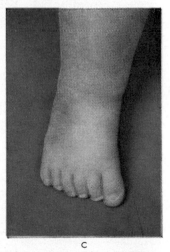

A   B   C

Fig. 589. Lawrence-Moon-Biedl syndrome. Note obesity causing knock-knee and polydactyly (supplementary little finger on left hand and six toes on the foot). (*Courtesy of the Gordon Photographic Museum, Guy's Hospital.*)

3. SOMNOLENCE. Somnolence is a common feature of lowered hypothalamic activity. It has been estimated that half the patients with narcolepsy become obese. An example from literature

it is suggested that chronic ventilatory insufficiency resulting from limitation of diaphragmatic respiration can cause haemodynamic embarrassment that will affect the cerebral circulation with a rise in the carbon-dioxide tension in the blood, leading to somnolence and transient disturbances of consciousness.

4. DIABETES INSIPIDUS. True organic diabetes insipidus results from bilateral interruption of the supra-optico-hypophysial tracts. Hypothalamic lesions may therefore be associated with both obesity and diabetes insipidus. The *Hand-Schüller-Christian syndrome* due to xanthomata involving the midbrain is not infrequently accompanied by diabetes insipidus.

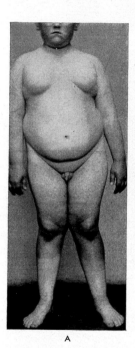 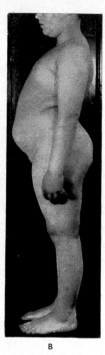

A   B

Fig. 590. A, Juvenile obesity. Note large breasts, knock-knees, and apparently small genitalia. Shaft of penis enveloped in pubic 'sporran'. Often described as 'Fröhlich's syndrome'. No evidence of endocrine disorder. Large appetite. B, Juvenile obesity. Note lumbar lordosis.

Apart from the conditions listed above and the accompanying classic features of the hypothalamic syndrome, it seems likely that the majority of cases of exogenous obesity are due to the loss of hypothalamic control of appetite, and there is evidence to show that in the early stages of derangement of the 'appestat' the increased appetite and food consumption go unnoticed, but by the time the appestat has been set permanently and irreversibly at a higher level the excessive weight can be maintained even on a substantially lower diet than the individual was accustomed to consume in the days when his weight remained steady and within the normal standard range.

Exogenous Obesity. The majority of obese patients eat too much, or drink a fair amount of beer, spirits, or 'fortified wines', and take insufficient exercise. These are cases of alimentary, *exogenous*, or gluttonous obesity. The distribution of fat is more or less generalized, though those parts of the body in which the muscles are especially active tend to become less obese. The small muscles of the hands and feet and the muscles of the forearms are in constant action, whereas the muscles of the abdominal wall and pelvic girdle are relatively idle. Thus the so-called 'generalized' obesity due to exogenous causes tends in reality to become a trunk obesity.

When the obesity is gross the distribution may become so bizarre as to suggest that it is not generalized and it used to be classified into different groups that might suggest various aetiological—and particularly endocrine, such as 'pituitary' and 'thyroid'—factors. An example of typical juvenile obesity—not Fröhlich disease—is shown in *Fig*. 590.

'Constitutional' Obesity. There are cases of obesity in which there is a strong family history, and these may be classified as *constitutional*. In rare instances what has been described as *familial congenital adiposa macrosomia* is accompanied by a high birth-weight and a ravenous appetite developing immediately after birth. Rapid growth and extreme obesity result but death usually occurs within the first year of life. In other cases, such as in the family illustrated in *Fig*. 591, obesity is not present at birth and overeating does not commence until some months later, nor is early death a feature. There is often a high incidence of obesity among normal members of families in which genetic disorders with hypothalamic involvement occur, such as the Laurence-Moon-Biedl and Morgagni-Stewart-Morel syndromes. This suggests that the obesity, which develops not only in affected members but also in the otherwise normal sibs, is of genetic origin. Furthermore, there is some evidence for true genetic transmission of excessive appetite. In a study of identical twins 8 pairs of obese identical twins were found, but no pair in which one twin was fat and the other thin. Since the members of some of these pairs of obese twins were reared in entirely different environments their similar habits of over-eating were most probably genetic. The constitutional factor, however, does not play as prominent a part in the aetiology of obesity as might be imagined. Fat parents often have fat children because they are brought up in the indulgent surroundings of a well-stocked larder and sedentary recreations which have made the parents themselves fat. On the other hand it has been observed that women who gain weight with each pregnancy, which they do not subsequently lose, tend to give birth to abnormally large babies, and that such women themselves tended to have an abnormal high birth weight.

Endocrine Obesity. Another group of cases is classified as endocrine.

Thyroid deficiency is sometimes associated with obesity, though not nearly so frequently as is popularly supposed. The oedema and myxoedematous deposits which lie beneath the skin

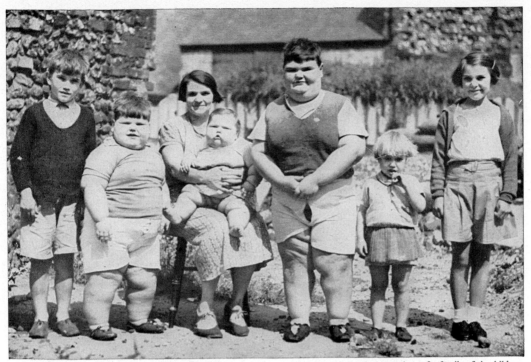

Fig. 591. 'Constitutional' obesity. To show the incidence of genetic adiposity affecting three members of a family of six children, the other children being normal. Ages from left to right are: 10½ years, 5¼ years, 11 months, 8½ years, 3¼ years, and 12 years. (*From 'Major Endocrine Disorders' (Oxford University Press), by courtesy of Dr. Leonard Simpson.*)

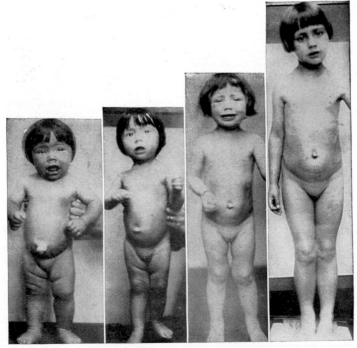

Fig. 592. Cretin. Pot-belly and umbilical hernia. Shows satisfactory effect of treatment with thyroid extract. (*H. G. Close, by kind permission of 'Guy's Hospital Reports'.*)

contribute largely to this excessive weight, as is dramatically shown in the first few days of thyroid therapy when the fluid pours from the body and the mucinous material melts away from the cutaneous tissues. Though the pot-belly and

region. The abdominal protuberance may suggest a full-term pregnancy, and is due to, or at any rate exaggerated by, the lumbar lordosis and

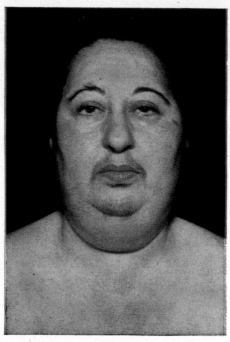

Fig. 593. Cushing's syndrome. Plethoric, 'moon-face' with hirsutism of upper lip and chin.

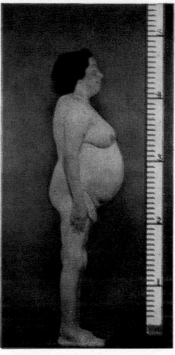

Fig. 594. Cushing's syndrome. Trunk obesity and wasted spindly legs: 'lemon-on-toothpick' distribution. (*Courtesy of the Photographic Department, Guy's Hospital. Dr. Peter Bishop's case.*)

umbilical hernia of the cretin (*Fig.* 592) may be typical features, obesity is not a characteristic finding in adult hypothyroidism.

Gonadal deficiency sometimes leads to a tendency to put on weight. In the eunuch the mammary region becomes prominent and flabby, and fat is deposited on the abdomen and around the pelvic girdle. On the other hand, the eunuchoid individual suffering from prepubertal testicular failure is usually lean and lanky. The 'middle-aged spread' of the menopausal woman may be to some extent associated with the waning ovarian function, though replacement therapy with oestrogen certainly has no slimming properties; indeed it may lead to increase in weight by causing fluid and salt retention.

Adrenocortical Obesity may vary considerably in its distribution. In classic cases of *Cushing's syndrome* (*Fig.* 593) it is confined to the face and neck, shoulder-girdle, and trunk. The pelvic girdle, hips, thighs, and legs are not involved and may even appear wasted owing to muscular atrophy (*Fig.* 594). The face becomes round like a full moon, and plethoric (*Figs.* 593, 595). The neck is thick-set, and there may be a cervicodorsal kyphosis—the buffalo hump—due to osteoporosis and even collapse of the vertebral column in this

the weakness of the abdominal muscles. The legs, thighs, and buttocks are wasted and spindly (*Fig.* 594) so that the bodily contours are those of a 'lemon-on-toothpicks', and the skin of the legs and shins is bruised and discoloured by the bursting of the superficial vessels under the thin and atrophied skin. A similar reason accounts for the purplish striae of the abdominal wall and axilla (*Fig.* 596). All these characteristic changes can be induced by exogenous administration of excessive amounts of corticosteroid (*Fig.* 597). In early and atypical cases of Cushing's syndrome, however, the obesity may be more generalized and it may be difficult to distinguish from simple obesity due to over-eating, especially as the appetite is characteristically increased in Cushing's syndrome. Indeed, in about 12 per cent of a large series of simple obesity striae somewhat resembling those seen in Cushing's syndrome were found, and in about 80 per cent of these there was biochemical evidence of adrenocortical over-activity. The cortisol production rate is higher than normal, and urinary metabolites of glucocorticoids and even the 17-oxosteroids are raised.

Pituitary Obesity: The over-quoted case of Fröhlich's patient with a tumour compressing the pituitary, and incidentally the hypothalamus, has established in the minds of some clinicians the concept of a condition of hypopituitary obesity

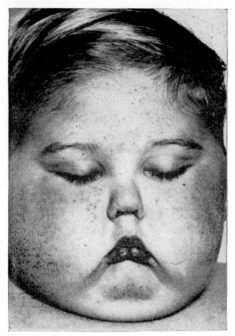

Fig. 595.—Cushing's syndrome in a child aged 2½ years. Note extreme moon-face producing 'sun-fish' mouth. It should be pointed out that though this facies is characteristic of Cushing's syndrome it may also occur in other children with extreme obesity—see 11-month child in Fig. 591.

or at any rate the idea that most cases of obesity are of endocrine origin, and many endocrinologists and other physicians spent much of their time dealing with fat women who demanded or were given prescriptions of pituitary, thyroid, and other endocrine extracts. More recently, the fashion has changed to slimming diets, though doctors who have to battle with the treatment of obesity which is an incurable disease admit that an attack on energy expenditure is more likely to lead to successful long-term results. Once obesity of alimentary origin has become well established it is beyond the strength of will to maintain a diet which will successfully control it, though a daily walk of a mile or two will sometimes achieve and maintain a reasonably successful result.

Obesity associated with Islet-cell Tumours of the Pancreas. It is not uncommonly found that islet-cell tumours of the pancreas are associated with obesity. This is primarily due to the hypoglycaemia produced by the excessive output of insulin. Patients suffering from hypoglycaemia, whatever its cause, often discover that they can relieve their symptoms by frequent eating and they therefore tend to put on weight.

Diabetes and Large Babies. Women who develop diabetes in later life—the 'fat' or 'lipoplethoric' type of diabetes—tend to give birth

to an unusually high proportion of large babies. This is probably due to excessive production of maternal growth hormone which may eventually give rise to diabetes, for it has been shown that a potent growth hormone extract can produce diabetes in dogs. This overactivity might give

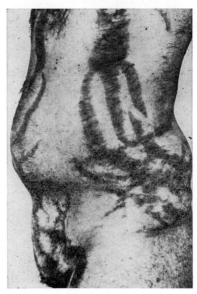

Fig. 596. Cushing's syndrome in a male. View of trunk and hips to illustrate striae.

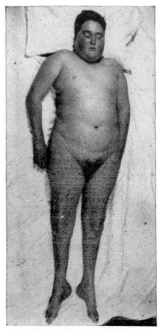

Fig. 597. Cortisone-induced Cushing's syndrome.

19*

rise to exceptionally large babies and a later tendency to diabetes in the mothers.

Lipodystrophy (*Fig*. 599). This curious condition is classified by some writers among the lipomatoses. The important feature, however, is

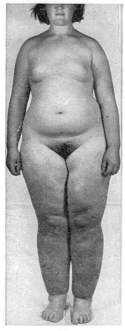

Fig. 598. 'Billiard table' legs. Possibly due to diffuse symmetrical lipomatosis of lower half of the body.

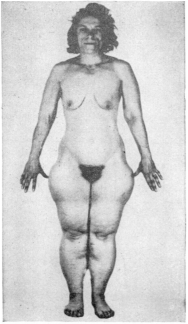

Fig. 599. Lipodystrophy: note loss of buccal pads, atrophy of breasts, contrasting with lower-body obesity.

probably not the obesity, which is typically of the lower body distribution, but the loss of subcutaneous fat from other regions, such as the cheek pads, breasts, etc. The aetiology is unknown. Many cases of lower-body obesity are probably due to diffuse symmetrical lipomatosis of these regions. It is characteristically found in these cases that even the strictest dieting has no effect upon the obese areas though flesh may be lost from the normal regions above the waist (*Figs*. 598 and 599).

Dercum's Disease. In this condition there is a distribution of obesity similar to that which occurs in the various types of 'exogenous' obesity. It is accompanied, however, by pain and tenderness in the more prominent fatty deposits. This may well be due to distension of the subcutaneous fatty lobules stimulating painful nerve-endings.

P. M. F. Bishop.

OBSESSIONS

Obsessions are thoughts and ideas which continually intrude into a patient's mind, despite efforts to keep them out. They are felt to have an alien quality and appear in consciousness against the patient's will. The patient, however, recognizes that the thoughts, however strange, are his. He does not, as the *schizophrenic*, believe they have been planted there by some outside agency. Obsessive thoughts tend to carry with them a compulsion to action which if not obeyed causes rising tension. This may lead the patient to strange and unaccountable behaviour from which he tries to desist but feels compelled to carry out. Thus, an obsession with the thought that his hands are contaminated and that some other person may come to harm thereby, by the transmission perhaps of some obsessively imagined form of contamination, may lead a patient into washing his hands a hundred times a day. Similarly a patient obsessed by the thought that everything he undertakes is certain to go wrong may feel that disaster cannot be averted unless he touches his desk three times before starting work and lays out his pens and pencils, etc., in a certain stylized way. The analogy between this and magical or superstitious ritual is patently apparent. Persistent thoughts and impulses in respect of a certain situation may lead the subject to avoid that situation and perhaps to develop a special fear of it, which itself resembles an obsession. Obsessive thinking (*rumination*) is that in which the patient is compelled constantly to turn some indifferent topic over in his mind, or to pursue some trivial question often of a metaphysical nature. It is characteristic of obsessive phenomena that the subject well knows them to be unreasonable, but cannot rid himself of them.

Some degree of obsessive behaviour is found in very many normal individuals, especially those who show some of the traits of the *obsessional* or *compulsive personality*; who are markedly orderly, precise, tidy, responsible, and scrupulous; who tend to have difficulty in making decisions; who over-adhere to routine, and tend to show undue irritability when this is disrupted in any way. Those who are obsessive by temperament tend to be guilt-ridden. If caught out, even in some minor lapse, their sense of shame may be disproportionate to the circumstance and such as to lead to an over-ready tendency to project the blame on to others. Certain traits, such as the checking and rechecking of facts and figures for accuracy, which spring from obsessive doubt, are in fact of some practical value, particularly in certain walks of life. Actions which have much in common with an obsessive pattern can often be seen in the play of children; for example, the careful arrangement of toys in a stereotyped manner. When, however, obsessive mechanisms have increased in range and obtrusiveness until the patient's daily life is cramped and hindered by them, the condition has passed beyond the limits of normal, and may be termed an *obsessional neurosis.*

An obsessional disorder can also occur as a manifestation of a *depressive* illness (*see* DEPRESSION, p. 209) and if so linked may disappear as the illness resolves. Similarly those who suffer from so-called *involutional depression* tend to be of somewhat obsessive pre-morbid personality. Severe obsessional symptoms are also common prodromata of *schizophrenic* reactions occurring either just before or together with the emergence of this psychosis. Obsessive rituals which become even more bizarre may be indicative of a schizophrenic development. Obsessional symptoms may also usher in a childhood psychosis of *autistic* type.

W. H. Trethowan.

OEDEMA, ASYMMETRICAL

While local oedema is nearly always due to a local cause, occasionally oedema resulting from a general or remote disease preponderates in one part and mimics the local variety. The possibilities are as follows:

A. LOCAL CAUSES:

1. *Congenital*—Amniotic bands, arteriovenous aneurysm.
   Hereditary—Milroy's (Meige's) disease (*see* p. 592).
2. *Traumatic*—Bruises, sprains, fractures.
3. *Infective:*
   a. Skin and subcutaneous tissues; boils, carbuncles, cellulitis, abscess, erysipelas.
   b. Deep tissues—osteomyelitis, infection by clostridia (gas-gangrene group).
4. *Venous Obstruction:*
   a. Thrombophlebitis: following pregnancy, surgical operation, or other conditions demanding recumbency.
   b. Weakness of wall causing back-pressure, not true obstruction: Varicose veins.
   c. Pressure from without: Glands, tumours, aneurysms. Also pressure from bands around limb; garters, ring of calliper, ligature by neurotics.
5. *Lymphatic Obstruction:*
   a. In the lumen: Filaria, metastatic carcinoma.
   b. In the wall: Previous cellulitis with resulting obliteration.
   c. Pressure from without: As for (c) *under* 'Venous Obstruction', *above.*
   d. Postoperative (*Fig.* 600).
   e. (Rarely) in rheumatoid arthritis.

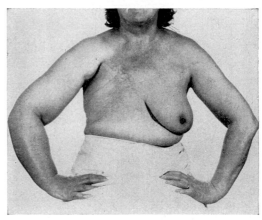

Fig. 600. Oedema of right arm following radical mastectomy.

6. The effects of stings, bites, and the like, caused by, for example, bees, wasps, ants, scorpions, tarantulae, snakes, jelly-fish, weaver fish, sea-cats, and nettles and other plants.

7. The local effects of excessive heat or cold: frost-bite; sunburn; scalds; burns.

8. The local effects of irritants and corrosives—from carbolic acid to mustard gas, not forgetting the possibility of unsuspected chemicals, for instance in artificially dyed furs.

9. Acute gout. Acute arthritis. Rheumatic fever.

B. GENERAL CAUSES:
Deficiency disease, including nutritional oedema.
Toxic, including drugs.
Allergic } Angioneurotic oedema to be grouped
Vasomotor } under one or both of these headings.

Oedema occurs in such diverse conditions and with such various significance that it is difficult to group the possible causes in a systematic manner. The oedema surrounding a carbuncle, for instance, is simply an integral part of the inflammatory reaction, has no separate existence, and has no diagnostic importance of its own, but only when considered with the lesion as a whole —a lesion easy to recognize. Although cardiac and renal oedema are seldom unilateral, the possibility should not be ruled out without examination of the two systems in order to avoid missing isolated cases when they do occur.

The pathological processes leading to the formation of oedema fluid are complex. Pressure inside the capillaries tends to push fluid out into the tissues, while the osmotic pressure of the plasma tends to draw it in. Changes in either of these forces upset the normal balance. Between the plasma and the tissues is the capillary wall, and defection of this also plays an important part in the production of oedema; even simple capillary dilatation alone may be sufficient cause. Experimental ligation of a vein such as the femoral does not result in oedema unless the main lymphatics are tied as well, and it is probable that some degree of thrombophlebitis, in which infected lymphatics may play a part, is necessary for the development of oedema.

In cases where the prime cause is back-pressure on the veins, seen perhaps in its purest form in cardiac failure, the oedema tends to pit readily on pressure, but where the lymphatics are blocked it is more solid. This may be helpful in diagnosis, but varying degrees of pitting are to be found between the two extremes, and much depends on the degree of the oedema and the tissues into which it occurs. There is a predilection for the fluid to gravitate into loose tissue and into dependent parts.

A. **Local Causes:**

1. *Congenital* causes are rare, and as a rule are identified easily.

2. *Trauma* is a common cause of localized oedema, occurring both at the time of the accident and sometimes for many months after; many people who have had an ankle sprain get recurrent oedema when they take exercise or remain standing for long. The same applies to fractures, especially those without displacement which have not been recognized at the time and have escaped treatment. Local blows and bruises also produce varying degrees of oedematous swelling. The diagnosis of a traumatic condition is usually obvious or can readily be made on the history; a radiograph should be taken in a doubtful case. Cases of traumatic oedema are often associated with a rarefying process of the adjacent bones, a condition commonly seen in the aged following sprained ankle or fracture of the lower ends of the tibia and fibula. This so-called 'Sudek's atrophy' may be accompanied by trophic skin changes and affects particularly the tarsal and metatarsal bones. It is a condition which is very unresponsive to treatment and may persist with crippling effects for years. Pressure to control the oedema and various methods for improving the circulation may be tried.

3. That an oedematous swelling is *infective* is suggested by the presence of local pain, redness, and heat, and by general symptoms of malaise and pyrexia; there may be leucocytosis. The skin infections such as boils and carbuncles can be recognized on inspection; the spreading raised red edge of erysipelas is characteristic, but the acute malady may be followed by a chronic oedema due to obstruction of the skin lymphatics which have been the seat of the inflammatory process.

Cellulitis may be difficult to diagnose from acute osteomyelitis; the latter causes graver general disturbance, while the presence of a possible septic focus on the overlying skin weighs the balance in favour of cellulitis. Cellulitis is frequently associated with lymphangitis and lymphadenitis of the regional lymph-nodes, whereas in acute osteomyelitis the paucity of lymphatics within bone and the fact that the infection is almost invariably with the *Staphylococcus* make these complications rare. It must not be forgotten, however, that once an osteomyelitis has burst through the periosteum a secondary cellulitis will develop, and lymphangitis or lymphadenitis may ensue. Radiographs may give help, but in an early case bone changes are not visible, and sometimes it is advisable to operate to settle the doubt; though a word of warning regarding acute gout is not out of place—acute gout may simulate acute cellulitis, and many cases have been operated on in error. Rheumatic fever, a post-infective condition, should also be borne in mind, especially when the oedema is in the vicinity of a joint. The 'flitting' nature of the affections and the presence of cardiac signs usually serve to distinguish this disease. Local asymmetrical oedema may occur in the region of any joint affected by acute or chronic inflammatory arthritis: although the joints are usually tender and obviously inflamed, in the ankles and feet swelling may be marked and resemble cardiac oedema. True lymphatic obstruction is rare in rheumatoid arthritis, the oedema being due partly to inflammatory changes in the adjacent joint, partly to stasis, the painful joint being moved less than usual. Chronic osteomyelitis may be the cause of some obscure cases of oedema, but once the possibility has been remembered the diagnosis can be made on the radiograph, and even without this in many cases thickening of the bone can be felt: while, if present, adherent scars indicating old sinuses or operations will provide the necessary evidence.

4. *Venous blockage* is commonly caused by thrombosis, in most cases more accurately called thrombophlebitis. It may arise during any prolonged debilitating malady such as typhoid fever, in which it is especially common, or with malignant cachexia, or one of the blood diseases such as leukaemia. The stasis and back pressure of varicose veins with or without thrombosis is a potent source of mild oedema. When none of these causes is present it is necessary to examine carefully to ascertain whether there is any *swelling pressing on and obstructing the veins*, such as an aneurysm in the popliteal space or a mass of malignant glands in the pelvis; and not only must the whole limb be examined, but also the rectum, vagina, and lower part of the abdomen, and the neck and upper thorax, in the case of the leg and arm respectively. For instance, there may

be a tumour, springing from some structure in the pelvis, causing pressure on the iliac veins; swelling of the arm may be caused by an aneurysm, subclavian or thoracic, or by a mediastinal new growth, in which case radiographic examination may be of material assistance in verifying the cause. Difficulty may arise where there is a thrombosis of one of the deep veins without any obvious reason. Sometimes this can be suspected by the noticeable dilatation of the superficial veins in setting up anastomotic channels to bridge the obstruction.

5. When the large *lymphatics are blocked* a condition of elephantiasis results which is probably in part due to concomitant attacks of inflammation. There is great thickening and induration of the tissues which may produce a grossly enlarged limb. The most striking examples are seen in filarial disease, which is uncommon in England. Lymphogranuloma venereum may produce a similar condition of the vulva, while it is sometimes seen in any part of the body as the result of repeated attacks of erysipelas—*see under* (3) *above.*

Carcinomatous spread along lymphatics by emboli or permeation is another important cause of lymphatic obstruction, and is typically seen in the breast where it gives rise to *peau d'orange,* and, if the axilla is invaded, to brawny oedema of the arm. In the case of the arm, venous obstruction due to pressure by the malignant glands probably plays an equal part.

The oedematous arm following radical mastectomy is, however, often due to an innocent fibrosis of the few remaining lymphatics and is simply caused by scar tissue at the site of the axillary dissection. X-ray therapy may aggravate this condition, and it is important therefore to be sure that the oedema is due to a recurrence of the carcinomatous process before this method of therapy is recommended. (*Fig.* 600.)

The conditions enumerated under headings (6) to (9), on p. 587, could be added to considerably, but in all the diagnosis depends upon the history and upon remembering the possibilities; there is nothing characteristic about the local oedema itself. The oedema of gout is part of the acute inflammation of the condition and is associated with great pain, redness, and heat of the tissues. The oedema in and around rheumatoid joints and in similar arthropathies is more often associated with a cold and clammy skin and is only occasionally red and warm to the touch.

When the diagnosis of the cause of the oedema of a limb is not obvious, lymphangiography and venography can be helpful.

B. **General Causes.** Angioneurotic oedema usually occurs on the face; it appears and disappears quite suddenly and is accompanied by irritation and burning. It is a vasomotor disturbance, probably allergic in nature and allied to the urticarias. It may occur in any situation, is commonly asymmetrical and occasionally afflicts several members of the same family. The other conditions mentioned in the list on p. 587 are diagnosed, not

by reason of the local oedema, but from the other symptoms presented by the case.

R. G. Beard.

OEDEMA, SYMMETRICAL

Oedema may be defined as an increase in the extravascular component of the extracellular body fluid. It results from derangement of the factors concerned in the circulation and character of tissue fluid. It will occur, therefore, in increased venous pressure; through diminution in the plasma proteins; by increased capillary permeability; and by obstruction to lymphatic drainage. To these must be added the influence of sodium retention and the action of the antidiuretic hormone secreted by the posterior pituitary.

Although the majority of cases can be explained by application of these principles, there remains a small group in which the pathology is little understood, a group consisting of otherwise healthy subjects whose sole complaint is swelling of the legs. These will receive consideration under an appropriate heading.

Owing to accidents of posture—such, for instance, as the patient sitting with one leg to the ground and the other supported upon a chair, or lying in bed turned well over to one side—it is possible for oedema which is in fact symmetrical to appear asymmetrical. Allowing for this source of fallacy, however, the causes of symmetrical oedema are different from those of OEDEMA, ASYMMETRICAL (p. 587). One may subdivide cases topographically into three main groups, namely: (1) *Those in which the oedema is universal;* (2) *Those in which the oedema involves the face, neck, and arms, but not the legs or the lower half of the trunk;* (3) *Those in which the oedema affects the legs, or the legs and the lower half of the trunk, but not the arms, neck, or face.*

Oedema of the legs is the commonest type; the important point in diagnosis is to decide whether this oedema is due to renal, cardiac, or to some other cause. The broad distinction between these groups is seldom difficult. The urine should be tested; if protein is present further urinary microscopical and bacteriological examination is necessary. If there is no protein in the urine, renal disease as a primary cause of oedema of the legs, although possible, is most unlikely. Estimation of the blood-pressure and other investigations will naturally be performed.

Failure of cardiac compensation is generally easy to diagnose, and the more common types of congestive cardiac failure will be considered and appropriately investigated. Other causes for oedema of the legs will be suggested by other symptoms or by the history but they cannot be diagnosed with certainty until both renal disease and heart failure have been excluded. Each of the main groups of symmetrical oedema may be discussed in greater detail as follows.

1. Cases in which Oedema is Universal. When the patient exhibits universal symmetrical oedema, the probability is that he is suffering from either *acute* or *chronic nephritis* or from one of the many causes of the nephrotic syndrome, such as syphilis, poisoning by heavy metals, renal vein thrombosis, diabetes (the Kimmelstiel-Wilson syndrome); systemic lupus erythematosus, and amyloid disease. The diagnosis is indicated by the occurrence of moderate to heavy albuminuria. The degree of oedema in different regions varies, partly by reason of inequalities in the looseness of the subcutaneous tissues in different places, and

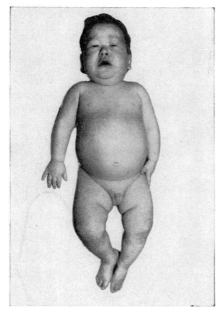

Fig. 601. Ascites and anasarca in nephrosis. (*Dr. P. R. Evans.*)

partly through the influence of gravity. Other things being equal, the oedema will be most evident in the legs, lumbar region (lumbar cushion), penis, scrotum, labia, eyelids, and face, though there may be some oedema in every tissue from scalp to toes (*Fig.* 601). The oedema is most marked in the legs when the patient is up and about, in the lumbar cushion and the genital organs when the patient is propped up in bed, or in the eyelids when the patient has been recumbent and asleep.

Other causes for universal oedema are rare. It may be due to *angioneurotic oedema*, though this is more often asymmetrical, or to overloading of the tissues with fluid—e.g., as the result of excessive transfusion or infusion.

Certain poisons may, though rarely, produce universal oedema. For instance, it is one of the effects of *snake-bite*, though as a rule the limb or other part bitten is very much more swollen

than is the rest of the body. In susceptible persons *food poisoning* causes generalized oedema, although urticaria is more usual. Shell-fish and strawberries are the commonest examples of foods responsible for such toxic or allergic reactions.

Aspirin affects certain individuals in a curious way, producing urticarial weals, transient as a rule, or lasting little more than twenty-four hours, though the reaction may be so severe that the whole face is swollen and bloated. The symptoms depend upon idiosyncrasy. *Potassium iodide* may produce a similar state of affairs. *Arsenic* is another drug which may cause universal oedema when given in excessive doses by the mouth; and organic arsenic administered intravenously has produced a state similar to generalized angioneurotic oedema.

Only in very rare cases and at the terminal stage does *heart failure* produce oedema of the hands and arms as well as of the legs.

Ancylostomiasis often causes oedema of the feet, ankles, and legs, as the result partly of the severe anaemia and partly of malnutrition. In the later phases of the disease generalized anasarca, similar to that of acute nephritis, is not uncommon, but by this time the nature of the malady has generally been diagnosed by reason of the progressive anaemia, eosinophilia, and the discovery of ancylostomata or their ova in the stools.

Chronic starvation, inefficient dietary, and circumstances of privation or want may cause a state of chronic oedema, but generally without proteinuria; such cases may be met with during conditions which lead to the description *war* or *famine oedema.* Hypoproteinaemia is the cause. Kwashiorkor is described elsewhere (p. 523). The generalized oedema of exceptional cases of *beriberi* comes into the same category since the condition is the result partly if not entirely of avitaminosis. Hypoproteinaemia and cardiac failure are the underlying features of such oedema.

It should be recalled that hypoproteinaemia may be produced by deficient intake, defective synthesis or absorption, or external loss of protein, so that oedema may result from a number of different conditions in which one or other of these may be concerned. Since the synthesis of plasma albumin is a function of the liver parenchyma, destruction of these cells as in hepatitis, cirrhosis, infiltration by leukaemia, or extensive destruction of liver tissue by other causes may cause a low level of albumin and consequent oedema. Similarly, any extensive loss of protein may be responsible, e.g., from the skin in exfoliative dermatitis. Defective digestion of protein may occur in chronic pancreatitis, or inadequate absorption of amino-acids may result from intestinal hurry, and in the steatorrhoeas the lowered osmotic pressure of plasma leads to loss of albumin, the so-called 'protein-losing gastro-enteropathy'. Serum-albumin may pass into the gut and so be lost to the body in diseases of the stomach and the small and large intestines ranging from post-gastrectomy syndrome to lymphoma, intestinal tuberculosis, and sclero-derma. Gross loss may also occur in high intestinal fistulae.

2. Oedema of the Face, Neck, and Arms, but not of the Legs or Lower Half of the Trunk, is nearly always due to obstruction of the superior vena cava or its main branches. The commonest causes of this obstruction are *mediastinal new growth*, *chronic mediastinal fibrosis*, *thoracic aneurysm*, and *thrombosis* spreading to the main trunk as from an axillary vein infected from a whitlow or other source of phlebitis in the hand or arm. Of these, obstruction of the superior mediastinum by a mass of tumour, together with secondary nodes, originating from bronchogenic carcinoma, is by far the most frequently seen. Acute nephritis may be simulated on account of the puffiness of the eyes; but further examination shows limitation of the oedema to the head and upper limbs, whilst albuminuria is not likely to occur. If the obstruction to the superior vena cava persists, evidence will be forthcoming of collateral circulation in the form of varicose veins upon the chest wall (*see* VEINS, VARICOSE THORACIC, p. 816).

Inflammatory lesions, although more usually asymmetrical, may sometimes produce almost symmetrical oedema of the face or neck. In this connexion may be mentioned *erysipelas, cellulitis, anthrax*, and *Ludwig's angina*, the differential diagnosis of which is based upon the history, the constitutional symptoms, the local appearances of the inflammation, and the results of bacteriological examination.

Similar symmetrical swelling may be produced in the face, hands, or arms by *angioneurotic oedema*. Swelling of the eyes and face suggestive of oedema can be produced by bouts of *crying*, prolonged attacks of *coughing*, as for instance in whooping-cough, or as the result of catarrh due to a *common cold, coryza*, or *measles*. In *trichiniasis* (a disease rarely encountered in Britain) oedema of the eyelids is a constant feature.

Oedema of face, neck, and hands may have its origin in an external irritant, such as impure *soap* upon sensitive skin, or the result of *occupational dermatoses*. The nature of the responsible irritant may in some cases be obvious—in satinwood workers, for instance, or in gardeners planting *Primula obconica* or *tulips*; or it may be more obscure—for instance, the effect of peeling bitter oranges in a jam factory. In the majority of such cases the development of vesicles, and other evidence of acute dermatitis, will generally be prominent. (*See also* BULLAE, p. 115.) Chemicals used in dyeing furs have been responsible for many cases of obscure oedema of the face and neck.

3. Oedema of the Legs and Lower Part of the Trunk, but not the Neck or Face, is suggestive of heart failure, of nephritis, or of cirrhosis of the liver, and the main points that arise in the differential diagnosis have been discussed above. If all these main groups of causes can be excluded, it should be remembered how often the legs may swell in any condition of anaemia. Various elements are contributory, such as venous stagnation, faulty muscular tone, anoxia from diminished blood-flow, increased capillary permeability, retention of sodium and water due to excess of the anti-diuretic principle of the posterior pituitary, as in premenstrual oedema. Some people are prone to oedema of the ankles on prolonged standing, and otherwise healthy persons suffer similarly in hot climates. Any of the severer types of anaemia may be responsible for oedema (*see* ANAEMIA, p. 25). *Cachectic conditions* such as result from carcinoma, sarcoma, syphilis, tuberculosis, starvation, malaria, and various tropical infections such as kala-azar may similarly operate. The differential diagnosis of these conditions will be found discussed under the heading of some other symptom arising from the particular malady.

Obstruction of the inferior vena cava may lead to extreme oedema of the legs. If due to *phlebitis*, the clotting of the inferior vena cava is nearly always preceded by that of the veins of one leg, so that even when the final result is symmetrical the history as a rule points to its having begun asymmetrically. When the inferior vena cava is obstructed by new growth or by a huge ovarian cyst, the diagnosis will depend upon the discovery of some abnormal abdominal mass. Pressure by the enlarged uterus is often responsible for oedema of the legs in pregnancy but other factors are contributory. Operative ligation of the inferior vena cava, in an attempt to prevent recurrent pulmonary emboli, may be followed by gross oedema.

A more innocent cause of oedema of the legs due to prolonged immobility in a sitting position with the legs dependent is represented by the so-called 'shelter oedema' during the last World War.

Interference with venous circulation may result from compression by the cross-bar of a deck-chair during prolonged sitting. The same effect is produced by lack of leg movement in long acroplane journeys.

The action of the vasomotor nerves in controlling the balance of fluid production and absorption in the legs is sometimes interfered with. One sees in this an explanation for the oedema which develops in the lower extremities in *convalescent patients* when after having been long in the horizontal position they begin walking. It is probable that even a perfectly normal person kept at rest in bed for three months would suffer from oedema of the legs in varying degree for some days or weeks after first resuming the erect attitude. Similarly oedema of legs, ankles, and feet is common in rheumatoid arthritics, who, because of involvement of weight-bearing joints, are unable to get about. Diseased conditions or functional disturbances of the vasomotor system may produce even more marked oedema, as seen in *elderly people*, some cases of *Raynaud's disease*, and other causes of trophoedema especially in young women, in *angioneurotic oedema*, and in association with *peripheral neuritis* in *beriberi.*

The condition of elephantiasis, well recognized in filariasis, is due to obstruction to lymph drainage from recurrent inflammation. Malignant nodes in both groins, e.g., from a penile cancer, may result in bilateral lymphoedema.

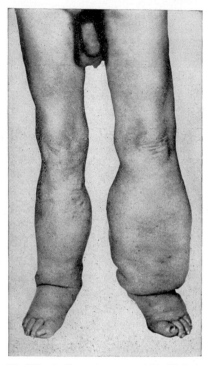

Fig. 602. Milroy's disease in a man of 74. He had never been abroad.

There is a peculiar hereditary disease in which oedema of the lower extremities, occurring in several members of a family, is a prominent feature (*Fig.* 602). This may present at birth (congenital lymphoedema) but much more often onset is delayed (lymphoedema praecox) and may not even occur until after the early thirties (lymphoedema tarda). In the early stages this oedema is asymmetrical, but sooner or later both legs become affected, so that if the family and personal history were not known the oedema of nephritis might be suspected. The affection is known as *Milroy's disease*. The abrupt demarcation between the swollen and the non-swollen parts at the level of a joint—ankle, knee, or hip—is distinctive. Associated with an increase in the swelling there is sometimes a history of periodic acute attacks of pyrexia. The swelling may cease at the ankle in the early stages; when a subsequent spread occurs it may reach almost suddenly up to the knee, ceasing there for a variable number of years until ultimately it reaches to the groin above which it seldom

extends. The scrotum, penis, or vulva may be implicated. At first pitting can be produced, later the swelling is semi-solid and fixed. The cause is a congenital anomaly of the draining lymphatics of the lower limbs. Lymphangiography demonstrates either aplasia, hypoplasia (commonest), or gross varices of the lymph-channels.

Myxoedema is a condition in which the swelling or thickening of the legs may closely simulate actual oedema, and in some cases the subcutaneous tissues of the feet and legs do pit on

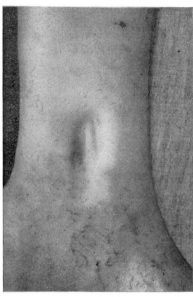

Fig. 603. Oedematous leg in cardiac failure showing deep pit produced by pressures. (*Dr. R. G. Ollerenshaw, Manchester Royal Infirmary.*)

pressure (*Fig.* 603). When there is true oedema as well as myxoedema, suspicion will arise of the co-existence of a cardiac or other factor. The diagnosis of myxoedema will be confirmed if the familiar symptoms and the abnormal state of the subcutaneous tissues disappear under thyroid medication.

A curiously localized pre-tibial myxoedema has been observed in subjects of past or present thyrotoxicosis. It is not relieved by thyroid administration but may spontaneously disappear. It may be uni- or bilateral.

In India and other countries in the East, sporadic outbreaks of *epidemic dropsy* arise. There is usually oedema of the legs with purple mottling of the overlying skin. Retinal haemorrhages, pyrexia, signs of bronchitis, and microcytic anaemia may be present. The condition affects those who habitually use mustard oil in the cooking of their food. Presumably some toxic product of this oil, possibly an impurity, is responsible.

Harold Ellis.

ONE EXTREMITY (LOWER), PARALYSIS OF

The diagnosis of the conditions in which paralysis of both legs occurs is dealt with under PARAPLEGIA (p. 618). It is, however, a common experience to find signs pointing to a bilateral affection when the patient is only aware of disability affecting one lower extremity. A common example of this is afforded by many cases of disseminated sclerosis. The patient complains of weakness in one leg, but there is exaggeration of both knee-jerks as well as extensor plantar responses on both sides. The various types of crural monoplegia may be divided roughly into two classes, one of which includes those cases without muscular atrophy; and the other those which present greater or less degrees of muscular wasting.

movements to the same extent. If the movements of the various joints are tested against the observer's resistance, it will generally be found that hip flexion, dorsiflexion of the ankle, and flexion of the knee are affected more than other movements; the patient tends to drag his toes more on the affected side than on the other, and evidence of this is often forthcoming in the fact that he wears away the toe of the corresponding boot. This is due to spasticity rather than weakness. The muscles of a spastic leg show no localized wasting, and present no alteration from the normal in their response on electromyography.

In diagnosing the level of the lesion which gives rise to spastic paralysis of one leg, certain considerations are of particular importance: if the lesion is situated immediately above the lumbar enlargement of the cord, the abdominal reflexes can be obtained; if the lesion is at the

Zone of Hyperaesthesia

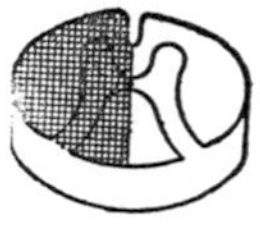

Local effects	Atrophic paralysis	No local effects
	Painful and thermal loss	
	Loss of all reflexes	

Spastic paralysis		No paralysis
Not constant	Loss of sense of position and passive movement	Loss of sensibility to painful and thermal stimuli usually only to within 4 or 5 segments of the lesion
	Loss of tactile discrimination	

Remote effects	Diminished skin reflexes	Normal skin reflexes
	Increased tendon reflexes	Normal tendon reflexes
	Ankle-clonus	No clonus
	Extensor plantar response	Flexor plantar response

Fig. 604. Diagrammatic representation of the results of a one-sided lesion of the spinal cord—Brown-Séquard syndrome.

Paralysis of One Leg without Muscular Atrophy. The cases in this class may be subdivided into two groups, the first comprising those in which the pyramidal tract is affected, and the second those in which there is no evidence of pyramidal affection.

Spastic paralysis of one leg may result from a lesion of the pyramidal tract in any part of its course, but for anatomical reasons it is more likely that the paralysis will be confined to one side when a lesion affects the opposite cerebral hemisphere above the pons, i.e., above the level at which the two pyramidal tracts run in close proximity. Spastic paralysis of one leg may, however, result from a lesion at any level, and the diagnosis of the level must be made from a consideration of other symptoms. In all cases the condition of the leg is qualitatively, if not quantitatively, the same. A spastic leg is characterized by a certain amount of weakness and rigidity, exaggeration of knee-jerks and ankle-jerks, and an extensor plantar response. The weakness in a spastic leg does not affect all the

level of the 10th dorsal segment, the lower abdominal reflex on that side will be absent, while the epigastric reflex remains intact. A lesion of any of the upper dorsal segments causes abolition of all abdominal reflexes on the corresponding side. A lesion above the cervical enlargement leads to some, even if slight, weakness in the corresponding arm, in which the tendon-jerks will be exaggerated. A lesion of the higher part of the pons or of any level between the pons and the cerebral cortex usually produces some asymmetry in the facial movements as well as weakness in the arm and leg.

Disseminated sclerosis has been mentioned already as a disease in which spastic paralysis of one leg may result from a lesion situated in the spinal cord. In all probability evidence of other patches of disease will be discovered in such cases if careful examination is made; intention tremor in one or both hands, nystagmus, diplopia, optic atrophy, and sphincter troubles are among the signs which may be forthcoming. Less commonly, a one-sided affection of the spinal cord above the lumbosacral enlargement is due either to some intramedullary disease, such as a *new growth*, a *gumma*, an asymmetrically placed *syringomyelia*, or an *extramedullary neoplasm*. When this occurs there may arise a symptom-complex to which the term *Brown-Séquard syndrome* is applied, in which there is spastic paralysis of the leg on the same side as the lesion together with loss of sensibility, especially of thermal and painful sensibility, in the opposite leg. The physical signs in Brown-Séquard syndrome are summarized in the accompanying diagrams (*Figs.* 604, 605).

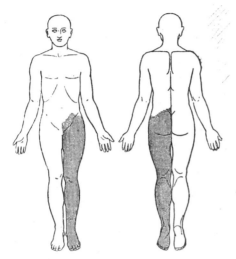

Fig. 605. Brown-Séquard syndrome due to an intramedullary one-sided lesion (right) of the lower thoracic cord. The shaded area was insensitive to pain and to all degrees of temperature, but sensitive to touch. The sense of passive movement and position and tactile discrimination were disturbed in the right foot. There was spastic paralysis of the right leg only.

Amyotrophic lateral sclerosis usually manifests itself by an initial wasting of muscles in the upper extremities, and this is followed by spastic weakness of the legs, but occasionally the pyramidal signs appear first, either in one leg or in both; in such a case it may be months before the onset of wasting in the upper limbs or trunk indicates the true nature of the malady.

A lesion of *the superior part of the precentral gyrus*, such as may be caused by a bullet wound, a meningioma or other tumour, thrombosis of the anterior cerebral artery, or a cortical venous thrombosis, will give rise to spastic weakness in the opposite leg; if the disease is situated on the medial aspect of the hemisphere, weakness may be greater in the thigh than in the foot. A tumour of this region—usually a meningioma arising from the falx cerebri—often causes bilateral signs, but unilateral weakness may be present in the early stages, and sphincteric symptoms are common.

Hysterical paralysis of one leg usually presents little difficulty in diagnosis. The affected limb may be either rigid or flaccid; there is no true muscular atrophy and no alteration in the muscular response to electrical stimulation. The reflexes provide most information; in hysterical paralysis the knee-jerks and ankle-jerks may be exaggerated, but they are never lost, true ankle-clonus is never obtained, and the plantar response is either absent or of the flexor type; as a rule the tendon reflexes in the opposite unaffected limb are found to be equally brisk. In contradistinction to spastic paralysis resulting from a pyramidal lesion, in which hip flexion, dorsiflexion of the ankle, and flexion of the knee are the movements most profoundly affected, the movements of the leg in a case of hysterical paralysis are more or less equally deficient at all joints and in all directions. Certain attitudes and certain types of gait are almost characteristic of hysterical paralysis of one leg; in one form the whole leg is kept rigidly extended, and the foot strongly inverted, so that the patient walks on the outer plantar edge with a stiff leg; in another form the leg is flaccid and is dragged behind the opposite limb with the toes scraping the floor; in some cases examination of the limb when the patient is at rest in bed reveals little or no paralysis, but in the attempt to stand or walk the limb appears to be quite useless. Hysterical paralysis of a leg may be associated with similar palsies of the opposite leg, or of the arm on the same side (hysterical paraplegia, hysterical hemiplegia). More often than not a leg which is the seat of hysterical paralysis also presents complete insensibility to all forms of stimulation, and the upper limit of such anaesthesia may correspond abruptly to some level for which there is no neuro-anatomical basis—to the line of the knee, for instance, or the groin. As in all cases of hysteria, diagnosis depends on (1) absence of 'organic' signs, (2) demonstration that the symptoms of which the patient complains can be altered by suggestion, (3) the presence of a psychiatric cause for the condition.

In the early stages of *paralysis agitans* a patient may complain of 'weakness' in one leg, and the diagnosis may present considerable difficulty if the characteristic tremor of this disease has not made its appearance. Examination of the limb may show little abnormal. Some slight stiffness to passive movements may be detected but no alteration in the character of the reflexes will be observed. The diagnosis depends more on the general aspect and the attitude and gait of the patient. Some loss of facial expression, the general slowness of his movements, and the tendency to shuffle with the affected leg, are points which may lead the observer to form a correct opinion.

Paralysis of the Leg with Muscular Atrophy. In a case which presents atrophic palsy of one leg, the first essential for making a diagnosis is to ascertain the exact distribution of the atrophied muscles, and to review this distribution in the light of the known central and peripheral innervation of the muscles of the lower limb.

Single-nerve palsies are not so common in the lower extremity as in the upper, but they may occur, especially as the result of injury. Isolated *paralysis of the femoral nerve* and of the *obturator nerve* is uncommon; they are generally the result of compression of the nerve within the abdominal cavity, either by a new growth or during the act of parturition. In affections of the femoral nerve the movements of flexion of the thigh on the trunk and extension of the leg upon the thigh may both be impaired or lost. Wasting of the anterior thigh muscles and diminution or loss of the knee-jerk are other signs of this condition. When the *obturator nerve is injured* the patient can flex his hip but cannot adduct the thigh, and so, when sitting, he can raise his knee but cannot throw it across the other leg. He can walk about with no obvious disturbance of gait, but he cannot rotate the thigh either outwards or inwards with any degree of force.

Paralysis of the main trunk of the sciatic nerve, which would include paralysis of all the muscles supplied by the tibial (internal popliteal) and common peroneal (external popliteal) nerves, points to disease or injury affecting the pelvis. It may be brought about by a fracture of the pelvis or of the upper end of the femur, or by injuries to the hip-joint; or the sciatic nerve may be compressed by a tumour, or by an inflammatory mass within the pelvis. Complete paralysis has been observed to follow difficult labour, from pressure upon the lumbosacral plexus by the foetal head. Sensory recovery is usually early and complete, but flaccid weakness of the 'sciatic' muscles persists and is particularly severe in the peronei and anterior tibial group. Such an extensive palsy has considerable effect on the patient's gait; he is unable to flex the knee, and consequently has to use the leg as a stiff, extended support; the disability is increased by the absence of all movements at the ankle-joint. The sensory loss in such a condition includes the outer side of the leg and the whole of the foot, except a small area on its inner and upper aspect.

Palsy of the *common peroneal (external popliteal) nerve* is the commonest isolated nerve palsy in the leg; the nerve is exposed to pressure and to direct injury as it winds around the fibula. It is liable to be picked out by lead poisoning and by leprosy, and is more severely affected than the tibial nerve in disease or injury of the sciatic nerve itself. Isolated paralysis of the external popliteal nerve has been observed frequently in tabes dorsalis. It may arise through prolonged squatting, as an occupational risk. Its most obvious result is a dropped foot and high-stepping gait to enable the patient to clear the ground with his toes.

Injury to the *tibial (internal popliteal) nerve* is less common. Paralysis of the calf muscles is the chief consequence, preventing the patient from extending his foot and standing on tiptoe, or from making any springing movement in an attempt to walk or run. The paralysis of the interossei and the unopposed contraction of the long extensors may lead to CLAW-FOOT (p. 162).

In addition to the peripheral nerve palsies of the lower limb, we have to consider weakness due to lesions of the nerve-roots, the cauda equina, and the anterior horn cells of the lumbosacral segments. As they pass through the intervertebral and sacral foramina, the roots are liable to be implicated by *fractures, dislocations, caries,* and *neoplasms* of the vertebral column. *Herniation of the L.4–5 intervertebral disk* may rarely compress both the 5th lumbar and the 1st sacral roots; as a rule, pain is more prominent than objective weakness or sensory loss, but exceptionally there is gross wasting and weakness of the glutei, hamstrings, and muscles below the knee. A similar condition—spreading sometimes to involve the quadriceps—is seen in severe *spondylosis* of the lumbar spine; here there is narrowing of the disk spaces between the vertebrae, and both degenerative and inflammatory processes in the intervertebral joints and the adjacent dural sheaths around the emerging roots. *Herpes zoster* is occasionally accompanied by a lower-motor neuron type of paresis in one or more muscles of the affected limb. *Infective radiculitis,* a disease of acute onset characterized by severe pain, the rapid onset of paralysis and wasting in muscles supplied by one or more roots, slight sensory loss of radicular distribution, and slow, partial recovery from paralysis, is usually seen in the upper limb and shoulder-girdle, but it may involve the leg. It occurs sporadically, with epidemic exacerbations, and almost always follows some febrile illness, or a sore throat, or inoculation or vaccination. It is liable to be mistaken for poliomyelitis unless care is taken to demonstrate the sensory loss. *Disease of the cauda equina* (tumours, meningitis serosa circumscripta, posterior herniation of intervertebral disks) usually affects both legs, but only one limb may be involved in the early stages of these conditions. *Poliomyelitis* furnishes the most common of all causes of flaccid weakness of the leg. The entire limb may be affected, or the distribution may be characteristically patchy; diagnosis is made by the history of the onset, and is often helped by the discovery of weakness, or an absent tendon reflex, elsewhere in the body. The weakness and wasting are not, as a rule, progressive, but they may appear to get worse if the limb is systematically overstrained. Thus a man who has had a wasted leg since boyhood may find the muscles wasting if he is called upon to undergo military training. *Tumours, syphilitic meningitis,* and *syringomyelia* will, on occasion, destroy anterior horn cells of the lumbosacral segments and so give rise to flaccid weakness of the leg; sphincter symptoms are the rule in such cases. *Disease of the muscles* is an exceptional source of unilateral weakness and wasting. The *progressive muscular atrophy* of motor neuron disease may sometimes first appear in the lower limb. *Peroneal muscular atrophy* is usually symmetrical, or approximately so, but it has been known to appear in a limb many months before the other was affected. Finally, weakness and wasting of peripheral distribution occur in association with peripheral sensory loss and loss of the Achilles reflex, as a result of *thrombosis of the femoral artery* in elderly subjects. The diagnosis is liable to be missed when, as sometimes happens, the collateral circulation is sufficient to maintain the health of the skin and gangrene is thereby avoided.

Ian Mackenzie.

ONE EXTREMITY (UPPER), PARALYSIS OF

The word 'paralysis' has come, by general use, to include the partial as well as the complete palsies, and to embrace all varieties of impaired voluntary movement. Accurate diagnosis is often difficult when the limitation of voluntary movement is only slight. Before discussing the various forms of paralysis met with in the arm, reference must be made to a few practical points which are important in the proper investigation of cases complaining of inability to use an arm. The medical man must not be satisfied with the patient's statement that he has lost power or that he is weak in his limbs. Tests must be employed to ascertain whether this is really the case. The movements at each joint, of flexion, extension, pronation, supination, must be investigated, and their power measured against the observer's resistance. It may be found that the grasp is powerful in a patient who is unable to use his hand on account of loss of control over the finger movements. In such a case there is not paralysis, but incoordination. Similarly, there is certain to be difficulty in carrying out delicate movements if there is loss of touch or postural sensibility. Without perfect sensibility it is impossible to handle a pen in a proper manner. Sometimes a patient will complain of loss of power, when investigation shows that the ability to execute movements is inhibited by the pain in a muscle or joint evoked by the attempt. In other instances mechanical limitation of movement by arthritic changes, without pain, may lead the patient to believe that there is loss of power. He finds he cannot lift his arm, and ascribes the disability to paralysis instead of to ankylosis of the shoulder-joint. On the other hand, pain and loss of power may be associated. If the patient says 'My arm is so painful that I cannot lift it', it must be ascertained whether the inability is due only to painful inhibition or to real paralysis in addition.

Stress must be laid upon the necessity for obtaining a careful history, and especially an accurate account of the duration of the trouble, whether its onset was sudden, rapid, or slow and progressive, and whether the loss of power was accompanied or preceded by pain, numbness, or tingling. The family and previous history must not be neglected. When examining the paralysed arm, care should be taken that the whole of the body is stripped, because it will also be necessary to carry out a full neurological examination. This is imperative even when no complaint is made of loss of power or other symptoms in any part of the body except one upper limb. The importance of this full examination is perhaps obvious, but it may be illustrated by reference to two points. A lesion of one internal capsule may give rise to paralysis of the opposite arm, but it will be likely to cause, in addition, some alteration in the abdominal and leg reflexes of the corresponding side. Similarly, a lesion of the 8th cervical and 1st dorsal spinal segments, or of their corresponding spinal roots, will also affect the fibres leaving the cord at that level and passing, via the cervical sympathetic, to the eye of the same side. In this way atrophic paralysis of the muscles of one hand may be associated with a small pupil and a ptosis on the same side, a coincidence which at once points to the cord or roots as the site of the lesion, and acquits the peripheral nerves of being concerned in the production of the palsy. In such a case the further investigation of the abdominal reflexes, the knee-jerks, and plantar responses will help to decide whether the lesion is intramedullary or extramedullary; in the former event the abdominal reflex on the same side would be absent, the knee-jerk would be increased, and the plantar response would be of the extensor type, while in the latter, *unless there was considerable pressure on the cord*, the reflexes below the arm would be normal.

For purposes of differential diagnosis, brachial palsies may be divided into two main groups: (1) *Those without*, and (2) *Those with*, *muscular atrophy*.

1. PARALYSIS WITHOUT MUSCULAR ATROPHY

This heading embraces: (1) Cases in which there is some affection of the upper motor neuron system (pyramidal lesions); and (2) Cases without a lesion of the pyramidal tract.

Paralysis due to Pyramidal Tract Lesions. The most familiar example of this group is afforded by cases of brachial monoplegia due to a *vascular lesion* (*thrombosis*, *haemorrhage*, or *embolism*) *in the internal capsule* or other part of the pyramidal tract in its course through the brain. In the diagnosis of this condition the points of importance are: The presence of some cardiovascular condition capable of producing the lesion, such as disease of the heart, kidneys, or arteries; the sudden or rapid onset of the symptoms, with or without loss of consciousness or other cerebral disturbance. The arm retains its natural contours, and the muscles are not atrophied, although they may appear, after some time has elapsed, to be smaller than those of the other arm. The paralysis may affect the whole limb and include inability to shrug the shoulder; or the movements of the hand and fingers may be more impaired than those of the elbow and shoulder. There is a tendency for the arm to exhibit more and more resistance to passive movement, that is to say, to develop spasticity. At the same time, if left to itself, the limb will adopt a fixed position, which includes adduction of the upper arm to the trunk, flexion and pronation of the forearm, and flexion of the wrist and fingers. If any movements are possible, they will be those of flexion rather than of extension at the various joints. The muscle tone is increased, and the tendon-jerks, such as the triceps, biceps, and supinator jerks, are exaggerated when compared with those of the opposite limb. Eventually contractures may develop, and it will be found impossible to extend the upper arm, forearm, hand, and fingers into one straight line. In elderly subjects, adhesions around the joints, especially the shoulder-joint, contribute to the immobility of the limb and interfere with recovery of movement.

Such is the clinical picture afforded by spastic paralysis of the arm, and one case will differ from another only in the degree of spasticity and the degree of paralysis; but the amount of spasticity and the paresis do not always correspond. In one patient the spasticity forms the chief obstacle to voluntary movement; in another the arm, though powerless, shows comparatively little increase in tone.

The fact that the pyramidal fibres destined for the face, trunk, and leg run in close proximity to those for the arm is sufficient reason for suspecting that, even if no other paralysis is complained of, there may be signs of disturbed function in other parts. The side of the face corresponding to the paralysed arm may not move so quickly or so powerfully as the other side in a voluntary effort to show the teeth, although no difference may be detected when the patient smiles. The corresponding abdominal reflexes may be found wanting, the knee-jerk may be increased, ankle-clonus and an extensor plantar response may be elicited: all on the same side.

The spastic arm, in all degrees of severity, may result not only from a vascular lesion in the brain but also from thrombophlebitis of cortical veins, cerebral abscess, tumour, or non-suppurative encephalitis. The arm will present identical features, so that the diagnosis must be made from a consideration of other data. Thus *cortical thrombophlebitis* and *cerebral abscess* only become likely when there is some infective process either in the bones of the skull (e.g., mastoid or frontal sinus disease) or in a distant part such as the heart or lungs (e.g., ulcerative endocarditis or bronchiectasis). Headache, vomiting, and papilloedema with a slow pulse, slow respiration, and subnormal temperature may help in the diagnosis, but are present only when the intracranial pressure has increased rapidly. In cases of *cerebral tumour* the development of the brachial palsy is nearly always slow and progressive, spreading from one part of the limb to another, and again there may be headache, vomiting, and papilloedema. It should be remembered, however, that these signs of increased intracranial pressure

are not always present, and that the presence of a tumour is always to be suspected when a spastic paralysis of one limb comes on in a slow and progressive manner. Some tumours grow at the expense of neighbouring tissues in such a way that pressure is raised little or not at all.

Encephalitis will need to be considered when there is a history of acute constitutional disturbance with fever, vomiting, headache, and perhaps convulsions preceding or attending the onset of the paralysis. The latter, however, is not progressive. It reaches its maximum in a few hours, and shows a general tendency to improve after the acute symptoms have passed off. In some cases of epidemic encephalitis the disease is ushered in by an attack of hemiplegia, the arm perhaps being the part chiefly affected.

Disseminated sclerosis is another disease in which a spastic monoplegia is not uncommon. The diagnosis is easy if it occurs as is usual late in the disease, when nystagmus, optic atrophy, spastic paraplegia, and sphincter trouble are already present, or if there is a history of previous transient palsies affecting other limbs. When, however, paralysis of one arm is the first symptom, diagnosis may be difficult. The gradual onset of the palsy in a healthy young adult, without constitutional disturbance, severe headache, or vomiting, and perhaps the discovery of absent abdominal reflexes and an extensor plantar response, should direct suspicion to the possibility of a patch of disseminated sclerosis being responsible for the trouble.

Diseases of the pons, medulla, and that part of the spinal cord which lies above the cervical enlargement, whether vascular, inflammatory, or neoplastic, may cause spastic palsy of the upper limb, but it is rarely a monoplegia. The arm and leg on one side, or both arms and both legs (quadriplegia), are much more likely to be involved in series, and the site of the lesion is inferred from the knowledge that the two pyramidal tracts are in close proximity in those regions.

Paresis in Extrapyramidal Lesions. It is not uncommon for a patient in the earliest stage of *paralysis agitans* to complain of loss of power in one arm. In early cases weakness is less obvious than rigidity, the limb is stiff and is slow in carrying out movements. The characteristic tremor may be absent or may only appear when the patient is nervous or excited; when present, the rigidity, as distinct from mild spasticity, is present throughout the full range of movement at a joint in both directions. A lack of expression in the face, absence of the natural swing of the arm in walking, and perhaps some hesitancy in the gait, should guide the observer to a correct diagnosis even if tremor is absent, as it often is, at this stage of the malady. This form of paralysis is unattended by changes in the reflexes. A somewhat similar form of plastic rigidity, with or without tremor, is seen in severe *arteriosclerotic cerebral degeneration*; it usually affects the neck, trunk, and limbs, and is often associated with paralysis of conjugate movements of the eyes in one or more directions, with bulbar palsy ('pseudobulbar palsy') and with intellectual loss.

A child suffering from *chorea*, and especially hemichorea, is often brought to the doctor with the complaint that he or she has lost the use of an arm. Examination will show that there is really some weakness of the affected limb, which is demonstrated, not so much by the poorness of the grasp, as by the fact that the child is unable to maintain a steady pressure. He will grasp the observer's fingers, but quickly release the pressure, although urged to continue the squeeze. In the same way, when asked to put out his tongue he will do so, but withdraw it at once. When required to extend his arm in front of him with the palm of the hand facing downwards, it will generally be noticed that the wrist is slightly flexed although the fingers are extended. These are points which may be useful in coming to a right conclusion when choreic movements are not conspicuous; but attention must also be paid to the condition of the heart and to any history of rheumatism. No information of value can be obtained from the reflexes unless perhaps the pendular form of knee-jerk is present.

Hysterical brachial palsy may resemble one due to a pyramidal lesion in presenting marked rigidity, or the whole limb may be flaccid and limp. Some general wasting of the muscles may be present, but there is no alteration in their electrical reactions. Organic pyramidal lesions must be excluded by an examination of the reflexes. The supinator, biceps, and triceps jerks may be elicited, but they will not be appreciably more brisk than those of the opposite limb. The abdominal and plantar reflexes will be normal. If the limb is rigid the observer will probably be able to overcome the rigidity by steady pressure, and to extend the arm, forearm, hand, and fingers into one straight line. When the patient is asked to perform a certain movement the observer can often see that in the effort to carry it out the antagonistic muscles are put into action rather than, or as well as, those which are necessary for its execution; thus, the triceps will contract as well as the biceps when the patient is requested to flex the elbow, with the result that the forearm is moved very little or not at all. This may also be demonstrated when the observer resists the movement of flexion by grasping the wrist and then unexpectedly relaxes his resistance; in an organic palsy this will be followed by further uncontrolled flexion at the elbow, whereas in a hysterical patient the contraction of the triceps maintains the forearm in its former position.

Another important point in distinguishing a palsy of cerebral origin from one which is hysterical is that in the organic case, even when no voluntary movement whatever can be carried out by the fingers, they may move involuntarily in association with energetic movements in the opposite limb. Thus, when the patient is asked to grasp some object as tightly as he can with the sound hand, flexion of the fingers may be detected on the paralysed side. The same phenomenon is seen in connexion with involuntary movements, such as yawning. In many, if not most, cases of hysterical palsy of an arm, the limb is also anaesthetic, and this anaesthesia can generally be recognized as hysterical on account of its complete character. In a cerebral palsy there is nearly always some impairment of postural sensibility, even if tactile, painful, and thermal sensibility is intact; but the hysterical patient is usually insensitive to all forms of stimulation, even pinching or a strong faradic current. Moreover, the distribution of the anaesthesia does not correspond to any form seen in organic disease, and is frequently of a glove or sleeve type with a very sharp line of demarcation.

Diagnosis depends on the demonstration of inconsistencies and the presence of psychoneurosis. Hysteria is a positive condition, and its clinical manifestations are the result of an emotional conflict. The somatic disability represents a subconscious attempt to avoid responsibility and to attract attention and sympathy; the inward conflict, so difficult to maintain, is converted into an outward and physical 'disease'.

2. PARALYSIS WITH MUSCULAR ATROPHY

In this category are included all cases of atrophic brachial palsy due to disease of the lower motor neuron or of the muscles themselves; weakness and wasting secondary to arthritis, periarticular disease, and bone lesions are excluded.

Destruction of the anterior horn cells or of their efferent fibres causes weakness, flaccidity, wasting, fibrillation, depression or loss of tendon reflexes, and changes in the electrical excitability of motor nerves and muscles. Affections of the larger mixed nerves are often complicated by paraesthesiae, sensory loss, and sympathetic paralysis with loss of sweating in the area of skin affected.

The Spinal Cord. *Poliomyelitis* is an extremely common cause of atrophic palsy of one or more muscles in the upper limb. The onset is rapid, usually with fever and pain, and paralysis of the affected muscles reaches its maximum very quickly, within twenty-four hours of the first feeling of weakness. Exceptionally, a second crop of paralyses occurs a few days after the first. Atrophy sets in rapidly, tendon reflexes are lost, sensation is normal, and sweating is unaffected. Contractures occur later in neglected cases. The reaction of degeneration is present in the weak muscles, and electromyography demonstrates the presence of fibrillation even if this is not visible to the naked eye, a fact useful in establishing subclinical degrees of motor impairment. The disease sometimes attacks only one limb, but it is more usual to discover that muscles or groups of muscles have been affected elsewhere as well. Progressive wasting does not usually occur after the initial three months, but excessive use of the weakened limb may appear to cause an increase of wasting and aggravation of weakness. Exceptionally, motor neuron disease starts in the weakened limb. *Motor neuron disease* occurs in adults and takes three forms—amyotrophic lateral sclerosis, with a lower motor neuron lesion in the arms and an upper motor neuron lesion in the legs, and secondly, progressive muscular atrophy, in which pyramidal signs are absent. The third variant of the disease, bulbar palsy, may be atrophic, spastic, or atrophic-spastic, and it often terminates the course of amyotrophic lateral sclerosis and progressive muscular atrophy. But they are all forms of the one disease. In *amyotrophic lateral sclerosis*, atrophic palsy of the upper limbs— usually starting in the small muscles of the hands —is accompanied by pyramidal signs in the legs. The wasting is accompanied by fibrillation, which may precede it. The tendon reflexes in the upper limb are brisk, and remain so *as a rule* until the muscles concerned in the reflex are completely paralysed. Sensory loss and sphincter disturbances do not occur. In *progressive muscular atrophy* there is weakness, atrophy, and fibrillation, with normal or depressed reflexes depending on the degree of wasting, normal sensibility, and a normal plantar response. Progress is usually slow and intermittent; the wasting may be confined to one arm for months or even years, but close examination of the muscles of the trunk and other limbs will often reveal fibrillation or a commencing atrophy which has escaped the patient's notice. Rarely, flaccid weakness comes on rapidly and spreads widely, with a fatal issue in a few months. A clinical picture similar to amyotrophic lateral sclerosis occasionally occurs as a result of a syphilitic meningomyelitis; the course of syphilitic amyotrophy is more rapid, the tendon-jerks and the jaw-jerks tend to be reduced rather than exaggerated, and the Wassermann reaction will be positive in the blood and spinal fluid. *Syphilitic pachymeningitis* of the cervical region may give rise to root pains, paraesthesiae, sensory loss, and atrophic palsies in one or both upper limbs, a condition which is clearly very different from syphilitic amyotrophy. *Syringomyelia* is an important cause of atrophic palsy in the upper limbs. It often starts in the small muscles of one hand, to which it may be confined for a long time. The tendon reflexes are lost, fibrillation is present, and there is the characteristic loss of pain and temperature sensibility, more or less symmetrically disposed in the two upper limbs and the upper part of the trunk and neck. Interference with the cervical sympathetic is often to be found, in the shape of a small pupil (spinal miosis) or in a fully developed Horner's syndrome. Expansion of the syringomyelic cavity may ultimately cause spastic weakness below the level of the lesion, by pressure upon the pyramidal tracts.

Tumours of the spinal cord are relatively uncommon. If intramedullary, and situated within the lower four cervical and first thoracic segments, they give rise to atrophic weakness of brachial muscles, with loss of tendon reflexes, fibrillation, and both motor and sensory signs below the level of the lesion; the clinical features may thus closely resemble those of syringomyelia, but are more rapid in evolution and progress. A lesion of the 6th cervical segment is accompanied by inversion of the supinator reflex; the normal response—flexion of the elbow and slight flexion of the fingers—is replaced by a simple flexion of the fingers. Extramedullary tumours are more likely to produce root pains, spastic weakness of the lower limbs, and a comparatively late onset of sensory loss, in that order; atrophic weakness of the muscles supplied by the segments directly involved by the tumour may or may not be obvious at an early stage. Wasting of the intrinsic muscles of the hands is an interesting feature of some tumours of the upper cervical segments in the region of the foramen magnum; this curious finding is perhaps the result of pressure upon the anterior spinal artery, whereby the anterior portion of the 8th cervical and 1st dorsal segments is exposed to a relative ischaemia. On theoretical grounds it should be possible to differentiate between intra- and extramedullary tumour of the cord, but experience shows that it is undesirable to place too much reliance on clinical evidence alone, and contrast myelography is indispensable for diagnosis. Even with radiological assistance, it is sometimes wiser to operate and inspect the tumour than to assume that it is intramedullary and therefore beyond the reach of surgery.

Peroneal muscular atrophy, a heredofamilial condition, is caused by degeneration of the ventral horns and, to a lesser extent, the posterior horns and peripheral nerves. Although it usually starts with wasting of the muscles of the feet, ascending to involve the distal portions of the peronei and anterior tibial group and ultimately attacking the intrinsic muscles of the hands and the muscles of the forearm, the upper limb is sometimes the first to be affected. There is wasting, weakness and fibrillation in the affected muscles and electromyography shows signs of denervation but since the proximal muscles of the arm are unaffected the tendon reflexes are preserved. Sensory loss is slight, peripheral, and often confined to impairment of vibration sense. The condition is usually symmetrical.

In *dystrophia myotonica*, a rare familial disease of children and of adult life, wasting and weakness of muscles is associated with myotonia, which is evoked by voluntary contraction and by percussion of affected muscles. Both wasting and myotonia occur in the face, sternomastoids, the muscles of the hands and forearms, the quadriceps, and the anterior tibial group (p. 557). The tendon reflexes are lost in advanced cases. Premature baldness, cataracts, and testicular atrophy occur in some cases and are seen by themselves in other members of the same family who escape the full brunt of the disease.

In *myotonia congenita* (Thomsen's disease) myotonia induced by voluntary effort exists from early life in several members of the affected family, but unlike dystrophia myotonica, muscular development is exceptionally fine and atrophy does not occur until late in the disease, and then only in a minority of cases. A curious feature of the disease is that sufferers therefrom are seldom aware—in the early stages—that there is anything wrong with their muscles, and the diagnosis is therefore liable to be missed unless the characteristic slowness of relaxation after effort, and the myotonia evoked by percussion, are deliberately sought for by the physician.

Amyotonia congenita (Oppenheim's disease) is a familial condition manifesting itself within the first months of life by the presence of extreme weakness, profound hypotonia, and absence of tendon reflexes. Some die from intercurrent infection; of those that survive, many appear to improve, but atrophy of muscles, which is hard to assess in plump infants, becomes more obvious; it is especially marked in the limb girdles and the proximal muscles of the limbs, in which respect it resembles the myopathies. *Werdnig-Hoffmann paralysis* is a rare condition which bears a close resemblance to amyotonia congenita in respect of weakness, hypotonia, and absent reflexes, but this disease is more rapidly progressive and is always fatal. Opinion is divided as to whether these two diseases are not in fact different manifestations of an identical pathology.

In fact diffuse muscular hypotonia with muscular weakness has a multiple aetiology, including hypotonia due to mental defect and a benign form, so that the term 'amyotonia congenita' is best discarded and an attempt made to identify the pathological process.

Disease of the Spinal Motor Roots is an important cause of atrophic palsy in the upper limb. Extramedullary tumours, fracture-dislocations, and spinal caries are liable to involve both the cord and the roots. Syphilitic infiltration of the meninges (*pachymeningitis cervicalis hypertrophica*) and *meningeal fibrosis* secondary to cerebrospinal meningitis are rare causes of damage to the motor roots and the anterior horn cells from which they spring.

Herpes zoster is occasionally accompanied by paralysis of one or more muscles within the affected segments; this is due to a spread of the inflammation to the meninges and the ventral horns.

Root lesions without involvement of the cord are seen in infective radiculitis, herniation of intervertebral disks, and spondylosis of the cervical spine. *Infective radiculitis* (syn. paralytic brachial neuritis, neuralgic amyotrophy) is a disease of acute onset which usually occurs some ten days or so after a cold, tonsillitis, or other febrile illness. It is probably identical with the 'serum neuritis' which causes paralysis of muscles five to twelve days after the administration of antitoxic or antibacterial sera. There is severe nagging pain in the muscles which are to become affected, and paralysis usually comes on after four to five days. It may involve any muscle or group of muscles, but the spinati, deltoid, serratus anterior, and biceps are most often affected. Slight sensory loss is found in the skin supplied by the affected roots, thereby distinguishing the condition from acute anterior poliomyelitis. Recovery is slow and sometimes incomplete. *Herniation of the C.5–6 or C.6–7 disks* causes pain, moderate weakness, and wasting, with reflex and less commonly sensory changes in the distribution of the affected root, which will be the 6th and 7th cervical root, respectively. Severe degrees of atrophic palsy are rarely caused by disk lesions of the cervical region. In spondylosis, the roots and their dural sleeves are liable to compression and inflammation; since the condition is not confined to one vertebra, several roots may be involved; pain and paraesthesiae therefore tend to be more diffuse than in simple herniation of a single disk. X-ray confirmation is usually available, but the incidence of spondylosis in elderly subjects is so high that it must not be too easily assumed that changes seen on the radiograph are necessarily the cause of the disability in the upper limb.

The Brachial Plexus is liable to injury at birth. Downward traction on the arm in a breech presentation may rupture the upper end of the plexus (C.5–6), with consequent paralysis and atrophy of the spinati, deltoid, brachialis, biceps, and brachioradialis. The arm hangs by the side internally rotated at the shoulder with the elbow straight, and the fingers flexed, the palm of the hand pointed backwards ('like a policeman taking a tip'). This is known as Duchenne-Erb paralysis. A similar condition resulting from falls on to the tip of the shoulder is referred to as Erb's paralysis. In both cases the motor disturbances are similar to those produced by a lesion of the 5th and 6th segments of the cervical cord, but there are none of the sensory and pyramidal signs which necessarily occur below the level of the lesion in the latter. A second form of obstetrical palsy, described as Klumpke's paralysis, results from injury to the lower cord of the plexus (C.8–D.1), by downward traction on the arm in a vertex or shoulder presentation. Atrophic palsy occurs in the intrinsic muscles of the hand and in the flexors of the wrist and fingers, and there is sensory loss in the medial border of the forearm and hand and in the ring and little fingers. Horner's syndrome may be present if the roots themselves have been torn. Atrophic paralysis and sensory loss of variable distribution are an obvious and common result of *gunshot wounds and stab wounds* of the brachial plexus. Wasting of the small muscles of the hand, with pain, paraesthesiae, and sensory loss of ulnar distribution, are occasionally caused by upward extension of *chronic inflammatory disease* from the apical pleura and by a similar spread of an *apical bronchial carcinoma* (Pancoast's tumour).

CERVICAL RIB. The brachial plexus and subclavian vessels cross the uppermost rib as they pass into the axilla. This may be a normal first rib, an ill-formed rudimentary first rib, or a cervical rib. The last may be a well-developed ossified structure or a fibrous band, but in either case it joins the first thoracic rib lateral to the insertion of the scalenus anterior, at the point where the brachial plexus and vessels pass into the axilla. Such a rib or band tends to angulate the nerves and vessels and to produce friction during respiration and in movements of the shoulder and upper limb, and this in its turn may give rise to pain and paraesthesiae in the ring and little fingers, and atrophic palsy of the small muscles of the hand (see below). But cervical ribs often give rise to no symptoms at all, and though they are present from birth symptoms are uncommon before middle life. It is apparent that some other factor or factors must be concerned in the production of symptoms. The most important, so far as is known at present, is descent of the shoulder-girdle, a normal feature of adult life but one which is aggravated by fatigue, thoracic scoliosis, weakness of the trapezius, and bad postural habits. The consequent drooping of the shoulder stretches the vessels and nerves over the abnormal rib, and the friction which then occurs may give rise to a reactionary fibrosis; the friction, plus the fibrosis, causes symptoms. Even in the absence of a supernumerary rib, similar clinical effects follow irritation of the neurovascular bundle by a normal first rib, or by a rudimentary first rib, when the affected shoulder sags, or as a result of the factors mentioned above. In some cases the descent of the shoulder appears to be associated with overaction of the scalenus anterior, which is thought by some to compress the lower part of the plexus between its lateral tendon and the first rib; whether this explanation is correct or not, it is certainly true that symptoms similar to those produced by a cervical rib, but occurring in its absence, are sometimes cured by freeing the scalenus anterior from its insertion and so allowing it to retract out of the way. Further, sagging of the shoulders so alters the anatomical relationships of the thoracic outlet that abduction and retraction of the arms cause compression of the neurovascular bundle between the clavicle and the uppermost rib. This costo-clavicular compression may itself produce symptoms and signs in the absence of a cervical rib, and will aggravate the condition if a rib is present. The clinical aspects of cervical ribs, the scalenus syndrome, and costoclavicular compression have both similarities and differences, and since the three mechanisms may exist in varying combination, the clinical picture may be complex.

Cervical ribs do not always cause symptoms. There may be pain behind the clavicle and down the inner aspect of the arm and forearm, with paraesthesiae in the ring and little fingers. These symptoms are aggravated by carrying heavy weights and by wearing a heavy overcoat. Friction on the plexus causes atrophy and weakness of the interossei, the thenar and hypothenar muscles, and the long flexors of the fingers and wrist (Fig. 606). Fibrillation may be seen in the affected muscles, and slight sensory loss is sometimes found in the medial two fingers and the ulnar border of the hand and forearm. To this essentially neurological picture there may be added symptoms and signs of vascular origin— Raynaud phenomena and chilblains, persistent

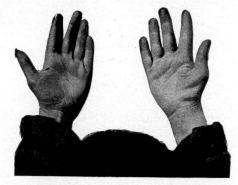

Fig. 606. Atrophic palsy of the right hand associated with a long 7th cervical rib of that side. Note the marked wasting of the abductor pollicis as compared with the other muscles of the thenar eminence. According to Dr. S. A. K. Wilson this is a common feature of these cases, but it is not pathognomonic. (Dr. P. W. Saunders.)

cyanosis of the hand, diminution or even loss of the radial pulse. The subclavian artery is subjected to friction and to costoclavicular compression, and this may lead to thrombosis or even to the formation of an aneurysm at the site of compression. If thrombosis occurs, ischaemia gives rise to pallor of the hand, paraesthesiae in all the fingers, claudication of the forearm and hand, and, in elderly subjects, to necrosis of the finger-tips.

Weakness and atrophy are uncommon in uncomplicated costoclavicular compression and in the scalenus syndrome. When they are present, they are usually similar to those of cervical rib, but of milder degree. In costoclavicular compression, vascular symptoms are predominant. There is aching pain in the shoulder, paraesthesiae in all the fingers, and a feeling of weakness in the limb. These symptoms are intensified by abduction of the arm, by using the hand above the level of the shoulder as in doing the hair or painting a ceiling, and by recumbency, so that paraesthesiae are worse at night. These symptoms may come on for the first time in middle age after a period of prolonged and unwonted physical work, and are more common in females than males. A troublesome form comes on in the late stages of pregnancy, usually disappearing after parturition and recurring in subsequent pregnancies; this behaviour is related to the postural readjustments which take place in pregnancy. Care must be taken not to confuse these symptoms with those due to compression of the median nerve in the carpal tunnel, for in the latter there are also complaints of paraesthesiae in the hand on waking in the morning, with or without wasting of the thenar eminence. In the carpal tunnel syndrome, however, the paraesthesiae rarely involve the ulnar distribution in the hand alone.

Atrophic Palsy in Peripheral Nerve Lesions. The circumflex (axillary) nerve is liable to injury by fractures of the neck of the humerus, by dislocation of the shoulder, by the use of an unpadded

which may be confined to a small patch over the first interosseous space. Inability to extend the wrist impairs the mechanical efficiency of the flexors of the fingers, so that the grasp is weakened, a circumstance which may lead to an erroneous diagnosis of a coincident lesion of the median nerve. Wrist-drop is a familiar feature of certain general affections—lead poisoning, leprosy, alcoholic neuritis—but in these

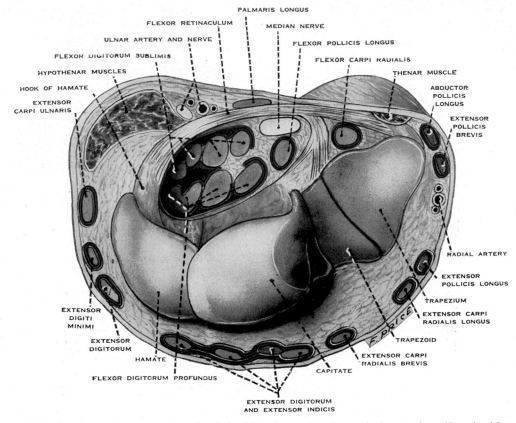

Fig. 607. Section through the carpus to show the relations of the flexor retinaculum to the flexor tendons. (*Reproduced from 'Textbook of Human Anatomy', by W. J. Hamilton, by kind permission of Macmillan & Co. Ltd.*)

crutch, and by penetrating injuries of the axilla and shoulder. The deltoid is paralysed and there is an area of sensory loss over the proximal half of the lateral aspect of the arm. Paralysis of the *radial nerve* occurs in fractures of the shaft of the humerus, pressure from callus, gunshot wounds of the axilla and arm, and not infrequently from sitting with the arm suspended over the back of a chair. With lesions in the neighbourhood of the shaft of the humerus, the triceps escapes, but there is paralysis of the brachioradialis and of the extensors of the wrist and fingers, with consequent wrist-drop and paralysis of finger extension. There is a somewhat variable loss of cutaneous sensibility over the radial border of the forearm and the radial half of the dorsum of the hand

conditions the weakness is not wholly confined to the radial distribution. Paralysis of the *median nerve* is usually due to penetrating injuries of the arm or forearm. If the lesion is above the elbow, atrophic palsy involves the pronator teres, flexor carpi radialis, palmaris longus, flexor digitorum sublimis, flexor pollicis longus, pronator quadratus, the inner half of flexor digitorum profundus, the muscles of the thenar eminence, and the lateral two lumbricals. Sensory loss and absence of sweating are limited to the median distribution in the hand. *Compression of the median nerve in the carpal tunnel (Fig. 607)* has long been known to cause wasting of the muscles of the thenar eminence, with paralysis of abduction and opposition of the thumb, and cutaneous sensory loss over the thumb, index, middle, and radial half of the ring finger. This florid picture is rare.

More recently it has been found that milder forms of compression are responsible for acroparaesthesiae in the hand even when signs are slight or absent. This is now referred to as the carpal tunnel syndrome.

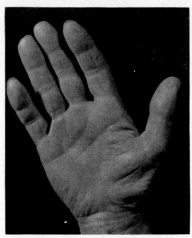

Fig. 608. Carpal tunnel compression showing wasting of abductor pollicis brevis.

It occurs mostly in women and usually for no apparent reason. In men there is likely to be a discoverable cause as, for example, arthritis of the wrist, ganglion of the wrist joint, acromegaly or myxoedema. These causes also operate, of course, in women in whom pregnancy may be an additional precipitating factor.

The early symptom is usually intermittent tingling of the fingers of one hand, often waking the patient from sleep. This tingling may spare the little finger and is sometimes most prominent in the ring and middle fingers. If the tingling is severe it may be accompanied by pain at the elbow or even in the shoulder.

As the condition progresses the patient may find in the morning that the fingers feel swollen and are numb. Later, symptoms may occur during the day and are brought on by use of the hands. Finally, abnormal signs may appear. These consist of weakness and wasting of the abductor pollicis brevis (*Fig.* 608) and sensory impairment within the distribution of the median nerve in the hand, both of which may be quite slight.

The condition is relieved by division of the flexor retinaculum at the wrist.

The *ulnar nerve* is frequently injured by penetrating wounds of the forearm, and it is particularly liable to pressure where it lies behind the medial epicondyle of the humerus. This occurs if the groove in which it lies is shallow, in which case it is subject to recurrent injury, as in clerks, telegraphists, and others whose occupation entails resting the elbow on a hard table. Cubitus valgus, whether congenital or as a result of fractures in the region of the elbow, predisposes to this traumatic neuritis. Pain is rare, but paraesthesiae and wasting of the interossei, the hypothenar muscles, and the medial two lumbricals cause discomfort and disability. Sensory loss of ulnar distribution, and a palpable thickening of the nerve at the elbow afford confirmatory evidence as to the nature of the condition. An *occupational palsy* of the muscles supplied by the deep branch of the ulnar nerve is seen in long-distance cyclists, who lean heavily on the handlebars, and also as a result of using a file—the instrument is held in one hand, and downward pressure is exerted by resting the hypothenar eminence of the other hand on the end of the file. Weakness and wasting are confined to the interossei and there is no sensory loss. Ulnar paralysis may be the sole manifestation of *leprosy*. *Polyarteritis* may cause atrophic palsy and sensory loss in the distribution of any peripheral nerve or combination of nerves and the neurological features are usually associated with the systemic signs of the disease. *Progressive hypertrophic neuritis* (Dejerine-Sottas disease) is a rare condition, often hereditary, characterized by the onset between the ages of 10 and 40 of a slowly progressive atrophic paralysis of the peripheral muscles of the limbs, with distal sensory loss, impairment of reflexes, and great thickening of the peripheral nerve-trunks. The hands may be affected before the legs, or vice versa. Weakness and wasting are late in appearance in *Friedreich's ataxia*, but a comparatively early wasting of the small muscles of the hands has occasionally been noted.

Diseases of Muscles. Atrophy and weakness of the muscles of the shoulder-girdle and upper arm occur in the heredofamilial *myopathies* (syn. muscular dystrophies). There is no sensory loss, and electrical reactions of the affected muscles remain normal for many years. *Dystrophia myotonica* (syn. myotonia atrophica) is characterized by prolonged relaxation of muscle after voluntary effort and wasting of the face, sternomastoid, the muscles of the forearm and hand, the quadriceps, and the anterior tibial group. The condition is familial, commences in or about the third decade, and is often associated with premature baldness, cataract, and testicular atrophy.

Ian Mackenzie.

OPHTHALMOSCOPIC APPEARANCES

PHYSIOLOGICAL VARIATIONS IN THE NORMAL FUNDUS

A Physiological Cup (*Fig.* 609) varies in size, but usually occupies the centre of the disk. The retinal vessels dip over the edge, which is usually steeper on the nasal side, the temporal slope being more gradual. At the bottom of the cup is seen the lamina cribrosa, which is mottled by the openings through which the retinal nerve-fibres pass.

The physiological cup may be absent altogether, or when present may be filled with

A physiological cup is distinguished from that caused by glaucoma (*Fig.* 624, p. 607) by the fact that it occupies only the centre and not the whole of the disk.

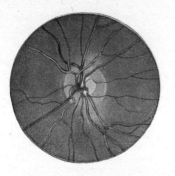

Fig. 609. Physiological cupping of the disk.

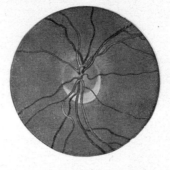

Fig. 610. Congenital crescent of the disk.

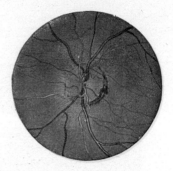

Fig. 611. Pigmented crescent at the disk margin.

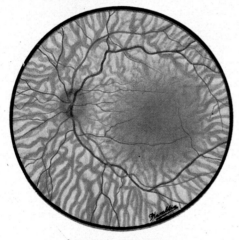

Fig. 612. Albinotic fundus, with cilio-retinal artery on nasal side.

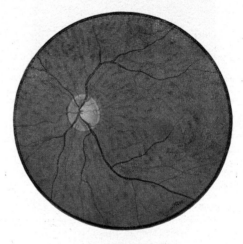

Fig. 613. Tigroid fundus.

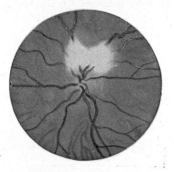

Fig. 614. Opaque nerve-fibres in the retina.

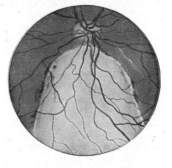

Fig. 615. Coloboma of the choroid.

embryonic connective tissue which blurs the details; the vessels may sometimes bifurcate before reaching the level of ophthalmoscopic visibility, when many are seen to enter and leave the disk instead of the single artery and vein.

Congenital Crescents (*Fig.* 610) are common, and usually situated at the lower part of the disk, in contrast to myopic crescents (*Fig.* 617), which are more usually seen on the outer side. They are probably due to an uneven distribution of connective tissue in the lamina cribrosa, and are often associated with hypermetropia. When the condition is marked and associated with evident

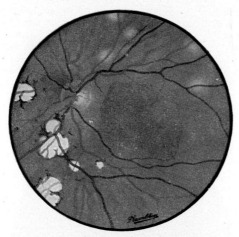

Fig. 616. Choroiditis, active and healed.

Pigmented Crescent at the Disk Margin (*Fig.* 611). The disk margin is often more or less pigmented, the amount varying from a small crescent to a complete ring. The pigment has no pathological significance.

The degree of pigmentation of the fundus varies considerably. When it is slight, the choroidal vessels are plainly seen—albinoid fundus (*Fig.* 612); when it is intense the appearance of tigroid fundus is presented (*Fig.* 613). The appearances often correspond to the complexion of the patient.

Cilio-retinal arteries and cilio-retinal veins are often seen. They enter and leave at the disk margin instead of the centre.

Opaque Nerve-fibres (*Fig.* 614) exist normally in the retinas of some mammals, e.g., the rabbit, and are occasionally present in man. They are due to the persistence of myelin sheaths in a patch of the nerve-fibres anterior to the lamina cribrosa; there may be a short interval between the disk and the opaque patch of the fibres.

The condition may be recognized by the brilliant white colour of the nerve-fibres, the

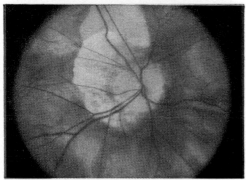

Fig. 617. Myopic crescent and chorio-retinal atrophy. (*Institute of Ophthalmology.*)

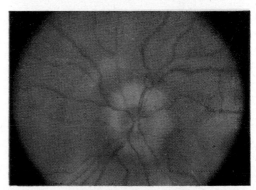

Fig. 618. Papilloedema. (*Institute of Ophthalmology.*)

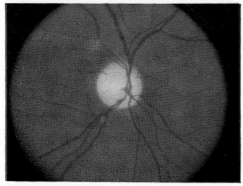

Fig. 619. Primary optic atrophy. (*Institute of Ophthalmology.*)

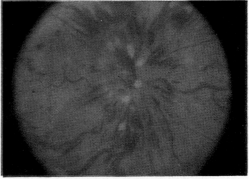

Fig. 620. Thrombosis of the central retinal vein. (*Institute of Ophthalmology.*)

distortion of the disk itself, it reaches the pathological and is referred to as *Fuch's coloboma*; astigmatism or hypermetropia is often high, and normal visual acuity unobtainable in spite of the correction of the refractive error.

striated appearance of the white patch, and the fact that the retinal vessels are more or less embedded among the nerve-fibres.

The retina may show congenital pigmentation, small oval or round greyish-black spots being found on ophthalmoscopic examination. They are similar to the melanomata of the iris. Colloid excrescences are seen as multiple oval or round yellowish spots, especially in the central fundus. They are so common in later life as to be justifiably considered a normal variation; they do not affect vision.

Pseudo-papilloedema. In marked hypermetropia the physiological cup may be absent, the disk pink, and the margin ill-defined; the vessels may be tortuous though not dilated, and unless the error of refraction is observed, the condition may be mistaken for papilloedema.

Choroiditis. A patch of active choroiditis shows itself as a greyish-white, ill-defined, slightly raised area. Vitreous opacities are commonly associated with active choroiditis. When healed, the patch is white, either from exposure of the underlying sclera or from the formation of fibrous tissue, and generally surrounded by pigment. Choroidal vessels may be seen in, and retinal vessels on, such areas (*Fig.* 616).

The Myopic Crescent (*Fig.* 617) is usually found on the outer side of the disk and may vary in size and extent from a thin crescent to a large atrophic area surrounding the whole disk

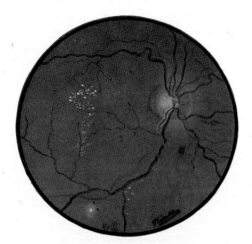

Fig. 621. Hypertensive retinopathy.

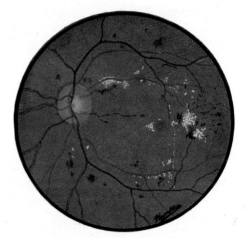

Fig. 622. Diabetic retinopathy.

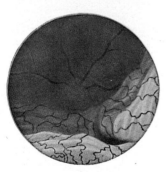

Fig. 623. Detachment of the retina.

PATHOLOGICAL APPEARANCES OF THE FUNDUS

Coloboma of the Choroid (*Fig.* 615) is a congenital defect, and it may be recognized by its situation, which is usually below the disk, as an oval area of exposed sclera, that may extend from the periphery and include the optic disk, the small amount of pigment at the edge of the white area, and the presence of healthy retinal vessels on its surface. It may be associated with other congenital abnormalities, such as coloboma of the iris, optic disk, or lens.

(posterior staphyloma). Usually the size of the crescent varies with the amount of the myopia and increases with age. Considerable difficulty may be experienced in viewing a highly myopic fundus even through a dilated pupil; a concave lens must be interposed behind the sight-hole of the ophthalmoscope corresponding to the refractive error.

Papilloedema and Papillitis (an anteriorly situated optic neuritis, in contrast to the more frequent 'retrobulbar neuritis') (*Fig.* 618) are characterized by the swelling of the disk and the blurring of its outline by retinal oedema. The retina is greyish and striated in appearance, owing to oedema between the retinal nerve-fibres, and the veins are dilated and tortuous. Flame-shaped haemorrhages may also be seen on the disk and in the surrounding retina, and numerous small retinal vessels on the disk, usually invisible, become dilated and apparent. In the later stages of the papillitis the haemorrhages may disappear, and the whole disk become greyer and paler, the condition ultimately terminating in 'consecutive optic atrophy'. The outline of the disk is lost and in severe cases the disk may be so swollen as to resemble a small mushroom in shape. The two conditions may be very difficult to distinguish ophthalmoscopically; but in a papillitis the visual acuity is lowered, while in a papilloedema due to increased intracranial tension there is usually only an enlargement of the blind-spot.

Optic Atrophy (*Fig*. 619) is characterized by the pallor of the disk, white or bluish-white, sharply defined lamina cribrosa, well-marked edge, and retinal vessels of normal size. When the atrophy follows a papilloedema (a 'consecutive atrophy'

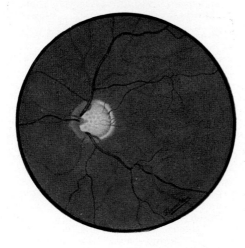

Thrombosis of the Central Retinal Vein (*Fig*. 620) makes the disk extremely swollen and oedematous, the edge being indistinct and blurred. All the retinal veins are enormously dilated and tortuous, and the fundus is covered with flame-shaped and petechial haemorrhages. The oedema of the retina from the obstruction of the venous

Fig. 624.   Glaucomatous cupping of the disk.

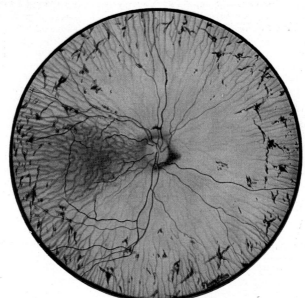

Fig. 625.   Retinitis pigmentosa.

-–*Fig*. 618), oedema residues may fill the physiological cup, the colour is then greyish-white, the retinal vessels are thin and tortuous, and the edge of the disk is irregular.

Sometimes a suitably situated space-occupying lesion will cause optic atrophy on one side by direct pressure and papilloedema on the other through the raised intracranial pressure—the Foster-Kennedy syndrome.

circulation may be so great that the vein may occasionally be hidden entirely. The condition occurs more commonly in the middle-aged or elderly, and is usually precipitated by an associated sclerosis of the central retinal artery.

Thrombosis of the Central Retinal Artery presents a pale grey retina, owing to the secondary retinal oedema. The macula itself does not share in the general retinal oedema, and appears as a bright cherry-red spot in contrast. The retinal arteries and veins are extremely narrow. The optic disk is blurred and pale.

Renal Retinopathy is characterized by the presence of flame-shaped haemorrhages in the nerve-fibre layer of the retina, and white patches. The white patches are of two kinds. Those seen in the early stages of the disease are ill-defined 'cotton-wool spots', scattered irregularly about the macular region. In the later stages, smaller white patches may be seen in lines radiating from the macula, well defined and glistening.

Hypertensive Retinopathy (*Fig.* 621) often resembles both renal and diabetic retinopathy, and evidence of vascular disease may be visible in all three. The arteries are small, show a heightened reflex (silver- or copper-wire arteries) and compress the veins at the crossings, which may show local deflexions at these points. They may show connective-tissue sheathing and some may be actually thrombosed, remaining as white streaks devoid of blood. The exudates are usually discrete, small, flat, and white, giving a 'hard' appearance.

Diabetic Retinopathy (*Fig.* 622) can usually be distinguished by the presence of micro-aneurysms, and by the punctate nature of the haemorrhages and often of the exudates too, though coalescence is common.

Detachment of the Retina (*Fig.* 623). The detached portion of the retina may be silvery grey in colour in a long-standing detachment, and is raised above the surrounding fundus. In early cases due to serous exudate the detached part of the retina is more transparent, arranged in billowy folds. When the detachment is due to an underlying growth, the retina appears smooth and opaque. The retinal vessels appear small, tortuous, and dark in colour. The diagnosis between a serous detachment and one due to a new growth or an exudate may be confirmed by transillumination of the eye from outside (in the sector overlying the detachment). In a serous detachment the interior of the eye is lit up, while in the case of a growth the light from the torch cannot penetrate this.

Eales's Disease. This manifests itself as recurrent intra-ocular haemorrhages in young adults and is generally attributed to retinal phlebitis. Sudden obscuration of vision results from haemorrhage into the vitreous. Recurrence is the rule, and retinitis proliferans may result, i.e., fibrous tissue organization in the vitreous from the recurrent haemorrhages; on the other hand, the haemorrhages may cease for no apparent reason.

Glaucomatous Disk (*Fig.* 624). The excavation of the optic disk may be distinguished from the physiological cup by the fact that it affects the whole of the disk, the edge often being surrounded by an atrophic ring. The retinal vessels bend sharply over the edge, and may disappear from view behind the overhanging margin of the disk, reappearing on the bottom of the cup. The lamina cribrosa is well marked, and the disk is white and atrophic.

Retinitis Pigmentosa ('Primary pigmentary retinopathy') (*Fig.* 625). This is a heredofamilial degeneration, usually affecting young adult males and leading to blindness in 20–30 years. In the earlier stages the patches of pigment, of typical bone-corpuscle shape, are found in the equatorial zone; in the later stages all but the central fundus may be involved, the disk is yellow and waxy in appearance, and the vessels very attenuated. The choroidal vessels are usually well seen.

P. Trevor-Roper.

OPISTHOTONOS

Opisthotonos is a condition in which the muscles of the neck, back, and legs are rigidly contracted in such a way that the body is overextended in the form of an arch, supported by the occiput above and by the heels below. This position may be continuously maintained; more often it is assumed intermittently with partial or complete relaxation between the tetanic seizures. Its chief cause is *tetanus*, but it may also be due to *strychnine poisoning*, *spinal meningitis*, or occur as a hysterical manifestation.

Tetanus. If there is the history of punctured wound during the previous one to six weeks, and if stiffness of the neck muscles and of the lower jaw (lockjaw or trismus, p. 802) has set in, to be followed within a day or so by generalized rigidity with severe paroxysmal exacerbations, the opisthotonos is almost certainly due to tetanus. The fixed smile—risus sardonicus—is, however, common to tetanus and to strychnine poisoning. In some cases there will be no obvious wound or contusion, but although the source of contagion will then be obscure, the early lockjaw and the course of the disease will point to tetanus.

In strychnine poisoning the paroxysms of opisthotonos are separated by intervals of more complete relaxation than is the case in tetanus. There may be evidence of the source of the poisoning, either accidental, suicidal, or homicidal, in the form of a bottle, packet, or a hypodermic syringe and needle. In some cases the diagnosis will depend on analysis of the gastrointestinal contents.

Spinal meningitis seldom causes difficulty in the diagnosis, for it is generally part of acute cerebrospinal meningitis of which the general symptoms and pyrexia will have existed for some days if not a week or more before opisthotonos is likely to occur. Optic neuritis may be found and bacteriological and cytological results of lumbar puncture, especially the discovery of the meningococcus, will establish the diagnosis.

Hysteria sometimes takes a form that may at first be difficult to distinguish from tetanus or from strychnine poisoning. Unlike malingering, hysterical contractions violent enough to cause opisthotonos do not always make the patient perspire, nor do they lead to fatigue in the way that similar voluntary efforts would certainly produce. Persistent lockjaw may be present, as in tetanus: but whereas in strychnine poisoning and in tetanus there is a great similarity between one exacerbation and the next, hysterical convulsions are apt to be polymorphous: the more the writhing and the change of attitude and position, the more likely is the attack to be hysterical. The mind is initially clear in tetanus and strychnine poisoning, though its outward expression may be prevented by the muscular paroxysms. In hysteria, the mental attitude is in one way or another abnormal. Knowledge of the patient's previous history may assist—there may have been similar hysterial outbursts on former occasions. As in all hysterical manifestations symptoms tend to be over-dramatic and rather too theatrical to be diagnostically convincing.

(*See also* TRISMUS (LOCKJAW), p. 802.)

F. Dudley Hart.

ORTHOPNOEA

A patient is said to have orthopnoea if he can breathe comfortably only when sitting upright. Although most breathless patients are more comfortable in the sitting position, a clear history of orthopnoea, often expressed as a complaint of intense dyspnoea in the recumbent position, is particularly characteristic of left ventricular failure, mitral stenosis, and other conditions causing pulmonary venous hypertension. Orthopnoea is also a common feature of asthma and pericardial effusion.

See also DYSPNOEA (p. 236).

P. R. Fleming.

OTORRHOEA

Otorrhoea or discharge from the ear may derive from the external auditory meatus itself, or may originate in the middle ear and pass into the meatus through a tear or perforation of the tympanic membrane.

Causes within the Meatus. The commonest cause of discharge is *wax* which is continually being secreted by the ceruminous glands and is normally so slight as to escape notice, but is removed in miniscule quantities when the ears are dried after ablution. Occasionally there is a more profuse secretion which is glistening and golden yellow, and may be mistaken for purulent discharge. It has a characteristic odour.

Blood escapes from the meatus when its wall has been damaged by the introduction of foreign bodies or instruments, or when a tear occurs as a result of a fracture of the temporal bone involving the bony meatus. In some fractures there may be a *bloodstained watery discharge* signifying the likelihood of a fracture of the

temporal bone with torn dura and cerebrospinal leak, and later this may cease to be bloodstained when clear cerebrospinal fluid drips from the ear. A *bloodstained serous discharge* is suggestive of *malignant disease* of the external meatus and examination will reveal ulceration and friable granulations. Histological examination is confirmatory.

In *acute eczema* such as that caused by sensitization to antibiotic drops there may be a profuse *serous* discharge, but more usually there is a scanty serous discharge in the common condition of *otitis externa*. Examination will reveal inflamed, and sometimes oedematous meatal walls and, if fungal infection is present, masses of moist white debris resembling wet blotting-paper fill the meatus. Black granules imply the presence of *Aspergillus niger*. Otitis externa is frequently bilateral, and there is likely to be a history of recurrence and perhaps some precipitating cause such as bathing. After the meatal canals have been cleared of debris the tympanic membranes are, in uncomplicated cases, found to be intact and the hearing good.

Boils of the external meatus cause a thick purulent discharge on bursting. The diagnosis is seldom in doubt as the boil will be seen in the outer part of the canal, and pressure on the tragus or movement of the pinna causes extreme pain. Another, though most uncommon, cause of purulent discharge which may appear to rise in the meatus is mastoid suppuration which has burst through the deep bony meatus. Finally, we may mention a salivary fistula in the anterior wall of the meatus. This is from the parotid gland and follows injury.

Causes in the Middle Ear. In *acute otitis media,* untreated, a little serous discharge is sometimes seen in the external auditory meatus prior to the rupture of the drum membrane. However, when the tympanic membrane does burst a copious discharge appears and at first this may be bloodstained. In young children it may be most profuse and appear at such a rate as to drip down the side of the face and neck. After the meatus has been cleaned the discharge is found to be pulsating and it may be possible to define the site of the perforation (*Fig.* 626 A). The discharge, which is yellow and green (the latter colour suggesting the presence of *Pseudomonas pyocyanea*), varies in consistency and is sometimes frankly mucoid.

In *chronic suppurative otitis media* of the so-called 'tubotympanic' type (*Fig.* 626 B and E) the discharge usually has a large mucoid content and after aural cleaning the perforation will be clearly seen. In the attico-antral type of chronic otitis media, on the other hand, the discharge is usually scanty, non-mucoid and often evil-smelling. On examination, a marginal posterior or attic perforation (*Fig.* 626 C) will be found and through it cholesteatoma may be seen, having a whitish appearance. Such a perforation is not infrequently accompanied by bright red friable granulations arising from the tympanic annulus or middle ear mucosa and on occasions a polyp may form obscuring part or all of the tympanic membrane. These polypi may be mistaken for the membrane itself but the use of the clinic otomicroscope and gentle probing will clarify the situation.

likely to be more profuse and cerebrospinal fluid is sometimes present. A cerebrospinal fluid leak from the middle ear is very rare following mastoid surgery and is also unusual in perilymph fistula following stapes surgery, as in the latter cases the tympanic membrane is usually intact

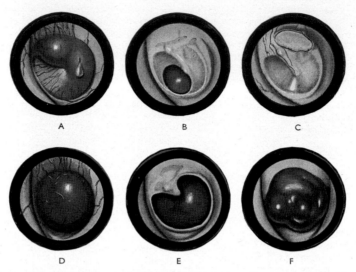

Fig. 626. A, Acute suppurative otitis media. B, Chronic otitis media, due to persistent tubotympanic infection. C, Chronic otitis, due to cholesteatomatous disease of the attic and mastoid antrum. D–F: Differential diagnosis of an inflamed area seen at the medial end of the meatus. D, The 'bulging membrane' of acute otitis media. E, The inflamed medial wall of the tympanum seen through a very large perforation, the result of chronic otitis. F, A polypus obscuring all details of the membrane. *(Illustrations by Sylvia Treadgold.)*

During an 'acute exacerbation' of chronic suppurative otitis media the discharge becomes more profuse and pulsation may be present. Such attacks are potentially dangerous and the presence of pain, pyrexia, vertigo, and particularly headache call for careful investigation in order to exclude intracranial extension of the infection.

Radiology is of importance in the diagnosis of infections of the middle-ear tract and, whereas opacity of the mastoid air cells is often seen in acute otitis media, the actual destruction of the cell outlines suggests mastoiditis with bony involvement. In chronic otitis media the mastoid is likely to appear sclerosed and a defect of any size is likely to indicate the presence of a cholesteatoma.

Bleeding from the middle ear may occur when the tympanic membrane is traumatized by an instrument or match-stick or by blast. The latter can occur in many different ways—a blow or a 'box on the ear', a loud noise, e.g., a bomb or shell explosion, deep-sea diving or descent in an aircraft—otitic barotrauma. In all these cases examination will reveal a tear of the tympanic membrane and in most instances the bleeding is very slight. In more severe degrees of trauma, for example fractures of the temporal bone with injury of the tegmen tympani, the bleeding is

and the C.S.F. passes down the Eustachian tube.

A *bloodstained discharge* from the middle ear is highly suggestive of *malignancy* and calls for microscopic examination and biopsy.

Miles Foxen.

OXALURIA

The normal excretion of oxalate in the urine is usually below 20 mg. per day, but occasionally normal adults may excrete up to 40 mg. per day. This amount is mainly dependent on the diet, but the rare syndrome of primary hyperoxaluria is also recognized. Foods containing much oxalate include rhubarb, strawberries, and spinach, but most of the ingested oxalate is destroyed in the body. An important dietary factor is the amount of calcium consumed, since this tends to precipitate the insoluble calcium oxalate in the bowel. If, therefore, it is desired to diminish the urinary excretion of oxalates a high milk intake is probably the most practical measure to adopt, particularly at meals in which an oxalate-rich food is taken.

The term 'oxaluria' refers to the appearance of calcium oxalate crystals in the urine; these crystals may appear in the familiar 'envelope' form (*Fig.* 627) or as 'dumb-bell' or 'biscuit' forms. The crystals appear most commonly in acid urines. They are soluble in mineral acid but not in acetic acid. They are seen in many normal urines and their relation to symptoms is very doubtful.

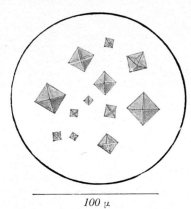

100 μ

Fig. 627. Calcium oxalate crystals.

Oxaluria has, however, been described as a cause of frequency of micturition, and of nocturnal enuresis. If symptoms are marked, and especially if red cells are also seen in the urinary deposit, the presence of oxalate calculus is a possibility, and it is probably wise not to attribute any urinary symptoms to oxaluria until all other causes have been excluded.

The rare condition of *primary hyperoxaluria* may be suspected if multiple oxalate calculi are formed during infancy; the urinary oxalate excretion will be increased about tenfold and deposits of calcium oxalate may occur in the kidneys and in other organs (oxalosis).

Affected patients usually die of chronic renal failure in adolescence. Renal transplantation is of no value as the donated kidney is soon affected by the disease. Continued intermittent haemodialysis is the only effective therapy if renal failure has occurred. The increased urinary oxalate output is due to an enzymatic deficiency and not to excess absorption of oxalate by the gut. A low calcium diet has been shown to delay development of oxalate calculi and oxalate deposits in the renal cortex by reducing urinary calcium.

Some patients may develop oxaluria and oxalate calculi after ileal resections, e.g., for Crohn's disease or ileal infarction. This causes an abnormally high absorption of oxalate in the jejunum, and therefore treatment should be by a low oxalate and high calcium diet.

M. D. Milne.

PAIN

Pain is a very important symptom. It is the main complaint in two of every three patients seeking medical attention. Like other sensory modalities, it is a phenomenon of considerable complexity: in particular there is no clear relation between disease severity and pain. Pain is often present without obvious disease and may be trivial or absent in patients with severe disease.

An accurate history is essential in the elucidation of pain.

The following properties of a pain should be noted:

Situation
Radiation
Severity
Character
Onset
Duration
Course
If intermittent, frequency, regularity, and duration of episodes
Precipitating factors
Aggravating and relieving factors
Associated symptoms.

The situation of pain is usually a guide to its origin though there are some obvious exceptions: pain arising from the hip joint may, for example, be felt in the knee and pain in the shoulder may arise from intrathoracic or intra-abdominal disease. Radiation of pain is sometimes helpful, for example in angina, the classic description of which includes radiation to the jaw and left arm. It is useful to note the severity and character of pain—colicky pains, for example, have a significance different from dull aching pains and imply involvement of a hollow visceral organ. Sharp stabbing pain is characteristic of pleurisy.

The onset of the pain may be characteristic, for example in gout, which often begins in the early hours with podagra. An insidious onset of pain makes gout unlikely. The subsequent time pattern of the pain is in some conditions the only clue to the correct diagnosis. In duodenal ulcer, for example, there are bouts of epigastric pain each lasting for a few weeks with months between in which there are no symptoms. In palindromic rheumatism the history of irregularly spaced attacks of arthritis, each lasting about 2 days, is often the only diagnostic feature. Obvious precipitating causes such as trauma must be elicited as well as those factors which aggravate or relieve pain whether time of day, meals, exertion, micturition, or defaecation. Aggravation by meals and exertion are characteristic features of peptic ulcer and angina; relief by rest and defaecation are characteristic features of angina and Crohn's disease. The effect of treatment such as alkalis may also help.

Associated symptoms often indicate the correct diagnosis. It is the paraesthesiae associated with pain in the arm which suggest carpal tunnel syndrome and the visual disturbances preceding a headache which suggest migraine.

The severity of pain in disease is related mainly to the severity of the disease process and the pain threshold of the patient. Patients with high pain thresholds have less pain, require less analgesia, and are more likely to be able to continue their occupation than those with low thresholds. Other factors, which may play some part include age, sex, race, fear and anxiety, suggestion, attitude, distraction, past experience, conditioning, and drugs.

Pain is of five main types:

Normal
Disease
Psychogenic
Psychosomatic
Disorders of the pain-producing mechanism.

Pain, like heat and cold, is an everyday experience which is beneficial as a protective mechanism. It is therefore not surprising that patients complain of normal pain. In addition, there are some very common pains, which are not due to disease—an example is Asher's precordial catch. In this condition there is a severe stabbing chest pain relieved after a moment of great agony by deep inspiration. Patients with conditions of this type need only to be told the nature of the pain, what it is not (heart trouble) and that most people have it.

Pain may be due to disease, either structural like peptic ulcer, or functional, like irritable bowel syndrome. Studies of patients with psychiatric disorders such as depression show that the incidence of complaints of pain is almost as high as in patients with organic disease. It therefore seems that pain may be a manifestation of psychological disturbance. There are many suggested ways of distinguishing organic and psychogenic pain, which is often very difficult; a selection of these is listed in the table. Pain may also be psychosomatic, for example the occipital headache which is caused by muscle spasm due to tension: and pain may be caused by disorders of the pain-producing mechanism, like causalgia.

Pains that arise in particular anatomical sites are considered separately.

E. C. Huskisson.

SOME FEATURES DESCRIBED AS USEFUL IN DIFFERENTIATING PSYCHOGENIC FROM ORGANIC PAIN

Incidence
 Younger age of onset than organic disease
 Lower social class, women, often aggressive
 Excess of single or divorced
 Family history of similar disorders.

Pain Pattern
 Dramatic description with similes such as 'like a knife turning. . . .'
 Site may be related to external factors
 Continuous and unvarying
 Analgesics have no effect
 Left-sided: not well localized.

Past History
 Appendicectomy and other unnecessary operations
 Frequent hospital attendance and investigation.

Other Symptoms
 Many
 Headaches and pains elsewhere
 Sexual difficulties.

Examination
 No evidence of disease
 Evidence of psychological disturbance.

Course
 Benign.

PALPITATIONS

Palpitations may be described as an abnormal awareness of the action of the heart. Thus they may be due either to an abnormality in the patient's action or, and much more often, to the patient's increased awareness. The commonest cause is *anxiety*. Most normal people have experienced palpitations briefly as a result of an alarming experience such as a narrow escape from an accident. More prolonged emotional disturbances, too, can produce palpitations; not only are such disturbances more common in the anxious but, once the palpitations have developed, they themselves can readily induce further anxiety by arousing suspicions of heart disease in the patient's mind. Thus a vicious circle is closed and *Da Costa's syndrome* results. In anxiety the mechanism of the palpitations is an increase in the force of cardiac contractions, often combined with tachycardia; both are mediated via catecholamine release. Palpitations as a whole can be considered according to whether they are due to an increase in the force, or more precisely in the type, of contraction or to a change in the rate or rhythm of the heart.

Palpitations are a feature of a group of cardiac lesions which have in common an *increase in the output* of one or other ventricle. Thus, in aortic incompetence, mitral incompetence, atrial and ventricular septal defects, and persistent ductus arteriosus, a complaint of palpitations is common. This is not the case, however, in uncomplicated mitral stenosis, hypertension, and ischaemic heart disease in which palpitations, if present, are due to superadded anxiety and not to the cardiac lesion itself. *High-output states*, in general, are also causes of palpitations which, as in the case of anxiety, are due both to the increase in the force of contraction and to tachycardia. In *thyrotoxicosis*, particularly, palpitations are a very common symptom but they may also be a feature of severe anaemia, arteriovenous fistula, beriberi, and cor pulmonale.

Catecholamine release as a cause of palpitations has already been mentioned. This is particularly prominent in *phaeochromocytoma*; both adrenaline and noradrenaline, but particularly the former, increase the force of ventricular contraction. Adrenaline also causes tachycardia but the release of noradrenaline, causing a sharp rise in blood-pressure, may be associated with a reflex bradycardia. It may be possible to distinguish between these two reactions from the patient's account of the paroxysms. Sympathomimetic *drugs* can produce similar effects and palpitations are commonly noticed by patients on ephedrine or isoprenaline. Palpitations may also be caused by other drugs. Most vasodilators, for example glyceryl trinitrate, produce a reflex tachycardia resulting from the fall in blood-pressure; atropine and similar drugs cause tachycardia by vagal blockade; hypoglycaemia, as a result of insulin administration or occurring spontaneously, causes catecholamine release; thyroxine in excess obviously simulates the effects of thyrotoxicosis. Digitalis and substances such as tea, coffee, and, particularly, tobacco can cause extrasystoles and palpitations resulting therefrom.

Paroxysmal disorders of the cardiac rhythm are an important cause of palpitations. *Extrasystoles*, either supraventricular or ventricular, are common and, very often, benign. By many, fortunate, subjects they are unnoticed; some, probably the majority, experience no more than a passing discomfort; in a few patients extrasystoles are disabling and a source of considerable anxiety. Unless the irregularity is present at the time of examination, the diagnosis depends on eliciting a history of a *momentary* disturbance of the action of the heart. A sensation of 'emptiness', a missed beat, or a sudden thump are often mentioned. Some patients seem to notice the feeble, premature, extrasystole itself, others the more powerful sinus beat following; this may become clear during interrogation.

Paroxysmal supraventricular tachycardia is not uncommon and occurs in patients with otherwise normal hearts whose only complaint is of attacks of palpitations. *Ventricular tachycardia* is usually, but by no means always, a manifestation of organic heart disease. The clinical and electrocardiographic features of such paroxysms are discussed in the section on TACHYCARDIA (p. 771). Usually the patient is seen in between attacks and careful history-taking is required in order to make a presumptive diagnosis. In the first instance an attempt should be made to determine the heart-rate in the attacks. The patient should be asked to try to reproduce the heart's action, as he felt it, by tapping on a table. Clearly no great precision is possible but, at least, significant tachycardia can be identified and distinguished from extrasystoles, for example. When this has been done, the important differentiation is between sinus tachycardia and an ectopic rhythm. The patient should be asked whether the attacks begin and end gradually or abruptly. Sinus tachycardia has a gradual onset and cessation whereas ectopic rhythms characteristically start and stop abruptly. In practice many patients with palpitations associated with sinus tachycardia will describe a sudden onset; as the rate gradually rises there comes a time when the patient notices it and interprets that moment as the sudden onset of tachycardia. For this reason more attention should be paid to the manner in which the attacks end; the patient can usually give an accurate account of this as, by that time, he is only too aware of the action of the heart. *Paroxysmal atrial fibrillation* also produces rapid palpitations which should be analysed in the same way; this condition should be strongly suspected if the patient taps out an obviously irregular rhythm.

Palpitations may be provoked by lesions such as *hiatus hernia* or *gastric distension* which may interfere mechanically with the action of the heart. In some such cases extrasystoles are found, in others one can only presume that an abnormality of the movement of the heart is responsible for the symptom. In addition, anxiety may well play a large part, as is certainly the case in palpitations associated with pectus excavatum.

Occasionally a complaint of palpitations refers to vascular throbbing, commonly in the neck. A patient with aortic incompetence, in whom Corrigan's sign is well developed, may well complain of palpitations, meaning a throbbing in his neck. Similarly, the large amplitude jugular venous pulse in tricuspid incompetence may be felt by the patient. In this connexion it is of interest that African patients with endomyocardial fibrosis, a condition in which mitral and tricuspid incompetence are often prominent features, may present with the scars of scarification over the apex beat and along the course of the jugular veins. These represent treatment by witch-doctors of the areas in which the patient has felt an uncomfortable sensation; similar scars may be seen over the enlarged, tender liver in such cases.

See also PULSE, IRREGULAR (p. 663), and TACHYCARDIA (p. 771.)

P. R. Fleming.

PAPULES

Papules are solid, circumscribed elevations of the skin up to the size of a pea. Similar lesions, if larger, are nodules or tumours. In many instances papules, especially those which are inflammatory, are transitional lesions, becoming vesicles or pustules or breaking down into ulcers. In shape they are usually round or oval, as in papular urticaria, but they may be irregular and in lichen planus are polygonal. The colour is also varied, being usually pink or red, but early in lichen planus they are lilac, in syphilis coppery, in xanthoma yellow, in milium white, in melanoma black or dark brown, and in warts skin-coloured. They may be discrete, as in prurigo, or may occur in patches, as in papular (lichenoid) tuberculide; sometimes they form round a hair follicle, as in follicular dermatitis and pityriasis rubra pilaris; or in connexion with the sebaceous glands, the sweat-glands, or the papillae. They may be inflammatory as in dermatitis, or non-inflammatory as in moles, or the result of retained secretion as in acne. Inflammatory papules usually cause itching.

The multiple small papules (*Fig.* 628) which occur in *dermatitis* are usually conical, with a rounded base, and of bright-red colour; when ruptured by scratching they are covered with a tiny blood crust and there is usually intense itching.

In *lichen planus* (*Fig.* 629) the papules are polygonal or irregular in shape, flat-topped, with a shiny surface and lilac in colour; white dots and lines on the surface of the papules are known as Wickham's striae (*Fig.* 630); there is no discharge or crust formation, and in spite of the intense irritation which is almost invariably present there are never any scratch marks. As the papules progress they become darker in colour and finally disappear, leaving temporary sepia-coloured stains. White striations are often present on the buccal mucosa and are an important diagnostic sign. When lichen planus affects the vulva and anal area the papules are larger and flatter and of a very pale pink colour,

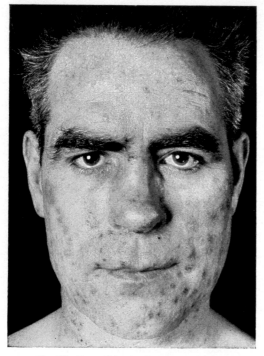

Fig. 628. Dermatitis, showing discrete papules. (*Dr. Peter Hansell.*)

sometimes nearly white, and when affecting either of these areas alone must be distinguished from leucoplakia, for which condition they are frequently mistaken. When the papules of lichen planus have become confluent they must be distinguished from areas of *lichenification* (*Fig.* 631) (neurodermatitis) by the presence of typical lichen planus lesions at the periphery of the patch and elsewhere, and by the colour. In patches of lichenification there are seldom individual papules to be seen and the colour is pink or pinkish-fawn. When there is a solitary patch the history is usually a long one, perhaps it has been present for many years, whereas in lichen planus the duration will probably have been weeks or months only. When dermatitis has become lichenified there will be signs of the primary disorder on other parts of the body. In Besnier's prurigo, a form of neurodermatitis, the prominent lesions are patches of lichenified papules. These occur most commonly in the bends of the knees and elbows and on the face and wrists. The disease usually follows infantile dermatitis, the transformation taking place within the first four years. It may persist throughout life and it is often associated with asthma, exacerbations of the two diseases alternating. *Hebra's prurigo* is an exaggerated form of this condition.

In the *papular* or *lichenoid tuberculide* there are numerous groups of minute follicular papules scattered over the trunk and extremities. They may be either reddish-brown or skin-coloured and are frequently topped by a tiny scale. There is no itching or other symptom and the rash may remain unnoticed for a long time. It may disappear and recur over a period of years. It is usually associated with tuberculosis of the bones and lymph-glands and affects children and young adults, being rare after the age of twenty. Owing to the absence of itching it must be distinguished

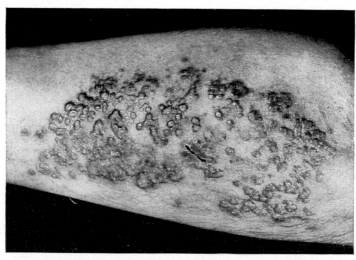

Fig. 629. Papules in lichen planus, showing their polygonal shape and flat shiny tops. (*Dr. Peter Hansell.*)

from secondary syphilis, which disease may be ruled out by a negative serology, the long history, and usually the youth of the patient.

In *keratosis pilaris* the papules consist of projecting cornified hair follicles of neutral colour.

In *ichthyosis hystrix* (linear naevus) there are numerous small warty papules with horny tops, running in lines or arranged in huge warty masses.

Warts (verruca vulgaris) should be obvious, but when round the finger-nails they may resemble

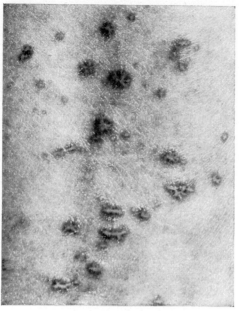

Fig. 630. Lichen planus showing Wickham's striae. (*Dr. Peter Hansell.*)

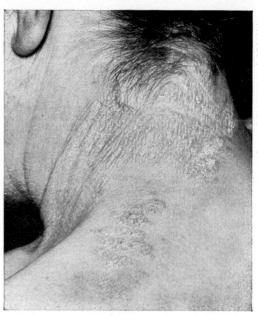

Fig. 631. Patches of lichenification, showing the confluence of round, dome-shaped papules. (*Dr. Peter Hansell.*)

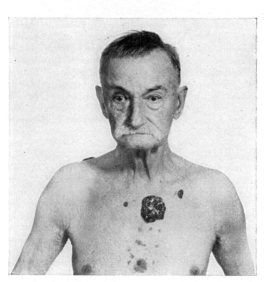

Fig. 632. Seborrhoeic warts. (*Dr. Peter Hansell.*)

It occurs on the extensor surfaces of the limbs, mostly the thighs and upper arms. When the area is stroked with the hand it feels like a nutmeg grater.

psoriasis or even dermatitis. The small flat wart (verruca plana) may sometimes suggest lichen planus, but it is smaller than the papule of that affection and is skin-coloured. It gives rise to no itching.

Seborrhoeic Warts (seborrhoeic keratoses) begin as small circumscribed papules, yellow or brownish in colour, and increase gradually in size. Some of the larger lesions may become dark brown or black (*Fig. 632*). Although they may be single, they are more often multiple and may occur in vast numbers especially on the back and front of the chest, though they may occur almost anywhere on the skin surface. They usually have a slightly greasy feel. Although they tend to develop late in life, they are probably genetically determined and are very common. They must be distinguished from moles, malignant melanomata, rodent ulcers, and common warts. They form part of the clinical picture of acanthosis nigricans (p. 729).

Dermatosis papulosa nigra (*Fig. 633*) is a common disease of Negroes in which lesions similar to seborrhoeic warts develop in large numbers on the face, starting in early adult life.

Senile keratomata (*Fig. 634*) must be clearly differentiated from seborrhoeic warts. They occur on exposed surfaces and are due to the action of sunlight on the skin. At first flat and slightly pigmented, they later become papular and may be covered with a crust. They are potentially malignant and may develop into squamous-celled epitheliomata.

In *pityriasis rubra pilaris*, papules form at the orifices of the hair follicles in the midst of scaly red patches. The papules, when they appear, are small, red, and dry, rough to the touch, more or less conical, and the centre of each is pierced by a single atrophied hair. The surface thus roughened is not unlike the skin of a newly plucked fowl. At first the papules are discrete but later they tend to run together into pale

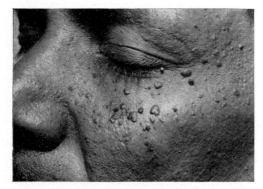

Fig. 633. Dermatosis papulosa nigra. (*Dr. Peter Hansell.*)

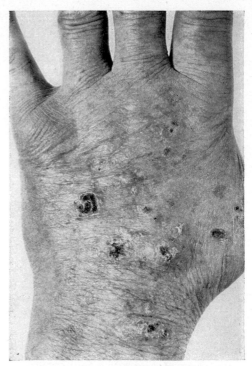

Fig. 634. Senile keratomata. (*Dr. Peter Hansell.*)

yellowish-red patches covered with papery scales. The limbs are mostly affected, especially where they are hairiest. Later the lower abdomen may be involved. Itching is absent or trivial. When the patches are scaly and occur on the tips of the elbows, fronts of the knees, and exterior surfaces, this condition may be confused with psoriasis; but at the edge of each patch the

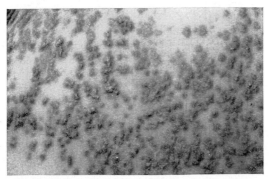

Fig. 635. Darier's disease: grouped greasy follicular papules. (*Dr. Peter Hansell.*)

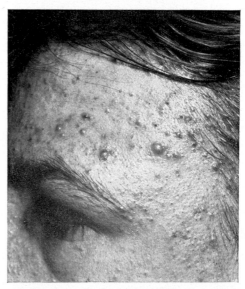

Fig. 636. Acne vulgaris, showing blackheads, papules, and pustules.

characteristic conical papule with its single hair plugging the mouth of a follicle is always to be seen. The best place to look for the papule is on the dorsal surfaces of the first phalanges of the fingers. In psoriasis the lesions grow by peripheral extension and not by the confluence of new papules. From lichen planus, pityriasis rubra pilaris is distinguished by its greater chronicity and the larger areas usually involved, and by the absence of itching and of the typical lilac, flattened papules which characterize the former disease.

Darier's disease (*Fig.* 635) is a rare congenital condition in which follicular papules appear in early life on any part of the body but especially the scalp, forehead, front and back of the chest, and the flexures. The papules, at first small,

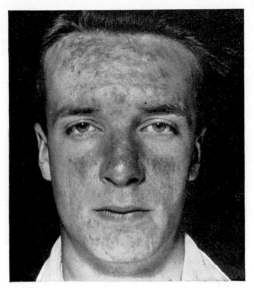

Fig. 637. Rosacea, showing multiple papule formation and redness on the nose and cheeks. Note the absence of black-heads. (*Dr. Peter Hansell.*)

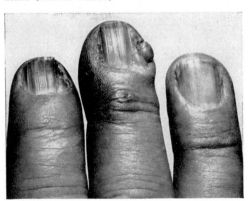

Fig. 639. Adenoma sebaceum: peri-ungual fibromata. (*Dr. Peter Hansell.*)

increase in size and have a greasy feel. They have a characteristic histology.

In *acne vulgaris* (*Fig.* 636) the papule is the predominant lesion, but there are also black-heads (comedones) blocking the sebaceous follicles and pustules caused by secondary infection of papules. Acne can usually be recognized by the distribution of the lesions, on the face, and sometimes on the back between the shoulders and the chest, the presence of comedones, and the patient's age, for the affection is one of puberty and adolescence. Usually, too, the several stages through which the lesions pass

20*

are present at the same time, the comedo, the papule, the pustule. An iodide or bromide eruption can resemble acne, but close inspection will show the absence of comedones. An acne-like eruption may occur on the forearms and thighs of workers in oily occupations, and this eruption sometimes occurs on the face as well. The history will be helpful here, but it must be

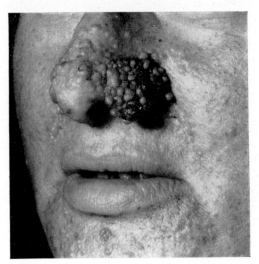

Fig. 638. Adenoma sebaceum. (*Dr. Peter Hansell.*)

remembered that a young man with acne, exposed to oil at his work (i.e., a mechanic), may have an existing acne considerably aggravated.

Rosacea (*Fig.* 637) differs from acne in that it chiefly affects the flush area of the face, is less often pustular, is marked by much congestion, and is most common in middle life. *Adenoma sebaceum* (*Fig.* 638) is a congenital affection, occurring on the cheeks and characterized by minute, closely aggregated papules, generally of a reddish colour, and due to hypertrophy of the blood-vessels and sebaceous glands; it is often associated with mental deficiency (epiloia). Fibromata around the nails are also characteristic of this condition (*Fig.* 639). *Erythema multiforme* (*see* p. 258) is sometimes mainly papular in character. *Papular urticaria*, in which the weals take the form of small papules, one of the commonest maladies of childhood, is usually easy to recognize. It is usually due to insect bites. It may, however, be difficult to differentiate from scabies, but careful search will usually discover a typical burrow in the webs between the fingers in the latter disease. Other characteristic features in scabies are a triangular group of papules at the lower part of both buttocks and a solitary papule on the glans or the shaft of the penis.

In the rash of *secondary syphilis* (*Fig.* 640) which occurs from two to ten weeks after the appearance of the primary chancre, papules are the predominating lesions; they may occur alone or in association with macules (maculo-papular eruption). They may appear as pseudo-vesicles or pustules; occasionally they ulcerate. The lesions are essentially pleomorphic—that is to say, they display a wide variety of characteristics. They may be of various shapes and sizes and are distributed over the whole body without any semblance of pattern. Constant features are: (1) Their colour, which is coppery or similar to the colour of raw ham; and (2) the complete

The skin changes of late syphilis may resemble those in many skin diseases, but in every instance the resemblance is not quite complete. Thus the psoriasiform syphilide is only superficially like psoriasis and closer inspection will reveal that the scaliness is minimal and the fine silvery scales of psoriasis are quite absent. In so-called 'pustular syphilides' there is no pus formation. Palmar and plantar syphilides may at first sight mimic dermatitis, but the lesions are quite dry

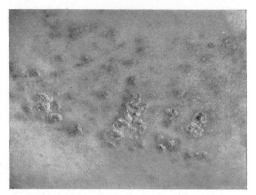

Fig. 640. Secondary syphilis, showing macules, maculo-papules, papules, and scaly lesions in close association. (*Dr. Peter Hansell.*)

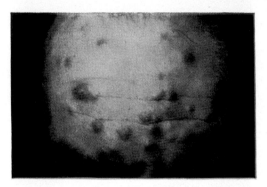

Fig. 641. Secondary syphilis: uniform large papules.

freedom from itching. No syphilitic eruption ever itches. There may be a predominance of one type of lesion (*Fig.* 641) or all types of lesion may go to make up the rash. In emaciated individuals papules with a pointed scaly top may occur, not unlike small barnacles set on the skin. This condition, which is rare, is known as *rupia*. Sometimes the papules are arranged in ring formation (*annular syphilide*) and sometimes there is a band of papules on the forehead at the hair margins (*corona veneris*). Round the anus or vulva, and in the groins in obese subjects, mucous patches occur; these papules are covered with white soggy epithelium. As a rule these lesions enlarge rapidly to form mucous condylomata (*Fig.* 563, p. 562). They are readily distinguished from warts in the same area by the absence of hyperkeratosis and by the presence of other signs of syphilis.

Secondary syphilis is readily diagnosed by the appearance of the eruption, the presence of other signs of the disease, such as a healing or healed chancre; polyadenitis; mucous patches in the mouth; snail-track ulcers on the tonsils. In women, syphilis is frequently only diagnosed in the secondary stage, as the commonest site for a primary chancre is on the cervix uteri where it may lurk unsuspected until the rash appears. In every case serological tests for syphilis are positive.

In *congenital syphilis* the appearance of secondary syphilis may occur from the third week of life onwards, when it in no way differs from that stage of the disease in the adult.

and of course there is no burning or itching. In every case of secondary syphilis serological tests are positive.

Itching is a feature of the reticuloses, especially Hodgkin's disease, and when severe may be accompanied by widespread excoriated papules.

P. D. Samman.

PARAPLEGIA

This term has come to be used for partial or complete paralysis of the legs caused by disease of the nervous system, and is not applied to cases in which there is inability to use the lower limbs on account of arthritis or other non-neurological affections, or to cases in which inability to walk is the result of mental deficiency. The latter group is distinguished from congenital paraplegia by the normality of tone, power, and reflexes which it exhibits. True paraplegia is usually due to disease of the spinal cord, less often to affections of the peripheral nerves, occasionally to intracranial lesions, and rarely to disease of the muscles. It may also be hysterical. The first step in diagnosis, therefore, is to decide from a consideration of the history and physical findings whether the condition is due to disease of the upper motor neuron (intracranial or spinal), of the lower motor neuron (cauda equina and peripheral nerves), of the muscles, or of the mind.

Affections of the corticospinal (pyramidal) pathways usually give rise to weakness, spasticity, increased tendon-reflexes, absence of the abdominal reflexes if the lesion is above the level of the 6th dorsal segment, and an extensor plantar response. To this there may be added sustained ankle-clonus. The legs are held in extension if the corticospinal pathway is incompletely severed, and in flexion if the lesion is complete, and contractures may develop in either position owing to shortening in muscles and periarticular fibrosis. There are, however, several reservations to be made in connexion with this general statement. In the first place, the paraplegia will be flaccid with reduced tendon-jerks for some days or weeks after the onset if this has been abrupt—a condition of neurological shock. Secondly, spasticity may be delayed, or abolished, by coincident sepsis from bed-sores, an infected bladder, or any other general toxaemia. In the third place, the degree of spasticity present varies greatly from case to case, irrespective of the factors noted above, and generally speaking its degree is inversely proportional to the amount of weakness in the legs. Very spastic legs are often very strong, and the incapacity complained of by the patients is then mainly due to the stiffness. The explanation of this phenomenon lies in the fact that lesions of the motor cortex proper, or of the pyramidal tracts proper, cause a flaccid paralysis, whereas lesions of the anterior portion of the motor cortex, or of the corticospinal fibres which arise from it, cause spasticity without weakness. In most cases of cerebral or spinal disease, both sets of fibres are involved, so producing both spasticity and weakness in varying combination, but cases are not rare in which there is spasticity without weakness, or vice versa. Finally, it is necessary to refer to the fact that in congenital diplegia, which is due to natal or prenatal disturbance of the corticospinal pathways to the legs, the plantar reflexes are not always extensor in type, although the limbs may be weak, spastic, and held in extension. The explanation is unknown.

Affections of the lower motor neuron, whether at the level of the anterior horn cells, or the cauda equina, or the peripheral nerves, are marked by weakness, flaccidity, atrophy, reduction or loss of the tendon reflexes, changes in electrical excitability including the reaction of degeneration, and in some cases by fibrillation in the affected muscles. It is to be noted that weakness is apt to be uneven in distribution, affecting some muscles more than others, in contrast to the weakness of group-movements which occur in upper-motor neuron lesions. Thus a tumour of the cauda equina, or poliomyelitis, may paralyse the muscles below the knee with the exception of one or two, which are either unaffected or but slightly weakened. In polyneuritis, on the other hand, it is more usual for the weakness to be generalized and more marked distally than proximally. There is flaccidity, absence of the tendon reflexes, and, if paralysis be complete, absence of any kind of response to plantar stimulation. Another point of value in determining that a paraplegia is of lower-motor

neuron type is the presence of sensory loss of peripheral or radicular distribution; it is present in the majority of cases, although it is often less marked a feature than the paralysis. There are important exceptions, however: anterior poliomyelitis and progressive muscular atrophy produce lower-motor neuron paraplegia without any sensory loss whatsoever. Lead palsy, which can cause considerable weakness of the legs, is also free from sensory involvement. Fibrillation of the muscles of the legs is an important sign of a lower-motor neuron affection, although it is often absent. It is particularly marked in motor neuron disease and in tumours of the cauda equina.

A third type of paralysis is sometimes seen in the condition known as *benign myalgic encephalomyelitis*, which has occurred in small localized epidemics in various parts of the world, as for instance in London, where it was almost but not quite confined to the nurses and doctors of the Royal Free Hospital. The onset is with depression, sore throat, severe headache and pain in the muscles, and slight pyrexia. Neurological disturbances usually appear at the end of the first or second week and may persist for many months. There may be upper- or lower-motor neuron weakness, with appropriate changes in the reflexes, and these may involve the arms or the legs, occasionally both. In some cases, however, there is a flaccid paralysis, e.g., of the legs, with intact tendon and plantar reflexes, without wasting or fibrillation, and with electromyographic changes which suggest disease of the spinal cord but *not* of the anterior horn cells. There may or may not be a slight peripheral sensory change in these cases, and the spinal fluid is always normal. Recovery is usually complete, but temporary recurrences are not uncommon, and the emotional disturbances seen at the onset may last for many months. The cause of the disease is not known, and a curious epidemiological feature is that prolonged personal contact in an institution appears to be necessary for 'infection' to occur. The combination of marked emotional disturbance and weakness or paralysis without appropriate reflex changes is apt to suggest an erroneous diagnosis of hysteria.

THE CAUSES OF PARAPLEGIA

1. Affections of the Upper Motor Neuron in the Spinal Cord:

a. INJURIES:

Penetrating wounds	Birth injuries
Fracture-dislocations	Electric shocks and
	lightning

b. COMPRESSION OF THE CORD:

Fracture-dislocations	Prolapsed disk
Tumours of:	Metastatic epidural
Cord	abscess
Meninges	Hydatid cyst
Roots	Meningitis serosa
Vertebrae	circumscripta
Spinal angioma	Leukaemic deposits
Pott's disease	Hodgkin's disease

b. COMPRESSION OF THE CORD (*continued*)

Paget's disease	Atlanto-axial
Severe kyphoscoliosis	subluxation in
Aortic aneurysm	rheumatoid
Spondylosis	arthritis and
	ankylosing
	spondylitis

c. INFECTIONS:

Syphilis:	Abscess of spinal cord
Transverse myelitis	in pyaemia
Erb's paraplegia	Benign myalgic
	encephalomyelitis

d. DEFICIENCY DISEASES:

Subacute combined degeneration of the cord	The captivity syndrome

e. DEMYELINATING DISEASES:

Disseminated sclerosis	Encephalomyelitis after acute specific fevers,
Neuromyelitis optica (Devic)	vaccination, and inoculation against rabies

f. CONGENITAL AND FAMILIAL CONDITIONS:

Myelodysplasia with spina bifida	Hereditary paraplegia
Syringomyelia, haematomyelia	Friedreich's ataxia

g. MISCELLANEOUS:

Amyotrophic lateral sclerosis	Spinal anaesthesia
Acute and subacute necrotic myelitis	Caisson disease
	Lathyrism

2. Affections of the Upper Motor Neuron in the Brain:

a. INJURIES:

Wounds of the motor cortex in the parasagittal region

b. INFECTIONS:

Thrombosis of superior sagittal sinus	Malaria
	General paralysis of the insane
Cortical thrombophlebitis	

c. TUMOURS:

Parasagittal neoplasms (mainly meningioma)

d. CONGENITAL:

Congenital diplegia	Congenital hydrocephalus

e. MISCELLANEOUS:

Schilder's disease	Thrombosis of unpaired anterior cerebral artery
Disseminated sclerosis	
	Paralysis agitans (advanced)

3. Affections of the Lower Motor Neuron:

a. INJURIES:

Injuries to cauda equina	Injuries to lumbosacral plexuses

b. INFECTIONS:

Acute anterior poliomyelitis	Diphtheritic polyneuritis
Leprosy	Polyneuritis of Guillain-Barré

c. POLYNEURITIS:

Alcohol	Hodgkin's disease
Beriberi	Malignant disease of lung, stomach, etc.
Diabetes	
Heavy metals	Polyarteritis nodosa
Porphyria	Sarcoidosis

d. COMPRESSION OF CAUDA EQUINA:

Tumours of cauda equina	Fracture-dislocation of lumbar spine
Tumours of meninges	Spondylolisthesis
Tumours of lumbar spine	Protrusion of annulus fibrosis
Pott's disease	Herniation of intervertebral disk

e. COMPRESSION OF LUMBOSACRAL PLEXUS:

Foetal head	Pelvic tumours

f. CONGENITAL ABNORMALITIES:

Myelodysplasia of lumbosacral cord	Meningomyelocele

g. MISCELLANEOUS:

Peroneal muscular atrophy	Progressive muscular atrophy
Hypertrophic polyneuritis (Dejerine-Sottas)	Bite of the wood tick
	Potassium intoxication

4. Affections of the Muscles. The heredofamilial dystrophies.

5. Hysteria.

Affections of the Spinal Cord. The diagnosis of *Closed Spinal Cord Injuries* from direct violence presents no difficulty when there is a clear history of injury; this may be absent when the patient is unconscious from concomitant concussion, so that careful clinical and radiological examination of the spine is important in such cases. *Penetrating injuries* will be less easily overlooked, but it is desirable to emphasize that a high-velocity missile which just misses the spinal cord may cause all the signs of transection. *Birth injuries* to the cord usually arise as a result of traction on the legs in a breech presentation. The infant is shocked and it is soon noticed that it is paralysed. Sensory loss below the level of the injury will differentiate the disability from congenital cerebral diplegia; survival is rare.

Electrical injuries, from live conductors or from lightning, occasionally cause paraplegia; care must be exercised to exclude the possibility of direct violence at the time of the shock, e.g., a fall to the ground from a ladder; lightning may hurl the victim several yards.

COMPRESSION OF THE SPINAL CORD may come on acutely, subacutely, or very slowly, and the resultant clinical picture varies between wide limits with the nature and situation of the lesion. If it happens suddenly (e.g., fracture-dislocation, myelitis, metastatic epidural abscess, haemorrhage into a syrinx, or from an angioma) paraplegia is at first flaccid, owing to spinal shock, and both the superficial and deep reflexes may be absent for days or weeks. There is dribbling incontinence, followed by retention of urine as the sphincter regains its tone. The upper level of the lesion is determined by the level of sensory loss

lesions. Manometric studies are often useful in establishing a compression lesion, but it is useful to remember that manometry may give no hint of any obstruction at all in cases of incomplete block, and that conversely, a very slow and incomplete rise or fall may be due to technical factors only. Examination of the spinal fluid may reveal xanthochromia and a high protein content

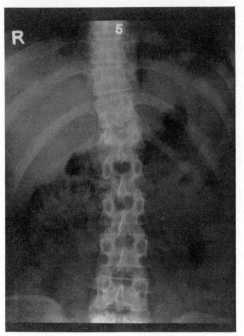

Fig. 642. A radiograph from a case of spinal caries involving the 11th and 12th dorsal and 1st lumbar vertebrae.

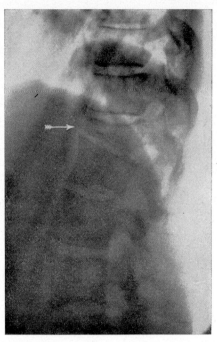

Fig. 643. A radiograph, lateral view, of the spine showing collapse of the body of the 12th dorsal vertebra, due to a deposit in it of carcinoma secondary to carcinoma of the breast. (Dr. J. H. Mather.)

and paralysis in the trunk. In slowly developing compression, motor paralysis will be more prominent than sensory loss—indeed both cutaneous and other sensibility may be quite unaffected in the early stages, though paraesthesiae in the legs will usually appear in the patient's story. Spinal tenderness must be looked for. Examination of the cerebrospinal fluid and both routine radiographs (Figs. 642–645) and contrast myelography are called for in every case of slowly developing paraplegia unless there are strong indications in the history or on physical examination of some non-compressive process such as disseminated sclerosis or motor neuron disease. When sensory loss is present, its upper limit is often, but not always, a good guide to the level of the compression. The nature of the sensory loss is not dependable in assessing whether the lesion is intra- or extra-medullary, for loss of pain and temperature sensibility with preservation of touch and proprioception does not invariably mean an intramedullary lesion, but may occur with pressure upon the cord from outside. In other words, dissociated sensory loss below the level of the lesion is not synonymous with intramedullary

which, together with complete block, characterizes the Froin syndrome, but here again it is necessary to recall that xanthochromia may be absent and the protein but little raised when compression is low down in the thoracic area, and that, on the other hand, a high protein content may occur in the absence of compression (e.g., subacute necrotic myelitis, disseminated sclerosis).

In rheumatoid arthritis and ankylosing spondylitis atlanto-axial subluxation may cause compression of the odontoid process on the spinal cord with slight and transient or more severe and lasting symptoms.

Infections—other than Pott's disease, epidural abscess, and hydatid cysts, which cause compression—play little part in the genesis of paraplegia. Syphilitic endarteritis of the spinal vessels can lead to a sudden softening of the cord—a transverse myelitis—while some middle-aged syphilitics exhibit a slowly developing spastic paraplegia without conspicuous sensory loss but with bladder symptoms (Erb's syphilitic spinal paralysis). It is useful to recall that the presence of a positive Wassermann reaction does not necessarily mean that the patient's paraplegia is due to syphilis. Intramedullary *spinal abscess* is a very rare condition which usually occurs in septicaemia or pyaemia and gives rise to rapidly developing paraplegia.

Of the *deficiency syndromes*, the one which is most common in civil life is *subacute combined*

signs of peripheral neuritis, but the plantars were often extensor and there was marked loss of vibration and position sense. The calves and feet were tender, and there was often visual loss in the shape of bilateral central scotomata with optic atrophy.

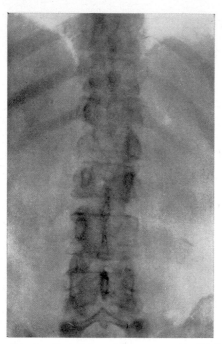

Fig. 644. A radiograph from the same case as *Fig.* 643, but taken in the anteroposterior position; to illustrate the point that gross change in the body of a vertebra may be missed if the spine is examined in the anteroposterior position only. (*Dr. J. H. Mather.*)

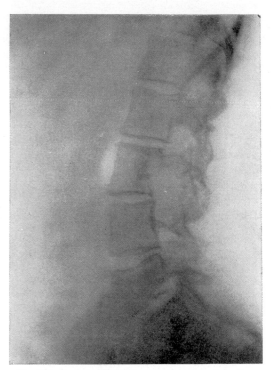

Fig. 645. A radiograph in lateral view of an hour-glass tumour of the spine; the neurofibromatous growth (Heuer's tumour) has led to considerable destruction of the posterior part of the body of the 3rd lumbar vertebra and similar but less destruction of the posterior part of the body of the 4th lumbar vertebra. (*Dr. J. H. Mather.*)

degeneration of the cord. This condition, which has become rare since the introduction of liver therapy and later the isolation and synthesis of cyanocobalamin, is found in association with pernicious anaemia and a histamine-fast achlorhydria, and may also accompany the gastrointestinal and cutaneous features of pellagra. Rarely, a similar condition occurs in the absence of achlorhydria, but is held in check by vitamin B_{12}. Whatever its causation, the disease is marked by a combination of paraesthesiae in the hands and feet, posterior column loss in the legs, tender muscles, weakness of the legs, spasticity, increased tendon-reflexes, and extensor plantar responses. In some cases, in which there is an additional element of peripheral neuritis, the weakness is a flaccid one and the tendon reflexes are reduced or lost, but the plantars remain extensor.

The captivity syndrome occurred mainly in prisoners of war in the Far East, and was due to a diet deficient in vitamin B and animal fats and proteins. There was weakness of the legs, with

Disseminated sclerosis is the most common cause of paraplegia in Europe, the United Kingdom, and North America. In most cases there will be a history, past or present, of symptoms indicating multiple lesions, e.g., diplopia, retrobulbar neuritis, paraesthesia of a limb, in addition to the paralysis of the legs, and the symptomatology will have been intermittent. In some cases, however, and particularly in middle life, the disease may take the form of a steadily progressive spastic paraplegia, with or without sensory loss below the level of the lesion, with a normal spinal fluid or with a paretic Lange curve in an otherwise normal fluid. Rarely such a case may rapidly progress to a condition resembling complete transverse myelitis. The latter is also seen in *neuromyelitis optica* (Devic), which is characterized by the rapid onset of paraplegia or quadriplegia, preceded, accompanied, or followed by bilateral retrobulbar neuritis, with consequent loss of the central fields of vision or complete visual loss. It is due to a more massive demyelinization than disseminated sclerosis, and it has a mortality-rate of some 50 per cent, but remarkable degrees of recovery are possible in non-fatal cases.

Encephalomyelitis may follow the acute specific fevers of childhood. It is marked pathologically by multiple patches of perivascular demyelinization in the brain and spinal cord, and clinically by evidence of multiple lesions coupled with fever, meningism, and prostration. Flaccid paraplegia due to multiple cord lesions of acute onset is an occasional finding. Similar symptoms may follow about ten days after vaccination against smallpox, after smallpox itself, and towards the end of a course of inoculation against rabies. The mortality is high, but those who escape death may ultimately recover completely. A few cases are left with persistent weakness of the legs, and—in children—mental defect.

CONGENITAL DEFECTS OF THE SPINAL CORD are usually associated with spina bifida, or with a meningocele, or with spina bifida occulta. Careful examination of the whole of the spine is necessary, for though the defect is usually in the lumbosacral region, it may be mid-dorsal or even cervical in situation. The cord may be normal, or the child may have a spastic paraplegia, or paraplegia in flexion with contractures, or slight stiffness of the legs with sensory loss in the feet, or—when the cauda equina is involved—a flaccid paraplegia with wasting of muscles, absent tendon-reflexes, and some degree of sphincter disturbance.

Syringomyelia is traditionally placed under congenital disorders, but it is doubtful whether it really belongs there. There is now some evidence that in some patients the primary lesion is a developmental anomaly or an acquired lesion in the region of the foramen magnum which obstructs the exit of the cerebrospinal fluid from the foramina in the roof of the fourth ventricle. The cerebrospinal fluid is thus forced down the central canal under pressure and eventually ruptures the ependyma and escapes into the central grey matter of the spinal cord. It is marked as a rule by spasticity of the legs, loss of arm jerks, loss of pain and temperature sensibility symmetrically in a 'jacket' distribution over the arms and thorax, and weakness and wasting of the upper limbs. If, as sometimes happens, the cavitation of the cord occurs in the thoracic segments, there is paraplegia with sparing of the arms, but with dissociated sensory loss on the abdomen, and ultimately in the legs, too. The condition evolves very slowly indeed, but may worsen abruptly if a haemorrhage occurs into the syringomyelic cavity. In either case, the picture is easily confused with an intramedullary tumour, which indeed it is, in the sense of an expanding mass.

Hereditary spastic paraplegia is usually familial, with or without a history of cases in previous generations, but sporadic cases occur. The symptoms are those of a slowly progressive degeneration of the pyramidal tracts starting between three and fifteen years of age, rarely later, and for a time there is only a spastic paraplegia, but gradually spastic weakness spreads to the upper limbs and ultimately to the bulbar muscles. There is no sensory loss but optic atrophy may occur. The disease takes many years to run its course, and is one of the heredofamilial group of which *Friedreich's ataxia* is the best known. In the latter, symptoms usually come on in childhood or adolescence, and the earliest complaints are of weakness and clumsiness of the legs. Ataxia of gait is apt to obscure the presence of weakness due to pyramidal degeneration, the more so as the tendon reflexes are diminished or absent and tone reduced. The ataxia is partly due to degeneration of the spino-cerebellar tracts, and partly to loss of position sense. Pes cavus and scoliosis are usually present. The reason for the loss of tendon reflexes is not known.

Amyotrophic lateral sclerosis is a fairly common cause of paraplegia in the second half of life. It is marked by a very slowly progressive spastic weakness of the legs, without sensory loss or sphincter disturbances, preceded or followed by weakness, wasting, and fibrillation in the upper limbs, shoulders, and trunk. The spinal fluid is normal. Early cases of this disease, and early cases of spastic paraplegia due to disseminated sclerosis, may be mistaken for spinal compression. It is this type of case which gave rise to the conception of 'primary lateral sclerosis', a diagnosis which has now fallen into disuse.

Acute and subacute necrotic myelitis are different forms of the same very rare disease. It occurs at any period of adult life and is characterized pathologically by scattered patches of necrosis in the spinal cord, such patches being caused by a primary hyaline sclerosis of the small meningeal and intramedullary vessels in the lower half of the spinal cord. Weakness of the legs comes on rapidly, but spasticity does not develop although the plantar reflexes are extensor. The tendon reflexes ultimately disappear, and sensory loss follows later. Pain, temperature, and deep sensibility are more affected than touch, and the level of the sensory loss usually ascends as the disease progresses. Sphincter disturbances occur early. There may be a slight rise in the protein of the cerebrospinal fluid. There is no block. The condition is steadily progressive, death occurring within months in acute cases and within two years in subacute types.

Haematomyelia—a haemorrhage into the substance of the cord—usually arises on the basis of some primary disease such as purpura, syringomyelia, or angioma of the cord, but in many cases the predisposing factor is not known. The symptoms are those of an abrupt transverse lesion of the cord, usually incomplete. The abruptness of onset is diagnostic. Most cases survive, and considerable recovery of function is to be looked for.

Caisson disease can cause a paraplegia, which is usually transient but may take months to clear up. Paraplegia has been known to occur following the administration of a *spinal anaesthetic*, which appears to give rise to a diffuse toxic myelopathy affecting both the cord and the spinal roots. *Lathyrism* is the name given to spastic paraplegia, without sensory loss, arising during famine conditions and ascribed to ingestion of the chick pea. A similar condition is encountered in persons who have been starved for prolonged periods but who have not eaten the chick pea, for which reason it is supposed that lathyrism may in fact be a deficiency disease akin to the captivity syndrome.

Affections of the Upper Motor Neuron in the Brain. These are a relatively uncommon source of paraplegia. *Injuries* to the parasagittal portion of the motor cortex are a fairly frequent occurrence in time of war, and in these cases there may be sensory loss as well as paralysis if the damage extends backwards to the sensory cortex. *Thrombosis of the superior sagittal sinus,* or of its cortical tributaries, may cause haemorrhagic softening of the 'leg area' on both sides, as for instance in the puerperium, in marasmic children, and in association with infected head wounds. *Cerebral malaria* has been known to cause a spastic paraplegia, usually transient, from cerebral softening. *General paralysis of the insane* produces widespread weakness and all the signs of pyramidal disease in advanced cases; in some instances the legs are more affected than the arms. The spinal fluid will invariably show an increase of globulin, a paretic Lange curve, and a positive V.D.R.L. reaction. *Parasagittal tumour*—usually a meningioma growing from the falx—may cause a slowly developing paraplegia as it expands laterally into the paracentral lobule on the medial aspect of each hemisphere. There may be early bladder symptoms in such cases, but sensory changes are rare. Plain radiographs of the skull, E.E.G., brain scan, and arteriography all have their place in the identification of a growth in this situation.

Congenital paraplegia, usually called *cerebral diplegia,* is not uncommon. The legs are spastic, adducted, and extended at the knee and ankle, the foot being often held in equinovarus, a position which gives rise to the 'scissors gait', if the child can walk. As a rule there is no sensory loss at all. The tendon reflexes are brisk, but clonus is often absent and in many cases the plantar responses equivocal. In more than half the cases the upper limbs are slightly affected, too; they are clumsy, stiff, and often afflicted by athetoid movements. In a few instances there is also a spasticity of the face, tongue, and pharyngeal muscles. Mental deficiency is common, and epilepsy frequent. The aetiology varies; in some cases it seems to be caused by faulty development early in pregnancy, while there is some reason to believe that in others the brain has been attacked by some unspecified condition, after it has been fully formed. Birth injury is rarely responsible, in contradistinction to its importance in congenital hemiplegia. Congenital diplegia sometimes accompanies *congenital hydrocephalus,* and such cases must be distinguished from the paraplegia which may occur in some hydrocephalics as a result of an associated myelodysplasia of the spinal cord or a meningomyelocele.

Another congenital condition, which can give rise to pyramidal and cerebellar signs, is the Arnold-Chiari malformation, in which a tongue of cerebellar tissue and an elongated medulla protrude downwards through the foramen magnum, compressing the cord. In some cases it interferes with the outflow of the spinal fluid from the fourth ventricle, so causing internal hydrocephalus. Unlike platybasia (p. 721) there is no invagination of the foramen magnum, but there are often associated abnormalities of the occipital bone, atlas, and axis, and a meningomyelocele may also be present. It is sometimes possible to relieve the hydrocephalus by suboccipital decompression.

Other causes of cerebral paraplegia are very rare. It has occurred as a result of *thrombosis of an unpaired anterior cerebral artery*—an anatomical abnormality which is not infrequent. *Schilder's disease* and *disseminated sclerosis* can pick out the corticospinal fibres to the legs only, but this is rare and in the case of the latter disease paraplegia is usually spinal in origin. There is no true weakness of the legs in the early phase of *paralysis agitans,* but as the disease advances enfeeblement of the limbs becomes more obvious and eventually it may be extreme; it is associated with severe rigidity of extrapyramidal type, and the plantar responses remain flexor to the end.

Affections of the Lower Motor Neuron cause a flaccid paraplegia with atrophy, loss of tendon reflexes and, in many cases, sensory loss and sphincter disturbances. The most common causes of a flaccid paraplegia are *acute anterior poliomyelitis, injuries to the cauda equina,* and certain forms of *polyneuritis.* The other conditions enumerated under this heading are all uncommon, but they will be discussed *seriatim* in the order of their classification. (*See also* the causes of muscular atrophy, p. 552.)

Injuries to the cauda equina or to the *lumbosacral segments of the cord* are commonly due to fracture-dislocation of the lumbar spine, while in war-time gunshot wounds are not unusual. A through-and-through wound of the pelvis may produce bilateral paralysis of sciatic distribution, the muscles innervated by the femoral nerve escaping. These conditions require no comment, for the diagnosis is plain.

Of the *infections* listed, *acute anterior poliomyelitis* is the most common. The sudden onset with fever and pain in the back and limbs, the rapid onset of a paralysis which reaches its peak in a few hours, and the objective findings of lower motor neuron paralysis with absent tendon-reflexes and normal sensation complete a picture which is almost diagnostic, and is made completely so if it is possible to demonstrate that individual muscles elsewhere in the body have been affected. Moreover, isolated muscles within the area of paralysis may be found to have escaped. Lumbar puncture in the acute stage commonly reveals a pleocytosis with a predominance of lymphocytes. *Diphtheritic polyneuritis* usually affects the legs more than the arms, which may even appear to have escaped. The diagnosis depends upon the rapid development of a polyneuritis, often preceded by weakness of accommodation and (in pharyngeal diphtheria) palatal paralysis, in a person who has had diphtheria and has received either no antitoxin or an insufficient quantity. Care must be taken not to miss cases in which polyneuritis supervenes on an unrecognized diphtheritic infection of wounds or sores of the surface of the body. Flaccid paraplegia of rapid onset is a common feature of the so-called *infective polyneuritis of Guillain-Barré*, which often comes on with a brief period of fever and usually affects all four limbs with a symmetrical paralysis of both motor and sensory functions, to which may be added cranial nerve palsies especially facial palsies on and in both sides. The protein content of the cerebrospinal fluid may be much raised, without any increase in the cells, but this finding is encountered in severe cases of polyneuritis of other types and cannot be regarded as specific. In some cases sensation is unaffected, and this may cause confusion with poliomyelitis, especially when—as sometimes occurs—the motor involvement is patchy in the legs. *Leprosy* may cause a paraplegia in the later stages of the disease, but the presence of cutaneous lesions, wasting of muscles in the upper limbs, and the palpable thickening of subcutaneous nerves will prevent errors.

Non-infective forms of polyneuritis are common, notably those due to *alcohol*, and (in Asia) *vitamin-B deficiency*. In most cases the upper limbs are affected as well as the legs, though to a lesser extent. Generally speaking the pattern of the signs is the same, whatever the cause, and differential diagnosis depends on specific features in the history or on physical examination— exposure to alcohol, or to *heavy metals* such as arsenic, or to a deficient diet; the presence in the urine of sugar or ketones in *diabetes*, and porphyrins in *porphyria*; the presence of enlarged glands in Hodgkin's disease; evidence of bronchogenic or gastric *carcinoma*; the cutaneous, glandular, skeletal, and ocular evidences of *sarcoidosis*; the fever, wasting, renal changes, and changes in the blood-vessels as determined by muscle biopsy, in *polyarteritis nodosa*—a condition in which muscle paralysis is usually patchy rather than universal. Rapidly advancing paraplegia, followed by weakness of the upper limbs, may occur, with fatal results, when the plasma-potassium is high, as in *renal failure*, or when the potassium level is too low, as in *Addison's disease* following over-enthusiastic medication with desoxycorticosterone. The disorders due to potassium are not a true polyneuritis, however, and are mentioned here only because they can be mistaken for the acute ascending form of the disease. The various forms of polyneuritis are more fully discussed in the section on muscular atrophy (p. 552).

Congenital abnormalities are rarely a cause of a flaccid paraplegia, but *myelodysplasia* of the lumbosacral cord, with or without a meningocele, is occasionally seen. The infant's legs are weak and flaccid, with absent reflexes, and examination of the lumbosacral area will usually disclose a meningocele or a sacral dimple, or a tuft of hair over the upper end of the sacrum. Hydrocephalus may be present.

There remain for consideration certain conditions which do not readily fit into any of the groups discussed above. *Peroneal muscular atrophy* (Charcot-Marie-Tooth's disease) is a heredofamilial disease characterized pathologically by degeneration of the motor nerves and loss of anterior horn cells, and clinically by the insidious appearance and slowly progressive development of wasting and weakness in the feet and distal portion of the legs, followed by a similar process in the hands and forearms. Involvement of the feet usually precedes that of the upper limbs by years. The atrophy affects muscles transversely rather than longitudinally, and ascends equally around the circumference of the limb. There may be slight superficial sensory loss in the feet, and the tendon reflexes are usually diminished or lost. Perforating ulcers may occur. The condition usually starts in late childhood, but may not appear until 40; it does not shorten life. *Progressive muscular atrophy* seldom starts in the legs, unlike amyotrophic lateral sclerosis, but it can do so. The combination of atrophy, fibrillation, and exaggeration of the tendon reflexes in the affected limbs is characteristic, and in most cases fibrillation or atrophy will be discovered elsewhere in the body. *Hypertrophic polyneuritis* (Dejerine-Sottas), a rare hereditary disease, is characterized by weakness and wasting of the feet and peripheral parts of the legs, peripheral sensory loss, and palpable thickening of the peripheral nerve-trunks.

Affections of the Muscles are rarely encountered as a cause of paraplegia. In *myasthenia gravis* the legs may fatigue to the point of paralysis as a result of exercise, but the swift recovery after rest, the usual presence of similar fatigue phenomena in the cranial nerves, and the immediate response to an injection of prostigmine or edrophonium will settle the matter. The *primary muscular dystrophies* are easily recognized when once they are fully developed, but difficulty may be experienced in the early stages when a child presents an ill-defined weakness of the legs, or in cases without a positive family history. Boys are affected much more often than girls, but it is generally inherited from the mother's side. Some members of the family may present atrophic myopathy, whilst others suffer from the pseudo-hypertrophic form. When fully developed the most striking feature of the case is the marked weakness of the legs notwithstanding the apparent firmness and great size of the calves (*Fig.* 646). The muscles are really atrophied, their apparent enlargement being due to extensive deposition of intramuscular interstitial fat. Ultimately, if the patient survives, all the muscles in the body become wasted and fibrous; but whereas some of them atrophy from the first, others exhibit marked pseudo-hypertrophy before they atrophy —particularly the gastrocnemii, the solei, the glutei, the deltoids, the supraspinati and infra-spinati, and portions of the triceps. The muscles of the hands and feet are generally unaffected; those most frequently atrophied are the lower

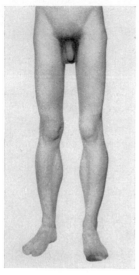

Fig. 646. Pseudo-hypertrophic muscular dystrophy ex-hibiting pseudo-hypertrophy of the calves. (*Professor W. J. H. Butterfield.*)

half of the pectoralis major, the latissimus dorsi, the serratus magnus, the biceps, and the flexors of the knee. There are no sensory or sphincter troubles. The weakness of the muscles of the pelvic girdle and thigh causes a waddling gait and a highly characteristic difficulty in getting up from a lying posture. The boy may be described as 'climbing up himself'. He first rolls over and rests on his hands and knees; then puts his head between his arms and raises the knees from the ground, so that he is now supported on his hands and feet; he next brings one hand nearer to his toes, and swinging his body over to the other side, places his opposite hand on the corresponding knee, straightens that leg, and repeats the performance on the first side, so that now, with his legs widely separated, he has one hand resting on each knee; he then works each hand alternately higher up his thighs, until finally, by a sudden backward movement of his shoulders, he attains the erect attitude. Another feature of the case is that if one tries to lift the boy up by putting one's hands under his armpits, his shoulders rise right up to his ears, and he slips through one's hands.

The *infantile* and the *juvenile* types of primary muscular dystrophy are both characterized by progressive wasting of the muscles without pseudo-hypertrophy; in the infantile form the muscles are atrophic from the first, whereas in the juvenile form the muscles develop in a normal way up to a certain point, and then gradually waste away. The disease is distinguished from peripheral neuritis by: The family history, the distribution of the wasting, the integrity of sensa-tion and the reflexes, the progressive course, and the electrical reactions. The primary muscular dystrophies receive different names according to the groups of muscles first affected. In the Lan-douzy-Dejerine (facio-scapulo-humeral) type, for instance, the face muscles are attacked first, the trouble spreading slowly to the shoulder and upper arm. It is probable, however, that what-ever groups of muscles may be the first affected, the differences are of degree and distribution rather than of kind, and that the muscular wast-ing, wherever it may begin, ultimately becomes widespread, and finally involves all of the muscles more or less.

Hysterical Paraplegia may be either 'spastic' or flaccid, but it is readily distinguished in recent cases by the absence of wasting, the normality of the tendon and plantar reflexes, normal electrical reactions, and the presence of positive evidence of psychological disturbance, whether it be an outspoken neurosis or the placid indifference of the successful hysteric whose paraplegia has resolved some personal difficulty. There is usually sensory loss in the feet, legs, or entire lower limbs. The upper level of this loss is usually transverse and clear-cut, and its extent can often be altered by suggestion. There are two features which may mislead: ankle-clonus can sometimes be main-tained for a considerable time in hysterics; and atrophy can be present in long-standing and neglected cases.

Ian Mackenzie.

PELVIC SWELLING

The following list tabulates the many swellings which may rise up out of the pelvis into the abdomen or which may appear to be pelvic when they are really primarily abdominal:

Bladder

Simple distension. New growth.

Vagina

Haematocolpos
Hydrocolpos.

Uterus

Pregnancy: normal or abnormal, or associated with tumours of the uterus or ovary
New growths: Fibromyoma. Adenomyoma. Sar-coma. Carcinoma. Chorionic carcinoma
Haematometra. Pyometra.

Ovary

Cyst. Solid new growths.

Fallopian Tubes

Salpingo-oophoritis
Hydrosalpinx
Pyosalpinx
Tubal gestation
Progressive extra-uterine gestation
Carcinoma.

Pelvic Peritoneum

Encysted peritoneal fluid
Haematocele due to extra-uterine gestation
Haematocele due to haemorrhage from a corpus luteum
Pelvic abscess
Ascites
Hydatid cyst
Retroperitoneal lipoma or sarcoma.

Pelvic Cellular Tissue

Cellulitis. Pelvic haematoma.

Appendix Vermiformis

Abscess. Appendicitis with pregnancy.

Pelvic Bones

New growths.

Omentum

New growths. Cysts.

Phantom Tumour

Pancreatic Cyst

Mesenteric Cyst

Kidney

Tumour. Hydronephrosis. Pyonephrosis. Pelvic kidney.

Spleen

Enlargement; displacement.

Urachus

Cyst.

Sigmoid Colon

Diverticulitis. Carcinoma.

Many of these lesions are not primarily pelvic, but they are included in the list because they are liable to be mistaken for pelvic tumours. Thus *renal, splenic,* or *pancreatic tumours* may reach the pelvic brim, but the history ought to show that they have grown down from above, not up from below. *Renal swellings* may be associated with urinary changes, or absence of urinary secretion on the affected side as detected by the cystoscope or an intravenous pyelogram. Malformations of the genital tract are associated with developmental abnormalities of the renal tract. It is not uncommon to find a solitary pelvic kidney in patients with congenital absence of the vagina and uterus. *Splenic enlargements* may be associated with blood-changes. *Pancreatic cysts* are the least likely to be mistaken for pelvic swellings, but they have been difficult to distinguish from ovarian tumours with long pedicles.

The commonest difficulty which arises in the diagnosis of pelvic swellings is to differentiate between the *distended bladder, pregnant uterus, ovarian cyst,* and *uterine fibromyoma,* and the commonest mistakes are made between these swellings. The *distended bladder* is the easiest to dispose of, the passage of a catheter settling the question; yet neglect of this simple procedure has led to the abdomen being opened.

The history is of value in differentiating the other swellings, for amenorrhoea is the rule in pregnancy, menorrhagia in fibromyoma, and no change in menstruation with ovarian tumours. These assumptions are correct in almost 99 out of every 100 cases, but exceptions do exist. The cardinal point in diagnosis is not to think of the possible fallacies until the common rule has been considered thoroughly. Normal menstruation during pregnancy is virtually unknown. It has been stated that menstruation is possible up to the 3rd month; that haemorrhages occur during the early months of pregnancy is true, but in most cases these haemorrhages represent threatened abortion, and not menstruation. Fibroids are associated with haemorrhages in the case of interstitial or submucous growths; but there may be no disturbance of menstruation with subperitoneal fibroids. Ovarian tumours only cause amenorrhoea when they are bilateral and destroy all ovarian tissue; as long as a small piece of ovarian tissue remains menstruation should occur normally. In the case of granulosa-cell tumours of the ovary irregular haemorrhage may occur from the uterus even after the menopause, or before puberty; these tumours secrete the follicular hormone, oestrogen, which causes the uterus to hypertrophy and the endometrium to undergo changes like those of the proliferative phase of the menstrual cycle; hence irregular haemorrhage after the menopause may be a symptom of this type of ovarian tumour.

Palpation of these tumours may be fallacious; in the early months of pregnancy the uterus may fluctuate like a cyst; a softened fibroid may do the same; or a tense ovarian cyst may feel so hard as to be mistaken for a fibroid. While the presence of the sound of the foetal heart is characteristic of pregnancy, its absence cannot be taken as evidence of a fibroid or of an ovarian tumour. It is not always possible to hear the foetal heart even in advanced pregnancy without the aid of an ultra-sonic device such as the 'Doptone'. If the pedicle of a tumour can be felt definitely attached to one uterine cornu it is strong presumptive evidence of an ovarian tumour. It is useful to pull down the uterus with a tenaculum, at the same time pushing up the tumour so as to make tense the pedicle, which might then be palpated by the vaginal touch. When small tumours are in question the first point which arises is: Can the tumour be separated from the uterus bimanually? If so, it can be neither a fibromyoma of the uterus nor a normal uterine pregnancy. This point can only be made out by careful bimanual examination, and requires considerable skill in some cases. A pedunculated fibroid is, of course, extra-uterine and may have the same anatomical arrangement to the uterus as an ovarian tumour. If it is a fibroid that has undergone cystic change the physical signs are identical to those of an ovarian cyst and only a laparotomy will reveal the true state of affairs.

Early pregnancy in a retroverted uterus should not give rise to diagnostic difficulties if it is remembered that the soft, cystic fundus is felt through the posterior fornix, that the cervix looks down the vagina or forwards to the symphysis, and that the posterior mass is continuous with the cervix. If the retroverted uterus is associated with vesical distension the picture is usually clear enough. The history of urinary retention followed by constant dribbling of urine (distension with overflow), amenorrhoea, other signs of pregnancy, the presence of two tumours—one in front, tense, tender, and elastic, the other behind, soft and cystic—and, finally, the passage of a catheter, will settle the question. The diagnosis of solid ovarian tumours is not always possible, for the pedicle is often short, and the tumour is then so close to the uterus that the two cannot be separated. They are therefore likely to be mistaken for fibroids of the uterus. They do not often cause menorrhagia, however, and this should be remembered as a cardinal point.

Large tumours arising in the pelvis are not often difficult to differentiate from one another, bearing in mind that ovarian tumours, uterine fibroids, and pregnancy are the common conditions met with. It cannot be repeated too often that amenorrhoea stands for pregnancy, and occasionally for ovarian tumours when bilateral; menorrhagia goes with uterine fibroids except in the case of subperitoneal tumours. Exceptions to these general statements are uncommon, and mistakes in diagnosis will occur but seldom if they are borne in mind. Ascites has to be differentiated from ovarian cysts, and occasionally from hydramnios. In general, ascites gives dullness in the flanks on percussion, with resonance over an area somewhere about the umbilicus, while ovarian cysts give dullness over the front of the abdomen, with resonance in the flanks. When ascites exists along with ovarian tumours the free fluid may be so large in amount that the tumour cannot be felt; as a rule, however, it can be touched on dipping through the fluid. Ascites with an ovarian tumour does not necessarily mean malignancy, but it may do so. Fibroma of the ovary, or a simple ovarian cyst with a twisted pedicle, may also be accompanied by some fluid. Ovarian fibromata may be accompanied by a large amount of ascites and bilateral pleural effusions (Meigs's syndrome).

When *pregnancy is associated with a tumour*, the diagnosis may be difficult. This does not lie in the recognition of the pregnancy; amenorrhoea, breast changes, foetal movements, and the foetal heart will usually make that clear enough; it lies in deciding the nature, or even the presence of a tumour along with the pregnant uterus. In the early months, when the presence of two tumours can be demonstrated, the diagnosis is easier, but in the later months the great size of the abdomen, and the way in which the swellings merge into one another, may obscure the picture. The relation to the uterus, whether a part of it, or attached to it by a pedicle; the feel of the tumour, whether solid or cystic, soft or hard; and the previous history, will assist in making out the nature of the growth. Fibroids are likely to soften and degenerate during pregnancy, so that they are liable to be mistaken for ovarian cysts.

In the case of *ovarian tumours*, it is often impossible to be sure of the exact nature of the growth until this has been decided microscopically after removal. Because of this doubt there should be no undue delay in the removal of an ovarian tumour larger than the size of an orange or one that is growing. Small follicular cysts may be left as they are harmless and eventually disappear. Fixation of the growth in the pelvis, obvious ascites, unilateral oedema of the leg, emaciation of the patient, abdominal pain, and rapid growth in size of the abdomen point to malignancy.

In the case of definitely *uterine tumours*, the diagnosis of malignant growths is not often difficult because they cause irregular bleeding in addition to uterine enlargement, but the diagnosis should always be confirmed by the microscopic examination of curetted fragments. Fibroids are only likely to be mistaken for malignant growths when they produce constant bleeding as a result of extrusion, infection, and sloughing. Rapid growth of a fibroid is more likely to be the result of degenerative changes, such as formation of cysts or necrobiosis, than to the development of a sarcoma or other malignant growth along with it. Growth of a fibroid after the menopause, however, should make one consider sarcomatous change in it.

With small tumours confined to the pelvis, or rising only a little above the brim, diagnosis is often a matter of difficulty. In practice, however, *extra-uterine gestation* and its resulting blood-tumour stand out pre-eminently as a swelling which must be recognized at once if treatment is to be successful. Before rupture or abortion has occurred a tubal gestation is essentially a small tumour in one posterolateral corner of the pelvis, attached to the uterus, indefinite in consistence, remarkably tender, and perhaps—though not always—associated with amenorrhoea of short duration and acute attacks of pain in the pelvis. Definite signs of pregnancy may be entirely wanting but a pregnancy test will be positive. It may be mistaken for a chronic salpingo-oophoritis, a small cystic ovary, a small pedunculated fibroid, or a small ovarian dermoid. The differential diagnosis may be difficult, but attacks of pain unassociated with menstruation are not likely to occur in any of the above conditions; the pains are usually the result of over-distension and stretching of the tube from haemorrhage into its wall or lumen around the fertilized ovum. Unless the swelling is tender (often very tender) it is not likely to be due to a tubal pregnancy. When tubal abortion has occurred, or tubal rupture, the signs of internal bleeding, accompanied by sudden pain and collapse, with haemorrhage from the uterus or the passage of a decidual cast, usually make an unmistakable picture. Intraperitoneal haemorrhage is more commonly severe and copious with tubal rupture than with tubal abortion. If the patient recovers from the initial bleeding the clinical picture may be that of a retro-uterine or peritubal *haematocele*. The uterus is pushed forwards and upwards against the symphysis pubis, and the mass of blood-clot can be felt posteriorly bulging the posterior fornix and also the anterior wall of the rectum. The tumour is usually semi-resonant in front, because intestine adheres to it. It is very tender. Tubal abortion is most likely to be mistaken for an ordinary uterine abortion; but the presence of a tender mass on one side of the uterus, with a closed cervix, and the absence of uterine contractions or extrusion of any products of conception, should make the case clear. Pain is much more severe but external bleeding is much less in extra-uterine pregnancy. The essential point in diagnosing an ectopic pregnancy is to approach every woman of child-bearing age who complains of irregular bleeding and abdominal pain with the possibility in mind. No two cases are alike and there are more exceptions to the rule in the symptomatology of this condition than in any other.

Progressive extra-uterine gestation is a rare occurrence, and is the result of continued growth of an embryo after a partial separation from the tube as a result of rupture, or extrusion from the fimbriated end (abortion). The continued enlargement of a mass beside the uterus, with amenorrhoea and progressive signs of pregnancy, are the most characteristic points. Abdominal pain in late pregnancy is a characteristic feature. The uterus may be felt in the pelvis separate from the foetal sac. The diagnosis, however, is difficult, because there is always some effused blood which obscures the outlines of the uterus, and makes it appear to be a part of the pelvic mass. The foetus is often situated high above the pelvis and it tends to lie transversely facing downward. A radiograph reveals the foetus adopting a position that is characteristically odd, the spine hyperextended or acutely flexed and the head and limbs at unusual angles to the trunk. If, on a lateral view, radiography shows foetal parts overlapping the maternal spine the pregnancy must be extra-uterine. A hysterosalpingogram will establish the absence of an intra-uterine gestation and also the size of the uterus, which never exceeds that of a 5 months' gestation even in the presence of a full-term extra-uterine pregnancy, and the cervix does not soften to the same degree. A hysterogram should only be undertaken when the diagnosis is virtually certain. In those cases where the foetus lies in the front of the false sac it will feel very superficial owing to the absence of uterine wall in front of it, and between it and

the examining hand. The foetus is, however, often difficult to palpate, due, perhaps, to the placenta in front, which may give rise to a loud vascular souffle just medial to the anterior superior iliac spine on the side from which it derives its main blood-supply (via the ovarian vessels).

The swellings due to *salpingo-oophoritis* are usually easy to distinguish. The form fixed tender masses in the pelvis, seldom of any definite shape, but occasionally presenting the characteristic retort shape, with its narrow end near the uterus, which the tube assumes when distended with fluid. The history is usually that of an acute illness at some period, with pain in the pelvis, rise of temperature, and peritoneal irritation. It is preceded, as a rule, by uterine discharge and menorrhagia. This inflammatory disturbance in married women is associated with long periods of sterility, owing to the sealing up of the tubes. In the chronic state pelvic pain, congestive dysmenorrhoea, dyspareunia, vaginal discharge, menorrhagia, and infertility are complained of. The signs of suppuration, pyrexia, leucocytosis, wasting, and daily sweating are usually absent and the pus in the tubes is sterile.

A large *pelvic abscess* may accompany salpingo-oophoritis, or may occur alone without infection of the tubes, as we see occasionally in puerperal septic infections. When it does occur, it is of course peritoneal; it fixes the uterus in a central position, bulges into the posterior fornix and rectum, tends to rupture into the rectum, before which occurrence there is a copious discharge of mucus per anum, is acute in onset, and accompanied by signs of local peritonitis. A swinging temperature, leucocytosis, sweats, and the symptoms of fever are present, all suddenly improving when the abscess discharges itself. It is likely to be confounded with *pelvic cellulitis*, in which the uterus is fixed in a laterally displaced position. This swelling bulges one lateral fornix and extends right out to the lateral pelvic wall, tends to burrow along the round ligament to the groin, and may point there like a psoas abscess, is slow in onset, chronic, and not accompanied by signs of local peritonitis. It always follows labour, or abortion, whereas pelvic abscess of peritoneal origin may occur with salpingo-oophoritis or appendicitis, quite apart from pregnancy. Pelvic cellulitis never bears any relation to salpingo-oophoritis. It may take many weeks to resolve, which it usually does without pointing.

Encysted peritoneal fluid, hydatid cysts, and *retroperitoneal lipomata* are generally diagnosed as ovarian cysts, and their true nature is only discovered at operation. There are no definite signs by which these conditions may be diagnosed, and as they all require operative treatment, postoperative diagnosis meets their requirements. Encysted peritoneal fluid due to tuberculosis may be suspected if tuberculous lesions are present elsewhere in the body. They lack the definite outline of an ovarian cyst and are often semi-resonant on percussion.

Distension of the vagina by menstrual fluid is not likely to be mistaken for anything else, if only on account of the absolute closure of the hymen which gives rise to it. Haematocolpos is practically the only central tumour met with between the rectum and the bladder reaching from the hymen to the pelvic brim. The uterus can usually be felt like a cork movable upon its upper extremity. The haematocolpos presents a blue-coloured swelling at the vulva. A similar swelling may be found on rare occasions in newborn girl babies: the vagina is filled with a milky fluid (hydrocolpos).

Urachal cysts occur in front of the uterus and in close relation to the bladder; but in spite of this they are usually mistaken for ovarian cysts. It is to be remembered, however, that ovarian cysts are only likely to get in front of the uterus when they are large, but dermoid cysts of the ovary of small size occasionally do so. Urachal cysts rarely attain a large size.

Appendicitis with pregnancy occurs occasionally, and may be mistaken for such a condition as torsion of an ovarian pedicle. The swelling due to appendix inflammations is, however, in close relation to the anterior superior spine of the ilium, and apparently adherent to the iliac fossa. The lump is ill-defined, and rarely fluctuates unless there is a large abscess. The acute onset may be similar to that of torsion of an ovarian pedicle. There is usually a definite fluctuating tumour when an ovarian cyst is present, and some interval between it and the iliac crest can usually be felt.

Phantom tumours are due to diaphragmatic contraction, causing the abdominal wall to bulge. They are usually mistaken by patients for pregnancy, but are not accompanied by any of the signs of pregnancy. Amenorrhoea must be excepted from this, however, because these cases usually occur about the menopause. Their true nature can usually be discovered by making the patient breathe normally, relaxing the diaphragm; but if any doubt exists, the protrusion will disappear under an anaesthetic.

Growths of the pelvic bones are very rare tumours, usually cartilaginous or sarcomatous. They are only likely to be mistaken for adherent inflammatory masses due to salpingo-oophoritis. They will be found to be continuous with the bones forming the pelvis, and when growing from the sacrum may have the rectum in front of them; all other pelvic tumours have the rectum behind them. In most cases of this nature the uterus and adnexa can be palpated bimanually, and shown to be free from disease and unconnected with the mass. When complicated by the presence of a pregnant uterus their true nature may be difficult to determine unless examination reveals that they are absolutely fixed and continuous with the bones of the pelvis.

T. L. T. Lewis.

PELVIS, PAIN IN

In practice, pelvic pain can usually be classified under four headings, namely: (1) *Deep-seated pain*; (2) *Referred pain*; (3) *Spasmodic pain*; (4) *Backache or sacralgia*; (5) *Mid-cycle ovulation pain (Mittelschmerz).*

1. Deep-seated Pain is aching in character, continuous, and may be acute in onset or chronic in duration. It is the result of congested blood-vessels and oedema of the pelvic organs, most commonly the result of inflammation. In acute inflammation the pain is severe, elicited by lower abdominal pressure and thereby made worse. Infection of the pelvic organs gives rise to *local peritonitis*, and hence the severe pain. Chronic dull aching pain is caused by chronic salpingo-oophoritis (pyosalpinx, hydrosalpinx, ovarian abscess, or chronic interstitial salpingitis), whether gonococcal, tuberculous, or pyogenic in origin or following labour or abortion, by endometriosis of the ovaries and by chronic pelvic appendicitis or diverticulitis. It may also occur as the result of infection of the pelvic cellular tissue, parametritis, following labour or abortion. More severe pain may be due to a twisted or infected or ruptured ovarian cyst or to a ruptured ectopic pregnancy.

Sometimes there is no evidence of infection or other disease to account for chronic pelvic pain. Although congestion due to unrelieved sexual stimulation is suggested as the reason there are not always good grounds for saying this. It is unlikely that retroversion or retroflexion of the uterus cause pelvic pain; they may occasionally give rise to backache. Culdocentesis (puncture and aspiration of the pouch of Douglas) and laparoscopy (visual examination of the pelvic contents through a laparoscope inserted through the anterior abdominal wall, usually at the umbilicus) are used to diagnose pelvic lesions, but generally a careful history and examination make such procedures unnecessary. When no lesion is found but the patient still complains these procedures may be used to exclude pathology.

2. Referred Pain may appear to arise in the pelvis when the true cause lies elsewhere, pain being referred through spinal segments D.10–L.3, as, for instance, from a spinal tumour, or in tabes dorsalis.

3. Spasmodic Pain in the pelvis is nearly always due to painful uterine contractions when it is of genital origin. The exception to this is the spasmodic pain which occurs in connexion with *tubal gestation*, as a rule in the few days which precede tubal abortion or rupture of the tube. The only way to diagnose between this tubal pain and that due to uterine contractions is by a careful consideration of the history of the case, and the finding of a definite tubal swelling by bimanual palpation. Even then the diagnosis may be difficult. Laparoscopy is indicated when doubt persists. Spasmodic pain due to *uterine contractions* is caused by: the onset of abortion or labour; spasmodic dysmenorrhoea (p. 230);

attempted expulsion from the uterus of a growth such as a fibromyoma; 'after-pains' following labour; the presence of a contraceptive in the uterus (e.g., an intra-uterine device such as a Gravigard copper-7, a Lippes loop, a Gynecoil, or a Dalkon shield).

The differential diagnosis of these conditions is easy, but it may be difficult to be sure that the pelvic pain has a uterine origin, for sometimes spasmodic pain may be referred to the pelvis from such relatively distant causes as appendicitis, intestinal, renal, or biliary colic, leaking gastric ulcer, ruptured tubal gestation, twisted ovarian pedicle, haemorrhage into a Graafian follicle, leakage or rupture of an ovarian cyst or pyosalpinx, dyspepsia, or flatulent distension of the bowels.

4. Backache, or **Sacralgia,** is a common complaint in many cases of pelvic disease, but as a sole symptom is most unlikely to be due to a pelvic lesion. It is true that in such cases the pain may be worse at the time of menstruation but the same applies to those cases which have an orthopaedic origin. Before the pelvic contents can be suspected there should be present other symptoms of pelvic disease, and it will be found, almost invariably, that the backache is only a secondary or minor complaint. The presence of such conditions as (1) a heavy congested retroverted uterus with prolapse; (2) large, or impacted ovarian or fibroid tumours; (3) a retroverted gravid uterus impacted in the pelvis; (4) a pelvic haematocele; (5) pelvic endometriosis or chronic salpingo-oophoritis make the association more likely, particularly if the backache is low down. Most backaches in women are at a high level in the small of the back or lumbar regions and are of orthopaedic origin; pain arising in the pelvic organs is at a lower level in the back, over the sacrum. Sometimes a large cervical erosion with surrounding parametritis is the only finding, and in many of these cases adequate treatment of the erosion cures the backache. Pelvic congestion, the result of coitus interruptus or other unsatisfactory sexual relationship, particularly if a retroversion is present, may be responsible. A backwardly displaced uterus, however, without some other complicating factor is hardly ever the cause of backache. In some cases where slight prolapse is present in addition, if the uterus is replaced and a ring inserted, the backache will be cured. Dyspareunia is often present in such cases owing to the prolapse of one or both ovaries. The back should be examined and any abnormal posture, limitation of movement, tenseness of the back muscles, or tender areas should be noted. In such cases an orthopaedic cause is more likely, although a pelvic cause may be responsible for the assumption of abnormal postures to secure comfort. In cases of impacted tumours the pain may be due to actual pressure on the sacral nerves at their exits, in which case pain will be felt down the inner sides of the thighs and back of the legs. In advanced cases of carcinoma of the cervix, backache is a complaint, but it is always associated with pain in the buttock, due to involvement of the sacral plexus, and the pain radiates down the legs. Secondary deposits in the lumbar spine may be the cause.

Probably not more than a very small minority of backaches are of genital origin. It may result from some urinary irritation due to oxalates or coli bacilluria; it may accompany a calculus in the ureter or some lesion of the renal pelvis, though as a rule, in renal cases, the pain is situated rather higher up. Caries of the spine low down, growth in the spine or in the spinal-cord membranes, might also cause it, or it may result from inflammation or strain of the sacro-iliac joint, displaced disk, rectal growth, haemorrhoids, proctitis, or scybala. Injuries to the lumbar spine, including strain and subluxation as well as damage of a minor character to the erector spinae and other muscles causing muscle fatigue, have to be remembered in this connexion. A correct diagnosis cannot be made without a complete examination of all adjacent structures, combined with careful urinary analysis.

5. Mid-cycle Ovulation Pain (Mittelschmerz). Some women habitually experience some dull pain in the midline or in one or other iliac fossa at about the time of ovulation about 14 days before the next period. In others the pain may be experienced for a few cycles only. Occasionally slight vaginal bleeding accompanies the pain. The timing of the pain and the absence of any abnormal pelvic findings usually make the diagnosis clear.

T. L. T. Lewis.

PENILE SORES

Sores on the penis may be present on the thin mucous covering of the glans or prepuce, or on the cutaneous surface of the body of the penis; they are more common in the former situation.

Ulceration in the neighbourhood of the glans penis may be due to:

> Balanitis
> Herpes genitalis
> Soft sore
> Granuloma venereum
> Lymphogranuloma inguinale
> Chancre
> Epithelioma
> Papilloma
> Gummatous ulceration
> Tuberculous ulceration.
> Injury, for example from a bite.

Balanitis. If inflammatory processes have been allowed to continue beneath the prepuce, ulceration and excoriation of the mucous membrane covering the glans penis or lining the prepuce will occur, accompanied by a stinking, purulent discharge. Multiple shallow ulcers are formed, rapidly coalescing and causing considerable discomfort. The prepuce often becomes swollen and oedematous, preventing retraction, so that a condition of phimosis occurs, or, if retraction has taken place, the analogous state of paraphimosis, almost strangulating the end of the penis and even causing it to become gangrenous. Care must be exercised in diagnosing a simple balanitis from one accompanying acute gonorrhoeal urethritis or an underlying syphilitic or soft chancre. The so-called balanitis circinata is part of Reiter's (Brodie's) disease, occurring in association with urethritis, arthritis, conjunctivitis (often slight and transient), and buccal ulceration. In Behçet's syndrome also ulcerative penile and scrotal lesions may occur in association with buccal ulcers. With an acute urethritis there will be a history of infection, pain along the course of the urethra during micturition, and, very rarely nowadays, chordee; the intracellular gonococcus may be identified in a Gram-stained smear of the discharge.

If a chancre exists under the swollen phimosed prepuce there is often a tender spot about the corona or at the fraenum. With a soft sore consecutive sores may appear about the orifice of the prepuce, while the inguinal glands are much more likely to be inflamed or to suppurate than with simple balanitis. A syphilitic chancre obscured by a phimosis can usually be felt distinctly under the skin, and causes a comparatively small amount of discharge, while the inguinal glands become enlarged but do not suppurate. The interval of about four weeks from the time of the possible source of infection until the appearance of the sore will suggest and the finding of spirochaetes (*Treponema pallidum*) in the fluid expressed from the ulcer will prove the diagnosis. In later cases, enlargement of the inguinal glands, secondary cutaneous rash, sore throat, and positive serological reactions will be present.

A form of balanitis which is frequently very obstinate to treatment may occur in patients with diabetes mellitus. Phimosis appearing in an adult male is often due to unsuspected diabetes; the urine should always be tested for sugar.

Herpes Genitalis. Herpes may attack the genital organs as part of a herpes zoster which is unilateral. This is a rarity compared with herpes simplex, which is now regarded as an important sexually transmitted disease. Recent work has implicated *Herpesvirus hominis* Type 2 in the aetiology of uterine cervical cancer. The disease begins as a patch of erythema on the inner surface of the prepuce or on the glans penis, followed by vesicles and pustules; the latter become rubbed by the clothes, and form small ulcers. Herpes of the genital organs tends to recur, so that a previous history of a similar attack is often forthcoming. If seen during the vesicular stage no difficulty will be met with in the diagnosis; but if suppuration has followed, it must be diagnosed from a venereal sore. Soft chancres are usually deeper, with marked edges; their bases are sloughing, and they are usually accompanied by a bubo, which is exceptional with herpes. A syphilitic chancre is usually single, indurated, and raised, and is accompanied by the typical multiple, discrete amygdaloid glands in the inguinal region. It should be remembered that syphilis may become inoculated upon a herpetic patch or that herpes may appear in an area already infected with syphilis.

Soft Sores or Chancroids of the penis occur almost invariably from infection during sexual connexion. The incubation period is short, a vesicle occurs in two days, and this breaks down rapidly to form a rounded or oval ulcer with undermined edges and a yellowish sloughing base. The ulcers appear usually on the mucous surface of the glans, fraenum, or corona, and are multiple, direct inoculation occurring from each ulcer to the contiguous part. They may cause rapid destruction of tissue, perforating the fraenum or spreading over the surface of the glans. The soft sore must be differentiated from others occurring on the glans, and above all from a syphilitic chancre, and serum from the edge of the lesion should be examined for *Haemophilus ducreyi* (Ducrey's bacillus) as well as by dark-ground illumination for *Treponema pallidum*. At the same time it must be remembered that besides the infection with chancroid, a simultaneous infection with syphilis may have taken place, so that a soft sore may ultimately become indurated and assume the character of a primary syphilitic lesion. The chancroids are multiple, are accompanied by a good deal of thin, purulent discharge, and by a painful swelling of the inguinal glands, usually of one side, which have a marked tendency to suppurate. On the other hand, a syphilitic chancre is single, is raised and indurated, has little discharge, and is accompanied by enlarged but firm and indolent glands in both inguinal regions; the incubation period of a syphilitic chancre is from twenty-one to twenty-eight days. The multiple ulcerations caused by herpes are more superficial, and rarely cause a bubo.

Granuloma Inguinale (granuloma venereum) is a chronic granulomatous ulceration which may affect the perineum and the inguinal regions as well as the penis. It occurs in tropical countries and is mildly contagious. The lesion on the penis starts as a papule which appears after a few days' or weeks' incubation period and breaks down to form a superficial ulcer. Examination of the discharge shows capsulated bacteria known as Donovan bodies, which are believed to be the causative organisms. Lymph-nodes are not involved.

Lymphogranuloma Venereum (lymphogranuloma inguinale) is also commoner in the tropics, and is a chronic condition characterized by a small initial lesion on the penis with marked glandular enlargement in the groins and severe constitutional disturbances. The glands tend to break down and form sinuses. The lesion on the penis appears, after an incubation period of about a week, as a vesicle, papule, or ulcer, and it tends to disappear by the time the lymphatic glands are enlarged. It is due to a filter-passing organism which is a member of the *Chlamydia* group and can be diagnosed by complement fixation re-actions, demonstration of specific skin reactivity, and a biopsy of primary lesion or lymph-node. It must be distinguished from chancroid and from granuloma venereum. Rectal stricture and effusions into joints are other lesions caused by this disease.

Chancre—the initial lesion of syphilis—generally appears on the penis, and is most common in the neighbourhood of the fraenum or coronary sulcus. A chancre appears about twenty-five days

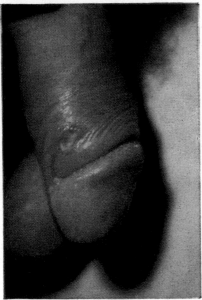

Fig. 647. Primary chancre of the penis.

after infection as a reddened patch, which becomes raised above the surface of the mucous membrane, with distinctly indurated margins. The central part breaks down into an ulcer (*Fig.* 647), discharging a thin, purulent fluid, and at the same time the inguinal glands of both sides become palpable, slightly enlarged, but discrete, and with no tendency to suppurate. The chancre increases but slowly in size, or may occasionally become smaller without any treatment, and after a further lapse of from four to six weeks the typical secondary symptoms make their appearance: namely, a roseolar rash (*Fig.* 522, p. 518) on the chest, abdomen, face, and thighs, general adenitis, and mucous patches about the faucial pillars and tonsils, accompanied by low pyrexia. The diagnosis of the primary lesion of syphilis frequently presents no difficulties, the indurated character of the sore, the date of its appearance after infection, and the presence of firm, indurated glands in the inguinal region being distinctive. If the character of the sore is not distinctive it is necessary to differentiate it from other lesions of the penis. Careful search must be made by dark-ground illumination for the *Treponema pallidum* in the serum expressed

from the sore; negative serological reactions in the early stage of the disease are not reliable. If the sore is syphilitic, the secondary manifestations of the disease will follow, provided that the doubtful ulcer is not treated as a chancre.

A chancre may be simulated by an inflamed soft sore; soft sores are, however, frequently multiple, appear within a few days of infection, and are accompanied by painful enlargement of the inguinal lymphatic glands, which are particularly prone to suppurate. It must not be forgotten that a double infection may have occurred, so that a soft sore may show little inclination to heal or, becoming indurated, may present the features of a chancre after about three weeks, followed later by the symptoms of constitutional syphilis.

Epithelioma of the penis in the early stage may be confused with syphilitic chancre. In epithelioma there is no history of infection; it occurs usually in elderly uncircumcised patients, and there is frequently a greater destruction of tissue than in syphilis. The inguinal glands are not enlarged until the sore has been present for some weeks, and there are no secondary lesions such as the faucial ulceration and cutaneous rash. Diagnosis is confirmed by histological examination of a biopsy specimen.

Perhaps the greatest difficulty in the diagnosis of a chancre is experienced when it is hidden beneath an inflamed and phimosed prepuce. There is a purulent and foul discharge from beneath the oedematous and swollen prepuce; the inguinal glands are enlarged from the associated sepsis. If a chancre is present it can frequently be felt as an indurated area under the prepuce, while if it has been present for some time the secondary lesions of syphilis may be present. If any doubt exists as to whether an indurated sub-preputial area is an early epithelioma or a syphilitic sore, the prepuce should be split up along the dorsal aspect under anaesthesia, the ulceration inspected, a small piece submitted to microscopical examination if necessary or some serum expressed from the ulcer examined on a dark stage for *Treponema pallidum.*

Epithelioma (squamous-celled carcinoma) is the commonest form of malignant growth of the penis (*Fig.* 648). It arises most frequently from the inner aspect of the prepuce, or from the mucous membrane of the glans, as a small, raised ulcer, with friable, irregular edges. It is rarely present before the age of forty, and frequently occurs on the site of previous ulceration or long-standing irritation; it is unknown where circumcision has been performed in infancy, although later circumcision does not confer this near-total immunity. An *epitheliomatous ulcer* increases in size gradually in spite of various forms of treatment, and with it is frequently associated glandular enlargement in the inguinal area. At first the glands may be enlarged from septic infection, but later from malignant infiltration. An epitheliomatous ulcer may in some cases be confused with a chancre; but the friable, irregular edges of the former, the liability to bleed, and the gradual progressive increase in size in spite of treatment, in an elderly patient, together with the extensive induration of the base, should give rise to grave suspicion of malignant disease. Microscopical examination of a small piece removed from the edge of the ulcer will give direct evidence of epithelioma.

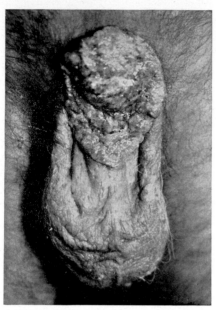

Fig. 648. Epithelioma of the penis.

Carcinoma of the penis may also occur in a *papillary form* which grows to produce a large cauliflower excrescence. In this type any enlargement of the inguinal nodes is more likely to be due to infection than to metastasis.
Papillomata (Venereal warts or Condylomata acuminata) occur on the glans and contiguous surface of the prepuce and are most frequently found on the corona. They are simple papillomata, usually multiple, and are distinguished from epithelioma by the absence of induration in the base.
Gummatous Ulceration of the penis occurs occasionally, resulting from the disintegration of a small gumma of the glans or prepuce, frequently in the position of an old scar. A gumma begins as a small, elevated nodule, which, if left untreated, softens and discharges its contents, leaving an ulcer bounded by thin edges and with a yellowish, sloughy base. A gummatous ulcer has been mistaken for a primary lesion of syphilis; but the absence of induration, the history of the onset and of a previous infection with syphilis, would be points against a chancre. A second infection with syphilis is by no means unknown, especially in those who, in years gone by, have had salvarsan alone in the treatment of the first attack, but it is rare. Occasionally the base of a

gummatous ulcer proliferates into a papillary tumour and has given rise to a suspicion of carcinoma: the diagnosis will be confirmed by a biopsy.
Tuberculous or Lupoid Ulceration of the penis is rare, and is generally associated with advanced

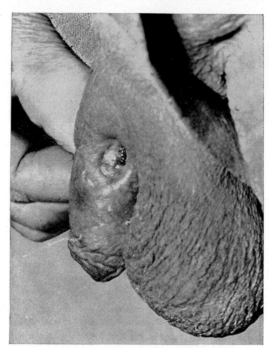

Fig. 649. 'Burrowing ulcer' on the shaft of the penis in a man of 84.

tuberculous infiltration elsewhere. Tuberculous ulcers are usually shallow, with thin overhanging edges, painful, and multiple. The infection has resulted from the rite of infantile circumcision by the Jewish method. The diagnosis is clinched by discovering tubercle bacilli in films made from the discharge.
A peculiar *burrowing ulcer* may occur on the shaft of the penis (*Fig.* 649). In the case illustrated there were intercommunicating tracts lined by squamous epithelium extending into the corpora cavernosa. There was no histological evidence of malignancy.
Injury is an uncommon cause of a penile sore but in one case under the care of Sir Eric Riches an epithelioma of the penis followed a bite from a pig!

Harold Ellis.

PENIS, PAIN IN

Pain in the penis is a symptom which occurs not only in association with lesions of the penis or urethra, but also as a referred pain from disease of the prostate, bladder, or kidney. Penile pain may be present either during or immediately after micturition, or may be entirely independent of the act. If pain is felt only during micturition there is probably some inflammatory lesion of the urethra or prostate; if it occurs immediately after the flow of the urine it suggests some lesion in the urinary bladder; pain present quite apart from micturition may be due to various diseases of the penis, bladder, ureter, or kidney.

The term 'pain', too, is a relative quantity, varying with the nervous susceptibility of the patient, for what is pain in one may be merely discomfort in another, so that the patient's description may have to be discounted to a certain extent by the clinician.

1. CAUSES OF PAIN IN THE PENIS EXPERIENCED DURING MICTURITION

1. *Diseases of Urethra*:

   Acute inflammation, gonorrhoeal or other. The passage or impaction of a calculus. Stricture of the urethra. Injury of the urethra. Foreign body in the urethra.

2. *Diseases of the Prostate*:

   Acute prostatitis. Prostatic abscess. Prostatic carcinoma. Prostatic calculus.

3. *Diseases of the Bladder*:

   Acute cystitis. Vesical calculus. Papilloma. Pedunculated carcinoma.

1. Diseases of the Urethra. The commonest cause of pain in the penis *during* micturition is acute inflammation of the urethra, usually gonorrhoeal, but may result from other organisms, and this is particularly common following catheterization. In the earliest stages of an acute urethritis, before any marked urethral discharge is apparent, there is usually a sense of smarting or tingling in the terminal urethra, more marked as the discharge increases, when it is of a burning or scalding character. This pain during micturition within a few days of sexual connexion is frequently the earliest symptom of urethral infection; a purulent discharge from the urethra is usually present when the patient comes under observation.

The *passage of a calculus* through the urethra causes a sharp, cutting pain along the urethra, the cause of which is apparent when the calculus is voided. Occasionally it may happen that micturition occurs in these cases in the dark, or that urine is not passed into a vessel, so that the calculus is not actually seen by the patient; but if there is a history of previous renal descent of a stone or symptoms pointing to vesical calculus, the sharp urethral pain during micturition occurring upon one single occasion is significant of the passage of a calculus. A stone may, however, pass into the urethra during micturition and become *arrested* at some narrowed portion of the canal, usually at the membranous portion or at the distal end, when a sudden, sharp pain is felt in the urethra, and at the same time the flow of urine is partially or completely stopped before the bladder has been emptied, further efforts to expel urine resulting only in a forceless stream; the whole length of the urethra should be examined by passing the finger along its course, when

a stone may be actually felt; or the calculus may be seen through an endoscope or identified on plain X-ray.

Occasionally a calculus may remain in the urethra, becoming gradually enlarged in size and causing pain on micturition. These calculi usually lie in the dilated posterior urethra behind a stricture in the bulb.

Urethral stricture occasionally causes pain in the urethra during micturition, especially if the calibre is small, and if there is septic infection or ulceration of the urethral mucosa behind the stricture, but as a rule stricture causes but little pain; gradually increasing difficulty in micturition, feeble stream, and dribbling of urine from the meatus after the stream has terminated, are common symptoms; the diagnosis will be confirmed by the obstruction offered to the passage of a full-sized bougie, or, better, by direct observation of the urethra through a urethroscope under air or water distension.

Injury of the urethra may cause pain during micturition. The urethra may be injured by a fall on the perineum, by a kick or blow, or by the faulty or careless passage of instruments; it may also be injured or lacerated in association with a fracture of the pelvis. The urethra may be merely bruised, lacerated on one aspect, or completely ruptured. If it is lacerated by direct injury blood usually appears at the external urinary meatus, together with a contusion in the perineum or along the course of the urethra; any attempt at micturition causes pain in the penis, while urine may or may not be expelled from the meatus, depending upon the extent of the injury, or may be extravasated into the perineal or scrotal tissues (*Fig.* 533, p. 540). As a rule there will be no difficulty in the diagnosis, but in any suspected case the greatest care should be exercised in passing an instrument into the urethra.

A *foreign body* in the urethra may cause considerable pain. In some cases the history will be clear; for instance the end of a catheter or bougie may have broken off within the urethra; but in others, especially in weak-minded individuals, no history of the insertion of a body into the urethra will be forthcoming. Direct endoscopic examination of the urethra with an irrigating urethroscope will show the foreign body; various articles have been found in the urethra, such as a wax taper, a seed of barley with its barb, a hairpin, a small shell, a nail and a glass tube used to contain hypodermic tablets.

2. Diseases of the Prostate. *Acute prostatitis* and *prostatic abscess* both give rise to pain during micturition in addition to increased frequency and difficulty during the act. Both are usually sequelae of an acute urethritis, and whereas an acute prostatitis is accompanied by a temperature raised to 100–101° F. (38° C.), a prostatic abscess causes the usual rise and fall common to septic processes. The diagnosis of the two conditions is made by careful rectal examination, the acutely inflamed gland presenting a much enlarged, smooth-surfaced prominence in the rectum, while if an abscess is present a softer acutely tender area in the inflamed gland can usually be detected. An acute prostatitis may accompany a haematogenous bacterial urinary infection as distinct from a venereal urethritis.

Adenomatous enlargement of the prostate gives rise to no penile pain during micturition; neither does the prostate containing tuberculous deposits; but pain in the penis is present during micturition occasionally in cases of *prostatic carcinoma*, owing to the direct infiltration of the urethral mucous membrane. Prostatic carcinoma is by no means uncommon (indeed, it is the sixth commonest cause of death from cancer in the United Kingdom), and while in its general symptoms it resembles those of prostatic adenoma, there is a marked difference found on digital examination of the gland per rectum. The carcinomatous gland presents rounded areas of densely infiltrated tissue, in contradistinction to the elastic, uniform feel of the adenomatous variety; the whole gland becomes fixed and immovable, and in advanced stages distinct infiltration of the lateral pelvic lymphatics and soft tissues may be felt extending laterally from the affected organ. It is often tender on palpation.

Care must be taken not to mistake the hard nodules felt in a prostate containing *calculi* for carcinoma; with calculous disease the gland is not fixed and is only slightly enlarged, whilst on gentle pressure with the examining finger the calculi may be felt to grate upon each other. During the passage of a catheter through the prostatic urethra distinct grating may be felt if any calculus has ulcerated the urethral wall. Radiography will distinguish the two conditions (*Fig.* 488, p. 478) but they may coexist.

3. Diseases of the Bladder may cause penile pain during micturition under certain circumstances, although it is much more common to find that pain in vesical disease follows the completion of micturition. In *acute cystitis*, penile pain is present throughout micturition, due to the intense congestion of the vesical mucous membrane of the trigone and around the internal urethral orifice. The other symptoms of acute cystitis, namely, suprapubic pain, pyrexia, increased frequency of micturition, and the presence of pus and blood in the urine, suggest the diagnosis.

Pain during micturition in other vesical lesions is caused whenever there is sudden obstruction to the normal flow of urine by the impaction of something against the internal urethral orifice. This may occur with a small *calculus* or with a *pedunculated tumour*, whether simple or malignant, when during micturition the flow is arrested suddenly, accompanied by a shooting pain in the urethra, while after an interval of a few seconds the stream may be re-established. With vesical calculus the urine may be normal or may contain pus and blood if the bladder has become infected; there is penile pain after micturition,

and the stone will be seen both on plain X-ray of the pelvis and with a cystoscope. With a simple villous papilloma there is no pain unless part of the fimbriated portion of the tumour engages in the urethral orifice during micturition, but there are usually recurrent attacks of profuse haematuria, while with a carcinoma there is increased frequency of micturition, with pain following the act and more frequent haematuria. Upon rectal examination the base of the bladder may be felt to be infiltrated, but by far the most valuable means of diagnosis between the three conditions is by cystoscopy, when a calculus or villous tumour is seen readily, whilst a pedunculated carcinoma appears as a dark red tumour covered with stunted processes. (*See Figs.* 365, 366, p. 346.)

II. PENILE PAIN FOLLOWING MICTURITION

This symptom is common to many lesions of the urinary bladder, more especially those in which there is ulceration or infiltration of the basal areas. The particular pain felt by the patient is described as a sharp pricking or tingling at the terminal part of the penis on the cessation of micturition, lasting some minutes and causing a desire to squeeze the glans. It was thought to be diagnostic of vesical calculus, but this is far from being the case, for it may be due to almost any affection of the trigone.

The common causes of pain in the penis following upon micturition are:

1. *Vesical*:
   Calculus. Tuberculosis. Tumour (carcinoma, papilloma). Acute cystitis. Bilharzia.

2. *Ureteric*:
   Calculus in lower end. Descending ureteritis. Descending tuberculosis.

3. *Prostatic*:
   Acute inflammation. Abscess. Calculus. Carcinoma.

4. *Vesicular*:
   Acute seminal-vesiculitis.

5. *Rectal*:
   Carcinoma.

6. *Anal*:
   Fissure or ulcer. Inflamed haemorrhoids.

1. Diseases of the Bladder

A *calculus* in the bladder, unless it is trapped in the pouch behind an enlarged prostate or in a diverticulum, causes pain in the glans penis after micturition. It may exist without causing cystitis, although commonly there is some degree of pyuria when the case is first seen. There is increased frequency of micturition during active exercise or during the jolting of travelling, but not during complete rest unless cystitis is marked. The terminal drops of urine during micturition are often tinged with blood, and on some occasions there may have been a sudden stoppage of the stream during micturition. In some cases there is a history of acutely painful colic due to the descent of a stone from the kidney without the subsequent passage of a calculus in the urine. Patients subjected to vesical stone have usually reached the later part of life in this country, although bladder stones in children are still common in tropical parts, and although the symptoms are as a rule sufficiently marked to render the diagnosis easy, sometimes they may be so few that vesical calculus is unexpected, or

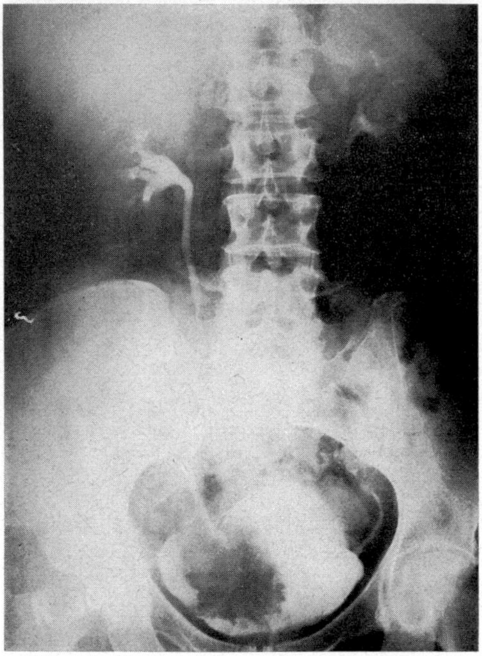

tuberculosis in which symptoms referable to the bladder are commonly present before the bladder is attacked by disease. In a young patient in whom increased frequency of micturition, pyuria, and penile pain are present, a search should be made for any tuberculous focus, especially in the kidneys by excretion urography, and in the epididymes, prostate, or seminal vesicles, or for

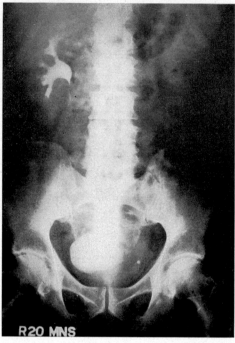

Fig. 650. An intravenous pyelogram and cystogram taken 20 minutes after injection. There is a filling defect on the right side of the bladder due to a large benign papilliferous tumour. Both kidneys are normal.

Fig. 651. An intravenous pyelogram and cystogram taken 20 minutes after injection. There is a solid defect in the left side of the bladder caused by an infiltrating carcinoma. The left ureter is obstructed and there is no function in the obstructed left kidney.

the symptoms are so like those caused by other lesions of the bladder that error is easy. The great majority of vesical calculi are radio-opaque and can be seen on a plain X-ray of the pelvis. In such a case it is advisable to examine the interior of the bladder with a cystoscope, by which means stones can be seen, their approximate size determined, and any other condition of the bladder accompanying or simulating calculus may be diagnosed with certainty. (*See Figs.* 369, 371, pp. 346, 347.)

Vesical tuberculosis is usually secondary to tuberculous disease in some other part of the genito-urinary tract, particularly the kidney. It causes marked penile pain after micturition, together with pyuria and a tinge of blood in the terminal drops of urine; the frequency of micturition is increased during both day and night, and is uninfluenced by rest, thus differing from the increased frequency of calculous disease. Vesical tuberculosis occurs in young adults and is usually associated with renal

marked thickening of the terminal ureter as felt per rectum, and a careful search should be made for tubercle bacilli in the urine. The deposit from three pooled, early morning specimens should be examined, and if this is negative, search should be continued by culture and by guinea-pig inoculation. A cystoscopic examination may be necessary to determine the extent of the disease (*Fig.* 685, p. 680), but, speaking generally, the less instrumentation that is carried out in these cases the better.

Vesical Tumours. Carcinoma of the bladder occurs in a papillary or a solid form. Papillary carcinoma is at first non-infiltrating, while the solid nodular and ulcerative types and adeno-carcinoma are infiltrating. They begin most commonly in the base of the bladder, except the urachal adenocarcinoma, which arises in the dome; the submucous coat and the muscular wall become infiltrated by malignant cells so that contraction of the bladder during micturition causes pain referred to the terminal portion of the urethra. All forms occur in elderly patients, mostly men, and give rise to increased frequency of micturition during both day and night, and to haematuria. They also often give rise to renal pain when the infiltration has extended to the ureteric orifice in the bladder.

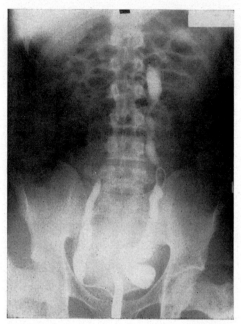

Fig. 652. Dilatation of the ureters following stricture of their lower ends in a case of vesical schistosomiasis. From a man of 20 who lived in East Africa.

The incidental cystogram of intravenous urography (*Fig.* 448, p. 478; *Figs.* 650, 651) may sometimes afford visual proof of the deformity the new growth is producing or of a filling defect in the otherwise regular contour of the bladder.

Under anaesthesia the base of the bladder may be felt per rectum to be thickened, or lymphatic infiltration may be felt in the lateral pelvic space, and a cystoscopic examination will usually clear up the diagnosis (*Figs.* 365, 366, p. 346).

Whereas solid infiltrating growths of the bladder give rise to penile pain after micturition from the direct infiltration of the vesical walls, the pedunculated papillary carcinoma and the simple villous papilloma may occasionally give rise to sharp penile pain during micturition from blocking of the internal urethral orifice by a process of growth. The occurrence of this, together with attacks of profuse haematuria, is suggestive of a pedunculated growth. On cystoscopic examination the carcinomatous pedunculated tumour is seen to be covered by blunt, stunted processes, whereas the innocent villous papilloma presents much more delicate fimbriae.

Acute cystitis causes tingling pain in the penis after micturition from the inflammatory infiltration of the trigonal area. The mode of onset, the character of the pain, and other symptoms of cystitis will point to the cause of the pain.

Bilharzia haematobia gives rise to clinical symptoms very similar to those of vesical tuberculosis. The history of residence in an infected district, microscopical examination of the urine

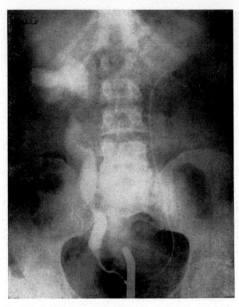

Fig. 653. Dilatation of the right ureter due to a calculus impacted at its lower end.

for ova, and the typical cystoscopic appearance of the bladder (*Fig.* 368, p. 346) establish the diagnosis.

X-rays may show calcification of the bladder or ureters and pyelography often demonstrates stricture formation and gross dilatation of the ureters (*Fig.* 652).

2. Ureteric Lesions not infrequently produce pain in the glans penis after micturition, and may cause considerable difficulty in the diagnosis from vesical disease.

When a *calculus* becomes impacted in the narrowed terminal or intramural portion of the ureter, symptoms are produced almost exactly similar to those of vesical calculus or tuberculosis, namely, increased frequency of micturition, pain in the glans penis after micturition, and a small amount of pus and blood in the urine. Intimate knowledge of the history of the illness will often be of value in these cases; the first attack of pain is usually described as being sudden, and felt in the renal angle posteriorly, passing forward above the iliac crest and spine, and finally becoming localized at the situation of the external abdominal ring. The calculus may become impacted in the terminal inch of the ureter, when, in addition to this pain, there will be increased frequency of micturition and penile pain, and possibly haematuria. With ureteric calculus there is usually aching pain in the kidney of the affected side from the dilatation of its pelvis. The diagnosis of these cases is not difficult if a careful inquiry is made into the history and symptoms, and so long as it is remembered that increased frequency of micturition and penile pain may be caused by ureteric impaction of a calculus; a good radiographic examination of the pelvic areas may show the shadow of a stone. Indeed, some 90 per cent of these calculi are radio-opaque but, when small, may mimic phleboliths or be obscured by gas shadows or underlying bony structures. (*Fig.* 653.) The stone itself may be felt occasionally as a small, painful nodule on pelvic examination, especially in women. A cystoscopic examination also affords valuable information, not only in excluding vesical lesions, but by giving a distinct indication of ureteric calculus by the marked congestion and dilatation of the blood-vessels in the immediate vicinity of the ureteric orifice. A small bougie passed into the ureter may meet with obstruction in its passage; a stereoscopic radiograph of the pelvis with an opaque bougie passed into the ureter will show the shadow to be in the immediate line of the ureter (*see Fig.* 63, p. 64).

Ureteritis descending from infection of the renal pelvis may give rise to slight penile pain and to increased frequency of micturition, and thus simulate vesical disease before the bladder is actually infected. This is seen most commonly in the *tuberculous* form, but is present in a less marked degree with infection by other organisms, of which the most common are *Bacillus coli communis* and *Streptococcus faecalis*. In the non-tuberculous form the ureter may be felt per rectum to be slightly thickened, but the cystoscopic appearance of the inflamed ureteric orifice is distinctive (*Fig.* 683, p. 680). In *descending tuberculosis* from the kidney, the ureter may be felt as a firm, infiltrated cord on the bladder base, the penile pain and increased frequency of micturition are more marked, the kidney may be felt enlarged and tender, and tubercle bacilli will be found in the urine. Apart from this, typical changes in the ureteric orifice are seen on cystoscopic examination, the orifice being pulled up or retracted or horseshoe shaped, and usually occupying a position slightly above and outside the situation of the normal orifice, due to the actual shortening of the ureter by infiltration of the submucous coats (*Fig.* 684, p. 680). The rigid 'golf-hole' ureteric orifice is a late manifestation caused by contraction of scar tissue around it and in the ureter above it.

3. Diseases of the Prostate often cause pain in the penis immediately following micturition. This is seen most commonly with acute inflammation or abscess in the gland as a sequela of acute gonorrhoea or septic urethritis. In either case there is penile pain, sometimes associated with erection, but little difficulty will be experienced in the diagnosis on due consideration of the symptoms and upon rectal examination.

Prostatic calculi are not uncommon; there may be a single calculus or a nest of them in the prostate. They may ulcerate into the urethra so that small calculi may be passed in the urinary stream, or some may pass back along the dilated prostatic urethra into the bladder. If a calculus projects from the prostate into the urethra it causes pain in the penis after micturition. A diagnosis of prostatic calculus is often made by the grating sensation imparted to a catheter in traversing the prostatic urethra, whilst on rectal examination the calculus may be felt as an isolated hard nodule in the gland (where it may mimic prostatic carcinoma), or, if more than one is present, by the crepitation of one upon another on digital pressure in the rectum. A radiograph of the pelvis will show the shadows of prostatic calculi at the level of the upper part of the pubic symphysis (*Fig.* 489, p. 478).

4. Diseases of the Seminal Vesicles are seldom present without accompanying disease of the prostate or bladder. Acute vesiculitis may follow urethritis and give rise to pain after micturition, but in most cases it will be associated with prostatitis. Similarly tuberculous nodules in the vesicle will be associated with foci in the epididymis, prostate, or bladder.

5, 6. Diseases of the Rectum and Anus may occasionally give rise to penile pain following micturition, apart from any infection of the bladder or prostate. Thus an infiltrating carcinoma in the anal canal, a rectal fissure, or an inflamed haemorrhoid may occasionally cause pain in the penis, but in each the local symptoms of the trouble will be the more marked, and little difficulty will be found in the diagnosis if a local examination is made with care.

III. PAIN IN THE PENIS APART FROM MICTURITION

Under the above divisions the symptom of penile pain has been considered in relation to the act of micturition, and it remains to consider some conditions giving rise to pain in the penis *apart from urination*. These include certain local lesions of the penis and urethra, and also the pains referred from disease elsewhere. Although a local lesion may cause little more than discomfort in many patients, in some it is described as pain, the degree of which depends upon the nervous susceptibility of the individual. Thus penile pain may be present with *acute urethritis*, with *balanitis* in association with *phimosis*, with *paraphimosis*, or with the *lymphangitis* of the organ due to a septic sore or abrasion of the skin or mucous membrane. In some instances *herpes* of the prepuce or penile skin causes distinct pain. Any infiltration of the cavernous tissue of the penis causes pain during erection of the organ; thus during an attack of acute urethritis the symptom known as *chordee* arises from this cause. It may occur in a chronic form in Peyronie's disease (chronic indurative cavernositis), a condition of unknown aetiology but similar to, and sometimes associated with, Dupuytren's contracture and retroperitoneal fibrosis. In this condition erection is not only painful but may be accompanied by lateral deviation of the organ. Another condition causing the same trouble arises from the organization of a haematoma in the cavernous tissues of the penis following upon a local injury, due either to external violence or arising during forcible attempts at coitus. A similar condition may arise spontaneously in blood diseases, especially *lymphatic* or *splenomedullary leukaemia*.

Epithelioma of the penis on rare occasions gives rise to pain in the organ.

Pain may be felt in the penis in some cases of *renal colic*, in which case it is classed as a referred pain. Thus in the acute colic accompanying the passage of a calculus, blood-clot, or debris of caseous material, aching pain may be felt in the penis quite apart from the increased desire to pass urine. Penile pain is, however, only a minor detail in the presence of the severe pain in the loin, and along the course of the ureter, and is often only lightly alluded to or revealed on direct questioning of the patient.

Pain in the penis was a prominent early symptom in two cases of *acute appendicitis*. In neither case was it associated with micturition, nor was there any increased frequency of micturition, but in both the appendix was found to occupy a very low position, turning down into the pelvis, which in one case contained a foul abscess.

Finally, pain in the penis may be based on an anxiety state or some other mental cause rather than organic disease.

Harold Ellis.

PERINEAL SORES

Ulceration may be present in the perineum as the result of:

1. Cutaneous inflammation or injury
2. Urethral suppurations or fistulae
3. Prostatic suppuration
4. Anal fistula
5. Syphilis
6. Granuloma venereum
7. Lymphogranuloma inguinale
8. Epithelioma and other cutaneous cancers
9. Carcinoma of the urethra.

1. Cutaneous Inflammation or Injury. An ulcer in the perineum may result from *direct injury* to the area, or from inflammatory *infection of the sebaceous* or *hair follicles*. An ulcer from these causes may be placed at the centre or to one side of the perineum, is movable on the deeper parts, and shows no track into which a probe can be passed. In women, ulceration of the perineal area may be associated with *gonorrhoeal* or *septic vaginal discharge*. It may also arise from severe scratching caused by the irritation of such skin infections as *tinea cruris* or *pruritus ani*.

2. Urethral Suppurations or Fistulae. During the progress of an acute urethritis a glandular follicle frequently becomes infected. The suppurative process leading from this in the bulbous urethra may extend towards the perineum and open externally, leaving a small fistula which may or may not discharge urine during the act of micturition. In a similar manner urinary fistulae may result from inflammatory processes behind a urethral stricture, and in an old-standing case it is not uncommon to find a urinary calculus in the dilated portion of the urethra behind the stricture. When the urethral suppuration is acute and an abscess bursts in the perineum, the diagnosis will be obvious, and the ordinary treatment for an abscess, in addition to that of the acute urethritis, will usually suffice to cure the condition. If the perineal wound discharges urine this occurs as a rule only during the act of micturition, as there is no interference with the vesical sphincter; a stricture of the urethra, not necessarily of sufficient degree to cause severe interference with micturition, will generally be seen on endoscopic examination, the sloughy granulations behind it denoting the position of the urethral opening of the fistula. Occasionally urine drains from a perineal fistula continuously, and not only during the act of micturition; in these cases there is constant soaking of the perineal skin, and frequently excoriation; that urine should leak constantly from the fistula denotes interference with the vesical sphincter, either by dilatation behind a tight urethral stricture, by the presence of a calculus in the prostatic or membranous urethra, or by actual division of the vesical sphincter following some operation, such as perineal prostatectomy or perineal lithotomy.

3. Diseases of the Prostate. An abscess or tuberculous focus in the prostate may occasionally discharge in the perineum, and remain as a sinus. An abscess in the prostate arises practically always from some infection in the posterior urethra, from venereal causes, or after septic instrumentation. It is accompanied by urethral discharge, or there is a history of a recent infection, whilst per rectum the prostate may be felt to be inflamed, or scarred from the shrinkage of the abscess cavity.

When a tuberculous cavity in the prostate opens in the perineum there is advanced tuberculous disease, so that little difficulty will be found in arriving at a diagnosis. A tuberculous prostate is very rarely a primary condition, but in most cases is secondary to disease in the kidney, epididymis, or bladder, so that examination of these organs will in nearly all cases give evidence of tuberculous disease and indicate the nature of the perineal fistula. Palpation of the prostate per rectum may reveal the rounded nodular deposit of tubercle in the gland.

4. Anal Fistula. An ulcer on the perineum may be present as the result of an anal fistula—commonly from perianal suppuration and occasionally as a tuberculous infection. The history of pain on defaecation followed by the rupture of a suppurating focus and the history of passage of flatus or faecal matter from the fistula is usually present, or a probe may be passed into the fistula and felt by a finger passed into the rectum. A tuberculous fistula is associated with considerable pain on defaecation.

Perianal and perirectal abscesses, fissures, and fistulae may occur in Crohn's disease, especially when the colon is involved, and less commonly in ulcerative colitis.

5. Syphilis may cause ulceration on the perineum either as a chancre or as mucous tubercles. A *chancre* at this site is rare. It forms a small ulcer with slightly indurated borders, indolent in character, and accompanied by slight enlargement of the inguinal lymphatic glands. A chancre of the skin does not possess the usual features of a genital chancre, and is not usually diagnosed with certainty until the secondary lesions of syphilis become apparent; but an ulcer with raised, infiltrated edges, which shows no tendency to heal under aseptic precautions, should always give rise to a suspicion of syphilis. The *Treponema pallidum* may be looked for, and the Wassermann test performed.

Condylomata may be present about the perineum in association with active syphilis. They may extend from the anal or vulval orifice, and form oval or rounded, flat-topped, sessile masses, covered by macerated greyish epithelium, or they may be ulcerated on the surface. The accompanying signs of syphilis will indicate the diagnosis.

Soft sores may occur in the perineum as well as on the scrotum or the vulva; they are generally venereal, but are not in themselves syphilitic; they are generally multiple, are apt to be foul, and cultures from them yield Ducrey's bacillus (*Haemophilus Ducrey*).

6, 7. Ulceration of Granuloma Inguinale sometimes attacks the perineum, and fistulae there can be caused by lymphogranuloma venereum (*see* PENILE SORES, p. 631).

8, 9. Epitheliomatous Ulceration of the perineum is seen as a direct spread of a growth of the anus or vulval area, when the diagnosis presents no difficulty. An epithelioma may develop in the scar of some former cutaneous affection, particularly in long-standing fistula in ano, in which case an ulceration may exist showing the usual characteristics of a cutaneous epithelioma. The inguinal glands may be enlarged early from inflammatory absorption, or later by invasion with malignant disease. Other cutaneous cancers, malignant melanoma, and basal cell carcinoma may also occur in this situation. In case of doubt a fragment may be removed for microscopical examination. In late cases of carcinoma of the urethra following urethral stricture malignant ulceration spreads to the perineum by direct extension.

Harold Ellis.

21

PERINEUM, PAIN IN

Pain in the perineum is a symptom often mentioned by patients in giving their history of some affection of the genito-urinary apparatus or of other organs, but usually only as a dull aching, of which little notice is taken, as it is generally of minor degree in comparison with other more striking symptoms. The complaint of perineal pain *per se* does not convey much information to the clinician, and it is practically never present as the only symptom in a case. It may be a manifestation of an anxiety state.

Aching in the perineum is frequently present in diseases of the following organs:

Prostate:
Acute or subacute inflammation
Abscess
Chronic prostatitis
Tuberculosis
Calculus
Adenomatous enlargement
Carcinoma.

Seminal Vesicles:
Acute inflammation
Tuberculosis.

Testicle:
Congenital misplacement in perineum.

Urinary Bladder:
Cystitis
Tuberculosis
Calculus
Carcinoma.

Urethra:
Gonorrhoea
Injury and rupture
Stricture with extravasation or urethral abscess
Fistula
Calculus impacted in bulbo-prostatic portion.

Anal Area:
Haemorrhoids
Fissure
Follicular abscess
Carbuncle
Ulcer
Carcinoma.

Vagina:
Acute inflammation
Inflammation or abscess of Bartholin's glands
Cystocele
Epithelioma.

Cutaneous Diseases
Intertrigo
Diabetic inflammation
Condylomata.

From the foregoing list it will be seen that aching in the perineum occurs with numerous different lesions, but other symptoms discussed elsewhere are in almost every case more marked. In prostatic disease it is an indication of inflammation rather than of enlargement. In clinical practice it is most commonly found to be due to chronic inflammation of the prostate gland. Examination of the secretion expressed after prostatic massage will show the presence of many pus cells.

Harold Ellis.

PERISTALSIS, VISIBLE

Usually visible peristalsis is pathological. However, in a number of conditions the normal

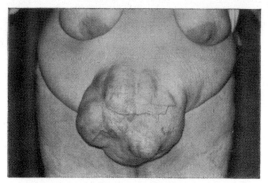

Fig. 654. Visible peristalsis was obvious in this large thin-walled umbilical hernia.

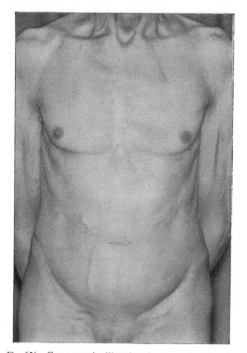

Fig. 656. Gross gastric dilatation due to a stenosing duodenal ulcer. The stomach was visible, with a loud splash, and showed typical gastric peristalsis.

movements of the bowel may be visible; these circumstances are divarication of the abdominal recti muscles, an incisional or massive umbilical hernia containing bowel, and extreme thinness of the abdominal parietes—the result of emaciation

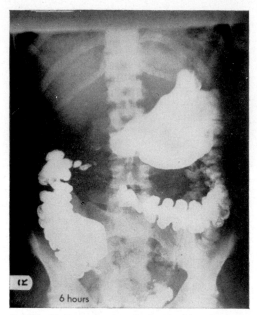

Fig. 655. Six hours after ingesting barium this patient, with gross pyloric stenosis due to duodenal ulceration and with obvious visible gastric peristalsis, still has considerable residue in the stomach. Note that the barium which has escaped through the stenosis has already reached the splenic flexure.

or, rarely, congenital absence of the recti. It is not uncommon to see visible peristalsis within the sac of a very large ventral or inguinoscrotal hernia (*Fig.* 654). In all these circumstances the diagnosis can be made at inspection and the patient is otherwise symptomless. In all other situations, visible peristalsis is pathological and may be of two types, gastric and intestinal.

Gastric Peristalsis takes the form of a comparatively large swelling in the upper abdomen showing slow waves of peristalsis which progress from under the region of the left ribs, slowly downwards and to the right. This swelling indicates obstruction to the gastric outlet. There may be other signs of gastric dilatation and distension, particularly a loud succussion splash (*Fig.* 656). Typically there is a history of the vomiting of large amounts of liquid in a projectile manner which may contain fragments of food ingested 24 hours or more previously. The diagnosis can be confirmed by the passage of a nasogastric tube which will yield a pint or more of fluid several hours after the last food or drink have been taken; the aspirate has a typical stale, unpleasant smell and may contain recognizable particles of food eaten even several days before. A barium X-ray examination will clinch the diagnosis by demonstrating the gastric retention and dilatation. An X-ray taken 6 or 8 hours after the ingestion of the barium is particularly valuable since this will confirm the extent of gastric hold-up (*Fig.* 655). In doubtful cases of visible gastric peristalsis, the sign may be accentuated by asking the patient to swallow several glasses of soda-water. In the normal subject no peristalsis is seen, but in cases of pyloric obstruction, previously invisible peristalsis may now become obvious.

In congenital hypertrophic pyloric stenosis of infancy not only can gastric peristalsis be seen after a drink from a bottle but the hypertrophied pylorus can often be felt. This interesting and eminently treatable condition becomes apparent not immediately, but some 4 weeks after birth. **Visible Intestinal Peristalsis** is a feature of advanced intestinal obstruction with the limitations discussed above. As a pathological entity it will not occur alone but is accompanied by colicky abdominal pain, abdominal distension, vomiting, and absolute constipation. The discussion of the differential diagnosis of the different causes of the symptoms will be found elsewhere. If the small intestine alone is involved, the waves are multiple and run more or less transversely across the abdomen—the ladder pattern; when the colon is obstructed, peristalsis takes the form of vertical waves, especially in one or both flanks, but this is much more rarely seen. Plain radiographs of the abdomen taken in the erect and supine positions are invaluable; the first demonstrate multiple fluid levels, the second the distribution of gas shadows within the dilated loops of bowel which will often enable the clinician to determine whether small or large bowel is obstructed. (*See also* p. 175 and *Figs.* 182, 183.)

Harold Ellis.

PHANTOM LIMBS

After amputation most patients feel that the missing limb is still there, and they affirm that they can move it about at will. The basis of the sensation is a sense of tingling, felt mainly in the non-existent fingers or toes, and to this may be added an impression of movement. As time goes on, the phantom usually becomes less prominent in the patient's mind, and it undergoes progressive shrinkage so that ultimately it may feel as if it is only a few inches long. In a few cases there are complaints of severe pain in the phantom. This pain has often been present before operation and the amputation may have been undertaken to relieve pain which it will not, however, do; nor will further local measures to the stump, except possibly cutaneous electrical stimulation to the painful areas. Pain can be relieved by cordotomy and if the painful phantom is the arm this will have to be in the high cervical region, but such relief is often transient.

Ian Mackenzie.

PHENYLKETONURIA (Phenylpyruvic Oligophrenia: Phenylpyruvic Amentia)

This is an inborn error of metabolism characterized by the appearance of phenylpyruvic acid in the urine and by a raised content of phenylalanine in the plasma (normal up to 1 mg. per 100 ml.). The basic metabolic abnormality is the absence of the enzyme phenylalanine hydroxylase in the tissues in affected individuals. The disease is inherited as an autosomal recessive character. Heterozygotes are clinically normal but may be detected by a phenylalanine-tolerance test. While the frequency in the general population is only about 1 in 50,000, the disease accounts for some 1 per cent of patients in mental deficiency hospitals.

The clinical picture is that of severe mental deficiency even to idiocy and a strong tendency to epileptiform convulsions. Those affected are usually of pleasant aspect and nearly 90 per cent have blond hair and light complexion even to the extent of albinism. Various skin rashes may occur and the patients are particularly susceptible to the effect of ultra-violet light, including sunlight, and they often suffer from eczema, profuse sweating, and dermographism. Walking is not learned as a rule until the fifth or sixth year of life and the gait is invariably clumsy. It is characterized by a certain jerkiness and stiffness, with a tendency to lean forward at the hips reminiscent of paralysis agitans. Athetoid movements are frequently seen.

Early diagnosis before any clinical signs have developed, and preferably within the first 2 weeks after birth, is of paramount importance, as a low phenylalanine diet will prevent mental retardation. A simple microbiological test for blood levels of phenylalanine (the Guthrie test) is preferable to the older test for phenylpyruvic acid in the urine using either a paper strip (Phenistix) or the addition of a few drops of a solution of ferric chloride. The low phenylalanine diet can usually be relaxed after the age of 8 years, although the biochemical abnormalities in blood and urine will persist. If, however, pregnancy occurs in a female phenylketonuric patient, a low phenylalanine diet must be reinstituted, as high concentrations of phenylalanine will be transported across the placenta to the foetal bloodstream, and will seriously interfere with normal intra-uterine cerebral development.

M. D. Milne.

PHOSPHATURIA

This is an indefinite term. Normally from 1 g. to 5 g. of phosphates (as P_2O_5) are excreted in the urine per day, the amount depending principally on dietary protein. The urinary phosphates are present as the sodium, calcium, magnesium, or ammonium salts, the last three being sparingly soluble. The term 'phosphaturia' is usually applied when the phosphates become visible as a turbidity, deposit, or as crystals visible microscopically.

A visible turbidity or deposit of phosphates may be seen in many normal urines after standing, and this deposit may occur in the bladder in normal subjects so that the urine is turbid when passed. This turbidity needs to be distinguished from that due to urates, pus, bacteria, and fat. This is easily done by adding dilute acetic acid. Only phosphates dissolve readily in the cold. Phosphates are less soluble in alkaline than in acid solution, and any condition causing an alkaline urine favouring precipitation. This explains the frequency of phosphaturia in urinary infection with urea-splitting organisms such as *Proteus vulgaris*. The resultant high ammonia content of the urine favour precipitation of 'triple

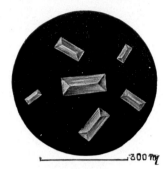

Fig. 657. Triple phosphate crystals.

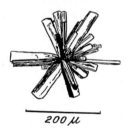

Fig. 658. Stellar phosphate crystals (calcium hydrogen phosphate).

phosphate' (ammonium magnesium phosphate), especially if there is some obstruction to urinary outflow. Such cases are particularly liable to the formation of phosphatic calculi.

Turbidity due to phosphates is also common when urine is boiled to test for protein: liberation of carbon dioxide during the boiling leaves the urine more alkaline, and the turbidity clears readily with dilute acetic acid.

Microscopical examination of the urinary deposit may show the presence of phosphate crystals in any alkaline urine. The commonest form of crystal observed is ammonium magnesium phosphate, $MgNH_4PO_4$ ('triple phosphate', *Fig.* 657), but calcium hydrogen phosphate, $CaHPO_4$ ('stellar phosphate', *Fig.* 658), may also be seen in acid urine.

From what has been said it is evident that 'phosphaturia' as here defined is not necessarily pathological but its occurrence should direct attention to the possibility of urinary infection with or without an obstruction to the urinary tract. Thus the ammoniacal urine with a heavy deposit of triple phosphate crystals is a very

typical accompaniment of conditions such as enlarged prostate.

Phosphate excretion may be increased secondarily to increased calcium excretion, whatever the cause. In these conditions it is the calcium that is of primary importance; hypercalcaemia should be sought and if found the cause should be determined and treated. 'Idiopathic hypercalciuria' may occur with normal plasma calcium levels, and be associated with calcium-containing renal calculi.

Joan F. Zilva.

PHOTOPHOBIA

Photophobia, or intolerance of light, needs to be carefully distinguished from blepharospasm (a reflex spasm of the orbicularis, usually due to some conjunctival or corneal irritant, which can be annulled by a drop of amethocaine).

Photophobia is found in albinos, who are dazzled by the excess of light reaching their retinas, in cases of acute iritis, keratitis and congestive glaucoma, and it can be allayed by dark-glasses or an eye-pad. A mild photophobia is usually noted in any conjunctivitis or (most commonly) a blepharitis. It should be emphasized that the vast majority of those who wear dark-glasses have no organic ocular lesion, and such glasses are generally worn for cosmetic or psychopathic reasons.

P. Trevor-Roper.

PILIMICTION

Pilimiction, that is the passage of hairs in the urine, a rare condition which almost invariably signifies that the patient has a pelvic dermoid cyst that has become inflamed, thereafter opening into the bladder and discharging its contents via the urinary passages, has been observed in men, but it is less uncommon in women. Subacute or acute cystitis accompanies the event with vesical pain, frequency of micturition, and pyuria. The obvious fallacy in diagnosis arises from the possibility of contamination in the urine of hairs which were not, as supposed, passed per urethram.

Harold Ellis.

PNEUMATURIA

The passage of gas per urethram, either with or independently of urine, is a rare but striking peculiarity, particularly when it occurs in males. It may be due to one or other of two distinct groups of causes, namely:

1. Communication between the rectum, caecum, vermiform appendix, or other part of the alimentary canal and the bladder, ureter, or renal pelvis, either directly or via an intermediate gas-containing abscess cavity.

2. Infection of the bladder or other part of the urinary tract by gas-producing micro-organisms.

When the cause lies in the first group, the patient is apt to pass faecal material as well as gas, and the differential diagnosis between the various possible lesions is discussed under FAECES PASSED PER URETHRAM (p. 804). It should be added, however, that the passage of gas without faeces per urethram by no means excludes a fistulous communication between some part of the alimentary canal and the urinary tract; the fistula may be of such a character that while gas can traverse it faeces cannot. It may also happen that a lesion such as appendicitis or, most commonly, acute sigmoid diverticulitis has led to the formation of a local abscess which, owing to infection by the *Escherichia coli*, contains gas; this abscess may open into the bladder and cause the discharge of pus and gas, but no faeces, per urethram. The same applies to similar abscesses which though not arising primarily in connexion with the bowel nevertheless contain gas from infection by the *E. coli*—for instance, a suppurating hydatid or ovarian dermoid cyst, or a pyosalpinx. Rectal, vaginal, abdominal, barium-enema X-ray, intravenous pyelographic, and cystoscopic examinations may yield the diagnosis, but on occasion doubt will persist whether the gas is finding its way into the urinary passages from some external source, or whether it is being produced in situ, for certain organisms, notably the *E. coli* and *Aspergillus aerogenes*, produce gas when they grow in urine, as may various *yeasts* in glycosuric cases.

If no sign of a fistulous communication between any part of the bowel or a gas-containing abscess cavity with the urinary tracts can be distinguished on cystoscopic examination, it may be with confidence presumed that the pneumaturia is due to infection. Such patients are usually elderly female diabetics with considerable glycosuria. The infecting organisms are usually *E. coli*, *A. aerogenes*, *yeasts*, or combinations of these.

The urine in such a case contains pus, sugar, and albumin. It may be acid, and not foul-smelling or ammoniacal; on the other hand, it may sometimes be so foul and faeculent as to arouse unwarranted suspicion of a communication between the colon and the bladder. A cystoscopic examination will serve to exclude a fistulous opening into the bladder, but it may be much more difficult to exclude a similar communication with the higher parts of the urinary tract, especially the renal pelvis. Such a condition is very rare, so that urinary infection is the more probable unless there is a known or recognizable cause for communication between the bowel and the renal pelvis, such as a carcinoma.

Harold Ellis.

PNEUMOTHORAX

Pneumothorax exists when gas is present in the pleural cavity. The gas enters either through a breach in the continuity of the chest wall and parietal pleura enabling air to enter from outside, or through a breach in the continuity of the visceral pleura allowing air to enter the pleura from the broncho-pulmonary air spaces; extremely rare causes are the action of anaerobic gas-forming organisms in putrid empyema, and rupture of the thoracic oesophagus. Pneumothorax may be *spontaneous*, when it arises without obvious external cause; *traumatic*, when it is caused by injury to the chest wall or lung; or *artificial*, when it is produced for therapeutic or diagnostic purposes. In spontaneous pneumothorax the air enters the pleura through a breach in the continuity of the visceral pleura; in traumatic pneumothorax it may enter either from without through a penetrating wound of the chest wall, or from the lung through a rupture of its pleural surface. Pneumothorax may be dry, without liquid effusion into the chest, or may be accompanied by either clear fluid (hydropneumothorax), pus (pyopneumothorax), or blood (haemopneumothorax).

Causes. In the artificial and traumatic groups the cause is obvious. It is important to note, however, that simple compression injuries of the chest, even without fractures of the ribs, may occasionally give rise to traumatic pneumothorax, by causing rupture of the visceral pleura or even, rarely, main bronchi.

Spontaneous pneumothorax may be divided into several groups according to the cause:

1. A large and important group is composed of those which occur in *apparently healthy persons* who display no other clinical evidence of pulmonary disease. In this group it is assumed that the cause is rupture of an insignificant emphysematous bulla, which may or may not be associated with previous inflammatory lung disease.

2. Closely related to group (1) is a group of cases of spontaneous pneumothorax associated with recognizable *emphysematous or cystic changes* of various sorts in the lung. In generalized emphysema pneumothorax is relatively rarely observed, probably because the intrapleural pressure in such cases approaches atmospheric. Patients who have localized emphysematous changes, for instance associated with obsolete fibrotic or calcified tuberculous lesions, may develop pneumothorax; localized cystic changes in the lungs may give rise to pneumothorax; and in the rare condition of 'honeycomb lungs' associated with eosinophilic granuloma (histiocytosis X), which is characterized by the presence of multiple small cysts throughout the lungs, spontaneous pneumothorax is a frequent complication.

3. Spontaneous pneumothorax may occur in the course of *pulmonary tuberculosis*.

4. *Pulmonary suppuration* may give rise to spontaneous pneumothorax by ulceration of intrapulmonary abscesses into the pleura; and occasionally *pleural empyema* ulcerates into the lung. Both these events lead to pyopneumothorax.

5. *Pneumonias*, especially of bronchopneumonic type and in infants, may give rise to spontaneous pneumothorax.

6. Very rarely, attacks of *asthma* may be complicated by spontaneous pneumothorax.

Symptoms and Signs. *The symptoms* of pneumothorax are seen in their pure form in group (1), in which they arise in a previously healthy person. They are very variable in severity, but

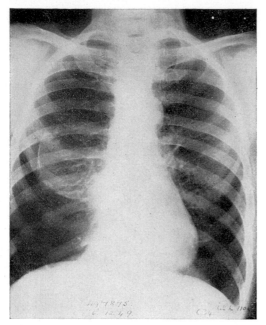

Fig. 659. Radiograph of chest showing simple spontaneous pneumothorax. In this case the causative emphysematous bulla is visible at the apex of the collapsed lung.

the essential features are sudden pain in the chest followed by progressively more severe dyspnoea. The initial pain may be so slight that it is hardly noticed, or so severe that it simulates an acute abdominal or cardiac catastrophe. The dyspnoea may become disabling within a few minutes or may be hardly noticeable at first and steadily increase over several days. The most severe dyspnoea is associated with tension pneumothorax, in which a valvular communication between the pleura and a bronchopulmonary air-space allows air to enter the pleura during inspiration but prevents it from leaving during expiration. In pneumothorax associated with trauma or with gross pre-existing disease, the picture will be modified by the symptoms of these conditions.

The physical signs of pneumothorax vary greatly with the size of the pneumothorax and according to the presence or absence of liquid effusion of various sorts. The one constant sign is weakness or absence of the breath-sounds on the affected side of the chest, or with loculated pneumothoraces over the affected part of the pleural space. A small pneumothorax in a free

pleural space may produce no other sign than weakness of the breath-sounds. A rather larger pneumothorax will produce absence of breath-sounds, a change in the percussion note which is often difficult to interpret, and slight displacement of the apex beat and of the cardiac dullness towards the opposite side. A large pneumothorax will produce hyper-resonance on percussion, with encroachment upon normally dull areas, such as the hepatic or splenic dullness, and gross displacement of the heart and trachea to the opposite side; the affected hemithorax will be observed to move less, and especially in

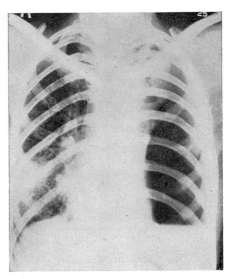

Fig. 660. Radiograph of chest showing spontaneous pneumothorax due to pulmonary tuberculosis. Note the presence of effusion in the pneumothorax.

younger subjects it may be inflated to more than its normal size. The presence of liquid, either clear effusion, pus, or blood, produces additional signs. Of these the most constant is dullness at the most dependent part of the hemithorax; the area of dullness is characterized by a horizontal upper limit, shifting in relation to the chest wall on movement, but always remaining horizontal. In a large hydropneumothorax a succussion splash may be elicited, but is more of interest than of practical value, since the diagnosis of hydropneumothorax should be obvious in such cases without the necessity for shaking the patient. If the effusion, either clear, purulent, or haemorrhagic, has been present for some time there will inevitably be some thickening of the pleura, and this will give rise to diminution in resonance over the chest generally, and to contraction rather than over-inflation of the affected side of the chest. In hydropneumothorax, and sometimes in a large dry pneumothorax, especially if it is under tension, a coin sound or *bruit d'airain* may be heard. This is elicited classically by placing a coin against the chest wall anteriorly and tapping it with another while auscultating over some other part of the hemithorax, preferably at the base or just above the level of any effusion which may be present. It may equally well be elicited by flicking the clavicle with the finger while auscultating similarly, and consists in a high-pitched bell-like sound. It is not a frequent sign in spontaneous pneumothorax.

Radiologically, pneumothorax is readily recognizable, the outline of the collapsed lung being clearly visible in an abnormally transradiant hemithorax (*Fig.* 659). The presence of effusion can be detected with certainty in films taken in the erect posture which will show a horizontal fluid level (*Fig.* 660).

Diagnosis. *Traumatic pneumothorax* should not be missed if the signs of pneumothorax are sought in all cases of trauma to the chest.

The diagnosis of *spontaneous pneumothorax* may be considered under two headings: (1) The diagnosis of pneumothorax from conditions which produce similar clinical pictures; and (2) The diagnosis of the cause of the pneumothorax.

1. Acute spontaneous pneumothorax produces very characteristic symptoms, and when these symptoms are typical little confusion should occur. However, occasionally a case is encountered in which the pain is of such severity, accompanied by a shock-like state, that acute abdominal emergencies, particularly perforation of peptic ulcer, may be simulated. This is especially the case when, as sometimes occurs, the pain is referred to the abdomen, presumably through the innervation of the peripheral part of the diaphragm from the lower intercostal nerves. More rarely, the onset of severe pain in the chest and dyspnoea may suggest a diagnosis of cardiac infarction. Careful examination of the chest should reveal the characteristic signs of pneumothorax and enable the differentiation to be made in either of these cases. The dyspnoea which is a feature of sudden severe spontaneous pneumothorax should also suggest the correct diagnosis. Occasionally a spontaneous pneumothorax may produce symptoms superficially resembling those of a pleurisy. The usual absence of fever in those cases not complicating inflammatory lesions of the lung will help in making this distinction; the physical signs should leave no doubt of the diagnosis.

There is one rather rare but important phenomenon which may occur in association with shallow left-sided pneumothorax and which is important in differential diagnosis. In such cases a peculiar clicking sound is sometimes observed in the region of the heart's apex beat, usually during the systolic part of the cardiac cycle. Very occasionally this sound may be so loud that it is heard by the patient and even by bystanders. It is very sensitive to changes of position, so that it may be clearly audible in one posture and quite a slight movement may lead to its disappearance. It is presumably due to the small bubble of air getting in front of the heart, which then produces the sound by sucking away from the chest wall

in systole, just as the tongue makes the sound 'T' against the hard palate. This sound may appear when a left-sided pneumothorax has nearly absorbed. Unless its possible association with pneumothorax is known, it may suggest an erroneous diagnosis of such serious conditions as pericarditis. The physical signs of pneumothorax are likely to be minimal, and the diagnosis depends upon radiological examination.

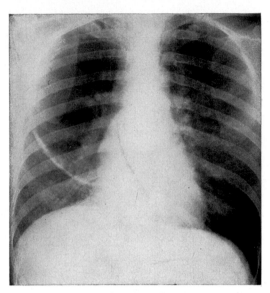

Fig. 661. Radiograph of chest, showing a large bullous cyst in the right lung, simulating a loculated pneumothorax.

Acute spontaneous pneumothorax must be distinguished from spontaneous mediastinal emphysema. This condition may rarely complicate any illness characterized by cough, such as bronchitis, bronchopneumonia, whooping-cough, and asthma, and has been recorded during parturition; it has also been observed to arise without obvious antecedent illness. Like spontaneous pneumothorax, it is characterized by sudden onset of pain in the chest and dyspnoea, but the pain tends to be central, and the characteristic physical sign of bursts of sharp crackling sounds synchronous with the heart-beat, audible all over the precordium, should suggest the diagnosis early; and later subcutaneous emphysema often appears, spreading out from the suprasternal notch into the base of the neck.

Chronic spontaneous pneumothorax, which occasionally results if the pleurobronchial communication which is responsible for acute spontaneous pneumothorax fails to close, must be distinguished from giant cysts and cavities in the lung, from diaphragmatic hernia, and from unilateral obstructive emphysema. The differential diagnosis from intrapulmonary cysts may be difficult, but radiology will usually provide a clue (*Fig.* 661). Bronchography may help. The introduction of a needle into the air space in order to investigate the pressure changes is not recommended, since if the condition is an intrapulmonary cyst and the pleura is free it may result in the addition of a traumatic pneumothorax to the patient's other troubles. Diaphragmatic hernia, especially on the left side and containing distended gas-filled stomach or coils of gas-filled intestine, may produce physical signs suggestive of chronic spontaneous pneumothorax, but radiological examination, aided if necessary by the administration of an opaque meal, will lead to the correct diagnosis.

2. The presence of pneumothorax having been established, the next step is the diagnosis of its cause. The most frequent problem is that of the spontaneous pneumothorax in a previously healthy young person, in which the question of a possible relation to tuberculosis arises. In most cases this question can and should be answered quite definitely. If a spontaneous pneumothorax (a) occurs in a person who has previously had no symptoms of ill health of any sort, (b) follows an afebrile course, (c) is not complicated by the appearance of clinically detectable amount of effusion, (d) is accompanied by a normal blood-sedimentation-rate, and (e) expands without incident, leaving a lung which is radiologically free from disease, it can be stated dogmatically that the pneumothorax is unrelated to tuberculosis, and the case should be treated accordingly. When a spontaneous pneumothorax occurs in a person suffering from pulmonary tuberculosis, the course is usually febrile, effusion usually appears, the sedimentation-rate is raised, and, of course, other clinical, radiological, and bacteriological evidences of pulmonary tuberculosis may be detected. When spontaneous pneumothorax complicates pulmonary suppuration and other acute respiratory illnesses, there is rarely any difficulty in deciding on its cause, since the symptoms and signs of the antecedent condition are usually obvious.

The problem of the diagnosis of the cause of chronic non-tuberculous spontaneous pneumothorax occasionally arises. It is commonly found to be due to localized or generalized cystic or emphysematous changes in the lung. Radiography in various planes and tomography may help by defining cystic changes. Thoracoscopy, however, permitting inspection of the greater part of the surface of the collapsed lung, is the most generally useful investigation.

J. G. Scadding.

POLYCYTHAEMIA

Polycythaemia denotes a significant increase in the body's total red-cell mass above the normal value of 25–35 ml. per kg. of body-weight. The diagnosis is suspected from the clinical appearance of the patient or from a routine-blood count which shows considerable increase in circulating haemoglobin content, red-cell count, and packed-cell volume. The increase in the haemoglobin content is usually rather less in proportion to the increase in the red cells, and it is not unusual to find the red cells reduced in cell volume. The total blood-volume is usually normal or increased and as a result of the increase in red-cell mass, there is an increase in blood viscosity. This may double in value with a rise in packed-cell volume from 45 to 55 per cent.

A *relative polycythaemia* results from a reduction in the plasma volume, the red-cell mass remaining constant, and may occur when, for any reason, there is a considerable loss of fluid from the circulation. It may also occur in pseudo-polycythaemia when for some unknown reason the regulating mechanisms controlling the plasma volume maintain it at a lower level than normal. An *absolute polycythaemia* may occur either as a primary condition (polycythaemia rubra vera) or secondary to some other abnormality, which is usually one which gives rise to chronic hypoxia, or a tumour producing excess of erythropoietin.

Classification of Polycythaemia

1. RELATIVE:
   Water depletion, vomiting, fever, diabetes, etc.
   Traumatic shock
   Pseudopolycythaemia.
2. ABSOLUTE:
   Primary (polycythaemia rubra vera)
   Secondary
      Chronic anoxia
         Congenital cyanotic heart disease
         Chronic lung disease
         Emphysema
         Fibrosing alveolitis
      Hypernephroma
      Hepatoma
      Cerebellar haemangioblastoma
      Uterine fibromata
      Methaemoglobinaemia
      Certain haemoglobinopathies.

Relative Polycythaemia. Loss of fluid from the circulation will occur (a) in severe vomiting, as in the *toxaemic vomiting of pregnancy*; (b) with insufficient fluid intake especially when associated with copious sweating, as in *prolonged high fever, hyperthyroidism*, or strenuous exercise in a hot atmosphere, or in association with polyuria due to *diabetes mellitus* or *diabetes insipidus*; and (c) in *traumatic shock* when there is a loss of plasma into the tissue fluids. Chronic reduction in plasma volume occurs in pseudopolycythaemia.

Pseudopolycythaemia. This is a condition common in middle age and benign in nature in which patients are usually found to have a high haemoglobin concentration and a corresponding increase in red-cell count and packed-cell volume but without the other clinical features of primary polycythaemia. The high cell-count in the peripheral blood is due to a reduction in plasma volume (normally 35–45 ml. per kg.), the cause of which is not known. These patients do appear to be particularly prone to thromboses and the condition is diagnosed by determining the reduced plasma volume. It is associated with an increased mortality rate.

Absolute Polycythaemia

PRIMARY POLYCYTHAEMIA OR POLYCYTHAEMIA RUBRA VERA. This is a disease of middle or late life affecting both sexes and characterized by plethora and cyanosis of the skin especially of the face and extremities. The common presenting symptoms are not specific but are frequently a fullness in the head or headache, dizziness, insomnia, pruritus (especially in a hot bath), and paraesthesiae. Occasionally there may be fits. The spleen is only palpable in about 50 per cent of patients but the retinae frequently appear dark red and show distension of the veins. The peripheral blood shows a variable increase in haemoglobin concentration, red-cell count, and packed-cell volume, the latter ranging from 50 to 70 per cent. The white cells are frequently increased in number as a result of a neutrophilia and may range between 15,000–30,000 per c.mm. and there is frequently an increase in the platelet count. The erythrocyte sedimentation rate (E.S.R.) is less than 3 mm. in 1 hour. The diagnosis is established by demonstrating an increase in the total body red-cell mass (normally 25–35 ml. per kg.) by the use of radio-active chromium-labelled red cells and by the exclusion of the various causes of secondary polycythaemia in which leucocytosis and thrombocythaemia are absent. The most important and common complications are thromboses and haemorrhages which may occur in any part of the body; thrombotic complications appear to be more likely to occur in patients with an increase in the platelet count. The absence of anaemia and of immature granulocytes in the peripheral blood should prevent the condition from being diagnosed as leukaemia, but primary polycythaemia may terminate as acute leukaemia and there is some evidence that this may be related to treatment with radioactive phosphorus. The disease runs a long course and may be readily controlled by venesection, radioactive phosphorus, or drugs such as busulfan or pyrimethamine. The median survival time is 11–13 years. Occasionally patients later develop anaemia which is of a leuco-erythroblastic pattern and are found to have myelosclerotic changes in the bone-marrow. In a few other patients, anaemia develops and is complicated by the appearance of numbers of primitive red cells in the peripheral blood which often have a megaloblastic appearance, similar cells being found in the bone-marrow; this condition is known as 'erythroleukaemia'. In patients with polycythaemia rubra vera it is unlikely that the association of the polycythaemia with hypertension constitutes a distinct clinical entity, although the association has gone under the name of 'Gaisböck's disease'.

SECONDARY POLYCYTHAEMIA. This most frequently results from persistent anoxia and may be a complication of congenital heart disease, chronic lung diseases, or residence at high altitudes. The type of congenital heart disease is that known as 'morbus caeruleus' in which there is marked cyanosis and clubbing of the fingers associated with the clinical signs of cardiac disease suggesting the presence of a shunt between the right and left sides of the heart which results in a partial dilution of arterial blood with venous blood. The most common type of cardiac defect is pulmonary stenosis with a patent septum or transposition of the arterial trunks. Such patients show plethora and cyanosis but no splenomegaly and, although the peripheral red-cell count is raised, there is usually no leucocytosis or thrombocythaemia. The diagnosis of anoxic polycythaemia can be made by demonstrating a low arterial Po_2. A similar type of anoxic polycythaemia complicates emphysema or idiopathic pulmonary fibrosis and is also associated with a low arterial Po_2; it may sometimes complicate silicosis and other fibrotic diseases of the lungs. During residence at altitudes over about 3000 metres polycythaemia is also common and may begin to develop after about 7 days at such a height—this type of polycythaemia is reversible on returning to sea-level and appears to be a result of the reduced partial pressure of oxygen in the atmosphere. Acute mountain sickness may be experienced by new arrivals at high altitudes but this disappears with the appearance of polycythaemia. Changes in the red-cell count and haemoglobin concentration are similar to those in other types of secondary polycythaemia and there is no leucocytosis or thrombocythaemia. Polycythaemia may complicate hypernephroma when it appears to be due to the production of an erythropoietin-like substance from the kidney tumour. The presence of proteinuria or haematuria and an unusual abdominal mass should suggest the diagnosis, especially if the E.S.R. is raised. Hepatoma is occasionally accompanied by polycythaemia probably also as a result of the production of an erythropoietin-like substance, and occasionally polycythaemia complicates the presence of a cerebellar haemangioblastoma or of uterine fibroids. The association of polycythaemia with other systemic lesions such as renal cysts and neurofibromatosis is probably not statistically significant.

METHAEMOGLOBINAEMIA. Various substances, but more particularly the *aniline derivatives*, convert haemoglobin into methaemoglobin and occasionally sulphaemoglobin and thus impair the oxygen-carrying capacity of the blood; if the condition persists a mild compensatory polycythaemia may develop. Since methaemoglobin is rapidly reconverted in the body back into haemoglobin, it will reach a concentration in the blood sufficient to cause cyanosis only when the offending substance is taken in large doses; even then the pigment will disappear completely from the blood after discontinuing the chemical. The drugs most likely to bring about this train of events are *phenacetin* and particularly *acetanilide*, which was a common constituent of many patent headache remedies; certain persons who complain of persistent headache may take these drugs almost daily over long

21*

periods of time. Some of the *sulphonamides* occasionally produce met- and sulphaemoglobinaemia, but they are unlikely to be prescribed long enough to produce polycythaemia.

Methaemoglobin may also occur in certain families in which a deficiency of the enzyme, methaemoglobin reductase, is lacking. Methaemoglobin then accumulates in the cells resulting in cyanosis and polycythaemia which is present soon after birth.

Certain abnormal haemoglobins (Chesapeake) have an increased oxygen affinity but do not form methaemoglobin. They do, however, produce tissue anoxia and secondary polycythaemia. Another abnormal haemoglobin (M) is unstable and spontaneously oxidizes to methaemoglobin and also gives rise to secondary polycythaemia. These haemoglobins can be identified by electrophoresis.

T. A. J. Prankerd.

POLYURIA

The term 'polyuria' signifies a larger than normal daily volume of urine. There is considerable variation from subject to subject in the amount of urine passed, but a urinary output of more than 2·5 litres per 24 hours is nearly always abnormal. Polyuria must not be confused with frequency of micturition due, for example, to prostatic hypertrophy or cystitis. Also, although polyuria will almost always lead to a complaint of nocturia, many individuals complaining of the latter have no increase in the total output of urine but show a reversal of the normal diurnal variation in urine flow; this is the case in most cases of sodium and water retention as in cardiac failure or the nephrotic syndrome, in suprarenal disorders, and in association with renal ischaemia. Polyuria may be due either to an increased solute load with obligatory water loss or to a primary water diuresis and will be discussed under these headings.

Polyuria due to Increased Solute Load. Any osmotically active solute will produce a diuresis if present in excess in the distal tubular fluid. For example, the massive protein breakdown occurring in a large haematoma may be associated with a diuresis, urea itself being the active solute. It is also the mechanism of *diuretic therapy* in which the solute concerned is sodium. *Diabetes mellitus* is much the commonest pathological condition in which this type of polyuria occurs. The daily urine volume is often 4 litres or more and polyuria and excessive thirst are the most common symptoms; in children, previously dry at night, enuresis may be an early symptom of diabetes. The diagnosis is usually straightforward and is discussed in the section on GLYCOSURIA (p. 320). In *chronic renal failure* the total solute load may be normal but the reduction in the number of nephrons results in a greater than normal load per nephron and consequent polyuria which is usually only of moderate severity. The polyuria which may follow the relief of chronic *urinary tract obstruction* is also partly due to this mechanism but some defect of concentrating power may also be present. Diuresis is also common during recovery from *acute tubular necrosis*; this is partly due to the elimination of water and electrolytes retained during the phase of oliguria and partly to incomplete recovery of tubular function.

Polyuria due to Water Diuresis. The simplest cause of this is an increased water intake which may reach pathological dimensions in the condition known as *compulsive water-drinking*. This is a hysterical manifestation and simulates diabetes insipidus. The differentiation is discussed below but, clinically, marked fluctuations in urine output would strongly suggest compulsive water drinking.

The urine is normally concentrated in the distal tubules and collecting ducts. Antidiuretic hormone (ADH) is secreted by the posterior pituitary in response to a rise in plasma osmolality; its action is to increase the permeability of the tubular epithelium to water. The effect of this is to increase the transport of water from the tubular lumen into the hypertonic renal medulla through which these tubules pass. Thus a pathological water diuresis may be due either to failure of secretion of ADH or to failure of the renal tubules to respond to its action.

Pituitary diabetes insipidus is often caused by an identifiable lesion of the hypothalamus or pituitary or both, but in about one-third of cases no such cause can be found. Tumours in that region are a common cause and include craniopharyngioma, pinealoma, glioma, and metastases from distant primary growths. Diabetes insipidus may also follow trauma to the skull (including operative), infections such as exanthemata in childhood, or be due to infiltration with granulomatous lesions such as sarcoidosis or histiocytosis X. Occasionally diabetes insipidus is complicated by a destructive lesion of the 'thirst' centre in the hypothalamus so that polydipsia does not accompany the polyuria; water loss is severe and hypernatraemia with brain damage may result.

Failure of the renal tubules to respond to the action of ADH is termed *nephrogenic diabetes insipidus*. A familial form is seen in males only, inherited as a sex-linked recessive. It may also be a part of other renal tubular defects such as the Fanconi syndrome with cystinosis and renal tubular acidosis in infants; it can also occur in renal amyloidosis, myelomatosis, and hyperglobulinaemia.

The differentiation of the two types of diabetes insipidus from each other and from compulsive water-drinking may be difficult. This is because a prolonged water diuresis from any cause may lead to partial resistance to the action of ADH. Thus deprivation of water in compulsive water-drinking may not cause immediate cessation of the polyuria although there will usually be a considerable reduction. In diabetes insipidus, nephrogenic or of pituitary origin, the polyuria will continue despite water deprivation and the patient become very thirsty and ill; the test is not without its dangers in this situation. Further information may be obtained from the administration of ADH. This will clearly have no effect in nephrogenic diabetes insipidus but will reduce the urine output in pituitary diabetes insipidus and in compulsive water-drinking; once again the result may not be clear-cut and the effect of ADH may not be apparent for several days. There is a danger that, in compulsive water-drinking, the continued ingestion of large amounts of water after the administration of ADH may cause water intoxication.

Failure of renal concentrating power is a feature of several other conditions which, although not usually classified as types of nephrogenic diabetes insipidus, are similar to that condition in several respects. Polyuria is a common feature of the renal lesion of *potassium depletion* or kaliopenic nephropathy; this condition might be suspected if muscular weakness is a prominent complaint or the deep reflexes are absent. Potassium depletion may be due to chronic diarrhoea, diuretic therapy, primary aldosteronism, excessive doses of corticosteroids, and alkalosis from any cause; it is particularly seen in the type of Cushing's syndrome produced by an ACTH-secreting bronchial carcinoma. The polyuria fails to respond to ADH but is reversible if the potassium balance can be restored to normal.

Hypercalcaemia also can cause a water diuresis and might be suggested by associated abdominal pain and vomiting. Thus polyuria may be a feature of primary hyperparathyroidism, vitamin-D intoxication, sarcoidosis, multiple bony metastases, or primary tumours secreting a parathormone-like substance. The renal lesion is reversible unless severe nephrocalcinosis has developed or renal calculi have produced irreversible damage. As in hypokalaemia there is no response to ADH.

Other conditions in which failure of urinary concentration occurs are *sickle-cell anaemia* and chronic *pyelonephritis* at an early stage. The polyuria due to the latter must not be confused with the osmotic diuresis of chronic renal failure discussed above.

Transient Polyuria. Polyuria lasting for a few hours only can occur in various circumstances. It is rarely of any great significance and indeed is often physiological. The diuresis which follows excessive water drinking needs no comment. The same applies to polyuria in the course of *diuretic therapy*, although the diuretic effect of such substances as tea or coffee may occasionally provoke a complaint from a patient who has not realized the association. *Cold* weather may also induce polyuria as a result of reduced fluid loss from the skin; travellers returning from a long stay in the tropics and accustomed to a large fluid intake may occasionally complain of polyuria on return to a colder country. It is this contrast with previous oliguria that partly explains

the polyuria following *fevers*; there may also be a temporary impairment of ADH secretion.

Polyuria can also occur following various stressful situations and has been described after attacks of *migraine, asthma,* and *angina.* A more striking polyuria may occur during and after attacks of *paroxysmal tachycardia.* Any dysrhythmia, supraventricular or ventricular, which lasts for more than half an hour may produce this effect.

P. R. Fleming.

POPLITEAL SWELLING

Popliteal swellings may be divided into:

1. Fluid Swellings:
Bursa
Morrant Baker's cyst
Varicose veins
Abscess
Aneurysm.

2. Solid Swellings not connected with Bone:
Enlarged glands
Malignant tumours
Innocent tumours.

3. Solid Swellings connected with Bone:
Exostosis
Sarcoma
Periostitis
Separation of the epiphysis.

1. FLUID SWELLINGS

Bursae. There are six primary bursae associated with muscles and tendons on the posterior aspect of the knee. Communications between two bursae and between a bursa and the knee joint are common.

The bursa that is underneath the insertion of the semimembranosus muscle into the posterior aspect of the inner tuberosity of the tibia is often enlarged. When the leg is extended it stands out as a tense fluctuating swelling on the inner side of the popliteal space; on flexion it disappears completely. It may be found enlarged in young athletes and cause no symptoms whatever. On account of its fairly frequent communication with the knee-joint it may be distended when that joint is the seat of an effusion. When much fluid is present fluctuation can be detected between the joint and bursa. Where the joint condition is an acute one the bursa may be very tender. When a communication does not exist the bursa will not of course be reducible at all by pressure. In rheumatoid arthritis it is common for fluid to pass from joint into bursa but not in the reverse direction, a ball-valve mechanism apparently operating.

The bursa under either of the two heads of the gastrocnemius muscle or those connected with the insertion of the semitendinosus may be enlarged similarly, but these are rare.

Morrant Baker's Cyst is a herniation of the synovial membrane and only occurs in connexion with chronic inflammatory changes in the joint, most commonly in rheumatoid arthritis. The extension from the joint tends to spread along fascial planes and may point at varying distances from its origin. The 'cysts' may be multiple. The condition of the knee-joint will indicate the nature of the lesion. Such extensions of the knee-joint may sometimes rupture and cause an inflammatory reaction in the calf muscles which may be mistaken for a phlebitis. Arthrography may be of help in diagnosis.

Varicose Veins are often present in the popliteal space; the diagnosis presents no difficulties, as the veins in the lower part of the leg will also be varicose.

These are the most common causes, the conditions which follow being much more rarely encountered.

Acute Abscess is recognized by the signs of acute inflammation; the skin is red and oedematous, the pulse and temperature are raised, and the swelling is very painful. The knee is kept flexed in order to minimize the tension of the part. The abscess may be caused by suppurating lymphatic glands or by suppurative periostitis or necrosis of the lower end of the femur. In the former case the abscess will be superficial, and in the latter deep to the popliteal vessels.

Aneurysm of the Popliteal Artery gives rise to an expansile pulsating tumour, the pulsation being synchronous with the heart's beat. Pressure on the femoral artery above will cause a diminution in size of the swelling and cessation of pulsation. The pulse at the ankle on the affected side may be smaller than that on the opposite, and delayed. If a stethoscope be placed over the swelling a distinct bruit can be heard. The complaint of the patient will probably be of pain, which may be referred down the leg if either popliteal nerve is pressed on, or in the site of the swelling if the bone is eroded. Varicose veins are almost always present on account of pressure on the popliteal vein. Owing to its pulsatile character an aneurysm is not often mistaken for anything else, but every swelling that pulsates is not an aneurysm. A soft vascular sarcoma growing from the end of the femur may be pulsatile, and over it a bruit may be heard, but the tumour is not as compressible as an aneurysm is and the effects on the distal pulse are not so marked. A radiograph will usually settle the question at once. Distinction must also be drawn between a tumour that pulsates and a tumour to which pulsation is communicated. For instance, an abscess or a solid swelling lying over the popliteal artery may appear to pulsate, but the movement is heaving in character and not expansile. In the rare event of an aneurysm having become filled with clot it might be taken for a solid tumour growing either from the soft parts or from the bone. Under this impression a leg has been amputated for sarcoma. Finally the aneurysm may present on the medial side of the lower end of the thigh, anterior to the tendon of the sartorius.

2. SOLID SWELLINGS NOT CONNECTED WITH BONE

Enlarged Glands. It is not common to find the popliteal glands enlarged from any cause. It is possible that they may become infected with pyogenic organisms from a sore on the back of the leg.

Tumours are rare. They may be innocent, e.g., *lipoma* and *neurofibroma*; or *sarcomatous*, starting in the connective tissue of the popliteal space, or attached to one of the muscles. The innocent tumours are of long history and well defined; the malignant, rapidly growing and infiltrating.

A lipomatous mass, either in the popliteal fossa or on the medial aspect of the knee, is not infrequently present in osteo-arthritis of this joint, and is part of the general fatty infiltration which gives rise inside the joint to the *lipoma arborescens* of the synovial membrane.

3. SOLID SWELLINGS CONNECTED WITH BONE

In all cases of bony tumour a radiograph should always be obtained.

Innocent Tumours. *Cancellous exostoses* may be found, generally in children and young adults, growing from the region of the epiphysial cartilage of the femur (*Fig. 98, p. 104*). There may be others in other parts of the skeleton, and sometimes several members of the family are similarly affected. The swelling is of slow growth, well defined, and rarely gives any trouble. It is most often found at the inner side of the popliteal space. There is one thing that may be confounded with it, namely, *ossification of the insertion of a tendon* or muscle. The adductor longus muscle is the one most commonly affected (rider's bone).

Medullary giant-cell tumour is prone to occur in the bones around the knee-joint and may cause an asymmetrical expansion of the cortex presenting in the popliteal fossa. Usually expansion of the bone can be detected on other aspects and the shell may be so thin in some places if the condition is advanced that 'egg-shell crackling' can be elicited. The radiographic appearances are typical—the expansion and thinning of the cortex, the absence of new bone formation, and the trabeculation.

Malignant Tumours include the osteogenic sarcomata, fibrosarcoma arising from the fibrous periosteum, and metastases from neoplasm elsewhere. Here, as in giant-cell tumour, enlargement of the bone is not usually confined to the popliteal space. The diagnosis from inflammatory lesions can be very difficult even with a radiograph, and is often impossible without. The type of *osteogenic sarcoma* which shows a palisade of bony spicules perpendicular to the line of the cortex is easily diagnosed by radiography, but it must be remembered that a sarcoma may present itself with an obvious clinical swelling and yet with little or no radiographic changes. This usually but not always denotes a *fibrosarcoma of* *the periosteum*, particularly if a thin line of periosteal new bone is laid down. Occasionally a small central area of erosion with a clinical swelling may indicate the presence of a bone sarcoma of the osteolytic type. Although there may be marked swelling, there is usually less effusion into the joint than is the case if the lesion is inflammatory. Serological tests and a biopsy of the diseased part should be done in all doubtful bone lesions. A *gumma* is indicated by dense sclerosis around the lesion, clear-cut central softening without erosion, and regular new bone formation. For further details and illustrations *see* the article on BONE, SWELLING ON (p. 101).

Periostitis. Popliteal necrosis with abscess formation may give rise to a big swelling. The signs of inflammation will usually be well marked and accompanied by constitutional symptoms and leucocytosis. Chronic periostitis, or chronic abscess of the bone, or central necrosis, may be extremely difficult to distinguish from a malignant growth. A radiograph should be taken, and if necessary an incision made down to the tumour for a piece to be removed for histological examination.

Separation of the Epiphysis. In the somewhat rare accident of separation of the lower epiphysis of the femur the lower fragment becomes displaced backwards, forms a prominence in the popliteal space, and presses on the vessels sometimes to a dangerous extent. It is unlikely that such a condition would present itself as a doubtful popliteal swelling for diagnosis.

R. G. Beard.

PORPHYRIAS

The porphyrias are a group of clinical syndromes, usually genetic in origin, in which symptoms are closely correlated with excess of circulating porphyrins, or with increased production of their precursors. Such excesses are due to abnormalities in the porphyrin synthetic pathway.

The iron-containing porphyrin, haem, is the major product of the pathway. Synthesis occurs mainly in the erythropoietic cells of the bone-marrow and in the liver. When production is excessive that produced in the liver is mostly excreted in the bile, while that from erythropoietic cells enters the circulation, mainly in erythrocytes, before it can reach the liver and kidney for elimination from the body. The pathway is complex, but is outlined in *Fig.* 662. The activity of the first enzyme in the pathway, ALA synthetase, controls the rate of synthesis of δ-aminolaevulinate (ALA) and of porphobilinogen (PBG): it is increased in some porphyrias. Normally the main route is via Type III porphyrins to haem. Type I porphyrins (only differing in the order of acetate and propionate side-chains on one ring) cannot be used for haem formation and are excreted in urine or bile.

The porphyrins, but not their precursors, are dark red, and fluoresce in ultraviolet light. Fluorescence is not only of importance in detection of porphyrins but, being associated with energy release, probably explains the typical skin photosensitivity associated with high circulating levels of porphyrins, but not with their precursors.

SCREENING TEST FOR PORPHYRINS AND THEIR PRECURSORS

Screening tests for porphyrias are usually performed on urine or faeces, but it must be remembered that in some conditions red cell levels are the most important, and that these can only be determined in the laboratory. Positive results should be confirmed in the laboratory, and the porphyrin typed, before a diagnosis of porphyria is made. Negative results do not exclude some types of porphyria in a latent phase.

Porphobilinogen in the Urine. The urine must be fresh, since PBG is labile. In the absence of porphyrins fresh urine will be of normal colour.

Tests depend on the red colour given by both porphobilinogen and urobilinogen with 2 per cent *p*-dimethylaminobenzaldehyde in 5N HCl (Ehrlich's aldehyde reagent). The colour given by porphobilinogen cannot be extracted by butanol. *Procedure.* Equal parts of fresh urine and of Ehrlich's reagent are mixed. If a red colour develops, 3 ml. of *n*-butanol is added to the mixture, the tube shaken well, and the layers allowed to separate. If the colour remains in the lower (aqueous) layer it indicates the presence of PBG; colour in the upper (butanol) layer is urobilinogen.

Porphyrins in Urine and Faeces. If much porphyrin is present in the urine the colour will be deep red, or reddish brown. Porphyrinogens and PBG are spontaneously converted to coloured porphyrins on standing (*Fig.* 663), especially in sunlight, and the urine may be colourless initially. The conversion may be speeded by boiling.

Tests depend on detection of fluorescence on exposure to ultraviolet light. Preliminary extraction is necessary to eliminate other fluorescing compounds which may be present.

The extracting solvent is equal parts of ether, glacial acetic acid, and amyl alcohol. Ten ml. of fresh urine, or a pea-sized piece of faeces, is shaken hard with 2 ml. of the solvent. A red fluorescence under an ultraviolet lamp confined to the upper (solvent) layer indicates the presence of porphyrins or, in faeces, chlorophyll. Further extraction of the fluorescing solvent layer from faeces with 1·5N HCl will remove porphyrins, but not chlorophyll.

There is no screening test for ALA. Excess is usually associated with excess of porphobilinogen, but in doubtful cases a urine specimen should be sent to the laboratory.

SYMPTOMATOLOGY OF PORPHYRIAS

Conditions associated with excessive amounts of ALA and PBG with little increase in circulating porphyrin are not associated with photosensitivity. Severe abdominal and neurological symptoms are

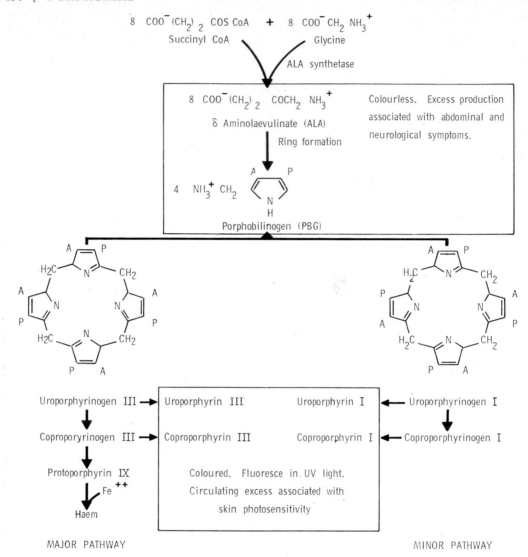

$$8 \quad COO^-(CH_2)_2 \; COS \; CoA \quad + \quad 8 \quad COO^- \; CH_2 \; NH_3^+$$

Succinyl CoA   Glycine

ALA synthetase

$$8 \quad COO^-(CH_2)_2 \; COCH_2 \; NH_3^+$$

δ Aminolaevulinate (ALA)

Ring formation

$$4 \quad NH_3^+ \; CH_2$$

Porphobilinogen (PBG)

Colourless. Excess production associated with abdominal and neurological symptoms.

Uroporphyrinogen III → Uroporphyrin III   Uroporphyrin I ← Uroporphyrinogen I

Coproporyrinogen III → Coproporphyrin III   Coproporphyrin I ← Coproporphyrinogen I

Protoporphyrin IX

↓ Fe^{++}

Haem

Coloured. Fluoresce in UV light. Circulating excess associated with skin photosensitivity

MAJOR PATHWAY   MINOR PATHWAY

Fig. 662. Pathway of porphyrin synthesis and metabolism. A, Acetate; P, propionate. Note different order in Type I and Type III compounds. Substances in capital letters, and enclosed in boxes, may be detectable in urine, faeces, or erythrocytes in the porphyrias.

common in such cases; the cause of this is not clear.

Subjects with very excessive amounts of circulating porphyrins (usually in the erythrocytes) are sensitive to even diffuse sunlight. In the worst cases severe blistering and scarring occur in exposed areas. This symptom is probably associated with the fluorescence and accompanying release of energy by porphyrins in ultraviolet light.

INHERITED PORPHYRIAS

Abnormalities of porphyrin synthesis may occur in the liver or in the erythropoietic cells of the bone marrow, and the porphyrias are classified according to the site of abnormality.

HEPATIC PORPHYRIAS

Acute intermittent (Swedish genetic) porphyria
Porphyria variegata (South African genetic porphyria)
Hereditary coproporphyria.

The first two are the least rare of the inherited porphyrias, acute intermittent porphyria being the commonest form in the British Isles, whilst porphyria variegata is relatively common in white South Africans. Coproporphyria is very rare. The three conditions have many features in common.

1. They are inherited as Mendelian dominant characteristics.

2. Acute attacks may occur in which severe abdominal pain may be misdiagnosed as, and operated on for, an acute abdominal emergency. Neuropathy may even cause respiratory paralysis. During attacks increased amounts of PBG and ALA are excreted in the urine: these abnormalities are due to increased activity of ALA synthetase (*Fig.* 662).

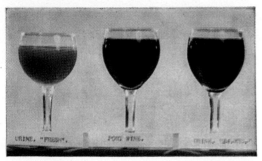

Fig. 663. Acute intermittent porphyria. Urine passed fresh (left) turns to dark red (right) after standing. Compare with port wine (centre). (*Courtesy of the Editor, Dr. F. Dudley Hart.*)

3. Attacks may be precipitated by barbiturates, oestrogens (including those in oral contraceptive preparations), sulphonamides, and griseofulvin.

4. Attacks are more common in women than in men, and are rare before puberty. This incidence may be related to oestrogen levels.

5. They may all have asymptomatic latent phases, when PBG and ALA may not be detectable in the urine.

Excess porphyrin of hepatic origin is likely to be excreted in bile and although porphyrins may sometimes be detectable in faeces, and less commonly in urine (especially after the latter has been standing for some hours), circulating levels appear normal. Only porphyria variegata, of the hepatic porphyrias, is associated with photosensitivity, usually relatively mild. The findings in urine and faeces can be summarized as follows:

	ALA and PBG	Urine Porphyrins	Faecal Porphyrins
Acute intermittent			
Attack	+	Variable (positive after standing)	—
Latent phase	Variable	—	—
Porphyria variegata			
Attack	+	Copro and uro	Proto
Latent phase	—	—	Proto
Hereditary coproporphyria			
Attack	+	Variable	Copro III
Latent phase	—	—	Copro III

ERYTHROPOIETIC PORPHYRIAS

Congenital erythropoietic porphyria (recessive)
Erythrohepatic protoporphyria (dominant).

These are both extremely rare. Because circulating red cell porphyrin levels are increased, the conditions are associated with photosensitivity. PBG and ALA are not detectable in the urine, and abdominal and neurological symptoms do not occur.

The highest circulating porphyrin levels are found in *congenital erythropoietic porphyria* in which severe photosensitivity is apparent from birth. Even the teeth and bones may be stained red, and may fluoresce in ultraviolet light, although this should *never* be used as a test. Patients are hirsute. There appears to be excessive production of Type I rather than Type III porphyrins, and this form is found in excess in the red cells. Both urinary and faecal porphyrins may be increased.

Erythrohepatic protoporphyria is so called because there is a tendency to cirrhosis of the liver, and because protoporphyrin is detectable in excess in red cells and faeces. Urine is usually normal.

ACQUIRED PORPHYRIAS

Asymptomatic porphyrinuria often occurs in liver disease. *Porphyria cutanea tarda* may be precipitated by severe hepatic damage, particularly due to alcohol and iron overload. An outbreak occurred in Turkey due to eating wheat treated with hexachlorobenzene. Photosensitivity, pigmentation, and hirsutism occurs. It may be due to impaired hepatic excretion of porphyrins, and urinary porphyrins are increased. In *lead poisoning* there is increased ALA, PBG, and coproporphyrin in the urine. Since acute abdominal pain and neuropathy occur in both hepatic porphyrias and lead poisoning, the differential diagnosis should be borne in mind.

Joan F. Zilva.

POST-PERICARDIOTOMY SYNDROME

In the early days of mitral valvotomy, relapses of 'rheumatic fever' were reported in many cases. After the immediately postoperative period, patients were developing an illness consisting of fever, pericarditis, arthralgia, and pleural effusion, and rheumatism certainly seemed a likely diagnosis. However, when an identical condition began to appear after surgery for congenital heart disease, it became clear that an alternative explanation was needed.

The post-pericardiotomy syndrome is one of a number of conditions which follow damage to the pericardium and subjacent myocardium. A few weeks after cardiac surgery, the patient complains of pericardial and, perhaps, pleural pain with arthralgia and myalgia. Variable fever appears, pericardial and pleural friction may be heard, and effusions may develop. Less often dysrhythmias and evidence of cardiac failure with raised jugular venous pressure, hepatomegaly, and gallop rhythm may be found. The sedimentation rate is always raised; leucocytosis, sometimes with eosinophilia, is common as is an unexplained anaemia. Spontaneous recovery is usually rapid and complete but, characteristically, one or more relapses may occur over the suc-ceeding months (*Fig.* 664). The aetiology is un-known but, in some cases, antibodies to heart muscle have been found. The suggestion that the condition is an auto-immune phenomenon is supported, to some extent, by the striking re-sponse to corticosteroids or other immunosup-pressive agents. The differential diagnosis in-cludes pulmonary infarction, infective endocard-itis, and genuine rheumatic fever.

is not, as was previously taught, necessary for the diagnosis. Ventricular septal defect also very often produces a thrill which, in the 'maladie de Roger' and with small defects in general, is strik-ingly long; abbreviation of the thrill from a ventricular septal defect is one of a number of signs which indicate that pulmonary hypertension of some severity has developed. A thrill is also frequently present in pulmonary stenosis. An innocent murmur is very rarely loud enough to

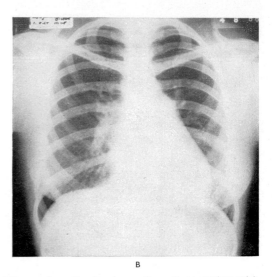

A   B

Fig. 664. Postero-anterior chest radiographs of a woman, aged 21 years, 8 months after closure of an ostium secundum atrial septal defect. In **A**, pericardial and left pleural effusions are seen which, **B**, had cleared spontaneously 1 week later.

A virtually identical condition can follow myo-cardial infarction (Dressler's syndrome) or be associated with the presence of a foreign body in or near the pericardium; it has been seen follow-ing gun-shot wounds and after the implantation of pacemaker electrodes. It is also worth noting that acute non-specific pericarditis, sometimes viral in aetiology, has the same relapsing course and it seems possible that, in certain patients, injury of any kind to the pericardium can release an antigen to which antibodies develop and pro-duce the characteristic syndrome.

P. R. Fleming.

produce a thrill, which must be assumed to indi-cate an organic lesion until rigorous investiga-tion has proved otherwise.

Heart-sounds, as well as murmurs, may be palpable. Among these the loud first sound of mitral stenosis, producing the characteristic tap-ping impulse at the apex beat, must be mentioned. Also at the apex, an atrial impulse may some-times be easily felt when the atrial sound is barely audible. This is a good illustration of the fact that low-frequency vibrations are more easily palpable than those of high frequency; it is the lower-pitched murmurs which, in general, are more commonly accompanied by thrills.

P. R. Fleming.

PRECORDIAL THRILLS

A thrill is nothing more than a palpable, and therefore loud, murmur and has the same diag-nostic significance as the murmur itself. Most thrills are more easily palpable when the patient is sitting up and holding his breath in full expira-tion. Almost any murmur may be loud enough to be accompanied by a thrill but in a few condi-tions they are very common. For example, a systolic thrill over the aortic area and transmitted into the carotid arteries is common in aortic stenosis but it must be emphasized that the thrill

PRIAPISM

Priapism signifies erection of the penis, per-sistent, of troublesome degree, and not necessarily accompanied by sexual desire. Though generally spoken of in connexion with the male sex, a precisely similar affection may occur in the female clitoris. The symptom is not often by itself of diagnostic importance. Though it may be due to a considerable number of different conditions, the ultimate cause is usually thrombosis in the vascular spaces in the cavernous tissue which are found to contain thick black grumous blood.

The more important causes are:

1. After injury to the upper dorsal region of the spinal cord. The damage may have produced fracture-dislocation of the spine with paraplegia, in which case the diagnosis will be obvious; short of this, however, a minor degree of injury, with contusion and small haemorrhages into the substance of the cord, may be followed by painful priapism, persisting sometimes for weeks before recovery occurs. Cerebrospinal syphilis or tumour may also be responsible.

2. In leukaemia; apart from obvious change in the penis—cavernous haemorrhage or the like —priapism has been noted in both myelocytic and lymphatic leukaemia even before the other symptoms and signs have led to a haematological diagnosis. The cause of the priapism in leukaemia is obscure, but the diagnosis is suggested by the concomitant splenomegaly and/or lymphadenopathy and is confirmed by the haematological findings (pp. 55 et seq.).

3. Sickle-cell anaemia.

4. New growths of the urethra, either primary or secondary to carcinoma of the bladder or testis.

5. Trauma with haematoma formation.

CHRONIC INTERMITTENT PRIAPISM is the term used to describe frequently repeated erections which are of long duration but lack the persistence of true priapism. The attacks occur in the night and are not associated with sexual desire. They are due to nerve irritation arising from lesions of the central nervous system or from local lesions in the posterior urethra, prostate, or seminal vesicles. In elderly men they are frequently associated with enlargement of the prostate.

Seldom will priapism be the only symptom in the case; the diagnosis will be made from the history and from the other symptoms.

Harold Ellis.

PROTEINURIA

Up to 0·08 g. a day of protein is normally excreted in the urine, although this amount is undetectable by the usual screening methods for proteinuria. On the other hand, negative results do not always exclude significant loss of protein other than albumin; for instance, Bence Jones protein may only be detected after concentration of urine and electrophoresis of the concentrated fluid.

Tests for Proteinuria

GENERAL POINTS

1. Apparent proteinuria may be due to contamination, especially from the vagina. Specimens should be collected after thorough washing of the area.

2. A *concentrated* (usually early morning) specimen offers the best chance of detecting slight proteinuria.

3. Bacterial growth may affect results, and

stale or heavily infected specimens should not be tested.

4. If quantitation is necessary it should be performed on a 24-hr. collection. The collection bottle, containing a suitable preservative, should be issued by the laboratory, who should also perform the test.

Albustix (*Ames*). This test detects albumin in concentrations greater than 0·3 g./l.

The strips ('stix') are impregnated with an indicator (tetrabromophenol blue), buffered to pH 3. This dye is blue in alkaline solution, but is normally yellow at pH 3. Albumin forms a complex with the dye, stablizing enough of it in the blue form, even at this pH, to give the strip a green colour.

Some important precautions should be remembered:

1. As its name implies, Albustix is most sensitive to the presence of albumin. *Other proteins, especially Bence Jones*, may give 'false' negative results.

2. Very acid or very alkaline urine may yield false negative or false positive results respectively, since the reaction depends on maintaining the strip at approximately pH 3. Acid should *not* be used as a preservative and a fresh urine specimen should be tested, since bacterial action may raise urinary pH.

3. Contamination with disinfectants and detergents may yield false positive results.

4. The strips should be stored in a cool, dry place, in a tighly capped bottle, and the manufacturers' instructions should be followed *exactly*.

Salicylsulphonic Acid Test. Turbid urine should be filtered. About 5 drops of 25 per cent salicylsulphonic acid are added to about 1 ml. of urine with mixing. Turbidity usually indicates protein at concentrations above 0·2 g/l.

False positive results may be given by radio-opaque media (from intravenous pyelograms), metabolites of tolbutamide, and large doses of penicillin.

Negative results may occur despite the presence of Bence Jones protein.

Boiling Test. Turbid urine should be filtered. The upper half-inch of urine in a half-filled boiling tube is carefully boiled, with the neck of the tube facing away from the operator. If the boiled section is turbid by comparison with the lower part a few drops of 10 per cent acetic acid are added; this dissolves phosphates, any remaining turbidity almost certainly being due to protein.

Bradshaw's test for globulins (including Bence Jones protein). Urine is layered gently onto a few millilitres of concentrated hydrochloric acid. A heavy white precipitate at the interface indicates the presence of globulins. Albumin *alone* gives a negative result.

Tests for Bence Jones protein. It must be stressed that the presence of Bence Jones protein should be confirmed, or excluded, by the laboratory. The classic heat test described by Bence Jones is unreliable, and the best 'screening' procedure is probably Bradshaw's test. A negative result does not exclude Bence Jones proteinuria. The diagnosis may be assisted by radiology (*Fig.* 665).

Causes of Proteinuria

HIGH CIRCULATING LEVELS OF PROTEIN. Proteinuria may be 'overflow' in type, associated with normal renal function and due to abnormally high amounts of circulating low molecular weight proteins. Haemoglobulinuria due to severe

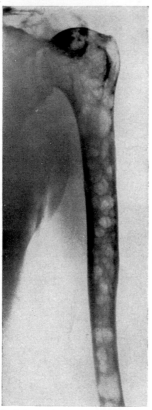

Fig. 665. The humerus in a case of multiple myelomatosis showing typical circular areas of rarefaction. (*Dr. T. H. Hills.*)

haemolysis and myoglobulinuria due to severe muscle damage cause coloured urine (*see* URINE, ABNORMAL COLORATION OF, p. 807). *Bence Jones protein* (monoclonal immunoglobulin light chain) is the only other protein with a molecular weight low enough to be cleared by the glomerulus, which is likely to be circulating in large amounts, and almost invariably indicates the presence of a malignant process, such as myelomatosis or, more rarely, macroglobulinaemia.

PROTEINURIA ASSOCIATED WITH DISEASE OF THE RENAL TRACT. If the above causes have been excluded, proteinuria indicates disease of the renal tract. *Haematuria* from any cause (for example calculi or tumours) will, of course, give a positive test for protein (*see* HAEMATURIA, p. 338) and microscopic examination will show erythrocytes. Similarly, in infection of the renal tract, when proteinuria also occurs, there may

be typical symptoms, pus may be present, and bacteriological examination will confirm the cause: renal tuberculosis should be remembered if there is apparently sterile pyuria (*see* PYURIA, p. 678).

The remaining causes are renal in origin. The protein may leak into the urine in abnormal amounts from the plasma because of increased glomerular permeability, or it may fail to be reabsorbed by damaged tubular cells. Slight proteinuria may be a non-specific finding in *severe illnesses*, such as those associated with pyrexia or in cardiac failure, and usually disappears when the disease remits. *Glomerular proteinuria*, due to increased permeability, can vary in severity. In the mildest ('selective') form proteinuria is mild, and only low molecular weight proteins (predominantly albumin, but also transferrin and other binding proteins) are found. In the severe form protein loss is massive, and although albumin is still quantitatively the main protein, higher molecular weight proteins (including immunoglobulins) increase in proportion with increasing severity ('non-selective'). A measure of selectivity can be made by comparing the clearances of low (for example, albumin) and high (for example IgG) molecular weight proteins. Massive proteinuria (more than 3 g. a day) is always glomerular in origin, and is known as the *nephrotic syndrome*. Consequences of severe albumin loss are hypo-albuminaemia, with consequent oedema. Plasma total calcium levels are low due to loss of albumin-bound calcium, but ionized levels are normal. Similarly, loss of such low molecular weight specific binding proteins as transferrin and transcortin cause low plasma iron and cortisol levels, which should not be misinterpreted. In severe cases loss of immunoglobulins leads to low γ-globulin levels and infection. *Plasma lipid levels (including cholesterol) are elevated*, and the α_2-globulin peak is increased in relation to other protein levels; it may even be raised in absolute terms. In the early stage, when glomerular permeability is high, plasma urea levels are normal. Later, as glomerular failure develops, uraemia supervenes; reduction of proteinuria under such circumstances does *not* indicate recovery. *Orthostatic (postural) proteinuria* is glomerular proteinuria occurring only in the erect posture. It is uncommon and often benign. However, it should not be assumed to be so until several years have passed.

Causes of Glomerular Proteinuria

  Most types of glomerulonephritis
  Secondary to non-renal disease such as:
    Diabetes mellitus
    Systemic lupus erythematosus
    Amyloidosis
    Malaria due to *Plasmodium malariae*
    Inferior vena caval and renal vein thrombosis
    Toxaemia of pregnancy.

Tubular Proteinuria is usually quantitatively mild, and the protein is predominantly the low molecular weight α_2- and β-globulins. It is associated with tubular damage, whatever the cause, and casts are often present. In acute oliguria following an episode of hypotension ('shock'), proteinuria and casts suggest true renal damage, rather than poor glomerular blood flow alone, as a cause of the oliguria and azotaemia. Infarction of the kidney, due to emboli, may be associated with loin pain.

Some other causes to be considered are:

Hypertensive renal damage
Pyelonephritis or, rarely, infestation by hydatids
Renal damage by:
    Hypercalcaemia
    Hyperuricaemia
    Heavy metal poisoning
    Many drugs, especially phenacetin.

Joan F. Zilva.

PRURITUS

Pruritus, or itching, may occur without visible lesions of the skin, save those due to scratching, or may be associated with various cutaneous eruptions. It is to the former condition that the word 'pruritus' should be restricted. Itching, either local or general, may be a symptom of psychoneurosis or of general disorders such as diabetes mellitus, jaundice, and renal disease; and it may occur in internal cancer, leukaemia, or lymphadenoma. Severe itching is also a constant symptom of mycosis fungoides; or the irritation may be set up by the attacks of lice, scabies, fleas, bugs, or other parasites, or by definite skin lesions. Itching varies in character; it may be interpreted by the patient as a tingling or pricking, or a formication, a feeling as of insects crawling on the skin. It varies in degree from a mild sensation which is welcome to the patient from the pleasure he finds in scratching, to an irritation so severe and persistent as to interfere with sleep.

The affections in which itching is slight are seborrhoea, erythema, psoriasis, pityriasis rosea, pityriasis rubra pilaris, and pemphigus; it is more severe, in varying degrees, in dermatitis, prurigo, dermatitis herpetiformis, dermatitis gestationis, occupational dermatitis (the itching caused by dermatitis in bakers and grocers is sometimes known as 'baker's itch' or 'grocer's itch'), lichen planus, lichenification, papular urticaria, mycosis fungoides, pompholyx, chilblain, prickly heat, tinea cruris, urticaria, scabies, the various kinds of pediculosis, flea-, mosquito-, and bug-bites, nettle, jelly-fish, and other stings. Even in the affections in which it is usually severe it varies much in degree in different cases. Itching seldom has any distinct diagnostic value, but in cases in which the cutaneous lesions may admit of more than one interpretation, its presence or absence may suffice to turn the balance; thus cutaneous syphilis never itches.

Pruritus proper may be general or local. Of general pruritus there are four varieties; pruritus universalis, pruritus hiemalis, pruritus senilis, and bath pruritus. The local varieties affect chiefly the anus, the vulva, and the scrotum, but it may affect any area. One of the most curious forms of pruritus is that which is associated with bathing. It affects most commonly the legs from the hips downwards; but the forearms also may be involved and it may have even wider range. It is an affection of adolescence and adult life and is more frequent in males than in females. A similar condition may be caused by air conditioning.

If no lesions of the skin are present except those due to scratching, the diagnosis of pruritus is fairly obvious, but itching caused by parasites must always be borne in mind. If the scratch-marks are across the backs of the shoulders or in the genital region, lice must be looked for; if on the wrists and between the fingers the burrows of the *Acarus scabiei* must be sought. Burrows are only found in human scabies but other mites may also cause itching in man. Thus animal scabies due to contact with a cat or dog suffering from scorbutic mange may produce an ill-defined pruritic rash usually on the hands and arms. The harvest mite is the cause of an urticarial reaction producing great irritation (harvest itch), while grain itch is due to a mite which lives in wheat fields and is also found in grain and straw.

Some patients, without developing actual urticaria, suffer from severe itching after the ingestion of certain foods, for example strawberries and shell-fish. While pruritus ani and vulvae are most commonly a symptom of psychoneurosis, both conditions may be secondary to organic diseases. Pruritus ani may occur with such local conditions as piles, fissure, fistula, or be the result of thread-worms or local infection with monilia or fungi; it may also be caused by a chronic discharge, as in gonorrhoeal proctitis. In long-standing diarrhoea itching is also sometimes set up. Pruritus vulvae may be caused by chronic vaginal and cervical discharge, and it has been known to occur in a case of cervical polyp. It occasionally arises in microcytic hypochromic anaemia. It is common in unbalanced diabetes mellitus, where it may be aggravated by superficial infection with *Candida albicans*, and may occur with leucoplakia. The condition known as lichen sclerosis is particularly liable to occur around the vulva and may give rise to intense itching. The skin is white, smooth and shiny, and with sharp margins. It may later cause atrophy and stenosis of the vaginal introitus, and leucoplakia may become superimposed on it. Although usually a disease of later life, it may start in childhood.

Itching may be the earliest symptom in exogenous dermatitis (q.v.), whether occupational or due to other external irritants.

Only when careful investigation fails to reveal any source of irritation, local or general, should a diagnosis of simple pruritus be made.

P. D. Samman.

PRURITUS VULVAE

Pruritus vulvae may be defined as an irritation of the vulva which necessitates scratching for its relief. In the majority of cases the patient is several years past the menopause; there are no detectable precipitating factors and the vulva shows either lichenification from scratching and rubbing or the thickened white skin of leucoplakia.

In some cases, in the absence of any abnormal physical signs, apart from scratch marks, the onset has seemed to follow some psychological shock or disappointment, following the discovery of marital infidelity, or other marital disharmony. In other cases, the pruritus may be due to simple uncleanliness, from the accumulation of sweat, sebaceous material or smegma, particularly in the obese, or to glycosuria.

Chronic congestion of the vulva, the result of sexual excess, masturbation, or even excessive walking or standing, may be responsible. In other cases the patient may be allergic to certain types of diaper or an article of underclothing, while the use of certain ointments or lotions to which she is allergic can be the cause. Examples are nylon or detergents used for washing. In the above cases the pruritus, though distressing, is rarely unbearable and can be cured by removing the cause as, for instance, glycosuria in a diabetic. *No case of pruritus vulvae, however, will be cured completely unless scratching is avoided.*

Monilia (*Candida albicans*) infections cause intense pruritus and may be recognized by the typical white curdy discharge which adheres to the vaginal wall.

Vaginal discharge from any cause may be responsible for some pruritus, as may infection of the urinary tract. The commonest cause of vaginal discharge, however, infection with the *Trichomonas vaginalis*, is more inclined to make the vulva sore than to itch.

Monilial infection is common in the diabetic, so that examination of the urine for sugar is essential. If sugar is absent, blood-sugar estimations should be done, and possibly glucose tolerance tests. An early diabetes may prove to be the underlying cause of the pruritus. The history of the birth of very large babies is often obtained in these cases, as is a positive family history of diabetes mellitus.

Certain deficiencies such as oestrogen deficiency at the menopause or vitamin-A deficiency may be the cause.

General diseases such as anxiety states, leukaemia, chronic nephritis, and Hodgkin's disease must be excluded.

Leucoplakia vulvae is a very common cause in later life, the itching being so intense that nothing less than excision of the affected parts gives relief. In a typical case the diagnosis is easy. The skin of the whole vulva excluding the vestibule is thickened and white with cracks and fissures. The lesion may involve the perineum, the perianal, and the perivulvar skin. Biopsy reveals characteristic histological changes.

A complete investigation of a case of pruritus vulvae will require at least (1) Examination of the blood; blood-count, blood-urea estimation, and blood-sugar estimations; (2) Assessment of presence or absence of an anxiety state; (3) Examination of the urine for sugar and organisms; and (4) Examination of the vaginal discharge for *Monilia trichomonas* and other organisms.

T. L. T. Lewis.

PTOSIS

Ptosis is the term applied to drooping of the upper eyelid with inability to raise it to the full

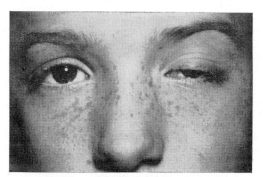

Fig. 666. Ptosis.

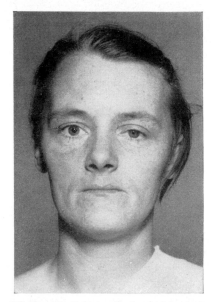

Fig. 667. Horner's syndrome affecting the left side showing ptosis, enophthalmos, and small pupil. (*Dr. R. G. Ollerenshaw, Manchester Royal Infirmary.*)

extent (*Fig.* 666). One of the commonest forms is a developmental defect, and if the pupil is in consequence covered surgical correction is indicated; the acquired kind is usually caused by *paralysis of the third nerve*, in which case it may also be associated with paralysis of other ocular muscles, either external or internal.

In *paralysis of the cervical sympathetic*, slight ptosis may be associated with diminution in the size of the pupil on the affected side, and retraction of the eyeball or 'enophthalmos'—Horner's syndrome (*Fig.* 667). Ptosis also occurs in *myasthenia gravis*.

Ptosis of the lids, associated with much oedema and infiltration of the lids, is also found in *inflammatory affections* of the conjunctiva and upper lids, in *angioneurotic* oedema (*see* p. 589), and is a very constant feature of *trachoma*. It also follows direct injury of the elevating muscle or its nerve-supply, as by wound or fracture.

Congenital ptosis is often bilateral, and associated with smoothness of the upper lids and absence of all the usual cutaneous folds. The levator palpebrae may be absent or ill developed, and efforts to open the eye are made by the occipitofrontalis muscle.

A slight ptosis is also present in the condition called 'jaw-winking', in which, on movements of the jaw, especially lateral movements, the lid rises.

P. Trevor-Roper.

PTYALISM

Ptyalism means excessive secretion of saliva. It is not always easy to determine if there really is excess, or if the patient is merely allowing the normal volume of saliva to dribble from the mouth. Thus the difficulty may be solely that of swallowing the normal secretion, as in bulbar paralysis. There may be both excess of secretion and difficulty in swallowing, as in mercurial stomatitis. In other instances there is too much secretion but no difficulty in swallowing, as in functional or hysterical ptyalorrhoea. The first step towards ascertaining the cause is to inquire as to any *medicine* or *drug* the patient may be taking orally or applying externally, especially:

Mercury
Pilocarpine
Iodide
Bromide
Arsenic
Antimony
Chlorate of potash
Copper salts.

Excessive smoking may perhaps be included under the description of 'drugs'.

Mercury was the most important of these when the drug was used in the treatment of syphilis; its effects are worst when the mouth is not kept clean.

If the salivation is not attributable to any drug it may be the result of one of the many forms of *general stomatitis*.

The nature of a severe stomatitis will be ascertained by local examination, ocular and digital, assisted by the history; by bacteriological examination of swabbings from the mouth; by serological tests for syphilis; or by microscopical examination of a fragment of the affected tissues. Tuberculous stomatitis is one of the rarer but severe forms; it may be primary but is more often associated with pulmonary phthisis.

If drugs and general stomatitis can be excluded, local examination may still serve to detect a cause acting by reflex irritation of the fifth nerve, especially:

A jagged carious tooth
A stump left beneath a dental plate
A broken or ill-fitting dental plate
A foreign body impacted in the gum
An ulcerating tumour of the oral cavity.

If appropriate examination serves to exclude these, the salivation, apparently rather than actually increased, may be found to result from *mechanical difficulties in swallowing* (*see* DYSPHAGIA). The excessive salivation seen in many cases of advanced carcinoma of the oesophagus results from the oesophago-salivary reflex; a constant excess flow of saliva is secreted in an attempt to 'swallow' the obstructing bolus of tumour in the gullet.

In the absence of obvious local structural lesion, apparent salivation may be due to inability to swallow, as in cases of:

Bulbar paralysis
Pseudo-bulbar paralysis
Bilateral facial paralysis
Myasthenia gravis
Hypoglossal nerve paralysis
Diphtheritic paralysis
Parkinsonism, especially the variety following encephalitis lethargica
Hydrophobia
Botulism.

The differential diagnosis of these conditions is discussed elsewhere. It is only in bulbar and pseudo-bulbar paralysis that the dribbling of much saliva is a prominent symptom. The sequence of events summarized by the term 'labio-glossopharyngo-laryngeal paralysis' is as a rule sufficiently characteristic; pseudo-bulbar paralysis, being of cortical instead of medullary nuclear origin, does not exhibit wasting of the tongue.

The salivation that results from *gastric reflexes* is almost physiological, as an attempt to neutralize acidity by an alkaline secretion. It is a prominent feature in duodenal ulceration (waterbrash). Other conditions in which it may occur are:

Dilatation of the stomach
Pancreatitis
Nausea from any cause including gastric and hepatic diseases.

Slovenliness and lack of cerebral control are responsible for the slobbering and salivation of some mentally defective patients.

Finally, a high degree of salivation can sometimes be attributed to nothing but functional disorder. It may occur in men as well as in women, generally in later life rather than at a time when hysteria is commonest. The condition is a neurosis, which may come on suddenly and without obvious cause, or as the result of some worry, shock, or mental emotion. It is sometimes prominent amongst the disturbances that may accompany pregnancy.

Harold Ellis.

PULSATILE SWELLING

When a tumour can be felt to be pulsating, the first point to decide, if possible, is whether the pulsation is expansile or whether it is merely transmitted by a non-expansile tumour which is in direct contact with large pulsating vessels. The distinction is sometimes obvious, especially when

not only when he lies on his back, but also in the knee–elbow posture, for sometimes a tumour which is in contact with the aorta in the former position falls away from it and ceases to transmit pulsation in the latter.

If it can be decided definitely that the tumour is itself pulsating, most probably it is either an *aneurysm* of an artery or else a very vascular *sarcoma*. Egg-shell crackling with pulsation in a tumour would suggest osteosarcoma, though it might also be felt over an aneurysm that had eroded adjacent bones extensively. Aneurysm will be the probable diagnosis when the markedly pulsatile swelling occurs directly along the course of a known artery. Absence of pulsation does

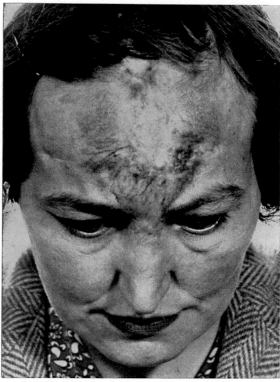

Fig. 668. Cirsoid aneurysm of the forehead. (Dr. J. F. Carter Brain.)

the tumour has developed in a place where there are no particularly large blood-vessels to transmit pulsation, for instance in the foot, or in direct connexion with a long bone at some spot not immediately adjacent to the main artery of the limb. The chief difficulty arises when the mass is either in the root of the neck or in the abdomen, and, to a less extent, when it is in the axilla, the inner aspect of the upper arm, in front of the elbow, in the groin, or in the popliteal space. Careful palpation is probably the best means of determining whether or not there is actual expansile pulsation; in the case of the abdomen it is important to examine the patient

not, however, exclude aneurysm, for either the latter may be situated too deeply for the pulsation to be felt, or else the sac may be filled partly or wholly by organizing clot.

Sometimes direct application of the ear to the part, in such a way that the pinna is in uniform contact with the patient's skin, will detect pulsation clearly when its amount, appreciable to the sensitive membrana tympani, is too slight for the hand to discern; this applies particularly to aneurysm of the first or second portions of the aorta.

On the other hand, marked pulsation may suggest aneurysm without any being present, particularly at the root of the neck and in the abdomen;

a normal subclavian artery may sometimes seem to be abnormal, particularly if it is pushed forward or displaced by a mass below or behind it, for instance an accessory cervical rib. Undue pulsation of the abdominal aorta, especially in women, is also to be remembered as a possible source of erroneous diagnosis.

It should also be remembered that normal arteries cause violent pulsation in cases of marked aortic regurgitation, and in severe cases of exophthalmic goitre, in which the whole neck, including the enlarged thyroid gland, may be seen pulsating vigorously.

Cirsoid aneurysm of the scalp (*Fig.* 668), a conglomeration of abnormally dilated arteries in the form of an arterial naevus, is rare but distinctive; its position on the scalp at once suggests the diagnosis.

A pulsatile orbital tumour will generally be due to an arteriovenous aneurysmal communication between the internal carotid artery or its ophthalmic branch and the cavernous sinus, in which case there is usually a prolonged bruit, with systolic accentuation, heard best over the upper lid, and which can be likened to a cannon booming in a canyon—a systolic bang followed by diastolic reverberations.

It is important not to mistake for the ordinary pulsatile tumours those which may move synchronously with respiration, for instance hernia pulmonalis, hernia cerebri, and certain congenital abnormalities of the brain and spinal cord, such as meningomyelocele.

It is unlikely that a pulsatile liver will be mistaken for any other kind of pulsatile tumour. It occurs in cases of chronic failure of cardiac compensation, generally from mitral stenosis and tricuspid stenosis, with oedema of the legs, lividity, orthopnoea, and ascites. It is not, however, every liver, seemingly pulsatile, that really presents expansile pulsation; an impression of pulsation is often given by the movements transmitted directly to the liver by the labouring hypertrophied right heart.

Rarely the cardiac pulsations may be transmitted direct to fluid contained in a pleural cavity, so that the bulging intercostal spaces may pulsate synchronously with the radial artery and simulate some more serious pulsatile tumour. The history and the physical signs, including displacement of the heart towards the opposite side, will generally indicate the correct diagnosis.

R. G. Beard.

PULSE, IRREGULAR

An absolutely regular pulse is rare. Even in normal sinus rhythm slight fluctuations in rate can be detected by measuring successive R–R intervals in the electrocardiogram. This can hardly be detected by palpation of the pulse, however, and this section will deal with irregularities which are apparent clinically. When examining the pulse, it is necessary first to determine whether it is regular or irregular and, if the latter, whether any pattern can be detected within the irregularity. Complete clinical analysis of an irregular pulse includes inspection of the jugular venous pulse and auscultation at the apex beat in addition to feeling the arterial pulse. The venous pulse provides evidence on the presence and frequency of atrial contractions; auscultation allows the detection of ventricular contractions too feeble to produce a pulse at the wrist. Many dysrhythmias can be diagnosed clinically but electrocardiographic confirmation is always desirable, if possible. In some cases the diagnosis can only be made from the electrocardiogram and, in a few, only with considerable difficulty.

There are two main mechanisms which can produce an irregular pulse. The first is a disorder of impulse formation in which, most commonly, an abnormal (ectopic) pacemaker drives the ventricles either directly or via the atrioventricular bundle. The other mechanism is a disorder of conduction in which a block develops somewhere along the long pathway from the sino-atrial node to the ventricular myocardium; if this block is intermittent, an irregular pulse is likely to result.

Disorders of Impulse Formation. The rate of discharge of the sino-atrial node can vary, more or less rhythmically, in many normal subjects; this condition, termed *sinus arrhythmia*, is quite benign and hardly justifies classification as a 'disorder'. The fluctuations in rate are most commonly in phase with respiration, the rate increasing during inspiration and slowing during expiration. This is very common in children and is due to reflex variations in vagal tone (*Fig.* 669). The *absence* of respiratory sinus arrhythmia is sometimes of some slight diagnostic significance in a child as this is a feature of a large atrial septal defect. There are also two, much rarer, types of non-respiratory sinus arrhythmia. In one the cycles of tachycardia and bradycardia are much longer and are quite unrelated to respiration; the P waves of the electrocardiogram are normal and constant in configuration. In the other type the P waves vary slightly in shape and the irregularity is believed to be due to changes in the site of the pacemaker within the sino-atrial node itself. The irregularity in respiratory sinus arrhythmia is exaggerated by deep breathing and, in all types, is abolished or markedly reduced by exercise or other cause of tachycardia.

Ectopic beats are a very common cause of an irregular pulse. They are due to the discharge of an abnormal pacemaker in the atria, atrioventricular junction (AV node and main bundle of His), or ventricles. Apart from their site of origin, they can be classified as escape beats, extrasystoles, and parasystoles. *Escape beats* should be regarded as a protective mechanism against asystole. They arise either from the atrioventricular junction or from the ventricles and occur whenever, for any reason, there is a prolonged pause in the activity of the sino-atrial node. Thus they may be seen in sinus brady-cardia and during the slow phase of sinus arrhythmia. They are difficult to recognize clinically but can be identified in the electrocardiogram by the abnormally long pause preceding an ectopic beat identified, as described below, as junctional or ventricular in origin.

Extrasystoles most frequently arise from the ventricles but atrial and junctional extrasystoles such as to indicate a momentary disturbance in the action of the heart; expressions such as 'my heart missed a beat' or 'my heart seemed to turn over' are not uncommon. In the electrocardiogram ventricular extrasystoles are identified by the bizarre configuration of the QRS complex and by the absence of a P wave (*Fig.* 670). The pause following the extrasystole is fully compensatory, that is the sum of the R–R intervals preceding

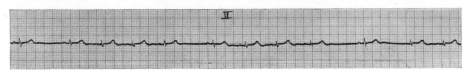

Fig. 669. Electrocardiogram showing gross respiratory sinus arrhythmia. The cycle lengths vary from 0·7 to 1·24 seconds.

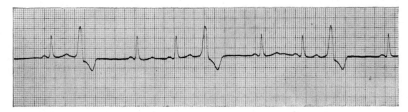

Fig. 670. Electrocardiogram showing ventricular extrasystoles producing pulsus bigeminus.

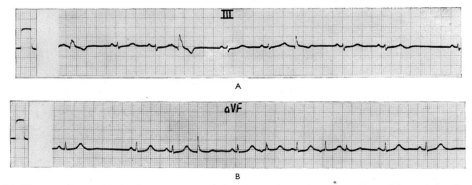

A

B

Fig. 671. Electrocardiogram showing frequent supraventricular extrasystoles conducted normally or with ventricular aberration. A, The first, fourth, and seventh complexes are supraventricular in origin, despite their abnormal configuration, as shown by the preceding P waves which deform the T waves of the previous complexes. The long pause at the end of the strip is preceded by an ectopic P wave which is completely blocked. B, The sixth and eighth complexes are supraventricular extrasystoles conducted normally, the fourth and ninth show ventricular aberration.

are also common. If a ventricular extrasystole occurs early in diastole, ventricular filling will be incomplete and the contraction may fail to open the aortic valve; even if it does so, the pulse may be so feeble that it does not reach the wrist. Thus, in the radial pulse a 'dropped beat' will be noticed; on auscultation the extrasystole will be heard either as the first sound only or as both sounds. Ventricular extrasystoles occurring later in diastole are more likely to produce a palpable impulse at the radial pulse. Often an extrasystole follows each sinus beat to produce pulsus bigeminus or coupled beats; this is often a result of digitalis overdosage. The patient with extrasystoles may have noticed no abnormality or he may complain of palpitations described in terms

and following the ectopic beat equals two complete cycles. Rarely, if the sinus is slow, interpolated ventricular extrasystoles occur—the only true 'extra' systole. Ventricular extrasystoles are usually benign and do not indicate organic heart disease; they are more common following overindulgence in tea, coffee, alcohol, or tobacco. They may be of more serious significance, however, particularly following myocardial infarction when, if they are multifocal, or appear in salvoes, or are so premature as to deform the T wave of the preceding complex (R-on-T), they may presage ventricular tachycardia or fibrillation.

Atrial and junctional (supraventricular) extrasystoles produce very much the same symptoms and signs as ventricular. The electrocardiogram shows abnormal P waves indicating the site of the ectopic focus; with junctional extrasystoles the P wave is typically inverted in Leads II, III, and aVF. The form of the QRS complex is usually normal as the impulse reaches the ventricles via the normal conducting pathways. Occasionally, however, if the supraventricular extrasystole is very premature, one or other branch of the bundle may still be partially refractory so that intraventricular conduction proceeds

helpful as cannon waves are a constant finding in junctional extrasystoles and may occur in other varieties also, if atrial and ventricular systole happen to coincide. A cannon wave implies an effective atrial contraction and therefore rules out atrial fibrillation.

Progressively more rapid rates of discharge of an ectopic atrial focus lead to atrial tachycardia and atrial flutter which can be regarded as series of atrial ectopic beats. In these conditions the

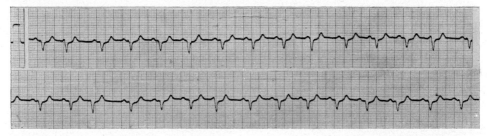

Fig. 672. Two strips of continuous record showing junctional parasystole with retrograde block. The sinus P waves continue uninterruptedly with a cycle length of 0·7 second. The second, tenth, and fourteenth complexes in the upper strip and the third and seventh in the lower are junctional in origin. The interectopic intervals are 5·76 seconds (=2 × 2·88), and 2·88 seconds. Later in the same record an interectopic interval of 31·5 seconds (=11 × 2·86) was found.

abnormally and the configuration of the QRS is bizarre, simulating a ventricular extrasystole. This phenomenon is known as aberrant ventricular conduction and can only be decisively distinguished from a ventricular extrasystole by the finding of an ectopic P wave preceding the QRS (*Fig.* 671). The pause following a supraventricular extrasystole is usually less than fully compensatory. Supraventricular extrasystoles are nearly always benign but if they are frequent, for example in a patient with mitral stenosis, they may indicate that atrial fibrillation is impending.

With extrasystoles in general, the interval between a sinus beat and an extrasystole—the coupling interval—is remarkably constant, implying that the discharge of the ectopic focus is in some way dependent on the preceding sinus beat. This is not the case in the phenomenon known as *parasystole*. In this situation an ectopic focus, most often in the ventricles but occasionally in the atria or atrioventricular junction, discharges at its own intrinsic rate regardless of the rate of the sino-atrial node or other dominant pacemaker. The ectopic focus is 'protected' from discharge by the normal sinus beats so that, whenever the ectopic discharge finds the ventricles in a non-refractory state, an ectopic beat appears. The diagnosis is made from the electrocardiogram by finding ectopic beats with varying coupling intervals and a succession of interectopic intervals all of which are multiples of a single shorter interval —the intrinsic cycle length of the ectopic focus (*Fig.* 672).

The clinical diagnosis of extrasystoles is usually easy but, if they occur frequently, they may be difficult to distinguish from atrial fibrillation. Exercise will usually abolish extrasystoles and, if anything, cause greater irregularity in atrial fibrillation. The jugular venous pulse may also be

ventricular rhythm is usually regular but when the rate of discharge of the ectopic focus exceeds about 400 per minute, co-ordinated atrial depolarization and contraction are impossible and *atrial fibrillation* results. The supraventricular impulses impinge, more or less at random, on the atrioventricular node, finding it and the remainder of the conducting tissue more or less refractory at any given time so that the ventricular response is totally irregular.

Atrial fibrillation is an extremely common finding in almost any type of heart disease. Probably the commonest cause is rheumatic heart disease, especially mitral valve disease; it is much less common, except as a terminal event, in isolated aortic valve disease. In thyrotoxicosis, also, it is a well-known complication, especially in the toxic nodular goitre of older subjects. It is not very common in uncomplicated angina, but it occurs quite frequently after myocardial infarction and when failure develops. In hypertensive heart disease, as well, it is rather unusual except late in the course of the disease. Other conditions characterized by chronic atrial fibrillation, as distinct from the transient type to be discussed below, are constrictive pericarditis, invasion of the pericardium by bronchial carcinoma or other mediastinal tumours, tumours of the heart itself, many varieties of cardiomyopathy and atrial septal defect, but not other types of congenital heart disease. Idiopathic or 'lone' atrial fibrillation, with no other evidence of heart disease, is well recognized but rather rare. Infections, particularly respiratory, can precipitate atrial fibrillation, especially in patients predisposed by rheumatic heart disease. Once the infection is over, sinus rhythm may be restored, either spontaneously or by direct-current shock. Return to sinus rhythm is also possible if atrial fibrillation has been caused by myocardial infarction and is almost the rule in thyrotoxic atrial fibrillation once the patient is euthyroid. Other causes of transient atrial fibrillation include pulmonary embolism, although it is rather unusual in chronic cor pulmonale, thoracotomy for any purpose, electric shock and hypothermia, either accidental or induced. It can rarely be caused by drugs such as digitalis, anaesthetic agents, and emetine.

atrial gallop rhythm if one had been heard previously. The electrocardiogram shows three diagnostic features: a totally irregular ventricular rhythm, absence of P waves, and their replacement by f waves, fairly large in amplitude if the atrial fibrillation is of recent onset and becoming smaller as the months and years go by (*Fig.* 674).

Atrial flutter, although usually associated with a regular ventricular rhythm, may produce an

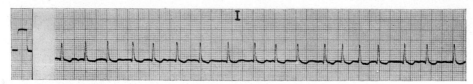

Fig. 673. Atrial fibrillation with a ventricular rate of 140 per minute. Recorded from a man, aged 51, with mitral stenosis who was in pulmonary oedema at the time. He became virtually symptom-free when the ventricular rate was controlled with digoxin.

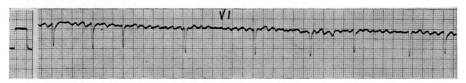

Fig. 674. Electrocardiogram showing atrial fibrillation with a ventricular rate of 60 per minute. The f waves are well shown as is usually the case in Lead V1.

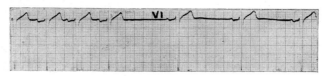

Fig. 675. Electrocardiogram showing the sudden development of 2 : 1 sino-atrial block. From a woman, aged 59, with severe hypertensive and ischaemic heart disease.

The development of atrial fibrillation will usually cause the patient to complain of palpitations, and failure may be precipitated in patients with severe heart disease. This is particularly the case in mitral stenosis in which the rapid ventricular rate, by restricting the time available for ventricular filling, causes a steep rise in left atrial pressure and may precipitate pulmonary oedema (*Fig.* 673). Once the ventricular rate has been brought under control by digitalis, most patients with atrial fibrillation have few, if any, symptoms attributable to the dysrhythmia. The pulse is totally irregular and rapid in uncontrolled atrial fibrillation. The true ventricular rate can be determined only by auscultation as many of the impulses fail to reach the radial pulse; it is usually around 160 per minute. The difference between the rates as determined at the radial pulse and by auscultation—the pulse deficit —is some measure of the lack of control. Once the ventricular rate is under control there is no pulse deficit and the irregularity of the pulse, although still present, may be less easy to detect. The other diagnostic feature is the absence of evidence of atrial systole; no a waves are seen in the jugular venous pulse and the presystolic murmur of mitral stenosis disappears as does an

irregular pulse if the degree of atrioventricular block is variable. Clinically this is very difficult to distinguish from atrial fibrillation and, indeed, at fast atrial rates the two conditions merge in so-called 'flutter-fibrillation'. This unsatisfactory term should be avoided if possible; if each of the varying R–R intervals is a multiple of the interval between two 'f' waves, flutter should be diagnosed. Atrial flutter is considered at greater length in the section on TACHYCARDIA (p. 771).

Disorders of Conduction. Failure of transmission of the impulse from the sino-atrial node to the ventricles causes 'dropped beats'. The ventricular rhythm will be regular only if every other beat is dropped as in 2 : 1 atrioventricular block or if the block is complete and a lower pacemaker is driving the ventricles. Any other pattern of failure of conduction will cause an irregular pulse.

Sino-atrial block is a rather rare conduction defect in which the impulse fails to pass from the sino-atrial node to the atrial myocardium. Clinically occasional dropped beats are noted or, if 2 : 1 sino-atrial block is present, a regular slow pulse (*Fig.* 675). The patients may be symptom-free but Stokes-Adams attacks can occur. The condition can occur in the absence of other evidence of heart disease but is quite often associated with ischaemic heart disease or, as a transient phenomenon, with acute rheumatic carditis. It can also be produced by digitalis.

Partial atrioventricular block can also produce an irregular pulse. In Mobitz Type I (Wenckebach) second-degree block conduction in the atrioventricular bundle becomes progressively more

it be confused with electrical alternans in which the QRS complexes alternate in amplitude; the two conditions may coexist, however. Though rather rare, pulsus alternans is an important sign of left ventricular failure.

Pulsus paradoxus is a feature of constrictive pericarditis, high-pressure pericardial effusion, and other, less common, conditions in which the primary abnormality is failure of the ventricles to

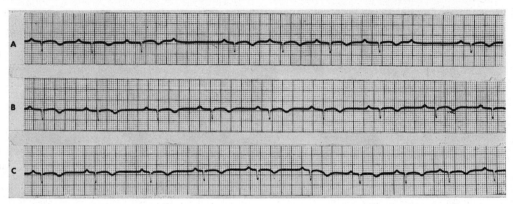

Fig. 676. Electrocardiogram showing Type I (Wenckebach) partial atrioventricular block. In A the P–R intervals progressively lengthen until conduction fails and a QRS complex is deleted. In B, recorded 1 min after 1 mg of atropine intravenously, the Wenckebach periods have ceased but the P–R interval is prolonged to 0·25 sec. In C, another minute later, atrioventricular conduction is normal.

impaired from beat to beat, as shown by an increasing P–R interval in the electrocardiogram, until conduction fails completely and a ventricular beat is missed (*Fig.* 676). Thus, in the radial pulse, every third, fourth, or fifth beat may be dropped; there is also a slight progressive increase in ventricular rate during the runs of conducted beats but this cannot be detected by palpation alone. This type of atrioventricular block is relatively benign and may be a transient occurrence in myocardial infarction or digitalis intoxication. Normal conduction is almost always restored by exercise, atropine, or any other measure which increases the atrial rate (*Fig.* 676). Mobitz Type 2 second-degree block is a much more serious condition. In its mildest form beats may be dropped intermittently, as in Type 1, but without any previous lengthening of the P–R interval; later 2 : 1 or 3 : 1 block with a slow regular ventricular rhythm is common. Increasing the atrial rate, by any means, increases the severity of the block. (*See also* BRADYCARDIA, p. 111.)

Two mechanical causes of a palpably irregular pulse should be mentioned. *Pulsus alternans* is characterized by a regular rhythm with alternation in amplitude of the equally spaced beats. It may be easily palpable but, more often, is detected by sphygmomanometry. As the cuff pressure is lowered, half of the beats are heard at the higher systolic pressure and, as the pressure of the smaller amplitude beats is reached, the rate seems suddenly to double. A run of pulsus alternans is often initiated by an extrasystole but it must not be confused with pulsus bigeminus. Nor should

fill adequately (restrictive cardiomyopathy, *see* p. 378). The normal tendency of the pulse-pressure to fall slightly during inspiration is much exaggerated so that, in a gross example, the arterial pulse may become impalpable during inspiration. At first the impression is of a grossly irregular pulse but there is little difficulty in relating the changes to the phases of respiration; the diagnosis is confirmed by finding other evidence of pericardial constriction. This includes a rise in the, already elevated, venous pressure on inspiration instead of the usual fall. This behaviour of the venous pressure, known also as Kussmaul's sign, is much commoner than a paradoxical arterial pulse and is truly paradoxical, or the opposite of the normal. The arterial changes are an exaggeration of, not opposite to, the normal; the term 'paradoxical' was applied because the heart's action appeared to have ceased during inspiration and yet, *paradoxically*, heart-sounds could still be heard normally at this time.

P. R. Fleming.

PULSES, UNEQUAL

A thorough physical examination should include palpation of all the easily accessible arterial pulses. The pulses on the two sides should be compared and, in the arms at any rate, inequalities should be confirmed by sphygmomanometry. It must be remembered that, in normal subjects, the blood-pressure in the right arm may be slightly higher than that in the left; this difference is, however, rarely palpable. It is always worth recording the arteries in which the pulse has been felt, if only for future reference; the significance of an absent pulse is much greater if it is known to have been present on a previous occasion.

The pulse in one or other radial artery may be reduced or absent as a result of a minor *congenital abnormality* in the course or calibre of the vessel. Other congenital conditions in which the radial pulses may be unequal include a few cases of *coarctation of the aorta*. In 2 per cent of cases the lesion is proximal to the left subclavian artery so that the pulses in the left arm are weaker than those in the right; in addition stenosis of the origin of a subclavian artery is a rare complication of coarctation. *Supravalvular aortic stenosis* is another, very rare, cause of unequal pulses; in this condition the blood-pressure in the right arm is often a good deal higher than that in the left and the difference may be palpable. There is no convincing explanation for this finding.

Inequality of pulses previously known to be equal is a most important sign. In the legs *atherosclerosis* of the larger arteries is the commonest cause and the level of occlusion should be sought by comparing the pulses in the femoral, popliteal, posterior tibial, and dorsalis pedis arteries. Another cause of unequal pulses, usually in the legs, is *Buerger's disease* although some authorities doubt the existence of this condition as a separate entity. Atherosclerosis is less common in the vessels of the upper limbs but can certainly involve the branches of the aortic arch and cause inequality of the brachial and radial pulses. Giant-cell *arteritis* and other inflammatory diseases of arteries occasionally cause occlusion of major limb vessels.

Arterial embolism is an important cause of unequal pulses in the upper or lower limbs. The three commonest sources of such an embolism are the left atrium in atrial fibrillation, particularly in association with mitral valve disease; vegetations in infective endocarditis of the mitral or aortic valve; and mural thrombus laid down on the endocardial surface of a myocardial infarct. Less common causes of systemic embolism are left atrial myxoma, left ventricular endocardial thrombus in a ventricular aneurysm or in congestive cardiomyopathy, thrombus detached from an atherosclerotic plaque in the aorta, and a so-called 'paradoxical embolus' passing from veins in the legs via a patent foramen ovale to the systemic circulation. This last occurs only if the pressures on the right side of the heart have been raised, often by a previous pulmonary embolism.

Frequent palpation of the arterial pulses is most important when *dissecting aneurysm* of the aorta is suspected. As the dissection proceeds along the length of the aorta the branches may be occluded one by one over a period of a few hours; the process may be capricious, branches past which the dissection has spread unexpectedly remaining patent. If re-entry occurs, the pulse may return in arteries previously occluded.

Takayasu's disease, or the 'pulseless disease', is a rare form of arteritis involving the branches of the aortic arch. Apart from inequality in the pulses in the arms or, perhaps more commonly, obliteration of the pulses in both arms, signs and symptoms of cerebral ischaemia are common. Takayasu's disease is one of the causes of so-called 'reversed coarctation', a not very satisfactory term implying diminished or absent pulses in the arms with normal femoral pulses. This situation can also occur as a result of *aortic aneurysm*, particularly of the arch, in which unequal pulses in the arms may be of diagnostic importance.

Occlusion of a subclavian artery by external pressure, as by a *cervical rib* or a *tumour* in that region, must be remembered. In cervical rib particularly, pain, paraesthesiae, and weakness and wasting of the small muscles of the hand, due to compression of the first thoracic root, are common associated features.

Finally, such obvious causes of unequal pulses as previous *subclavian–pulmonary anastomosis* for cyanotic congenital heart disease or brachial *arteriotomy* must be mentioned. An experienced cardiologist may be puzzled, momentarily, by unequal radial pulses until he recalls, with some embarrassment, an inexpert arteriotomy performed when he was less experienced.

P. R. Fleming.

PUPIL, ABNORMALITIES OF

Abnormalities of the pupil may be classified into: (1) *Irregularities in shape*; (2) *Irregularities in movement and size*.

1. Irregularities in Shape. The normal pupil is circular, or slightly oval with the longer axis horizontal. Its outline may become irregular owing to an adhesion between the iris and the lens, the result of preceding *iritis*; these adhesions are most evident when the pupil is dilated (*see Fig.* 280, p. 265). A similar irregularity sometimes occurs in association with the *persistence of a pupillary membrane*—a congenital affection; the adhesions due to this cause are distinguished from inflammatory adhesions by the fact that they arise from the anterior surface of the iris at a slight distance from the pupil, and not from the posterior surface or the extreme edge.

The pupil may also become irregular in shape as the result of *injury*, such as rupture of the sphincter and tearing of the root of the iris from its ciliary attachment (*iridodialysis*); or dislocation of the lens; or of partial adherence to an old perforated corneal ulcer. A concussion injury may cause a dilatation of the pupil, regular or irregular, with or without associated loss of reflex movement; rarely a traumatic miosis is seen. Irregularity of shape after injury may give an important clue as to whether perforation of the globe has occurred, since incarceration of the iris in a corneal wound necessarily causes distortion of the pupil.

The circular shape of the pupil is lost in *coloboma*, either congenital or operative. The conditions are differentiated by the fact that in the former the normal pigmented margin extends along the pillars of the coloboma, while in the latter it does not.

2. Irregularities in Movement and Size. Before considering the irregularities in the movement and size of the pupil it is desirable to remember that its normal size varies during life. In extreme infancy it is small. It becomes larger during young adult and middle life, and ultimately becomes small again in old age. It is also, as a general rule, smaller in hypermetropic and larger in myopic eyes.

There are also four main normal pupillary reflexes: (i) The light reflex; (ii) The near reflex; (iii) The reflex to sensory stimulation; (iv) Psychic reflexes. The reflexes to light and for near are both constrictive; the sensory and psychic reflexes are both dilatations, the dilatation being caused by either sudden sensory stimuli or some sudden emotion such as fright or terror.

The pathological variations in the pupil may be classified as follows:

a. LOSS OF THE PUPILLARY LIGHT REFLEX, either with or without constriction of the pupil, but with persistence of the reaction to accommodation, constitutes the Argyll Robertson pupil. It is observed most frequently in *tabes dorsalis*, to an extent varying from 70 to 90 per cent of all the cases. The condition is usually permanent. It also occurs in *general paralysis of the insane*, in which there is also liability to pupil inequality. The pupil is constricted in nearly all tabetic cases, and the affection is most commonly bilateral. The Argyll Robertson pupil may also occur in epidemic encephalitis, in certain cerebral tumours, and in disseminated sclerosis, though in the last disease, as in encephalitis, the pupil affections are very variable and are never a reliable guide.

b. IN ANY CONDITION IN WHICH THERE IS A LESION OF THE OPTIC NERVE on one side, between the chiasma and the globe, there may be, as a result, a loss of direct light reflex in that eye, and of the consensual light reflex in the opposite eye.

c. LOSS OF SENSORY OR PSYCHIC REFLEX results from lesions of the dilator pupillary tract, such as *paralysis of the cervical sympathetic*, in which condition it is associated with ptosis, enophthalmos, and diminished tension of the globe. Such a condition may be seen in syringomyelia.

d. ABNORMAL CONSTRICTION OF A PUPIL, WITH RETENTION OF THE LIGHT AND CONVERGENCE REFLEXES (MIOSIS), may occur from abnormal stimuli of the sphincter, or paralysis of the dilator pupillae as the result of acute *encephalitis, syringomyelia, intracranial abscess*, or *growth* in which the lesion irritates but does not destroy the centre for constriction. In all cases of brain disease the constriction is ultimately replaced by dilatation.

e. ABNORMAL DILATATION OF THE PUPIL, WITH RETENTION OF THE LIGHT AND CONVERGENCE REFLEXES (MYDRIASIS), is met in cases of stimulation of the cervical sympathetic, for instance by an aortic *aneurysm*, or by a *mediastinal sarcoma* or *lymphosarcoma* or *Hodgkin's disease*, or by a *pulmonary carcinoma*, in the early stages when the growth has not destroyed and therefore paralysed the nerve. The diagnosis may be afforded by X-ray examination of the chest. It may also be observed in certain mental states, such as *acute mania* or *catalepsy*. In epileptic seizures the pupil is dilated, and in all except the mildest cases is inactive to light.

f. INEQUALITY IN THE SIZE OF THE PUPILS (ANISOCORIA) is observed frequently, and may have no pathological significance; but pronounced difference in the size of the pupils may be symptomatic of some organic lesion. In cases where the abnormal pupil is the smaller, the condition is usually due to hyperaemia of the iris, such as occurs in *iritis*; *paralysis of the cervical sympathetic*; or the use of a miotic drug such as *eserine* or *pilocarpine*. In cases where the abnormal pupil is the larger, the dilatation is usually due to *stimulation of the sympathetic*, the use of a mydriatic such as *atropine* or *homatropine*, *paralysis of the fibres of the 3rd nerve*, or increased ocular tension, such as may occur in *glaucoma*. In cases of marked inequality of the pupils one may suspect tabes, general paralysis of the insane, a unilateral lesion of the 3rd nerve or cervical sympathetic, trigeminal neuralgia, carotid or aortic aneurysm, a unilateral intracranial lesion, glaucoma, or Adie's syndrome. One needs to beware of overlooking an *artifiicial eye*.

P. Trevor-Roper.

PURPURA

Purpura signifies haemorrhage into the skin, and, according to the size of the extravasation of blood, the lesions are spoken of as petechiae or small patches, ecchymoses or bruises. The lesions cannot be obliterated by pressure with the finger, so distinguishing the effused blood from mere congestion. The diagnosis of the actual fact of purpura is seldom difficult; the persistence of the discoloration under pressure differentiates it from erythematous lesions, and the colour generally serves to distinguish it from pigmentation of the skin other than that due to haemorrhage. In a case of doubt the fact that the lesions presently alter in colour and then disappear serves to distinguish purpura from capillary naevi and from pigmentation of the skin, which persist. It may be more difficult, however, to decide what is the nature of the purpura in any given case; the following is a list of its better-recognized causes:

CAUSES OF PURPURA

A. Due to Vascular Damage (Symptomatic Purpuras):

LOCAL
    Blows
    Bug-bite

Flea-bite
Leech-bite
Pediculosis
Punctures by hypodermic needles
Rupture of a muscle
Rupture of a vein, especially a varicose vein
Sprains
(*See also* Senile Purpura)

GENERALIZED

1. *Associated with Drugs and Chemicals:*
   Antihistamines
   Arsenic
   Barbiturates★
   Belladonna
   Benzol
   Bismuth
   Chloral hydrate
   Chloramphenicol★
   Chlorothiazides★
   Corticosteroids
   Ergot
   Gold★
   Iodides
   Isonicotinic acid hydrazide (INH)
   Meprobamate★
   Mercury
   Oestrogens
   Penicillamine★
   Penicillins
   Phenacetin
   Phenylbutazone and oxyphenbutazone★
   Phosphorus
   Potassium chlorate
   Quinidine,★ quinine★
   Salicylates★
   Sedormid★ (Apronal)
   Streptomycin
   Sulphonamides★
   Sulphonyl ureas★
   Tetracyclines
   Thiouracils
   Toluene derivatives
   Troxidone★

★ May be associated with thrombocytopenia.

2. *Associated with Infections:*
   Bacterial endocarditis
   Blackwater fever
   Cerebrospinal fever (meningococcal)
   Cholera
   Dysentery
   Infectious mononucleosis
   Miliary tuberculosis
   Measles
   Plague
   Rubella
   Rocky Mountain spotted fever
   Kedani disease
   Scarlet fever
   Septicaemia
   Variola and varicella
   Typhoid fever
   Typhus
   Weil's disease, leptospirosis
   Yellow fever

3. *Associated with Metabolic Conditions:*
   Amyloidosis
   Chronic liver disease
   Collagen diseases—S.L.E., polyarteritis nodosa
   Cushing's syndrome
   Dysproteinaemias—cryo- and macroglobulin-
       aemias

4. *Associated with Allergic States (Anaphylactoid Purpura):*
   Purpura simplex
   Henoch-Schönlein purpura

5. *Associated with Vitamin-C Deficiency:*
   Scurvy

6. *Associated with Mechanical Factors:*
   Convulsions
   Orthostatic purpura
   Suffocation
   Whooping-cough

7. *Senile Purpura.*

8. *Von Willebrand's Disease.*

B. Due to Platelet Deficiency:
   1. *Primary Thrombocytopenia:*
      Congenital thrombocytopenia
      Idiopathic thrombocytopenic purpura (ITP)
   2. *Secondary Thrombocytopenia:*
      Blood transfusion
      Bone-marrow failure: aplastic anaemia
      Disseminated lupus erythematosus
      Drug-induced thrombocytopenia (marked★ in
          A. 1)
      Hypersplenism
      Megaloblastic anaemias
      Septicaemia
      Thrombotic thrombocytopenia

C. Due to Coagulation Disorders:
   Circulating anticoagulants
   Factor VIII
   Factor IX
   Fibrinogen deficiency (defibrination)
   Prothrombin factors (II, V, VII, X)

D. Due to Platelet Abnormalities:
   Thrombasthenia
   Thrombocythaemia

The coagulation of blood is mainly dependent on the formation of an active complex 'thromboplastin' according to the scheme in *Fig.* 677. 'Thromboplastin' may thus be formed by two different mechanisms. One is relatively slow and depends on the activation of factor XII by contact with abnormal surfaces, after which a sequential activation of subsequent factors occurs and results in the formation of 'thromboplastin'. The other system occurs much more rapidly; activation is initiated by the release of tissue factors after damage, which also leads to the formation of 'thromboplastin'. Certain steps are common to both processes and the various factors involved are summarized in the Table (p. 672) as is the consequence of any deficiency of each factor, and the tests upon which a diagnosis of the deficiency depends.

An estimation of the bleeding- and clotting-times is of importance in patients suspected of haemorrhagic diatheses. For the bleeding-time it is necessary to make certain that the hand or ear is warm; and in cold weather it is better to immerse the finger for a few minutes in hot water. The finger or ear is then pricked in the usual way and a drop of blood is removed every half-minute with a piece of blotting paper without touching the skin until the bleeding has stopped. The normal bleeding-time is generally between 2 and 5 minutes. In conditions in which the platelets are much reduced or in which the capillaries are abnormal the bleeding-time may be grossly lengthened. The clotting-time is very sensitive to changes in temperature and should

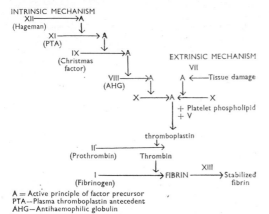

A = Active principle of factor precursor
PTA—Plasma thromboplastin antecedent
AHG—Antihaemophilic globulin

Fig. 677. Coagulation system.

therefore be determined by one of the methods by which the temperature of the blood can be controlled by a water-bath, such as that of Dale and Laidlaw or Lee and White. Lee and White's method is the more reliable as, with it, the clotting-time of the patient's blood is compared with that of a control sample; the normal value is between 5 and 11 minutes at 37° C.

If the clotting-time of a patient's blood approaches twice as long as that of the control, it may be regarded as significantly prolonged. In some cases of haemophilia it may be many times as long as that of the control. The commonest causes of a definitely prolonged clotting-time are haemophilia and Christmas disease, in which antihaemophilic globulin (VIII) and Christmas factor (IX) respectively are missing from the blood. These are two of the factors in normal blood which are necessary for the formation of an active 'thromboplastin'. A rare cause of extreme prolongation of the clotting-time is a gross deficiency or even absence of fibrinogen. In patients receiving heparin for the treatment of thrombosis the clotting-time is increased and the test can serve to control the efficiency of the treatment. The whole blood clotting-time is a crude test and is frequently normal in mild disorders of blood coagulation. A more sensitive but more elaborate test is the partial thromboplastin time in which the clotting-time of blood is measured at 37° C. after the addition of kaolin, which provides a maximum contact factor, and cephalin, which provides a maximum platelet factor. By this means two variables in the clotting-time are made constant and the average clotting-time is reduced to about 60 seconds. The partial thromboplastin-time is quite a sensitive test and is abnormal in most coagulation disorders.

In some patients a haemorrhagic tendency may exist but the bleeding- and clotting-times are

normal. In these cases the abnormality in the coagulation mechanism may be a deficiency of one or more of the three clotting factors—prothrombin, factor VII, and factor V. Such conditions include haemorrhagic disease of the newborn, the haemorrhagic tendency in long-standing obstructive jaundice, and treatment of a patient with dicoumarin derivatives for thrombosis. In these the ordinary clotting-time, as described above, will not be appreciably increased until the haemorrhagic tendency has advanced to a dangerous degree, and it is necessary to estimate the so-called 'prothrombin-time' for the coagulation abnormality to be detected. This method is actually a determination of the clotting-time of the plasma after the addition to it of a fully active 'thromboplastin' and calcium. It therefore gives a normal figure in haemophilia and in Christmas disease, but is prolonged when prothrombin, factor VII, or factor V is deficient, and also in afibrinogenaemia. The method is particularly useful in the control of therapy with dicoumarin derivatives. It must be remembered that the clotting-time is increased in heparinized patients. If, during the first few days of oral anticoagulant therapy the patient is also receiving heparin, the blood for the test must not be collected until the ordinary clotting-time has returned to normal, which will mean waiting for 4–6 hours after the previous dose of heparin.

Other more sophisticated tests may be required for the specific identification of a missing coagulation factor. Specific assays for factors VIII and IX can be made, and as a screening test the thromboplastin generation test is useful. By intermixing the three components, serum, aluminium-hydroxide-treated plasma, and platelets, from a normal person and from the patient it is possible to find in which fraction the defect lies; for example, serum contains factors IX and X whilst aluminium-hydroxide-absorbed plasma contains factors VIII and V, and a lengthening of the clotting using the patient's serum or plasma indicates which factors are likely to be deficient. Factors X and V also prolong the one-stage prothrombin-time whilst factors VIII and IX do not.

Owing to the many technical difficulties it is essential that the determination and interpretation of clotting-times be left to experienced hands.

The Table on the next page identifies the specific factors with their clinical disorders and appropriate diagnostic tests.

Little is known about the mechanism of many forms of purpura. The view that the conditions listed under A are due to increased permeability of the capillary wall is little more than a working hypothesis. With regard to the conditions listed under B (1) and (2) we are on somewhat surer ground. In the first group we can say definitely that the purpura is associated with a marked reduction in the number of platelets (usually less than 100,000 per c.mm.), and that the severity of the purpura is roughly paralleled by the extent of their reduction. In the second group, bleeding in obstructive jaundice, the new-born, and in dicoumarol therapy is definitely the result of a deficiency in prothrombin factors; bleeding in haemophilia is due to a deficiency of factor VIII; while bleeding in heparin therapy is due to an excess of that substance interfering with the normal action of thromboplastin.

It will be noticed that many drugs produce purpura in one of two ways, either by damaging the vascular endothelium or by producing thrombocytopenia. With some drugs the thrombocytopenia is the result of marrow aplasia whilst in

The haemorrhage around a *leech-bite*, with its triangular central puncture, is characteristic. Scratching may produce petechiae which are linearly distributed.

Blows and *sprains*, if sufficiently severe, produce purpura even in the healthy, in whom the history gives the diagnosis; some normal individuals bruise with such ease that there may be no clear evidence of injury unless careful inquiry is made, when some trivial stumble or knock may be recalled to mind by the patient. Such easy bruising may also occur in any of the blood

Factor	Clinical Effects	Detection
XIII Fibrin stabilizing factor	Very rare. Mild bleeding	Poor clot. Soluble in 5 M urea
XII Hageman factor	No clinical disorder	Lack of contact activation
XI Plasma thromboplastin antecedent	Mild bleeding. Familial	PTT+ PT± TGT-plasma and serum+
X Stuart Prower factor	Severe bleeding. Familial	PTT+ PT+ (corrected by normal serum) TGT-serum+
IX Christmas factor	Mild/severe bleeding. Familial	PTT+ PT± TGT-serum+ Specific assay
VIII Antihaemophilic globulin	Mild/severe bleeding. X-linked. Familial	PTT+ PT± TGT-plasma+ Specific assay
VII	Mild/severe bleeding. Familial/acquired	PTT± PT+ TGT-plasma and serum+
V	Mild/severe bleeding. Familial/acquired	PTT+ PT+ TGT-plasma+
II Prothrombin	Mild/severe bleeding. Familial/acquired	PTT+ PT+ TGT-plasma and serum+
I Fibrinogen	Mild/severe bleeding. Familial/acquired	No clot with thrombin
Inhibitors/anticoagulants	Mild/severe bleeding. Acquired	PTT+ PT+ (not corrected by normal plasma) TGT+ or ± (plasma and serum) May have heparin-like activity or factor specificity

PTT = Partial thromboplastin-time. PT = Prothrombin-time. TGT = Thromboplastin generation-time.
+ = Prolonged. ± = Marginal change.

others it is the result of the production of a platelet antibody and increased destruction of platelets in the circulation. In some conditions, such as Von Willebrand's disease, hereditary haemorrhagic thrombasthenia, and thrombocythaemia, the cause of the purpura is complex. Increased capillary fragility may exist with a factor-VIII deficiency as in Von Willebrand's disease, or there may be a failure of platelet agglutination as in hereditary haemorrhagic thrombasthenia.

A. Vascular Damage due to Local Injury. *Flea-bites* are a common cause of purpura and they may sometimes be so numerous as to raise a misleading suspicion that the patient is suffering from some serious disease. The relatively small haemorrhagic foci, and their prevalence on the parts covered by the clothes rather than upon the hands, face, or exposed parts of the legs, serve to indicate the diagnosis; a magnifying glass reveals the central puncture of the bite.

Bug-bites will also be suggested by the central puncture; in susceptible individuals the purpuric areas may be as large as 10 mm., or larger.

diseases. A case of *epilepsy* may sometimes come under observation for multiple bruises simulating some other kind of purpura, but due to injuries produced during the attacks, which may themselves be unsuspected if they occur during the night. Very extensive purpura on the legs or other parts has sometimes been produced by multiple self-injury in girls suffering from *hysteria*, or by *malingerers*; serious organic disease may be feared unless other factors in the case or the distribution of the purpura suggest an artificial origin; the haemorrhagic spots and blotches may be abundant on the fronts and sides of the legs, for instance, and not down the backs of them; organic purpura seldom has so selective a distribution.

Spontaneous *rupture of a muscle* leads to extensive purpuric extravasation of blood, but the diagnosis is not difficult if the history is clear. The *purpuric discoloration of the skin around varicose veins* in the legs, together with its resultant dark-brown pigmentation, is familiar.

B. Generalized Capillary Damage

1. DRUGS AND POISONS. As regards *drugs*, the list above indicates that there are many which may sometimes produce purpura; but none does so commonly. The possibility should be borne

So characteristic is the purpura in some cases that the malady has earned the title of spotted fever, which sometimes occurs in epidemic form. The diagnosis may be clinched by bacteriological examination of the cerebrospinal fluid.

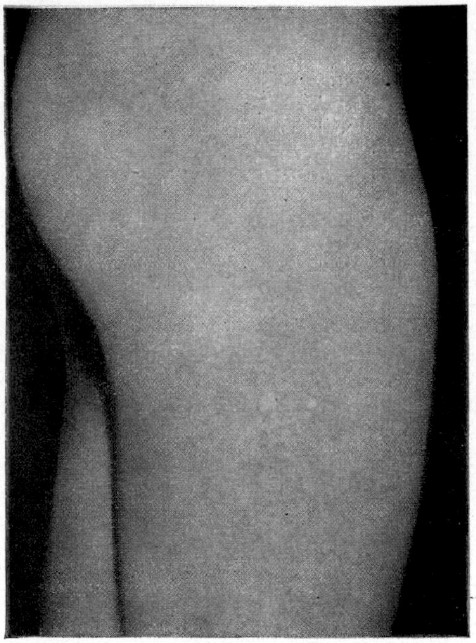

Fig. 678. Purpuric rash on thigh.

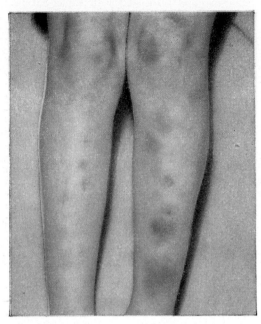

Fig. 679. Purpura and ecchymoses of unknown origin.
(*Dr. Philip Evans.*)

in mind, and inquiry made as to the remedies the patient may have been taking. Individual susceptibility is undoubtedly an important factor, for whereas most of these drugs can be given with impunity in normal doses to the majority of patients, a comparatively small dose may produce purpura in others. Prolonged treatment with corticosteroids is a common cause of purpura. Most drug purpuras are due to sensitization and are thus allergic in nature. The patient may be taking the drug for months before sensitization causes purpura. It will then occur after every dose.

2. INFECTIONS. In the majority of *acute fevers* the occurrence of purpura is of prognostic rather than of diagnostic value. The two fevers in which purpura is of essentially diagnostic value are *typhus* and *cerebrospinal fever*. The former is now very rare in Great Britain, but when it was common and typhoid fever began to be differentiated from it, the point upon which greatest stress was laid was that in true typhus fever there is always more or less purpura, whereas in typhoid fever all the red spots fade upon pressure; if flea-bites are excluded, purpuric spots are rare in typhoid fever. Cerebrospinal fever presents many characters that are common to it and to other forms of acute meningitis; but a purpuric eruption differentiates it from the others, though the absence of purpura does not exclude the disease.

Smallpox may present cutaneous haemorrhages of three different kinds; there may be haemorrhage *into the pustules* in a late stage, *between the pustules*, vesicles, or papules; and there may be a haemorrhagic eruption either all over the body or in the bathing-drawers region in the *prodromal* stage of the disease. Purpura may also occur in severe chicken-pox.

Almost any condition in which there are pyogenic micro-organisms or their toxins circulating in the blood-stream may be associated with extensive purpura, and this applies to *pyaemia* and *septicaemia* in general. The purpura may be very severe, when it is known as 'purpura fulminans', and it may be associated with extensive peripheral intravascular clotting, defibrination, and platelet consumption with gangrene of the peripheral tissues. This syndrome which resembles the Schwartzmann reaction is often associated with hypotension and vascular collapse. The diagnosis will be confirmed best by obtaining cultures from the blood. *Bacterial endocarditis* is a variety of pyaemia or septicaemia. Seeing that it is rare to get purpura in association with ordinary chronic valvular disease of the heart, the occurrence of purpura in a heart case (*Figs.* 678, 679) may be one of the earlier symptoms indicating that bacterial endocarditis has supervened. The purpura in acute bacterial endocarditis may have a similar mechanism to that in

22

septicaemia, but in subacute bacterial endocarditis the purpura is usually the result of minute peripheral emboli giving the typical splinter haemorrhages in the finger-nails, the conjunctival haemorrhages, and minute petechiae in the skin. Osler's nodes may be associated with some purpuric staining.

The remainder of the fevers mentioned above are diagnosed, not from the purpura, but from the other symptoms, from the general circumstances, and from the geographical incidence of each. *Rocky Mountain spotted fever* is due to infection from the bites of ticks, *Dermacentor andersoni seu venustus*, a similar disease being met with in the Himalaya mountains and probably in other regions, but not in England; *kedani disease* or *Japanese river fever* is caused by a mite (*Trombicula pseudoakamushi*) analogous to the harvest-mite of England; the illness has a high mortality, is associated with pyrexia lasting an average of about two weeks, and is characterized by the development of multiple small haemorrhages appearing on the face at the end of the first week, spreading thence to the trunk, and sometimes to the extremities—a generalized purpura.

3. METABOLIC CONDITIONS. In the late stages of renal failure, when the blood-urea is greatly raised, extensive purpura with large ecchymoses may occur. Though this usually happens in a patient who is known to be suffering from chronic nephritis, it may occasionally be the first indication of the presence of advanced renal disease. In such cases examination of urine and blood will settle the diagnosis.

The cause of the purpura in chronic renal failure is unknown. Deficiencies of prothrombin factors may arise in cirrhosis of the liver, especially from chronic alcoholism, and are also a feature of the malabsorption syndromes. Purpura may also be seen in Cushing's syndrome as a result of the atrophy of the elastic supporting structures of the capillaries in the skin, and is frequently seen in the collagen diseases such as systemic lupus erythematosus, when many factors may operate to produce purpura. In certain rare disorders of protein production, especially if the protein is a macroglobulin or cryoglobulin, purpura may be an important feature, but then it is sometimes found only around the peripheral aspects of the retina.

4. ALLERGIC CONDITIONS. These forms of purpura are usually known as 'anaphylactoid'. It seems probable that they are all the result of capillary damage produced by some protein to which the patient has become sensitized. The responsible protein may be introduced via the patient's diet or by injection, or it may be bacterial. When a person takes food, such as shell-fish, to which he is sensitive he is more likely to develop an urticarial rash or oedema, but occasionally a typical purpuric rash may result, frequently arising in the urticarial weals. The same is true of the serum rash which may occur nine to ten days following the injection of antidiphtheritic or other sera. When the offending protein is bacterial it is usually the streptococcus that is to blame. Often a sore throat precedes the attack of purpura. The mildest cases, in which the manifestations are limited to the appearance of numbers of fine purpuric spots, are classed as *purpura simplex*. This and the two following types of purpura are commonly associated with urticaria and other allergic symptoms.

Schönlein's purpura (*purpura rheumatica*) was formerly regarded as related to acute rheumatism; but it is rare for a patient affected by it to present unmistakable valvular heart disease, though there may be a local systolic bruit at the impulse. In addition to the extensive purpura, which appears in successive crops and may affect any part of the body, though it is commoner upon the lower limbs than elsewhere, there is considerable pain, redness, and swelling of many joints, which may become affected successively; the temperature rises during an attack to 39 or 40° C., the throat generally being sore at the same time. The swelling of the joints is usually due to a simple effusion and not to a haemarthrosis.

The diagnosis is not difficult when the purpura, the joint pains, and the pyrexia are present together. The disease is little influenced by sodium salicylate; it may be associated with more or less erythema as well as purpura; the malady affects young persons, especially between the ages of 10 and 30, of either sex; the prognosis is good.

Henoch's purpura is met with chiefly in children; the patient may suffer from recurrent attacks. In addition to haemorrhages beneath the skin there is generally some tendency to joint pains not unlike those of Schönlein's purpura, but in addition to this the child is seized with more or less acute abdominal symptoms, varying from simple vomiting and stomach-ache to severe prostration with agonizing cramp-like attacks of colic, some of which may be followed by the passage of blood and mucus per rectum to such an extent as to simulate acute intussusception; the abdominal attacks are the result of submucous intestinal haemorrhages. There is every degree of the affection, from mild to very severe, but the association of the purpura with the abdominal attacks in childhood suggests the diagnosis at once, especially if there has been a similar attack previously. Occasionally changes may be found in the urine, proteinuria and haematuria occurring. When this happens it is difficult to distinguish the condition from acute nephritis, but the association of anaphylactoid purpura and evidence of renal damage is usually regarded as having a more serious outlook than if the purpura occurs without urinary changes.

Although Schönlein's and Henoch's purpura have been differentiated as separate entities, it is common to find symptoms of one or more types of purpura overlapping in any particular individual.

5. VITAMIN-C DEFICIENCY. *Scurvy* in an adult is rare, but is sometimes met with in those who have been obliged by poverty to live upon a diet containing no fresh vegetables, in which case

typical scurvy may develop, with the spongy heaping up of the gums both inside and outside the teeth, and with the knotty haemorrhagic swellings in the muscles of the calves, as well as purpura. Children fed on patent foods without sufficient fresh milk or vegetable food or fresh meat not infrequently develop a milder form of scurvy, with marked tenderness of the periosteum of the long bones, pasty pallor, mouth bleeding from spongy gums, and possibly purpura; this is *infantile scurvy*, or *Barlow's disease*, which should not be confused, as it is apt to be, with rickets, though it has been called scurvy rickets. The diagnosis of scurvy can usually be made by an estimation of ascorbic acid saturation or of the concentration of ascorbic acid in white cells.

6. MECHANICAL FACTORS. Purpuric spots or large extravasations of blood may occur in *convulsions*, in *epileptic fits*, in the coughing spasms of *whooping-cough*, or in partial *suffocation* or *strangulation*. Orthostatic purpura occurs in the lower limbs of some people as a result of prolonged standing; this is presumably due to the increased hydrostatic pressure associated with an exceptional weakness of the capillaries.

Petechiae may appear as a result of wearing certain types of clothing to which the individual may show skin sensitivity.

7. SENILE PURPURA is probably the commonest of all purpuras. It is seen usually on the dorsum of the hands in conjunction with the atrophic skin and reduced subcutaneous fat of the aged. Slight leakage from capillaries unsupported by connective tissue can spread freely and give rise to quite large bruises. Probably minor traumata initiate this form of purpura.

C. Due to a Haematological Abnormality

1. PLATELET DEFICIENCY. This is the commonest haematological abnormality causing purpura but bleeding is not usually seen until the platelet count has fallen below about 100,000 per c.mm. The normal range of platelet count varies between 200,000 and 500,000 per c.mm. In idiopathic thrombocytopenic purpura (ITP) (*essential thrombocytopenic purpura*, *Werlhof's disease* or *purpura haemorrhagica*) the deficiency in platelets is the primary abnormality, the white cells usually being normal and the red cells altered only in so far as there is anaemia from the blood-loss due to the purpura. Occasionally a haemolytic anaemia with a positive antiglobulin test may occur. The disease may be acute or chronic. In the chronic type the symptoms usually first appear in childhood or adolescence, though they are sometimes delayed until later in life. It then either runs a continuous but fluctuating course or takes the form of attacks, which may be mild or severe and separated by symptomless intervals of months or even years. The fluctuations or attacks follow closely the variations in the number of platelets in the blood, purpura only appearing if they fall below the critical level of about 100,000 per c.mm. If the platelets fall very much below this figure there may occur in addition to the simple

purpuric rash a general oozing of blood from one or more of the mucous surfaces, particularly of the mouth, nose, and bowel, and less commonly of the urinary passages—purpura haemorrhagica. An exacerbation or an attack may prove fatal or merely give rise to a mild degree of anaemia. Some patients may be perfectly fit between attacks, others may be more or less permanently incapacitated.

In the acute type an attack starts suddenly, usually with fever, in a previously healthy individual: sometimes it is fatal, sometimes it clears up completely in a few days; sometimes it passes over into the chronic type of the disease. The diagnosis depends on finding a significant reduction in the platelets, and on being able to exclude the various other diseases listed above under (7) which may give rise to a *secondary* thrombocytopenic purpura. The spleen may be palpable in either the acute or chronic type of purpura but this is not commonly so.

Thrombotic thrombocytopenic purpura is a very rare and fatal disease of unknown aetiology in which thrombocytopenia is associated with a severe anaemia (probably haemolytic in type), transient focal neurological lesions, and fever. This condition is probably mainly due to an inflammatory change in the small peripheral vessels where a primary coagulation process ensues consuming platelets and fibrinogen, which is frequently found to be deficient in the plasma. The resulting fibrin strands in the small vessels probably result in red-cell fragmentation and haemolysis.

The other conditions listed under this heading are either associated with some specific blood disease or produced by a definite poison. In the former case the blood-picture will practically always point to the presence of some general disorder of the haemopoietic system even though it may not indicate the precise nature of that disorder. The majority of drugs which produce thrombocytopenia as a result of bone-marrow failure often have an effect on the red cells or the white cells or both, and though the effect may not always be sufficient to produce the clinical signs of an anaemia or of an agranulocytosis, it will usually be obvious from the blood-picture. The most important drugs of this type are the *organic arsenicals*, *gold*, *benzene*, and much more rarely the *sulphonamides*. There are, however, certain drugs—*apronal (Sedormid)*, *quinidine*, *quinine*, *phenobarbitone*, *carbromal*, *bromvaletone*—which are peculiar in having in susceptible individuals a completely selective effect on the platelets. This effect is often due to an increased destruction of platelets in the peripheral circulation as a result of the production of a platelet antibody brought about by the particular drug. The blood-picture they produce shows only a gross reduction in platelets, unless the severe bleeding has produced a superimposed haemorrhagic anaemia. The picture is thus identical with that of essential thrombocytopenic purpura, while clinically the two conditions are essentially similar. In adults the possibility of drug poisoning should always be considered even though the history is negative, for it often may be so in the case of drug addicts.

If a drug is to blame, then after stopping the drug the symptoms may disappear and the platelet count rise to normal levels within a week or so.

In the treatment of thrombocytopenia with severe bleeding, fresh blood transfusion and even the administration of concentrated platelets may be required to control haemorrhage. In the absence of any severe bleeding and any obvious cause for the thrombocytopenia, steroids may produce a remission of the thrombocytopenia in a week or two. If they fail, or the patient relapses after they are stopped, splenectomy should be considered. In thrombocytopenic purpura, whether essential or secondary, and with increased capillary fragility, the bleeding-time is prolonged to a greater or less degree, while the clotting-time, partial thromboplastin-time, and prothrombin-time remain normal. Bone-marrow examination is helpful. In ITP there are usually increased numbers of megakaryocytes, often of juvenile form; they are usually present in excess in other forms of immune thrombocytopenia due to drugs. In marrow depression, on the other hand, megakaryocytes are scanty or entirely lacking.

2. CLOTTING ABNORMALITY. *Haemophilia* (factor VIII deficiency) and *Christmas disease* (factor IX deficiency) occur almost invariably in males and are usually manifested in early childhood. The diseases are sex-linked and are transmitted through the female, so that one should look for other cases occurring in the family among the patient's brothers, his maternal uncles, his maternal grandfather, and great-uncles. The female carrier of haemophilia never shows any evidence of the disease, but in Christmas disease some female carriers show slight deficiency of factor IX and are mildly affected. Both diseases are characterized by excessive bleeding from cuts, bleeding into joints, and subcutaneous, submucous, and intramuscular haemorrhages, following comparatively slight trauma. Spontaneous purpura is not common. If the intra-articular haemorrhages, which are specially liable to occur when a child begins to crawl, are frequently repeated, serious permanent changes take place in the joints. The clotting-time is prolonged, sometimes greatly so, as also is the partial thromboplastin-time, but the bleeding-time and prothrombin-time are normal. Both the clotting-time increase and the tendency to bleed may undergo variations from time to time.

In *obstructive jaundice, haemorrhagic disease of the newborn, the malabsorption syndromes*, and in overdosage with *dicoumarol-type drugs* the underlying defect is a deficiency of prothrombin factors with a resulting increase in the prothrombin-time. Vitamin K is present in the diet and is normally absorbed from the intestine and built up into 'prothrombin' in the liver. As it is a fat-soluble vitamin any disorder which leads to a defect in fat absorption may result in deficiency of this vitamin. Usually obstructive jaundice must persist for several weeks before deficiency occurs, and it is important to appreciate that a patient with obstructive jaundice, who has as yet shown no signs of spontaneous bleeding, may well bleed if operative interference is resorted to. In all such cases the prothrombin-time must be determined, and if this is increased, injections of vitamin K must be given and the operation postponed until the prothrombin-time is normal. In the presence of these conditions severe deficiencies may occur and a haemorrhagic state set in. The deficiencies can usually be remedied by the injection of vitamin K. In severe liver disease, however, they are not usually reversible.

Haemorrhagic disease of the newborn appears two to three days after birth, with spontaneous bleeding into the skin or various internal organs or from the umbilical cord, vagina, alimentary canal, or renal tract. If the true nature of the condition is suspected in time, the cessation of bleeding which may occur within a few hours of injecting vitamin K or its synthetic substitutes will substantiate the diagnosis.

The blood-prothrombin as well as other clotting factors are purposely reduced in the treatment of postoperative and other forms of thrombosis with dicoumarin or its derivatives. The treatment has to be carefully controlled by daily estimations of prothrombin-times. The first signs of a haemorrhagic state are usually a few red cells in the urine, slight oozing from the site of venepuncture or, if there has been an operation, from the operation site, a mild epistaxis, or a few purpuric spots. These are not necessarily of serious import, but should the prothrombin-time increase much further, extensive purpura and generalized bleeding may endanger the patient's life or even prove fatal. A prothrombin ratio in excess of three should be regarded as a danger signal. The bleeding that occurs as a result of excessive anticoagulant therapy with these drugs can usually be reversed within 6 hours by injection of vitamin K_1 intravenously, but if large doses are used, there may be some difficulty in restarting anticoagulant therapy subsequently.

In all these conditions in which the prothrombin-time is increased the ordinary clotting-time is sometimes also prolonged. Unfortunately this latter determination, which is so much the easier one to carry out, does not provide a sufficiently delicate index of the degree of altered coagulability of the blood.

The treatment of thromboses with *heparin* may lead to a haemorrhagic condition essentially similar to that produced by dicoumarol. Heparin, however, has no constant effect on the prothrombin-time, and its dosage is regulated by determinations of the ordinary clotting-time. If dangerous haemorrhage occurs with heparin, the drug can readily be neutralized by the intravenous injection of protamine sulphate, or if that is not available by *fresh* blood transfusions. Very rarely a haemorrhagic diathesis has been found to be due to a congenital deficiency of one or other of the three clotting factors, prothrombin, factor V, and factor VII. In all three conditions there is a prolonged prothrombin-time.

Fibrinogen deficiency may result from the activation of the normal fibrinolytic mechanism in the blood (*Fig.* 680) or as the result of the consumption of fibrinogen by diffuse intravascular

Tissue products
Plasma urokinase   Fibrin
Bacterial kinases

Plasminogen——→ Plasmin ————————→ |
                                    ↓
                          Fibrin degradation
                          products
                          (FDPs)

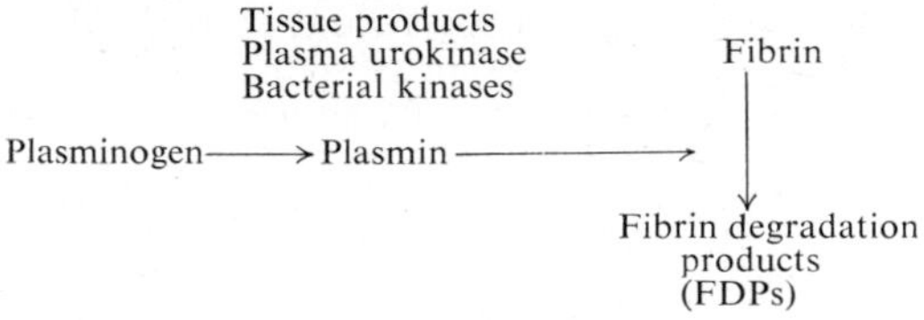

Fig. 680. Defibrination system.

coagulation. Both these processes may complicate various diseases and result in a haemorrhagic state, 'the defibrination syndrome'. Fibrinolysis may complicate prostatectomy, severe trauma, and burns, also incompatible blood transfusions, whereas defibrination from diffuse intravascular coagulation may complicate septicaemia, malignant disease when it may be a chronic process, and premature separation of the placenta and septic abortion. The distinction between these two processes is not sharp and either may complicate any of these conditions. Laboratory tests reveal a prolonged partial thromboplastin-time with deficiency of fibrinogen and, in the case of consumption coagulopathy, a decreased platelet count and the presence of fragmented red cells in the peripheral blood. In the case of pure fibrinolysis, a platelet count is usually normal and degradation products of fibrinogen (FDP) are found in the plasma. In addition *in vitro* fibrinolysis can be demonstrated by clot-lysis. Fibrinogen infusions and amino-caproic acid may be used in the treatment of the condition if it is essentially fibrinolytic, whereas heparin has been used with success when the process has been mainly one of intravascular coagulation. Rarely, a haemorrhagic disease may be due to the development of a circulating anticoagulant. These inhibitors occasionally complicate pregnancy, malignant disease, and collagen disorders and occasionally arise without cause. Their presence can be demonstrated by showing a prolongation of the clotting-time of normal blood when the patient's plasma has been added to it.

Von Willebrand's disease is inherited as an autosomal dominant and resembles mild haemophilia in its clinical course. However, it can be diagnosed by the presence of a prolonged bleeding-time associated with a mild deficiency of factor VIII. Frequently increased capillary fragility can be demonstrated by the Hess test. Excessive bleeding can often be controlled by the use of factor VIII substitutes.

3. PLATELET ABNORMALITY. *Hereditary Haemorrhagic Thrombasthenia* is a rare familial disease occurring in either sex and characterized by spontaneous bleeding, most often from the alimentary tract and nose, and sometimes, though rarely, by purpura. The platelets are normal in numbers but show defective agglutination; coagulation tests are normal but the bleeding-time is prolonged.

T. A. J. Prankerd.

PUSTULES

A pustule is an elevation of the skin containing pus, differing from a vesicle or bulla only in its contents. It may be unilocular or multilocular and usually starts as a papule, vesicle, or bulla. It may develop so rapidly that its origin cannot be observed. A pustule may arise in any of the skin layers or in the subcutaneous tissues and it may also start in a follicle. In colour pustules are usually yellow, but they may be grey or brown, the latter when blood is present as well as pus.

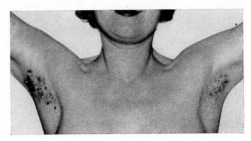

Fig. 681. Hidradenitis suppurativa. (*Dr. Peter Hansell.*)

Pustules are mostly the result of staphylococcal infection, and various forms of staphylococcal folliculitis are common. In these disorders the organism may be introduced from the outside, especially by friction, but it may also be blood-borne from a distant latent focus. Probably local lowered resistance to the ubiquitous staphylococcus is the commonest origin.

A *boil* (furuncle) is an acute staphylococcal infection of a follicle in the skin; on the scalp it starts in a hair follicle, and on the eyelid, where it is known as a *stye* (hordeolum), in the follicle of an eyelash. The resulting inflammation is very acute, and after the formation of a hard painful papule necrosis rapidly sets in in the centre and a pustule is formed. There may be intense local reaction around the lesion, which ultimately becomes boggy, fluctuates, ruptures, and discharges pus. In many cases a hard central 'core' of necrotic material is extruded before healing takes place. The neck, buttocks, and face are the commonest situations for boil formation. Occasionally the contents of the pustule are absorbed before rupture occurs and the lesion regresses. This is known as a blind boil. After poulticing a boil a ring of small satellite boils may form around the original lesion. In the axillae and groins especially the apocrine sweat-glands may become infected and this produces an intractable condition known as hidradenitis suppurativa (*Fig.* 681).

A *carbuncle* resembles a boil, but the infection spreads to the deeper tissues and when rupture occurs there may be several openings in the skin. Boils may follow one another in series for many months, when the condition is known as *chronic furunculosis*.

A superficial *multiple staphylococcal folliculitis* of the skin is known as follicular or Bockhart's impetigo. It affects the thighs and forearms, especially when they are hairy, but it may occur anywhere on the body. The lesions are groups of yellow pustules. Friction is the main cause and it may occur in certain dirty trades, particularly in workers whose skin is in contact with oil-soaked clothing (oil acne).

Small pustules occurring in the scalp around the bases of hairs either in groups or scattered are known as *acne necrotica*. These may terminate as minute ulcers which heal rapidly.

Sycosis barbae is staphylococcal folliculitis of the hairy parts of the face, including the eyebrows. It differs in no way from the other forms of staphylococcal folliculitis; it may be localized to small areas or it may affect the whole of the face and neck. The pustules are grouped on a bright erythematous base and in the centre of each pustule there is a hair which pulls out easily. It must be distinguished from the more common seborrhoeic sycosis in which the predominating lesions are red diffuse papules with little or no pustule formation. In all forms of staphylococcal folliculitis the diagnosis is fairly simple. Other organisms, e.g., streptococcus and *Pseudomonas aeruginosa*, sometimes produce similar lesions.

In acne the pustule is often a late stage in the development of individual lesions.

In *acrodermatitis perstans* numerous pustules appear under the skin of either the palms or soles, or both; these are usually sterile and the cause of the disease is obscure. It has been considered to be a bacterid. The disease runs a protracted and intractable course. An alternative name for this condition is *pustular psoriasis*. Probably about 25 per cent of cases are associated with psoriasis elsewhere on the body.

Groups of pustules in the webs of the fingers and on the wrists, with single lesions scattered about both hands, are sometimes a feature of neglected scabies.

Anthrax infection of the skin in its localized variety takes the form of a carbuncle-like inflammatory lesion caused by the *Bacillus anthracis*. It is contracted from cattle, their hides, or hairs, or rarely from shaving brushes. It affects an exposed area of the skin and the incubation period is from one to three days. The first sign is a small itching red macule not unlike a flea-bite. Within two days a papule forms which rapidly becomes a pustule; this soon ruptures and sometimes blood as well as pus is extruded. There results a gangrenous ulcer which in a simple case heals in a few weeks. In severe cases there may be grave constitutional symptoms, with septicaemia and death, and sometimes there

are multiple skin lesions. It must be distinguished from carbuncle and extragenital syphilitic chancre. Scrapings from the lesion contain the causal organism in large numbers. As anthrax is mostly an occupational disease in handlers of hides or wool ('wool-sorters' disease), the diagnosis is usually easy.

Glanders is a disease of horses, mules, and donkeys, which very rarely affects man and then only those in constant contact with these animals. The main lesion is an ulcerating pustule. It is not unlike a carbuncle in its early stages and occurs on the exposed areas of the skin. The general symptoms are those of septicaemia, and there is always a purulent nasal discharge. The presence of *Bacillus mallei* in this or in material from the ulcers or pustules is diagnostic. The disease is almost invariably fatal.

The pustule is an important manifestation of *smallpox*. After an incubation period of from eight to twelve days the disease begins with fever, headache, backache, and vomiting. On the third or fourth day there is macular erythema, and after a few hours shotty papules develop; these become vesicles and by the fifth day they pustulate. The rash is most profuse on the head and limbs and there is only one crop of lesions, which mature in order of their appearance. The vesicles are tough, firm, and often multilocular, and show definite umbilication. By the time the pustules have formed the umbilication is less well marked. In severe cases there may be confluence of the pustules, particularly on the face. The mucous membranes are usually involved as well. As a rule the temperature falls slightly with the eruption, but rises again when on the eighth or ninth day rupture of the pustules occurs. In the final stage the pustules dry up to form brown crusts. Pitting or scarring is the rule. Previous vaccination may modify the course of the disease considerably and there is a mild type of the disease known as *alastrim*.

Smallpox is distinguished from *chicken-pox* by the usually milder nature of the latter disease, which is vesicular rather than pustular, and by the fact that the rash is as a rule more profuse on the trunk than on the extremities. In chicken-pox the eruption comes out in successive crops and the vesicles are unilocular, fragile, and do not exhibit umbilication. In spite of these differences, mild smallpox and severe chicken-pox may be difficult to differentiate.

Other viral diseases causing pustules are vaccinia, cow-pox, and orf.

In the so-called *pustular syphilides* there are no true pustules, their resemblance to pustules being only superficial; on incision they will be found to be solid and to contain no pus.

P. D. Samman.

PYURIA

Pus appears in the urine in all suppurative conditions affecting the urinary tract, and occasionally from the rupture of an extra-urinary abscess into the urinary apparatus. It may be present in large or in microscopic quantities; when in bulk it forms a thick, greyish, tenacious sediment which must be distinguished from a deposit of phosphates or of urates; urates, though they may be colourless, are generally of a pinkish or even of a brick-red colour, and they clear up on warming the specimen to body temperature; phosphates clear up on the addition of acetic acid; pus, on the other hand, will remain unaltered by either of these tests.

In alkaline urine pus cells tend to run together into a dense viscid deposit, leaving the upper layers of the urine slightly turbid. Microscopically each pus cell is multinuclear, rounded, and about twice the size of a red blood-cell. The contents are granular, but the addition of acid clears the cell and makes the nucleus stand out distinctly. Urine containing pus always contains at least traces of albumin, and frequently epithelial cells from some part of the urinary tract. The best test for its presence is the microscopical examination of the centrifuged deposit in the urine.

The following is a classified list of the causes of pyuria:

I. From Diseases of the Urinary Organs:

1. RENAL:
   Pyelitis
   Pyelonephritis
   Renal abscess
   Renal papillary necrosis
   Pyonephrosis
   Tuberculosis
   Calculus
   Medullary sponge kidney.

2. URETERIC:
   Calculus
   Megaureter.

3. VESICAL:
   Cystitis
   Tuberculosis
   Calculus or foreign body
   Ulcer—simple, epitheliomatous
   Tumour—sloughing papillary or solid carcinoma
   Diverticula
   Bilharzia haematobia
   Trichomoniasis.

4. URETHRAL:
   Urethritis—gonorrhoeal, septic
   Stricture
   Calculus or foreign body.

5. PROSTATIC:
   Prostatitis, acute or chronic
   Prostatic abscess
   Calculus.

6. VESICULAR:
   Seminal vesiculitis, acute or chronic vesicular abscess.

II. From Diseases outside the Urinary Organs:

Leucorrhoea
Balanitis with phimosis

From the extension of inflammatory processes to the bladder, or the rupture into the bladder or urethra of an abscess such as:
   Prostatic abscess
   Appendicular abscess
   Iliac or pelvic abscess
   Abscess due to colonic diverticulitis
   Psoas abscess
   Pyosalpinx
   Carcinoma of the uterus, rectum, caecum, sigmoid, or pelvic colon
   Ulceration of the small intestine—tuberculous or dysenteric.

It is impossible to determine the lesion producing pus in the urine simply by the examination of the latter. Due consideration must be given to the history and the other symptoms of the individual case, and particular care be taken not to lay too much emphasis upon any symptom which may point to a vesical lesion when in reality the trouble is in the kidney. This is perhaps most likely to occur in a haematogenous infection of the kidney by micro-organisms, in which increased frequency of micturition is a marked symptom, while the bladder may remain free from disease. Occasionally, after pus has been present continuously in the urine for some time, it may disappear entirely, the change being accompanied by increase of pain in the side, by an elevation of temperature, or enlargement of the kidney in a case of pyonephrosis when the obstruction to the flow of urine from that side has become temporarily complete. Very little help is derived from the character of epithelial cells accompanying pus in the urine. The shapes of the cells of the renal pelvis, ureter, and deeper layers of the bladder are so much alike that it is usually impossible to differentiate them.

Some assistance in the determination of the origin of the pus in the urine may be gained by instrumental or radiological examination:

BY CATHETER. If a catheter is passed and the bladder washed out with clear solution of boric acid or normal saline, it will be found that the medium is soon rendered clear if the pyuria is of renal origin, but that it is much more difficult to obtain a perfectly clear medium if the bladder is the seat of the suppuration. If the medium is cleared quickly, but yet after some ten minutes' retention in the bladder it is again found to be turbid, the pus is almost certainly descending from the kidney.

THE CYSTOSCOPE. Much more certain evidence is gained by a careful cystoscopic examination. By this means it can be determined in the great majority of cases if the bladder is infected or if any ulceration is present. In a few cases the bladder may be so affected that only a small distension is possible, or bleeding is produced so easily that cystoscopy is rendered difficult; in these cases there will be little need for an inspection of the bladder. If the bladder is found to be normal, evidence of a suppurative lesion in the kidney may be obtained from the appearance of the ureteric orifices or by the variations in the character of the urinary efflux from them.

Instead of the normal forcible flow of clear urine from each orifice, mixing with the medium in the bladder in a characteristic swirl, urine containing pus may be seen emitted, appearing in the field as a small smoky puff from the orifice (*Fig.* 682); pieces of mucopus may be seen to pass

diseases in which the ureter is thickened, the whole ureteric orifice is drawn upwards and outwards from its normal situation (*Fig.* 684), and is seen at the apex of a conical retracted area in the bladder base. In cases of old-standing pyelitis the ureteric orifice of the affected side appears as a

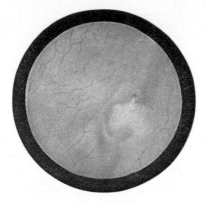

Fig. 682. Purulent urine issuing from the ureter.

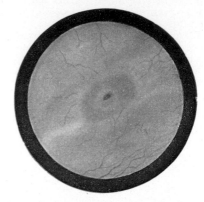

Fig. 683. Congestion around a ureteric orifice in calculous pyelitis.

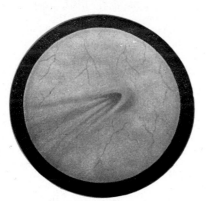

Fig. 684. The retracted ureter common with descending renal tuberculosis.

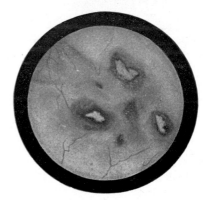

Fig. 685. Tuberculous ulceration around the ureteric orifice in descending renal tuberculosis. (*Dr. C. F. Walters.*)

from the orifice, or the turbid urine may be seen to leave the orifice in a gentle trickle instead of a jet if the renal secreting function is impaired or if renal dilatation is present. In cases in which the renal secreting tissue is much destroyed, a firm worm-like cast may be seen to be slowly exuded from the ureteric orifice and to fall to the base of the bladder, resembling the expression of tooth-paste from a collapsible tube.

Apart from the alterations in the urinary efflux from an orifice, the actual appearance of the orifice may show changes which indicate renal disease. Thus, in pyelitis the margins of the orifice are slightly oedematous and congested, and appear to pout into the bladder (*Fig.* 683); the mucous membrane of the bladder, immediately below and internal to the orifice, is frequently congested or granular. If the renal pelvis and ureter are dilated, the orifice is usually elongated and patulous, while with tubercle or in

rounded, patent opening, with rigid margins showing none of the rhythmic movement of the normal orifice accompanying the efflux into the bladder.

I. PYURIA CAUSED BY DISEASES OF THE URINARY ORGANS

Renal Disease—Diseases of Inflammatory Origin. The distinction between *pyelitis* and *pyelonephritis* is arbitrary, for it is certain that in many cases of so-called 'pyelitis' there is also infection of the interstitial tissues of the kidney. Recurrent attacks of 'pyelitis' in childhood or during the puerperium are often the precursors of chronic pyelonephritis in later life.

Infection may reach the kidney by the bloodstream, or from the bladder via the lumen of the ureter if the uretero-vesical valve is incompetent. Infection by the peri-ureteric lymphatics may take place, and direct spread in the submucous tissue of the ureter is also possible. Infection of the kidney is much more likely to occur if there is obstruction at any level in the lower urinary tract. Thus it is common in cases of prostatic

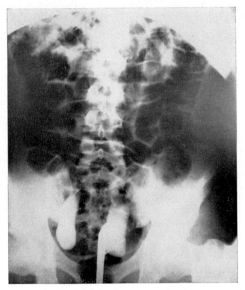

Fig. 686. Bilateral megaureter in a boy.

enlargement and stricture. When cystitis is present it is usually bilateral, although one kidney may show more advanced disease than the other. Any growth in the bladder which involves the

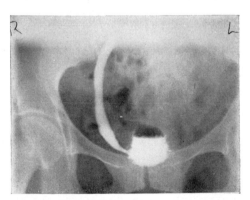

Fig. 687. Vesico-ureteric reflux shown during a voiding cystogram.

ureteric orifice, or the direct involvement of one or both ureters in the spread of uterine carcinoma, may set up pyelonephritis in the kidney from *ascending infection*. In this group of cases the primary cause of the disease has usually advanced to a sufficiently late stage to be obvious and the symptoms of ascending infection of the kidney may be overshadowed by those of the disease causing the obstruction. Infection is also particularly likely to occur in a kidney which is

22*

the seat of some congenital anomaly which interferes with its free drainage, for example a horseshoe, pelvic, hydronephrotic or duplex kidney.

Normally the uretero-vesical valve prevents regurgitation of urine into the ureter during the act of voiding, but if it becomes incompetent *vesico-ureteric reflux* may occur and infected urine can reach the kidney. Whether such incompetence is the effect as well as the cause of infection is still doubtful. It is accompanied by the formation of a small saccule above the ureteric orifice which produces traction on and straightening of the intramural part of the ureter; peristalsis now stops short at the lower end of the former juxtavesical ureter and the ureter above dilates. The effects are now those of obstruction, although there is no occlusion of the ureter or alteration of its orifice and a ureteric catheter can still be passed.

In children the resulting dilatation produces the condition of *megaureter* with the constant appearance of a narrow supravesical segment (*Fig.* 686). Stasis predisposes to infection; pyelonephritis with pyuria follows. Older patients, particularly women who get recurrent attacks of urinary infection, are frequently found to have ureteric reflux which may be the result of structural damage in childhood. In men of prostatic age reflux may occur in association with urethral obstruction. In all these cases if there is infection in the bladder it will be transmitted to the kidneys.

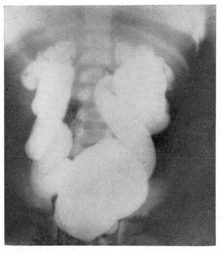

Fig. 688. Bilateral vesico-ureteric reflux with gross hydroureter due to congenital valve of the posterior urethra in a boy of 5 years.

Reflux can be demonstrated by a cystogram made during voiding, or by cinefluoroscopy (*Fig.* 687). It may be present during acute infection but absent when the infection has been controlled. In some cases of obstruction at or below the bladder neck, *such as congenital urethral valve*, there is gross reflux on filling the bladder from below (*Fig.* 688). A similar state results in the *megaureter megacystis* syndrome where the ureteric orifices are widely patent (*Fig.* 689).

Haematogenous pyelonephritis may arise apart from any other disease in the urinary tract. It is not uncommon in acute fevers, or with mild forms of suppuration in other parts of the body, or in association with pregnancy or typhoid fever. 'Catheter fever' is due to bacteriaemia from an infected urethra or prostate and is one form of pyelonephritis.

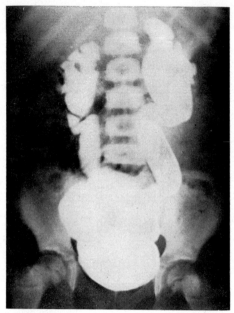

Fig. 689. Bilateral vesico-ureteric reflux in the megaureter megacystis syndrome.

The organisms responsible are most frequently *Escherichia coli* and less often the staphylococcus (especially in calculous cases), *Streptococcus faecalis*, pneumococcus, typhoid bacillus, *Pseudomonas pyocyaneus*, or *B. proteus.*

In *acute pyelonephritis* the symptoms are severe. There is pain in the loin, increased frequency of micturition with dysuria and urgency. There may be a rigor at the onset and a temperature reaching 104° with a rapid pulse. The urine is turbid and opalescent; it contains a little albumin and many bacteria with some pus cells. The white cell-count and E.S.R. are raised; excretion urograms show little loss of function but may reveal any stones present. The condition must be treated by appropriate chemotherapy or antibiotics until the urine is sterile; otherwise it may become chronic.

Chronic pyelonephritis is a more serious condition because it leads to destruction of the kidney and death from uraemia. It is often associated with ureteric reflux and with causes of urinary stasis such as stone, hydronephrosis, carcinoma of the bladder or ureter, prostatic obstruction, and neurogenic disorders.

Unless there is an acute exacerbation there are few symptoms in the early stages. There may be only mild dysuria and renal aching, but there is more often general poor health, anaemia, and low-grade fever: hypertension is sometimes present. When the condition is bilateral the first symptoms are often those of uraemia. The urine is of low or fixed specific gravity; it may contain only a few pus cells and bacteria with a trace of albumin and some granular casts. The blood-urea is raised and other renal function tests will show a gradually increasing degree of renal damage. Excretion urography shows irregularity and blunting of the calices or dilatation in a later stage with poor concentration. The retinal vessels may be narrowed and show flame-shaped areas of haemorrhage.

SPECIAL DIAGNOSTIC TESTS. The diagnosis of chronic pyelonephritis can be difficult and as the outlook is serious and prolonged treatment is likely to be needed use may be made of some special tests to confirm it.

1. *Urinary White-cell Excretion* after provocative pyrogens or steroids. It has been found that the intravenous injection of a pyrogen ('Pyrexal') or of prednisolone produces an increase in the number of white cells in the urine in most cases of chronic pyelonephritis. The pyrogen produces some side-effects and it is better to give prednisolone phosphate, 40 mg. in 10 ml. of saline injected slowly intravenously over a period of 3–5 minutes. The urine is collected with full aseptic precautions for a fixed period ($1\frac{1}{2}$–3 hours) and the excretion rate of white cells per hour is determined. A doubling of the number of white cells to more than 400,000 per hour is highly suggestive of chronic pyelonephritis, and a doubling to a figure less than 400,000 per hour does not exclude it. There is also a rise in acute pyelonephritis if the patient is not having treatment.

The bacterial count in the urine is also increased. The test is more often positive after an acute exacerbation and the rise is greater in chronic pyelonephritis with gross urinary infection. There may be an exacerbation of infection on the day after the injection. A negative finding does not exclude pyelonephritis and repeated examinations and culture of the urine should be performed.

2. *Renal Biopsy.* Percutaneous needle biopsy of the kidney is used in many medical centres to establish a diagnosis of chronic pyelonephritis and distinguish it from the nephrotic syndrome, glomerulonephritis, and amyloid disease.

Precautions. Although it is a safe procedure, there are some hazards of which haemorrhage is the greatest. The patient should be in hospital; an excretion pyelogram is made, provided the blood-urea is less than 100 mg./100 ml. Any bleeding tendency should be excluded by estimations of the prothrombin concentration, platelets, bleeding and clotting time and capillary fragility. If oral anticoagulants are being taken they should be stopped at least ten days before the test. Intravenous heparin should be discontinued for 24 hr.

The urine should be examined bacteriologically and any gross infection treated.

The procedure is carried out under sedation with the patient prone, lying over a firm sandbag. The position of the kidney is marked on the radiograph and a measurement taken from the vertebral spines to the lateral border of the kidney where it is crossed by the last rib. A vertical line is marked on the back through this point. The site of puncture is chosen in the lower and outer part of the kidney.

After infiltration with a local anaesthetic an exploring needle of the same length as the biopsy needle is introduced until it meets the resistant renal tissue, the patient holding his breath. When he resumes gentle breathing the correctness of the puncture is shown by the excursion of the butt of the needle.

A Franklin Vim-Silverman biopsy needle or other suitable type is then introduced along the needle track to the required depth and the specimen is taken.

The patient should stay in bed for 24 hours and be given copious fluids. The urine should be examined for blood.

For satisfactory interpretation the specimen should contain both cortical and medullary tissue and at least five glomeruli. It is also possible to culture the biopsy material and sometimes to obtain evidence of a specific infecting organism which was not found on urine culture.

The success rate varies with the experience of the operator but does not reach 100 per cent. A method of open biopsy through a 2-cm. incision, made under general anaesthesia, has been described. It is claimed that adequate tissue is always obtained and that the needling and aspiration under vision enable focal as well as diffuse disease to be picked out.

RENAL ABSCESS. In some cases of acute haematogenous infection suppuration may occur to form an abscess, with the resulting general symptoms of suppuration. An abscess may also result from injury when an effusion of blood in the renal tissues becomes infected by pyogenic organisms, or by the breaking down of a renal infarct.

RENAL PAPILLARY NECROSIS is not unlike renal abscess but it occurs in some diabetics and in others after the prolonged use of certain drugs, particularly analgesic compounds containing phenacetin; this is a constituent of about a quarter of the many analgesic and antipyretic tablets on the market. The renal papillae undergo necrosis and separate from the kidney; they are passed as sloughs or may be retained in the renal pelvis where they are liable to undergo calcification. There is often bacterial infection as well as pyuria. The condition usually has an acute onset with renal pain or colic and frequency. There is leucocytosis and there may be diabetic ketosis.

Pyelography sometimes shows the sloughing papillae or the cavities resulting from their separation. If the condition is bilateral there will be progressive renal failure and death from uraemia. It is important in taking the history to find out if analgesic tablets have been taken regularly and to inquire into their composition. Those containing phenacetin should be forbidden.

A condition known as *renal carbuncle* occasionally occurs in which a suppurative focus exists in the kidney, frequently following an acute skin or bone staphylococcal infection. It remains for a time localized in the renal tissue and tends to spread to the perinephric tissues, where it gives rise to a perinephric abscess, rather than into the renal pelvis. There is tenderness or enlargement of the kidney, but the urine contains only a minute trace of pus and albumin; it is often sterile on culture, although a blood culture may yield a growth of staphylococci.

PYONEPHROSIS—or dilatation of the pelvis and calices of the kidney with pus and urine—is caused when suppuration has occurred in a kidney which is at the same time subjected to some form of obstruction to the normal exit of the urine. Pyonephrosis is caused most commonly by renal calculus or tuberculosis or infection of a hydronephrosis but is by no means uncommon with chronic cystitis complicating urinary obstruction from an enlarged prostate or stricture. Carcinomatous ulceration affecting a ureteric orifice, either primary in the bladder or by direct extension of uterine carcinoma, is also an important cause of pyonephrosis. In contradistinction to suppurative pyelonephritis, the symptoms of pyonephrosis are less severe; at first they are those of the obstructive lesion causing the disease, to which are added the general symptoms of suppuration with increased tenderness in the loin on bimanual examination. Pyonephrosis causes a renal tumour of variable size, a decrease being associated with the discharge of a larger amount of pus in the urine. In pyonephrosis due to calculous disease the urine may contain a large amount of pus, but there may be no lumbar pain suggesting a renal stone. In these cases a large calculus will usually be found in the renal pelvis, and will be shown on X-ray examination (*see* KIDNEY, ENLARGEMENT OF). A pyelographic examination will demonstrate the renal dilatation, although if there is severe destruction of renal tissue there may merely be the soft-tissue shadow of the enlarged, non-functioning kidney.

The urine in suppurative disease of the kidney and its pelvis requires careful examination. It may be normal with a localized cortical renal abscess or with closed pyonephrosis; in all other lesions it contains pus and micro-organisms. If the pus-cells are in the form of casts of the renal tubules, infection of the renal parenchyma is present; in this case the protein in the urine is in excess of that due to the pus present. Polyuria, with a diminution of the total solids of the urine, is common with inflammatory lesions of the renal tissue.

RENAL TUBERCULOSIS. The miliary form of tuberculosis occurs in children as part of a general dissemination of tubercle, and causes no urinary symptoms. The kidney is, however, attacked not infrequently by microscopic tuberculous infection, beginning as a deposit of small tuberculous nodules. One or more of these foci enlarge and coalesce to form a caseating area, which eventually opens into the renal pelvis by direct ulceration into a calix; the lining membrane of the renal pelvis and ureter become infected with tubercle and thickened by submucous infiltration. At first, before ulceration into the renal pelvis has occurred, the symptoms of the disease are very slight; there may be aching in the loin and slight albuminuria, but as soon as the renal pelvis is involved more marked symptoms occur—persistent pyuria, lumbar aching, increased frequency of micturition, and polyuria. The urine is pale, acid, of low specific gravity, and of opalescent turbidity; on careful examination after centrifuging, the tubercle bacillus is usually found. A small amount of blood is generally present. The increased frequency of micturition occurs before any descending vesical infection has occurred and this symptom, accompanied by pyuria, has frequently given rise to a diagnosis of vesical disease. The occurrence in a young adult of persistent pyuria with 'sterile' acid urine should always be looked upon with grave suspicion, and a careful search made for the tubercle bacillus; should this not be found by the microscope, diagnosis by culture or by inoculation of some of the urinary deposit into a guinea-pig should be resorted to, but it must be remembered that 6 weeks may be required before positive results are obtained. A careful cystoscopic examination of the bladder should also be made, when early vesical tuberculosis may be seen (*Fig.* 685, p. 680), or the characteristic changes in the ureteric orifice may show the presence of renal infection (*Fig.* 684, p. 680). By digital examination per rectum or per vaginam the lower end of the ureter may be felt to be thickened and rigid in renal tuberculosis. An intravenous pyelogram usually shows a partial failure of excretion of contrast medium by the affected kidney with some dilatation of the ureter (*Fig.* 362, p. 343), while an ascending pyelogram (not usually required) shows a lack of definition and irregular outline of the renal calices (*Fig.* 500, p. 483).

Renal tuberculosis is often confounded with renal stone, and the colic which is usually associated with stone may be present in tuberculosis if a piece of caseous debris is passing down the ureter. A radiographic shadow of a calculus shows well-defined margins (*Fig.* 483, p. 475), whereas a tuberculous focus in the kidney may give rise to a faint, blurred, indistinct shadow in the renal area. The presence of tubercle bacilli will, however, determine the existence of tuberculosis, while tuberculous lesions elsewhere in the body, most frequently in the epididymes, prostate, or vesiculae seminales, or evidence of former disease in spine, joint, or chest, may also serve to confirm the diagnosis.

The symptoms of *renal calculus* vary with the position of the stone and the changes that have taken place in the kidney in consequence of its presence. It may be situated in a calix, and cause no symptoms beyond lumbar aching; or in the renal pelvis, when, if movable, it may cause acute renal colic, due either to the attempted passage of the stone by the pelvic outlet or to the increased intrarenal pressure from blockage of the ureter. So long as the kidney remains aseptic the urine contains but traces of albumin, and only microscopic quantities of blood; but if it becomes infected with micro-organisms, pyelitis, pyelonephritis, or pyonephrosis may result, with their attendant symptoms. Pus occurs in the urine in a case of renal stone only when infection of the kidney has occurred.

MEDULLARY SPONGE KIDNEY. This is probably a congenital defect allied to congenital polycystic kidney. Small saccular dilatations occur at the tips of the calices which often contain stones. Renal pain is present and there is pyuria and often bacterial infection. The condition is generally bilateral but unilateral cases are sometimes seen and it is occasionally localized to a small area of the kidney. The histological changes are those of pyelonephritis (*Fig.* 690). The condition is diagnosed by plain radiography and excretion pyelography; it is not usually detected on a retrograde pyelogram.

Ureteric Calculus. A small renal calculus may become impacted during its passage along the ureter, and may cause some difficulty in diagnosis. The usual situations of the obstructed calculus are in the upper few inches of the ureter, at the pelvic brim, or at the vesical end of the tube; in most cases the previous history of renal colic and symptoms of renal stone will be sufficient to indicate its partial ureteric descent. A calculus may, however, be present in the upper end of the ureter or at the pelvic brim, and give very few symptoms beyond a fixed pain in the course of the ureter; in this situation it has frequently been mistaken for ovarian pain or for appendicitis.

If the stone blocks the ureter completely, the kidney of the same side—in the absence of septic infection—becomes functionless and atrophies; but if the calculus occludes the lumen of the tube only partially, renal distension will occur with resulting hydro- or pyonephrosis. If, however, the calculus becomes impacted in the vesical segment of the ureter a train of symptoms occurs simulating vesical stone or vesical tuberculosis—namely, increased frequency of micturition, penile pain following micturition, and often a small amount of blood and pus in the urine, in addition to the aching pain in the loin. A ureteric calculus impacted in this situation may be felt in the ureter upon rectal or vaginal examination. It may be demonstrated by X-rays (*Fig.* 63, p. 64; *Fig.* 487, p. 477); while the changes seen around the ureteric orifice, and the absence of a vesical lesion on cystoscopic examination, will confirm the diagnosis. A stereoscopic X-ray examination, especially after a radioopaque catheter has been passed into the ureter, is of great assistance in these cases (*Fig.* 63, p. 64).

Megaureter has already been described.

Vesical Diseases. Pyuria may be met with in any lesion of the bladder which is associated with inflammatory changes. The fact that urine is retained in the bladder renders the latter liable to septic infection, so that cystitis is common with urethral stricture or prostatic obstruction. Any ulceration of the bladder, simple, tuberculous, or malignant, is accompanied by inflammatory changes, and pus will be present in the urine.

nearly all cases, is preceded by acute urethritis; the presence of swelling of the gland, elevation of temperature, and acute pain on rectal palpation, will determine the existence of prostatic inflammation.

Sterile cystitis (abacterial pyuria) is a condition in which all the symptoms of cystitis come on acutely but with no evidence of bacterial infection either on direct smear or on culture, although there is considerable pyuria. There may

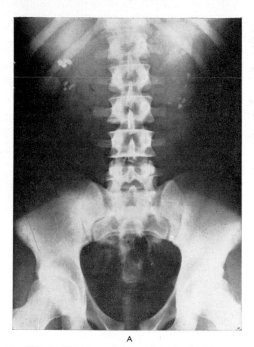
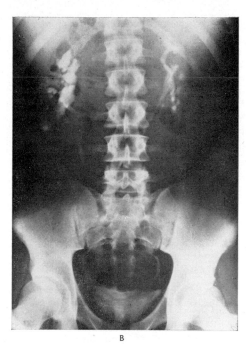

A   B

Fig. 690. A, Multiple small bilateral renal calculi in a case of medullary sponge kidney. B, Excretion pyelogram in the same case showing caliceal saccules which contain the stones. From a boy of 16.

CYSTITIS may be acute or chronic, and the essential factor of either form is infection of the bladder by some micro-organisms; any agent which produces either congestion of the bladder or retention of urine acts as a predisposing cause.

With *acute cystitis* the mucous membrane of the bladder becomes oedematous and highly congested, and epithelial desquamation and formation of pus follow. Haemorrhage may occur from the congested mucosa, or small abscesses develop in it, rupturing into the bladder to leave small areas of ulceration. In severe cases patches of the mucous membrane may become gangrenous. The symptoms of acute cystitis are usually distinctive: frequent and painful micturition, pain in the perineum and suprapubic area, with the presence of pus and blood in the urine, which is commonly of acid reaction. Usually the cause of the acute cystitis is apparent, such as some form of acute urethritis, or previous instrumentation, and there is little difficulty in the diagnosis. The same symptoms are, however, produced by an acute inflammation of the prostate which, in

be a preceding urethral discharge which is also sterile. This condition is especially seen in young women and is often precipitated by sexual intercourse ('honeymoon cystitis').

Chronic cystitis may succeed an acute attack. The symptoms are less marked, but increased frequency of micturition is always present. The urine is alkaline, contains pus and mucus, and the disease is commonly associated with some form of urinary obstruction or with retention or incontinence due to some nervous disease, such as multiple sclerosis, tabes dorsalis, or transverse myelitis or to traumatic transection of the spinal cord. The association of pyuria and increased frequency of micturition, which is present in chronic cystitis, must be distinguished carefully from that due to pyelitis or pyelonephritis, for increased frequency of micturition may be present without any vesical infection. In pyelonephritis the urine is usually acid in reaction, pale in colour, and shows a general turbidity, with little inclination to a deposit. The urine of chronic cystitis is alkaline, and rapidly deposits a greyish sediment of pus together with ropy adherent mucus. In pyelitis and pyelonephritis, the urine contains more albumin than the pus would account for, and on microscopical examination renal or pus casts are found; in cystitis the albumin is less, and vesical cellular elements are present, without casts unless the kidneys are affected also. Intravenous pyelography is invaluable in demonstrating a renal source of infection. Further evidence may be obtained by the use of the cystoscope. In cystitis the bladder wall is thickened, has lost its normal iridescent appearance, looks reddened and velvety, and the vessels of the mucous membrane are obscured. With pyelonephritis the bladder wall is normal, but the ureteric orifice of the affected side shows thickened or pouting lips and a slightly raised area of thickened mucous membrane, whilst the urine flowing from the orifice may be seen to be turbid or to contain small particles of mucopus.

Tuberculous cystitis occurs usually in young adults, and is almost always secondary to tuberculous disease of a kidney or of the generative organs. The characteristic symptoms are increased frequency of micturition during both day and night, pyuria, with pricking pain in the glans penis at the end of micturition, and the appearance of a few drops of blood in the last drops of urine. The same symptoms are often present with vesical calculus and with vesical carcinoma when ulceration has taken place. Vesical calculus is usually present in older patients, and during the early part of the illness, before cystitis has set in, the calculus only gives rise to penile pain and desire to micturate during movement. When cystitis supervenes, the frequency of micturition will be marked during both day and night. Vesical carcinoma also occurs in older patients, and when ulcerated may cause haematuria; sometimes the diagnosis may be made by palpation per rectum of an indurated area in the bladder base, or of infiltration in the pelvic lymphatic space. Tuberculous cystitis in the early stages, when the disease is characterized by the deposition of greyish tubercles in the submucous coat of the bladder, may give rise to increased frequency of micturition without other symptoms, but in the progressive advance of the disease the tubercles enlarge, coalesce, and ulcerate, by which time pus and blood will be present in the urine, tubercle bacilli should be found, and the patient may be unable to hold urine for more than twenty minutes or half an hour. It may be taken as a general rule that in any patient of young adult life with increased frequency of micturition and pyuria in a 'sterile' acid urine, a careful search should be made for tubercle bacilli in the urine, and for other tuberculous lesions, especially in the epididymes, prostate, or vesiculae seminales.

Tuberculous cystitis is rarely a primary disease and is usually secondary to tuberculous disease of the kidneys, when, after the primary focus has ruptured into the renal pelvis, the lining membranes of the latter, of the ureter, and of the bladder become affected successively. It may be due to tuberculous disease of the epididymis, via the vas deferens, seminal vesicle, and prostate; on rare occasions a prostatic focus ulcerates directly into the bladder. With renal disease, persistent pyuria, increased frequency of micturition, and penile pain at the termination of urination may be present before the bladder shows any sign of disease; blood is usually present in a small quantity in the urine, but its amount is not so definitely greater in the urine passed at the end of micturition as is the case in vesical disease. In renal tuberculosis there may be tenderness in the loin, the kidney is slightly enlarged, and the lower end of the ureter can occasionally be felt distinctly thickened upon rectal or vaginal examination. Primary vesical tuberculosis should not be diagnosed unless complete examination of the kidneys by excretion and ascending pyelography and by examination of the separate kidney urines has proved negative. The two conditions cannot always be distinguished even by careful examination. In either the deposition of submucous tubercles, together with the shallow ulceration in the bladder mucous membrane, may be seen (*Fig.* 685, p. 680), while in renal tuberculosis changes may be seen in the ureteric orifice of the affected side (*Fig.* 684, p. 680): at first the orifice becomes thickened, oedematous, and slightly patulous; but later it is rigid and patent, or drawn up by the shortening of the ureter to occupy a position above and outside the normal situation in the trigonal area of the bladder, or drawn up to the apex of a conical retraction of the bladder base. Intravenous or ascending pyelography (p. 474) may be necessary.

VESICAL CALCULUS may give rise to pyuria when it is accompanied by cystitis, but may be present a long time before any inflammatory infection occurs. When cystitis is present the urine shows no features which will distinguish it from that of patients suffering from some other form of cystitis, except that there may be a constant presence of crystals, or an increased amount of blood after exercise. The constant symptoms of vesical calculus are vesical irritability during the day time, penile pain after micturition, and haematuria, especially after any exercise. If a calculus in the bladder is suspected, examination by the X-rays (*Fig.* 371, p. 347) or the cystoscope will reveal it; the cystoscope may detect a stone that is in a diverticulum, partially encysted or lying in the pouch behind an enlarged prostate; X-rays may fail to show a shadow of a uric acid calculus.

ULCERATION OF THE BLADDER, apart from tuberculosis and epithelioma, may occur as a simple ulcer, consecutive to chronic cystitis, or as the result of injury or perhaps due to radionecrosis following treatment of malignancy in or close to the bladder. A single non-tuberculous ulcer, similar to gastic ulcer, has been described as occurring in women (Hunner's ulcer) in the neighbourhood of the ureteric orifices, causing haematuria and painful frequent micturition. Later, the surface of the ulcer may become encrusted with phosphatic material, when the urine contains mucopus, and often small flakes of phosphatic debris from the surface of the ulcer. This single ulcer is rare, and can be diagnosed only by the use of the cystoscope. Typically, the bladder capacity in this condition is very small. The aetiology remains the subject of speculation. Ulceration may also occur in the bladder as a result of severe cystitis when necrosis has occurred in the mucous membrane. This condition is present occasionally in a case of obstinate cystitis, giving rise to painful and frequent micturition, and may be diagnosed by means of the cystoscope. Both the simple and the consecutive ulcer must be differentiated from tuberculous ulceration of the bladder; in the latter, haemorrhage is usually slight, and occurs at the termination of micturition; tubercle bacilli may be found in the urine, or other deposits of tubercle found in the epididymis, prostate, or seminal vesicles. The cystoscopic appearance of tuberculous disease, and its more generalized distribution in the vesical wall, will afford confirmatory evidence, and in case of doubt cystoscopic biopsy is usually conclusive.

MALIGNANT ULCERATION OF THE BLADDER occurs in two main forms: (a) papillary; (b) solid.

a. The *papillary carcinoma* of the bladder is more common, and it gives rise to irregular profuse haemorrhages. The tumour is attached to the bladder by a broad pedicle or may be entirely sessile and covered by blunt villi, presenting a coarsely mamillated surface. It occurs in elderly patients, and the tumours are frequently multiple. The surface is often necrotic, giving rise to pyuria. The diagnosis is not difficult, the frequently recurring haematuria, associated with increased frequency of micturition, pain, and pyuria in an elderly patient, being fairly distinctive. Not uncommonly there is unilateral renal aching from the interference, by the position of the growth, with the flow of urine from one ureteric orifice, so that renal disease may be suspected; but in all cases a careful cystoscopic examination will show the nature of the disease. Difficulty may be experienced in obtaining a satisfactorily clear medium for a cystoscopic view, but in most cases this can be accomplished by gentle manipulations or by the use of an irrigating cystoscope. Difficulty may be found in distinguishing cystoscopically between a benign papilloma and villous-covered pedunculated carcinoma; the broad attachment of the latter to the bladder, the stunted villi covering it, the increased congestion of the bladder at the attachment of the growth, and the multiplicity of the tumours, will be signs of malignant disease (*Fig.* 365, p. 346). In rare instances a *benign papilloma* may begin to slough on the surface or may be accompanied by cystitis, when pyuria will be present. A cystoscopic examination will reveal the diagnosis. Microscopical examination of the urinary deposit may show distinctive fragments of new growth; in the method of *exfoliative cytology*

the centrifuged deposit is stained by the Papanicolaou technique. In a positive case clumps of malignant cells can be recognized by the expert pathologist (*Fig.* 360, p. 340). The removal of a fragment of growth by cystoscopic biopsy, especially if it includes part of the base of the tumour, will show whether there is infiltration and will give information as to the nature and degree of malignancy of the tumour. A cystogram may show a mottled filling defect in the bladder typical of papillary carcinoma (*Fig.* 650, p. 637).

b. Solid carcinoma is a much less common variety. It is a nodular, sessile, transitional-cell growth usually solitary and involves the base or lower reaches of the bladder, but may be multiple and can involve the dome. In contrast to the papillary tumours it tends to extend into the wall of the bladder rather than into the lumen. It is commonly a high-grade carcinoma and rapidly invades and ulcerates. It can be felt on bimanual examination as a hard and often fixed mass and gives rise to blood and pus in the urine associated with symptoms of cystitis.

A cystogram will show a typical bite deformation of the bladder.

A *diverticulum of the bladder* may give rise to intermittent or persistent and excessive pyuria accompanied by increased frequency, pain, and difficulty in micturition. A diverticulum usually indicates some form of urinary obstruction, but may be present as a congenital defect when no obstruction exists. The diagnosis is best made on cystoscopic examination, when the rounded opening into the bladder may be seen. Its size is best shown radiographically by a cystogram (*see Fig.* 691) or in the bladder pre-micturition film taken during pyelography.

Bilharzia haematobia may cause pus in the urine in advanced cases. When the small nodules in the submucous tissues (*Fig.* 368, p. 346) of the bladder ulcerate, small fungating masses are found in the bladder. The typical ova in the urine, in addition to pus and blood, will be found on microscopical examination of the urinary sediment and living or dead ova will be found on rectal biopsy. X-ray examination may show calcification in the bladder or ureters, while pyelography shows the presence of dilatation and strictures (*Fig.* 652, p. 638). In late cases there is often a carcinoma of the bladder.

Trichomoniasis, although predominantly affecting women, may be found in men whose partners are infected. The urine contains pus, and trichomonads may be found on staining, or as motile organisms in the centrifuged deposit. They can also be found sometimes in the urethral discharge or in the semen.

Urethral Causes. Any condition which sets up a purulent urethritis will cause pyuria. If the urethritis is recent or profuse, the local condition will be enough to indicate the diagnosis, but it must be remembered that cystitis may complicate a case of urethritis by direct backward infection. If, in addition to urethral discharge, there is increased desire to urinate, suprapubic pain, or haematuria, acute cystitis is probably present. Pyuria is commonly present in cases of stricture of the urethra, from the coexisting urethritis or cystitis. A urethral calculus or foreign body will also cause purulent urethritis.

Prostatic Causes. The onset of acute prostatitis complicating urethritis gives rise to increased desire to micturate, and to perineal and suprapubic pain, in addition to pyuria, or may cause retention of urine. An enlarged and very tender prostate will be felt on rectal examination.

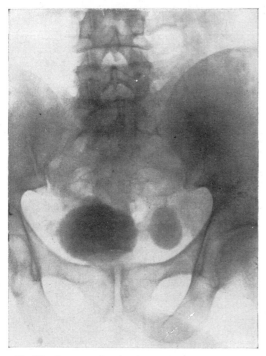

Fig. 691. Cystogram showing three vesical diverticula. That on the left is connected to the bladder by a narrow isthmus; the posterior one is partly superimposed on the bladder; the sac on the right is small. The prostate was enlarged.

Prostatic abscess is most frequently a sequela of acute urethritis which has infected the posterior urethra and caused an acute prostatitis. It may be due to a gonorrhoeal infection, or may result from septic instrumentation in the urethra. An acute prostatitis is prone to result in the formation of an abscess which may rupture into the urethra, bladder, or rectum, unless appropriate surgical measures are undertaken. The onset of acute prostatitis is marked by increasing desire to micturate, pain in the perineum and hypogastric areas, and raised temperature, while per rectum the prostate is felt to be uniformly enlarged and very tender. If an abscess results, there may be rigors, pyrexia, and increased difficulty in micturition, even retention of urine, while a soft area may be felt in the prostate from the rectal aspect. As a rule, however, the tenderness is so exquisite that this can only be done under

anaesthesia. A prostatic abscess may occur more rarely in connexion with a *prostatic calculus*; it may be present in advanced *genito-urinary tuberculosis*, when a prostatic focus may caseate and ulcerate into the trigonal area of the bladder, a condition which is usually accompanied by a sharp attack of haematuria. A tuberculous focus in the prostate is commonly a comparatively late feature in the disease, and the presence of nodules in the epididymis or seminal vesicles, or the previous knowledge of vesical tuberculosis, will assist largely in the diagnosis. Some degree of pyuria usually follows operations on the prostate, particularly transurethral resection and prostatectomy. The urine may be kept sterile by the use of antibiotics, but temporary pyuria is unavoidable.

Vesicular Causes. Inflammation of the seminal vesicles commonly accompanies prostatitis and they are a frequent source of residual infection after gonorrhoea. Acute vesiculitis may follow prostatectomy or endoscopic resection of the prostate and sometimes abscess formation occurs. The vesicles may be the seat of tuberculosis.

Seminal vesiculitis should be suspected if the patient complains of low backache or of pain in the perineum or rectum. Pyuria may be microscopic or profuse, and haemospermia is not infrequent; acute epididymitis is a common sequel. On rectal examination the inflamed vesicle will be palpable and tender, and pus may be expressed from it into the urethra on gentle massage.

II. PYURIA CAUSED BY DISEASES OUTSIDE THE URINARY ORGANS

Pus may be present in the urine, apart from any disease in the urinary apparatus, either by accidental contamination of the urine, or by the direct spread of inflammatory or carcinomatous processes from neighbouring organs to the urethra, the bladder, or more rarely the ureter. In the male, the accumulation of pus behind a *phimosis* may account for pyuria; in the female a *leucorrhoeal discharge* may contaminate the urine. In the latter case, if there is doubt about a coexisting urinary infection, the vulva should be cleansed well with an antiseptic, and a catheter passed to obtain a specimen for examination.

The spread of inflammatory processes, or the actual rupture of an abscess into any part of the urinary tract, will cause pyuria, and may create considerable difficulty in diagnosis. If symptoms pointing to urinary trouble, such as markedly increased frequency of micturition or slight haematuria, are followed by the sudden appearance of a quantity of pus in the urine, there is strong probability of the *rupture of an extra-urinary abscess* into the bladder or urethra, or very rarely into the ureter, provided that the sudden emptying of a renal abscess or a pyonephrosis can be eliminated. Frequently the history will give some indication of the primary troubles, of which the most frequent are prostatic abscess, appendiceal abscess, pyosalpinx, psoas, iliac, and pelvic abscess, and an abscess around a carcinoma or diverticulitis of the colon, this last being most common of all.

Pyuria in inflammation of the vermiform appendix. In the usual position of the appendix the bladder is commonly not affected; but if the appendix passes downwards across the pelvic brim it is not uncommon to find that, should it become inflamed. the patient complains of frequent and painful micturition. The appendix may be adherent to the bladder, which will show on cystoscopic examination a localized area of acute congestion on the right lateral wall, and both pus and blood may be present in the urine. Further, a small abscess may be formed in the adhesions between the appendix and the bladder, ulcerating into the latter and giving rise to pyuria; a ureteral calculus may be simulated, but cystoscopic examination will show a normal ureter, and a small ulcer in the right lateral wall of the bladder surrounded by an area of acute cystitis. The diagnosis of these cases is by no means easy; the situation of the pain is lower in the pelvis than is usual with appendicitis, and the association with urinary symptoms points to vesical disease; but the character of the onset of the trouble, with elevation of temperature and pulse-rate, and right-sided abdominal rigidity, will make one think of alternative acute intra-abdominal lesions. An abscess resulting from appendicular suppuration may track down into the pelvis and, if unopened, may rupture into the

bladder. In these cases there will be the usual history of acute appendicitis, followed by a tumour in the right iliac fossa or pelvic space, with a continuance of pyrexia, or even rigors, which subside on the appearance of a large quantity of pus in the urine. Examination per rectum may show inflammatory thickening behind the bladder or in the right pelvic space.

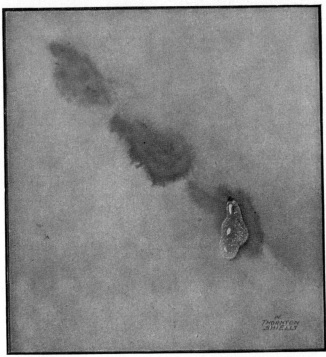

Fig. 692. A case of abdominal actinomycosis, showing granules in the sero-pus exuding from a chronic sinus in the groin.

A *pyosalpinx* may rupture into the bladder or cause cystitis from direct spread of the inflammatory process to the bladder. There will usually be a history of leucorrhoea, with constant aching or dragging pains in the lumbo-sacral region, with more severe attacks of pain and malaise at intervals. The periods may be profuse and associated with more pain than usual, and on vaginal examination a distinct fullness or tumour may be felt in one or both fornices.

Psoas or *iliac abscess* may rupture into the bladder, and a psoas abscess has been known to open into a ureter; the swelling in the iliac fossa or the inguinal region, together with signs of spinal caries, will point to the condition.

Diverticulitis of the pelvic colon may become adherent to the bladder, and if suppuration occurs may ulcerate into the bladder, causing pyuria together with the formation of an intestino-vesical fistula and the passage of flatus and faeces per urethram; the patient may notice a hissing or whistling sound, rather like a soda-water siphon, as the bubbles of gas pass in the urine. The formation of such a fistula is more frequent with diverticulitis than with carcinoma of the colon, so that care should be taken before giving the graver prognosis.

Carcinoma of the neighbouring organs in the pelvis frequently attacks the bladder by direct spread of the growth. This is most common with carcinoma of the uterine cervix and of the rectum, but may result from carcinoma of the pelvic colon, sigmoid, or caecum. The spread of the disease to the bladder occurs late; symptoms of the primary trouble have generally pointed to the diagnosis before pyuria ensues. The implication of the bladder is shown first by an increased desire to pass urine, and by pain during the act; later, when the growth has actually infiltrated the vesical mucous membrane, ulceration into the bladder occurs, with the passage of pus and blood in the urine. If the growth has extended from the uterus or vagina, there may be a leakage of urine into the latter; or if from the rectum or colon, some faeces or flatus may be passed per urethram.

Tuberculosis or *dysenteric ulcers of the intestine* have in some instances become adherent to the bladder wall and caused cystitis by direct spread, or have even perforated into the bladder.

A very rare cause of pyuria is *actinomycosis of the caecum*, which, instead of infiltrating the skin and pointing in the groin externally (*Fig.* 692), may extend into the pelvis and open into the bladder or rectum or both; the diagnosis may be missed entirely unless ray fungi are discovered in the urine as a result of routine and thorough bacteriological investigations. *Actinomycosis of the kidney* is even rarer; it is apt to be mistaken for tuberculosis until the laboratory investigations discover the characteristic ray fungi in the urine.

The commonest causes of the intermittent appearance of a large amount of pus in the urine are pyonephrosis, diverticulum of the bladder, and vesico-colic fistula.

Harold Ellis.

RECTUM, ABNORMALITIES FELT PER

Method of Examination. The patient is placed in a good light on a high couch. The gloved finger should be lubricated throughout its length, pressed gently on the anal orifice, and inserted farther only when the sphincters relax. The standard position is the left lateral, with the hips and knees well flexed, for in this the right index finger of the examiner slips easily along the backward curve of the rectum. Other positions have advantages for certain examinations: for feeling the prostate and vesiculae seminales the knee–elbow position is best; for bimanual palpation the patient should lie on his back with the right hip flexed so that the examiner's left hand can be placed over the hypogastrium while the right index finger is in the rectum; to reach as high as possible along the posterior wall it is

sometimes helpful to examine the patient sitting upright.

The average index finger is 7·5 cm. long from web to tip, but sense of touch is well developed in the last phalanx only; the finger should therefore be inserted to begin with as far as the first joint, and should examine the lower inch of the bowel thoroughly, but the examination must not be concluded till it has passed up as high as possible and explored the whole of the rectum within reach, as well as the coccyx, sacrum, ischiorectal fossae, and adjoining viscera. Though the rectum is 15 cm. long, it is usually possible by pressing up the pelvic floor to reach its upper limits with the finger, or even to palpate the colon just above it. The rectal speculum and the sigmoidoscope may also be needed to complete the examination.

If any abnormality is felt, the first thing to ascertain is: (I) *Whether it lies free in the lumen or is attached to the wall of the rectum*; (II) *Whether it is some abnormality of an adjoining structure or viscus that can be felt through the rectum.*

I. ABNORMALITIES LYING FREE IN THE LUMEN OR ATTACHED TO THE WALL OF THE RECTUM

Foreign Bodies. Though faeces can hardly be considered as foreign to the rectum, yet a hard, scybalous mass, enterolith, or hair-ball may amount to an abnormality. True foreign bodies include those that have been introduced through the anus, and those that have been swallowed. Examples of the first class are met with in children, persons of weak intellect, and thieves who sometimes employ the rectum as a hiding-place for stolen goods—diamonds for instance. The majority of foreign bodies felt per rectum have been swallowed—fishbones, pins, needles, splinters of wood. Their importance lies in the fact that they may cause a rectal or ischiorectal abscess, and in treating such a case their discovery and removal are essential for a complete cure.

Swellings of the Rectum projecting into the Lumen

INTERNAL HAEMORRHOIDS are rarely palpable unless chronically inflamed, thrombosed, or gangrenous. If palpable they will be felt immediately inside the anus, and can be hooked out through the anal orifice for inspection. The existence of piles having been diagnosed, an effort should be made to see if there is any causative condition, such as a carcinoma in the bowel above.

ABSCESS (submucous) gives rise to a more or less elongated, smooth, elastic swelling in the rectal wall. It is intensely tender, the slightest pressure causing great pain. The mucous membrane may feel hot, and pit on pressure. If the abscess has burst or bursts during examination, the finger on withdrawal will be covered with pus. An abscess that has already emptied itself feels like a small pea or bean in the submucous tissue.

GRANULAR PROCTITIS. This condition, often mistaken for 'piles' because its predominant symptom is bleeding, gives rise to a hypervascular, dull appearance of the rectal mucosa when viewed through the proctoscope, the passage of which often causes the mucosa to bleed. The pathology and bacteriology of this not uncommon condition are unknown, although it is now thought to be related to ulcerative colitis into which it may develop.

POLYPUS is a term used to designate, without reference to its histological characteristics, any benign tumour that is pedunculated. Almost all innocent tumours in this position, even if sessile at the beginning, ultimately become pedunculated owing to the downward drag of the faeces. A polypus may not be easy to feel, because its consistence is much the same as that of the mucous membrane, and because its pedicle may allow such free movement that it may easily be mistaken for a small mass of faeces. The best way of fixing these growths is to sweep the finger around the whole circumference of the rectum up to the highest point attainable; the growth is then arrested by the pedicle, and the finger can be hooked around it, so as to draw it down and perhaps make it protrude through the anus. If the polypus is large, a rectal speculum may be of service. Polypi are often multiple.

ULCERS, unless malignant or chronically inflamed, can rarely be felt with the finger; they must be viewed with the speculum or the sigmoidoscope. They may be tuberculous, gummatous, traumatic, or due to ulcerative colitis or dysentery.

CARCINOMA. Malignant tumours usually occur in people over 40, but in the rectum they may be met with in the twenties or even earlier. The commonest site of a carcinoma is in the upper half of the rectum, or at the rectosigmoid junction. Its extent varies with its stage; it may involve only part of the circumference of the bowel, or may extend right round the lumen. A carcinoma of the rectum has a hard irregular nodular feel that is usually unmistakable, but its exact characters vary with the age and configuration of the growth. Two types are commonly encountered, the proliferating and the constricting. The first leads to discharge of blood and mucus and is therefore commonly found at an earlier stage than the second. The edges are hard, the surface friable, bleeding easily, and the growth often involves part of the circumference only, or if it encircles the bowel does not constrict it completely, so that the upper limit may sometimes be ascertained by inserting the finger through it. The constricting type bleeds little, but causes increasing constipation and a sense of incomplete evacuation. The growth completely encircles the bowel, and this cylinder, with its everted edges encircling a small rigid lumen no bigger than a pencil, feels something like a very hard cervix uteri. In both types there is usually a belt of normal mucosa between the internal sphincter and the neoplasm, and in the constricting type this normal surface extends round the projecting edges like the vaginal fornices, so that the tumour in the middle may not at first be felt. Another point to

be gauged by a rectal examination is the degree of infiltration as measured by the fixity of the tumour to the neighbouring structures, the sacrum and coccyx behind, and the bladder and prostate in front. Following the rectal examination, the abdomen should be palpated for evidence of infection of the inguinal, pelvic, or lumbar glands, and the existence of secondary deposits in the liver.

The clinical symptoms of carcinoma of the rectum are suggestive. The patient describes a recent and progressive alteration in the bowel habit, in the direction of either constipation or diarrhoea. Periods of constipation, accompanied by abdominal distension with wind pains, alternating with diarrhoea controlled with difficulty, are common. Diarrhoea is more frequently the outstanding complaint: the bowels are open five to twenty times a day, but the total amount of faeces passed on each occasion is small and no satisfaction is obtained by the patient after stool. Often there is a sensation that something still remains behind. An urgent evacuation first thing in the morning is a common symptom. Blood and mucus may be noticed in the motion, but this is not constant. Wasting is not as common as it is in cases of carcinoma of the colon, and far less common than it is with gastric carcinoma. Pain is usually a late feature and takes the form of dull aching in the rectum and at the bottom of the back, not made much worse by the passage of a motion, quite unlike the sharp temporary excruciating pain associated with an anal fissure or ulcer.

Carcinoma of the rectum is unlikely to be overlooked except through the omission of rectal examination. It cannot be insisted too strongly that any alteration in bowel habit in a middle-aged person previously healthy demands such an examination, and if nothing is felt with the finger, a sigmoidoscope should be used. A barium enema, invaluable in the colon, may fail to show even a large growth in the rectum. Difficulties may arise in the differentiation between carcinoma and an adenomatous polypus or ulceration, either traumatic, colitic, dysenteric, venereal, or tuberculous, around which much long-standing inflammation has caused thickening. The facts that a carcinoma is hard, the surface often excavated, and the edges nodular and everted are generally sufficient. As the treatment of this condition usually involves a permanent colostomy, most authorities recommend that the diagnosis should in all cases be confirmed unequivocally by taking a piece of the ulcer for section, and submitting this to histological examination. Only in this way can the differential diagnosis from the extremely confusing 'amoeboma' of amoebic dysentery be made with certainty. If the histological report is 'negative' and the clinical evidences are strongly suggestive of neoplasm, this biopsy should be repeated until the diagnosis has been established.

VILLOUS TUMOUR OF THE RECTUM. These uncommon tumours have the naked-eye appearance of a sea anemone, and are columnar-celled papillomata. They are confined to the mucous membrane and entirely innocent, but may attain the size of an orange. The history is one of the passage of large quantities of pure mucus per rectum over many years, and occasional large haemorrhages, in a patient who is otherwise well and not constipated. To the finger they feel raised from the surrounding mucous membrane, soft and almost jelly-like, and freely movable; they tend to bleed when an attempt is made to hook them through the anus.

INTUSSUSCEPTION. Occasionally a piece of intussuscepted bowel may come down so far as to be felt per rectum. This condition is associated with the passage of blood and mucus, and therefore might be mistaken for a disease of the rectum proper. The fact that intussusception occurs nearly always in children, especially at the age of nine months or thereabouts, and causes intestinal obstruction, should make such a mistake easily avoidable. Chronic intussusception in an adult is uncommon; when it does occur it results as a rule from a pre-existing polyp, carcinomatous polyp, or submucous tumour.

Stricture due to carcinoma is dealt with above, but a few words remain to be said about fibrous stricture. This may be present at the anal orifice, at the level of the upper border of the internal sphincter, or 7–9 centimetres up the rectum. It may be annular or tubular. The finger meets with a firm cord-like constriction, which perhaps will not allow the entrance of more than its tip; there will be no bleeding unless the finger is forced through the stenosis and the mucous membrane is torn.

Since many of these strictures are the result of lymphogranuloma inguinale, particularly in women, inquiry should be made for a previous history of genital sores and inguinal buboes: the diagnosis can be established by the Frei intradermal allergic reaction. Other benign strictures are the result of trauma. This trauma may have been physical, following a foreign body or the careless passage of the nozzle of an enema syringe; thermal, as after the administration of a scalding enema; or chemical.

Fistulae, either recto-vaginal or recto-vesical, whether congenital or acquired, may be felt with the finger. The passing of urine or faeces by abnormal passages indicates the complaint.

Malformations of the Rectum. Some children are born without an anus, or without the lower portion of the rectum, or the finger introduced may be stopped by a membrane separating the upper from the lower portion of the bowel. The diagnosis is obvious.

II. ABNORMALITIES OF NEIGHBOURING STRUCTURES FELT PER RECTUM

It does not lie within the scope of this article to give the differential diagnosis of all the morbid conditions that can be felt through the rectum; it suffices to take the structures within reach of the finger, and indicate the varying conditions in which a diagnosis may be aided by a rectal examination.

Structures lying Outside the Abdominal Cavity in relation to the Rectal Walls

ON THE ANTERIOR WALL. The structures that can usually be felt are the prostate in the male, and the cervix uteri in the female.

The Prostate. The normal prostate has a flat surface opposed to the rectum, and is slightly grooved in the midline. Any enlargement is easily felt; an *adenoma* is the commonest form; it is soft and elastic, rounder than the normal prostate, and the median groove may be distorted; a *carcinoma* or *sarcoma* is hard, fixed, and nodular: lateral extensions along the vesiculae seminales may be felt; a *prostatic abscess* causes a soft protrusion into the rectum which is hot and very tender. In thin patients an enlarged prostate may be felt bimanually and in adenoma the degree of intravesical projection may be thus estimated.

The Vesiculae Seminales are not palpable normally; when they can be felt the fact is almost sufficient to declare them diseased; they are affected most commonly in connexion with tuberculous epididymitis or from present or past gonococcal vesiculitis.

The Bladder is not felt if healthy. If greatly distended it may form a tense resistance in the anterior wall of the rectum. Rarely a large stone or a malignant growth of the floor may be felt.

The Cervix Uteri forms such an obvious projection on the anterior wall of the rectum that it is sometimes mistaken by the inexperienced for a tumour. It varies so much in size, direction, outline, consistency, and level in the parous woman that it should always be identified first as a guide to the relationship of other structures that may be felt.

The Vagina cannot be felt unless it is occupied by a foreign body such as a pessary, or is the seat of a growth.

ON THE POSTERIOR WALL. The only normal structures that can be recognized are the coccyx and sacrum. The *coccyx* may be found bent in and pressing on the rectum; in coccydynia any movement of the coccyx may cause great pain. The *sacrum* may be the seat of a growth or an abscess, which causes a bulging into the posterior rectal wall. Tumours arising from postanal gut or the notochord may occur between the sacrum and rectum.

On the two lateral surfaces no structures are normally recognized. The ischiorectal fossae are common sites for abscesses, and these can be felt as tense swellings pushing in the wall. Rarely an aneurysm of the internal iliac artery or a stone in the lowest portion of the ureter may be felt. The sciatic nerve may be found to be very tender in cases of sciatica, or it may be surrounded by malignant deposits. Rectal examination should never be omitted in a case of sciatica.

Structures in the Abdominal Cavity felt through the Pouch of Douglas. The peritoneum covers the front of the rectum in its upper two-thirds, and is then reflected on to the posterior vaginal fornix in the female, and on to the base of the bladder between the seminal vesicles in the male. This reflection is called by clinicians the pouch of Douglas in both sexes, though in anatomy the term is only applied to the female pelvis. The pouch of Douglas is the lowest part of the coelomic cavity, therefore that to which fluids and malignant deposits tend to gravitate, but it may be occupied by many organs under normal or abnormal conditions. The top of the index finger when fully inserted reaches about an inch above the floor of the pouch of Douglas in the female, about half that distance in the male.

Pus. Any infection in the abdominal cavity tends to gravitate to the pelvis, and even if early and minimal will give rise to tenderness there. It is important to distinguish between true tenderness at the level of the peritoneum, and the inevitable discomfort of a rectal examination. Tenderness per rectum may be the deciding factor in the diagnosis of an obscure abdominal emergency. Later on, established peritonitis is recognized by a general sense of rigidity and thickness in the structures around the rectum in addition to tenderness. Later still, an abscess will be recognized as a soft and tender swelling on the anterior rectal wall above the peritoneal reflection.

BLOOD, coming from a ruptured or leaking ectopic gestation, gives an elastic doughy feeling and tenderness.

MALIGNANT DEPOSITS. Some tumours, particularly those of the stomach and ovary, show a tendency to metastasize by free cells in the coelomic cavity. These cells may start secondary tumours anywhere, but are particularly prone to do so in the ovaries and on the floor of the pouch of Douglas. Such deposits can be felt from the rectum as a firm shelf, constricting the rectum in front and on both sides and extending forwards and laterally, and quite unlike a growth or stricture of the rectum itself.

THE UTERUS is easily palpable. Enlargement or retroversion or a pelvic fibroid can be recognized; the pressure of a foetal head may occlude the rectum.

THE OVARIES, if enlarged by cystic disease or by new growth, may come within reach of the finger; pyosalpinx is often a bilateral affection in which the inflammatory masses can be felt per rectum in Douglas's pouch; they can be detected more readily by vaginal examination, however, when this route is permissible.

THE INTESTINES. The pouch of Douglas is normally occupied by pelvic colon and coils of ileum. A carcinoma of the colon can often be felt through the rectal wall as it lies in the pouch of Douglas, or can be manipulated by a hand on the abdomen into a position where it is within reach. The ileum, normally impalpable, may be felt if it is affected by strangulation, chronic infection, Crohn's disease, or new growth. An inflamed pelvic appendix may also be accessible to the examining finger.

R. G. Beard.

REFLEXES, ABNORMALITIES OF

Reflex activity—loosely defined as an involuntary response to the passage of nervous impulses through a reflex arc—enters into a wide range of somatic and visceral functions both in health and disease. A comparatively small number of these reflexes are used in the practice of clinical neurology, and of these only the more important will be considered here: (1) The stretch reflexes, usually referred to as the tendon-jerks. (2) The superficial reflexes—the abdominal, the cremasteric, and the plantar reflexes (*see* p. 84). (3) The pupillary reflexes (*see* p. 669).

THE TENDON REFLEXES

In normal man muscles contract momentarily when stretched by a sharp tap on the tendon of insertion. Anatomical factors limit the application of this test to the masseters, triceps, biceps, brachioradialis (formerly called supinator longus), flexors of fingers, quadriceps, adductors, and gastrocnemius. The reflex pathway ascends from the muscle through the posterior roots, passes forward to the anterior horn cells of the same segment, and descends to the muscle or muscles concerned via the motor nerve. Although each muscle is supplied by fibres from more than one segment of the cord, damage to a single root can abolish the reflex.

Exaggeration of Tendon Reflexes occurs in excitement, anxiety, and certain intoxications, e.g., benzedrine and strychnine poisoning. In these conditions the increased activity of the reflexes is generalized. Asymmetrical or localized exaggeration of tendon reflexes is a valuable sign of disease affecting the pyramidal tract, in which case it may be associated with loss of the abdominal reflexes and an extensor plantar response if the pyramidal fibres to the abdominal and leg muscles are also involved. It follows that normal abdominal and plantar reflexes may be found when the pyramidal lesion is limited to the portion of the tract which supplies the upper limb.

Depression or Loss of Tendon Reflexes occurs as a transient event in shock, haemorrhage, cerebral and spinal concussion, deep anaesthesia, severe general infections, diabetic ketosis, potassium intoxication (in uraemia), and overdosage with drugs which depress the central nervous system. A slow relaxation of the ankle reflex is said to be constant in myxoedema. General depression of reflexes, occurring as a by-product of a more important disaster, is of less diagnostic importance than localized or generalized loss of reflexes due to local disease affecting the reflex arc itself. Such disease may affect the muscles, the afferent fibres in the peripheral nerve or sensory root, the spinal segment, the motor root, or the peripheral motor nerves.

1. DISEASE OF MUSCLES. Depression or loss of the reflexes occurs as a late event in myotonia dystrophica, in the non-myotonic muscular dystrophies, and in dermatomyositis. They are

absent in amyotonia congenita and in the paralytic incidents of periodic paralysis and potassium intoxication.

2. DISEASE OF THE AFFERENT PATHWAY—between the muscles and the spinal cord—usually affects the motor or efferent part of the reflex arc concurrently, as in the many forms of toxic and infective polyneuritis, but it is interesting to recall that loss of tendon reflexes is sometimes found without demonstrable motor or sensory loss as the sole objective sign of a mild polyneuritis. *Tabes dorsalis* is the outstanding example of areflexia arising from disease of the afferent pathway, the lesion being in the posterior nerve-roots. Rarely, generalized loss of reflexes is seen in the sensory 'polyneuritis' occasionally associated with comparatively small malignant growths of the lung, stomach, or elsewhere.

3. DISEASE OF THE SPINAL CORD may abolish tendon reflexes, either by interrupting the reflex path as it passes from the root entry zone to the anterior horn cells (e.g., syringomyelia, haematomyelia, intramedullary tumours) or by destroying the anterior horn cells, as in acute anterior poliomyelitis, tumours in the ventral horns, thrombosis of the anterior spinal artery, compression of the spinal cord, and advanced cases of motor neuron disease.

4. DISEASE AND INJURY OF THE MOTOR NERVES usually affect the afferent fibres as well, but a predominantly motor polyneuritis is sometimes seen in diphtheria, beriberi, and lead poisoning. Herniation of cervical or lumbar intervertebral disks is a common cause of depression or loss of a single tendon reflex but it is often difficult to know whether the interference is in the motor or the sensory part of the reflex arc. The segments concerned in the most important tendon reflexes are listed below.

REFLEX	MUSCLE
Biceps	Biceps
Triceps	Triceps
'Supinator'	Brachioradialis
Patellar	Quadriceps
Achilles	Gastrocnemius

PERIPHERAL NERVES	ROOT AND SEGMENT
Musculocutaneous	C.5 and 6
Radial (to Triceps)	C.7
Radial (to Brachioradialis)	C.6
Femoral	L.4
Tibial (medial popliteal)	S.1

Sometimes the reflexes are lost in relation to a myotonic pupil. This occurs almost exclusively in women, coming on in the third or fourth decade. The disorder is usually unilateral, of sudden onset and accompanied by some discomfort in the eye or difficulty in 'focusing', but at times the attention of the patient is drawn to the pupil which is larger than the other. A myotonic pupil does not respond to an ordinary light stimulus, although it may constrict slowly in sunlight, but it reacts slowly and completely to convergence so that it may become smaller than the normal pupil, dilating again slowly when convergence is relaxed. A myotonic pupil will constrict if a few drops of 2·5 per cent mecholyl are instilled into the conjunctival sac but this will not affect a normal pupil. Sometimes the knee- and ankle-jerks are lost, less commonly the arm-jerks, in association with such a pupil.

In acute cerebellar lesions the hypotonia of the affected side is reflected in a notable depression of the tendon reflexes, but this is not seen in chronic cerebellar disease. Moreover, if the knee-jerk is elicited with the leg hanging down, the jerk is succeeded by a few pendulum-like swings of the leg, an expression of the hypotonia. This 'pendular' jerk is occasionally seen in chorea.

Finally, it may be impossible to elicit the tendon-jerks when there is apparently no associated abnormality.

Ian Mackenzie.

RIGORS OR CHILLS

Rigors, or chills, are common at the onset of various febrile disorders and may occur at regular or irregular intervals. The cardinal feature of a rigor is shivering. The extremities are chilled superficially, the patient sits or lies huddled up complaining of the cold, but the internal temperature is raised. More or less violent shaking movements appear during which the teeth chatter, the bed shakes, and even the muscles of the face twitch involuntarily. This shivering lasts for perhaps an hour, gradually dying away as the patient feels warmer and presently over-hot. Thus the initial stage of the fever passes into the second stage in which the complaint is of sweating, thirst, and sensation of undue heat, the body temperature rising still higher. In children, general convulsions, with partial or complete coma, may occur at the onset of an acute infection in conditions that would give rise to a rigor in adults.

Hysterical shivering may sometimes lead to diagnostic confusion. Here, however, the patient has no fever, does not look systemically ill, has a normal skin, and the chill has the usual over-dramatic qualities typical of hysteria. Also, a history or the identification of other hysterical phenomena may be obtainable.

Rigors may be classified as single or multiple. **Single Rigors.** The occurrence of a *single rigor* at the outset of an acute infective disorder is not unusual; it may occur with any fever of sudden onset, but with acute urinary infections in particular. Once common in lobar pneumonia it is now less often seen in this condition. A mismatched blood transfusion, injection of T.A.B. or other vaccines, or a serum reaction may be responsible, and in some cases the passing of a catheter.

Recurring Rigors. The occurrence of a *series of rigors* often gives information of more definite value, for they are seen in but a limited number of local or general infections most of which have some characteristic or localizing signs. In themselves these rigors are no more than evidence of the severity of the infection. The following are the chief disorders in which may occur a series of rigors:

Malaria: quartan, tertian, subtertian, aestivo-autumnal, or malignant
Relapsing fever
Pyaemia
Acute leukaemia
Portal pyaemia
Septicaemia
Puerperal fever
Bacterial endocarditis
Acute osteomyelitis
Suppurative pylephebitis
Pyelonephritis
Cystitis
Cholelithiasis and cholecystitis
Bronchiectasis
Infective sinus thrombosis
Pulmonary tuberculosis
Abscess formation:
  Lung
  Pleura (empyema)
  Hepatic (amoebic)
  Appendicular
  Subphrenic
  Perinephric
  Pelvic
  Prostatic
  Cerebral
  Endosteal
Erysipelas
Rat-bite fever
Neoplasms.

Multiple rigors are always of serious significance. They may be due to some deep-seated abscess that produces but scanty physical signs. When no explanatory abnormal physical signs can be found, several blood-cultures should be taken. Blood-cultures are more likely to be positive if the patient's temperature is 102° F. (39° C.) or higher at the time the blood is taken than when the patient's temperature has fallen below this level.

In *malaria*, the rigors tend to recur at regular intervals of forty-eight or seventy-two hours (*Fig.* 315, p. 297) in the benign tertian and quartan infections; at shorter intervals if the infection is mixed. In the aestivo-autumnal form, the rigors and also the course of the fever are less regular. (*See* FEVER, PROLONGED.)

In *relapsing fever*, the onset is acute with a rigor or a series of rigors. A fortnight later, during which the patient has been convalescing for a week or ten days, relapse and a second rigor or series of rigors occurs (*Fig.* 321, p. 299). A second relapse may occur at the end of the third week, and, in a very few cases, a third relapse. Relapsing fever is met with in Egypt, India, and other subtropical countries. It occurs in epidemics, especially during periods of distress, famine, and privation, circumstances in which infection is spread by lice or ticks carrying the infecting spirochaetes of the genus *Borrelia*. Relapses are much less common now that antibiotics are available for therapy. Blood-films

examined repeatedly will show the infecting organism.

Multiple rigors occur exceptionally in the course of *acute blood diseases*, such as acute leukaemia. Severe and progressive anaemia, wasting, fever, heavy sweats, and haemorrhage from the mucous membranes are likely to occur in these cases, with characteristic haematological changes.

Multiple rigors are commonest in the various forms of *acute blood infections*. Thus *puerperal fever* occurs after childbirth, due to bacterial infection of the uterus and its spread to the blood-stream; the patient will probably have a thin sero-purulent or offensive vaginal discharge as well as the evidences of septicaemia or pyaemia. In *acute bacterial (malignant) endocarditis* the attention is directed mainly to the condition of the heart, to the presence of valvular murmurs, and to emboli. In *acute infective osteomyelitis*, the first complaint is directed to the acute inflammation occurring in a bone. *Portal pyaemia* or suppurative pylephebitis is seen in patients with various acute inflammatory intra-abdominal lesions and is due to the spread of bacterial infection to the liver through the portal vein; the commonest precursor is appendicitis. The blood in the portal vein clots, the clot is invaded by bacteria, softens and breaks up, to be dispersed throughout the liver in the form of infective emboli. Multiple hepatic abscesses result, with pain, swelling, and tenderness in the hepatic region; jaundice is present in less than half the cases, vomiting and diarrhoea are frequent, and there is hectic fever. *Pyaemia* is characterized by the formation of metastatic abscesses, most often in the subcutaneous tissues or in the lungs in consequence of the lodgement there of multiple infected emboli. Pyaemia is today infrequent and when it does occur is secondary to a severely infected wound, to septic phlebothrombosis, or to deeply seated abscesses that are not amenable to surgical treatment, often in association with an inoperable carcinoma. Occasionally it seems to be idiopathic, when it is probably some infective lesion that escapes discovery. Pyaemia is generally of sudden onset. The main symptoms and signs are hectic fever, rigors, leucocytosis, diarrhoea and vomiting, heavy sweats, prostration, and the formation of secondary embolic abscesses. When the lungs are the site of multiple abscesses, the breathing becomes rapid, and signs appear of bronchitis, pleurisy, or pulmonary consolidation. Abscesses in the more superficial tissues or joints advertise themselves by local pain, swelling, redness, and heat; in the deeper tissues, by pain and disturbances of function.

Multiple rigors are commoner in pyaemia— where several may occur daily—than in *septicaemia*, in which growth of bacteria in the blood is not accompanied by the formation of metastatic abscesses.

Multiple rigors may result from *acute localized inflammatory infections* if the inflammation is sufficiently extensive and the infecting micro-organism virulent. If situated in the genito-urinary tract, as they often are, these inflammations produce specific pathological changes in the urine (haematuria, pyuria, proteinuria) or difficulties in micturition. If the gall-bladder or bile-ducts are the seat of the inflammation, jaundice and pain in the hepatic region will probably

In *amoebic abscess of the liver* malaise, fever, sweating, and rigors are the most usual symptoms; a pleural effusion may develop secondarily to spread of infection through the diaphragm with nothing particularly suggestive of implication of the liver. As a rule, complaint will be made of dull pain in the right hypochondrium, axilla, or shoulder. The liver is usually enlarged and tender

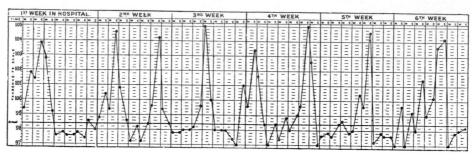

Fig. 693. Temperature chart in a severe case of rat-bite fever. Only part of the chart is shown; the recurrent attacks extended over a period of four months.

be observed with fever and rigors, and possibly a history of gall-stone colic may be obtained. In *suppurative cholecystitis* the gall-bladder is enlarged and tender; in *suppurative cholangitis* the liver as a whole is swollen. Charcot's hepatic intermittent fever is due to *chronic cholangitis*, with intermittent biliary obstruction due to a ball-valve stone lying in the ampulla of Vater. *Infective sinus thrombosis* occurs mainly in patients with otorrhoea and indicates that the bacterial infection has spread from the ear to one of the cranial venous sinuses. Its symptoms are general—that is to say those of septicaemia or pyaemia, often with an initial rigor and vomiting followed by high fever, more rigors, and sweating, and local very severe pain about the ear, excruciating headache, and venous congestion of the optic disk. Other symptoms and signs vary with the site of the thrombosis. If the sigmoid sinus is thrombosed, oedema and tenderness appear over the mastoid process, and should the clotting spread downwards a thrombus may be felt in the internal jugular vein. Thrombosis of the cavernous sinus is accompanied by squint, exophthalmos, and oedema of the orbit and eyelids. Thrombosis of the superior longitudinal sinus may cause oedema of the scalp near the sagittal suture. The diagnosis must be made from cerebral or cerebellar abscess, in which repeated vomiting is likely to occur and the localizing signs and symptoms suggest brain disease, and from meningitis, in which rigors are rare. In other patients, some acute inflammatory disorder may result in definite *abscess formation* when rigors may develop. The virulence of the particular organism causing the inflammation is the chief factor in determining whether rigors occur or not; in many cases the rigors are due to secondary and sometimes terminal septicaemia or pyaemia.

and pressure applied to the lower right ribs in the axilla is resented. The intercostal depressions may be filled in, the flank bulging somewhat. A high polymorphonuclear leucocytosis is the rule.

Multiple rigors may occur in various subacute diseases of the lungs, particularly *lung abscess*, *bronchiectasis*, and advanced *pulmonary tuberculosis* with secondary pyogenic infection, also of pleura (empyema). A bronchial carcinoma may be the underlying pathological process in many cases.

High or irregular fever with recurring rigors has been recorded in a few unusual cases of *enteric fever* and in *erysipelas*.

Rat-bite fever is probably commoner than is generally supposed; many cases escape recognition. It occurs in persons who have been bitten or deeply scratched by rats, or by ferrets, cats, or weasels that have recently killed rats. The rat-bite heals slowly and imperfectly, and after an incubation period of from 1 to 6 weeks the patient begins to suffer from a series of acute febrile attacks at fairly regular intervals of a few days. These attacks continue for from two to ten months (*Fig.* 693). The onset of each is abrupt, with a rigor, headache, fever up to 102–106° F. (39–41° C.), malaise, severe pain and swelling in some of the muscles, recurrence of inflammatory but rarely suppurative phenomena about the original wound, and urticarial, measly, patchy erythematous rashes on the face, limbs, and trunk. Each attack lasts for 1–4 days, the patient being fairly well in the intervals: during the attack some degree of leucocytosis is common. Rat-bite fever is not fatal; it is due to infection by a spirochaete (*Spirillum minus* or *Spirochaeta muris*) which responds to antibiotic therapy.

Neoplasms. Rigors may sometimes occur in patients with lymphoma, hypernephroma, myeloma, or other malignant conditions.

F. Dudley Hart.

RISUS SARDONICUS

Risus sardonicus is a fixed unmirthful grin resulting from spasm of the muscles of the face. The angles of the mouth are drawn outwards and the eyelids raised by tonic contraction of the muscles that are employed in the production of a smile, but the spasm is maintained in a way that at once excludes natural smiling (*Fig.* 694). The chief causes of the condition are *tetanus, strychnine poisoning, malingering, hysteria, catalepsy.*

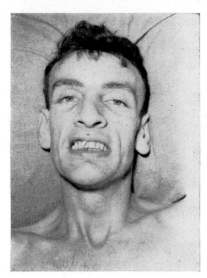

Fig. 694. Risus sardonicus in tetanus. (*Dr. R. G. Ollerenshaw, Manchester Royal Infirmary.*)

Strychnine Poisoning and **Tetanus** are the two chief causes of risus sardonicus. The main point of distinction is the history if this is obtainable— the injection of an overdose of strychnine hypodermically or the taking of a rat-paste, on the one hand, the occurrence of some small but penetrating wound by a rusty nail or earth-soiled knife or stick during the preceding fortnight, on the other. The absence of a visible wound does not necessarily exclude tetanus. If lock-jaw and stiffness of the neck are prominent accompanying features, tetanus is more probable than strychnine poisoning. In strychnine poisoning, either the patient will die quickly or the symptoms will subside rapidly, whereas in tetanus they may persist unabated for several days before death or recovery ensues. In a few instances the diagnosis may only be settled by the discovery of strychnine in the gastric contents, or of tetanus bacilli in anaerobic cultivations from the infected wound.

Malingering may take the form of imitated convulsions, during which the features may be kept fixed in one position or another, sometimes in that of smiling. The fixed voluntary contractions cannot be maintained for long on account of fatigue so that the deception is as a rule easily discovered. The patient is usually a man who has something to gain by malingering, a night's lodging in a hospital, for instance.

Hysteria sometimes takes a form that may for a while raise doubts as to strychnine having been taken, but as a rule the multiformity of the contortions points to the correct explanation. The features may be kept fixed for a time, but sooner or later they become twisted into all sorts of shapes and the tonic and clonic spasms of the body and limbs do not exhibit the regularity of those exhibited in strychnine poisoning and tetanus. Another distinguishing feature is that during a quiescent interval it may be found possible to stroke or touch the patient without bringing on a convulsion, whereas in strychnine poisoning and in tetanus the slightest touch will almost certainly evoke a violent and generalized spasm, even opisthotonos.

Catalepsy. The differential diagnosis is not, as a rule, difficult. The chief characteristic of this condition is the maintenance for hours at a stretch of some attitude that would rapidly fatigue an ordinary person. The facies is by no means always that of smiling, but if it should be then the smile is a fixed one. The history and the associated mental symptoms of melancholia or dementia point to the diagnosis. Tetanus and strychnine poisoning would be excluded by the absence of tetanic spasms.

A few cases of *facial scleroderma* may simulate risus sardonicus, though more often there is complete smoothness of the features and lack of expression. There are no spasmodic contractions, the condition comes on gradually, is permanent, and the diagnosis becomes obvious when the hard smooth skin is palpated.

Ian Mackenzie.

SALIVARY GLANDS, SWELLING OF

The salivary glands are subject to swelling due to inflammation and new growth in the same way as any other organ. In common with other externally secreting glands they are also subject to swelling resulting from retention of secretion. This most commonly occurs as a result of blockage of a duct by a stone. Parotid swelling with fever, often with lacrimal adenitis and uveitis (Mikulicz's syndrome) may occur in leukaemia, Hodgkin's disease, tuberculosis, systemic lupus erythematosus, and sarcoidosis. Confusion in diagnosis may result from the close proximity of the lymphatic glands; in the case of the submandibular the lymphatic nodes may be right in the centre of the salivary tissue. The different glands do not exhibit the same liability to each lesion, the submandibular for instance being the most liable to calculus formation, while inflammatory lesions are only common in the parotid. Mumps is the commonest cause of all salivary swellings; it may occasionally involve other glands than the parotid, but this is a rare exception and usually occurs only after the parotid is first attacked. Here, as in all diagnosis, it is important to decide

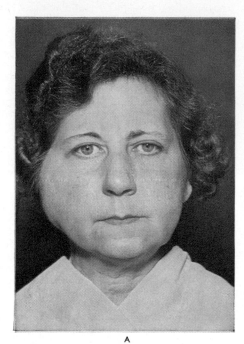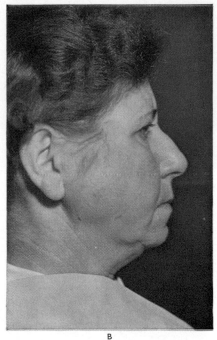

A   B

Fig. 695. Mixed parotid tumour. (*Courtesy of the Gordon Museum, Guy's Hospital.*)

The lesions of the salivary glands may be summarized as follows:

SALIVARY GLAND	ACUTE UNILATERAL ENLARGEMENT	ACUTE BILATERAL ENLARGEMENT	CHRONIC UNILATERAL ENLARGEMENT	CHRONIC BILATERAL ENLARGEMENT
Parotid	Non-specific infective parotitis (rarely bilateral)	Mumps. (One side usually appears first, second commonly appears 24–36 hours later, but occasionally up to 4–5 days later.)	(1) Progressive—growth or inflammation. May involve part of gland only; differentiate from preauricular adenitis by searching area drained, etc. (*see below*) (2) Intermittent—(calculus rare)	Sarcoidosis
	Both of these show signs of inflammation with much pain. In both, orifice of Stensen's duct is red and pouting			
Submandibular	As for parotid, but both very rare. *N.B.* Inflammation of submaxillary lymphatic glands common		(1) Progressive—growth (rare) (2) Intermittent—stone. Swelling occurs at mealtimes when the flow of saliva is stimulated, but the gland is permanently swollen when condition is of long standing. Stone may be palpable in duct and will show on X-ray. Orifice of duct inflamed	
Sublingual	Uncommon. Ranula was originally thought to be due to retention of secretion in this gland, but retention in adjacent simple mucous glands is the more probable explanation.			
All Glands	Mikulicz's syndrome—characterized by chronic painless swelling of all the salivary glands and the lacrimals. This occurs in Hodgkin's disease, tuberculosis, leukaemia, sarcoidosis, and systemic lupus erythematosus.			

the exact anatomical site of the lesion before considering its pathology. For example, swelling of the loose tissues over the jaw from alveolar inflammation may mimic parotitis. A useful point in this connexion is that a generalized parotid swelling tends to lift the auricle away from the head and inspection of the orifice of Stensen's duct within the mouth will usually reveal some abnormality. If lymphatic nodes are suspect as a site of swellings, the presence of others enlarged or of a primary lesion should be sought.

Sialography may prove helpful. Radio-opaque material is injected into the appropriate orifice (Wharton's or Stensen's, the lingual ducts are not suitable for injection). The branching system of ducts is well visualized in the radiograph. Blockage by a stone or by growth, or the presence of a fistula, is the lesion most likely to be demonstrated in this way.

Parotid Tumours. The histology of salivary tumours is complicated and will not be discussed. It is sufficient to mention the so-called 'mixed tumour' (*Fig.* 695) which is benign as a rule although locally recurrent owing to inadequate removal. Characteristically the tumour arises as a lobulated mass, noticed first when about the size of a cherry, and of variable consistency. If there is much myxomatous degeneration, the lump will appear to be fluctuant; if chiefly composed of fibrous tissue it will be hard yet elastic. The lump is painless and is typically situated between the ascending ramus of the mandible and the mastoid process, although no part of the parotid is exempt from this change and these tumours may be found as low as an inch below the angle of the mandible. Women between the ages of 30 and 50 and men between 45 and 60 are the usual sufferers, and a frequent history is that the lump, over a period of years, shows alternating periods of growth and quiescence. Involvement of the facial nerve or fixity to the skin indicates that the growth is a carcinoma.

Sarcoidosis. In sarcoidosis asymptomatic enlargement of the parotid, sublingual, and submaxillary glands occurs in about 6 per cent of cases. Spontaneous resolution often occurs. The glands are not tender. Facial palsy may occur with parotid enlargement. The syndrome of fever, uveitis, and lacrimal and salivary gland enlargement is known as 'uveoparotid' fever or 'Heerfordt's' syndrome.

R. G. Beard.

SALPINGO-OOPHORITIS, CHRONIC (TUBO-OVARIAN ABSCESS, PYO-SALPINX, HYDROSALPINX)

Tubo-ovarian abscess may develop as the result of an attack of pelvic inflammation. The ovary is usually secondarily infected from the Fallopian tube; the ovary is particularly resistant to infection of its substance owing to its thickened capsule (tunica albuginea), but if small thin-walled cysts are present on its surface, or it is

the time of ovulation, infection from a diseased Fallopian tube is liable to take place. However, it is surprising how often extensive salpingitis may be present with little evidence of ovarian involvement. The causal organism is either the gonococcus, which reaches the Fallopian tube by surface spread via the endometrium, or the pyogenic organisms, following infection after childbirth or abortion, when infection spreads via the lymphatics through the parametrium to the ovary, where an ovarian abscess may form. In these cases the Fallopian tube may only show a mild perisalpingitis with no distension, while in the gonococcal variety the tube as well as the ovary is distended with pus. Tuberculosis of the pelvic organs occurs as the result of blood-borne spread nearly always from a focus in the lung.

Occasionally a suppurating appendix may be the cause of a right-sided tubo-ovarian abscess, or a perforated colonic diverticulum may be responsible on the left side. Both these conditions are rare. In all other types the pelvic infection is bilateral, although a tubo-ovarian abscess may only be present on one side. The symptoms are lower abdominal pain, bearing-down feeling, backache, dysmenorrhoea of the congestive type, vaginal discharge, menorrhagia, and a general impairment of health. Bilateral tender fixed masses will be felt on both sides of the uterus, usually larger on one side than the other. If the condition is an acute one the swellings will be very sensitive. The uterus may be displaced backwards, or may be in its normal position, but it cannot be moved separately from the pelvic swellings. Unless the mass is fluctuating it cannot be said with certainty that a tubo-ovarian abscess is present, but a tender mass in the pelvis, with a marked leucocytosis and high temperature in the acute stage, is suggestive. Fluctuation cannot be detected in a chronic abscess owing to induration around it.

1. Suppurating Ovarian Cyst. In this condition the swelling has a more defined outline, and is unilateral. Furthermore, the swelling can be felt when the attack of pain first begins. It takes at least a week for a tubo-ovarian abscess to develop from the time of the start of the attack.

2. Ectopic Gestation. The history of a few weeks' amenorrhoea followed by slight bleeding vaginally is uncommon in tubo-ovarian abscess. The pain is much more colicky and severe, and tends to occur in bouts in an ectopic gestation, and the pelvic mass is unilateral. In an ectopic gestation a pregnancy test may be positive; a negative result is of no value.

3. Pelvic Endometriosis. Differential diagnosis may be impossible, but constitutional symptoms are as a rule absent. The pelvic mass has a more nodular feel; if small nodules can be felt in the utero-sacral ligament, the diagnosis of endometriosis is most probable. The decision is often made only at laparotomy.

4. Pelvic Tuberculosis. Occasionally a tuberculous tubo-ovarian abscess will be found. The characteristic cheesy contents at operation will make the diagnosis obvious, but the diagnosis should be made before operation if possible by examination of the uterine curettings for tuberculous endometritis. Even at operation their nature may not be suspected until microscopically sectioned. They may be suspected if the patient is known to be virgo intacta, or has tuberculosis elsewhere in the body.

Since the use of penicillin and the sulphonamides in the treatment of pelvic infection tuboovarian abscesses are much less frequently encountered.

T. L. T. Lewis.

SCABS

The scab or crust is a secondary lesion of the skin and is produced by inspissation of serous exudate, pus, or blood, or a mixture of any of them. In addition it may contain dirt and the remains of local applications. As a rule scabs constitute the last stage of vesicles, bullae, pustules, ulcers, and erosions, and may be the result of scratching. They vary considerably in thickness, from the light crust in exudative dermatitis to the thick barnacle-like scab of rupia. The colour is determined by the constituents, and in severe impetigo in a dirty individual they may be dark green or black from admixture with grime. It may sometimes be necessary to remove a crust before a diagnosis can be made; an epithelioma of the skin may be so heavily crusted over that its nature is disguised.

In *herpes simplex* the vesicles dry up to form fine yellowish crusts, which separate after a few days leaving no mark, but it is not uncommon for this disease to become secondarily impetiginized and exhibit the weeping and heavier crusting of that disease.

In *herpes zoster* the same thing may occur, but more often there is a deeper secondary septic infection which may give rise to pustules and ulcers; in the latter case there will be scarring.

The crusts in *sycosis barbae*, which affects the hairy parts of the face, are brown or yellow and thin and adherent. It is around the mouth that scab formation mostly occurs.

In *impetigo contagiosa* (*Fig.* 121, p. 116) scabs are formed by the rapid drying of the discharge. They are usually of a characteristic amber colour. At first loosely attached, the scabs in impetigo contagiosa later become so firmly adherent that their removal may need some force, which in turn may cause bleeding. The reddish stain that appears when the lesion heals is not permanent.

In *ecthyma* the flat irregular scab formed from the ruptured vesicle is surrounded by a more or less pronounced hyperaemic areola.

In *pemphigus vulgaris* the crusts into which the bullae dry are brownish-yellow and when they fall off the surface beneath is not raw, as in impetigo, but is covered with newly formed epithelium. In *pemphigus foliaceus* (*Fig.* 123, p. 118),

the crusts are yellowish, and as the disease proceeds large scales are formed. In the vegetating type (*pemphigus vegetans*) the foul-smelling secretion from the patches of affected skin forms a thin crust which can be stripped off easily, revealing moist vegetations.

In the rare rupial form of secondary syphilis the crusts are greenish or blackish and consist of

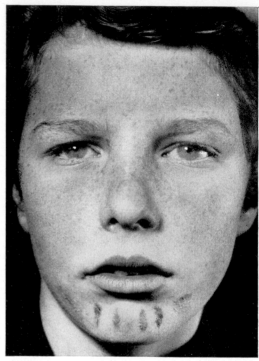

Fig. 696. Typical self-produced lesions with scabbing.

several layers, each smaller than the one immediately below it, so that a pyramidal structure is formed resembling a barnacle. Removal of these crusts exposes a foul-smelling ulcer. As a rule rupia occurs only in undernourished individuals.

One of the features of *yaws* (framboesia) is the heavy crusting which occurs on the top of the granulations of that disease. Occasionally crusts form on a patch of lupus vulgaris; they are greenish in colour and probably due to secondary infection. The long history and the presence of 'apple-jelly' nodules will identify the disease.

Keratodermia blennorrhagica is the skin eruption of Reiter's syndrome. It is chronic and is characterized by a symmetrical eruption of nodules, pustules, and crusts on any part of the body, but particularly on the palms and soles. It may have to be distinguished from arthropathic psoriasis.

Brown crusts accompany the pustules on palms and soles in pustular psoriasis.

In *smallpox* the formation of scabs on the pustules begins in the centre and causes a secondary 'umbilication'; it is generally attended by intense itching; in from three to four weeks from their appearance the crusts fall off, leaving a reddened surface, made uneven by scars or 'pits'. The true nature of the disease will have been discovered, even in doubtful cases, before the crust stage is reached (*see* PUSTULES, p. 677).

In the diagnosis of *ulcers* the crust is of little importance; these are dealt with under FACE, ULCERATION OF (p. 272), FOOT, ULCERATION OF (p. 304), *and* LEG, ULCERATION OF (p. 489).

It should not be forgotten that dermatitis, scabs, and ulcers may sometimes be produced deliberately by malingerers or by neurotics (*Fig.* 696).

P. D. Samman.

SCALP AND BEARD, FUNGOUS AFFECTIONS OF

Ringworm of the Scalp (tinea tonsurans) is mainly a disease of childhood. It is contracted by direct contact. In England the greatest number of cases are caused by the small-spored *Microsporum audouini* and *M. canis*, and the remainder by large-spored trichophytons. The small-spored infections only occur in children, the large-spored may occasionally be found in adults.

The hair follicles are at first infected, causing a small, red, scaly patch on which the hairs are broken off short: some of these hair stumps are bent or twisted, rather like downtrodden stubble. The patch extends at the periphery and further patches soon appear on other parts of the scalp. Itching of the patches may or may not be present and the degree of scaliness varies from a fine branny desquamation to heaped-up masses of soft scales (*Fig.* 7, p. 16).

Diagnosis is determined by examining a few stumps soaked in liquor potassii under the microscope, when the spores of the fungus may be readily seen. Cases of small-spored ringworm of the scalp when examined in a darkened room with ultra-violet light filtered through Wood's glass (glass containing nickel oxide) show a characteristic greenish fluorescence of affected hairs. Other features are the age of the patient and a possible history of contact with a known case; but it must be remembered that the disease is relatively uncommon today.

It must be distinguished from alopecia areata, in which the patches are uniformly bald and smooth, and in which there is no redness or scaliness. Patches of alopecia areata may, however, have been rendered temporarily red and scaly by the application of strong stimulating lotions.

In psoriasis of the scalp there are heaped-up masses of scales. In seborrhoea of the scalp there is a diffuse fine scaling with no broken hairs. In impetigo of the scalp there are loose amber-coloured crusts and often pediculosis as well. In chronic streptococcal dermatitis there are red, scaly patches, some loss of hair but no stumps, and a tendency for the scales to climb up the hairs.

Very rarely in large-spored ringworm of the scalp the infection is so severe that multiple abscesses form in the hair follicles, which run together and invade the underlying tissues. This is known as a *kerion* and its appearance is very similar to that of a carbuncle, the lesion being boggy and tender, with pus exuding from the follicles. This eventually causes patches of permanent baldness.

These infections are usually due to fungi of animal origin, *Trichophyton verrucosum* (*T. discoides*) or *T. mentagrophytes*. *T. sulphureum*, on the other hand, is a fungus found only in human beings and produces a very mild reaction with minimal scaling. There may be little hairfall so that it is difficult to trace contacts and confirm the presence of infection as the hairs do not fluoresce under Wood's light. The most satisfactory way of tracing the infection is to examine hairs and scales on the hairbrushes of suspected patients and to make cultures direct from the hairbrush. Black dot ringworm is another condition due to a fungus found only in man (*T. violaceum* in most cases). Here the hairs break off close to the scalp and it is necessary to remove some of the short stumps for examination to confirm the diagnosis. A number of other fungi may infect the scalp, including *T. soudanense* and *T. gourvilli*.

Favus is a rare fungous infection of the scalp, in which other parts of the body may be affected. It is caused as a rule by the *Achorion schönleinii*, and in a small number of cases by the *Achorion quinckeanum* or mouse favus. It first appears as tiny yellow disks or cups (scutula), each of which is pierced by a hair. These increase in size and become crusted, but at all times at the edge of the crust scutula may be seen. The hairs are not broken but are easily pulled out, and there is a characteristic musty smell associated with the disease. The disease causes scarring and patches of permanent baldness. Diagnosis is easy when there are scutula, and in all cases identification of the parasite on microscopical examination of hairs is relatively simple.

Ringworm of the Beard is a rare disorder confined almost exclusively to agricultural workers who contract the disease from infected animals. It may take the form of superficial crusted bald patches with folliculitis or more usually a deep suppurative type (*see* KERION *above*). It is distinguished from sycosis barbae by its situation on the hairy part of the neck and along the jaw, whereas the chin and face are more usually involved in sycosis. The nature of the patient's work, a history of contact with infected cattle, and finally the presence of fungus in hairs examined under the microscope will determine the nature of the disease.

P. D. Samman.

SCALP, TENDERNESS OF

Tenderness of the scalp may be due to local disease of the skin, pericranium, skull, or meninges. It may be a referred phenomenon, caused by disease of the upper cervical spine, the nuchal muscles and fascia, the eye, teeth, accessory sinuses, and (perhaps) the viscera. And finally, it is a common symptom of an anxiety state.

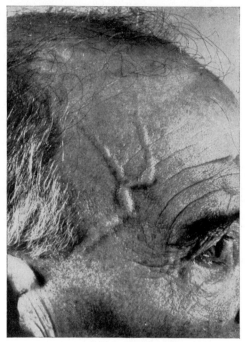

Fig. 697. The superficial temporal artery in a case of giant-cell arteritis which was enlarged, pulseless, and tender.

Diseases of the skin which are accompanied by an inflammatory reaction give rise to local tenderness—*pediculosis, ringworm* (when infected: kerion celsi), *seborrhoeic dermatitis, favus, furunculosis, infected sebaceous cysts, impetigo, acne decalvans, erysipelas, dermatitis herpetiformis, lupus erythematosus.* In *Von Recklinghausen's disease* subcutaneous neurofibromata may cause tender nodules in the scalp, whereas the nodules of *molluscum fibrosum* are not tender. *Scleroderma* of the scalp may occasion much tenderness in the early stages; it is a chronic diffuse infiltration of the skin, ending in atrophy, and supposed by some to include the *pseudopelade* of Bracq, an atrophic indurative affection of the scalp, giving rise to depressed areas of permanent baldness that adhere to the underlying skull. *Herpes ophthalmicus* may cause extreme superficial tenderness within the territory of the affected division of the trigeminal nerve: the history of an eruption, the severe pain, and the scar of healed vesicles will make clear the diagnosis. *Giant-cell*

arteritis, a cause of intense pain and local tenderness of the temple, often involves the arteries of the rest of the scalp and elsewhere. They are distended, hard, and tender. (*Fig.* 697). There may be accompanying visual disturbances owing to a similar affection of the vessels supplying the optic nerve. There may be unformed visual hallucinations followed by rapid loss of vision in one or both eyes. Complete blindness can occur within a few hours, and recovery is unusual. Diplopia occasionally occurs in cases without visual loss and, unlike those with visual loss, prognosis for recovery is good. It is a disease of the elderly, and is pathologically distinct from polyarteritis nodosa.

Diseases of the pericranium and skull bones are uncommon. Local tenderness at the site of an *injury* is of course a common occurrence, but it seldom persists for long and when present months or years after the injury it is usually associated with psychoneurosis; occasionally it is due to a small neuroma at the site of the scar. Tenderness of the skull is found in *rickets*, in congenital or acquired syphilitic periostitis, gummata of the pericranium, and primary or secondary tumours of the cranial bones. The value of X-ray examination of the skull in such cases needs no emphasis.

Affections of the meninges—meningitis, subarachnoid haemorrhage, subdural haematoma, cerebral abscess, meningioma, invasion of the membranes by malignant gliomata or by carcinomatosis—may cause tenderness, but it is important to remember that this is the exception rather than the rule. Strictly localized tenderness sometimes occurs over a superficial tumour, but only if the meninges are involved. Significant tenderness of the scalp is seldom found in cases of raised intracranial pressure.

Referred tenderness of the anterior half of the scalp on one side is seen in *tic douloureux*; a light touch to the hair may precipitate a paroxysm of pain, but firm pressure is not painful. On the other hand, when trigeminal neuralgia is due to irritation of the trigeminal nerve by tumour or inflammation within the skull, there may be persistent cutaneous tenderness associated with impairment of sensation and an early loss of the corneal reflex. Hyperalgesia of the posterior part of the scalp—in the distribution of the second cervical root—is very common in *cervical spondylosis*; there is an associated tenderness of the cervical muscles. Some authorities believe that *fibrositis* of this area is an important source of occipital pain and tenderness. The writer regards such muscular tenderness as the result of spondylosis, since proof of the existence of 'fibrositis' as a pathological entity is lacking. Other examples of referred tenderness are seen in *diseases of the eye, frontal sinusitis, otitis media, mastoiditis,* and *disease of the upper teeth.* Thus glaucoma, iritis, and refractive errors occasionally cause pain and tenderness over the anterior half of the scalp; frontal sinusitis acts in similar fashion. Disease of the ear causes tenderness over the same side of the head. Dental disease may give rise to considerable hyperalgesia in the temporal region. *Visceral disease* is rarely associated with referred tenderness of the scalp. Sir Henry Head taught that disease of the heart, lungs, or stomach may cause pain and tenderness in the temporal region, but this observation has little practical value except in so far as it stresses the need for a complete history and a thorough examination in all cases of headache and tenderness of the scalp.

Finally, tenderness of the scalp is often complained of in psychoneurosis. In such cases there are often complaints of additional sensations— 'pins and needles', a sensation of cold or heat, a feeling as if a nail were being driven into the skull, and so on. Diagnosis is suggested by the bizarre nature of the symptoms, the absence of organic disease, and the presence of satellite symptoms of psychoneurosis.

Ian Mackenzie.

SCALY ERUPTIONS

The scale is a dry laminated exfoliation of the skin and is the result of either an inherent dryness of the skin, as in ichthyosis, or of hyperaemia and inflammation; the latter is the usual cause in most scaly skin diseases.

As a rule scales consist of dead cells of the horny layer, but in psoriasis the shedding of these cells is so rapid that their nuclei are still present. The latter process is known as 'parakeratosis'.

Scales vary in size and colour and may be dry, moist, or greasy. In all inflammatory disorders of the skin the final stage is scaling, and as a rule the more acute the inflammation the more severe the scaling will be. Examples of this are found in acute *toxic erythema*, *dermatitis*, and *scarlet fever*. In *fungous affections of the skin* (q.v.) there is always considerable scaliness, and when ringworm of the toes has spread to the feet it must be distinguished from dermatitis due to contact with a skin irritant such as rubber footwear, chemicals, medicaments, or other substances; the late stage of pompholyx; or the hyperkeratotic plantar syphilide (*Fig.* 698). In the last case the lesion is frequently unilateral and the serological tests will be positive. In no instance should a diagnosis of foot ringworm be made unless a fungus is found in scrapings.

Psoriasis of the palms and soles (*Fig.* 699) is usually accompanied by typical lesions elsewhere. The same applies to *lichen planus* (*Fig.* 700), in which, when the palms and soles are affected, there is considerable desquamation.

In *xeroderma* and *ichthyosis*, which are congenital conditions, there is dryness and scaliness of the skin, but the fact that the skin retains its normal colour, and the history of the case, will usually make the diagnosis obvious. In *ichthyosis serpentina* the scales are coarser and darker. It has a sex-linked inheritance. In *tylosis* there is congenital hyperkeratosis of the palms and soles only.

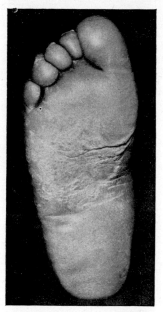

Fig. 698. Late syphilide affecting one sole. (*Dr. Peter Hansell.*)

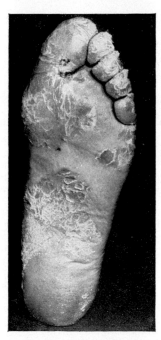

Fig. 699. Psoriasis of the sole. (*Dr. Peter Hansell.*)

In *lupus erythematosus* (*Fig.* 701) there are areas of scaly erythema of varying degree, from the superficial type in which the scales are thin and lightly adherent to an erythematous base, to the fixed type in which there is marked induration and thick and more firmly adherent scales.

This disorder affects the light-exposed areas and in its commonest form takes on a butterfly-wing shape over the nose and cheeks. On removing a scale little plugs may be seen on the under-surface where the sebaceous follicles have been blocked. The diagnosis is usually simple but occasionally, as when it is confined to patches on the scalp or on the fingers, it may present real difficulty. When what are apparently chilblains persist through warm weather, the possibility of lupus

of erythema and even weeping. It is likely that these acute outbreaks are due to secondary infection. This disorder has to be distinguished from *streptococcal dermatitis of the scalp* (acute or chronic), *lupus erythematosus*, and *psoriasis*. In the first condition there are localized patches of scaly erythema as opposed to seborrhoeic dermatitis, which is uniformly spread over the whole scalp. Acute seborrhoeic dermatitis may spread to the face, particularly around the eyes

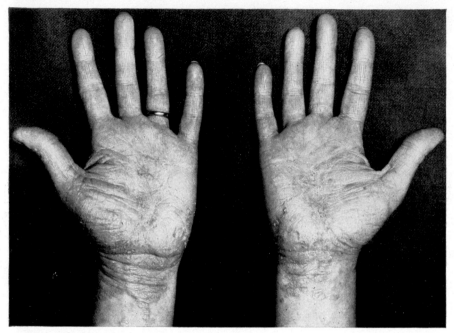

Fig. 700. Lichen planus of the palms. Note typical lichen planus lesions on the wrists.

erythematosus should be considered. Lupus erythematosus, including disseminate lupus erythematosus, is discussed more fully under ERYTHEMA (p. 257).

Lupus vulgaris (*Fig.* 702) is often scaly, but when it affects the face it usually ulcerates early. The patches are brown rather than red, and on pressure under glass the so-called apple-jelly nodules become apparent. Scarring is also a feature of this disease. (*See also Fig.* 577, p. 574.)

In *pityriasis sicca* or *alba* there are dry, scaly, white, yellowish, or skin-coloured patches on the face, mostly around the mouth. Children are chiefly affected. The cause is unknown but it is more common in atopic individuals, i.e., children with a personal or family history of infantile dermatitis or asthma.

In *seborrhoea of the scalp* the chief symptom is the perpetual scaling which takes place (dandruff). The scales are made up of exfoliated epidermic cells together with inspissated sebum and varying amounts of surface dirt. From time to time the disease may take on an acuter phase (*seborrhoeic dermatitis*), when there will be areas

and ears and on to the pinnae, where there will be considerable local oedema and erythema associated with the scaliness. *Psoriasis* may affect the scalp alone, and this is a far from uncommon form of the disease. When this occurs the patches are thick and feel lumpy and the scales are much more silvery than those of seborrhoea. In *ringworm of the scalp*, which rarely occurs after puberty, there are red scaly patches partly devoid of hair. On them short stumps will be found and examination of these stumps microscopically will reveal fungus.

When *seborrhoeic dermatitis* affects the trunk there are dry, pinkish-yellow, scaly patches, and these may occur without seborrhoea of the scalp being present. Itching is often minimal. Favourite sites for these patches (seborrhoeides) are over the sternum (*Fig.* 703) and between the shoulders.

In *pityriasis rosea* the eruption, which consists of numerous round or oval, pinkish or fawn, scaly patches, is confined to the trunk, the neck, the arms down to the elbows, and the legs down to the knees. The diagnosis is usually simple, as the eruption is normally preceded by a 'herald patch' which occurs somewhere on the trunk from 10 to 14 days before the main eruption. This patch may be confused with a patch of animal ringworm, but the absence of fungus from the scales will rule out this condition. When the scales begin to separate they do so from the centre, leaving a fine collarette of scales as a surround, with the free edge pointing inwards.

Psoriasis (*Figs.* 704–706) is one of the commonest of skin diseases and is also the most scaly. The scales are of distinct diagnostic importance, for when not at once apparent they may always be produced by lightly scratching

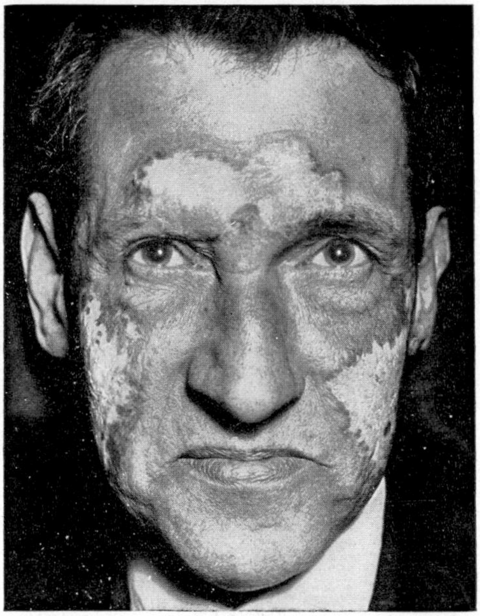

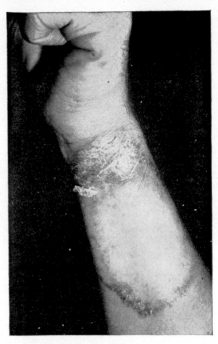

Fig. 701. Lupus erythematosus. Fixed type with marked scarring.

Fig. 702. Lupus vulgaris, showing marked scaliness of the active edge and scarring in the centre.

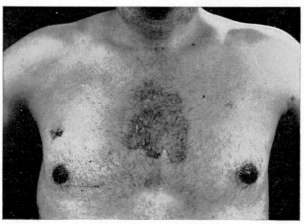

Fig. 703. Patch of seborrhoeic dermatitis.

This is the only disease in which this method of scale separation occurs. Pityriasis rosea is frequently confused with secondary syphilis, but there is no real occasion for this. In *secondary syphilis* the lesions are always characteristically copper-coloured, indurated, not confined to the trunk and upper parts of the limbs, and are associated with other signs of that disease.

the surface of a lesion. In character the scales are silvery or asbestos-like and profuse. In some instances they are heaped up into dense concrete-like masses. The lesions are of all sizes from that of a pin's head to vast sheets, even up to a foot across on the trunk. The initial lesion is a scaly, dark-red papule which may remain small or rapidly grow in size. Later, individual patches

23

may run together or they may fade in the centre and spread at the periphery. The commonest sites to be affected by psoriasis are the extensor surfaces of the knees, elbows, and the scalp, but any part of the body may be involved. The disease may start at any age, but most commonly

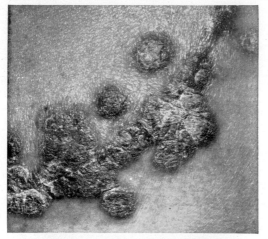

Fig. 704. Psoriasis showing heaping up of the scales.

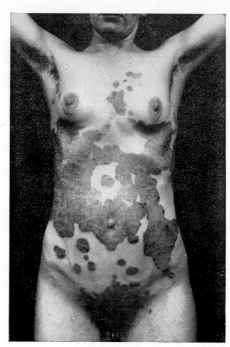

Fig. 705. Psoriasis.

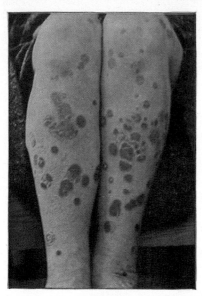

Fig. 706. Psoriasis.

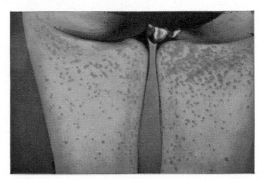

Fig. 707. Acute guttate psoriasis. (Dr. Peter Hansell.)

the initial cause is unknown, it is generally recognized that exacerbations of the disease occur under emotional stresses, and it is under extreme mental tension that the rapidly generalizing form of the malady occurs. When this takes place rapidly it may be temporarily transformed into

in childhood or adolescence. It tends to break out in bouts and sometimes disappears spontaneously and does not recur for months or years. The first attack of psoriasis is sometimes an acute generalized eruption consisting of minute lesions which enlarge quickly, but there may be no true scaling for several days. This type is often preceded by streptococcal infection of the throat and has therefore to be distinguished from exanthematic eruptions in the early stages. It is known as *acute guttate psoriasis* (*Fig.* 707). While

what is, to all intents and purposes, an acute exfoliative dermatitis; but even in the worst type of this form of the disease careful search will show true elements of psoriasis. The diagnosis in all but the last form of the disease is usually easy, but in doubtful cases the characteristic pitting of the nails (p. 558) should be looked for and the scalp carefully examined. When psoriasis occurs in the flexures there is considerable erythema and the scales are usually larger and duller in character. There is a psoriasiform type of *late syphilide* when the lesions may strongly resemble psoriasis. Scratching of the surface, however, will not produce the typical scales of psoriasis. There is an arthropathic form of

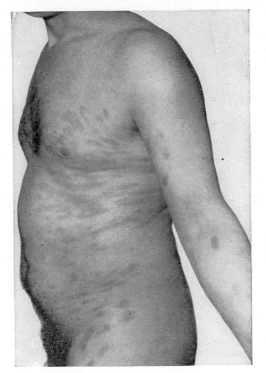

Fig. 708. Parapsoriasis *en plâques*. (*Dr. Peter Hansell.*)

psoriasis associated with the rheumatoid type of arthritis.

There are several forms of *exfoliative dermatitis* including: (1) a primary idiopathic form (pityriasis rubra); (2) a form resulting from the toxic effect of drugs, such as novarsenobillon or gold salts; and (3) a type complicating other skin diseases, such as dermatitis, erythema multiforme, lichen planus, and above all, psoriasis. Overtreatment may be a cause, especially in psoriasis, but it may also be the result of an extra acute attack of that disease. Clinically the whole cutaneous surface becomes red and inflamed and this is rapidly followed by profuse branny desquamation; there is no induration of the skin and no exudation. Itching is a variable symptom. In the primary idiopathic form the prognosis is poor as it may progress to a fatal termination after a few years. In the other types recovery takes place sooner or later, but the attack may last many months. The diagnosis is usually easy, especially in view of the continual branny desquamation and absence of weeping. In a minority of cases exfoliative dermatitis is a symptom of a reticulosis, e.g., Hodgkin's disease or leukaemia. In any case of long-standing exfoliation there may be signs of malabsorption.

Pityriasis rubra pilaris (p. 616) is often associated with a good deal of scaliness of the patches. Sometimes this disease produces a generalized exfoliation and may be difficult to distinguish from psoriasis.

There is a group of diseases which are often described as the *erythemato-squamous eruptions*. These include seborrhoeic dermatitis of the trunk (the seborrhoeides), pityriasis rosea, secondary syphilis, pityriasis lichenoides acuta, pityriasis lichenoides chronica, and *parapsoriasis en plâques*. Three of these have already been described above.

Parapsoriasis en plâques (*Fig.* 708) is an uncommon affection presenting with patches which are erythematous and covered with a fine scale. The patches may be round or oval or arranged in finger-like processes. They affect trunk and

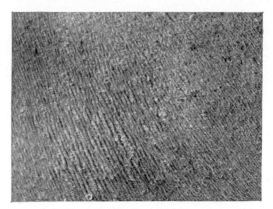

Fig. 709. Poikilodermia vasculare atrophicans. (*Dr. Peter Hansell.*)

limbs. They are extremely stubborn and last for years, gradually increasing in numbers. Treatment may remove them temporarily but they always return and are more prominent in winter than summer. There is little itching but the patient may complain that the patches feel dry. The condition known as *poikilodermia vasculare atrophicans* (*Fig.* 709) (or atrophic parapsoriasis) is another chronic and intractable condition showing patches of reticular pigmentation, telangiectasia, and atrophy. The skin surface in the affected areas shows a fine wrinkling which gives the appearance of scaling, although no true scaling is present. The condition may affect any area but especially the flexures and the breasts. A high percentage of these cases progress to a reticulosis.

Pityriasis lichenoides chronica (previously known as *parapsoriasis guttata*) is another uncommon condition. It presents with widespread small erythematous patches covered with a fine scale which may be picked off intact, unlike the scales of psoriasis which come away in layers. It may occur at any age. In children it usually lasts about three months but in adults may persist for years, individual lesions only lasting for a short time but being constantly replaced by others.

Pityriasis lichenoides acuta is a variant of the above in which larger erythematous patches appear in addition to the smaller ones and show a marked tendency to break down and ulcerate, leaving varioliform scars. Vesicles may precede the ulcerations and this phase has to be distinguished from chicken-pox. The 'acute' phase may last for a few weeks or persist with remissions for years. A few of these cases show abnormal mononuclear cells histologically closely resembling a reticulosis.

P. D. Samman.

SCROTAL SORES

Ulceration of the scrotum occurs in association with:

1. New growth:
   Epithelioma
   Papilloma
2. Fistulae
3. Syphilis
4. Testicular disease:
   Inflammatory
   Tuberculous
   Syphilitic
   Malignant growths
5. Suppurating cysts
6. Infected haematocele
7. Irritants and corrosives, such as mustard gas
8. Behçet's syndrome, herpes simplex, candidiasis.

1. New Growth. *Epithelioma of the scrotum,* formerly known as 'chimney-sweep's cancer', or 'tar-worker's cancer', is by no means limited to these occupations, but is certainly more common in men engaged in work in which they are exposed to much irritation from solid particles or from noxious fumes. Hence the disease is, or was, most commonly seen amongst chimney-sweeps, employees in gas works, paraffin, tar, and chemical works, and coal mines, and in mule-spinners in the cotton trade. It often begins as a small subcutaneous nodule, over which the skin is thinned and adherent; the nodule enlarges slowly, and the thinned covering gives way, to form an ulcer with thickened irregular edges and a tendency to bleed on slight injury. The ulcerated area extends both radially and into the tissues of the scrotum, later involving the testes. The inguinal lymphatic glands become enlarged soon after active ulceration begins, at first from inflammatory causes, later from malignant infiltration and, untreated, themselves ulcerate; this indeed is the common mode of death in this condition, from repeated haemorrhages. In other cases a scrotal epithelioma begins in a *wart* or *papilloma,* which may have been present for years with only slight increase in growth (*Fig.* 710). These soft papillomata are not unusually the starting-point of malignant change, when they become more vascular, while the surface epithelium becomes thinned and easily excoriated. A small amount of foul discharge is present, often

encrusted into a scab, which on removal leaves an ulcer with indurated, everted edges, with the gradual progress of a cutaneous epithelioma. Any ulcer on the scrotum, especially if indurated

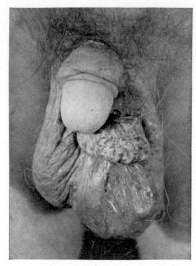

Fig. 710. Epithelioma of scrotum.

or readily caused to bleed, must be looked upon with extreme suspicion and immediately subjected to biopsy for microscopic examination. It is not unusual, however, for a large mass of glands to be found in the groin when the primary lesion is very small and almost imperceptible. The scrotum must be examined very carefully in such cases lest the primary lesion be missed.

Epithelioma may occur in the scrotal area as a localized recurrence after removal of a malignant growth of the penis or testicle or rarely the bladder. Knowledge of the previous condition for which operation has been performed would give the diagnosis.

2. Fistulae may occur in the scrotum and cause ulceration. Sinuses occur in association with tuberculous or syphilitic disease of the testes, but fistulae may follow urine extravasation, or burrowing from rectal suppuration. An abscess may form and open through the scrotal skin from a peri-urethral abscess accompanying an acute urethritis or formed by septic infection behind a urethral stricture. In either case a small amount of urine may leak through the opening during micturition while the history of urethral discharge, or of difficulty in micturition and other symptoms of stricture, will point to the diagnosis.

3. Syphilis of the Scrotum may be present either as a primary chancre or as a mucous tubercle. A *primary chancre* in this situation is by no means easy to recognize unless other signs of syphilis are present; but the presence of a cutaneous sore which does not show much inclination to heal under antiseptic dressings should always give a suspicion of syphilis. There is often only slight induration of the ulcer compared with that of a penile chancre, but the edge is raised and of a rolled appearance. The inguinal lymphatic glands are enlarged and discrete, and some five to six weeks after the commencement of the ulcer the usual secondary symptoms of syphilis become manifest.

Mucous tubercles may be present on the scrotum, usually on the femoral aspect. They may extend directly from the anal area. No difficulty will be met with in the diagnosis, as other signs of syphilis are obvious.

4. Testicular Disease. In some cases extension of disease in the testicle may involve the coverings of the scrotum, and may even perforate them to form a scrotal sore. This sequence occasionally occurs with: (1) A testicular abscess; (2) Tuberculosis of the epididymis; (3) Gumma of the testis; (4) Malignant disease of the testis.

A *testicular abscess* is somewhat uncommon, but may arise from direct extension from the urethra via the vesiculae seminales and vasa deferentia or by a haematogenous infection during the course of a specific fever, such as scarlet fever, mumps, or typhoid fever. With urethral disease, the primary trouble may be due to gonorrhoea, or more frequently to a septic urethritis from the introduction of infected instruments, and is thus not infrequent in cases of prostatic enlargement in which the patient is passing his own catheter. In cases in which the infective process extends from the urethra the epididymis is affected first, while in the metastatic cases the body of the testis usually shows the first sign of enlargement. If the vas has been divided as part of the operation of prostatectomy, the swelling and possible abscess will occur in the upper part of the scrotum at the site of the division. These acute inflammations of the testis occasionally suppurate, when the scrotal tunics become inflamed and adherent, whilst softening occurs later, and unless surgically relieved the abscess opens through the skin, leaving an ulcer, and a sinus discharging pus. An unusual form of abscess of the testicle is caused by a *suppurating dermoid cyst* of the testicle, and may discharge through the scrotal coverings to form an ulcer.

Tuberculosis of the testicle rarely occurs as a primary disease but more often as a secondary deposit in association with tuberculosis elsewhere in the genito-urinary tract. Testicular tubercle almost always begins as a nodule in the epididymis, but in the later progress of the disease may extend into the testis proper. If the tuberculous nodule progresses rather than undergoes cure, the scrotal skin becomes adherent, thinned, and finally perforated, leaving a shallow ulcer with thin, undermined edges, and discharging thin pus. The ulcer in this case is most likely to be on the posterior aspect of the scrotum. Occasionally the necrotic epididymis fungates through the opening in the scrotum, appearing as a greyish, sloughy projection from the cutaneous opening—the so-called 'hernia testis'.

A *gumma of the testis* causes a swelling in the body of the testis rather than in the epididymis.

A gumma which remains unrecognized or untreated may soften and ulcerate through the scrotal skin in a manner similar to tuberculous disease, leaving a clearly defined ulcerated area with sharply cut margins and a wash-leather-like sloughy base. Such ulcers are usually placed on the front of the scrotum. The gummatous granulation tissue may fungate through the scrotal aperture, forming a yellowish necrotic mass.

The diagnosis of these three conditions may produce some difficulty in the earlier stages (*see* SCROTAL SWELLING, p. 710), but in the advanced stage now under consideration, when an open scrotal sore is present, the diagnosis is easier. The *opening of a testicular abscess* on the scrotum leaves a small sinus discharging pus and accompanied by a general enlargement of the organ. Preceding the rupture of the abscess there is acute pain in the testicle, with rise of temperature, rigors, and general signs of suppuration, which are much diminished as soon as the abscess bursts or is incised. There is often a urethral discharge, which, however, is frequently much lessened with the onset of the acute epididymitis, with distinct thickening of the cord and aching pain in the neighbourhood of the external abdominal ring. In metastatic cases the abscess occurs during the progress of an acute fever. The general history is one of acute pain beginning in the testicle, with rapid and extremely tender swelling of the organ, followed by abscess formation.

In *tuberculosis of the testis* the progress is much more gradual. A nodule may have been present in the epididymis for some time, gradually enlarging, but causing very little pain; in some cases a nodule may have been present for months without any apparent change, and then it may enlarge rapidly, involve the scrotal tunics, and discharge its contents. By the time the disease has reached this stage it is probable that evidence of tuberculous trouble will be found in other organs, particularly the other testis, prostate, seminal vesicles, or bladder. The affected testicle usually presents several nodules in the epididymis, tender on pressure, whilst small nodules may also be felt in the vas deferens.

The opening remaining from the discharge of a *gummatous orchitis* is usually a rounded ulcer with sharply cut edges and yellowish base. The whole testis is enlarged and practically painless. The cord is not thickened, and there is no evidence of disease in the other testicle, prostate, or seminal vesicles. There is probably a history of syphilis, and other tertiary syphilitic lesions may be present elsewhere, such as gummatous periostitis.

A *hernial protrusion of necrotic testicular tissue* may be present either with tuberculous disease or from a gumma. In tuberculosis the mass is greyish and necrotic, discharging thin pus, and there will be evidence of tuberculous disease in the underlying testis and other genital organs. Tubercle bacilli very rarely may be found in the discharge. A distinctive feature of the gummatous hernia testis is found in the appearance of the cutaneous opening; if the fungating mass is pushed aside the opening in the scrotal skin will be seen to be cleanly cut and to encircle the protruding tissue tightly. The fungating hernia testis of tubercle or syphilis must also be diagnosed from other conditions producing a raised tumour on the scrotum. An epithelioma of the scrotum has raised borders, but the centre is

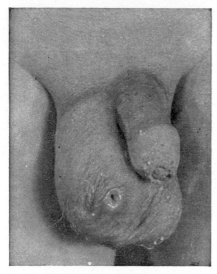

Fig. 711. Infected haematocele.

excavated, and there is rarely any enlargement of the testis. A sloughing papilloma of the scrotum may more nearly reproduce the appearance, but the tumour and the skin are freely movable on the underlying testis, while in hernia testis the mass is connected with the testicle, and the tubular structure of the latter is often apparent on picking up a small fragment of the fungating tumour.

New growths of the testis seldom cause ulceration of the scrotum because they have generally been removed by operation before so late a stage is reached; any variety, however, whether seminoma or teratoma, may cause local recurrence in the scar, with ulceration; the diagnosis depends upon histological examination either of the tumour previously removed, or of snippings from the edge of the recurrence. Occasionally fungation of the tumour is seen through the scar of the biopsy site in the scrotal skin when there has been delay in carrying out definitive treatment, a state of affairs which should never be allowed to happen.

5. Cysts of the Scrotum. As an exceptional occurrence, a sebaceous cyst in the scrotal skin may suppurate and leave an open sore. The areas remaining present raised borders, and are easily mistaken for an early epithelioma. An accurate history of the previous swelling in the skin is of little assistance in these cases, but microscopical

examination of a piece removed from the margin of the ulcer will exclude malignancy. A suppurating cyst in the scrotum is less common than epithelioma.

6. A Haematocele which becomes infected may form an abscess which bursts through the scrotal coverings (*Fig.* 711). It may have a superficial resemblance to a gumma.

7. Mustard Gas caused most troublesome ulceration of the scrotum, as of other parts, during the war of 1914–18; but the diagnosis is easy if the correct history of exposure to this or some other irritant is available.

8. Behçet's Syndrome causes painful ulcerative lesions of the scrotum as well as the penis, unlike the lesions in the vulva and vagina, which are often painless and therefore often missed. Behçet's syndrome may be accompanied by abscesses or herpes-like lesions of the scrotum. Herpes simplex, both types I and II, may cause vesicular lesions less commonly, and very rarely candidiasis.

Harold Ellis.

SCROTAL SWELLING

It is first essential to prove that the swelling is really scrotal. This is done by grasping the root of the scrotum between the thumb and index finger to determine whether any of the swelling extends along the cord into the inguinal region. True scrotal swellings may arise in: (1) Skin; (2) The various connective-tissue coverings of the testicle; (3) Tunica vaginalis; (4) Testicle; (5) Epididymis; (6) The lower end of the spermatic cord; (7) The urethra; (8) The bones of the pubic arch. Of these the swellings in the cord, testicle, epididymis, and tunica vaginalis are the commonest and most important.

1. Swellings affecting the Skin. The nature of these is usually obvious. The only common ones are boils, soft sores and chancre, sebaceous cysts, warts, and epithelioma. The last-named soon ulcerates and commonly occurs in sweeps or in those who work in tar, tar products, or petroleum; the groin glands soon become enlarged.

2. Swellings of the various Connective-tissue Coverings are rare, but occasionally a fibrosarcoma may occur. These swellings are movable upon the testicle. The symmetrical enlargement called *elephantiasis scroti* (*Fig.* 712), due to the *Filaria sanguinis hominis*, is limited to the tropics, though sometimes a similar state of scrotal distension and overgrowth results in Great Britain from lymphatic obstruction due to pelvic cellulitis or to congenital abnormality. The enlarged scrotum resulting from acute generalized oedema in acute or chronic renal disease is seldom difficult to recognize; the penis and prepuce are generally distended by oedema at the same time as are the legs, loins, eyelids, and other parts, and the diagnosis is confirmed by the albumin and tube-casts in the urine.

Gross oedematous scrotal swelling also occurs with ascites or inferior vena caval thrombosis, and may accompany the abdominal swelling of pellagra and infantile kwashiorkor.

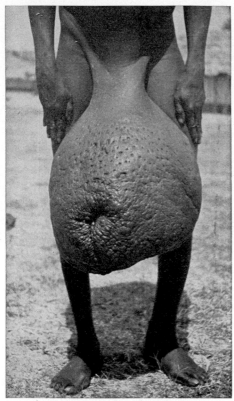

Fig. 712. Elephantiasis of the scrotum due to filariasis. (*Dr. C. J. Hackett, Wellcome Museum of Medical Science.*)

Neurodermatitis affecting the scrotum may produce a considerable amount of scrotal oedema, as does moniliasis (candidiasis).

3. The Tunica Vaginalis may become distended with serous fluid, blood, or pus: distension with fluid may be primary, the ordinary vaginal hydrocele, or secondary to disease of the testis or epididymis. *Vaginal hydrocele* usually arises slowly, though some follow injury and give a short history. The patient is well, with no pain or urinary complaint, and merely complains of the lump or of the drag it causes. The swelling is large, heavy, ovoid, tense, and elastic rather than fluctuating, though fluctuation can be proved if the swelling is fixed by an assistant or the patient; neither testis nor epididymis can be felt apart from the swelling. A hydrocele can be transilluminated, but it needs a dark room and a strong light: when transilluminated the testicular shadow will be noticed at one edge of the swelling, usually behind. Tapping withdraws a golden fluid of soapy feel, with a specific gravity of about 1030, that coagulates solid on boiling. *Secondary hydrocele* follows disease of the testis

or epididymis: the amount of fluid is usually small, and the swelling lax, so that the finger can be passed through it to touch the testis. The complaint is of the causative disease rather than of the hydrocele, which is usually discovered on examination. Transillumination will confirm the presence of fluid. A *haematocele* has the physical characters of a hydrocele except that it is not translucent. Vaginal hydroceles vary very much in this respect, for their wall becomes thicker from fibrosis or deposition of fibrin, particularly after repeated tapping, and the fluid becomes stained with blood-pigment and hazy with cholesterin crystals, so that the strongest light may only just be perceptible across them. Tapping may be required to establish the presence

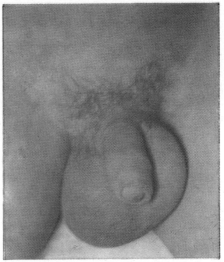

Fig. 713. Torsion of the testis. (*Courtesy of the Gordon Museum, Guy's Hospital.*)

of blood. Haematocele is due to injury, torsion, or growth of the testis, and its discovery is therefore the indication for exploration, unless the history of trauma is recent and definite. A *pyocele* is merely part of a suppurative process arising in the testis or the epididymis. The differential diagnosis of hydrocele is from translucent swellings in the epididymis and cord—spermatocele and encysted hydrocele.

4. Swellings of the Testicle usually affect either the body or the epididymis, rarely the two together. The first group includes torsion, mumps, gumma, and new growth; the second tuberculosis, gonorrhoea, *Bacillus coli* infection, and cysts. Determination of the anatomical site of the swelling will therefore go some way towards settling its pathological nature. Some acute blood-borne infections, however, produce a simultaneous infection of body and epididymis—an *epididymo-orchitis*. Such acute infections are seen in staphylococcal septicaemia and in debilitated children after measles or scarlet fever. In children tuberculosis may also affect the body as well as the epididymis.

SWELLINGS OF THE BODY OF THE TESTICLE

	MUMPS	SYPHILIS	GROWTH
Age	Puberty or adolescence	Any age, but usually 18 to 30	Any age, commoner after 50
History and other symptoms	Short history with pyrexia. Previous contact with mumps. Parotids enlarged	Previous history of exposure to venereal disease; usually has had chancre and rash. Gummata or tertiary rashes may be found elsewhere	Onset insidious. History of months
Scrotum	Normal or red and hot	Normal or adherent in front. Later, ulcer with sharp edges and slough at base, or hernia testis	Normal or merely stretched till growth is size of tennis ball, when it may be invaded
Testis Size and shape	Moderately enlarged, shape normal	Enlarged up to two or three times normal. May be nodular	Increases steadily and may reach diameter of 10–13 cm. First smooth, later nodular
Sensation	Tender and painful. Testicular sensation present	Not tender or painful. Testicular sensation lost	Painful, but not tender. Testicular sensation lost late in disease
'Weight'	This test is hoary with tradition, but it is quite valueless. It will be found that the specific gravity of a cubic centimetre of each of the pathological tissues is identical		
Tunica vaginalis	Slight hydrocele in most	Hydrocele in 60 per cent	Hydrocele in early stages; later haematocele
Epididymis	Unaltered	Usually unaltered	Flattened
Cord	May be tender	Normal	Usually normal, but may have nodules of growth in lymphatics
Glands	Not characteristically enlarged	Not characteristically enlarged	Drainage to para-aortic glands at kidney level. These may form very large mass. Inguinal glands not enlarged unless scrotal skin is invaded

SWELLING OF THE BODY OF THE TESTICLE. Torsion is met with as an acute condition accompanied by abdominal pain and vomiting, and it often occurs in the undescended testis (*see* INGUINAL SWELLING, p. 424). Torsion of a fully descended testis, giving rise to a scrotal swelling, is seldom seen except in small boys; the local signs, in addition to the abdominal pain and vomiting, are moderate enlargement of the testicle, tenderness, the presence of a small haematocele, and the appearance after a few hours of a cold oedema of the scrotal wall on the affected side. Recurring subacute torsion of the testicle is not uncommon, and in these cases the signs and symptoms are less pronounced than in the acute variety into which they eventually pass. *Chronic torsion* which is occasionally seen in adults is the result of a blow or an injury in the saddle. (*Fig.* 713.)

The main points of distinction between the less acute enlargements of the corpus testis may be tabulated as above.

It is often difficult to distinguish syphilitic enlargement of the testicles from that due to growth; but a course of anti-syphilitic therapy and the serological reactions may settle the matter. Malignant new growth nearly always grows steadily, and being entirely within the tunica albuginea it maintains the shape and smooth surface of the testicle until it reaches a size much larger than that of a syphilitic testicle.

The pathology of malignant tumours of the testicle has proved a fertile ground for debate, but nothing can be gained by discussing their classification since the differentiation depends upon examination of sections from the removed specimen and is impossible on clinical grounds. Both the teratomata, which may contain structures representing the three layers of the embryo, and the seminomata, supposedly derived from the germinal elements, may give rise to metastases in the lymphatics or by the blood-stream. In many teratomata and some seminomata the anterior hypophysial sex hormone (Prolan A) is

INFLAMMATORY SWELLINGS OF THE EPIDIDYMIS

	TUBERCULOSIS	*Esch. coli* AND 'NONSPECIFIC'	GONORRHOEAL	SEPTIC
History	Previous tuberculous infection, especially urinary	Usually none	Recent infection, with gleet, and pain on micturition	Recent catheterization or operation on bladder or prostate
Other signs and symptoms	? Cough, wasting. ? Evidence of phthisis in lungs. ? Tubercle bacilli in urine	Usually none. Urine may smell fishy and contain *Esch. coli*	Ureteral discharge. Gram-negative diplococci: other manifestations such as joints	Pus in alkaline urine
Scrotum	May be adherent behind. May have sinus discharging thin pus	Normal	Red, hot, swollen, and tender	Red, hot, swollen, and tender. May suppurate
Testes	Usually normal	Normal	Normal, but outline obscured by surroundings	Normal, but outline obscured by surroundings
Tunica vaginalis	Hydrocele in 30 per cent	Normal	Small hydrocele usually present	Hydrocele or pyocele
Epididymis	Nodular enlargement of globus minor, less commonly globus major or whole epididymis. Nodules, hard and very tender. Later break down to abscess, with sinus	No local nodules or much enlargement, but affected part hard and tender. Changes usually involve globus minor or whole epididymis. Does not break down	Whole epididymis large, hard, and broad; hot and tender	Globus minor or whole epididymis enlarged and broad; hot and tender
Cord	Oedema of cord. Vas may be thickened. Beading of vas excessively rare	Normal	Whole cord tender and swollen	Whole cord tender and swollen
Prostate and seminal vesicles	Vesicle on affected side may be hard and tender	Normal	Prostate may be hot and tender. Tenderness along vesicles	Swollen and tender. Vesicles may be felt

present in the urine in sufficient quantities to give a positive Aschheim-Zondek test—a positive finding, with enlargement of the testicle, being virtually pathognomonic of malignant growth, a negative finding being of little value. Sarcoma, formerly considered common, is very rare.

5. The Epididymis may become enlarged as the result of inflammation, new growth, or cystic degeneration. Primary new growth of the epididymis is excessively rare and need not give rise to much concern in differential diagnosis; it will generally be regarded as tubercle until after operation and microscopical examination of the tissue excised.

Inflammatory swellings are characterized by being elongated in a vertical direction; by their relation to the testicle, which they overlap at its posterior border and its upper and lower poles; and by being flattened from side to side. Inflammatory swellings may be (*a*) tuberculous, (*b*) due to *Esch. coli* (certain cases of epididymitis, indistinguishable clinically from *Esch. coli* infection, are of very obscure aetiology: some say that

they are due to irritation by urine passing by reflux up the vas, others that a virus is responsible; they are grouped as 'non-specific' epididymitis, and they tend to settle spontaneously in about three to four weeks), (*c*) gonorrhoeal, (*d*) septic, secondary to some infection of the urethra. The main points of the distinction are shown in the above table.

It will be seen that *Esch. coli* epididymitis may bear a close resemblance to a tuberculous lesion, but lacks any distant or constitutional evidence of the disease. Support of the testicle in a suspensory bandage and the administration of suitable therapy will cause marked improvement in a few days and thus settle the diagnosis. Apart from the history and an increased liability to suppuration in septic epididymitis, there is little to distinguish the latter from the gonococcal variety.

Cysts of the epididymis are solitary cysts, or spermatoceles, and multiple cysts. A *spermatocele*, being a large single translucent swelling, is sometimes mistaken for hydrocele, but there should be no difficulty in making the distinction.

A spermatocele is placed above and behind the testicle, from which it is distinct; though attached to the epididymis, it is rounded, but being thin-walled it does not feel as tense as a hydrocele; it tends to have several rounded projections rather than a simple surface; and the fluid withdrawn by tapping is milky or opalescent, of low specific gravity, containing little albumin but showing numerous cells under the microscope, some of which may be spermatozoa. *Multiple cysts* occur in men past middle age, and are probably analogous to cystic degeneration of the breast. They are painless and increase in size very slowly. These swellings are usually strikingly trans-lucent.

6. Swellings of the Lower End of the Cord. The most important swelling of the lower part of the spermatic cord is *varicocele.* It is apt to be mistaken for omental hernia, but this mistake should never be made, because of the characteristic feel of the varicocele (like a bag of worms), and the reappearance of the swelling after it has been completely reduced and the finger is firmly pressed on the external abdominal ring. Varicocele is far commoner on the left than the right.

7. Urethral Conditions. Occasionally a *peri-urethral abscess* may form a swelling in the scrotum. Tenderness, oedema, and fluctuation, together with the history and evidence of urethral disease, serve to make the diagnosis clear. *Primary epithelioma of the urethra* is distinguished by the great pain and urethral obstruction that it engenders.

8. Diseases of the Pubic Bones. Inflammatory products may travel into the scrotum from diseases of the bones of the pubic arch, especially from the neighbourhood of the symphysis pubis. *Acute necrosis* of these bones is sufficiently indicated by the grave constitutional symptoms which always accompany it. *Caries* gives rise to more difficulty.

R. G. Beard.

SCROTUM, SURFACE AFFECTIONS OF

The skin of the scrotum may be involved in any generalized or widespread eruption such as that of an exanthematous fever or exfoliative dermatitis, or it may be attacked in common with other parts of the body by dermatitis or psoriasis. On the other hand it may be the only part of the body to be affected. Owing to the heat, moisture, and mobility of the part, it is particularly liable to become chafed. In a bedridden patient it may be irritated by urine or faeces. Acute dermatitis and intertrigo are common affections here. *Acute dermatitis* of the scrotum frequently follows the over-treatment with strong remedies of such disorders as pediculosis pubis or groin ringworm. *Seborrhoeic dermatitis* of the scrotum may be confused with ringworm (tinea cruris), but the latter nearly always affects the neighbouring skin of the groin, has a well-defined wavy edge, and shows mycelium when the scales are examined under the microscope; moreover patches of white macerated or scaly skin produced by the same fungus may be found elsewhere, often between the toes. It is when a seborrhoeic dermatitis of the groin and scrotum is mistakenly treated for ringworm that a particularly acute and painful dermatitis is set up.

Erythrasma occurs as a discoid patch or patches of a brownish-red colour covered with fine scales; unlike tinea cruris these do not undergo involution in the centre, are uniform in appearance, and have no vesicular margin. It fluoresces pink under Wood's light.

In *psoriasis* of the scrotum the skin is dry, and covered with flaky scales; there is little itching, and generally it is associated with psoriasis of some other part of the body.

Syphilis gives rise to moist papules or serpiginous erythematous patches and ulcers; the whole of the scrotal skin is not affected as in dermatitis, itching is absent, and the Wassermann reaction will be positive. Hard and soft *chancre* may affect the scrotum as well as other parts of the genitals; their differential diagnosis is discussed in the section SCROTAL SORES (p. 708). Boils, warts, sebaceous cysts, and epithelioma are referred to under SCROTAL SWELLING (p. 710).

Ulceration of the scrotum may be a feature of Behçet's syndrome, the characteristics of which are recurrent ulceration of the genital area, recurrent ulceration of the mouth, together with iritis and keratitis.

Tuberculous ulceration sometimes follows tuberculous epididymitis, and the ulcer is indolent with thin undermined edges, contrasting with the clean-cut edge and slough of a breaking-down gumma. In the rare cases in which the skin of the scrotum is affected by *Paget's disease* the ulceration is superficial and the ulcer has a well-defined spreading edge with a red granular surface. *Ulcerating granuloma of the pudenda* (granuloma inguinale), a disease of the tropics, may invade the scrotal skin by extension.

Small angiomata are very common on the scrotum in elderly persons; they are called the Fordyce type of angiokeratoma, although a keratomatous element is usually not apparent clinically.

Small nodules on the scrotum are characteristic of scabies.

P. D. Samman.

SENSATION, SOME ABNORMALITIES OF

Sensory disturbances are so intimately woven into the fabric of clinical medicine that they are necessarily referred to in many sections of this book, but it is convenient to consider the subject as a whole under the present heading. Pain, paraesthesiae, tenderness, sensory loss, and sensory agnosia will be dealt with; phantom limbs are described on p. 643.

Terminology. The inaccurate application of an exact terminology gives rise to so much confusion in the literature that it is often preferable to describe sensory experiences and sensory findings in plain language. 'Paraesthesiae' is used for sensations of tingling, 'pins-and-needles', subjective numbness, and feelings of cold and heat whether they appear spontaneously or as a result of touching or manipulating the part. Since the term covers so many different sensations, it should be avoided when precise descriptive work is required, as for instance in case histories.

Anaesthesia means 'without feeling', but neurologists use it for loss of sensibility to light touch; reduction of such sensibility is called 'hypo-aesthesia' or 'hypaesthesia'. Analgesia (loss of pain) and hypo-algesia or hypalgesia (reduction of pain sensibility) are useful terms, free from ambiguity. Thermanaesthesia and therm-hypaesthesia (loss of, and reduction of, temperature sensibility) are explicit if inelegant. This cutaneous sensibility with that derived from the special senses is called 'exteroceptive'. 'Proprioceptive' sensibility is concerned with information received from the labyrinths and from muscle and joint sense. Vibration sense is difficult to classify and is of no apparent value to the patient, but its loss may help to localize a lesion, especially of the spinal cord.

Hyperaesthesia, hyperalgesia, and hyperthermaesthesia refer to increased sensibility to touch, pain, and temperature respectively. Increased sensibility to proprioceptive stimulation has not been described.

Anatomy and Physiology. Fibres conveying touch, pain, and temperature pass via cutaneous nerves to mixed nerves, where they are joined by fibres carrying impulses from joints, ligaments, and muscles, which accompany motor nerves. It follows that lesions of cutaneous nerves will not cause proprioceptive sensory loss, whereas interruption of mixed nerves and 'pure' motor nerves will do so. All sensory fibres have their cell station in the ganglia of the cranial nerves or the posterior spinal roots. The spinal roots enter the posterolateral aspect of the cord in the root entry zone. Fibres conveying touch and postural sensibility pass upwards in the posterior columns to the nuclei gracilis and cuneatus in the medulla, those from the lower half of the body lying medially and those from the upper half occupying the lateral half of the posterior column. These fibres then cross the midline as the sensory decussation and form the medial lemniscus, so passing upwards through the brain-stem to reach the thalamus. Some proprioceptive impulses are conveyed from the dorsal roots to the dorsal and ventral spinocerebellar tracts on the same side of the cord; these end in the cerebellum, which is thus provided with information as to muscular tone and the position of the limbs, head, neck, and trunk. The fibres of the posterior root which convey pain and temperature end around cells in the posterior horn, where a fresh relay crosses the midline in front of the central canal of the cord to ascend in the spinothalamic tracts. In the lower levels of the cord, these fibres cross transversely, but the decussation becomes increasingly oblique at higher levels, so that it occupies three segments in the upper thoracic region and from four to five in the cervical cord. The spinothalamic tracts, ventral and lateral, pass upwards in the cord, on their way to the lateral nucleus of the thalamus, whence all sensory impulses are relayed to the postcentral gyrus. The separation of fibres conveying light touch (dorsal column) affords an opportunity for the surgeon to cut the pain tracts, leaving touch and proprioception intact. This form of cordotomy is useful for the relief of intractable pain in the lower limbs, pelvis, and abdomen, but owing to the obliquity of the decussation in the cervical region it is an unsatisfactory operation when the cause of the pain lies in the upper limb or the upper part of the chest, for it is difficult to get high enough through a cervical laminectomy; the alternative, brain-stem section, carries considerable risks. It is worth noting that the pain fibres of the trigeminal nerve descend through the pons and medulla into the upper three cervical segments, whereas the touch fibres end in the pons itself. It is therefore possible to cut the pain fibres, leaving tactile sensibility intact (and therefore preserving the corneal reflex), as in the case of tic douloureux of the upper two divisions; pain fibres from the mandibular division descend hardly at all and medullary tractotomy should not be attempted when pain is felt in this division.

Pain. The majority of all forms of pain are due either to tension, to chemical stimulation of pain-fibres and receptors, or to both. The mechanism causing *central pain*, which occurs in rare cases of disease in the spinothalamic tracts and the lateral nucleus of the thalamus, is not known.

Pain is felt at the site of the lesion when the latter is situated superficially—in the skin, subcutaneous tissue, superficial bones, and joints (e.g., tibia, knee-joint). If the affected tissue is deeper, there may be an ill-defined ache in the region, together with pain referred to a distance. In some instances there is no local pain, all the discomfort being felt peripherally. Thus pain from a diseased hip may be felt solely in the knee, and a root pain may be felt solely in its peripheral distribution. Pain from deep structures is referred to other structures having the same segmental innervation. Thus the pain from disease affecting the gall-bladder or the central portion of the diaphragm may be felt in the tip of the shoulder (C.4), and sciatica from a lesion of the 5th lumbar root is felt in the glutei, hamstrings, and peronei of the affected side. This segmental reference is *not* in terms of the segmental zones of the skin, but of other deep structures, including muscles. When the area of skin and the deep structures innervated by a common segment happen to coincide anatomically, as in the intercostal spaces, no difficulty arises, but when this is not so, errors in interpretation are likely to arise. A common instance is the pain felt in the pectoral region in disk herniation affecting the 7th cervical root. The reference of pain to this site is inexplicable in terms of the dermatomes (T.4), but becomes intelligible when it is remembered that the underlying lower pectoral muscles are innervated by the 7th cervical segments. Another familiar example is reference of renal pain to the testicle (L.1–2), not, be it noted, to the scrotum (S.3–4).

The distinction between pain referred from a sensory root, on the one hand, and from an extra-neural lesion, on the other, can be difficult. From both, reference is segmental. In both, the referred pain may be limited to a small area within the segmental zone. For example, disease of the 8th dorsal vertebra, or of the 8th dorsal root, may give rise to pain in the epigastrium without any discomfort in the line of the 8th intercostal space and—occasionally—without any pain in the back.

Fortunately for the clinician, there is usually a linear radiation of pain throughout the seg-mental area, but exceptions are sufficiently common to demand care in the interpretation of an apparently local pain in both visceral and somatic disease. There are few symptoms which give so much diagnostic information as pain provided that sufficient attention is given to its precise distribution and qualities. It is a considera-tion of these factors that enables the clinician to recognize the site and, at times, the nature of disease. There are five types of pain, however, which deserve special mention. *Tic douloureux* is dealt with elsewhere (p. 268); its situation in the distribution of one or more divisions of the tri-geminal nerve, its peculiar quality, its intermittent occurrence and its provocation by certain stimuli such as touching the face, blowing the nose, eat-ing, talking, laughing, impart to the condition an easily recognized label. The *lightning pains* of tabes are equally distinct and equally unlike any other form of pain; they consist of stabbing pain, occurring intermittently, without relationship to movement or any other factor. They are usually felt in the limbs, but the neck and face may also be involved. Each stab of pain appears to the patient to be at right angles to the body, 'like a knife'; exceptionally, the pain shoots down the long axis of a limb. They are momentary, but repetitive. Though easily recognized, their identity may be missed if a patient's references to 'rheu-matism' are accepted uncritically. Lightning pains also occur in diabetic neuropathy and in subacute combined degeneration of the cord.

Causalgia is the third type of pain which de-serves special mention. As the name implies, it is a burning pain, and it is this quality which identifies it. It results from incomplete section of mixed nerves such as the median and sciatic, and is felt in the skin of the periphery, usually in the hand or foot. It is aggravated by superficial stimuli such as touch, or cold air currents, and also by emotional factors. Partial relief is some-times obtained by wrapping the limb in cold wet bandages, and by keeping it absolutely still. It is associated with pallor of the skin, increased sweating, trophic changes in the skin and nails, and by such motor, sensory, and reflex changes as are appropriate to the nerve lesion. A charac-teristic feature of this particular form of pain is that it is immediately abolished by sympathec-tomy (D.1–5 in causalgia of the arm, and L.2–4 when it affects the lower limb). Causalgia occurred in less than 2 per cent of all peripheral nerve lesions during the 1939–45 war; this was an im-provement on the results in the First World War and is thought to be due to the lower incidence of sepsis and scar tissue formation owing to the use of antibiotics.

Central pain occasionally occurs in disease of or injury to the lateral nucleus of the thalamus or the spinothalamic tracts in the cord. The pain is felt in the limbs and trunk, is paroxysmal, and has an intense sickly quality. The paroxysms sometimes appear to be spontaneous, but may also be induced by ordinary sensory stimuli applied to the affected side. Owing to the presence of the central lesions in the sensory system, there will be some degree of sensory loss, so that light stimulation may not be felt. But if the threshold is reached, the sensations aroused are excessive and have a peculiar sickly quality. Thus a pin-prick may cause severe pain, and stroking the skin with a warm hand may give rise to an un-reasonable degree of pleasure. Central pain is seen in vascular lesions of the thalamus, and less often in injury or disease of the spinothalamic tracts in the cord. The *thalamic syndrome of Dejerine and Roussy* consists of central pain, the 'thalamic' response to peripheral stimuli already described, some degree of hemianaesthesia, and involuntary movements and hemiparesis—all these symptoms being on the side of the body opposite to the side of the thalamic lesion.

Girdle pains and feelings of constriction both around the trunk and in the limbs are discussed elsewhere (p. 319).

Paraesthesiae is a term that signifies abnormal and inappropriate sensations which are evoked by a normal stimulus; for example, tingling in the skin when it is subjected to light touch. In clinical practice the term is also used for apparently spontaneous sensations of tingling, numbness, 'pins-and-needles', coldness, formi-cation, etc., for it is believed that such paraes-thesiae are not truly 'spontaneous' but are the result of factors such as the pressure of clothes or bedclothes, cold or heat. The presence of paraesthesiae always indicates an affection of the sensory system, whether peripheral or central. They are never caused by extraneural lesions. They are felt in the area of skin corresponding to the sensory pathways which are affected, and are therefore of great localizing value. In *peripheral vascular lesions* such as Raynaud's syndrome, Buerger's disease, atheroma with thrombosis, surgical ligature of a major artery, and costoclavicular compression of the sub-clavian artery, ischaemia of the peripheral nerves cause paraesthesiae which are uniformly distributed over the periphery of the affected limb. On the other hand, lesions of sensory nerves and of the posterior roots give rise to paraesthesiae within the limits of the area they supply, a fact which is of great value in determining which nerve or root is involved. The situation of paraesthesiae is of particular importance in distinguishing the identity of the affected root in sciatic and brachial pain caused by prolapse of an intervertebral disk. Disease of the *spinal cord* is often heralded by the early appearance of paraesthesiae—they occur in the hands and feet in subacute combined degeneration of the cord, and are also present, without objective signs of organic damage, in microcytic hypochromic anaemia of women. The presence of 'pins-and-needles' in both hands and both feet should always direct attention to those two possibilities. Tingling in the feet, or in the saddle area of the buttock, is common in tumour of the cauda equina; feelings of intense cold, of 'deadness' and of numbness in the legs may appear early in the development of pressure on the spinal cord itself. Intramedullary lesions may give rise to similar sensations; disseminated sclerosis and tumours are familiar examples. Disease of the brain-stem, lateral nucleus of the thalamus, and the sensory cortex itself is sometimes accompanied by paraesthesiae; a sensory *Jacksonian fit* usually takes the form of a sensation of tingling, followed by numbness, which marches rapidly from the fingers to the shoulder, thence to the face, and lastly to the leg on the affected side; or, in the case of a lesion in the 'leg' area, the march may be from foot to thigh, spreading thence to the face and the upper limb. A special form of paraesthesiae described as an unpleasant tickling or tingling which marches slowly from hand to face is occasionally experienced as the aura of *migrainous headaches*; it has been likened to 'the march of a thousand cold-footed insects', and takes about half an hour to spread from the fingers to the head.

Allocheiria is a rare condition in which a sensory stimulus applied to a spot on one side of the body is felt at the corresponding spot on the opposite side. As a rule it occurs in association with objective sensory disturbances in diseases affecting the sensory pathways, as in tabes, disseminated sclerosis, transverse hemisection of the cord, and so on. This must not be mistaken for the confusion between left and right which occurs in the mind of patients with body agnosia, i.e., disturbance of the body image, a condition found without objective sensory loss in lesions of the parieto-occipital cortex.

Tenderness signifies a reduction of the threshold to painful stimuli; this is often, though by no means always, associated with a comparable reduction of the thresholds to touch and temperature, but it is with hyperalgesia rather than with hyperaesthesia or hyperthermaesthesia that the clinician is mainly concerned. Increased sensitivity to joint and vibration sense does not appear to have been studied at all.

Hyperalgesia may be superficial or deep, and it may be of local origin or referred from a distance. *Its interpretation as a clinical sign requires knowledge as to its precise situation in depth and in area.* Failure to appreciate these two points is responsible for many diagnostic errors and for much confusion in medical literature; they will therefore be considered in some detail.

Tenderness of the skin is elicited by the reaction to pin-prick; of the subcutaneous tissues by pinching a fold of skin; and of deep structure by deep pressure. It follows that the presence of superficial hyperalgesia, in the skin or subcutaneous tissues, will mask any deep tenderness which may be present. Fortunately, superficial tenderness is very much less common than deep tenderness and it is usually possible to distinguish between them if ordinary care is exercised. The distinction is of little interest when there is unequivocal evidence of local disease in the tender areas, but is of great practical importance when we are dealing with referred hyperalgesia. For instance, tenderness in the region of the sacro-iliac joint may be due to disease of the joint itself, or it may be referred to the overlying fibres of the gluteus maximus from an irritative lesion of the 5th lumbar root (e.g., prolapse of the L.4–5 disk), or it may be referred to the skin of the area which is supplied by the 3rd lumbar root and, inferomedially, by the 3rd sacral root. Similarly, tenderness below the middle third of the clavicle may be cutaneous (3rd and 4th cervical roots) or muscular (6th and 7th cervical roots) or, rarely, it may lie deeper, in disease of the 1st rib. Similar care is needed in distinguishing between the abdominal tenderness of visceral disease and tenderness referred to the abdomen from disease of the lower thoracic parietes and spine.

Cutaneous hyperalgesia is an obvious accompaniment of inflammation or injury to the skin. It may also be referred from distant lesions to the tip of the shoulder in disease within the phrenic distribution, to the skin of the right iliac fossa in acute appendicitis, to the dermatome supplied by an irritated sensory root (herpes zoster, disk lesion, spinal tumours and abscesses), and to the skin immediately above the zone of sensory loss in transverse lesions of the spinal cord.

Subcutaneous hyperalgesia is uncommon except in the presence of local inflammation or injury; a curious condition, sometimes known as *panniculitis*, occurs in middle-aged women, who are afflicted by the presence of tender masses of lobulated fat, especially about the shoulders, the upper arms, the buttocks, and thighs. These collections are intensely tender, and since they appear to be part of a general obesity, the tenderness is apt to be mistaken for evidence of some serious disease, whereas its cause lies in the fatty masses themselves. Extreme cases, in which obesity is generalized and vast, are known as Dercum's disease or adiposis dolorosa (p. 586).

Deep tenderness may be local or referred. It is usually due to local disease when present in ligaments, bones, and superficial joints. In muscles, it may be local or referred. In the abdomen, it is usually due to visceral disease, but it provides a pitfall when it is referred from thoracic or spinal disease within the territory of the lower six dorsal segments; the danger of mistaking such referred tenderness for evidence of local disease is enhanced by the presence of the muscular rigidity which may accompany referred pain.

Tenderness of muscles contributes a physical sign of great diagnostic importance. Of local causes, direct injury, torn fibres, and unwonted exertion are obvious and common. It occurs in muscles around diseased and injured joints and bones. It is an important feature of ischaemia, as in Buerger's disease, atheroma with thrombosis, and arterial injuries. Postural abnormalities—inequality in the length of the legs, scoliosis, kyphosis, and bad postural habits—impose a strain on muscles, and thereby produce the tenderness of muscular fatigue, a condition which is all too liable to be regarded as 'rheumatic' if the postural factor is not appreciated. The exquisite tenderness usually found in polyneuritis is probably of local origin; it is seen in alcoholism, arsenical poisoning, the polyneuritis of Guillain-Barré, vitamin-B deficiency, and acute diabetes. In rheumatic fever most of the pain and tenderness occurs in and around joints, but the inflammatory process also occurs in the larger muscles and this contributes to the deep hyperalgesia. Trichiniasis, dermatomyositis, and suppurative myositis are rare causes of local tenderness. In McArdle's syndrome—a phosphorylase-deficient myopathy—the most constant symptoms are muscle pain and stiffness. The pain and stiffness are usually provoked by more than moderate exercise but this varies from patient to patient. The exercise tolerance tends to be decreased with infection or depression of mood.

Referred hyperalgesia of muscles is common. It is seen in the presence of meningeal irritation, as in meningitis, subarachnoid haemorrhage, and the early stages of poliomyelitis. Of greater importance is the large group in which it is due to implication of the sensory pathways. It is a curious fact that referred tenderness is uncommon in lesions of the spinal cord and brain, whereas it is an important feature of disease of the larger plexuses and the posterior roots; further, it is more likely to occur in slowly progressive disease than in acute affections. The lumbosacral plexus is particularly liable to be involved by malignant disease in the pelvis, and rarely by an extension of inflammatory disease of the pelvic adnexa and of the sacro-iliac joint. The brachial plexus, on the other hand, is more liable to the mechanical irritation of cervical rib and costo-clavicular compression; it is occasionally involved by the spread of malignant disease of the breast and from the lung (*Pancoast's tumour*), and exceptionally by inflammatory fibrosis from the apical pleura. There is acute tenderness of the muscles of the shoulder-girdle in the acute phase of infective radiculitis (syn. neuralgic amyotrophy), a condition of unknown aetiology and characterized by the sudden onset of acute pain in the shoulder region, tenderness of the muscles, the rapid appearance of flaccid paralysis with wasting, and comparatively slight sensory loss.

Irritative lesions of the posterior nerve-roots are by far the most common cause of referred tenderness of muscles. It is seen in herniation of intervertebral disks, spondylosis, spondylitis ankylopoietica, and in gross inflammatory and neoplastic conditions of the spine. The tenderness is found in muscles supplied by the affected root or roots, but its distribution is not uniform. Thus, when the 6th and 7th cervical roots are affected, it is usually present in the pectoralis major, the triceps, and the extensors of the wrist and fingers, but not in the biceps or the long flexors. Similarly, implication of the 5th lumbar and 1st sacral roots gives rise to tenderness in the glutei, hamstrings, and calf muscles, but not in the peronei or the anterior tibial group. The tenderness is largely due to a lowering of the sensory threshold, but electromyographic studies have shown that involuntary spasm of small groups of muscle-fibres plays a subsidiary part in its production.

Sensory Loss. The pattern and the nature of sensory loss depend on the site and the size of the causal lesion. Illustrations of the more common forms are given in *Figs*. 714–719.

PERIPHERAL NERVES. When a cutaneous nerve is cut, there is loss of all superficial sensibility in the central portion of the affected area, together with incomplete loss along its margins where there is a collateral supply from adjacent nerves. There is loss of sweating, the hair falls out, nails become brittle and deformed, and indolent ulceration may follow injuries to the part. Deep sensibility is unaffected unless a mixed or a motor nerve has been cut. Regeneration, which takes from three months to two years to attain whatever degree of completion is possible in any given case, is heralded by the return of sensibility to pain and temperature. At first, the threshold is high, the response when attained is excessive and unpleasant, and localization is faulty. Later, the threshold returns to normal, fine gradations of stimuli are appreciated, localization becomes accurate, and sensibility to light touch returns.

In *polyneuritis*, sensory loss (1) always involves more than one limb, (2) is usually symmetrically disposed, (3) usually involves all the sensory nerves within the affected area, and (4) is greater in the periphery of the limb than it is proximally. All forms of sensibility may not be affected equally. Light touch is usually more affected than pain; superficial pain may be lost, but deep pain may be increased. Proprioceptive loss may be slight or severe. Such dissociations are found in many forms of sensory disturbances, and they may alter with the evolution of the disease in any given case, so that the conventional use of the term 'dissociated' in describing the cutaneous sensory loss in syringomyelia by no means

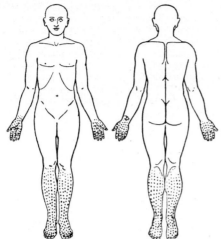

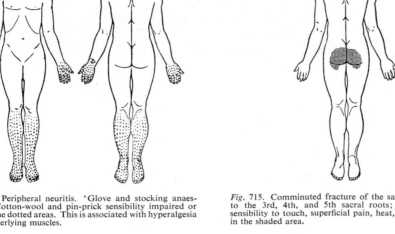

Fig. 714. Peripheral neuritis. 'Glove and stocking anaesthesia'. Cotton-wool and pin-prick sensibility impaired or lost over the dotted areas. This is associated with hyperalgesia of the underlying muscles.

Fig. 715. Comminuted fracture of the sacrum, with injury to the 3rd, 4th, and 5th sacral roots; complete loss of sensibility to touch, superficial pain, heat, and cold resulted in the shaded area.

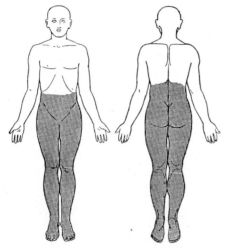

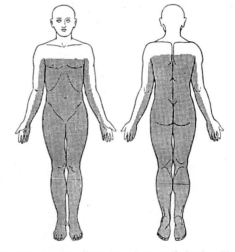

Fig. 716. Dorsal myelitis affecting the cord as high as the 9th dorsal segment. The shaded parts are insensitive to touch, deep and superficial pain, and all degrees of temperature.

Fig. 717. Fracture-dislocation of the cervical spine. The shaded area represents the loss of sensibility to touch, pain, heat, and cold.

describes an isolated example. It is seen in many forms of polyneuritis; in tabes; in the analgesia without anaesthesia of leprotic macules; and in the loss of light touch and the retention of pain sensitivity following ischaemia of nerve-trunks from occlusion of a major artery. A dissociation also occurs frequently in disseminated sclerosis when vibration sense is lost and postural sense is unaffected, both sensations being thought to travel in the posterior columns. There is, however, reason to believe that vibration sense travels in the medial part of the lateral columns.

MONONEURITIS MULTIPLEX. Any involvement of a single nerve is sometimes referred to as a neuritis and this is usually traumatic, often due to pressure, as in ulnar neuritis at the elbow.

There are, however, certain conditions not due to pressure in which there may be involvement of more than one nerve in the same pathological process in a completely random way. This is, therefore, something less than a polyneuritis and is referred to as a mononeuritis multiplex. The conditions which may give rise to this clinical picture are polyarteritis nodosa (probably the commonest), diabetes, alcoholic poisoning, and leprosy. With the possible exception of leprosy these conditions can all, of course, also give rise to a polyneuritis.

CARCINOMATOUS NEUROPATHY. There is a group of neurological syndromes which are now recognized as appearing in the presence of a carcinoma, usually of the lung and less frequently of the breast, the ovary, the gut and elsewhere, of which the appearance does not depend on the presence of metastases.

The neuropathy may appear before the carcinoma is discovered, may be present at the time the carcinoma is diagnosed, or may appear later. Its appearance, the nature of the neuropathy and its extent bear no relation to the size of the carcinoma. It runs a variable course, sometimes

objective changes are usually limited to a reduction of sensibility situated on the lateral surface of the ankle, the lateral and dorsal aspect of the foot, and the great toe. Joint and vibration sense will be reduced slightly (if at all) in the great toe. In many cases the area of sensory loss is a less reliable guide than the zone of paraesthesiae. A second point of importance in the interpretation of radicular sensory abnormalities is the fact that

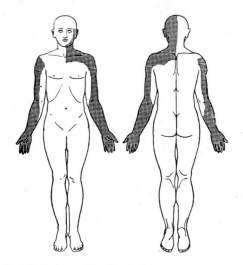

Fig. 718. Syringomyelia. The shaded parts show the areas of dissociated anaesthesia, i.e., of thermo-anaesthesia and analgesia. This was associated with atrophic palsy of the upper extremities.

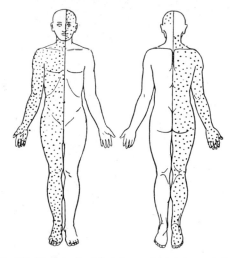

Fig. 719. Thrombosis of the left posterior inferior cerebellar artery. The dotted areas show the regions of dissociated anaesthesia, i.e., loss of sensibility to pain and temperature of all degrees.

undergoing partial remission, but not greatly influenced by removal of the primary growth.

Syndromes so far recognized include polyneuritis, often predominantly sensory; neuromyopathic pictures with muscle wasting and weakness which is often variable and may demonstrate features of myasthenia gravis, even to responding to neostigmine; tremor, ataxia, and dysequilibrium resulting from cerebellar degeneration and a clinical picture resembling subacute combined degeneration of the cord. Sometimes two or more of these clinical pictures are combined and the very fact that the manifestations are so bizarre suggests the diagnosis.

LESIONS OF POSTERIOR ROOTS AND THE ROOT ENTRY ZONE should, theoretically, abolish all sensibility, superficial and deep, within the area supplied by the root. In practice, both the area and the severity of the sensory loss are very much reduced by overlap from the adjoining segments. Thus the 5th lumbar root supplies sensory fibres to a strip of skin extending from the lateral aspect of the thigh, down the outer surface of the leg and foot, and into the dorsum of the foot and the great toe; it also conveys proprioceptive sensation from the anterior tibial muscles, the peronei, the ankle, and the joints of the great toe. Section of this root may produce an unpleasant subjective sense of numbness in the whole of this area, but

whereas on the head, neck, and trunk the disposition of the dermatomes is simple and relatively constant, there is considerable variability in this distribution in the limbs, and these differences are embarrassingly clear in the segmental 'maps' published by various authorities. Nevertheless, in practice it is usually possible to identify the root at fault, because the sensory loss is maximal in the periphery, and in the central part of the dermatome, i.e., it is greatest in the area about which there are no conflicting views. Difficulty may arise in deciding whether an area of sensory loss is radicular or peripheral in origin. Thus, the 2nd cervical root has the same distribution as the great occipital nerve, and there is a similar correspondence between the twelve thoracic roots and the intercostal nerves. The distinction can only be made on other evidence. In the limbs, not only are there differences in the patterns of sensory loss, but sweating is reduced in the areas of sensory loss caused by peripheral lesions and is normal in root lesions because the sympathetic fibres do not emerge in these roots but join the brachial and lumbar plexuses from the cervicodorsal and lumbar sympathetic chains respectively.

LESIONS OF THE SPINAL CORD. In complete transection (injuries, tumours, transverse myelitis) there is loss of all sensation below the level of the lesion; the upper level of loss may be marked by a band of hyperalgesia.

Section of one half of the cord—a rare occurrence in pure form—causes impairment of touch, loss of proprioceptive sensibility, and upper-motor neuron paralysis on the side of the lesion, and loss of pain and temperature sensibility on the opposite side (Brown-Séquard syndrome).

An intramedullary lesion situated near the central canal of the cord interrupts the decussating fibres carrying pain and temperature sensation, giving rise to loss of pain and temperature sensibility. If the lesion extends laterally, it may give rise to pyramidal and spinothalamic signs at lower levels, and it may also interrupt the fibres serving the stretch reflexes, with loss of tendon reflexes at the level of the lesion. This combination of signs occurs in syringomyelia and in tumours of the central part of the cord. If the lesion is situated in the upper cervical region, the descending root of the trigeminal nerve may be implicated on one or both sides, with a resultant loss of pain and temperature sensibility in the face.

Dissociated anaesthesia of this type, distributed more or less symmetrically and extending over several segments, is usually due to a central lesion, but it must not be inferred that such loss is necessarily and always due to intramedullary disease; on the contrary, loss of pain and temperature sensibility with relative preservation of touch and proprioception sometimes occurs as a result of pressure upon the cord from without, as in extramedullary tumours, especially when situated in the upper cervical region. Indeed, tumours in the region of the foramen magnum may superficially resemble syringomyelia by giving rise to dissociated sensory loss, pyramidal symptoms, and—curiously enough—wasting of the small muscles of the hands. A similar pattern of sensory loss is encountered in *platybasia*, a condition in which the basi-occiput is displaced upwards so that the medulla and the cerebellar tonsils lie within the foramen magnum and thus cause compression of the cord at that level. It occurs as a congenital anomaly, as a part of the Klippel-Feil syndrome, and in Paget's disease. The Klippel-Feil syndrome is a rare condition in which the cervical vertebrae are reduced in numbers and fused together. Spina bifida occulta is usually present. The neck is very short and its movements are limited, while the scapulae are elevated. There may be an associated dysplasia of the cord, with increasing spastic weakness of the arms and legs, and inability to dissociate the movements of the two hands.

SENSORY LOSS IN INTRACRANIAL DISEASE. In cases of thrombosis of the posterior inferior cerebellar artery there is ataxia and loss of pain and temperature sensibility in the face on the same side as the lesion, and spinothalamic loss on the opposite side of the body. The brain-stem is a favourite site for the plaques of disseminated sclerosis, but whereas such lesions almost invariably produce pyramidal symptoms or diplopia, sensory disturbances are usually confined to paraesthesiae in the limbs, or fleeting and incomplete interference with cutaneous or proprioceptive sensibility in the opposite side of the body. This illustrates the general rule that when both motor and sensory tracts are involved by the same lesion, motor symptoms are more pronounced than sensory, whether we are dealing with peripheral nerves, the spinal cord, or the brain.

Destruction of the lateral nucleus of the thalamus causes complete and total sensory loss on the whole of the opposite side of the body. In slowly progressive lesions, such sensory loss is often partial; the limbs are more deeply involved than the trunk and the trunk more than the face; moreover, the discriminative forms of sensibility are more affected than crude touch, pain, and temperature, although this distinction is more clearly seen in cortical lesions. In cases of rapid destruction of the internal capsule, such as occurs in gunshot wounds and cerebral thrombosis or haemorrhage, sensory loss is likely to be complete in the first few hours, but there is, as a rule, some degree of improvement thereafter. It is unusual for a capsular lesion to be confined to the sensory fibres; the corticospinal (pyramidal) fibres which lie in front, and the visual fibres which are situated behind the sensory tract, are often implicated as well.

The sensory area of the cortex has complex functions. The appreciation of light touch, different degrees of pain and temperature, vibration sense, and joint sense is a function of the postcentral gyrus, and destruction of this area by injury or by disease causes loss of these sensations in the opposite side of the body. In acute lesions limited to this gyrus there is an initial deeper loss, especially in the hand, forearm, foot, and leg, which is so markedly peripheral in distribution that it sometimes resembles the 'glove and stocking' loss of hysteria, but after the acute phase is past it is only the more discriminative form of sensibility which remains defective. The posterior portion of the postcentral gyrus and the adjacent superior parietal lobule, the supramarginal gyrus and the angular gyrus, are concerned with a still higher level of discrimination; the sensations appreciated at the cortical level are subjected to critical appraisal in the light of sensory memories; their nature and intensity are accurately judged, and their spatial relationships are recognized. Consequently, it is possible to identify the nature, form, and intensity of sensory impressions, and, by matching them with sensory memories, to identify without visual aid the nature of peripheral stimuli such as an object placed in the hand, the position of a limb in space, or the distance between two points simultaneously applied to the skin. Lesions limited to this area of the sensory cortex destroy this capacity, with a resulting astereognosis. Sensations are appreciated, but their total significance is not understood. It will be seen that the sensory cortex is closely related anatomically and functionally to the cortex behind the postcentral gyrus, and that disease of the sensory cortex can interfere with the appreciation of sensation as such or with the higher functions of interpretation and recognition. Astereognosis is one form of sensory agnosia, and is comparable to auditory agnosia (known as sensory aphasia), in which the sounds of speech are heard but their meaning is not understood, a condition found in destruction of the superior and middle temporal convolutions of the dominant (usually left) hemisphere. Similarly, destruction of the parieto-occipital cortex may not interfere with vision as such, but it may prevent a recognition of what is seen—a visual agnosia. Astereognosis occurs in disease of both hemispheres, whereas auditory agnosia is only seen when the dominant (usually left) hemisphere is marked; visual agnosia as regards the written symbols of speech (alexia) is similarly associated with disease of the major hemisphere, although visual agnosia for other objects is not necessarily thus limited.

Ian Mackenzie.

SEXUAL PRECOCITY

Puberty is initiated by the release of the gonadotrophins, follicle-stimulating hormone (FSH) and luteinizing hormone (LH) or interstitial-cell-stimulating hormone (ICSH) as it is sometimes called, from the pituitary. LH/FSH–RH ('releasing hormone') is secreted by the hypothalamus and is responsible, by maintaining cyclical secretion of LH and FSH in the female, for causing ovulation and menstruation and secretion of ovarian hormones to induce secondary sex characteristics in fertile girls and women. In the male the ICSH and FSH are secreted continuously, but not cyclically, to produce adolescence and virile and fertile manhood under the influence of androgen.

When androgen (testicular or adrenal) is secreted precociously its protein-anabolic effect leads to rapid skeletal growth. A similar effect is caused by oestrogen. Early closure of the epiphyses, however, terminates this growth prematurely, and during the second decade a mild degree of dwarfism becomes evident. As the long bones are principally affected the upper measurement may considerably exceed the lower measurement and the individual may even slightly resemble an achondroplasiac.

Precocious puberty should be distinguished from sexual precocity. In the former, puberty is normal though advanced, so that the menstrual cycles will be ovulatory, spermatogenesis will take place and the testicle will achieve adult size. In sexual precocity excessive production of androgen or oestrogen will suppress pituitary gonadotrophin with secondary gonadal atrophy.

'*Constitutional*' *precocious puberty* is by far the commonest type, especially in girls, in whom it comprises about 90 per cent of all cases. Frequently there is a history of early puberty occurring in many members of the family of the same sex as the patient. Sexual development may occur at a very early age, even during the first year of life. Enlarged ovaries can often be palpated per rectum; the enlargement is due to the presence of follicular cysts, probably resulting from excessive secretion of pituitary gonadotrophin. They should not be confused with granulosa-cell tumours. *Premature pubarche* (sometimes referred to as *premature adrenarche*) indicates that pubic hair begins to grow at an early age and the height and bone age may be advanced by 2 years, though there are no other signs of premature development of a secondary sexual character and full puberty develops at the normal ages. Similarly, *premature thelarche* refers to very early breast development as the only sign of pubertal change. It commonly develops between 6 months and 2 years of age and often subsides gradually during a further 6 months to 2 years.

Precocious puberty due to neurogenic causes occurs rarely in girls but much more commonly in boys in whom neurological investigations should always be undertaken. It is produced by a lesion of the corpora mammillaria or posterior hypothalamus. This may be a neoplasm, such as a tumour of the pineal encroaching on the hypothalamus (true pinealomas seldom, if ever, cause precocious puberty of their own accord), or it may be inflammatory, or due to congenital brain defects. The diagnosis may be aided by the presence of other features of the hypothalamic syndrome, such as excessive thirst, polyuria, a voracious appetite, obesity, or disturbances of sleep, temperature, or pulse-rate. Pressure on the corpora quadrigemina may give rise to neurological signs such as Argyll-Robertson pupils or squints. Optic atrophy, visual-field defects, papilloedema, spasticity, ataxia, convulsions, attacks of rage, or hydrocephalus are other features which suggest a neurogenic cause.

Albright's syndrome is usually associated with precocious puberty. One of the characteristic features is polyostotic fibrous dysplasia which tends to be unilateral. Though the typical lesion is osteitis fibrosa, there are some areas of increased bone density, especially at the base of the skull where the thickened bone may cause pressure on the hypothalamus. There are pigmented areas of the skin roughly corresponding with the underlying bony lesions. The condition is almost entirely confined to girls and is very rare.

Hypothyroidism has very rarely been reported in association with precocious puberty sometimes accompanied by increased skin pigmentation and galactorrhoea. It is assumed that the hypothyroidism interferes with hypothalamic function and reduces the secretion of melanocyte-stimulating-hormone release-inhibiting hormone (MRIH) and the prolactin release-inhibiting hormone (PIH).

Sexual precocity is due to excessive production of androgen by the testis or adrenal cortex, or of oestrogen by the ovary. Gonadal sexual precocity is caused by an interstitial-cell tumour of the testis, or a granulosa-cell tumour of the ovary; adrenocortical sexual precocity by congenital adrenal hyperplasia, an adrenocortical tumour, or postnatal hyperplasia.

Interstitial-cell tumour of the testis occurring in childhood and giving rise to sexual precocity is extremely rare. The tumour is usually palpable, but occasionally is so small that the diagnosis is difficult. In most cases the condition is fully established by the age of 6. Precocity is marked: the physique is strong and muscular, body-hair growth is considerable, the voice is strikingly gruff and manly, the penis and prostate are abnormally large, though the unaffected testicle is small and atrophied. In about half the cases psycho-sexual precocity is so strongly developed as to be embarrassing. In the majority of cases 17-oxosteroid excretion is not outside the normal adult range, though occasionally it may be very high. It usually depends on how soon the tumour is detected and removed. The clinical features of sexual precocity produced by an interstitial-cell tumour of the testis are indistinguishable (apart from the palpably enlarged testis) from those produced by adrenocortical over-activity.

Congenital adrenal hyperplasia due to a defect of certain enzymes, usually 21-hydroxylase, preventing the biosynthesis of cortisol but not of adrenal androgens and developing in foetal life, gives rise to sexual precocity in the form of *macrogenitosomia precox*. Owing to the defective biosynthesis of the adrenocortical hormones the abnormal metabolite pregnanetriol appears in the urine and helps to distinguish the condition from that produced by a *postnatal adrenocortical tumour*. (Postnatal adrenal hyperplasia very rarely develops during the first decade.) It is often very difficult to distinguish between these two conditions clinically, for enlargement of the penis and growth of pubic hair may not be noticeable until the age of 2 or 3 in cases of congenital adrenal hyperplasia, whereas a tumour may develop as early as the first year. In both cases the clinical picture is the same. These tumours are almost always malignant, though the prognosis is good if the tumour is still completely encapsulated on removal. Malignant adrenocortical tumours are autonomous and the quantity of cortisol they produce does not depend on corticotrophin control. Thus, in addition to the absence of pregnanetriol, the tumour can be differentiated from congenital adrenal hyperplasia by the corticotrophin stimulation (Synacthen) test and the dexamethasone suppression test. In cases of hyperplasia the already raised 17-oxosteroid and 17-oxogenic steroid levels are further markedly increased by corticotrophin stimulation, whereas the administration of dexamethasone (8 mg. daily for 2 days) will suppress adrenocortical activity, so that the urinary metabolite levels will be greatly diminished. In the case of an autonomous tumour there will be little variation from the pretreatment levels of 17-oxosteroids and 17-oxogenic steroids following these two tests. Congenital adrenal hyperplasia may also occur in females, when it gives rise to female pseudohermaphroditism (p. 224).

Granulosa-cell tumour of the ovary (or occasionally other types of ovarian tumour giving rise to precocious output of oestrogen) has to be distinguished from constitutional precocious puberty though it very rarely occurs in the first decade. In many cases the tumour is palpable, though it may be necessary to examine the patient under an anaesthetic. In most cases of precocious puberty the menstrual cycle is regular and ovulatory and this can be demonstrated either by finding a secretory type of endometrium, taken by biopsy during the second half of the cycle, or by observing the characteristic 'biphasic' basal temperature pattern, the early morning temperature being significantly lower during the pre-ovulatory phase than after ovulation has taken place or by having serum progesterone levels equivalent to those of post-ovulatory phases. In contrast, in cases of granulosa-cell tumour, uterine bleeding, which is the first clinical sign, tends to be irregular, with episodes of prolonged metropathic haemorrhage alternating with phases of amenorrhoea, and endometrial biopsy may reveal cystic glandular hyperplasia. The basal temperature records will fail to show the biphasic pattern and serum progesterone will not be detected. The clinical features of the two conditions will be identical. Apart from the menstruation there will be adult mammary development and growth of pubic and axillary hair.

P. M. F. Bishop.

SHOULDER, PAIN IN

Pain in the shoulder (*see also* LIMBS (UPPER), PAIN IN, p. 500) may be due to two entirely different groups of causes, namely: (1) *Direct causes*, lesions of the shoulder-joint itself, or of the nerves, tendons, blood-vessels, ligaments, muscles, fasciae, bursae, close to it; and (2) *Indirect causes*, when the pain is referred to the shoulder region from some remote seat of disease, as in the case, for instance, of angina pectoris, or gastric or hepatic or diaphragmatic disorders.

1. Direct Causes:

Injury
Occupational strain
Arthrosis or arthritis of glenohumeral or acromio-clavicular joints
Synovitis and capsulitis
Subacromial bursitis
Tendinitis and tenosynovitis
Apical bronchial carcinoma
Dermatomyositis
Muscular paralysis, local

Polymyalgia rheumatica
Vasculitis
Shoulder–hand syndrome (*see* p. 468).

2. Indirect Causes:

  a. CARDIOVASCULAR LESIONS:

    Ischaemic heart disease
    Pericarditis
    Aortic aneurysm.

  b. PLEURAL, PULMONARY, OR MEDIASTINAL LESIONS:

    Pleurisy and pleuro-pneumonia
    Pulmonary tuberculosis
    Intrathoracic new growth
    Pneumothorax.

Primary disease, e.g., multiple sclerosis
Syringomyelia
Psychogenic
Pachymeningitis, syphilitic, cervico-dorsal.

  h. CERVICO-DORSAL VERTEBRAL LESIONS:

    Degenerative disease of cervical spine
    Tuberculous disease
    Ankylosing and other types of spondylitis
    Rheumatoid arthritis
    Still's disease
    New growth.

1. Direct Causes. *Injury* not only produces immediate symptoms but in some cases goes on to cause the shoulder–hand syndrome described on

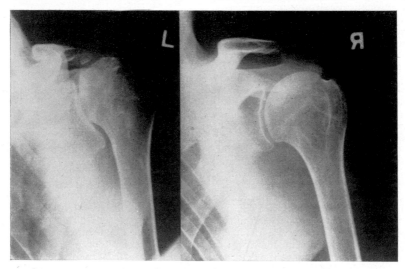

Fig. 720. Unilateral rheumatoid arthritis in the left shoulder-joint.

  c. GASTRIC AND DUODENAL LESIONS AND DISORDERS:

    Hiatus hernia
    Gastric ulcer
    Gastric carcinoma
    Duodenal ulcer.

  d. HEPATIC LESIONS:

    Gall-stones
    Cholecystitis
    New growth
    Liver abscess.

  e. PANCREATIC DISEASE:

    Chronic pancreatitis
    Stone in the pancreas
    Carcinoma of the pancreas.

  f. AFFECTIONS OF THE UNDER-SURFACE OF THE DIAPHRAGM:

    Local peritonitis from leaking gastric or duodenal ulcer or from hepatic abscess
    Subdiaphragmatic abscess.

  g. NERVOUS LESIONS:

    Hemiplegia
    Herpes zoster
    Vascular disease of brain or cord
    Trauma to brain or cord
    Neoplasm of brain or cord
    Cervical osteophytosis and disk disease

p. 468. Severe injuries, such as dislocations and even fractures, are not infrequently overlooked, particularly in the elderly and the non-complaining. Minor musculotendinous and ligamentous capsular tears around this joint are by no means rare, particularly when the joint is already restricted by previous disease. Lifting patients incorrectly up the bed with the nurse's hands in the axillae will readily traumatize such shoulders. *Arthritis* of the shoulder (glenohumeral) joint occurs commonly in rheumatoid arthritis (*Fig.* 720), ankylosing spondylitis, and less commonly in any other inflammatory arthritis. *Osteo-arthrosis*, however, more commonly affects the acromio-clavicular joint, unless it is secondary to injury, when it may affect the true shoulder-joint also —it is a common cause of shoulder pain at night from pressure on the bed and pillow. *Tendinitis* may affect biceps or supraspinatus, and calcification may occur in the muscles (*Fig.* 721). *Occupational strain* of this highly mobile joint is common in, for example, painters, sportsmen (fast bowlers, tennis players, or baseball pitchers), and others. *Subacromial bursitis* may present as an agonizing pain relieved only by incising the tense, distended bursa and releasing the enclosed sterile gelatinous material, or as a milder persistent ache with diminished range of movement because of pain. This same bursa becomes involved frequently in rheumatoid arthritis. On occasion a *paralysed shoulder*, as in acute anterior poliomyelitis, is acutely painful at onset. *Polymyalgia rheumatica* (p. 465), often due to giant-cell arteritis, typically gives painful stiffness in the shoulders, worse in the morning on awakening.

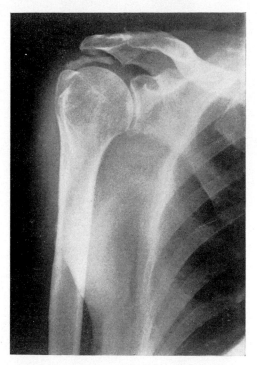

Fig. 721. Pains in shoulder due to calcification in supraspinatus tendon with adjacent calcification probably in subacromial bursa.

It will be noted that only a small percentage of shoulder pains are due to actual arthritis of the shoulder-joints; although arthrosis (degenerative disease) is more common, most painful conditions arise in the soft tissues around the joint—the so-called 'periarthritis'.

The commonest intrinsic soft tissue lesions are:

1. Calcareous tendinitis
2. Subacromial bursitis
3. Adhesive capsulitis
4. Lesions of the musculotendinous cuff
5. Bicipital tenosynovitis

or combinations of some or all of these components.

2. Indirect Causes. *Cardiovascular lesions.* X-ray examination of the thorax may reveal an unsuspected aneurysm of the aortic arch which by pressure on the lower part of the right brachial plexus may be responsible for acute pains in the right deltoid region. Pain from disease of the ascending arch of the aorta is usually felt at the right side of the neck and shoulder, the transverse or descending parts of the arch to the left side of the back and shoulder. *Ischaemic heart disease*, either due to angina of effort, coronary thrombosis, or the much rarer syphilitic arteritis, may be the explanation for very acute pain in the left shoulder region. The nature of the attacks, and the spread of the pain from the precordial region, where it tends to be tight, oppressive, and constricting, to the left shoulder and down the left arm, are generally but not always characteristic. The pain of pericarditis may be referred also to the left shoulder.

Pleural, pulmonary, or mediastinal lesions. Pleurisy of the central portion of the diaphragm may be referred to either shoulder, and an apical and subapical consolidation, whether tuberculous, pneumonic, or malignant, may on occasion cause shoulder pain. An *intrathoracic new growth* may not be apparent until X-rays and possibly tomographs are performed; invasion of pleura and other structures adjacent to the joint may produce intense and persistent agony. In *spontaneous pneumothorax*, the sudden onset of unilateral chest pain and dyspnoea, with diminished breath-sounds on the affected side, are characteristic.

Less common are the referred pains of *gastric, hepatic*, and *duodenal* lesions in the subscapular region rather than in the region of the shoulder-joint itself—stomach disorders on the left side, hepatic and duodenal on the right.

In *chronic pancreatitis* serum and urine amylase levels are elevated. Pancreatic calcification may be seen on X-rays. *Carcinoma* of pancreas should be suspected strongly if there is loss of weight and increasing icterus.

A special variety of pain referred to the shoulder-joint region (Kehr's sign) results from acute or subacute *inflammation of the under-surface of the diaphragm*. If the front part of the under-surface of the diaphragm becomes acutely inflamed, pain may be referred to the front of the shoulder-joint on the corresponding side. If the centre of the diaphragm is affected, the pain is referred to the tip of the shoulder-joint region under the acromion process; if the back of the diaphragm, the referred shoulder pain is posterior, under the hinder part of the deltoid muscle. It is sometimes possible to determine from these considerations whether a subdiaphragmatic abscess is located more to the front or more to the back. Such subdiaphragmatic lesions may be caused by a leaking gastric ulcer, a perforated duodenal ulcer, a ruptured spleen, a hepatic abscess with local peritonitis, or spread of infection from cholecystitis or gall-stones. In appendicitis, perinephritis or pyosalpinx, or other pelvic inflammation, infection may spread up the back of the right side of the abdomen to the under-surface of the diaphragm rather than to the peritoneum generally.

A ruptured ectopic gestation is a possible cause of such pain in the shoulder region.

Of the nervous causes, *herpes zoster* will be recognized by the characteristic eruption (p. 820): the pain nearly always extends down the arm. Severe pain may occur before the appearance of the vesicles and persist subsequently for a considerable time.

The *hemiplegic* arm is sometimes the site of great pain, especially in the shoulder; the pain is probably referred from the sensorimotor cortex of the cerebrum. Cervico-dorsal *pachymeningitis* of syphilitic origin may cause no symptoms other than ill-defined though acute pains in various parts of the neck, shoulder, arm, or hand.

Cervical and upper dorsal vertebral lesions may cause pain to be referred to the shoulder, the commonest being *cervical spondylosis*. Degenerative disease of the cervical spine tends to be maximal at the C.5, 6, and 7 areas, with disk narrowing and considerable degenerative changes. In *ankylosing spondylitis* the whole spine tends to be involved with characteristic radiological changes. In *rheumatoid arthritis* the neck is less often involved than in Still's disease, pain being occasionally referred to the shoulder. *Tuberculous* and *malignant* involvement of the cervical spine may give similar pain reference.

F. Dudley Hart.

SKIN, FUNGOUS AFFECTIONS OF

Ringworm of the Body Skin (tinea circinata) (*Fig.* 722) starts as a small circular red, raised patch with a spreading scaly edge. At the edge small vesicles are usually present. As the edge spreads slowly, healing occurs in the centre. One type is contracted from domestic pets affected with ringworm mange and the cause is the ringworm fungus specific to the cat or dog (*Microsporon felineum, M. canis*). Another group of cases occurs in agricultural workers, when one of the cattle trichophytons is the cause. In this latter group the inflammation is much more severe and *kerion* (q.v.) formation is almost the rule. Microscopical examination of a small piece of scale from the spreading edge will always reveal the presence of fungus. Diagnosis is usually simple, as there will be a history of contact with infected animals. In cases of doubt it is advisable to examine household pets. It may be very difficult to find fungous infection in a cat unless the examination is made under Wood's light.

The herald patch of *pityriasis rosea* (q.v.) is commonly mistaken for ringworm on the trunk, but a microscopical examination will settle the matter beyond dispute.

Ringworm of the Groin (tinea cruris, dhobie itch) (*Fig.* 723) is a common contagious fungous affection, epidemics occurring in schools and institutions. The causal fungus may be the *Epidermophyton floccosum* or one of the trichophytons, *Trichophyton mentagrophytes* or *T. rubrum*. The main characteristics of this disease are very itchy, red, scaly patches with a sharply demarcated

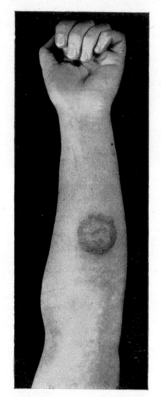

Fig. 722. Tinea circinata in a laboratory worker. (*Dr. Peter Hansell.*)

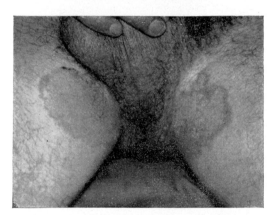

Fig. 723. Tinea cruris. (*Dr. Peter Hansell.*)

spreading edge affecting both groins symmetrically. It must be carefully distinguished from seborrhoeic dermatitis occurring in the same area. In the latter disorder the patches are more fawn in colour and less itchy. There may also be patches of seborrhoeic dermatitis on other parts of the body. The presence of fungus in scrapings from the lesions when examined under the microscope will determine the diagnosis. *Candida albicans* can produce a very similar condition but it is usually moister and there are small flaccid vesicles near the margin. Microscopical examination will establish the diagnosis.

Ringworm of the Feet and Toes (athlete's foot) (*Fig.* 724) is the commonest of all fungous affections, and in England the predominant parasites

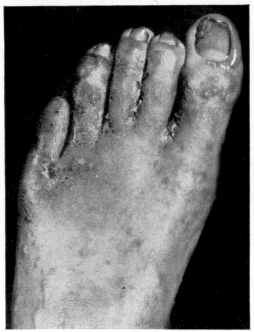

Fig. 724. Acute interdigital ringworm of the toes. (*Dr. Peter Hansell.*)

other parts of the body; it is now much commoner in England than it was a few years ago.

Tinea Versicolor (pityriasis versicolor) (*Fig.* 725) is caused by *Melassezia furfur* and takes the form of sheets of fine branny scaliness affecting the trunk. The patches are a fawnish-brown colour and have to be distinguished from leucoderma, in which disease the patches of hyperpigmentation surrounding the white areas are somewhat similar in colour to the patches of tinea versicolor. In leucoderma, however, there is no scaliness.

Tinea Imbricata is a tropical form of body ringworm in which the scaly patches are arranged in closely set concentric circles. In countries where it is endemic the diagnosis presents no difficulty

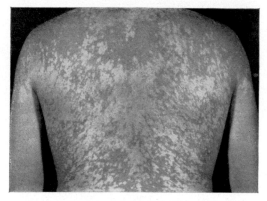

Fig. 725. Pityriasis versicolor. (*St. John's Hospital.*)

are the *T. mentagrophytes* and the *T. rubrum.* The former causes an acute inflammatory state, with vesicle formation and maceration. It starts between the toes, most commonly in the cleft between the fourth and fifth toes. From there crops of vesicles may spread over the soles and on to other parts of the feet. The early stage of the disease is accompanied by a great deal of burning and itching. Later there is crusting and secondary infection of the ruptured vesicles and occasionally ulceration takes place. It must be distinguished from acute dermatitis such as that produced by rubber footwear or the dye of socks, and from podopompholyx. *Trichophyton rubrum* is responsible for a relatively non-inflammatory type of eruption. It is invariably chronic and is characterized by faint erythema and a great deal of scaliness. It may be confined to the interdigital spaces and the nails, but may spread over the soles of the feet. It must be distinguished from psoriasis of the soles and chronic dermatitis. The diagnosis must always be confirmed by microscopical examination of scrapings. If possible cultures of the fungus should be made to determine which trichophyton is present. For while cases due to *T. mentagrophytes* respond readily to treatment, those due to *T. rubrum* are less easily treated. *Trichophyton rubrum* infections may spread widely from the feet to the hands and

and scrapings will disclose the presence of *Trichophyton concentricum,* the causal fungus.

Erythrasma, for long thought to be a superficial fungous infection, is now known to be bacterial and is an infection with *Corynebacterium minutissimum,* an organism highly sensitive to erythromycin. It causes reddish brown patches with slight scaliness, usually in the groins. The patches fluoresce pink or red under Wood's light.

P. D. Samman.

SKIN HARDENING

Hardening of the skin is the principal feature of scleroderma. In localized scleroderma (morphoea) there are usually small areas of hardening and in the early stages these are surrounded by a bluish halo. After a time the skin gradually softens again, but the sites are often marked by pigmentation which persists for years. Occasionally scleroderma appears in linear form, most often on the scalp and forehead (*coup-de-sabre*) (*Fig.* 12, p. 18) but at times involving a whole limb which then becomes greatly deformed. The linear type shows little tendency to spontaneous resolution.

The progressive type of scleroderma is a systemic disease. It starts with symptoms of

Raynaud's phenomenon and gradually the skin of the fingers and hands hardens and loses its mobility (*Fig.* 726). The feet are affected similarly and the skin of the face may become hard, tight,

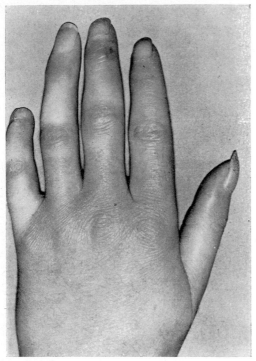

Fig. 726. Scleroderma (acrosclerosis). (*Dr. Peter Hansell.*)

and immobile. Systemic manifestations follow later in many cases involving the digestive system, kidneys, lungs, and heart. The skin of the extremities often shows areas of pigmentation and patches of calcification may occur.

In addition to scleroderma hardening of the skin may occur in various other conditions. Tense oedema especially of the legs may give the impression of hardness and true hardening may be a late manifestation of the post-thrombotic syndrome (pseudo-scleroderma). A pseudo-scleroderma picture is also seen on the limbs in the rare Rothmund's syndrome. The end stage of chronic dermatomyositis may closely simulate scleroderma. Pseudo-scleroderma of the lower legs is also an important sign of iron overload (i.e., excess ingestion of iron) in the South African Bantu.

Patchy hardening may be due to callosities and corns and also to Dupuytren's contracture.

P. D. Samman.

SKIN, PIGMENTATION OF

Increase in pigmentation of the skin may be considered under three main headings: (1) That due to increase in the production of melanin;

(2) Coloration caused by the deposition of haemoglobin or its derivatives in the skin; (3) A small group where the skin is coloured by a variety of other substances.

1. Increase of Melanin in the skin occurs after many forms of irritation or inflammation, for example sunburn and dermatitis. The persistent areas of pigmentation on the lower part of the legs that follow varicose dermatitis exemplify this. After prolonged friction or scratching,

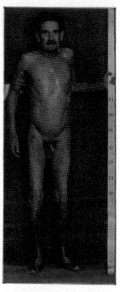

Fig. 727. Vagabond's discoloration in lice-infested vagrant suffering from scurvy.

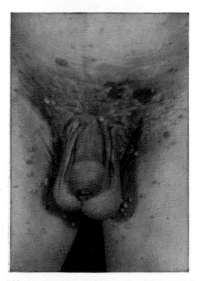

Fig. 728. Acanthosis nigricans. (*St. John's Hospital.*)

areas of pigmentation are often seen, e.g., vagabond's disease (*Fig.* 727) due to louse infestation. It occurs in *dermatitis herpetiformis* and is a regular late phase of *lichen planus* where the patches are sepia in colour. In the raindrop pigmentation due to chronic *arsenical poisoning* the colouring is due to melanin or some closely allied substance. In tar and pitch workers there is a tendency to hyperpigmentation.

Patchy increase in pigmentation in Indians and allied races is common. It is known that some

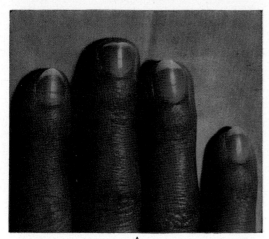

of these cases are due to vitamin-B_{12} deficiency when the increased pigmentation is particularly well marked on the backs of the hands overlying the joints.

In nearly every case of *leucoderma* (*Fig. 521*, p. 517) there is a zone of hyperpigmentation around the white patches. Patches of pigmentation form, especially on the face, during pregnancy (chloasma uterinum) and may occur in women taking the contraceptive pill; and freckles, X-ray dermatitis, xeroderma pigmentosum, urticaria pigmentosa (*Fig. 807*, p. 837), and the macular pigmentation of old age are further examples of localized increase in pigmentation. *Café-au-lait* patches are a constant feature in *von Recklinghausen's disease*. *Acanthosis nigricans* occurs in juvenile and adult forms. The juvenile form is of little importance but the adult form (*Fig. 728*), although uncommon, is important because it is always associated with carcinoma, usually of the intestinal tract. There is patchy increase in pigmentation in various sites but especially in the axillae, groins, and neck. The skin of the affected areas also shows an increase in skin markings and increase in thickness. Multiple seborrhoeic warts and other warty lesions are also common. The skin of the palms and soles may be much thickened and there may also be involvement of the mucous membranes.

Diffuse melanoderma is a feature of certain systemic diseases, especially when the endocrine glands are involved. Thus in *Addison's disease* (*Figs. 729A*, B) there is bronzing of the skin together with increased pigmentation of the

mucosae. To a lesser extent there may be hyperpigmentation in malaria, pellagra, diabetes mellitus, hyperthyroidism, lymphadenoma, abdominal carcinomatosis, and cachexia.

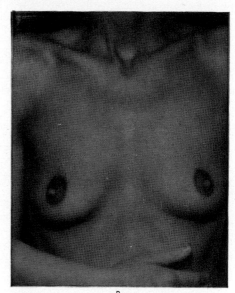

Fig. 729. A, Addison's disease.   B, Addison's disease showing pigmentation of areolae, neck, and anterior axillary fold.

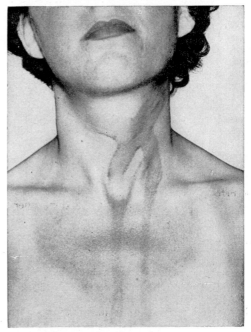

Fig. 730.   Berlocke dermatitis from eau-de-Cologne showing where it has trickled down from the neck.

In *Riehl's melanosis*, after a period of itching, redness, and peeling of the skin, patches of pigmentation appear on various parts of the body, especially the face and neck. The pigmentation is spotty rather than uniform, and while it usually fades in time it may be permanent. It is the result of a combination of the use of cosmetics and exposure to sunlight.

Berlocke (perfume) dermatitis (*Fig*. 730) is a rare artificial discoloration of the skin of the neck and other parts, and is caused by exposure of the skin to sunlight after the application of eau-de-Cologne. The causal agent is bergamot oil, the essential oil of eau-de-Cologne. Oil of lemon, orange peel, and lavender have also occasionally produced this effect. The pigment itself is melanin.

varicose dermatitis, and purpura annularis telangiectodes, which is similar.

A purpuric dermatitis, especially over the lower limbs, is a characteristic drug eruption due to carbromal. It has to be distinguished from Schamberg's disease and varicose pigmentation (*Fig*. 732).

Patches of pigmentation may follow the use of intramuscular iron in the treatment of anaemia. The pigmentation is usually over the site of the injection, but occasionally is far removed from it.

3. Pigmentation from Other Causes. Deposition of fine metallic particles in the skin may cause

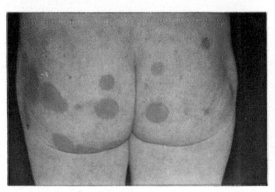

Fig. 731. Fixed drug eruption. (*Dr. Peter Hansell.*)

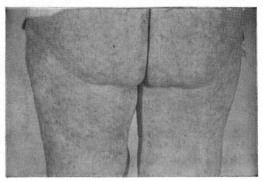

Fig. 732. Carbromal eruption. (*Dr. Peter Hansell.*)

In *poikilodermia climactericum*, brownish patches of pigmentation occur on the face and neck of women during the menopause. This disease is probably identical with the form of poikilodermia originally described by Civatte. Accumulations of melanin are present in *pigmented naevi* and *melanocarcinoma*.

Following the spontaneous resolution of patches of localized scleroderma (morphoea), the sites may be marked by pigmentation which persists for years. Pigmentation is also an important feature in scleroderma of the progressive type.

Patchy pigmentation of short duration and sometimes surmounted by a blister is the characteristic feature of a fixed drug eruption. Phenolphthalein is the drug most often involved. The pigment is a dusky blue or black (*Fig*. 731).

2. Deposition in the Skin of Haemoglobin or its derivatives occurs in ecchymosis, purpura, and haemorrhagic diseases, as well as in haematochromatosis (bronzed diabetes), where the pigmentation is due to haemosiderin.

Schamberg's disease, or progressive pigmentary dermatosis, runs a slow course. It occurs only in males and starts as patches of red punctate lesions which appear in crops on the shins, ankles, and dorsa of the feet. After a month or two the lesions fade to a characteristic cayenne-pepper colour. The pigment is probably haemosiderin. The condition is of no clinical significance and must be distinguished from purpura, angioma serpiginosum, the pigmentation due to

pigmentation. In *argyria* a slaty discoloration is caused by the presence of silver, which is carried in the blood-stream chiefly to the light-exposed areas of the skin, where it is found in the form of the albuminate. There is always a history of prolonged administration of silver preparations.

In some cases after *gold therapy* a gold salt is deposited in the skin on the light-exposed areas. It varies in colour from lilac-grey to fawn or brown, and is often seen at the edges of patches of lupus erythematosus which have been so treated.

Very rarely *bismuth* or *mercury*, internally administered for the treatment of syphilis, may form a slate-coloured deposit on the eyelids or other parts of the face. A blue line at the margin of the gums is nearly always present as well, although this is apt to be more pronounced in the presence of dental sepsis.

In *ochronosis* there is blue-black pigmentation of skin, nails, cartilage, ligaments, and tendons, and pigmented spots may be found on the sclerotics of the eyes. It results from alkaptonuria (homogentisic aciduria). Freshly voided urine is normal in appearance but darkens slowly from the exposed surface downwards on standing and rapidly when made alkaline.

In *carotinaemia* there is yellowish discoloration of the skin, most noticeable on the palms (*Fig*. 733) and soles. It has been observed in diabetes, but is more usually due to the over-ingestion of carrots and some other vegetables and fruits. Excess of carotene may be demonstrated in the blood-plasma and urine. The normal level is 50–200 μg. per 100 ml. Plain xanthomata may at times cause extensive yellowing of the skin, as, of course, may jaundice from any cause.

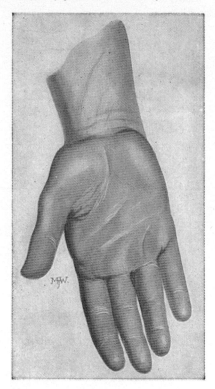

Fig. 733. Carotinaemia in a female who was consuming 15 tangerine oranges daily. The blood carotene level was 693 μg. per 100 ml. (*Drawing by Miss M. Waldron*.)

The blue marks in the skin of coal-miners due to tattooing with coal, and the tattooing of asphalt into the skin after road accidents, require no comment, nor do powder marks caused by fireworks or other explosions.

P. D. Samman.

SKIN SIGNS OF INTERNAL CARCINOMA

There are a number of skin markers of malignancy. Acanthosis nigricans of the adult type is almost always a sign of carcinoma of the digestive tract.

Dermatomyositis appearing in adult life indicates the presence of internal carcinoma in about 50 per cent of cases. The carcinoma may be in various sites including breast, intestine, ovary, and larynx.

Pemphigoid not infrequently occurs in association with internal malignancy.

A few of the rare cases of gyrate erythema appear to be caused by internal carcinomata, as they clear as soon as the malignancy has been treated.

The true relationship of the carcinoma to the skin lesions is at present uncertain in these cases, but in dermatomyositis an immune reaction to the tumour cells and some other tissues may be demonstrated. There is, however, one other association and that is between patches of Bowen's disease (intra-epidermal epithelioma) on the skin and internal carcinoma, especially of the lung, where both are probably due to the same cause, namely the ingestion of arsenic over a period of months or years many years previously.

P. D. Samman.

SKIN, TUMOURS OF

Many types of malignant disease may form secondary deposits in the skin, with ultimate ulceration. Direct extension from structures immediately under the skin also occurs. A notable example of this is the so-called *carcinoma en cuirasse*, which is an infiltration of the skin of the chest with breast-cancer cells. A not dissimilar state occurs when secondary malignancy of the axillary or inguinal lymph-nodes infiltrates the overlying skin. The skin is often infiltrated in leukaemia and in reticulum-celled sarcomata.

One of the commonest primary malignant diseases of the skin is *epithelioma* (squamous-cell carcinoma). It is usually single and as a rule of fairly slow growth, extending peripherally and infiltrating deeply while ulcerating at the centre. Sooner or later the lymphatic glands draining the affected area become involved. Usual sites for epitheliomata are the lips, the glans penis, and the exposed areas. Senile keratomata, moles, X-ray scars, and lupus vulgaris may all undergo epitheliomatous changes. The main diagnostic features of epithelioma are its origin as a single growth, its craggy hardness, its slow development, and the metastases in neighbouring glands. In all cases of doubt a biopsy will give the answer.

Molluscum sebaceum is dealt with under NODULES (p. 573).

Malignant melanoma (naevocarcinoma) (*Fig.* 734) may arise anywhere on the skin surface at any age, often in what was previously thought to be a simple pigmented or non-pigmented mole. It may occur in the hairy scalp or under a nail. Characteristic of this tumour are its rapid development and growth, its deepening in colour, its ulceration, bleeding, and crust formation, and its speedy adenopathy. Sometimes multiple metastases occur in the skin itself. The disease is highly malignant, but if diagnosed early and widely excised the prognosis is good especially in women and when situated on arm or leg.

Rodent ulcer (basal-cell carcinoma) usually affects the face and is dealt with on p. 273. Occasionally in its ordinary form it is found in other areas. On the trunk, where it may occur in multiple patches, the *benign erythematoid epithelioma* (superficial rodent ulcer) is not uncommon in the middle-aged or elderly. The patch is red and scaly, but close examination of the growing edge will show it to be heaped-up or rolled, an important diagnostic sign in basal-cell carcinoma. These tumours do not metastasize and are of very low malignancy.

Paget's disease is a rare epithelial carcinomatous disease affecting the nipple or areola. At first it looks like dermatitis of the same area; later it becomes keratotic, infiltrated, and finally ulcerated. It is accompanied by carcinoma of the mammary duct. In the early stages it must be distinguished from dermatitis; the latter disorder, however, nearly always affects both sides. If there is the slightest suspicion of Paget's disease a

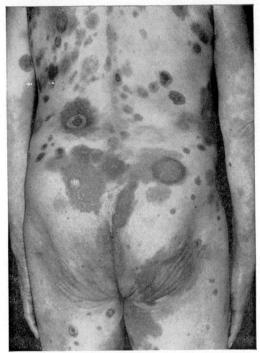

Fig. 735. Mycosis fungoides, early tumour stage. (*St. John's Hospital.*)

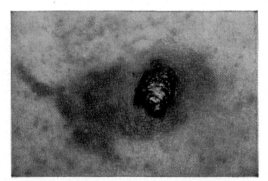

Fig. 734. Malignant melanoma. (*Dr. Peter Hansell.*)

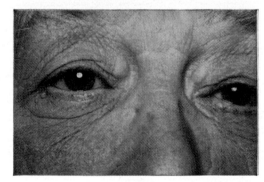

Fig. 737. Xanthelasma palpebrarum. (*Dr. Peter Hansell.*)

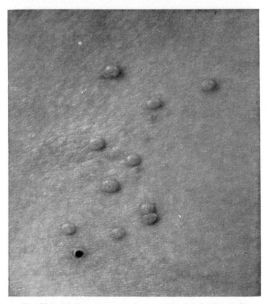

Fig. 736. Molluscum contagiosum. (*St. John's Hospital.*)

biopsy must be performed, when collections of large, round, clear-staining 'Paget's cells', often undergoing mitosis, will be found in the rete pegs, which in themselves are considerably widened.

Bowen's disease (pre-cancerous dyskeratosis) is an intra-epidermal squamous-cell carcinoma which later develops into a true squamous-cell carcinoma. The lesions are single or multiple, dull red, crusted papules affecting the skin and mucous membrane anywhere on the body. When the crusts are removed a dull red, moist, hard surface is exposed. Biopsy is essential for a final diagnosis.

The *erythroplasia of Queyrat* is similar to Bowen's disease, but affects the glans penis only. At first there is a slowly growing, circumscribed, moist, shiny patch; later this gives place to a typical squamous-cell carcinoma. A very similar but entirely benign condition is called *plasma-celled balanitis*. The sharply marginated red patch on the glans penis in this condition is apparently due to the plasma-cell infiltration.

Mycosis fungoides (*Fig.* 735) is a rare chronic fatal disease which is characterized in its final stage by tomato-like tumours which ulcerate and fungate. At first there may only be a severe generalized pruritus; this is followed, perhaps after several years, by what is called the 'premycotic stage'. This may be *poikilodermia vasculare atrophicans* (Jacobi) (*Fig.* 709, p. 707) or it may occur as a dry scaly eruption which superficially looks eczematous. Sometimes there is a generalized exfoliative erythrodermia (*homme rouge*). In the early stage an accurate diagnosis is sometimes impossible, but where there is chronic long-standing disease of one of these types associated with severe itching, the possibility of its being the premycotic stage of mycosis fungoides should be borne in mind. When the typical tomato-red tumours appear the nature of the disease is obvious. Biopsy is often helpful and may establish the diagnosis at a relatively early stage. The so-called *tumour d'emblée* type, where the tumours appear before other evidence of disease, is probably never a true example of mycosis fungoides but a variety of sarcoma.

Xeroderma pigmentosum is an extremely rare disorder starting in childhood and affects the light-exposed areas. It is due to an inherent hypersensitivity to ultra-violet light. At first there is a simple increase in freckles, then follow patches of hyperkeratosis, atrophy, telangiectasia, ulceration, and the formation of squamous-cell carcinomata and malignant melanoma. Death ensues early, but before this there may be destruction of the nose, eyes, ears, or mutilation of the fingers and toes.

The diagnosis of the numerous benign tumours affecting the skin is usually a simple matter. *Warts* and *moles*, pigmented or non-pigmented, occur anywhere on the body. *Sebaceous cysts*, commonest on the back, face, scalp, and scrotum, are of various sizes, cystic on palpation, and with a minute orifice to be found somewhere on their surface. Histologically they are usually keratin rather than sebaceous cysts. *Lipomata*, usually solitary, can be identified by their texture as also may be fibromata and papillomata. *Multiple papillomata* on the trunk must be distinguished from von Recklinghausen's disease (p. 577). Rarer lesions are *myoma* and *myxoma*. In cases of doubt excision of a lesion and microscopic examination will give the answer. Seborrhoeic warts are extremely common. They start as papules but may develop into tumours. They are described in detail under PAPULES (q.v.).

Molluscum contagiosum (*Fig.* 736) is a viral infection in which numerous small, hard, pearly tumours form anywhere on the body. They are flat on top, with a largish opening out of which white caseous material may be expressed. This substance when examined microscopically contains numerous large, non-nucleated, cell-like structures (molluscum bodies) which are diagnostic of the disease. The diagnosis is usually easy, but there may be confusion with warts and simple papilloma.

Xanthelasma palpebrarum (*Fig.* 737) is a common disease of the middle aged and elderly wherein soft yellow plaques appear on the eyelids, looking as if small pieces of chamois leather have been inserted superficially in the skin. Apart from their unsightliness they are usually

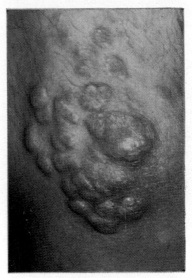

Fig. 738. Xanthoma tuberosum multiplex. (*Dr. Peter Hansell.*)

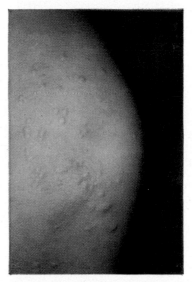

Fig. 739. Xanthoma eruptiva. (*Dr. Peter Hansell.*)

of no significance, but may be associated with types II and III hyperlipoproteinaemia.

Xanthoma tuberosum multiplex (*Fig.* 738) is an infiltration lipoidosis in which numerous round, yellow, flat plaques or nodules form in the skin. They may occur anywhere, but are usually found over the joints, particularly the elbows. They occur in types II, III, and IV hyperlipoprotein-aemia. Eruptive xanthomata (*Fig.* 739) are smaller and are usually found on the buttocks. They appear rapidly and fade just as quickly. They occur in types III and IV hyperlipoprotein-aemia but also, rarely, in severe diabetes.

Xanthomata unassociated with increased lipo-proteins may be found in histiocytosis X but also as small self-resolving lesions in juvenile xan-thoma and in xanthoma disseminatum (*Fig.* 740).

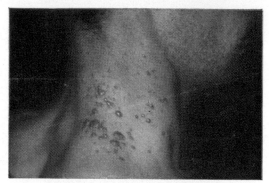

Fig. 740. Xanthoma disseminatum. (*Dr. Peter Hansell.*)

In *colloid milium* small, soft, yellow, cyst-like, minute tumours containing a gelatinous sub-stance appear in the skin around the eyes and on the upper part of the cheeks; they must be distinguished from *epithelioma adenoides cysti-cum*, in which multiple, small, round, smooth, shiny papules occur on the face, scalp, neck, and chest. They are hard and yellow or reddish and tend to coalesce. Middle-aged women are particularly affected.

Lymphocytomata are small glistening tumours which occur mainly on the face. They may be single or multiple and are often more prominent after exposure to sunlight.

P. D. Samman.

SLEEP-WALKING

Sleep-walking (*somnambulism*) is a common disturbance of childhood. If it only occurs occasionally it is of no significance whatsoever. But if it happens frequently it should be regarded as a symptom of a neurotic disorder and efforts made to trace its cause.

Although it is often said that there are no disturbed children, only disturbed parents, this is a statement which, while possibly somewhat far-fetched, obviously contains an element of truth. The child who sleep-walks, who wets the bed, who has temper-tantrums, is the child who is reacting to a family disturbance. As the treat-ment of the child, therefore, is the treatment of the family, it is the investigation of the family which is a necessary prerequisite of diagnosis and of treatment. The child who sleep-walks or who exhibits some other neurotic symptom of

childhood often does so in response to rows between parents and the anxiety occasioned thereby.

Apart from this, sleep-walking, either in child-ren or adults, is of great interest in that it demonstrates a mechanism occurring spon-taneously which is precisely similar or very closely analogous to a hypnotically induced trance in which a patient may sometimes perform a whole series of more or less complicated actions without, apparently, any awareness of what he is or has been doing. It lends support to the theo-retical concept of *dissociation* in which certain mental elements are apparently able to operate independently of the main stream. Somnam-bulism is also closely akin to a *hysterical* or *depressive fugue*, which does not necessarily begin while the patient is asleep in bed but may take place by day. As in the case of sleep-walk-ing, the patient, in a *fugue*, wanders in a state of clouded consciousness and later is usually amnesic for what has occurred.

W. H. Trethowan.

SMELL, ABNORMALITIES OF

Abnormalities of the sense of smell fall into three main categories, namely: (1) *Too great sensitiveness to smells which actually exist* (hyper-osmia); (2) *Deficient sensitiveness to smells which actually exist*; (3) *Subjective sensations of smells which do not exist externally*.

Too great sensitiveness to existing smells is some-times a nuisance to the individual, but is not a sign of disease. There are great differences in the powers of perception of different sensations in different persons, and just as some can appreciate very slight differences in sounds more than others, so can some detect smells that are not discernible by others. This is a natural idiosyncrasy, and is sometimes experienced in pregnancy. In general, sensitivity is reduced in heavy smokers.

Deficient sensitiveness to actual smells is often but the obverse of the above and no sign of disease, although it may be a detriment to the individual, especially in certain commercial pursuits in which the varying qualities of products are judged partly by smell. When the power of smell, having been normal, becomes deficient or totally absent, the change may affect one nostril only, or both. The condition may be transient or persistent. The commonest cause of transient anosmia is *acute nasal catarrh*, whether the result of an ordinary *cold*, or of other affections such as *hay fever* (coryza e feno), oncoming *measles*, or the effects of drugs such as *iodide of potassium* or *arsenic*. Transient anosmia is occasionally present during an attack of migraine.

Persistent anosmia may be due to:

a. PARTIAL OR TOTAL BLOCKAGE OF THE NOSE:

Adenoids	Deflected septum
Polypi	Syphilis
Hypertrophic rhinitis	Tumour

b. DISEASE OF THE OLFACTORY MUCOUS MEMBRANE, the airway being intact:

Atrophic rhinitis	Paralysis of the 5th
Leprosy	nerve, leading to dryness of the mucosa

c. ABNORMALITIES OF THE OLFACTORY NERVES AND UNCUS:

Congenital absence	Tumour of the frontal
Rupture of nerve filaments from a head injury	lobe and uncus; meningioma of the olfactory groove
Tabes and general paralysis	Raised intracranial pressure
Basal meningitis	

d. HYSTERIA.

There is little need to discuss the above table in detail, for each heading speaks for itself. When a case is being investigated the history is important; it is next necessary to examine the nose carefully through a speculum, and to test the airway through each nostril; if there is any local lesion it will generally be obvious, and only after local affections have been excluded should conditions in groups (*c*) and (*d*) be considered. Anosmia due to any cause other than local affection of the nose is nearly always associated with other symptoms which attract attention more than does the anosmia itself.

Parosmia is a perverted sense of smell, often unpleasant, which occurs after damage to the olfactory nerves and is usually transient.

Subjective sensations of smells which do not exist externally may be due to:

a. Offensive or purulent inflammation of the nose or of the air-cells communicating with it, especially empyema of the antrum of Highmore, or of a frontal, ethmoidal, or sphenoidal sinus—cacosmia.

b. Local irritation of the hippocampus by cerebral or pituitary tumour, basal meningitis, or aneurysm of the circle of Willis.

c. An aura preceding an epileptic seizure.

d. Insanity.

In arriving at a diagnosis, it is chiefly important to exclude purulent affections discharging into the nose; if it is possible to state with certainty that the abnormal sensations have no such organic basis it is not difficult as a rule to decide between the other causes. Subjective abnormalities of smell are apt to be associated with delusional insanity, in which the prognosis is not free from acute dangers—suicide or homicide.

Ian Mackenzie.

SNEEZING

Sneezing (or sternutation) is usually produced by irritation of the nasal mucosa and is characterized by the violent expulsion of air through the nose and mouth. It is essentially a reflex from the nasal endings of the 5th cranial nerve and serves to rid the mucosa of dust, dirt, and other irritants, e.g., snuff. In some persons hyperalgesia of the nasal mucosa will encourage sneezing from a change of temperature. Strong sunlight may have the like effect through stimulation of other endings of the trigeminal nerve. Of the local causes, *coryza* is the commonest, and sneezing is often the first symptom of a common cold. When running at the nose is fully established, sneezing usually subsides. Bouts of sneezing are common in *nasal allergy* and during the hay fever season sufferers from pollinosis may be incapacitated and exhausted by a bout of a dozen or more violent and rapidly recurring sneezes often associated with profuse watery rhinorrhoea, lacrimation, and conjunctival injection. Such a picture is in fact almost pathognomonic of pollinosis and is a useful means of distinguishing the latter from non-specific vasomotor rhinitis. In vasomotor rhinitis there is often copious rhinorrhoea but sneezing is usually absent and ophthalmic symptoms do not occur.

Sneezing is not common in true *influenza*, but when it does occur it is usually after the first two days of the disease, and is caused by a developing nasal catarrh. Sneezing is common in the prodromal stage of *measles* and *smallpox*. The presence of *foreign bodies* in the nasal cavities, particularly when in a finely divided state, causes intense sneezing to those persons who are not habituated to their presence, and there are various plants whose emanations or powdered leaves, or sawdust, may similarly produce sneezing: for instance, sneezeweed (*Helenium autumnale*); Tasmanian aster (*Centipoda orbicularis*); South African sneezewood sawdust (*Ptaerxylon utile*); English sneezewort, a species of yarrow (*Achillea ptarmica*); and ordinary *pepper*. Certain *poison gases*, many of which are not true gases but finely particulate liquid or solid, have such a powerful sternutatory effect that they are used as harassing agents in warfare; examples are the lacrimatory gases (tear gases) bromo-benzyl-cyanide (B.B.C.) and chloro-acetaphenol (C.A.P.); the lung irritants chlorine, phosgene, and chloropicrin; and the special nasal irritants chloro-dihydrophenarsazine (D.M.) and diphenyl-cyanoarsine (D.C.). Touching the septum with a probe opposite the middle turbinal is prone to cause sneezing.

Miles Foxen.

SNORING

The noise of snoring is produced by vibration of the soft palate and adjacent structures including the faucial pillars, tonsils, and tongue.

Nasal obstruction is an important factor in many cases of snoring, and the commonest conditions causing this obstruction are adenoids (in young children), deflections of the nasal septum, nasal polypi, nasal allergy, and collapse of the alae nasi. The view is widely held that nasal obstruction is the *only* cause of snoring but this is not so, for in some cases of loud snoring there is no evidence of an impaired nasal airway. Large tonsils may be responsible, or enlargement of the lateral bands of pharyngeal lymphoid tissue, and palatal paresis must be excluded. In some patients it is difficult to trace a definite cause of the symptom and it is probable that the general shape of their jaws, skull, and neck, and the flabbiness of their soft tissues, summate to produce the disorder.

Miles Foxen.

SPASTIC STATES

'Spasticity' refers to the increase of tone which results from agenesis or interruption of the upper motor neuron. The hypertonicity which occurs in disease of the corpus striatum is spoken of as 'rigidity', a useful convention to which proper attention is not always paid.

In spastic hemiplegia, which ordinarily results from a lesion in the internal capsule, the muscular tone is unequally distributed, with the result that the parts affected tend to adopt and maintain a highly characteristic posture. The upper limb develops flexor spasticity: it is adducted, flexed at the elbow, wrist, and finger, and the forearm is pronated. The leg is adducted at the hip, extended at hip and knee, and the foot is inverted.

Passive alteration of this posture is met by an increase of tone in the affected muscles, but if this is overcome the resistance gives way quite suddenly—'clasp-knife spasticity'. Spasticity of the face, tongue, and bulbar muscles is not obvious in unilateral lesions, but bilateral hemiplegia is usually associated with spastic weakness of the face, a spastic tongue, and spastic dysarthria. Transverse lesions of the spinal cord below the cervical enlargement give rise to spasticity in the legs which differs in no way from the condition produced by bilateral lesions of the corticospinal tracts at a higher level.

The degree of spasticity varies with the cause. It is most marked in slowly progressive and chronic cases, but is often absent for some days after sudden interruption of the motor pathway, as for instance after a cerebral thrombosis, a gunshot wound, or a fracture-dislocation of the spine with compression of the cord. It may be abolished by severe general toxaemia, and is reduced in the presence of a coincident affection of the peripheral motor nerves, such as occurs in the combination of pyramidal, posterior column, and peripheral nerve damage of subacute combined degeneration of the cord.

Interruption of the pyramidal tracts gives rise to increased tendon reflexes on the affected side or sides of the body; the abdominal reflexes are usually lost, and an extensor plantar response is present if the fibres to the lower limb are involved. Clonus is often but not invariably present at the ankle and knee. Contractures tend to perpetuate the abnormal position of the limbs, so that physiotherapeutic measures are essential in cases where recovery is to be expected.

Disturbances of the sphincters—precipitancy, incontinence, and retention—are common in bilateral pyramidal lesions, but are usually absent in unilateral cases. The retention of urine which is so constant a feature of transverse lesions of the cord requires immediate attention, for stasis of urine paves the way for infection of the urinary tract, with all its discomfort and danger.

The pathological causes of spastic states are numerous and important; they extend over the whole range of neurological disease, and they are discussed in the sections on HEMIPLEGIA (p. 391) and PARAPLEGIA (p. 618).

Ian Mackenzie.

SPEECH, ABNORMALITIES OF

Disorders of speech fall into three classes—psychogenic, aphasic, and dysarthric. In the first, the abnormality is a by-product of an emotional conflict (as in hysteria), or of a psychosis (as in schizophrenia), and normal speech is possible *during* the period of illness. In aphasia the abnormality is due to organic disease of the major (usually the left) cerebral hemisphere, and although the severity of the defect may fluctuate from day to day or from hour to hour, the abrupt recovery of function seen in psychogenic cases cannot occur, for the mechanism of speech is impaired although the will to speak is present. The third class of defect, dysarthria, involves inability to articulate clearly; in extreme instances, no articulation is possible—anarthria.

Functional (Psychogenic) Disorders. *Stammering* occurs in highly strung and obsessional individuals; it dates from early life and grows less in adult life, but is apt to recur with anxiety and after psychological shocks. It is said to be particularly common in left-handed children who have been forced to use the right hand. Lisping is encountered in persons who have not reached emotional maturity. In *lalling* speech there is difficulty in the pronunciation of certain consonants, R being replaced by W, Th by V, K by T, and so on. This is a normal feature of infancy and it is seen in some mental defectives; also, occasionally, in otherwise normal persons. In *idioglossia*, this substitution of consonants is on a scale which amounts to a new and personal language. It is sometimes associated with high-tone deafness. Idioglossia, which affects all words, must be distinguished from the occasional neologisms invented by schizophrenics; the general pattern of speech is normal apart from the recurrent use of a word or words of the patient's own making; these often represent a combination of words which have a special meaning for him. *Perseveration* (the repetition of a word or sentence)—and echolalia (the repetition of words heard) are usually seen in schizophrenia, but both also occur in organically determined aphasia.

Mutism may be an expression of schizophrenic catatonia, or of extreme depression, or of emotional conflict in hysteria, but it may also be the result of complete motor aphasia whether congenital or acquired. The differentiation between organic and functional disturbances of speech will depend in such instances upon a study of the case history and satellite symptoms and signs.

Aphasia. A definition of aphasia is difficult to supply in a few words. The term is used to denote that loss of speech which does not depend on mental deficiency or upon paralysis of the motor

With these physiological and anatomical data as a basis, we can proceed to consider the chief varieties of aphasia and the points in their differential diagnosis. Before doing so, it is well to sound a note of warning with regard to the complications which are constantly being met with by the clinician in attempting to analyse cases of aphasia. In the first place, a diagrammatic anatomical definition of the cerebral 'centres' is apt

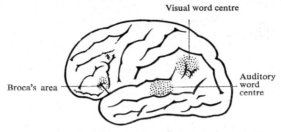

Fig. 741. A diagrammatic representation of the left cerebral hemisphere, showing the chief centres concerned with speech.

mechanism of articulation. Such a negative description requires, however, some modification, because aphasia is frequently associated with impairment of the capacity to think, resulting from disturbance of internal language. This plays an important part in all intellectual processes, and any lesion of the cerebral centres connected with it must necessarily interfere with mental activities. This is particularly the case in what is called 'receptive' aphasia, that variety which depends upon a lesion of the auditory and visual word centres situated in the cortex near the posterior part of the left Sylvian fissure of the brain (*Fig.* 741). In right-handed persons the chief speech centres are placed in the left cerebral hemisphere, and it is customary to consider them as being three in number. The posterior part of the first temporal convolution is the area in which the auditory memories of spoken words are stored and recalled; it plays an important part in the development of speech, because it is largely through the sense of hearing that the child first learns to associate objects with their names, and expressions with their meanings. The cortex of the angular gyrus has a similar function in regard to the storage of visual word memories, a function which bears the same relationship to written language as the auditory word centre has to spoken language. These two portions of the cortex constitute the sensory speech centres. A third important centre is located in Broca's area, in the posterior part of the third frontal convolution. In this situation are stored memories of afferent impulses excited by the motor activities associated with speech. Unless this centre is intact the conversion of internal into external language is imperfect or impossible. In the opinion of some authorities there is a similar centre in the posterior part of the left second frontal convolution, which plays a part in connexion with written language comparable to the part played by Broca's area in relation to spoken language.

to give a wrong impression. These centres are more diffuse in their function than they appear to be on a map of the brain, and they are much more interdependent than their topography would suggest. Communicating nervous tracts bind them together in such a way that a destructive lesion of one must necessarily upset the function of another, and so modify the clinical picture of any particular case profoundly. Aphasia is, in most instances, the result of a vascular lesion and all the centres referred to lie in the area supplied by one artery—the middle cerebral. Consequently even when the main brunt of a vascular disturbance falls on one of the special speech centres, the others may also suffer more or less, temporarily or permanently, from disturbances of nutrition. In any case of aphasia, therefore, we may have to be satisfied if we can arrive at a conclusion as to the site of the chief defect, without being able to define the exact limits of the cerebral lesion.

Again, due allowance must be made for the fact that the right cerebral hemisphere may gradually acquire some degree of speech activity, especially in cases of aphasia occurring during the earlier years of life, and may tend to replace the loss caused by the defective action of the left. Moreover, there is evidence that the right hemisphere is concerned with 'emotional' speech—a completely aphasic subject may be able to swear with fluency or to make appropriate comments if frightened or otherwise stirred.

Word-deafness is the result either of a lesion of the auditory word centre in the temporal cortex or of one which isolates that centre from the periphery—a subcortical lesion cutting off the centre from auditory impulses. In either case the patient who is word-deaf is unable to recognize the meaning of spoken language, although he may hear perfectly the sounds by which it is conveyed. He fails to understand anything which is said to him, and does not obey simple commands so long as they are not accompanied by gestures suggestive of their meaning. If the visual word centre has not been affected at the same time, he will still be able to read and to understand what is written. He will depend upon writing and reading for his means of communication with others. The amount of interference with spontaneous speech will depend upon whether the lesion is cortical or subcortical. If the latter, the integrity of the auditory word centres preserves internal speech, and so permits the patient to speak spontaneously with fluency and probably with accuracy, and his power of writing will be unimpaired. When the cortical centre is itself destroyed, internal language is thoroughly disorganized, and although some spontaneous speech may be possible it is certain to be more or less unintelligible. According to the extent of the lesion it will vary between a speech containing inaccuracies of minor importance and one which is a jargon incapable of interpretation. Characteristic of this defect is the fact that the patient himself does not appreciate the mistakes he makes. His written language is likely to be more accurate and more intelligible than his spoken language, but it will probably not reach a very high standard. He may copy with accuracy but be quite unable to write from dictation. Such are the usual chief attributes of word deafness in its pure form. Clinically, word-deafness is usually accompanied by word-blindness, to a greater or less extent.

Word-blindness, or *alexia*, is produced by a lesion of the left angular gyrus, and may or may not be accompanied by a defect in the field of vision. As in the case of word-deafness it may result from a cortical or from a subcortical lesion, and it is in association with the latter class of case that HEMIANOPIA (p. 387) is most common. In cortical word-blindness the patient is unable to read, although he sees the letters clearly and may even be able to copy them in the same way as a child copies letters when learning the alphabet. Writing conveys no meaning to his mind, although in the less severe cases the patient may still recognize familiar words, such as his name. There are, in fact, varying degrees of word-blindness, some of which are difficult to understand and to analyse. The word-blind patient suffers in his spontaneous speech to a greater or less extent according to whether he uses his visual or his auditory memories chiefly in the process of internal language. Should he be a 'visual' his spontaneous speech will suffer much more than if he is an 'auditive'. Spontaneous writing is likely to be lost completely, but writing from dictation may be carried out with more or less accuracy. In word-blindness due to a subcortical lesion, although hemianopia is most certain to be present, spontaneous speech and spontaneous writing are preserved perfectly, although the power of reading and of copying hand-written sentences to printed capitals is entirely in abeyance.

When word-blindness and word-deafness co-exist the condition is called *receptive aphasia*.

Cortical motor aphasia results from a destructive lesion of Broca's area, the part of the cortex which stores memories of the afferent impulses excited by speech, and in which such memories must be revived if spontaneous speech is to be carried out perfectly. This form of expressive aphasia may be present without any paralysis, but it is usually accompanied by some disturbances of internal speech, and perhaps even by some defective understanding of spoken and written language, which, however, never amounts to complete receptive aphasia.

Much more common is the *subcortical motor aphasia* which is due to a lesion cutting off Broca's cortical area from the motor mechanism connected with articulation. In this form intellectual processes and internal language may be perfectly intact, but in most cases the inability to speak is associated with right hemiplegia in right-handed persons, or with left hemiplegia in left-handed individuals. The imperfect speech of the patient who is partly aphasic from a subcortical motor lesion may resemble to some extent that of the patient who is word-deaf; but the former is conscious of his mistakes and the latter is not. Subcortical motor aphasia may perhaps be described better as an articulatory rather than a speech defect.

Agraphia results usually from a lesion of the visual word-centre, or in some cases from a lesion of the posterior part of the left second frontal convolution. In the former case the power of writing may be lost, although there is no paralysis of the arm or hand. In the latter case the agraphia is usually associated with right hemiplegia, and in order to test whether the power of communicating thoughts by written language is preserved, the patient must be asked to use the left hand for the purpose. There is some doubt as to whether *isolated* motor agraphia occurs.

We have now considered the various forms of aphasia and have indicated their points of distinction. This will serve as a basis for diagnosing the site of the lesion responsible for the speech defect, but the nature of the lesion must be determined from other considerations. Vascular lesions, for instance, are usually acute in their onset, sudden in the case of *embolism*, less precipitate as a rule in cases of *haemorrhage* or *thrombosis*. With *cerebral tumour* or *abscess* the onset of symptoms is more gradual and local signs such as aphasia may be eventually accompanied by headache and papilloedema. But aphasia is not always the result of a gross and permanent lesion. Transitory aphasia may be observed after epileptiform convulsions, or may be in itself a seizure equivalent —a form of minor epilepsy. Temporary aphasia occurs also in connexion with *migraine*, in transient ischaemic attacks and as a symptom of *hypertensive encephalopathy*.

Dysarthria is an obvious result of extensive disease of the lips, tongue, palate, and pharynx, but the term is usually employed for defects of articulation which have a neurological origin, and it is this conventional usage which is accepted as the basis for the present account. As is the case with voluntary movements elsewhere in the body, dysarthria may be caused by muscular weakness, spasticity, rigidity, ataxia, or involuntary movements.

1. Weakness of the lips, tongue, soft palate, and larynx, due to disease of the bulbar nuclei or their efferent fibres, causes a slow, slurring dysarthria with a notable deficiency in the pronunciation of consonants. It is seen in congenital facial diplegia, acute poliomyelitis of the bulbar nuclei, polyneuritis (e.g., the infective form of Guillain-Barré, diphtheria, uveoparotid polyneuritis), the atrophic form of bulbar palsy in motor neuron disease, gummatous meningitis of the posterior fossa, botulism, and thrombosis of the posterior inferior cerebellar artery.

Spastic dysarthria results from bilateral involvement of the pyramidal fibres to the bulbar nuclei. This is seen in motor neuron disease, general paralysis of the insane, some cases of disseminated sclerosis, congenital and acquired double hemiplegia, and in the pseudo-bulbar palsy of progressive cerebral arteriosclerosis. Speech is thick and often slow. Spasticity of the vocal cords interferes with the conservation and regulation of the air blast as it passes through the larynx, with the result that the normal 'stops' of the voice are lacking and words and sentences are telescoped into each other. To get as many words as possible into each expiration the patient may speak very quickly, truncating words and ignoring the pauses of normal speech.

2. Extrapyramidal rigidity of the muscles of articulation, seen in Parkinson's disease, post-encephalitic Parkinsonism, and hepatolenticular degeneration, gives rise to a slow, monotonous, slurred speech, in which the normal modulations of voice are absent and the 'stops' between words are lacking.

3. Myasthenia gravis is marked by the extreme fatigability of voluntary muscles. Early manifestations are usually ocular, but bulbar symptoms are not uncommon. Speech is normal after rest, or after the injection of neostigmin, but a slurring dysarthria develops during conversation. Permanent paralysis, with persistent 'bulbar' speech, occurs late in the disease.

4. Cerebellar ataxia of speech occurs in disseminated sclerosis, cerebellar neoplasms, Friedreich's ataxia, and vascular lesions of the pons and cerebellum. Speech is slurred and slow; attempts to circumvent the difficulty by enunciating words syllable by syllable give rise to the 'scanning speech' often found in disseminated sclerosis. Severe cerebellar dysarthria is sometimes marked by explosive utterance, and an unevenness of diction comparable to the irregularity of voluntary movement seen in the limbs.

5. Involuntary movements of the tongue, lips, larynx, and respiratory muscles interfere with speech in chorea and congenital bilateral athetosis. Speech is jerky, irregular, and explosive.

6. Dysarthria occurs when the muscles of articulation are involved in the myopathies and in myotonia dystrophica, but this is a late event, and diagnosis is made easy by the myopathic facies and the wasting elsewhere in the body.

Ian Mackenzie.

SPINAL CURVATURE

The first thing is to distinguish between curvature in the lateral and in the anteroposterior plane. Though in a certain number of cases lateral curvature (scoliosis) is accompanied by some anteroposterior deformity (kyphosis or lordosis), and in a few instances of angular kyphosis due to tuberculous disease there is lateral deviation as well, the main direction of the curvature is always apparent. Lateral curvature is usually due to congenital malformation, posture, poliomyelitis, or compensation for a short leg, and is seldom the result of bone disease; whereas anteroposterior deformity with the concavity forwards (kyphosis) is suggestive of osteoporosis, tuberculous or malignant disease of the vertebral bodies, and in the opposite direction (lordosis) of nerve disease or some affection of the hip-joint.

LATERAL CURVATURE—SCOLIOSIS

Lateral curvature rarely takes the form of a single curve; owing to the necessity for maintaining the general alinement of the head and trunk in order to preserve equilibrium, a lateral deviation in one part of the spine is usually compensated by another above or below it in the opposite direction, so that two or even three curves are commonly seen. Curvature in the lateral plane is nearly always accompanied by rotation of the spine, the vertebral bodies moving towards the convexity of the curve. This rotation has two important results; that the apparent curve as judged by the line of the spinous processes is always less than the real one: and that the ribs are carried round with the vertebrae, backwards on the side of the convexity, causing a visible 'hump' and elevation of the scapula and point of the shoulder, and forwards on the side of the concavity, giving rise to flattening behind and prominence of the breast in front.

A similar effect is produced by the transverse processes in the lumbar region, and the lump so caused, together with the pain from the scoliosis, has been mistaken for a perinephric abscess.

Scoliosis can usually be recognized when the patient is examined from behind, standing stripped to the hips in a good light: the curve can be demonstrated by marking the spinous processes with a skin pencil. When the curve is not obvious, it may often be suspected when it is noticed that one scapula is raised or prominent, one hip projecting more than the other, or the angle between the arm and the chest wall more open on one side. The deformity is often noticed first by a dressmaker. When the patient is made to bend forward, the rotation is brought into prominence. A radiograph is valuable in confirming the diagnosis, and showing the degree of rotation of the vertebral bodies. The following are the most important varieties of lateral curvature:

CONGENITAL. Wedge-shaped deformity of a vertebra.

ACQUIRED:

Habitual or postural, due to deficiency in muscle tone, often associated with faulty habits of standing or sitting, or occupations involving carrying heavy weights. It has been suggested, not unreasonably, that some of these so-called 'postural' cases may be consequent on an abortive attack of poliomyelitis which has picked out the small muscles of the back.

Compensatory, the result of wry-neck or shortening of one leg.

Paralytic, following poliomyelitis, peripheral neuritis, and some of the muscular dystrophies.

Rachitic.

Reflex, to relieve pain, especially in sciatica and renal disease.

Hysterical.

Congenital Scoliosis can usually be recognized from the history of a deformity existent from birth, and should be suspected when the lateral deviation is abrupt. A sharp angulation to one side or the other is noticed, usually in the mid-dorsal region, and a more gradual curve in the opposite direction above and below it. Other congenital malformations, especially Sprengel's shoulder (congenital elevation of the scapula), and cervical rib, are often present in addition. A radiograph will show a wedge-shaped half-vertebra, and an uneven number of ribs on the two sides, one being absent on the concave side or an additional one appearing on the side of the convexity.

Genetic abnormalities predisposing to the development of scoliosis include neurofibromatosis, Marfan's and Ehlers-Danlos syndromes, osteogenesis imperfecta, Morquio's disease and gargoylism (Hurler's syndrome), possibly by a combination of abnormal vertebral development and altered muscular action.

Idiopathic or so-called **Postural Scoliosis** is the type most commonly encountered. It is much commoner in girls than boys, and usually appears between the sixth and tenth years, though in a large proportion of cases the deformity is not noticed until about the age of puberty. In the early stages the error is one of posture only, and the curve disappears when the patient is lifted by the head; later, structural changes in bones and ligaments supervene, and only partial correction is possible by suspension. The basic cause is unknown, but poor health, insufficient fresh air or exercise, or rapid growth of the skeleton in proportion to muscular power, faulty habits of standing or sitting, ill-designed school desks, and sagging beds are all possible contributory causes. Idiopathic scoliosis can usually be recognized without difficulty by the age and sex of the patient, the symptomless onset, and the absence of any bone deformity or shortening of one leg.

Characteristically two curves are seen, convex to the left in the lumbar region and to the right in the dorsal region, and rotation is more marked than in any other type of scoliosis; the right shoulder is raised and the right hip prominent.

Compensatory Scoliosis when due to *wry-neck* is usually slight, and involves the dorsal spine. The curve is convex to the side to which the head is inclined, and tends to bring the head upright. The wry-neck usually attracts attention, and the spinal curvature is only noticed during the course of examination. *Unequal length of the lower limbs* may be a cause of lateral curvature, and in the investigation of any case the legs should be measured. Lateral curvature due to a shortened limb takes the form of a sharp curve in the lumber region convex towards the side of the short leg, and a gradual curve of the upper part of the spine in the opposite direction. In its early stage the curvature disappears when the shortening is corrected or the patient sits on a level surface; after many years, however, the deformity becomes fixed.

Paralytic Scoliosis is generally due to *poliomyelitis*, and the diagnosis is usually obvious, not only on the history, but on the presence of a typical lower neuron paralysis with vascular changes involving the limbs. The disease rarely attacks the trunk muscles alone, and both legs, and often the arms as well, are usually affected in cases with scoliosis due to it. The curvature varies in severity with the degree of muscle atrophy, may involve any part of the spine, and may show any combination of lateral with anteroposterior bending. *Peripheral neuritis* as a cause of scoliosis is nearly always due to diphtheria. The history may indicate this, or there may have been other postdiphtheritic paralyses, notably that of the soft palate, with nasal voice and regurgitation of fluid through the nose. In an early case throat swabs may be positive. Scoliosis is often seen in the various *muscular dystrophies* (p. 625) and in Friedreich's *hereditary ataxia* (p. 623).

Rachitic Scoliosis is associated with a history going back to infancy, and typical changes will be found in the skull, thorax, and long bones of the limbs. Spinal curvature in rickets is more often anteroposterior than lateral.

Reflex Scoliosis is a response to some painful affection—sciatica, or disease of the hip, kidney, or appendix; the cause is brought to light by an analysis of the history and physical signs.

Hysterical Scoliosis is recognized by the general stigmata of the affliction, by the changing character of the deformity, and by its disappearance during sleep or under anaesthesia.

EFFECT OF SCOLIOSIS

Generally speaking the higher the site of the scoliosis in the spine the greater the deformity and the likelihood of it causing cardiorespiratory dysfunction. Lumbar scoliosis is relatively benign. The large majority of patients suffer only psychological upset from their deformity.

ANTEROPOSTERIOR CURVATURES

These may take the form of *kyphosis* or *lordosis*.

Kyphosis (Hump-back or Hunch-back). This means a bending forward of the upper part of the back on the lower. The curve may be: *Angular*, limited to a small portion of the back; or *Diffuse*, involving a large portion or the whole. ANGULAR KYPHOSIS. Due to collapse of the bodies of one or more vertebrae.

The causes of angular kyphosis are:

Tuberculous caries of the vertebral body.
Crush fracture of the vertebral body.
Growths of the spine, either primary sarcoma or secondary deposits of carcinoma.
Hydatid disease of the vertebrae.

Angular kyphosis appearing in a child is probably due to tuberculosis, in a healthy adult male to fracture, and in a patient over 50 to malignant disease.

Tuberculous caries usually appears first before the age of 10. It is very important to recognize the disease before the deformity becomes well marked, but unfortunately the wrong diagnosis may initially be made as pains are often referred to the abdomen or lower ribs rather than the back. The child looks ill and is disinclined to play: he walks carefully and steadies himself by grasping articles of furniture; when asked to pick a coin from the floor he will not stoop, but bends the hips and knees, keeping the trunk upright. On examining the back a prominence in the line of the spinous processes will be noticed, usually in the lower dorsal region. The degree of angulation depends on the amount of bone destruction, and the number of vertebrae involved. The spine is tender at the level of the deformity on percussing the affected vertebrae, or jarring the head. The diseased segment is held rigid in bending or in making lateral movements of the trunk. In later cases a cold abscess may be discovered in the erector spinae or psoas muscles. Radiographs, especially those taken in the lateral plane (*Fig.* 81, p. 89), will confirm the diagnosis by showing destruction of the bodies of the vertebrae, and in some cases the fusiform shadow of a paravertebral abscess.

The comparative frequency of *crush fracture of a vertebral body* as a cause of angular curvature has been recognized recently owing to the greater attention which is paid to minor industrial accidents, and the invariable use of X-rays. Sudden and forced flexion of the trunk causes fracture-dislocation of the spine with paraplegia, but lesser degrees of the same violence may lead to a cancellous fracture of a vertebra without obvious deformity. If the injury is not recognized and treated at the time, the cancellous tissue yields to the weight of the trunk, the injured vertebral body is compressed into a wedge shape, and an obvious angular kyphosis appears. The diagnosis will be suggested when a sharply localized angulation is found in a healthy man above the usual age of tuberculosis

and below that of cancer. The patient rarely presents himself because of the deformity, but complains of a 'weak back' or 'girdle pains' due to irritation of the spinal roots. A history of an accident some months or even years previously can often be elicited. A radiograph taken in the lateral plane will show a wedge-shaped vertebra without evidence of bone absorption—an appearance sometimes termed Kümmell's disease.

Neoplasm of the spine is a rarer cause of angular curvature. The invasion of the vertebra may be heralded by intractable girdle pains; collapse of the diseased body may occur suddenly, and be accompanied or followed shortly by paraplegia and death. The surgeon should, however, inquire carefully into the history of every case of rapidly developing angular curvature in a patient over middle age, and examine every possible source of primary carcinoma, particularly the breast, prostate, lungs, thyroid, and kidneys. A radiograph will in most cases demonstrate abnormality of a vertebra (*see* Figs. 643, 644, pp. 621, 622).

Hydatid disease is a rare cause of spinal curvature, and the diagnosis may be impossible unless there is collateral evidence of hydatid disease elsewhere. In the absence of a history of probable infection, the condition is usually mistaken for tuberculous caries or new growth. Pathological fractures may occur. The discovery of eosinophilia or a positive indirect haemagglutination test in the blood-serum will suggest the correct diagnosis. Casoni's skin reaction is less specific and less reliable.

DIFFUSE KYPHOSIS due to an increase in the normal forward curve of the spinal column is partly the result of weakness in the muscles supporting the trunk, but also of disease of the bones or joints of the spine.

The commonest causes of diffuse kyphosis are:

Muscular weakness in: idiocy; muscular dystrophy; congenital spastic paralysis
Adolescent kyphosis
Rickets
Osteoporosis and osteomalacia
Hyperparathyroidism
Osteitis deformans
Ankylosing spondylitis
Osteoarthrosis.

Spinal curvature due to *muscular weakness* involves the whole column in a gradual curve and is characterized by an entire absence of rigidity. The distinguishing features of the causative disease will be apparent.

Adolescent kyphosis usually appears between the ages of 14 and 20. It is associated with poor health, rapid growth, or overwork, allowing the normal kyphosis of the dorsal spine to become exaggerated. Short sight, stooping over desks, or occupations which involve carrying weight upon the shoulders may all contribute to produce the deformity. The curvature is most marked in the dorsal spine, giving the familiar appearance of round shoulders said to betoken the student. Adolescent kyphosis is at first often a matter of faulty posture only, but the curve is later fixed by secondary changes in the bones and joints. Radiographic findings include irregularities of the epiphyses which appear in a lateral radiograph as wedge-shaped slips of bone applied to the upper and lower borders of the vertebral bodies at their ventral margins. Well-defined notches (first described by Scheuermann)

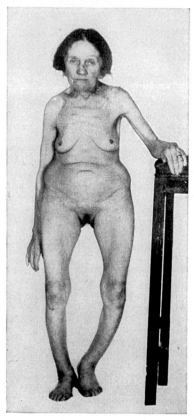

Fig. 742. Paget's disease, showing the kyphosis, bowing of the legs and apparently over-long arms, with increase in the size of the head. (Dr. C. Baker.)

are sometimes found in the same position, while prolapse of the nucleus pulposus (Schmorl's nodes) may be seen. The exact significance of these findings is uncertain, but it may be that in a proportion of cases there is a definite change in the bone from the beginning.

The kyphosis of *rickets* develops in the first and second years in rickety children who are allowed to sit up. At this age the lumbar lordosis has not appeared, and the back in the sitting position assumes a long curve most marked in the lumbar region. The rickety deformity is an exaggeration of this position—a rounded prominence of the lower part of the spine. Other indications of the disease will be found in the skull, ribs, and extremities of the long bones. In later life this lumbar convexity is usually compensated by obliteration of the dorsal curve, so

that the whole spine is abnormally straight. The so-called 'vitamin D resistant rickets' (familial hypophosphataemia and the rare inherited hypophosphatasia) may give a similar picture.

Osteoporosis is the commonest cause of the rounded bent back of the elderly, and is more common in females than males. It is the main cause of the shortening of body length seen in those over 60 years of age. Usually painless, acute pain may occur after a crush fracture develops in the body of a vertebra. Anti-anabolic hormones, such as the corticosteroids, may aggravate the condition and speed the tempo of a process which occurs to some extent in all elderly subjects. In *osteomalacia* gross deformities may occur with considerable chronic discomfort, due often to chronic intestinal malabsorption. In *hyperparathyroidism*, usually due to the presence of a benign parathyroid tumour, considerable kyphosis may occur in a porotic spine in which many vertebral bodies become wedged and narrowed.

Kyphosis due to *osteitis deformans* (Paget's disease—*Fig.* 742) takes the form of a uniform curve, with consequent stooping, without compensatory lordosis, and is irreducible. The curvature first makes its appearance after middle age, and there is usually evidence of the disease in other parts—a progressive increase in the size of the head, and thickening and bending of the tibiae and femora. The disease is pronounced in the long bones, especially the tibiae, long before the spine is affected. The diagnosis is suggested at once by the stance. (For radiographic changes *see Fig.* 743.)

In *ankylosing spondylitis* some patients have straight, stiff spines and look like guardsmen on parade; others are bent forwards with greater or lesser degree of kyphosis, sometimes with scoliosis also. The patients, usually males, have sacro-iliac involvement and often a stiff neck. Hips and shoulders are involved in about 40 per cent of cases. It is more common in younger men than older, usually starting in the 20s. *Rheumatoid arthritis* in adults and *Still's disease* in children lead less commonly to milder degrees of kyphosis.

Osteoarthrotic changes in the vertebral bodies appear with advancing years, and are accepted as so characteristic of age that a fixed stoop is essential to the make-up of an actor playing senile parts. The whole back, especially in the dorsal region, becomes bowed forwards, and its movements are diminished. Trauma, laborious occupations, or faulty posture will accentuate the deformity due to osteoarthrosis.

Porters carrying heavy weights on the upper part of the back—*deal porters* for instance—develop prematurely a kyphosis analogous to that of old age; they frequently have a bursa over the 7th cervical spinous process ('porter's hummy') (*Fig.* 744).

Lordosis (Hollow-back). This is common only in the lumbar and lower dorsal regions, and is an exaggeration of the natural hollow of the loins.

The chief causes of lordosis are:

Muscular weakness
Forward projection of the spine above or below the lumbar region (kyphosis above; spondylolisthesis below)
Flexion deformity of the hip
Congenital dislocation of the hips.

In each case the lordosis is compensatory, and has for its purpose the maintenance of the erect position of the trunk.

Weakness or *paralysis of the muscles of the back* provokes a backward inclination of the upper

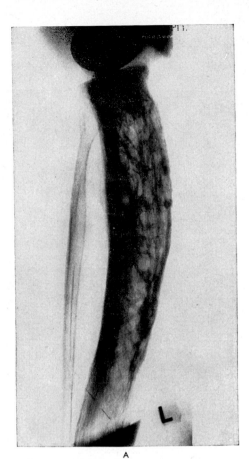

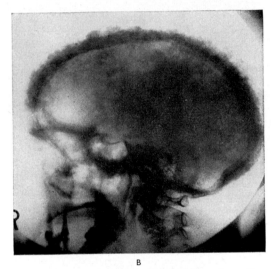

Fig. 743. A, Paget's disease of the tibia, showing patchy sclerosis and rarefaction. B, Paget's disease of the skull. Note the woolly appearance of the tables. (*Dr. J. D. Dow.*)

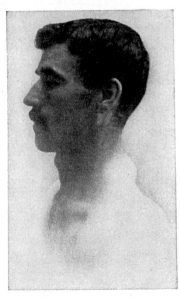

Fig. 744. 'Deal porter's bursa' over vertebra prominens.

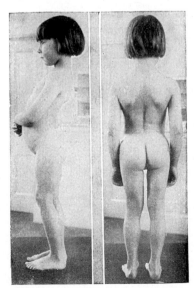

Fig. 745. A case of congenital dislocation of the hips, showing the stance and pronounced lordosis. (*Dr. Hawarth.*)

part of the trunk to maintain balance. When no cause for a compensatory lordosis has been discovered, a search should be made for evidence of muscular dystrophy or poliomyelitis.

Spondylolisthesis, a slipping forwards of the 5th lumbar upon the 1st sacral vertebra, and/or

can be restored to its natural shape by placing the patient in the supine position and flexing the thighs.

R. G. Beard.

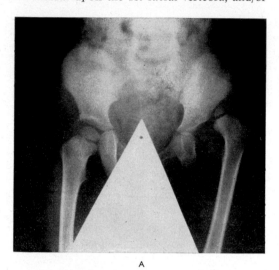
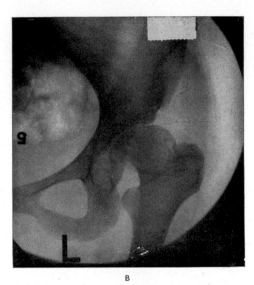

A   B

Fig. 746. A, Congenital dislocation of the hips. The upper femoral epiphysis is displaced laterally and upwards in relation to the acetabulum, which is poorly developed. (*Dr. John D. Dow.*) B, Old congenital dislocation of the hip with malformation of the head of the femur and false acetabulum. (*Dr. T. H. Hills.*)

the 4th on the 5th lumbar vertebra, can sometimes be recognized by the abnormal prominence of the upper part of the sacrum, which forms a marked and visible projection. The deformity is usually seen in women. In most cases radiography gives the only positive evidence that the condition is present. It is often, if not usually, symptomless.

Lordosis is often secondary to the flexion of *hip disease*, which must not be overlooked. Limitation of movement in the hip-joint, especially of rotation, and wasting of the thigh serve to demonstrate the existence of this disease.

Lordosis and waddling gait may be the first indication of *congenital dislocation of the hips.* In this condition, which is more commonly seen in girls (*Fig.* 745), the erect position is maintained only by throwing the trunk backwards to an unusual degree in order to bring it into line with the heads of the femora, which are dislocated backwards. The suspicion of congenital dislocation of the hip may be confirmed by the unnatural width of the hip, the hollow appearance of Scarpa's triangle, by palpation of the head of the femur upon the dorsum ilii when the thigh is flexed, adducted, and inverted, by the gliding movements of the head of the femur upon the pelvis, and by radiography (*Fig.* 746).

Contortionists usually have a good deal of lordosis owing to the unusual suppleness of the lumbar spine and the elongation of the hamstrings.

In all these conditions the back is supple, and

SPINE, TENDERNESS OF

Tenderness of the spine is usually due to local disease of or injury to the tissues at the site of tenderness. Such tenderness is always deep, but may be associated with cutaneous hyperalgesia as well. In a second and less important group the tenderness is partly or entirely cutaneous, and is a referred phenomenon found in visceral disease. In testing for spinal tenderness it is therefore desirable to differentiate between cutaneous and deep tenderness, and, in the case of the latter, between tenderness elicited by pressing upon the spinous processes and tenderness in the adjacent muscles, since spinal disease is usually accompanied by local muscular spasm, and the muscles thus affected become tender although they are not themselves the site of the disease. Failure to allow for this fact is the usual explanation of the mistakes—sometimes serious —which are so often made in attributing muscle tenderness to a strain or to a rheumatic condition when in reality it is due to local spasm in response to disease of the vertebrae, intervertebral disks, or the spinal cord and its membranes.

The chief morbid conditions in which spinal tenderness occurs are summarized in the following table:

1. Diseases of the Overlying Skin and Subcutaneous Tissue. These are rare and clinically obvious.

2. Diseases of the Vertebral Column:

a. INFLAMMATORY:

Pott's disease	Spondylitis
Staphylococcal	ankylopoietica
spondylitis	Actinomycosis
Typhoid spine	Hydatid cyst
	Paget's disease

b. DEGENERATIVE:

Spondylosis	Herniation of nucleus
Osteochondritis	pulposus
(rare)	

c. NEOPLASTIC:

Secondary deposits	Myelomatosis
Sarcoma	Leukaemic deposits

d. TRAUMATIC:

Fractures	Disk herniation
Dislocation	Spondylolisthesis

e. EROSION BY AORTIC ANEURYSM.

3. Diseases of the Spinal Cord and Meninges:

Metastatic epidural	Meningitis serosa
abscess or tumour	circumscripta
Meningioma	Tumour of the spinal
Neurofibroma	cord
Herpes zoster	Syringomyelia

4. Hysteria and Malingering: Compensation Neurosis.

5. Metabolic Disorders: Osteoporosis, Osteomalacia, Hyperparathyroidism.

The investigation of spinal tenderness requires an exhaustive case history, a careful examination, and certain special investigations. The history is of particular importance, because not only will it disclose the duration, site, and severity of the spinal symptoms, but it will also indicate whether the spinal cord or nerve-roots are involved (root pain, girdle sensations, paraesthesiae in the limb, muscular weakness or stiffness, sphincter disturbances). A systematic interrogation as to general health, previous diseases, and symptoms referable to the other systems of the body may bring out facts relevant to the spinal condition. There is no laboratory procedure which can give this information, and a further advantage of the historical approach is that it provides a guide to the patient's mental and emotional conditions which is invaluable in assessing the reality and severity of the spinal symptoms. The second step, physical examination, must cover the whole body in a search for factors which may throw light on the spinal tenderness. Reference has already been made to the need for care in determining that the tenderness is really in the spine itself, and not in the adjacent muscles or the overlying skin. The extent of the tenderness and the presence or absence of limitation of movement must be established. Acute tenderness of organic origin is always associated with limitation of movement in one or more directions. The examination of sensation, power, and reflexes below the level of tenderness is important, for significant neurological abnormalities may be found in the absence of any subjective symptoms. Attention must be paid to the chest, cardiovascular system, abdomen, and prostate. The long bones should receive attention, and the skull must not be forgotten, because in carcinomatosis painless secondary deposits may be found in the latter. Of the special investigations, X-ray examination of the spine takes the first place, but evidence of local disease may be long delayed and it is dangerous to assume that a negative finding is conclusive; further radiographs, taken at a later date, may tell a different tale. X-ray examination of the chest, aorta, skull, and long bones may be necessary. The blood sedimentation-rate may be raised before any other evidence of Pott's disease becomes apparent. The cerebrospinal fluid should be examined, not only to see whether there is a pleocytosis or a raised protein such as may be present in disease within the spinal canal, but also to exclude the possibility of a spinal block (Queckenstedt's test). A rise in the acid-phosphatase of the serum will suggest the presence of a secondary growth from the prostate, and a high alkaline-phosphatase is found in Paget's disease. A raised serum calcium may suggest hyperparathyroidism.

Pain and tenderness in the spine are sometimes functional. There is usually an organic nucleus to this form of hysteria, either in the form of a long-past injury to the back or some minor physical abnormality. The frequency of this condition after railway accidents a hundred years ago earned for it the title of 'railway spine', a common subject for protracted and profitable litigation. Features to be looked for are: (1) absence of clinical or radiological evidence of injury, (2) the presence of hysterical features in the patient's past history and present personality, (3) the existence of a profit motive, which need not necessarily be financial, but may be an escape from domestic, personal, or professional problems. The neuroses which crystallize around an injured spine are similar in origin and characteristics to those encountered after injury to other parts of the body. The same applies to arthritic and other disorders of the spine. Patients with spinal osteoarthrosis and ankylosing spondylitis, for instance, are seldom tender over the spine unless anxiety or other mental overtones becomes superimposed.

TENDERNESS IN THE SPINE DUE TO DISEASE IN OTHER PARTS OF THE BODY: Superficial tenderness over the spine is a common association of visceral disease, and the tenderness is situated over the portion of the spine corresponding to the segmental innervation of the affected viscus. The tenderness is not associated with local rigidity, and there is invariably well-marked evidence of the visceral disease, so that such tenderness is unlikely to be taken for a manifestation of spinal disease. The boot is more likely to be on the other foot, for spinal disease which gives rise to local tenderness and to a root pain in the chest or abdomen is easily mistaken for visceral disease.

Ian Mackenzie.

24*

SPLEEN, ENLARGEMENT OF

Enlargement of the spleen is almost always a sign of some underlying disorder; sometimes simple and benign, sometimes infective and sometimes neoplastic or due to a disorder of the blood. Rarely is it found in normal people, and so-called 'splenoptosis' is excessively rare. By the time a spleen has become palpable it has become enlarged more than two or three times its normal size. **The Physical Signs of Enlargement of the Spleen.** If the organ is only slightly or moderately enlarged there is no alteration in the size or shape of the abdomen. On occasions when very considerable enlargement occurs, the abdomen may be distended to an extent that simulates ascites, but on closer inspection the distension is found to be by no means uniform and the left side of the abdomen to be more conspicuous. The inner border of the spleen may be tilted forward so that a distinct edge or ridge may be seen pushing the abdominal wall, this ridge running downwards and inwards from the left costal margin near the anterior axillary line towards the umbilicus; in a few cases a notch can be identified in this edge or ridge. When the patient takes a deep breath the prominence may be seen to move distinctly downwards, though occasionally the spleen may be so enormously enlarged that its lower end becomes impacted in the pelvis, when downward movement is impossible.

Palpation is the best means of detecting splenic enlargement. If the organ is but little enlarged it may not be felt until the observer, standing on the left-hand side of the recumbent patient and supporting the lower left ribs posteriorly with his right hand, steadily but firmly presses the fingers of his left hand under the left costal margin just in front of the anterior axillary line; when the patient now takes a deep breath a definite sense of increased resistance may reveal splenic enlargement when the organ is comparatively soft, as, for example, in many cases of typhoid fever; in more obvious cases a firm mass with a distinct edge may be felt. When the enlargement is considerable the splenic tumour will be felt descending from beneath the left ribs close behind the abdominal wall; and, unless there is a very large liver or some other cause preventing the viscus from following its natural direction as it enlarges, it tends to reach and ultimately cross the middle line at or just below the level of the umbilicus. It is generally smooth and firm, and the characteristic notch can be felt in its anterior border. Except in very rare cases of ptosis of the spleen it will not be possible to insert a hand between it and the left costal margin or define its upper limit by palpation. Many clinicians prefer to palpate when standing on the patient's right and, of course, reversing the hands in the above description. In some cases the spleen can only be felt with the patient lying on his right side, the examining physician kneeling at the side of the couch, palpating upwards with the right hand.

Percussion over the mass yields a dull note, which is continuous with an increased area of dullness in the thorax extending upwards as high as the 7th rib in the mid-axillary line, the 6th rib in the nipple line or even higher, and including the ordinary area of splenic impairment of resonance behind. Percussion of the left loin may elicit resonance, indicating that the colon is not displaced as is usual in the case of a renal tumour. Percussion, however, is much less helpful than palpation, and rarely gives any additional reliable information.

Auscultation seldom affords evidence of value in these cases, but when the splenic enlargement is associated with local perisplenitis, as for example, in cases of infarction, a loud rub may be heard over the mass when the patient takes a particularly deep breath.

Distinction between an Enlarged Spleen and other Tumours in the Left Hypochondrium. These are: (1) Kidney tumours or perinephric abscess; (2) Suprarenal tumours; (3) Carcinoma of the splenic flexure of the colon; (4) Pancreatic cyst or carcinoma; (5) Carcinoma or sarcoma of the stomach; (6) Ovarian tumour; (7) Tuberculous peritonitis; (8) Faecal accumulation in the colon; (9) Pathological rarities.

DISTINCTION FROM A RENAL TUMOUR (*see also* KIDNEY, ENLARGEMENT OF, p. 470). Distinction may sometimes be extremely difficult. Both may cause local prominence or bulging of the left side of the abdomen; in the case of splenic enlargement the expansion is more forward and inward: in a kidney enlargement the loin is more likely to be bulging out. The notch is the most characteristic feature but this is not evident in the case of most splenic enlargements. Either tumour may move downwards when the patient takes a deep breath. A renal tumour being situated more deeply in the abdomen seldom approximates closely to the anterior abdominal wall unless the enlargement is very great, in which case the loin will be filled out and feel very firm and resistant on bimanual examination. A renal tumour generally slopes away as it approaches the ribs so that it is less difficult to get one's hand between its upper pole and the costal margin than is the case with the undislocated spleen.

The colon may be identified over the anterior surface of a renal tumour (which is never the case with splenic enlargement) when percussion may yield a resonant note in front or, in typical cases, a vertical band of colonic resonance down the centre of an otherwise dull mass, the loin being dull posteriorly. With a splenic tumour the loin is resonant and the anterior aspect of the mass dull. A local bruit or rub would make renal tumour unlikely.

MALIGNANT DISEASE OF THE LEFT SUPRARENAL GLAND may form a mass difficult to distinguish from either a splenic or a renal enlargement. Owing to the close proximity of the suprarenal capsule to the kidney and the liability for the capsule of the kidney to become infiltrated by growth of the suprarenal, the physical signs are practically the same as those of a renal tumour except that it may be more difficult to pass the hand between the mass and the costal margin. Since the growth may infiltrate the capsule of the kidney, anatomical differentiation may be impossible and, indeed, laparotomy alone will reveal the diagnosis, though X-ray studies, including angiograms, are often very helpful.

CARCINOMA OF THE SPLENIC FLEXURE of the colon is usually annular, giving rise to no definite tumour but to distension of the transverse colon with symptoms of intestinal obstruction. Occasionally, however, the growth may be more voluminous, or it may have caused leakage and inflammatory matting from local perforation through or above the growth, with the result that a fairly large tumour may be felt in and below the left hypochondrium. This mass is generally resonant to percussion, has no well-defined edge or notch, and may vary somewhat in position from day to day: it will usually be associated with intestinal symptoms, especially constipation alternating with diarrhoea and the passage of mucus and occasionally blood per rectum. There may be obvious secondary deposits in the liver or the left supraclavicular lymph-nodes. Radiographs of the colon (Fig. 184, p. 177) will help to establish the diagnosis.

PANCREATIC TUMOURS are usually situated between the ensiform cartilage and the umbilicus more in the median line of the abdomen than is a spleen. A very large cyst may cause difficulty in the diagnosis. Such a cyst is seldom primarily within the pancreas but is really a cyst of the lesser omental sac with the pancreas spread out over and incorporated in its wall. A feature of importance is that no edge and no notch can be felt. The stomach generally lies in front of a pancreatic cyst and the relative positions will be established by radiography after an opaque meal. A splenic tumour rarely extends to the right of the middle line unless the enlargement is great, in which case it crosses at or below the umbilicus, whereas a pancreatic cyst extends across to the right of the middle line above the navel. Pancreatic new growth has a similar position but the outline of the mass, if any at all, is more nodular. Jaundice and a palpable gall-bladder are familiar accompaniments, with, in addition, glycosuria and fatty stools.

MALIGNANT GROWTH OF THE STOMACH may be mistaken for enlargement of the spleen, especially gastric sarcoma, which though very much rarer than carcinoma is more likely to involve the whole of the stomach and give rise to a very large tumour occupying most of the upper part of the left side of the abdomen. The following features will serve to distinguish a gastric new growth from an enlarged spleen. The mass is apt to shift its position slightly during the course of an examination or from day to day; it does not present a well-defined edge with a notch or notches; it may extend a considerable distance to the right of the middle line although its lower limit may not be below the level of the umbilicus;

it is likely to be resonant in front, though the percussion note over it may be impaired; there may be anaemia and leucocytosis, but the blood changes would not be characteristic of any positive blood disease; vomiting of altered blood and of other material suggestive of new growth will generally be a prominent symptom and pain is associated with taking of food; secondary deposits, especially in the liver or in the left supraclavicular lymph-nodes, may be identified. Radiography or gastroscopy may confirm the diagnosis (Figs. 356, 357, p. 335).

OVARIAN TUMOURS have been mistaken for enlargement of the spleen, and vice versa, distinction being particularly difficult in cases in which the spleen has become dislocated or is so large as to reach down into the pelvis. The differential diagnosis depends on the following points. An ovarian tumour rarely extends upwards into such close contact with the left costal margin that the hand cannot be placed between it and the ribs; downward movement during deep inspiration is very slight; its pelvic origin may be evident on vaginal examination; it is usually more globular than a splenic tumour and has no well-defined edge with notches in it even when covered with projecting bosses of new growth; it usually extends more to the right of the middle line than does an enlarged spleen; amenorrhoea is probable.

TUBERCULOUS PERITONITIS may produce various forms of abdominal tumours including a mass occupying the left hypochondriac region, the result of matting together of the intestines, thickening of the omentum, or thickening and infiltration of the peritoneum. The tumour does not as a rule extend close up under the ribs so that the hand can be placed between it and the costal margin, but it may feel somewhat rounded, with a more or less well-defined edge, and when there are two or more separate masses united together a notch may be closely simulated. The mass itself may be dull to percussion but there is generally resonance between it and the normal splenic dullness. Ascites is often present and there may be palpable lumps in other parts of the abdomen. In advanced cases there may be redness and oedema of the abdominal wall or a purulent or faecal discharge from the umbilicus. Signs of tuberculosis may be recognized elsewhere, for instance in joints or lymph-nodes. The tuberculin skin test is strongly positive. The presence or absence of pyrexia may not be helpful in the differential diagnosis except perhaps that in a young subject an evening pyrexia with a subnormal temperature in the morning is an additional argument in favour of tubercle. The rarely encountered 'inverted' type of pyrexia—morning rise and evening fall—has been regarded as typical of tubercle.

FAECAL ACCUMULATION IN THE SPLENIC FLEXURE or adjacent parts of the transverse or descending colon may upon a first examination be mistaken for an enlarged spleen, but this source of error is usually removed when the patient is re-examined after an action of the bowels. A history of severe constipation with possibly attacks of temporary obstruction is not unusual. The mass is generally irregular, more or less cylindrical, and in thin persons it may be possible to modify its shape by manipulation. In cases of extreme constipation it is as well to think of neoplasia, and, in cases of very long duration, megacolon. (*See Fig.* 186, p. 178.)

HAEMATOMA DUE TO INJURY OR TO LEAKAGE FROM AN ABDOMINAL ANEURYSM is a rarity, but it may be mistaken for an enlargement of the spleen or the kidney; the history, the blanching due to the amount of blood lost, or possibly the pulsation of an aneurysm, may point to the diagnosis.

CAUSES OF SPLENIC ENLARGEMENT

There are various ways in which the different causes may be classified; from a diagnostic point of view the following is serviceable (it must be emphasized that in childhood splenic enlargement occurs more readily, and is more common than in adults):

I. Chronic Enlargement of the Spleen

1. VERY GREAT ENLARGEMENT (TO OR BELOW THE UMBILICUS):

   Chronic myelocytic (myeloid) leukaemia
   Chronic malaria
   Tropical splenomegaly syndrome
   Kala-azar
   Myelofibrosis
   Polycythaemia rubra vera
   Tuberculosis
   Portal hypertension (chronic congestive splenomegaly)
   Gaucher's and other lipid storage diseases
   Thalassaemia major in children.

2. MODERATE ENLARGEMENT. All conditions mentioned in Group 1 at an earlier stage of enlargement. In addition, moderate enlargement of the spleen may be exhibited in cases of:

   Chronic lymphatic leukaemia
   Malignant lymphoma (Hodgkin's disease, lymphosarcoma, reticulum-cell sarcoma, follicular lymphoma)
   Acute leukaemia (late)
   Amyloidosis
   Anaemias: megalo- and normoblastic
   Haemolytic disorders
   Idiopathic thrombocytopenic purpura
   Thalassaemia and some haemoglobinopathies
   Biliary cirrhosis
   Chronic active hepatitis
   Haemochromatosis
   Sarcoidosis
   Acute and subacute bacterial endocarditis
   Essential hypertriglyceridaemia
   Multiple myeloma (occasionally).

II. Acute Enlargement of the Spleen, the Enlargement as a rule being Slight

1. ACUTE INFECTIVE FEVERS:

   Malaria
   Infectious mononucleosis
   Acute viral hepatitis
   Typhoid
   Paratyphoid
   Relapsing fever
   Undulant fever (brucellosis)
   Septicaemia
   Typhus
   Trench fever, etc.
   Generalized (miliary) tuberculosis
   Histoplasmosis
   Trypanosomiasis
   Schistosomiasis intestinal
   Psittacosis
   Tularaemia

2. CONNECTIVE-TISSUE DISORDERS:
   Systemic lupus erythematosus
   Polyarteritis nodosa
   Felty's and Still's diseases.

3. INJURY:
   Haematoma
   Rupture.

4. VASCULAR CAUSES:
   Infarction
   Thrombosis of the splenic vein
   Passive hyperaemia from torsion of the pedicle
   Embolism.

5. CYSTS AND BENIGN TUMOURS:
   Hydatids
   Dermoids
   Haemangioma
   Lymphangioma
   Endothelioma
   Polycystic disease.

It will be noted that no mention has been made of abscess, gumma, carcinoma (whether primary or secondary), sarcoma (primary or secondary), or hydatid cyst of the spleen, for all of these are exceedingly rare and very unlikely to be encountered. It is exceptional for back pressure in congestive cardiac failure to produce enlargement of the spleen. So true is this, that in a case of chronic heart disease with failing compensation a palpable spleen is evidence of more than mere mechanical heart failure—probably superimposed subacute bacterial endocarditis.

I. CHRONIC ENLARGEMENT OF THE SPLEEN

1. Chronic and Very Great Enlargement of the Spleen. When the spleen is so large as to occupy half the abdomen or more the field of probable causation is relatively restricted. The largest of all spleens are those due to *chronic myeloid leukaemia* (*Fig.* 747). Blood-counts and sternal biopsy will confirm the diagnosis. There is a great variability in the degree of splenomegaly in chronic lymphatic leukaemia. In some cases enlargement is hardly recognizable, in others it may be considerable (*see* ANAEMIA, p. 25 et seq.). CHRONIC MALARIA is the commonest cause of gross enlargement of the spleen in most parts of the East. The history usually makes the diagnosis self-evident. The *tropical splenomegaly syndrome* is a term given to unexplained big spleens in the tropics. It seems that it is essentially due to malaria, though only a few people exposed to malaria get it. Such people are often immigrants from a low to a high malarial endemicity. Intermittent exposure may be the cause. It is commonest in young adults, though it may appear in childhood. The liver is also usually enlarged and portal hypertension may be present.

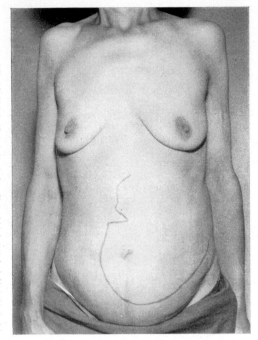

Fig. 747. Gross splenomegaly in chronic myelogenous leukaemia.

On specific therapy immunoglobulin IgM levels, initially high, drop and the spleen after some six months diminishes in size. If these two things fail to happen it is likely that malaria is not the cause and that the diagnosis is incorrect—leukaemia, lymphoma, or some other disorder being responsible.

Kala-azar is diagnosed chiefly by the discovery of the Leishman-Donovan bodies in the fluid obtained by splenic or by sternal puncture.

In MYELOFIBROSIS fibrosis and osteosclerosis of the marrow cavity occur with extramedullary haematopoiesis in spleen and lymph-glands with leucoerythroblastic changes in the peripheral blood. The patient is middle-aged or elderly, both sexes being affected equally. Most occur idiopathically, though some are due to poisons, such as benzene or phosphorus, or chronic irradiation, and some are late phases of another blood disorder, as described below in polycythaemia rubra vera. Anaemia develops. Normoblasts and myelocytes are present in the circulating blood. A trephine bone biopsy should be performed if the diagnosis is in doubt.

POLYCYTHAEMIA RUBRA VERA is characterized by more or less cyanosis and polycythaemia amounting perhaps to seven, ten, or even twelve million red corpuscles per c.mm. In most cases the spleen, though enlarged and firm, extends for only a few finger-breadths below the ribs; great enlargement is unusual, but occurs more frequently as the patient begins to become anaemic, when lymph-nodes and spleen become haematopoietic and enlarge very considerably.

TUBERCULOSIS of the spleen may rarely cause gross enlargement. In such cases the tuberculous disease appears essentially confined to this organ and there is usually no apparent pulmonary disease or lymphadenopathy.

PORTAL HYPERTENSION (chronic congestive splenomegaly) occurs in Laennec's (alcoholic) and post-hepatitis cirrhosis and in intestinal schistosomiasis. The spleen is usually only moderately, but occasionally greatly, enlarged. These intrahepatic causes are usually associated with hepatic enlargement, often of considerable degree. Extrahepatic causes, such as thrombosis or cavernous change of portal vein, compression from pancreatic tumour, or fibrosis, or from an aneurysm of the splenic artery, are often not associated with hepatomegaly. Epistaxes, haematemeses, or melaena and anaemia, are common diagnostic pointers, but splenomegaly may be the presenting sign and occurs sometimes long before any other manifestation of portal hypertension.

GAUCHER'S DISEASE occurs in adults and children. The spleen may become very large, sometimes rapidly in childhood, but usually gradually. Pigmentation of exposed surfaces of skin occurs and sometimes becomes generalized. Brown wedge-shaped pinguecula, thickenings of the subconjunctival tissues, often appear, first on the nasal sides. Diagnosis is by bone-marrow biopsy, where the typical, pale Gaucher cells are seen.

Another rare disorder characterized by abnormal storage of lipoids in the reticulo-endothelial cells is the genetically determined disorder NIEMANN-PICK DISEASE (*lipoid histiocytosis*). It is diagnosable with certainty only by microscopical examination of marrow aspirates or tissue biopsies, the foam cells being typical, though further chemical tests will show an increase of sphingomyelin in the tissues and prove the diagnosis. The patients are infants dying before the age of two; the clinical symptoms are enlargement of the liver and spleen, ascites, oedema, moderate leucocytosis. Jaundice does not occur. The Jewish race is particularly affected and females preponderate.

HAND-SCHÜLLER-CHRISTIAN DISEASE, starting in early childhood, is characterized by bony softening, exophthalmos, and diabetes insipidus, caused by accumulation of lipoid material in bone, with formation of granulation tissue and fibrosis and deposition of cholesterol crystals. X-rays show cystic lesions in bones. The liver and lymph-nodes are enlarged in addition to the spleen. The *Letterer-Siwe* syndrome is a more acute variant.

2. Chronic Enlargement of the Spleen, the Enlargement being of Moderate Size. Conditions which produce great enlargement of the spleen must go through a process of gradual enlargement and a stage must therefore occur in which all those diseases that have just been discussed will come into the present group. In chronic lymphatic leukaemia the spleen is enlarged, often markedly, but not to the degree seen in the chronic myeloid variety.

PORTAL HYPERTENSION is described above. Splenic enlargement is variable but is almost always present.

The spleen of a small child being relatively large and readily accessible is sometimes palpable in the absence of any disease. *Rickets* and *congenital syphilis*, once not uncommon, are today extremely rare causes of splenomegaly.

A large number of *blood disorders* cause a moderate degree of splenomegaly and full haematological studies will be required to differentiate the different types of megaloblastic, haemolytic, hypochromic, and other types of anaemia and to differentiate the different types of thrombocytopenic disorders. In thalassaemia major in childhood splenic enlargement may be great. The severely anaemic child often has a mongoloid appearance. In thalassaemia minor splenomegaly is less marked.

HODGKIN'S DISEASE is generally associated with considerable and progressive LYMPH-NODE ENLARGEMENT (p. 513), especially those of the neck, and later those of the axillae, groins, thorax and abdomen, together with moderate but seldom very great enlargement of the spleen. Anaemia is not present in the early stage but may be progressive and with variable features in the leucocyte count (*see* p. 44). Splenomegaly is not present in all cases. The spleen may be enlarged in a large number of the reticuloses (lymphomata) and also in lymphosarcoma and follicular lymphoma. The diagnostic boundaries between these different disorders are not always well defined, even after biopsy, which is always required.

CIRRHOSIS OF THE LIVER has already been discussed under PORTAL HYPERTENSION, but there are a number of *biliary cirrhoses* characterized by chronic obstructive jaundice and marked hepatomegaly with interference of some kind with the flow of bile. Splenomegaly and lymphadenopathy follow. Such cases may have an obvious cause, in the shape of an obstructive lesion in the biliary tract, such as stone, cysts, fluke infestation, or haemochromatosis, or none at all, as in primary biliary cirrhosis. Cholangiography, liver biopsy, biochemical and antimitochondrial antibody studies are necessary aids to diagnosis, though exploratory laparotomy may be necessary. The diagnosis of *sarcoidosis* is suggested by fever, erythema nodosum, and cervical or hilar lymph-node enlargement. The tuberculin test is usually negative or only weakly positive. The Kveim test is usually positive (50–80 per cent of cases), but a biopsy may be necessary for histological proof.

AMYLOID DISEASE (*Amyloidosis*). This condition results from long-continued suppuration. At one time discharging sinuses from empyema or spinal caries, purulent cavities in phthisis or bronchiectasis, or tertiary syphilis were not uncommon causes. Today they are relatively rare and conditions such as rheumatoid arthritis and, more rarely, ankylosing spondylitis and Reiter's disease are the primary disorders, or, overseas, leprosy and familial Mediterranean fever. It may occur secondarily to Hodgkin's disease, malignancy, ulcerative colitis, and a number of other disorders. It may, however, be a primary system disease. The amyloid material (swollen, waxy) stains brown with iodine, a feature that gives rise to the name. In secondary amyloidosis the commonest sites to be affected are the spleen, kidney, liver, and adrenal cortex, but lymphnodes, pancreas, gastro-intestinal tract, prostate, and thyroid may be affected; in primary amyloidosis the cardiac, skeletal, and smooth muscles. The heart, particularly in men over 50, may be enlarged and go into failure, but many other systems may be involved, including the skin. Macroglossia may be mistaken for carcinoma. If the intestines are implicated diarrhoea will occur, albuminuria when the kidneys are diseased. There is also the rare condition of primary generalized amyloidosis (*see* p. 509). Amyloidosis may also be associated with multiple myelomatosis. Diagnosis is by biopsy: renal, rectal, or hepatic.

ACUTE AND SUBACUTE ENDOCARDITIS are nearly always associated with palpable enlargement of the spleen which may attain considerable size. Ordinary heart disease with failure of compensation does not give rise to splenic enlargement that can be recognized clinically. The enlargement in fungating endocarditis may be due to embolism and infarction, in which case a history is probable of acute pain low down on the left side of the chest accompanied by a rub due to perisplenitis over the infarct. Fungating endocarditis sometimes develops in the absence of any cardiac murmurs; the diagnosis is then exceedingly difficult unless the patient exhibits multiple emboli—cerebral, renal, intestinal, splenic, peripheral. An embolus may on occasion be followed by the development of an aneurysm—femoral, popliteal, or cerebral, for example. A cerebral embolism of this kind has sometimes resulted in sudden transient coma and hemiplegia. The patient after apparent recovery has relapsed into coma and died, the cause of the relapse and fatal ending being the development of a cerebral aneurysm at the site of the embolus, rupture of this aneurysm, and death from the resultant haemorrhage. Progressive anaemia, without high leucocytosis, is another feature of these cases. The diagnosis must always be uncertain when there is no cardiac murmur.

Thrombotic infarction may cause acute splenic enlargement in almost any of the blood diseases, particularly Hodgkin's disease and leukaemia.

ESSENTIAL HYPERTRIGLYCERIDAEMIA is a disorder in which low-density lipoproteins are present in greatly increased concentrations, as are the serum triglycerides. Eighty per cent of children have hepatosplenomegaly, adults far less frequently. Xanthomata occur in about half the patients, usually on buttocks, trunk, and on extensor surfaces of the extremities.

II. ACUTE ENLARGEMENT OF THE SPLEEN

Acute Infectious Fevers. The spleen may to a greater or less extent become enlarged in any of the acute specific fevers.

MALARIA. Apart from the chronic enlargement which results from recurrent attacks of malaria, the spleen becomes enlarged and soft during an acute attack. For the characters of the fever, *see* p. 296. The nature of the malady will be suggested by geographical considerations, but the only conclusive proof is the discovery in stained blood-films of the malaria parasites (*Figs.* 318–320, p. 298).

INFECTIOUS MONONUCLEOSIS (GLANDULAR FEVER) is a common condition today particularly in children, where there may be a rash, and in young adults, where a rash is usually absent. In addition to fever, generalized lymph-node enlargement, and splenic enlargement, there may be a marked sore throat with a form of tonsillitis which may somewhat resemble diphtheria. The characteristic blood-count during the second or third week of the illness and, then or later, the Paul-Bunnell blood test help to prove the diagnosis. A highly specific and rapid slide test (the Monospot) is now in common use.

ACUTE VIRAL HEPATITIS A (INFECTIOUS HEPATITIS) AND B (SERUM HEPATITIS). Slight or moderate splenic enlargement may occur, sometimes before the jaundice has appeared, when the patient is febrile and nauseated. Mild leucopenia or neutropenia at this stage may suggest typhoid fever.

TYPHOID FEVER. In *typhoid fever* the spleen is usually so soft that no more than an increased sense of resistance may be noted on palpating close under the left ribs. The enlargement may be so slight that the organ is felt only when the patient takes a deep breath so as to push it down from under the costal margin, or it may be considerable enough for its lower border to reach several finger-breadths below the ribs. If the spleen is found to be enlarged in a case of obscure fever in which a continued pyrexia (*Fig.* 307, p. 289) is associated with a relatively slow pulse-rate, the diagnosis of typhoid fever should be considered. The onset is usually gradual with anorexia and lassitude accompanied by headache and sometimes epistaxis. The temperature generally rises in staircase fashion—that is, a rise of about two degrees every night, with a fall of one degree the following morning, until step by step it reaches 39° C. or 40° C., or even higher. The characteristic rash in the form of small rosy-red flattened papules which fade on pressure appears on the sixth day, and later in successive crops. Serum agglutinations do not become significantly raised until the second week.

Leucopenia (p. 495) is usual, and unlike many febrile illnesses typhoid fever produces a relative increase not in the polymorphonuclear cells but in the small lymphocytes. Typhoid bacilli may be recovered from the blood quite early in the illness. The ratio of the pulse-rate and temperature is often of considerable value in diagnosis; for instance, with a temperature of 40° C. the pulse-rate may be only 90 per minute, when the average ratio for this temperature is 120.

PARATYPHOID FEVER is closely related to typhoid fever in clinical features; the differentiation depends on agglutination tests.

RELAPSING FEVER causes considerable enlargement of the spleen. It is characterized by an acute onset, with chills, pains in the back, and a sudden rise of temperature that persists for six or seven days and then falls by crisis. The temperature remains normal for about a week then rises as before, several such remissions and relapses succeeding each other (*Fig.* 321, p. 299). The pulse is frequent and there is profuse sweating. Enlargement of the spleen occurs early in the illness. The diagnosis is eablished by identification in the blood of *Treponema recurrentis*.

BRUCELLA ABORTUS AND MELITENSIS INFECTIONS (UNDULANT FEVER) give rise to splenomegaly. In spite of high fever the patients may remain surprisingly well. These infections may last for many months, even years. Diagnosis is by blood-culture (often difficult) and agglutinations. Tissue or marrow cultures may be positive where blood-cultures are negative.

SEPTICAEMIA. In some cases of chronic or subacute septicaemia, enlargement of the spleen may be considerable and suggest the diagnosis of infective endocarditis. Whether or not the heart valves are affected in these cases, the ultimate diagnosis depends on discovery of infective organisms in blood-cultures.

TYPHUS FEVER. The spleen becomes soft and moderately enlarged but less constantly so than in typhoid fever. The disease sets in more acutely than enteric, with chills, early prostration, and a high temperature which ends by lysis less marked as a rule (*Fig.* 748) than that of typhoid fever (*Fig.* 307, p. 289), and sometimes almost by crisis at the end of the second week (*Fig.* 749). The rash which appears on the fifth day differs from that of typhoid fever in consisting of petechiae and of dark-red groups of subcutaneous macules in addition to rose-red papules on the surface. The first lesions appear on the trunk and later spread to the extremities, sparing the face, palms, and soles except in severely ill patients, a point of distinction from Rocky Mountain spotted fever. Nervous symptoms are conspicuous especially after the first week, the so-called 'typhoid state' being an expression employed to denote, not the condition that occurs in typhoid fever but that which develops in typhus. There may be severe vomiting and retention of urine, features rare in typhoid fever. The causal organism, *Rickettsia prowazeki*, may in the patient's blood be inoculated into experimental animal or chick embryo, or diagnosis, initially and essentially a clinical one, confirmed by a rising agglutination titre (*Proteus* OX 19) and by specific complement-fixing antibodies which first appear in the serum between the seventh and twelfth days of the disease.

INTESTINAL SCHISTOSOMIASIS may give rise to marked splenomegaly, the so-called 'Egyptian splenomegaly', which may be associated with other signs of portal hypertension. It carries a poor prognosis. Diagnosis rests on finding ova in the stools or rectal mucosa.

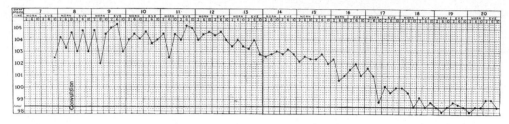

Fig. 748. Temperature chart from a typical case of typhus fever ending by rather unusual lysis.
(*Figs.* 748, 749 *kindly supplied by Dr. Turner, Medical Superintendent of the South-Eastern Fever Hospital, London.*)

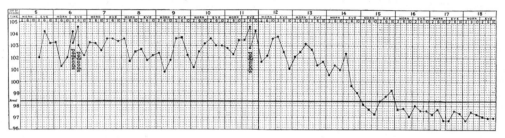

Fig. 749. Case of typhus fever, showing termination by crisis at the end of the second week. The majority of the cases exhibit a less abrupt ending to the pyrexia although the above type is characteristic in some epidemics.

TRENCH FEVER, a rickettsial disease spread by body lice, is an influenzal-like acute febrile disorder, in 70–80 per cent of cases associated with splenomegaly and a red macular rash.

GENERALIZED TUBERCULOSIS, today a rare disorder, may also simulate typhoid fever in certain details including enlargement of the spleen from the development of tubercles. The headache may be equally severe in both, but with tuberculous meningitis vomiting is more severe and retraction of the head, optic neuritis, and perhaps choroidal tubercles, may be conspicuous. In some cases generalized tuberculosis provides a clinical picture that may be almost indistinguishable from typhoid fever.

HISTOPLASMOSIS is caused by a fungus, *Histoplasma capsulatum*, which multiplies in the cells of the reticulo-endothelial system. Symptoms are nil or slight in some cases, fatal and disseminated in others. Diagnosis is made on cultures of bone-marrow, blood or tissue biopsy, or in sputum or exudate from an ulcer.

In TRYPANOSOMIASIS diagnosis depends on finding the causative organism, *Trypanosoma brucei*, in the blood, lymph-node, or cerebrospinal fluid, in Gambian or Rhodesian sleeping sickness. *T. cruzi*, the cause of Chagas disease (American Trypanosomiasis), is easily grown in blood broth in acute cases, but in less than half the chronic ones, where a complement fixation test (Machado-Guerreiro) may prove helpful.

IN PSITTACOSIS splenomegaly is not uncommon. When acute pneumonitis and splenomegaly co-exist this condition should be suspected.

IN TULARAEMIA 80 per cent of cases start as a lesion of the skin or mucous membranes with enlarged and tender regional lymph-nodes. Splenomegaly is often present.

Connective-tissue Disorders. The spleen in *rheumatoid arthritis* in adults is seldom palpable, some 3–5 per cent of cases; in *Still's disease* around 16 per cent, and in *Felty's syndrome* (by definition) 100 per cent. This last is merely a variant of rheumatoid arthritis where splenomegaly and lymphadenopathy are associated with a neutropenia and a liability to suppurative infection. There may also be diffuse skin pigmentation and leg ulcers. In *systemic lupus erythematosus* splenomegaly is present in about 25 per cent of cases.

Injury: or Strangulation by Twisting of the Pedicle. A blow in the splenic region may cause a rupture in the pulp of the spleen without bursting its capsule and without obvious injury to the chest wall or abdomen. The bleeding that occurs within the capsule of the spleen causes enlargement of the organ with great pain; the diagnosis can seldom be more than guessed at unless laparotomy is performed. Strangulation of the spleen seldom occurs if the organ is in its natural position, but when there has been previous dislocation an abdominal injury or a sudden effort has led to its becoming twisted on its own hilum; the symptoms, although by no means indicative of the occurrence, at any rate suggest an acute intra-abdominal condition requiring immediate laparotomy.

A pneumoperitoneum, therapeutic or accidental, may displace a normal spleen from its usual site and render it palpable.

F. Dudley Hart.

SPUTUM

Sputum may be defined as material expelled by coughing from the lower respiratory tract. Normally, a considerable amount, about 100 ml. daily, of bronchial secretion is removed by ciliary action from the airways of the lung, through the larynx, and disposed of into the alimentary tract by unconscious acts of swallowing. Sputum may thus consist of bronchial secretions in excess of the amount that can be disposed of in this way; of pathological secretions, exudates, and pus from abnormal bronchi, bronchioles and alveoli, or from abscesses, cavities, or cysts in the lung; or of material derived from morbid processes in pleura, lymph-nodes, mediastinum, oesophagus, subphrenic space, and liver which have ulcerated into the lung. It may be mixed with saliva and secretions from the upper respiratory tract, but should be distinguished from these.

Much may be learnt from the study of the sputum. The patient's account of its mode of production, quantity, and quality, and the physician's observations, especially the naked-eye appearances of the material expectorated, are essential parts of this study, and often give information at least as important as that derived from laboratory procedures.

Although the production of sputum is usually associated with cough, some chronic bronchitic patients deny cough, regarding the expectoration of mucus or even mucopus in the mornings as so 'normal' that they refer to it as 'clearing the throat'. Other patients, who evidently raise excess secretions from their lower respiratory tracts by cough, deny producing sputum because they habitually swallow the material expectorated. In such cases, exhortation may result in the production of a sample of sputum; but it may be necessary for some purposes—e.g., for the isolation of tubercle bacilli—to obtain a specimen of gastric contents early in the morning before food or drink has been taken, which will contain the material expectorated and swallowed during the night.

In questioning a patient who produces sputum, attention should be directed to a number of points, including the duration of this symptom, the time of day or night at which it most often occurs, if long-standing whether it is persistent or recurrent, and whether cough or sputum-production is the more troublesome symptom. The patient will generally indicate clearly if sputum is either scanty or profuse; otherwise some idea of the daily volume can be obtained by inquiring whether expectoration occurs principally in the mornings and, if not, how many times a day it occurs. It is useful also to find out whether the patient can produce a specimen of sputum to order: this also may give an immediate opportunity to assess its appearance and physical qualities.

Sputum arising from the bronchi may be mucoid, mucopurulent, or frankly purulent. It is important to record these appearances, and a number of brief codes for this purpose has been devised. Most of these depend upon assessing how much of the specimen is white or colourless and how much yellow. It is important to remember that in asthmatic patients a yellow sputum does not necessarily indicate the presence of pus—i.e., neutrophil polymorphs; it may be due to eosinophil polymorphs, associated with antigen–antibody reactions rather than infection.

In acute pulmonary oedema the material expectorated is derived largely from the oedema fluid transuded into the alveoli; it is thin, frothy, and may be pink from uniform blood-staining.

When sputum is profuse and purulent, giving rise to suspicion that it may arise from a localized abnormality, such as bronchiectasis, lung abscess, or empyema with pleurobronchial fistula, inquiry should be made about the effect of posture upon it. The patient may have noticed that certain postures lead to cough and expectoration; the posture which he adopts for sleeping may be significant, since it may have been chosen because it does not lead to cough. The sudden production of a large volume of sputum suggests the evacuation of a localized collection of liquid into a bronchus from a pleural empyema, a cyst (infected or otherwise), a lung abscess, or a mediastinal subphrenic or intrahepatic abscess. An episode of this sort may be followed by persistent expectoration, or may cease temporarily when the bronchial communication becomes occluded, and recur later. Rupture of a hydatid cyst in the lung may result in the sudden expectoration of a large amount of thin watery material, which may be accompanied or followed by an anaphylactic reaction.

The uniformly purulent sputum of a patient with a localized source of suppuration in the lungs or pleura is generally distinguishable from that of a patient with a diffuse mucopurulent bronchitis with or without bronchiectasis; it is often evidently thinner with little or no viscid mucoid secretion mixed with it, and flows easily.

Diseases giving rise to malodorous sputum include some types of lung abscess, empyema with pleurobronchial fistula and severely infected bronchiectasis. The pus in acute specific lung abscesses due to *Staphylococcus aureus* or *Klebsiella pneumoniae* and in empyemas due to these organisms, or to pneumococcus, or to *Streptococcus pyogenes* is not malodorous. When the sputum is foul-smelling, mixed bacterial infection including anaerobic organisms is generally present. The sickeningly offensive odour associated with anaerobic infection in putrid lung abscess, empyema, and bronchiectasis is now encountered less frequently than formerly, partly because all forms of intrathoracic suppuration are less frequent, and partly because the organisms responsible for it are usually susceptible to antibiotics, especially to penicillin.

In addition to the yellow of pus or eosinophil pseudopus, other colours may be observed in the sputum. A uniformly purulent sputum may be green rather than yellow, either because of degeneration of leucocytes in specimens that have been left standing, or because of infection by *Pseudomonas aeruginosa*. The ulceration of an amoebic liver abscess into the lung gives rise to the expectoration of reddish-brown so-called 'anchovy-sauce' pus. Sputum may be stained with fresh or altered blood, or mixed with larger quantities of blood; this is considered under HAEMOPTYSIS (p. 352). The sputum of those exposed to dust will contain the dust that has settled on the bronchi, often aggregated by ciliary streaming to give a mottled appearance. The commonest example of this occurs in town-dwellers, especially during periods of heavy air-pollution—e.g., at times of 'smogs' due to temperature inversion during the winter, the sputum of chronic bronchitics usually presents a mottled black appearance. The sputum of coal-miners similarly contains coal-dust. In coal-miners with complicated pneumoconiosis, the confluent collagenous masses incorporating coal-dust that constitute progressive massive fibrosis sometimes liquefy centrally; when this occurs, the liquid black contents are expectorated, resulting in an episode of expectoration of inky black material, or 'melanoptysis'.

Formed elements may be visible in sputum. Although careful search by floating the sputum in water may reveal fragments which are evidently casts of small parts of the peripheral bronchial tree in patients with asthma or with diffuse bronchitis, large casts with multiple branching are rarely seen. They occur in the very rare plastic or fibrinous bronchitis; the patient, often an asthmatic, suffers recurrent febrile illnesses with collapse–consolidation of a lobe or lobes of the lung, re-expanding after expectoration of the cast. Much more frequent is allergic broncho-pulmonary aspergillosis, in which the sputum may contain 'plugs', generally about 4–5 mm. in diameter and 15–20 mm. long. Usually they are roughly spindle-shaped, without the multiple branching of bronchial casts, though occasionally there is a single bifurcation at one end. They consist mainly of tough mucus, containing many eosinophils, and with a little *Aspergillus mycelium* in the centre, usually demonstrable only by special staining. This disease occurs in extrinsic atopic asthmatics, and the sputum may also have the microscopic features seen in asthma (*see below*). Careful search in the sputum of asthmatic patients suspected of allergic aspergillosis may be required to demonstrate the 'plugs', but patients on inquiry will often be found to have noticed the presence from time to time of a tough fragment in the sputum. Very rarely, a patient with a bronchial carcinoma coughs out a gross fragment of the tumour. Another rare event is the expectoration of a fragment of calcified caseous material from an old tuberculous focus, either in lung or in a bronchopulmonary lymph-node. If a previous chest radiograph is available, it is sometimes possible to see that one of the calcified foci evident in it has disappeared in a subsequent film.

The principal laboratory examinations to which sputum should be submitted are microscopy and bacteriological culture.

The presence of pus can be microscopically confirmed by the finding of large numbers of neutrophil polymorphs. As already noted, it is important to distinguish the eosinophil pseudopus which appears in the sputum of some asthmatics from true pus. Additionally, in the mucoid sputum of asthmatics, many eosinophils may be present. This finding is of especial importance in the differential diagnosis between late-onset intrinsic asthma and chronic bronchitis. The sputum of asthmatic patients may also contain Curschmann's spirals and Charcot-Leyden crystals. Curschmann's spirals consist of whitish, twisted threads of mucus, often including eosinophils; Charcot-Leyden crystals are colourless, elongated octahedrons, up to about 50 μ in length, and appear to be associated with eosinophils. Occasionally, small clumps of desquamated bronchiolar epithelial cells, the so-called 'Creola bodies', may be seen in the sputum of asthmatic patients, especially after a severe attack or during a prolonged attack.

Examination of the sputum for cancer cells can make an important contribution to the diagnosis of bronchial carcinoma. This is a specialized procedure, its reliability depending very much upon the skill and experience of the cytologist. Clinicians should be aware of some possibly confusing factors. In asthmatic patients a report that clumps of adenocarcinoma cells have been seen should be interpreted in the knowledge that the 'Creola bodies', mentioned above, may mimic such cells very closely; and in patients with chronic tuberculous or other cavities in the lung, which may be lined with metaplastic squamous cells, these cells may be desquamated and prove difficult to distinguish with certainty from squamous carcinoma cells.

After haemoptysis from any cause and in the presence of pulmonary congestion associated with heart disease, iron-containing macrophages or siderocytes may be seen in the sputum. They also appear in the sputum in idiopathic pulmonary haemosiderosis, but are not of specific significance in this disease.

Persons who have been exposed to asbestos dust produce 'asbestos bodies' in their sputum. These consist of very thin, needle-like fibres of asbestos surrounded by a clear brownish coating of proteinaceous material containing iron, often arranged in an irregular beaded distribution or with a terminal bead or beads causing the whole to resemble a drumstick or dumb-bell. The presence of these bodies indicates only exposure to asbestos and is not necessarily associated with pulmonary asbestosis. Apart from this, microscopy of the sputum gives no specific information in pneumoconioses. Similarly, although oil-containing macrophages may be found in the sputum of patients with exogenous oil-aspiration pneumonia, they may also be found in persons who have been exposed to oil aspiration—e.g., users of oily nasal drops—but without pathological consequences in the lungs.

Finding elastic fibres in sputum suggests inflammatory breakdown of lung tissue, e.g., in actively progressive tuberculosis or acute lung abscess.

In pulmonary alveolar proteinosis microscopy of the sputum shows amorphous eosinophilic PAS-positive material, and electron microscopy shows the presence of lamellar bodies, presumably derived from type II pneumocytes, which may be diagnostic.

Microscopy of suitably stained sputum-smears is an essential part of the examination of the sputum for tubercle bacilli. It has been estimated that sputum specimens must contain as many as 100,000 bacilli per ml. if acid-fast bacilli can be reliably demonstrated in them by microscopy after Ziehl-Neelsen staining. Examination by fluorescence microscopy after suitable staining has a somewhat higher sensitivity. Appropriate methods of culture can demonstrate tubercle bacilli in specimens containing far fewer organisms, but delay of several weeks is inevitable before the result can be available. For this reason, persistent attempts should be made to find acid-fast bacilli by microscopy in any patient who is acutely ill with an inflammatory process in the lung that might be tuberculous. In the interpretation of negative findings it is important to remember that failure to find acid-fast bacilli in a scanty mucoid sputum in a patient with acute pneumonic changes without cavitation militates very little against a diagnosis of tuberculosis: whereas in a patient with a cavitated inflammatory process and frankly purulent sputum, repeated negative findings are much more significant.

Microscopy of Gram-stained smears of sputum may be of value in indicating the morphology of the prevailing bacterial flora. This may be helpful in acute pneumonias—e.g., a preponderance of Gram-positive diplococci suggests a pneumococcal infection, or of clumps of Gram-positive cocci a staphylococcal infection—but in bacterial infections culture is generally required both to identify organisms and to provide information about their sensitivity to antibiotics. In general, the results of sputum culture must be interpreted in the light, not only of the known pathogenicity of the organisms isolated but also of their possible relevance to the clinical and radiological aspects of the case.

The production of sputum is an essential feature of chronic bronchitis, and the presence of pus in the sputum is the criterion by which mucopurulent is distinguished from simple chronic bronchitis. It has been established that the change from mucoid to mucopurulent sputum can be correlated with bacterial infection, principally with *Haemophilus influenzae*, sometimes with pneumococcus, and only occasionally with other organisms. For this reason, inspection of the sputum of chronic bronchitic patients usually gives a satisfactory indication of the need for treatment by antibacterial drugs, especially as those most frequently used are effective against both *H. influenzae* and pneumococcus.

It should be remembered that in the sputum of patients receiving broad-spectrum antibiotics organisms other than the original pathogens often become predominant. These may be organisms that rarely become pathogenic, such as *Proteus* and coliform organisms, as well as some that can assume independent pathogenicity, such as *Pseudomonas pyocyanea* and *Monilia*. Even with the latter, it is often difficult to be certain whether or no in an individual case of chronic mucopurulent bronchitis they are truly pathogenic.

Sporing organisms, such as *Aspergillus* species, whose spores are frequently present in the air, appear as contaminants in a proportion of all sputum cultures. For this reason, the finding of an *Aspergillus* species in the sputum is of no significance unless supported by clinical and immunological evidence.

J. G. Scadding.

SQUINT

Squints may be classified according to their *direction*, into convergent, divergent, or vertical; and according to their *cause*, into paralytic and non-paralytic (concomitant). The diagnosis between paralytic and non-paralytic squint is, as a rule, easy. In a paralytic squint the degree of deviation of the two eyes varies, as the farther the eyes are moved over in the direction of the action of the paralysed muscle the greater will be the deviation from parallelism. In a concomitant squint the eyes always bear the same relative position to each other in whatever direction they are turned. Concomitant squint is characteristically a disorder of childhood, while paralytic squint more frequently occurs later in life.

The diagnosis of the cause of a paralytic squint is discussed under DIPLOPIA (p. 214).

Concomitant squints are usually the sequel to dysharmony in the accommodation–convergence synkinesis (as with high hypermetropia), poor development in the power of fusion, or faulty anatomical setting of the eyes—all of which may have an hereditary basis. They may be aggravated by any sensory or central impediment to the acquisition of the binocular fixation reflex (e.g., poor vision from a congenital cataract, etc., or poor co-ordination from mental deficiency or emotional disturbances).

P. Trevor-Roper.

STEATORRHOEA

A daily faecal excretion of 'fat' (as fatty acid) of more than 18 mmol (5 g.) a day is defined as 'steatorrhoea'. If very large amounts are excreted the stools look greasy and, because of the low specific gravity of fat, tend to float on water.

Faecal fat estimation is commonly used to indicate malabsorption of all nutrients, but in some conditions causing steatorrhoea protein and carbohydrate absorption is normal.

Normal Triglyceride Absorption. Normally almost all the dietary triglyceride (fat) is absorbed, and faecal fat excretion, which is almost independent of dietary intake, is derived from desquamated mucosal cells.

other micellar components, in the form of chylomicrons. The absorptive area is very large, being considerably increased by the folding of the intestinal mucosa into villi. Reduction of this area by flattening of villi, or disease of the mucosal cells, may cause steatorrhoea.

Direct Consequences of Steatorrhoea. Certain long-term effects are common to all forms of steatorrhoea. Depletion of fat-soluble vitamin D may cause calcium deficiency, with hypocalcaemia, hypophosphataemia, and osteomalacia, and the presenting symptom of steatorrhoea may be bone pain. The proliferating osteoblasts of osteomalacic bone release alkaline phosphatase, causing an increase in plasma levels of the enzyme. Vitamin K, another fat-soluble vitamin,

Table 1. Differential Diagnosis of Steatorrhoea

	Upper Small Intestinal Disease	Pancreatic Disease	Biliary Obstruction	Blind Loop Syndrome
Carbohydrate absorption	Oligo and polysaccharide impaired	Polysaccharide impaired	Normal	Normal
*Xylose	*Impaired	*Normal	Normal	*Usually normal
Glucose tolerance test	May be flat	May be diabetic	Usually normal	Usually normal
Protein absorption Plasma albumin	Impaired Significantly low in advanced cases, with oedema	Impaired Non-specific	Usually normal Non-specific	Usually normal Non-specific
Anaemia	*Mixed megaloblastic and iron-deficiency common	*Rare as consequence of malabsorption	*Rare as consequence of malabsorption	*Megaloblastic common
*Intestinal biopsy	*Flattened villi or other cause	*Normal	Not usually indicated (normal)	Usually normal
*Duodenal enzymes and bicarbonate (in gastro-intestinal units)	Normal response to secretin and pancreozymin	*Impaired response to secretin and pancreozymin	Not usually indicated (impaired response if pancreatic duct involved)	Normal response
Other relevant findings	—	—	*Obstructive jaundice predominant	—

* Most useful tests in differential diagnosis.

Triglycerides consist of glycerol combined with fatty acid. Dietary fat cannot be absorbed until it has been partially hydrolysed by pancreatic lipase to a mixture consisting mainly of monoglycerides and fatty acids. The action of lipase is facilitated by emulsification of large fat globules by bile-salts. Both lipase and bile-salts enter the duodenum by the common bile-duct, and disease of the pancreas, or biliary obstruction, impairs digestion of dietary fat.

The mixture of bile-salts, monoglycerides, and fatty acids, together with cholesterol, phospholipid, and the fat-soluble vitamins A, D, and K, aggregate to form a micelle which is 100–1000 times smaller than the emulsified fat particles. The micelles pass through the microvillous spaces in the luminal surface of the epithelial cells. Triglycerides are resynthesized within these cells, and enter the bloodstream, together with the

may also be deficient; as a consequence the prothrombin time may be prolonged, but returns to normal if vitamin K is given parenterally (*see* p. 512). In advanced cases haemorrhages and bruising may occur. Hypocholesterolaemia is an incidental finding of no diagnostic importance.

Intestinal Steatorrhoea. Steatorrhoea may be due to impaired absorption of digested fat by a diseased small intestinal mucosa.

CAUSES. Flattening of villi occurs in three important conditions.

Coeliac disease usually occurs in children, and is due to gluten sensitivity which is associated with damage to the villi. Subjects respond to a gluten-free diet.

Tropical sprue responds to administration of broad-spectrum antibiotics, together with folate. A bacterial factor is probable.

Idiopathic steatorrhoea responds neither to withdrawal of gluten from the diet nor to antibiotic therapy.

The absorptive area may be reduced by *surgical resection* of the gut.

Infiltration or inflammation of the small intestinal wall extensive enough to cause steatorrhoea may occur in:

Crohn's disease
Intestinal tuberculosis
Intestinal amyloidosis
Intestinal scleroderma
Malignant infiltration of the intestinal wall.

Accelerated passage of gastric contents through the small intestine may cause steatorrhoea. This is usually mild after partial gastrectomy, but may be severe in the very rare cases associated with the carcinoid syndrome.

CONSEQUENCES. In intestinal steatorrhoea absorption of nutrient other than fat is also impaired.

In advanced cases amino-acid malabsorption causes muscle wasting, osteoporosis, low plasma protein and even low urea levels. If hypoalbuminaemia is severe there may be oedema, and the reduction of physiologically inert albumin-bound calcium may give an exaggerated impression of the severity of true (ionized) hypocalcaemia when total calcium levels are measured. Low immunoglobulin (γ-globulin) levels may predispose to infection.

Anaemia, which may cause the presenting symptoms, may be multifactorial, due to protein, iron, and vitamin B_{12} deficiency, with a mixed hypochromic and macrocytic blood film.

Malabsorption of carbohydrate may be reflected in a flat glucose-tolerance curve; this is a non-specific finding, which may be due to causes other than malabsorption, and which may even occur in some normal individuals. Malabsorption of the pentose, xylose, is more specific for intestinal disease, although, if the upper small intestine is spared, absorption may be normal.

Pancreatic Steatorrhoea. The steatorrhoea of pancreatic failure is due to impaired digestion rather than true malabsorption: small molecules can be absorbed. It is a less common cause than intestinal disease.

CAUSES. Pancreatic damage must be extensive to cause steatorrhoea, and may be due to chronic pancreatitis, to extensive carcinoma of the gland (in which case involvement of the bile-duct often causes obstructive jaundice), or, very rarely, to deposition of iron in haemochromatosis. In children and young adults with chest symptoms and signs, cystic fibrosis should be considered: the diagnosis is likely if the sweat electrolyte concentration is higher than 70 mmol/l.

CONSEQUENCES. Absorption of fat and protein is impaired because of impaired digestion by lipase and trypsin. Although polysaccharide digestion is also impaired by pancreatic amylase deficiency, mono- and disaccharides can be normally absorbed. The glucose-tolerance curve is often diabetic due to destruction of islet cells. Xylose absorption is normal.

Anaemia is relatively rare, since iron and vitamin B_{12} are absorbed without prior digestion.

Demonstration of reduced pancreatic secretion of enzymes following injection of pancreozymin, and of bicarbonate following injection of secretin, depends on duodenal intubation. The validity of the test depends on accurate positioning of the tube by an expert; wrongly positioned tubes may result in completely misleading results.

Steatorrhoea due to Biliary Obstruction. Reduced entry of bile-salts into the duodenum may cause steatorrhoea, with the usual consequences. Protein and carbohydrate (including xylose) absorption are unaffected. The presence of severe obstructive jaundice points to the cause, and steatorrhoea is rarely of sufficiently long-standing for the long-term effects to develop.

'Blind Loop Syndrome' and Neomycin Therapy. These syndromes cause fat malabsorption by altering the bacterial flora; bile salts may be metabolized to bile acids. The 'blind loops', in which stagnation and bacterial overgrowth occur, may be diverticulas, or 'backwaters' in loops resulting from surgery. Neomycin also alters bacterial flora, and possibly itself combines with bile-salts. In both conditions bile-salt deficiency causes steatorrhoea, without malabsorption of protein or carbohydrate. Megaloblastic anaemia is common, due to increased bacterial requirements for vitamin B_{12} and folate.

The differential diagnosis of steatorrhoea is summarized in *Table 1*.

Joan F. Zilva.

STERILITY

May be defined as inability to conceive when attempts have been made over a reasonable length of time, variously defined as between one and four years, according to the particular circumstances. Ten per cent of all marriages are barren and less than 10 per cent of pregnancies occur after the end of the second year of marriage.

The differential diagnosis of the causes of sterility is often difficult, and although there are many well-defined conditions which give rise to it, there are numbers of cases in which no definite cause can be found. There are many cases in which the sterility is due to a number of minor 'infertility factors' unimportant in themselves, but which in aggregate result in sterility.

In 20 per cent of cases a single cause for the unfertile marriage will be found, furthermore in 30 per cent of cases the husband is responsible, therefore we must not consider investigation complete until the husband has been examined. If the examination of a fresh ejaculate of semen shows it to be within normal limits with regard to volume (2–4 ml.) and number of spermatozoa (above 80 million per ml.), 60 per cent showing motility, and in addition there are not more than 20 per cent of abnormal forms, the husband should be regarded as fertile. Repeated checks must be made as the male counts vary much according to the state of health. Any fever depresses spermatogenesis. The effect appears over weeks after the start of fever and attains its maximum in six weeks' time. Spermatogenesis may not return to normal for several months. If also live spermatozoa can be found in the cervical mucus after coitus about the time of ovulation the male can be excluded as the cause of the infertile marriage. Four active progressing spermatozoa to the high-power field is the average. Providing there are some spermatozoa in the ejaculate it is not possible to say that a man is infertile no matter how low is the semen count. Pregnancies seem to occur in the face of very low counts indeed.

The causes of sterility are as follows:

1. Male Factors. Impotence, oligospermia, necrospermia, aspermia, varicocele, premature ejaculation, and failure to ejaculate during coitus.

Constitutional diseases such as tuberculosis, diabetes, anaemia, syphilis, alcoholism, and dietetic deficiencies. *Overwork* of a mental nature. *Endocrine factors* such as hypothyroidism or hyperthyroidism. Hypopituitarism suggested by underdevelopment of the penis, and obesity.

Men suffering from the chromosomal anomaly, Klinefelter's syndrome (XXY), have undeveloped genitalia with small soft testes and are infertile.

The commonest cause of complete sterility in the male is blockage of the epididymis due to gonorrhoea. Atrophy of the testes following orchitis as a complication of mumps (about 10 per cent of males contracting mumps develop orchitis) may be responsible. The male with both testes undescended is almost certainly sterile.

Failure of the male to ejaculate during coitus is a not infrequent cause when both partners are found to be normally fertile.

2. Female Factors:

LOCAL:

  a. Gross Pelvic Lesions:

  Absence of uterus, vagina, Fallopian tubes, or ovaries
  Infantile and pubescent uterus
  Hyperinvolution of the uterus
  Closure of hymen, vagina, or cervix
  Fibroids, polypi, carcinoma
  Cystic ovaries
  Tuberculosis of the endometrium
  Endometriosis.

  b. Cervical Lesions:

  Cervicitis
  Abnormalities of cervical secretion
  Stenosis of cervix
  Abnormal position of cervix.

  c. Tubal Lesions:

  Inflammatory lesions
  Tuberculosis
  Rudimentary tubes.

  d. Vaginal and Vulval Lesions:

  Dyspareunia
  Vaginismus.

  e. Endocrine Lesions:

  Gross Disorders:
    Fröhlich's syndrome, myxoedema
    Simmonds's disease
    Adrenocortical tumours
  Menstrual Disorders:
    Amenorrhoea, hypomenorrhoea
    Metropathia
  Anovular menstruation.

  f. Chromosomal Anomalies:

  Turner's syndrome (XO)
  Super-female (XXX)

GENERAL:
  Old age
  Obesity
  Anaemia
  Nutritional: Vitamin A, B deficiency
  Occupational.

3. Combined Male and Female Factors present together:

  a. Subnormal sperm count with abnormal cervical secretion in the female
  b. Incomplete penetration
  c. Profluvium seminis
  d. Defective germ plasma.

The above list shows that some causes of sterility are primary, others secondary. Thus absence of the uterus or infantile uterus means primary sterility, while hyperinvolution, salpingitis, etc., may occur in women who have had children, and only secondarily become sterile on account of these lesions.

Congenital Lesions. Some of the congenital lesions are diagnosed easily, such as *imperforate hymen*, *absence of the vagina*, or *stenosis of the cervix*, while absence of the essential organs often requires an anaesthetic in order that a bimanual examination may be made satisfactorily. The *infantile uterus* and *small adult type* are difficult to differentiate; but in the former the body forms only one-third of the total length of the organ, while in the latter it forms two-thirds, both types of uterus being small in the anteroposterior and lateral dimensions, and only slightly shortened in the vertical. *Pseudo-hermaphroditism* usually shows itself by shortness of the vagina, elongation of the clitoris, and the presence of glandular masses in the groins, which are almost always testes, proving that the subjects of it are really undeveloped males.

Acquired Lesions. The differential diagnosis of the acquired lesions can only be made by complete examination of the patient by inspection, bimanual examination, and the use of the microscope to elucidate doubtful growths. *Blockage of the Fallopian tubes* as a result of a past salpingo-oophoritis, the cause of many cases of absolute sterility, may be demonstrated by insufflation of the tubes via the uterus with carbon dioxide (Rubin's test for patency of the tubes) or injection into the uterus and tubes with a substance opaque to X-rays such as lipiodol or a more quickly absorbable aqueous substitute. An anaesthetic is often given for hysterosalpingography, but a more accurate assessment is obtained with the patient awake using a fluorescent screen and an image intensifier. These tests may have to be repeated after the inhalation of amyl nitrite to exclude tubal spasm as the cause of the blockage of the Fallopian tubes (*Figs.* 750–752).

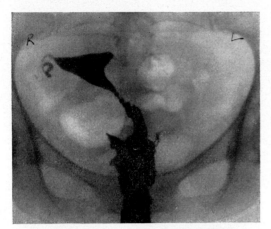

Fig. 750. Radiograph of the uterus and Fallopian tubes after intra-uterine injection of lipiodol. The left tube is closed at the uterine end. The right tube is stenosed.

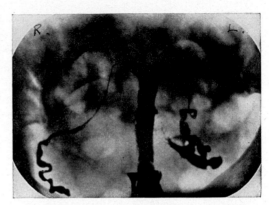

Fig. 751. Radiograph of the uterus and Fallopian tubes after intra-uterine injection of lipiodol. The left tube is patent. The right tube is closed at its outer end.

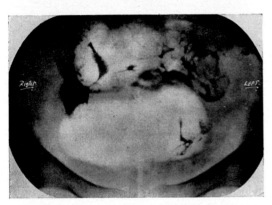

Fig. 752. Radiograph, taken 24 hours after injection of lipiodol, showing a 'free spill' in the peritoneal cavity. Both tubes patent.

Before embarking on salpingostomy the blockage of the tubes revealed by X-rays should be confirmed by direct vision, the surgeon using a laparoscope and an assistant injecting dye into the uterus and tubes. *Dyspareunia* as a cause is dealt with under this heading (p. 231).

Sterility of endocrine origin is now believed to be the common type, in which no gross abnormality of the pelvic organs can be found. Amenorrhoeic women or women who menstruate at long intervals are always of low fertility. Defective corpus luteum or absence of luteinization leads to reduction or absence of the luteal hormone progesterone, and consequently hypertrophy of the endometrium is imperfect, so that in spite of fertilization of the ovum embedding in the endometrium does not occur. Estimation of the blood

progesterone done in these cases about the twenty-first day of the cycle will often show their true character. Oestradiol measurements at the time of ovulation are also helpful. The test is by radioimmunoassay following ether extraction. About 1 ml of blood is required for a progesterone measurement and 5 ml for oestradiol. The underlying factor in some of these cases is anterior pituitary failure as described in pituitary amenorrhoea (p. 22). *Smears of vaginal cells* in the hands of the expert cytologist accurately reflect the hormonal changes. They can be taken easily by the patient herself and provide evidence of the hormonal balance throughout the menstrual cycle, including ovulation and the length and character of the luteal phase. Lesser aberrations of the anterior pituitary function affecting the thyroid and ovarian activity may be responsible as indicated by an abnormal metabolic rate and blood cholesterol levels. A diagnostic curettage of the endometrium, taken on the first day of menstruation to establish that ovulation is taking place, is necessary. Repeated monthly curettage or serial vaginal smears may have to be taken before anovular monthly bleeding can be diagnosed, as ovulation may not occur every month. If ovulation has occurred the endometrium shows marked secretory activity, the glands having crenated margins with fern-like tufts projecting into the lumen of the glands (Opitz-Gebhard glands). The finding in the cervix of the typical clear elastic mucus at the time of ovulation is a further proof that ovulation has taken place. As the result of normal oestrogen secretion by the ovary the cervical mucus can be drawn into long threads up to 10 cm. in length. This phenomenon is known as *Spinnbarkeit*. From about the sixth to the twenty-second days of the menstrual cycle cervical mucus spread thickly on a glass slide rinsed in distilled water and allowed to dry will show a characteristic pattern resembling a fern leaf. This 'ferning' of cervical mucus due to crystallization occurs as the result of oestrogen secretion and disappears under the influence of progesterone in the second half of the cycle.

The occurrence and time of ovulation can often be verified by taking the oral or vaginal

than sleep, e.g., coma, and it may also occur when there is a partially obstructive lesion of the oropharynx as in a quinsy, oedematous uvula, retropharyngeal abscess or tumour of the tonsil or posterior part of the tongue.

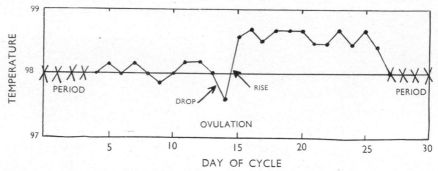

Fig. 753. A typical basal temperature chart.

temperature on waking in the morning before partaking of food or drink, and before getting out of bed. A characteristic drop followed by a rise in temperature will be detected at the time of ovulation. In about 60 per cent of women ovulation occurs on the 14th day preceding the onset of the period. (*Fig.* 753.) Absence of ovarian activity must be the true cause in the general conditions which are outwardly shown by *obesity, anaemia,* and *disturbances of nutrition*; some women do not conceive as long as they remain too fat, while loss of weight has in some cases been followed by conception. *Sexual incompatibility* between husband and wife may lead to there being no baby, but it is difficult to prove. It is very doubtful whether such a condition exists. It is more likely that both partners are subfertile. Should the marriage be dissolved and marriage with a more fertile partner take place, a pregnancy often results. *Absence of sexual feeling* or the sexual orgasm is not a cause of sterility, for conception takes place normally in women who are absolutely devoid of these feelings. On the other hand, most authors quote the case of a woman who conceived as a result of the only coitus at which an orgasm was experienced. The influence of *age* on child-bearing must not be forgotten, the liability to conceive falling rapidly every year over thirty.

T. L. T. Lewis.

STERTOR

The term 'stertor' or 'stertorous respiration' implies that variety of noisy breathing arising from causes in the region of the oropharyngeal isthmus. Thus it might be regarded as synonymous with the term 'snoring', which is caused by vibrations of the soft palate in sleep. It is, however, usually reserved for the breathing present in a deeper plane of unconsciousness

It should not be confused with the term *stridor* which is higher pitched, more marked on inspiration, and caused by an obstructive lesion in the larynx, trachea, or main bronchi.

The cause of the stertorous breathing usually becomes evident upon examination of the buccal cavity and pharynx.

Miles Foxen.

STIFF-MAN SYNDROME

This syndrome, as originally described in 1956 and as since confirmed by others, is characterized by a tautness of striated muscles, usually of the trunk but sometimes involving the arms and legs, more severely proximally. Superimposed on this are painful muscle spasms. Apart from the stiffness neurological examination is normal except for the occasional discovery of extensor plantar responses. Associated metabolic disturbances have been reported especially in relation to glucose metabolism. The clinical picture tends to be gradually progressive but the condition may become arrested.

Ian Mackenzie.

STOMACH, DILATATION OF

Dilatation of the stomach presents itself clinically under two totally different aspects: (1) *Acute*; (2) *Chronic*.
1. Acute Dilatation of the Stomach. This is generally a serious complication or even a fatal catastrophe arising in the course of some other condition, especially after operations (notably laparotomy), or after abdominal injury.

The diagnosis is generally easy. The abdomen is distended and tympanitic; there is constant effort to bring up wind, sometimes in vain, sometimes with copious and recurrent eructations, often with intractable hiccoughs. Sometimes immense quantities of blackish-brown or greenish-brown fluid flow effortlessly from the mouth and nostrils. The dilatation itself is of the nature of an acute paralysis of the stomach. Diagnosis is confirmed, and indeed treatment initiated, by the passage of a stomach tube which deflates the gastric dilatation.

2. Chronic Dilatation of the Stomach. This is due to conditions which cause stenosis at, or more commonly on either side of, the pylorus.

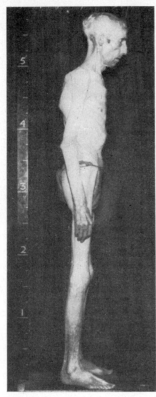

Fig. 754. Typical appearance of a patient with long-standing pyloric stenosis due to a duodenal ulcer. The patient demonstrates the drawn, anxious facies, gross dehydration, and wasting.

Causes of Stenosis:

Peptic ulcer, particularly of the duodenum, although much less commonly a benign gastric ulcer at the pylorus or in the antrum may be responsible

Carcinoma of the pylorus or antrum

Other tumours in this region; these include leiomyoma, leiomyosarcoma, infiltration with Hodgkin's disease or lymphosarcoma, or invasion from an adjacent carcinoma of pancreas or gallbladder

Congenital pyloric septum

Adult hypertrophy of the pylorus

Heterotopic pancreatic tissue

Adhesions of the duodenum to the liver bed following cholecystectomy.

The history in an established case of pyloric stenosis may be absolutely typical. In the case of a peptic ulcer there may be a long preceding story of ulcer pain. Vomiting is an important symptom and occurs in at least 9 out of every 10 patients. Typically copious amounts of vomitus are produced in a projectile manner and the patient will recall (but often only on direct questioning) that he has noticed fragments of food, particularly vegetable or fruit debris, which had been ingested one day and vomited up the next, or even two or three days later. There is really no condition other than obstruction to the gastric outlet in which this state of affairs obtains. Obstruction due to carcinoma, in contrast, often has a shorter history perhaps of only a few months, and pain is completely absent in about one-third of patients. Examination of the patient often reveals features of importance. There may be evidence of dehydration and loss of weight; indeed the classic 'ulcer facies' applies only rarely to uncomplicated examples of peptic ulcer but is perfectly mirrored in the usual appearance of the victim of long-standing stenosis (*Fig.* 754). A gastric splash is present 3 or 4 hours after a meal or drink is elicited in two-thirds of patients with benign stenosis. Often the patient when asked directly will agree that he himself has noticed a splashing sound when walking or moving about. Visible gastric peristalsis, passing from left to right, is present much less frequently, and still less often the loaded and hypertrophied stomach may actually be palpable as well as audible and visible. About half the patients with malignant obstruction will reveal a palpable tumour at the pylorus. Such a mass may, it is true, be felt rarely in the benign case, when a large inflammatory mass is present around the first part of the duodenum. Because of the more rapid progression in the malignant case, gross dilatation of the stomach is much less often seen than in benign obstruction, so that a gastric splash and visible peristalsis may not be elicited. (*See Fig.* 636, p. 642.)

Radiological investigation in these cases is mandatory. The findings can be divided into two groups: the first confirms the presence of an obstruction at the gastric outlet and the second indicates its pathology. A plain radiograph of the abdomen may itself be at least suggestive of pyloric stenosis by demonstrating a large gastric gas bubble with considerable quantities of retained food particles as demonstrated by patchy translucent areas. A sign of obstruction at the gastric outlet on the barium meal is the large residue of food within the stomach shown after taking a few mouthfuls of barium. Instead of the normal appearance of the barium running down the lesser curvature, the particles of barium can be seen to sink through a layer of fluid and then to rest at the bottom of the greater curve like a saucer. In the erect position three layers can be seen; the air bubble above, then the layer of gastric juice, and finally the lowermost layer of barium (*Fig.* 755). In the early phase of pyloric stenosis giant peristaltic waves may be seen passing along the gastric wall, but in late decompensated obstruction the stomach is a large atonic bag. Obstruction of the gastric outlet is confirmed by taking further films at 4–6 hours when it will be seen that a large residium of barium remains in the stomach (*Fig.* 757). Under normal

responsible is given by the presence of an active ulcer crater or severe scarring in the duodenal cap. If the obstruction is situated in the antrum of the stomach it is most probable that the diagnosis

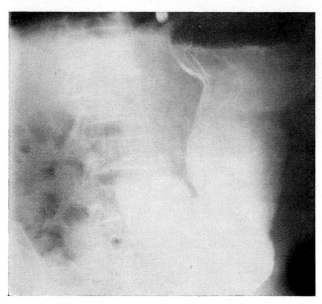

Fig. 755. Pyloric stenosis due to chronic duodenal ulcer. Note three layers: air, gastric juice, and barium.

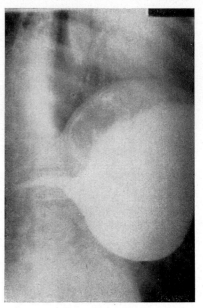

Fig. 756. Pyloric obstruction due to extensive antral carcinoma.

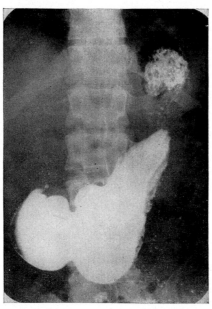

Fig. 757. Pyloric stenosis due to chronic duodenal ulcer. The picture was taken 3 hours after a barium meal. (*Dr. Keith Jefferson.*)

circumstances the stomach is all but empty at the end of 2 hours. It is not always easy to tell the exact cause of the pyloric obstruction. Radiological evidence that a duodenal ulcer is

is cancer (*Fig.* 756) but occasionally a similar appearance is given by a penetrating benign gastric ulcer. A further sign of duodenal bulb obstruction that we have found to be useful is abnormal dilatability of the pyloric canal which may be seen on screening to dilate up to 2·5 cm. or more in width and then contract down again to its usual size proximal to the point of stenosis.

The less common causes of pyloric obstruction mentioned above which may be associated with chronic dilatation of the stomach are rarely diagnosed before laparotomy. However, since obstruction of the gastric outlet almost invariably requires surgical intervention the elucidation of the exact cause preceding operation is a luxury rather than a necessity for the experienced surgeon.

Harold Ellis.

STOMACH, TESTS OF FUNCTION OF

Although these tests have become less popular in recent years, many refinements of technique are now available for testing gastric function.

Motility. Stomach motility as tested by *radiology* is very variable in normal subjects and in this connexion radiologists are mainly concerned with the demonstration of frank pyloric stenosis. This diagnosis may also be made by detection in the vomit of food known to have been eaten more than 12 hours previously or by the finding of starch or obvious food residue in the stomach contents obtained by intubation after 12 hours' fast. Such contents usually have a foul or rancid odour and contain much lactic acid produced by fermentation.

Secretion. These tests also involve the passage of a stomach tube in the fasting state and the quantitative collection of juice usually after administration of a powerful stimulus of gastric secretion. Continuous collection by suction is used for night specimens. The manipulation of the tube is a skilled procedure and misleading results may be obtained if this is done by untrained staff. The following stimulants may be used: *betazole hydrochloride* (100 mg.) or *pentagastrin* (6 μg. per kg. of body-weight) are injected intramuscularly, antihistamine cover being desirable with the former. Basal secretion is collected for 1 hour before injection and four 15-minute specimens thereafter. Normal secretion is up to 40 mEq. of HCl per hour. *Insulin* (0·2 unit per kg.) is an alternative stimulant which depends on vagal stimulation due to hypoglycaemia. The procedure is similar to that described above but specimens are collected for up to 2 hours after injection. A positive response is shown by an acid secretion exceeding 2 mEq. in any 1 hour. In this test it is essential that the blood-glucose should fall below 2·2 mmol/l (40 mg. per 100 ml.), and that the patient should be clinically hypoglycaemic.

Secretion of *intrinsic factor* may be tested by the administration of ^{58}Co-labelled vitamin B_{12} and the subsequent estimation of urinary radioactivity (Schilling test). Low absorption may be due either to intestinal malabsorption or to lack of intrinsic factor, but a repetition of the test with the simultaneous administration of intrinsic factor will show a normal response if the absence of this substance was the cause of the impaired absorption.

Cytology. Examination of gastric washing to detect malignant cells is of value only if the material is correctly obtained and the laboratory is skilled in its interpretation. The early morning resting juice must be aspirated as completely as possible but is valueless for cytology. One should inject about 300 ml. of normal saline down the aspiration tube and then place the patient for 2 minutes each in the prone position, the left lateral, the right lateral, and the supine positions, and then reaspirate saline. Probably not more than 150 ml. will remain for reaspiration. This should be sent immediately to the laboratory. If it is impracticable to arrange immediate transport, it should be placed in a large test-tube in a Thermos packed round with ice. Examination more than 2 hours after taking is likely to be valueless as the acid present rapidly destroys cell morphology.

Applications. It is now recognized that gastric function tests are only useful in a few well-defined situations. They are clearly relevant to the diagnosis of *pyloric stenosis* as indicated above. The demonstration of hypersecretion is an important feature of the *Zollinger-Ellison syndrome* (q.v.). A milder degree of hypersecretion is common in patients with duodenal ulcer who also show a continued night secretion of acid in high concentration. The test has no diagnostic value in this condition but the degree of hypersecretion has been used by some surgeons as a guide to operative treatment. The *insulin test* is mainly used after vagotomy to establish the completeness of the operation. Tests for *intrinsic factor* are appropriate in some cases of macrocytic anaemia of uncertain origin.

Achlorhydria (pH above 3·5) by itself is of relatively little significance as it occurs in a proportion of normal subjects. It is almost invariably present in pernicious anaemia but its presence is not essential for diagnosis. Achlorhydria is also common with gastric carcinoma but is usually a late finding. In this condition *gastric cytology* is of value if available.

Gastrin is a hormone normally secreted by the G cells of the gastric antrum in response to the presence of food; it is carried in the bloodstream to the parietal area of the stomach where it stimulates acid secretion. A low pyloric pH inhibits gastrin release.

Plasma gastrin levels may be measured by radio-immunoassay by special centres. The high acid secretion of the Zollinger-Ellison syndrome is due to excessive production of gastrin, usually ectopically by pancreatic islet tumours. In the syndrome levels of plasma gastrin are very high (5–30 times the upper limit of normal), despite the very acid gastric contents which should normally cut off hormone secretion.

Joan F. Zilva.

STOOLS, MUCUS IN

Mucus in the stools is not pathognomonic. It occurs in *malignant disease of the colon* as a clear glairy substance often blood-stained, and it has the same character in *intussusception*; the obstruction in both these conditions accounts for the absence of faecal colouring. Large amounts of mucus may be secreted by extensive *benign papillomatous tumours* of the colon and rectum. Since this material is rich in potassium, profound potassium depletion may occur in this condition, leading to weakness, paraesthesiae, and even paralysis and vascular collapse. The volume of fluid passed may amount to 2 or 3 litres daily. Mucus is often seen with *constipated motions*, the hard faeces having led to irritation of the large bowel with consequent increased secretion of mucus as a defensive mechanism against misguided therapy, especially intestinal lavage. In severe cases a motion may consist almost entirely of coagulated shreds with little faecal matter. With less retention in the bowel, mucus takes the form of a jelly outside the motion, or it may have the appearance of uncooked white of egg, sago, or tapioca. In other cases, complete casts of the bowel formed of coagulated mucus are passed; they may be a foot or more in length. They may have become broken into fragments which the patient describes as skins, looking not unlike segments of tape-worm for which indeed they are on inadequate examination easily mistaken. Patients passing this variety of mucus are said to have *membranous* or *spastic colitis*, an incorrect term, for no inflammatory process occurs. The term 'irritable colon syndrome' is also used for this disorder, which is characterized by colonic abdominal pain, abnormal stools, and alteration in bowel habits. It is commoner in females aged 15–45 years but may occur in either sex under conditions of emotional tension. The patients on examination often appear anxious and tense and perspire excessively. Curiously enough, this hypersecretion of mucus has almost disappeared during the past thirty years, although the general symptomatology is still recognized. It may be added that the popular treatment of lavage to remove the mucus will be responsible for its continued secretion as a protest against irritation of the mucosa. In the more acute varieties of inflammation of the bowel the mucus passed is jelly-like and semi-liquid, of varying colour according to the amount of faecal staining. In *polyposis coli* and severe cases of *enteritis* and *dysentery* the motions consist of nothing but mucus and blood. One cannot differentiate between the numerous varieties of enteritis and colitis upon the basis of the mucus in the stools alone.

Harold Ellis.

STOOLS, PUS IN

Pus in the stools in sufficient amount to be recognizable by the naked eye indicates the rupture of an abscess into the intestinal tract. Such recognition is, however, unusual; for even when a large appendicular abscess perforates into the caecum the pus becomes indistinguishable either from admixture with the faeces, the patient believing he simply has diarrhoea, or on account of digestion and decomposition. The less the pus is mixed with other intestinal contents, the nearer to the anus must the site of rupture have been; but the diagnosis of the source of the abscess needs to be determined upon other grounds, particularly the history and the results of examination including that of the rectum and vagina. Abscesses most apt to cause a discharge of pus with the stools are of the appendicular, pericolic, pelvic, or other local peritoneal types; of prostatic or perirectal origin; or a pyosalpinx.

Microscopical quantities of pus in the stools may be due to any of the causes already mentioned and, in addition, to affections of the mucous membrane itself. These comprise acute or chronic ulcerative colitis, Crohn's colitis; dysentery; cholera; dengue; malignant, tuberculous, typhoidal, carcinomatous, or venereal ulceration of the bowel. The pus cells may be recognizable as such under the microscope. Examination with the sigmoidoscope (*Figs.* 65–70, p. 69) is invaluable in deciding the diagnosis.

Harold Ellis.

STRANGURY

Strangury differs somewhat from mere pain on micturition, in that, in addition to severe pain before, during, or after the act, the patient is troubled constantly by urgent and repeated necessity to pass his urine, sometimes as often as every few minutes, yet without satisfactory relief to his discomfort. The condition is also spoken of as 'vesical tenesmus'. Very little urine is passed each time; sometimes the desire and the necessity are urgent when there is no urine in the bladder at all. The causes resolve themselves into five groups, as follows:

1. Nervous Conditions, especially:
Hysteria
Anxiety state
Tabes dorsalis (vesical crises).

2 Obstruction to the Urine Outflow:
Urethral stricture
Enlarged prostate
Prostatic calculus
Carcinoma of the prostate
Retroverted gravid uterus
Uterine fibroid
Ovarian cyst } impacted in the pelvis
Ovarian carcinoma
Extreme prolapse of the uterus and bladder
Calculus impacted in the urethra
Inflamed urethral caruncle
Gonorrhoea
Urethritis other than gonococcal
Periprostatic abscess
Ischiorectal abscess.

3. Local Affections of the Bladder Wall:
Injury
Acute cystitis
Chronic cystitis
Interstitial cystitis (Hunner's ulcer)
Tuberculous cystitis
Calculus irritating the trigone
Papilloma vesicae
Carcinoma vesicae
Bilharziasis
Infiltration by—
    Carcinoma of the uterus
    Carcinoma of the rectum
Acute vesiculitis.

4. Reflex Conditions:
Inflamed haemorrhoids
Tuberculous kidney, before the bladder is involved
Coli bacilluria } even before there is infection of the
Pyelitis } bladder wall.

5. The Effects of Certain Drugs, especially:
Cantharides
Oxalic acid
Turpentine
Hexamine and its derivatives.

Most of the conditions mentioned above, and the methods of distinguishing between them, are discussed in the article on MICTURITION, ABNORMALITIES OF. The vesical crises of *tabes dorsalis* merit special mention. The patient's sole complaint may be that he can never be far from a lavatory because of acute and painful calls to empty his bladder at frequent intervals; sometimes he has no sooner passed what is in his bladder than he has to run back and try to do it again, though there is no urine whatever to pass, and his vesical pains may be extreme. From loss of sleep his general health suffers, and he becomes wasted to such an extent that carcinoma of the bladder or genito-urinary tuberculosis are simulated, or acute cystitis may be diagnosed erroneously. The true diagnosis will be made by cystoscopy, which shows the fine trabeculation, sacculated bladder, and funnel-neck deformity characteristic of the disease. These changes often precede objective signs in the central nervous system, but the diagnosis will be suggested when it is discovered that the ankle-jerks are absent, tendon sensation is lost, and the pupils give the Argyll Robertson reaction; in some cases, however, the nature of the malady may be difficult to decide for a time, because crises of all kinds, like the lightning pains, may develop in the earlier stages of tabes when the knee-jerks may as yet not be absent. Both ankle- and knee-jerks should be tested, for there are cases in which one knee-jerk is still present when the other has disappeared. A thorough examination of the urine and bladder should be carried out even if the patient is known to have tabes dorsalis, for he may have a gross lesion of the bladder in addition to his nervous disease. Actual cystitis resulting from retention of urine with overflow is generally a late symptom, and not a relatively early one like the vesical crises; as time goes on the bladder crises may cease spontaneously, just as the lightning pains, the rectal crises, and the other painful phenomena of tabes are apt to do.

Interstitial cystitis (Hunner's ulcer) is probably not an infectious disease. Histologically there is inflammatory infiltration of the bladder wall, unifocal or multifocal with mucosal ulceration and scarring, leading to contraction of smooth muscle, diminished capacity and frequent painful micturition with haematuria. The patients are usually middle-aged women.

Another point that merits attention is the strangury produced by certain drugs. *Cantharides* is familiar in this respect, but more from its prominence in textbooks upon forensic medicine than from its occurrence in actual practice. The same applies to *oxalic acid* and to *turpentine*. Hexamine and similar drugs derived from it are important. These have been employed in the treatment of pyuria, as well as other conditions, but have now been largely replaced by sulpha drugs and antibiotics. If given for pyuria, when there may have been frequent and painful micturition already, the increased frequency and pain that sometimes ensue when any of the above drugs are administered are apt to be attributed to an increase in the cystitis or other genito-urinary lesion, and the dose of the drug may be increased instead of diminished. The important point is that hexamine and other drugs of like nature may be responsible for such strangury as may simulate local disease of the bladder, and unless this is borne in mind an erroneous diagnosis is liable to be made.

Harold Ellis.

STRIDOR

Stridor is the harsh noise produced as respired air passes through a partial obstruction of the main air-passages. In general it will be produced only if the obstruction is so placed that all the air going into the lungs has to pass the obstruction. Thus obstruction in the pharynx, the larynx, the trachea, or, more rarely, both main bronchi, is required to produce stridor. Obstruction to one main bronchus, the other being patent, results in most of the respired air passing in and out of the unobstructed lung, and the noise produced by air passing through obstructed bronchi can be heard only by special manœuvres such as making the patient inspire very deeply with the mouth open. If the obstruction is more than very slight, stridor will be accompanied by signs confirmatory of respiratory obstruction, such as inspiratory recession of the intercostal spaces and action of the accessory muscles of respiration. Especially in children these signs may be very obvious. There are many possible causes of stridor; they may be classified as follows:

1. Causes above the Larynx:
  Retropharyngeal abscess
  New growths of the pharynx.

2. Causes inside the Larynx or Trachea:
  Mucus or mucopus in patients enfeebled by illness or in whom a defect of the cough mechanism (laryngeal palsy, respiratory muscle palsy) leads to inability to expel these secretions.
  Foreign body.

3. Affections of the Wall of the Larynx or Trachea:
  a. INFLAMMATORY:
    i. Acute: *Diphtheria*; *Acute laryngitis*, including acute catarrhal laryngitis, acute laryngo-tracheo-bronchitis of infants, and acute laryngitis due to exposure to *irritant gases*.
    ii. Chronic: *Tuberculous* or *syphilitic* laryngitis with stenosis.

  b. TRAUMATIC OR POST-TRAUMATIC:
    Injuries of larynx or trachea
    Post-traumatic stenosis of larynx or trachea, e.g., after tracheostomy, after attempted suicidal 'cut-throat', and after prolonged use of a cuffed endotracheal tube, with or without tracheostomy.

  c. NEOPLASTIC:
    Carcinoma of larynx
    Carcinoma of trachea
    Benign tumours of larynx or trachea.

  d. ALLERGIC:
    Oedema of the glottis in angioneurotic oedema.

e. CONGENITAL:
> Congenital web of larynx
> Congenital laryngeal stridor.

f. ANKYLOSIS OF CRICO-ARYTENOID JOINT IN RHEUMATOID ARTHRITIS.

4. Compression of Larynx or Trachea from without:

> *Goitre,* especially haemorrhage into an adenomatous goitre. Hashimoto's disease, intrathoracic goitre.
> *Riedel's thyroiditis*
> *Carcinoma of the thyroid*
> *Aneurysm* of the arch of the aorta.
> *Malformations of the aorta*—double aortic arch.
> *Mediastinal new growths,* including metastatic involvement of mediastinal lymph-nodes.
> *Mediastinal Hodgkin's disease* and other reticuloses.
> *Carcinoma of oesophagus* invading the trachea.
> *Malignant disease of lower cervical lymph-nodes*
> *Cellulitis of the neck*
> *Ludwig's angina*
> *Tuberculous lymph-nodes in mediastinum.*

5. Laryngeal Nerve Palsies (p. 400):

> *Bulbar or pseudobulbar palsy*
> *Bilateral lesions of recurrent laryngeal nerves.*

6. Laryngismus Stridulus—in rickety children; a manifestation of underlying tetany.

7. Narrowing of Both Main Bronchi:

> *Bronchial carcinoma,* either starting in one main bronchus and extending into the other, or metastasizing to subcarinal lymph-nodes.
> *Mediastinal new growths*
> *Tuberculous strictures of main bronchi*
> *Strictures of main bronchi in sarcoidosis.*

In many cases the cause of stridor is obvious, for instance when it is caused by secretions lodging in the larynx or trachea in seriously ill patients, or in patients in coma from any cause. In others local examination of the upper respiratory tract or larynx will provide the diagnosis without much difficulty. The greatest difficulty is likely to be encountered in children in whom the possibility of stridor of acute onset being due to diphtheria should never be forgotten, and in less acute cases retropharyngeal abscess must be borne in mind. Foreign bodies in the larynx or the main air-passages are also a possible source of difficulty in children. Acute upper respiratory infections may cause stridor more readily in childhood (croup) than in adults; the so-called *laryngitis stridulosa,* for example, occurs suddenly in children under 4 years of age, without warning in the night, usually subsiding in a few days. In adults stridor is much more likely to be associated with chronic illness. In any case of doubt inspection of the larynx by indirect or direct laryngoscopy, and of the trachea and main bronchi, if indicated, by bronchoscopy, should be carried out.

J. G. Scadding.

STUPOR

Stupor is a state in which there is complete or almost complete cessation of activity, with a corresponding reduction in response to external stimulation. While it may be possible to rouse the patient to some extent by a forcible command or by painful stimulation, thus differentiating the condition from *coma,* stupor can sometimes be so profound as to render the subject completely non-responsive. In contrast to coma the patient in stupor may stare with open eyes. Thus although his state of consciousness may be clouded, unlike coma he appears to be at least partially awake.

Stupor may be due to *intoxication* by narcotic drugs, or may precede coma in *diabetes* and *uraemia.* Stupor may also occur in a variety of cerebral diseases where it may either precede coma or follow upon it, when consciousness starts to return. Otherwise, the term *stupor* is more properly applied to those states in which the disorder appears to be mental in origin, the chief forms being those due to *catatonic schizophrenia,* severe *depression,* certain *hysterical states,* and to *emotional withdrawal* which is rare to the point of stupor, usually short-lived, and follows some profound psychological trauma.

The *catatonic* form of schizophrenia shows two phases, one of *excitement* and one of *stupor;* these may occur singly or may alternate. In the stuporous state the patient sits or lies in a fixed position, often a cramped or uncomfortable one; his face may be expressionless, although his lips are often protruded in a curious static pout (*schnauzcrampf*). The nature of this state can only be inferred, since the patient is quite inaccessible; he does not respond to questions—or even to painful stimulation. He may appear to be listening and may in fact be experiencing vivid hallucinations. There may be incontinence, or alternatively retention of urine and faeces. His mouth may fill with saliva which he is too apathetic to swallow, so that drooling occurs. This sign is most uncommon in other forms of stupor. The limbs may be rigid, or may retain the posture to which they are placed or may strongly resist an attempt to move them (*catalepsy; flexibilitas cerea*). This resistance, which is one form of *negativism* is also found in some cases of hysterical stupor. Catatonic stupor may at any time be suddenly interrupted by a phase of intense and purposeless activity, with violent and impulsive actions which may portend homicidal or suicidal intent. The diagnosis of catatonic stupor is supported if there is a clear history of delusions, hallucinations, or unaccountable and bizarre behaviour. It is as well to remember that although catatonic patients appear to be quite out of touch they may in fact be fully aware of everything going on around them. Remarks made within their hearing should therefore be guarded. It should also be noted that true catatonic stupor has, for some obscure reason, become much rarer during the past two decades. Thus the occurrence of catatonic symptoms in a patient with no previous schizophrenic history may suggest the more likely possibility of some other cause, e.g. *encephalitis* or an *epileptic* condition.

In *depressive states* the depression may be so intense and *retardation* so marked that activity is brought to a halt and the patient remains silent, motionless, and withdrawn. His posture and facial expression may be eloquent of his extreme misery and dejection, or his expression may be blank. If he makes any spontaneous movements at all, he does so slowly and reluctantly. Withdrawal is seldom so complete as in catatonic stupor and is not accompanied by catalepsy. The prodromal symptoms and signs are those of an illness with gradually increasing depression and retardation, ideas of guilt and despair or hypochrondiacal notions, restriction of normal activity, interference with sleep and bowel function. There is often a history of previous similar depressive attacks lasting a few weeks or months.

Manic stupor, which is an extremely rare condition indeed, resembles depressive stupor in that gross retardation is present and the patient remains silent, despite the fact that it subsequently transpires that his thoughts are racing round his head. But although he says and does nothing, he appears far from depressed; his face may bear a broad grin or a general expression of elation. So puzzling is this discrepancy that those inexperienced are inclined to misdiagnose the condition as being of schizophrenic origin. Other *mixed affective states* are similarly prone to misdiagnosis.

Overwhelming emotional experience may induce in subjects of *hysterical* personality, a stuporous, semi-stuporous, or trance-like state. This may be recognized by consideration of the circumstances of the attack. The *Ganser syndrome* is a rare condition of hysterical or depressive origin, often a combination of both, in which the patient lies semi-stuporous, may experience *pseudo-hallucinations*, and if he can be got to answer questions at all, exhibits *pseudodementia* in that his replies are never correct but near-miss answers.

As already indicated, *functional stupor* has to be distinguished from certain *organic states*. Profound apathy can accompany severe *frontal lobe* damage or appear in the later stages of severe dementia. A midline tumour in the *corpus callosum* can also give rise to a complete arrest of activity. Finally, a so-called *epileptic twilight state* which in actual fact is a prolonged *psychomotor seizure* which may persist for days, even for a week or two, may resemble stupor in that the patient may lie withdrawn, motionless, and speechless, although if disturbed he may suddenly become violently aggressive. In the absence of a history of epilepsy, an electro-encephalogram may clarify the diagnosis.

W. H. Trethowan.

SUCCUSSION SOUNDS

Succussion sounds may be heard when a viscus or cavity that contains both liquid and air or gas is shaken whilst the ear or the stethoscope is applied over it. The sounds may be loud enough to be audible at a distance from the patient. A good example of succussion is often afforded by the normal stomach after a quantity of liquid has been swallowed. Gastric succussion sounds are not necessarily evidence of abnormality, they merely indicate that the viscus contains liquid and gas, and although the gas may be due to fermentation, it is more usually air that has been swallowed during drinking. The chief value of gastric succussion sounds is that they afford some indication of the rate of emptying.

Succussion sounds may be heard in the chest in cases of *hydropneumothorax* when the patient oscillates his trunk to and fro. Less often, succussion sounds may be produced by a pyopneumothorax or a haemopneumothorax, the difference between these being decided by exploratory needling.

Succussion sounds other than those due to the stomach, or to gas and liquid in the pleural cavity, are uncommon.

The following is a list of all possible causes:

1. Causes of Succussion Sounds in the Thorax:

Hydropneumothorax
Pyopneumothorax
Haemopneumothorax
Diaphragmatic hernia
Subdiaphragmatic abscess communicating with the stomach or duodenum, or infected with *E. coli*: in either case, gas and pus are present
Hydropneumopericardium
Pyopneumopericardium

2. Causes of Succussion Sounds in the Abdomen:

The normal stomach
Dilatation of the stomach
Gross dilatation of the caecum
Gross dilatation of the colon
Pneumoperitoneum induced as a therapeutic measure in pulmonary tuberculosis or due to: (*a*) Perforated gastric ulcer; (*b*) Perforated duodenal ulcer; (*c*) Perforated typhoid ulcer of the intestine; (*d*) Perforated tuberculous ulcer of the intestine; (*e*) Perforated carcinoma of the colon; (*f*) Production of gas by *E. coli*, either in a local abscess (e.g., appendicular or subdiaphragmatic) or in the general peritoneum
Subdiaphragmatic abscess communicating with the interior of the stomach
Air and urine in the bladder (*see* PNEUMATURIA, p. 644)
Gas-production by *E. coli* in a large pyonephrosis
Infection by a gas-producing micro-organism of an ovarian cyst or other collection of liquid.

Succussion Sounds in the Chest. It is almost unknown for a *tuberculous cavity* to give succussion sounds. Should it do so, the situation would be subapical rather than basal, and thus distinguishable from most cases of hydro- or pyopneumothorax. *Hydro-* and *pyopneumopericardium* are also rare: they are identified by the churning sounds made by the heart beating within the mixture of air and liquid. The cause is generally a new growth of the oesophagus or bronchus opening the pericardium from behind, a foreign body such as a dental plate ulcerating through from the oesophagus, the opening of an air-containing subdiaphragmatic abscess through the diaphragm into the pericardium, or infection of the pericardial sac by a gas-producing organism.

A *subdiaphragmatic abscess* containing air due to communication with a hole in a gastric or duodenal ulcer may push the diaphragm up so high that the condition may be mistaken for hydro- or pyopneumothorax. Decision may be impossible until the position of the diaphragm is ascertained, either by the use of X-rays or at operation. When the trouble is subdiaphragmatic the tendency is to displace the heart upwards rather than towards the opposite side of the chest; the contrary is usual in the case of pneumothorax.

Diaphragmatic hernia, if large and if the stomach is herniated into the thorax, will show the effect of eating and drinking upon the physical signs and may point to the diagnosis. X-rays will demonstrate the condition after the administration of a barium meal.

In most cases of *hydropneumothorax* there is little difficulty in diagnosing the condition itself, although it may not be easy to ascertain its cause. If the onset has been sudden with acute pain in the affected side of the chest, cyanosis, and dyspnoea, the most likely cause is *phthisis*. In some instances, an injury or a ruptured emphysematous bulla may have been responsible, but injury seldom produces hydropneumothorax unless a tuberculous or other lesion in the lung was present at the time of the accident. Hydropneumothorax may result from *paracentesis thoracis*; if bleeding occurs during the puncture, *haemopneumothorax* will be produced. This too is common after bullet wounds of the chest. Either a hydro- or a haemopneumothorax may become infected with pyogenic organisms and converted into a *pyopneumothorax*. Pyopneumothorax may develop in cases of gangrene of the lung, obstruction of a bronchus by a foreign body or a new growth, the breaking down of an infective bronchopneumonia or pulmonary infarct, or the conversion of a pleural haematoma into a mixture of pus and gas as the result of infection by gas-gangrene organisms after gunshot or other wound of the chest. Fluid often collects in the pleural cavity when an artificial (therapeutic) pneumothorax has been induced, giving succussion sounds.

Succussion Sounds in the Abdomen. The first point in the differential diagnosis of succussion sounds in the abdomen is to decide whether the sounds are or are not of gastric origin. This is usually obvious but any doubt can be at once resolved by a barium meal. Dilatation of the stomach has three causes, namely atony, non-malignant pyloric or duodenal obstruction, especially by a healed simple ulcer, and malignant pyloric obstruction by primary gastric carcinoma (*see* p. 761). The presence of visible peristaltic waves or the occurrence of vomiting will indicate some degree of pyloric obstruction. Such obstruction will usually result in periodic vomiting, when the particles of food eaten a day or more previously can be recognized. Visible peristaltic waves corresponding to the stomach are another confirmatory feature. The most certain method of detecting pyloric stenosis is by means of a barium-meal examination.

If there are well-marked abdominal succussion sounds that can be definitely shown to be of non-gastric origin there are generally other signs and symptoms to assist the diagnosis. Succussion sounds in the peritoneal cavity are exceedingly rare, for even though this cavity should contain both gas and liquid—for instance after perforation of a typhoid ulcer—the coils of bowel prevent the sounds from being readily produced. The most common cause is iatrogenic, occurring either when air is introduced into the peritoneum, when ascites is tapped, or when carbon dioxide is introduced at laparoscopy in the presence of ascites. It would clearly be next to impossible to diagnose most of the conditions listed above unless the previous state of the patient were known or without resort to laparotomy. *E. coli* produces gas so that intra-abdominal abscesses, appendicular and otherwise, are occasionally resonant; the occurrence, however, of marked non-gastric succussion sounds in the abdomen of a patient who is not acutely ill will support the conclusion that there is distension with gas and liquid of some part of the large bowel, especially the caecum or the sigmoid colon. This distension is generally the result of either chronic constipation or intestinal stenosis. In cases of idiopathic dilatation of the colon, volvulus of the sigmoid colon, or Hirschsprung's disease, the sigmoid dilatation may be so extreme that this part of the intestine bulges up as far as the diaphragm.

C. Wastell.

SUICIDE, ATTEMPTED

Attempts or apparent attempts at suicide (*parasuicide*) are now so common as to present a constantly recurring problem of psychiatric assessment in the casualty department of any major general hospital. Whilst at present about 3000 persons per annum in England and Wales actually commit suicide, it is believed that about ten, or more, times this number make unsuccessful attempts or gestures. While there is an overlap and some common ground, suicide and attempted suicide are not otherwise identical phenomena. Indeed, from an epidemiological point of view there are several very distinct differences. The incidence of successful suicide in younger persons is rare on the whole and, corrected for age, rises constantly with advancing years, reaching a peak in the old. Attempted suicide, in contrast, rises to a peak incidence between 20 and 35 years of age and declines thereafter. More women attempt suicide unsuccessfully; more men succeed, although this sexual difference has now started to diminish. Suicide is more frequent among those who are socially isolated; unsuccessful attempts, on the other hand, are more prone to occur as a result of fairly immediate disturbances of interpersonal relationships, having a less contemplative and a more sudden, explosive, or *short-circuit* quality. Indeed, in attempted suicide the intention appears often to be more of a '*cry for help*' or an effort to draw attention to an immediate problem rather than a true act of self-destruction.

Among those who commit suicide a high proportion are overtly mentally ill. About a quarter also suffer from some disabling physical illness, such as *cancer, chronic bronchitis*, or *arthritis*. Younger persons who attempt suicide unsuccessfully tend, in contrast, to be physically healthier and to suffer more often from personal problems and personality disorders than from severe, overt mental illnesses of psychotic proportions.

In assessing the seriousness of a suicidal attempt, attention must be paid to the *circumstances* under which the attempt has occurred, the *method* used, the subject's expressed *intention*, his or her *mental* and *physical state, social background*, and so on. And yet, no one of these is likely in itself to be a reliable indicator of the seriousness of the attempt. Whilst jumping from a height or trying to kill oneself by hanging or drowning are clearly highly dangerous and must be taken seriously, judgement may be much more difficult in cases of self-poisoning. While one subject may take a small amount of a relatively innocuous substance apparently believing that its effect may be fatal; others will expose themselves to greater risk with seemingly lesser intent. Expressed intention is still harder to assess. A statement following resuscitation that an 'overdose' was taken merely to obtain a good night's sleep must obviously arouse suspicion. But even if this is regarded, often rightly, as dissimulation, the examiner may be left with the impression that the underlying motive was not, after all, very strong. Many subjects appear to be considerably confused about their intentions at the time of making a suicidal attempt and can or will give no satisfactory information regarding this. There is a danger here also. In a small number of those who are genuinely depressed, the emotional catharsis, brought about by the suicide attempt itself, has a beneficial though temporary effect upon their condition. This may lead to the attempt being regarded less seriously than it should be, and the patient's overall condition likewise. If, as a consequence, supervision is over-abruptly terminated and relapse occurs, a second and possibly successful attempt at suicide may soon follow.

The circumstances of occurrence may possibly be a guide. Suicidal attempts which have a domestic or histrionic quality and those which take place in front of others in a setting of domestic or marital strife and under the influence of alcohol (all very common) may be less seriously regarded than those which possibly occur without such acute prodromata in subjects who are cut off from family and friends and in whose cases there may be evidence of more or less careful preparation. The significance of suicide notes is obscure. On the whole, they should probably be taken as indicating some degree of serious intent though in many instances this is patently not so. It is not known, of course, how many of those who actually commit suicide leave a letter behind which, if found, may be destroyed without its presence ever being revealed.

On the whole the surest indication of the seriousness of a suicidal attempt is provided by a detailed assessment of the subject's mental state both following resuscitation and as it seems likely to have been before the attempt was made, given sufficient time for a degree of equilibrium to be reached. In those who are *depressed*, particularly when this is accompanied by *insomnia, loss of weight, appetite*, and *libido*, together with *feelings of failure, inadequacy*, and *hopelessness* as regards recovery (*see* DEPRESSION, p. 269), an attempt at suicide should be taken seriously with due regard to possible recurrence. The matter is even more serious if *delusions* of worthlessness, guilt or—in particular—*hypochondriacal delusions* (particularly of cancer, etc.) are present. In *schizophrenics* there is also a real risk which, in those who are younger, is hardly less than in depression. Indeed *schizophrenia*, together with concealed sexual problems, is probably one of the commoner causes of suicide in relatively young persons. As the risk of suicide is increased in *epileptics, alcoholics*, and *homosexuals* attempts among those in whom these complaints are identifiable should probably always be taken seriously.

While all attempts at suicide merit thorough psychiatric investigation this at present is largely impossible to implement. Of those who attempt suicide unsuccessfully about 5 per cent kill themselves within the next 3 or 4 years. The long-term prognosis is unknown. Like many other endemic disorders prevention is, in the long run, likely to prove more fruitful than cure. It is known that those who intend to take their lives (and who may well succeed) often visit their doctors on some or other relatively vague pretext a short while before. Although vague, this pretext, if correctly identified, may indicate an oncoming depressive state which may include among its symptoms a suicidal attempt, and possibly a successful attempt at that.

W. H. Trethowan.

SWEATING, ABNORMALITIES OF

Hyperidrosis or excess of sweating may be either general or local.

Generalized sweating is normal when due to exercise or excessive heat. Occasionally there is sweating during menstruation. The degree is variable and depends upon the individual concerned. It may be produced by drugs such as alcohol, the salicylates, or pilocarpine. Sweating is a feature of rickets, pink disease, infantile scurvy (Barlow's disease), and hyperthyroidism. Night sweats occur in tuberculosis. It may also be a feature of anxiety states when profuse sweating can occur even in a cold room. Hyperidrosis is also caused by pain of any sort and by motion sickness.

Localized hyperidrosis may occur in organic diseases of the nervous system, such as brain tumour, injury to the spinal cord, or to a peripheral nerve. A localized area of continuous sweating may be a symptom of post-encephalitic Parkinsonism. The parts most commonly affected are the palms and soles or the areas profusely supplied with sweat-glands such as the axillae and genital regions. In palmar and plantar hyperidrosis, which is frequently a form of psychoneurosis, the skin of the affected area becomes pink and shiny. Emotional sweating is almost confined to palms, soles, and axillae, but hyperidrosis of the hands may occur in otherwise normal subjects. Cold, clammy extremities are a feature of active rheumatoid arthritis even when no salicylates are being given. The Immersion Foot syndrome is also associated with local hyperidrosis.

In *granulosis rubra nasi*, a rare disease, there is profuse sweating of the tip of the nose associated with diffuse erythema and the formation of minute dark-red papules. The disorder must be distinguished from rosacea, lupus erythematosus, and lupus vulgaris.

In *miliaria* or sudamina (sweat rash) small vesicles occur on the skin of the trunk. It is caused by obstruction of the sweat-ducts. *Miliaria papulosa* or *rubra* (prickly heat) is a tropical disease, and the predominant lesions are papules which appear in crops on any part of the body. It usually occurs in Europeans freshly exposed to tropical heat. It is due to escape of sweat through the walls of blocked sweat-ducts into the surrounding tissues. Hydrocystoma is a miliary eruption which occasionally occurs on the faces of those exposed to extreme heat. It consists of small groups of vesicles due to blocking of the sweat-ducts.

In *anidrosis*, which is much rarer than hyperidrosis, sweating may be either diminished or totally suppressed, and either the whole skin or only some particular area may be affected. It may be present in *ichthyosis* or in *congenital ectodermal defect*, when there is associated lack of development of the sweat apparatus. Suppression of sweating is a characteristic of heat stroke. Destruction of certain areas in the hypothalamus by tumours, vascular lesions, trauma, or surgery may result in complete anidrosis.

Bromidrosis, or foul-smelling sweat, nearly always accompanies hyperidrosis and may occur in connexion with such general affections as acute rheumatism, uraemia, scurvy, or pneumonia. Occasionally generalized, it is much more frequently limited to particular parts, such as the feet, axillae, and the perineum. The foul smell is due to the growth of bacteria in the sweat after excretion. Imaginary bromidrosis is a well-recognized psychological condition.

In *chromidrosis* the sweat is coloured, generally some shade of blue, but occasionally red, green, yellow, and even black. It is caused by pigment-producing bacteria. Occasionally workers in certain chemical industries suffer from coloured sweat. There is no such disorder as 'haematidrosis' (bloody sweat); this term has been erroneously applied to the red form of chromidrosis. Bromidrosis and chromidrosis are affections of the apocrine sweat-glands, the remainder are affections of the eccrine glands.

P. D. Samman.

TACHE CÉRÉBRALE

Tache cérébrale is the term used to denote that condition in which, after the finger-nail has been

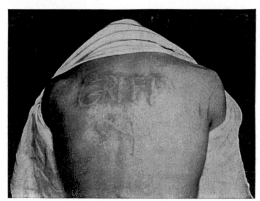

Fig. 758. Factitious urticaria, or dermatographia, in a man who seemed to be in perfect health. (*Dr. Wilson.*)

drawn with moderate firmness across the patient's skin, the line along which it has passed becomes of a bright red colour from dilatation of the superficial arterioles and capillaries; the phenomenon develops within thirty seconds or a minute of the finger stroke, and the red mark remains evident for two or three minutes or more. If letters or figures are marked out on the skin in this way, they appear as though they had been written in red; the condition differs from factitious urticaria or dermatographia (*Fig.* 758) in that in the latter the central part of the local vasomotor reaction is white and the margins are red, as in a weal, instead of the whole reaction being red as in tache cérébrale. The latter is seen characteristically in cases of tuberculous meningitis, but it is not pathognomonic, for not only is it sometimes absent in cases of the latter, but it is also present occasionally in a number of other different conditions, and sometimes in perfectly healthy people. All forms of meningitis may give rise to it, so that it is not even a means of distinguishing one type from another. A similar condition is observed sometimes in the later stages of other severe febrile illnesses.

Ian Mackenzie.

TACHYCARDIA

In normal adults the resting pulse-rate varies widely, from about 40 to 100 per minute. Rates faster than this are common in children; at birth the average rate is around 120 and falls to reach adult levels at about puberty. At a first consultation a rate of 120 would not necessarily be remarkable but persistent tachycardia at this rate or above certainly requires explanation.

Tachycardia may be due to an increased frequency of discharge of the sino-atrial node—sinus tachycardia—or to the activity of an abnormal (ectopic) pacemaker. Ectopic rhythms causing an irregular or slow pulse are discussed under PULSE, IRREGULAR (p. 633) and BRADYCARDIA (p. 111) respectively. In this section only those ectopic rhythms producing a rapid regular pulse will be discussed in any detail.

Sinus Tachycardia. Tachycardia is present in most *febrile conditions*, due to a direct effect of the pyrexia on the sino-atrial node. In a few infections, such as typhoid, the rise in pulse-rate may be rather less than expected from the degree of fever; this relative bradycardia may be of some slight diagnostic significance. The sino-atrial node is affected directly in a number of other situations in which tachycardia is prominent. These include *thyrotoxicosis* in which there is also the reflex effect of the high cardiac output discussed below, *phaeochromocytoma* secreting predominantly adrenaline, *anxiety states*, and other conditions, such as severe pain, in which there is a raised level of circulating catecholamines. In the latter group *Da Costa's syndrome*, known also as cardiac neurosis, effort syndrome, and neurocirculatory asthenia, is an important cause of moderate tachycardia persisting sometimes for many years. Various *drugs* including atropine and sympathomimetic agents such as ephedrine and isoprenaline also produce tachycardia by a direct action.

Sinus tachycardia can also be caused by reflex mechanisms. In conditions causing a rise in right atrial pressure the sinus rate is increased via the Bainbridge reflex. Hypotension from any cause, or, more precisely, a fall in pulse-pressure, also causes tachycardia via baroceptors in the aortic arch and carotid sinus; this is the mechanism, for example, of the tachycardia during the straining period of a Valsalva manœuvre. In *high-output states* the tachycardia is probably secondary to the tendency of the right atrial pressure to rise as a result of the increased venous return.

The pulse-rate is rapid, therefore, in thyrotoxicosis, severe anaemia, pregnancy, beriberi, widespread Paget's disease, and arteriovenous fistula. If such a fistula is accessible, the effect of the high cardiac output can be convincingly demonstrated by the abrupt fall in pulse-rate which results from digital occlusion of the fistula. In *cardiac failure* the tendency to a reduction in pulse-pressure, acting on the aortic and carotid baroceptors, combines with the rise in right atrial pressure to produce considerable tachycardia in most, although not all, cases. Tachycardia is also a feature of *severe myocardial disease*, even in the absence of frank failure; thus it is seen in most cases of myocarditis and in some cases of ischaemic heart disease. Hypotension due to extracardiac factors is also a cause of tachycardia, which is seen in *shock* and as a result of the administration of *vasodilating agents* such as glyceryl trinitrate.

Disproportionate tachycardia on exertion, with a normal resting pulse-rate, is seen in patients less severely affected by the conditions discussed above and is also a measure of an individual's lack of training. Physical fitness can be roughly quantified by the amount of work which can be done at any given heart-rate.

The sleeping pulse-rate is often recorded as an aid to the diagnosis of thyrotoxicosis. Tachycardia persisting during sleep certainly favours the latter as against nervous tachycardia, but it must be remembered that, in most organic diseases causing tachycardia, it is likely to persist during sleep.

Lesions of the vagus nerves may occasionally cause tachycardia, which has been described with subtentorial tumours and in various types of peripheral neuropathy including alcoholic and diphtheritic.

Ectopic Tachycardia. This is very often paroxysmal, with the notable exception of atrial fibrillation, and the abnormal pacemaker may be in the atria, atrioventricular junction, or ventricles. *Paroxysmal atrial and junctional tachycardia* are common in otherwise normal individuals and do not, by themselves, indicate organic heart disease. The attacks begin abruptly, sometimes as a result of sudden alarm but often without apparent cause, and the patient complains, with more or less emphasis depending on his or her temperament, of palpitations and lightheadedness. The associated anxiety may cause hyperventilation, and paraesthesiae in the fingers or even frank tetany may occur; in such cases it is clearly important to distinguish cause and effect in the manifestations. The attack may last for minutes, hours, or, rarely, for days and ends abruptly as it began. Prolonged attacks, lasting for a week or more at a very fast rate, can cause cardiac failure even in normal individuals but this resolves rapidly and completely once the attack is over. In older patients more serious symptoms may occur; in particular, ischaemic pain is common even though the associated coronary artery disease may be quite mild.

There are some varieties of paroxysmal tachycardia requiring special comment. Repetitive paroxysmal tachycardia, which may be either atrial or ventricular in origin, is characterized by around 180–200 per minute in all types of paroxysmal tachycardia and does not help in differentiating the various sites of origin. If an electrocardiogram can be recorded during an attack a

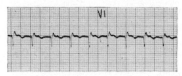

Fig. 759. Supraventricular tachycardia at 160 per minute, probably junctional as P waves cannot be certainly identified, in a patient 1 week after inferior myocardial infarction.

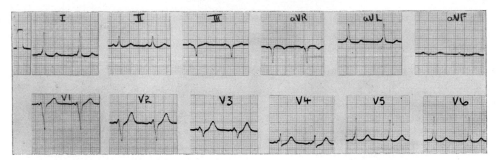

Fig. 760. Wolff-Parkinson-White syndrome showing short P–R interval and broad QRS complexes. The slowly rising initial part of the QRS complex (the delta wave) is well shown in Leads aVL and V6.

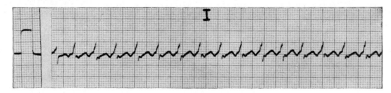

Fig. 761. Atrial flutter with 2 : 1 atrioventricular block; the atrial rate is 340 per minute and the ventricular 170 per minute. The baseline is nowhere iso-electric.

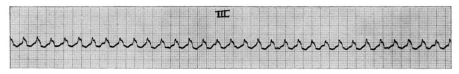

Fig. 762. Ventricular tachycardia at 190 per minute in a patient a few hours after a myocardial infarction. Low-amplitude deflexions which are probably P waves at a slower rate can be seen between some of the ventricular complexes; this confirms the ventricular origin of the dysrhythmia.

multiple short runs of tachycardia separated by sinus rhythm with extrasystoles. This condition, which produces a most alarming appearance in the electrocardiogram, can be quite benign and may continue for many years without deleterious effects. A similar situation can, of course, arise after myocardial infarction, in which case the dysrhythmia is much more serious. Paroxysmal tachycardia, usually atrial, is a rare complication of pregnancy; though each attack may be disabling, the ultimate prognosis is good and the paroxysms cease abruptly after delivery.

The diagnosis of supraventricular tachycardia can sometimes be made clinically by finding regular cannon waves in the jugular venous pulse; this is a characteristic, though not pathognomonic, feature of junctional tachycardia. The rate is often

precise diagnosis can nearly always be made. In atrial and junctional tachycardia the QRS complexes are usually normal, although they may be bizarre as a result of aberrant ventricular conduction; the P waves are abnormal both in their timing in relationship to the QRS and in their shape (*Fig.* 759).

In a few patients with paroxysmal atrial tachycardia the resting electrocardiogram will show the features of the Wolff-Parkinson-White syndrome. In this the P–R interval is pathologically short and the initial part of the QRS rises or falls slowly to form the so-called 'delta' wave (*Fig.* 760). In paroxysms of tachycardia in such cases the QRS assumes a normal configuration. This condition is nearly always benign and is occasionally familial.

Faster atrial rates than those found in atrial and junctional tachycardia produce *atrial flutter*. The atrial rate is often around 300; this is faster than the bundle can conduct and some degree of atrioventricular block is almost invariable. A 2 : 1 ratio is most common, producing a regular ventricular rate of about 150 per minute. This particular rate is rather characteristic of atrial flutter as it is faster than most sinus tachycardias and slower than many atrial and nodal tachycardias. It may be possible to see atrial waves at twice the rate of the arterial pulse in the jugular venous pulse but this requires a good deal of experience—or imagination! The diagnosis can be made with near-certainty by studying the effect of pressure on the right carotid sinus. In atrial flutter the degree of atrioventricular block is increased with, characteristically, an abrupt halving of the pulse-rate. In sinus tachycardia carotid sinus pressure produces a more gradual slowing and in supraventricular tachycardia the attack is either terminated or continues unabated; junctional tachycardia is more likely than atrial to be terminated by carotid sinus pressure. In atrial flutter the electrocardiogram shows rapid regular flutter waves with QRS complexes at half or a quarter of the atrial rate. The atrial rate is so rapid that, in most leads, the flutter waves produce a continuous 'saw-tooth' appearance of the baseline (*Fig.* 761). The absence of any isoelectric segments in the baseline has been suggested as a diagnostic criterion of flutter. There is, however, no real justification for this view and many authorities prefer to use the term 'flutter' for all atrial dysrhythmias with an atrial rate of 250–350 per minute. The causes of atrial flutter are similar to those of atrial fibrillation (*see* p. 665) except that it is not so common in mitral valve disease or thyrotoxicosis.

Atrial fibrillation presents with an irregular tachycardia and is discussed at length in the section on PULSE, IRREGULAR (p. 663).

Ventricular tachycardia is a much more serious affair than its supraventricular counterpart. Although it can occur in patients with otherwise normal hearts, either as paroxysms, lasting for several minutes or hours, occurring rather infrequently or as repetitive paroxysmal tachycardia, there is usually serious underlying organic heart disease. Much the commonest cause is ischaemic heart disease and it is particularly common after myocardial infarction when it can cause a serious deterioration in the patient's condition and may be a forerunner of ventricular fibrillation. The rate is very variable; most commonly around 180 per minute, it may be as low as 100, in which case some prefer to use the term 'idioventricular rhythm' rather than tachycardia. The rhythm may be slightly irregular, unlike that in atrial tachycardia which is almost always completely, even pathologically, regular. The electrocardiogram shows broad, often notched, QRS complexes with no preceding P waves. Sometimes it may be possible to identify P waves separately at a slower rate, in which case the diagnosis of

ventricular tachycardia is certain (*Fig.* 762). Otherwise there can be confusion with supraventricular tachycardia with aberrant ventricular conduction. This is a difficult diagnostic problem as the certain identification of P waves in such a record may be impossible.

See also PULSE, IRREGULAR (p. 663) and PALPITATIONS (p. 612).

P. R. Fleming.

TASTE, ABNORMALITIES OF

The appreciation of taste is a function of the tongue; fibres from the anterior two-thirds pass via the chorda tympani to the geniculate ganglion, passing from there to the pons by the nervus intermedius. Fibres from the posterior third pass centrally via the glossopharyngeal nerve. In the pons taste fibres pass into the tractus solitarius and from the nucleus of this tract a gustatory lemniscus is formed which, after decussating, passes upwards near the midline to the thalamus and from there to the cortical centre for taste at the foot of the postcentral gyrus. The 'taste' of food is made up of a combination of smell and taste proper; a patient with anosmia will complain that food is 'tasteless', because the normal tongue can only distinguish sweet, salt, sour, and bitter. Consequently, both the sense of smell and the sense of taste must be tested in every case. Both may be lost in acute upper respiratory infection with a coated tongue and inflamed nose. Loss of taste proper is found in disease of the tongue itself, of the chorda tympani, of the glossopharyngeal nerve, and of the glossopharyngeal nucleus in the medulla. Loss of smell by itself occurs in inflammatory conditions of the nose, in tumours of the anterior fossa which compress the olfactory nerves, and frequently as a result of fractures of the cribriform plate (*see also* p. 734).

1. Impairment or Loss of Taste (Ageusia):

   a. AFFECTIONS OF THE MOUTH:

Coated tongue	Epithelioma
Glossitis	Sjögren's syndrome

   b. AFFECTIONS OF THE NERVES:

Lesion of lingual nerve	Lesion of glossopharyngeal nerve
Lesion of chorda tympani	Bell's palsy

   c. DRUGS, e.g., D-Penicillamine

2. Perverted Taste (Parageusia):

Pregnancy	Glossitis
Hysteria	

3. Hallucinations of Taste:

Insanity	Lesion of uncus

4. Foul Taste of Mouth (Cacogeusia):

   a. LOCAL CONDITION OF THE MOUTH:

Caries	Stomatitis
Gingivitis	Epithelioma
Glossitis	Gumma

b. Gastro-intestinal Disease:

Gastric carcinoma	Pyloric stenosis
Gastritis	

c. Septic Lung Condition:

Bronchiectasis	Abscess or gangrene
T.B. cavity	

From the diagnostic point of view, impairment of taste sensation is important only when it is persistent or recurrent, and even then it is usually a symptom of secondary interest due to a more obvious primary condition of the mouth, nose, lung, or gastro-intestinal tract. In the absence of some such explanation, diagnosis becomes difficult, and the cause must be looked for in the central nervous system.

The most common neurological cause of loss of taste is Bell's palsy, in which it often occurs as an early and transient feature, the loss being confined to the anterior two-thirds of the tongue on the same side as the facial paralysis.

A similar but more permanent combination of facial palsy and loss of taste may result from spread of inflammatory disease from the middle ear to the Fallopian canal. Taste may disappear as a result of gummatous meningitis around the pons and medulla or as a result of bulbar disease, but in such cases it is overshadowed by more important symptoms and signs. Organic lesions of the uncinate gyrus (glioma, pituitary tumour, syphilis, perhaps arterial thrombosis) give rise to *uncinate fits*, characterized by episodic attacks in which the patient experiences a hallucination of smell or taste, usually unpleasant, followed by salivation, champing or sucking movements of the mouth and jaws, and a disturbance of consciousness which usually amounts to little more than a 'faraway' feeling but may go on to unconsciousness, with or without a generalized convulsion. The uncinate hallucination may occur by itself—a brief, discontinuous experience which is repeated from time to time, and in such a case it may be mistaken for the hallucinations of smell which are a significant symptom of delusional insanity. In the latter, however, the hallucination is more persistent and less episodic, the other features of the uncinate fit do not occur, and there are usually other features of a primary psychological illness. The perversions of taste which occasionally occur during pregnancy are neither delusional nor hallucinatory, but their origin is not understood. The sensation of taste is no exception to the rule that anything can occur in hysteria, but disturbances of smell or taste are uncommon manifestations of hysteria. Complete loss of taste and smell occasionally occurs during an attack of migraine; it is analogous to the hemiplegia and other focal disturbances which sometimes occur in this condition. Patients taking D-penicillamine may lose their sense of taste, which returns some little time after stopping treatment.

Ian Mackenzie.

TEETH, GRINDING OF, DURING SLEEP

This is a symptom in itself of little importance to the patient but disturbing to those who sleep with him. It is popularly held that grinding of the teeth at night, especially in children, is an indication of the presence of intestinal worms, particularly *Oxyuris vermicularis*. The faeces should be examined for parasites and their ova, but the popular belief in the association of intestinal parasites with the teeth-grinding habit is seldom verified clinically. Very often teeth-grinding is rather a rattling of the upper teeth against the lower owing to lateral movements made by the lower jaw as the individual when half roused turns over in bed; actual gritting of the teeth during sleep is less common.

Ian Mackenzie.

TESTICLE, PAIN IN

Pain in the testicle of varying degree may be present in many conditions, which may be discussed under separate headings as follows: (I) *Diseases of the body of the testis or epididymis*; (II) *Affections of the coverings of the testicle*; (III) *Affections of the spermatic cord*; (IV) *A retained or misplaced testicle*; (V) *Pain from lesions remote from the testis*.

I. DISEASES OF THE BODY OF THE TESTIS OR EPIDIDYMIS

Inflammatory Lesions may attack the testis proper, or, as is more common, may begin in the epididymis. The investing tunica vaginalis distends with inflammatory exudate to form a secondary hydrocele. This tender mass may be mistaken for a swelling of the testis proper and the condition is frequently labelled an 'acute epididymo-orchitis'. However, surgical exploitation and histological study reveal that the testis proper is rarely implicated and it is accurate, therefore, to speak of 'acute epididymitis'. An inflammatory affection of the testicle may be acute, subacute, or chronic, the last often being the terminal result of the others.

An acute epididymitis arises most commonly by spread of infection to the organ from the urethra via the vas deferens or by the lymphatics accompanying the vas. When any inflammation has reached the prostatic portion of the urethra the orifices of the vasa deferentia may become infected, and inflammation spreads along the duct to the epididymis.

Causes of Acute Epididymitis:

Causes of Urethral Origin:
    Gonorrhoeal urethritis
    Septic urethritis
    Passage of catheters
    Urethral instrumentation
    Infection behind a stricture

Ulceration about an impacted calculus or a pro-
static calculus
Injections into the posterior urethra
After operations on the prostate
Urinary infections
Non-specific epididymitis.

CAUSES OF ACUTE ORCHITIS:

Fevers:
Parotitis (mumps)
Typhoid
Brucellosis
Leptospirosis
Chicken-pox
Lymphocytic choriomeningitis
Scarlet fever
Injury

Causes of Chronic Epididymitis:
Tuberculosis
Resolving acute epididymitis

Syphilitic Disease of the Testis:
Diffuse interstitial orchitis
Gummatous orchitis

Other Diseases:
Malignant tumours of the testis
Torsion of the testis
Cysts of the epididymis.

Acute epididymitis begins as a painful thickening of the epididymis associated with febrile
symptoms. Before any actual pain is noticed in
the testis there is often a sense of discomfort and
weight over the external abdominal ring and
inguinal canal due to the inflammatory process
extending along the vas deferens. The swelling
of the epididymis increases, and with it there is
a secondary effusion of exudate into the tunica
vaginalis (secondary hydrocele), causing swelling
of its body and increase of pain. The whole organ
thus becomes enlarged, and it is often exquisitely
tender, the touch of the clothes or the most
gentle examination causing pain. The swollen
gland is often flattened on the outer and posterior
aspect from pressure against the adductor
muscles of the thigh; the vas deferens and tissues
of the spermatic cord are thickened.

By far the most common cause of an acute
epididymitis was formerly an *acute gonorrhoeal
urethritis*; under the more effective modern treatment of gonorrhoea it occurs less often. During
the disease the prostatic portion of the canal
frequently becomes infected, when the orifices
of the ejaculatory ducts may share in the inflammation, and infection be conveyed by the vas
deferens to the testicle. Infection may arise
similarly, but less frequently, from a *septic
posterior urethritis*, contracted during connexion
with a woman the subject of a vaginal leucorrhoea. The gonorrhoeal form of acute epididymitis usually resolves slowly, and shows little
liability to suppurate, whereas the inflammation
resulting from a staphylococcal or a streptococcal infection may break down into a testicular
abscess.

Acute epididymitis may also arise from septic
processes in the urethra following the *passage
of catheters*, of *instruments* for vesical operations,

transurethral prostatic resection or lithotrity for
example, from infection behind a *urethral stricture* or about a *calculus* in the prostatic urethra,
occasionally after the *instillation of strong solutions* into the posterior urethra in the treatment
of a chronic urethritis, or after operations on
the prostate, especially prostatectomy, or as a
complication of a urinary infection by *Bacillus
coli* or other organisms. It may follow prostatic
massage. In any case the onset of pyrexia with
pain and rapid swelling of the testis should lead
to suspicion of a urinary tract infection. Bacteriological examination of any urethral discharge and
of the urine is essential (*see* URETHRAL DISCHARGE,
p. 805).

In *non-specific epididymis* there may be no
evidence of urethral infection and bacteriological
studies are entirely negative; the condition sometimes arises after unaccustomed exercise and has
been attributed to a reflux of urine down the vas.
The testicle becomes painful, and enlarges rapidly
in the same manner as in acute inflammation
from urethral infection, and under appropriate
conservative treatment by means of a scrotal
support gradually resolves. Less frequently
testicular inflammation may occur after a direct
injury to the organ, such as a *blow* or *squeeze*.

The pain in an acute inflammation is generally
of an aching character at first, felt not only in the
testis but also at the external abdominal ring, and
often as a heavy dragging pain in the inguinal
or iliac areas of the affected side. As the testis
enlarges the local pain becomes more severe, so
that the swollen gland is exquisitely tender to
pressure or to the touch. After a few days the
pain subsides to a large extent, but remains as a
dull ache until the swelling becomes greatly
reduced, and it usually does not disappear
entirely until the organ returns to the normal
size. In a few cases in which a fibrous scar
remains in the epididymis pain may remain and
cause some difficulty in the diagnosis from an
incipient tuberculous lesion, but the earlier
history of acute inflammation will help in forming an opinion. In other cases the persistence of
the pain and swelling may indicate the formation
of an abscess in the testicle, when, after decreasing
at first, the swelling increases, the skin covering
it becomes reddened and oedematous, and a soft
area becomes evident in one aspect of the
organ.

Acute Orchitis may complicate *acute specific parotitis* (mumps), especially when this occurs in
adolescents or adults. Both testes may be affected
and the result may be testicular atrophy. Much less
often the testis may be affected in *typhoid, scarlet
fever* or *influenza*.

Tuberculosis of the Testicle is comparatively common today in many parts of the world, including
India and the Far East, but is comparatively rare
in this country. It arises with extreme rarity as a
primary disease but more commonly as secondary
to tuberculous disease of the kidney, bladder,
prostate, or seminal vesicles. It is most frequently
seen in young adults. It begins as a localized

deposit in almost all cases, causing a rounded, firm nodule in the epididymis, usually in the lower pole. This nodule may remain unaltered for many months, or may enlarge, soften, become adherent to the skin and coverings of the testicle, or actually ulcerate through them to form a discharging sinus in the scrotum. The small nodule in the epididymis is usually painless at first and may be found by accident, but later, as it gradually enlarges, it causes an aching pain in the organ. There may be an associated hydrocele of the tunica vaginalis. Other nodules may be formed in the epididymis, or the body of the testis may become involved, while commonly small shot-like thickenings may be felt in the course of the vas deferens, or a progressively increasing thickening as it is traced down to the epididymis. In the more advanced stages nodules may be felt upon rectal examination in the seminal vesicles or prostate, or there may be some in the epididymis of the other side.

Tuberculous disease of the testicle usually presents some difficulty in its diagnosis from non-specific epididymitis, particularly when it has an acute onset, as sometimes happens. In an early case the occurrence of one or more nodules in the epididymis, which are painful on pressure and which have not resulted from a preceding acute epididymitis, should always suggest a tuberculous focus, and a careful search should be made for other tuberculous lesions in the body. If none is found the gradual subsidence of the lesion under careful observation will indicate that it was a non-specific epididymitis. In later stages the diagnosis is less difficult; the gradual enlargement of the nodules, their craggy or bossy feel, the infection of the vas or other genito-urinary organs with tuberculosis, and above all the tendency of the focus in the epididymis to soften and to become adherent to the scrotal coverings and to produce an indolent sinus, are points to be looked for.

Syphilitic Disease of the Testis causes very little pain in the organ, but there is often a sense of dragging or heaviness. Syphilis may attack the testicle in several different ways, producing:

IN ACQUIRED SYPHILIS:

Diffuse interstitial orchitis
Localized gummatous orchitis.

IN CONGENITAL SYPHILIS:

Interstitial orchitis
Localized gummatous orchitis.

The outstanding feature of syphilitic disease of the testicle is that it affects the body of the testis rather than the epididymis, thus differing in a marked degree from tuberculous disease. In the interstitial form there is thickening of the intertubular connective tissue, with an infiltration of spindle cells, which, forming young connective tissue, yield fibrous tissue. The subsequent contraction of this fibrous tissue may cause atrophy of the testis. The testis may, on section, show small gummata in addition to the diffuse orchitis, or if the inflammation is more localized, gummata may be the main feature, these varying in size from that of a pea to that of a walnut, or larger. The epididymis is affected but rarely, though cases are on record of a nodular swelling in the epididymis during the secondary stage of syphilis which disappears rapidly under anti-syphilitic treatment.

In congenital syphilis, both the interstitial and gummatous forms exist; they usually occur in childhood or in young adult life, and in many cases the affection is bilateral. Syphilitic inflammation of the testicle may be accompanied in either the acquired or the congenital form by a vaginal hydrocele. A gummatous testis may ulcerate through the scrotum, usually in front, producing a circular 'punched-out' ulcer with a slough in the base.

There is a sense of weight in the scrotum rather than pain, and often an aching or dragging feeling in the inguinal or lumbar region. On palpation, the body of the testis feels enlarged and nodular with the gummatous deposits, but the epididymis can usually be distinguished from the testis and be found to be unaffected. Testicular sensation is lost. The tissues of the cord remain unthickened. Tertiary syphilitic lesions of the testicle give rise to very little tenderness on palpation.

The diagnosis of syphilitic disease of the testis is usually simple. There may or may not be a history of syphilis, but other signs of the disease should be looked for—thus, in the acquired form, any scar of previous ulceration or periosteal thickening, or, in the congenital variety, signs in the teeth, eyes, or ears. Syphilitic disease is distinguished from *tuberculous disease* of the testis by the fact that the epididymis is usually free; that the cord, prostate, and vesicles remain normal; and that pressure applied directly to the testicle gives little or no pain. Tuberculous deposits tend to soften and to involve the scrotal coverings in spite of treatment. From haematocele it is differentiated by the history of injury or by the absence of the history or signs of syphilis. From *malignant tumours of the testis* it is distinguished by the history of syphilis, the tendency of syphilitic disease to be bilateral, the slow enlargement, and a positive Wassermann reaction. In malignant disease, the increase in the size of the testicle is more rapid, while the tumour often shows areas of varying consistence; the cord is often thickened in malignant or in tuberculous cases, but seldom in syphilitic.

It should be pointed out that gumma of the testis is so rare in this country today, compared with its former frequency, that it is safer to regard any solid swelling in the testicle itself as the much commoner and more likely malignant tumour of the testis, and treat it as such by orchidectomy. In the unlikely event that a gumma is thus removed, the surgeon can comfort himself with the fact that a functionally useless organ has been excised.

Malignant Tumours of the Testis may give rise to pain in the organ, but as a rule pain is experienced only in the later stages of the disease, as testicular sensation is completely lost. Although benign tumours of the epididymis may occur, nearly all tumours of the testis are highly malignant. They fall into two main pathological

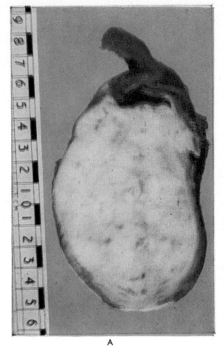

gonadotrophic hormone is sometimes found in the urine. Either type may follow injury in a significant proportion of cases although it is likely that trauma merely draws attention to the testicular mass, and the undescended testis is more prone to develop malignant disease than is the normally placed one. The testis which has been initially undescended and subsequently brought down into the scrotum maintains this higher tendency to malignant change, estimated at about ten times that of the normal organ.

A testicle that is the seat of a malignant growth enlarges slowly or rapidly, but as pain is at first absent there may be nothing to arouse the patient's suspicions. As long as the tunica albuginea remains intact the swelling retains the shape of the testis, but when perforation of the fibrous covering takes place nodular projections appear and render the tumour irregular. These projections are softer than the remainder of the growth, and form a valuable point in the diagnosis. A

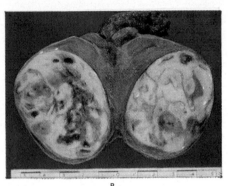

A   B

Fig. 763. A, Seminoma and B, teratoma of the testis.

varieties, *seminoma* and *teratoma*, the latter including the sub-groups of *chorionepithelioma*, *dermoid*, and *fibrocystic disease*. The *seminoma* (*Fig.* 763 A) is a soft vascular solid growth composed of large spheroidal cells derived from the germinal epithelium of the seminiferous tubules. It occurs at about the age of 40 and is less malignant but more radio-sensitive than teratoma. It tends to retain the shape of the testis as it enlarges. The *teratoma* (*Fig.* 763 B) or mixed tumour is a solid or multilocular cystic growth in which one or other of the germinal layers may preponderate. Dermoids, containing hair or teeth, are less common than in the ovary but sometimes occur in childhood and are relatively benign.

Fibrocystic disease pursues an even more benign course and may be present for ten or more years before exhibiting its malignant characteristics by sudden rapid growth and the formation of metastases. Most cases of teratoma occur at the age of 25–30; they give a short history, are more resistant to X-ray treatment, and show early metastases. There may be enlargement of the breasts and chorionic hormone may be present in the urine, giving rise to a positive Aschheim-Zondek reaction; in seminoma the pituitary

rapidly growing malignant tumour of the testis may be so soft as to appear to be a fluid collection in the tunica vaginalis. Generally, however, although a growth may be accompanied by a small amount of fluid in the tunica vaginalis, the more solid mass can be felt through the fluid on careful examination; this fluid is often blood-stained. The epididymis may become incorporated in the growth so that it cannot be distinguished, and the tissues of the cord become thickened. The coverings of the testis become stretched over the tumour; the mass does not become adherent to the scrotal skin until late in the disease. Clinically it is impossible to distinguish between a teratoma and a seminoma. In both types the para-aortic lymph-nodes become enlarged, and may be felt in a thin subject to one or other side of the epigastric area, and pain due to the pressure of these glands upon nerve structures may become marked. The inguinal nodes are usually not enlarged unless the scrotal skin is affected; retrograde spread may then occur to the iliac nodes which may be felt at the brim of the pelvis. In advanced cases, the left supra-clavicular lymph-nodes are involved and become palpably enlarged. Mediastinal or pulmonary metastases are frequent, the latter giving the characteristic radiological appearance of 'cannon-ball' secondaries. The diagnosis of malignant disease of the testis may be quite easy in the case of rapidly growing tumours, but in others, especially in the early stages, it may present great difficulty. Rarely an *interstitial-cell tumour* occurs in a child and produces sexual precocity.

GUMMATOUS ORCHITIS may be confused with the more slowly growing forms of tumour. In both the swelling may have followed an injury, and in both there may be a syphilitic history. Gummatous orchitis is, however, either more acute or more chronic; it retains more the oval shape of the testis, and does not present the rounded, slightly raised bosses which are commonly present in a malignant testis. In orchitis the epididymis is usually distinguished more easily, and the cord is not so thickened as with a growth. In any case of doubt it is a wise course to advise exploration. (*See above.*)

TUBERCULOUS DISEASE is usually diagnosed easily from malignant disease by the tendency of tubercle to attack the epididymis, to caseate, suppurate, and to become adherent to the scrotal skin comparatively early. Tuberculosis occasionally attacks the body of the testicle first, however, forming an oval, smooth tumour of the organ; the epididymis and vas deferens may be unaffected for a time, and if no deposit is found in the prostate or vesicles the differential diagnosis between tubercle and growth may be far from easy before operation. Tuberculosis most frequently occurs in young adults.

HAEMATOCELE. The diagnosis between a haematocele and a malignant tumour of the testis may present considerable difficulty. In both, the swelling may date from an injury, while the indistinct fluctuation obtained in the soft areas of a growth, accompanied sometimes by some fluid in the tunica vaginalis, may simulate a haematocele. The latter feels heavy to the hand, but is usually softer in its whole mass and more regular than a growth. Care must be taken not to place too much reliance upon the withdrawal of a few drops of blood from the tumour by means of a trocar and cannula, a result which may happen equally with growth or haematocele. A haematocele may cease to enlarge, or even diminish in size, whereas, in growth, increase in size in progressive. The cord remains unaffected with haematocele, and testicular sensation is more likely to be lost in growth. If any doubt exists it is advisable to excise the testis, dividing the cord at the internal ring. Incision into a testis which is the seat of a growth is almost invariably followed by rapid recurrence. If necessary, a radical operation can be done after the histology is known, or radiotherapy can be given.

HYDROCELE. A hydrocele of very long standing with an irregular, nodular surface, and absence of translucency due to the thickened tunica vaginalis and the thick contents of the sac, may simulate a new growth, but the long history of the case, and the absence of progressive increase in size of the swelling, will prevent a mistake of this kind.

Torsion of the Testis on its vascular pedicle may occur in a testis which has a mesorchium or in one which is ectopic. It occurs most commonly in youths soon after puberty, or in infants; the exciting cause may be some mild exertion or movement such as crossing the legs or turning over in bed. There may be a history of repeated minor attacks before complete torsion takes place, and the other testis may have suffered similar incomplete attacks or be found to be unduly mobile or horizontally placed. At the moment of torsion there is severe sickening pain which may be felt at first in the abdomen but is quickly localized to the testis; the boy may even say that his testicle has twisted. There is usually nausea and sometimes vomiting. The

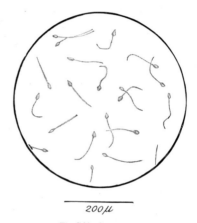

200 μ

Fig. 764. Spermatozoa.

testis forms a tense tender swelling in the upper part of the scrotum or at the external abdominal ring, and the scrotum below is empty. This sign serves to distinguish the condition from a strangulated hernia or an inflamed lymph-gland. In acute epididymitis the testis is in its normal position and there may be evidence of urethral discharge or of a urinary-tract infection. Because of the initial abdominal pain and vomiting the condition has been mistaken for acute appendicitis, but adherence to the rule of examining the scrotal contents in all abdominal cases should prevent this error.

Cysts of the Testis occur most frequently in connexion with the epididymis, very rarely with the body of the testis. These cysts are quite different from hydrocele of the tunica vaginalis, and are often spoken of as a spermatocele, although all do not contain spermatozoa and the term is thus better avoided. They cause a swelling of varying degree in the scrotum, and usually an aching in the testicle, groin, or lumbar region. They may arise as retention cysts of the tubules of the epididymis or from one of the foetal remains which occur about the globus major of the epididymis, namely the organ of

Giraldés, the hydatid of Morgagni, or the vas aberrans of Haller. These cysts are usually placed above and to the outer side of the testis, occasionally behind it. They move with the organ, and can usually be distinguished from the latter by the test of translucency. They may be multiple and are frequently bilateral. Their increase in size is very slow, but they may cause aching pain in the testicle by pressure upon, or stretching of, the tissues of the epididymis. They can be distinguished from hydrocele of the tunica vaginalis by the position of the swelling relative to the testicle, and by the fact that the fluid contained in them is colourless or slightly opalescent from the contained spermatozoa (*Fig.* 764), in distinction from the straw-coloured clear fluid of a vaginal hydrocele.

II. AFFECTIONS OF THE COVERINGS OF THE TESTIS CAUSING PAIN IN THE ORGAN

The only common lesions of the coverings of the testis are *hydrocele* and *haematocele*: new growths of the testicular tunics are so rare as to render them surgical curiosities and they rarely cause pain.

Hydrocele may occur occasionlly as an acute affection accompanying an acute epididymitis, injury to the scrotum, or in the course of acute specific fevers such as smallpox, rheumatism, or mumps. Acute hydrocele has been described in conjunction with acute lesions of other serous membranes—polyserositis or polyorrhymenitis. The more usual form of hydrocele is the chronic variety, which may be due to some disease of the testicle, but for which, in the majority of cases, no ascertainable cause can be found (primary or idiopathic hydrocele).

A hydrocele may cause some aching in the testicle, but more frequently it causes a dragging sensation in the inguinal or iliac areas from the mechanical effect of its weight. It forms a swelling on one side of the scrotum, oval with smooth uniform surface; it gives a distinct sense of fluctuation. The swelling is limited above from the cord or external abdominal ring, and gives no sense of impulse on coughing; with a good light it can be found in most cases to be translucent, the testicle occupying a posterior and low position in the swelling. The diagnosis of hydrocele is usually easy, but difficulty may be experienced in old-standing cases in which the walls are much thickened. A hydrocele must be diagnosed from: (1) A scrotal hernia, (2) Haematocele, (3) New growth, and (4) A cyst of the epididymis.

SCROTAL HERNIA. Usually a hernia gives an impulse on coughing, can be reduced into the abdomen with a sudden slip or gurgle, and varies in size with the position of the patient. A hernia comes from above and descends into the scrotum. In a large irreducible hernia, some part of it is usually resonant from the contained intestine, the swelling is not limited above, and the testis can be distinguished at the bottom of the scro-

tum. A hydrocele is distinctly limited above so that the examining fingers can meet above it, gives no impulse on coughing, is translucent, and the spermatic cord can be distinguished easily. The testis in a hydrocele cannot usually be distinguished in the scrotum as in a hernia. Difficulty may arise between the two conditions when the hydrocele extends along the funicular process in the inguinal canal and thus gives an impulse on coughing, or if the translucency is lost owing to the thickness of the walls of the sac. A scrotal hernia in an infant may be translucent.

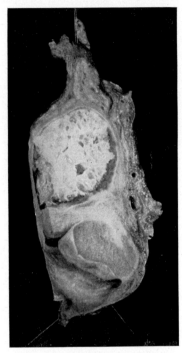

Fig. 765. Organizing haematoma of epididymal cyst which formed a solid tumour.

Haematocele is distinguished from hydrocele by the absence of translucency and the rapidity of the onset, usually after an injury or puncture.

NEW GROWTHS OF THE TESTIS. A hydrocele is of much slower rate of increase in size, of smooth surface and uniform consistence, and is translucent.

CYST OF THE EPIDIDYMIS. (*See above.*)

Haematocele may occur from puncture of a vein in the sac or of the testicle as the result of tapping a hydrocele, or by the occurrence of bleeding into a hydrocele. It may occur quite independently of a hydrocele, usually after direct injury. As a rule there is a rapid onset of swelling in the scrotum following the injury, with ecchymosis of the scrotal skin; the resulting tumour resembles a hydrocele in its clinical symptoms, save that it is not translucent. In other cases the swelling arises more slowly, when a pyriform or oval swelling is present in one side of the scrotum covered by normal skin; the surface of the swelling is smooth, and gives a sense of fluctuation and elasticity. There is no translucency, and, on tapping, dark blood-stained fluid is withdrawn.

The diagnosis in the less acute cases often presents a difficulty, especially with regard to *malignant disease of the testicle (see above)*; this is particularly so when the haematoma is organized (*Fig.* 765). From *hydrocele* it is distinguished by the absence of translucency; from *hernia* by the same points, except translucency, mentioned above in the diagnosis between hydrocele and hernia.

III. AFFECTIONS OF THE SPERMATIC CORD CAUSING TESTICULAR PAIN

An inflammatory affection of the cord secondary to urethral infection is not uncommon. Tuberculous infection of the cord is practically never present without corresponding infection of the epididymis. New growths of the cord, lipomata, sarcomata (extremely rare), and hydroceles of the cord, cause no pain in the testis. A *varicocele*, especially if large, in a pendulous scrotum, is a frequent cause of a dull, aching pain in the testicle; it is nearly always left-sided, although the reason for this is obscure. The characteristic feel of the enlarged veins in the erect position, and the slight impulse and thrill on coughing, will readily point to the correct diagnosis.

IV. RETAINED OR MISPLACED TESTIS

This, in its various situations, may give rise to pain. A testis may be arrested in its descent at the external abdominal ring, in the inguinal canal, may remain inside the abdomen, or may pass upwards and outwards from the external abdominal ring into the superficial inguinal pouch where it can be felt readily. It is doubtful if a testis retained within the inguinal canal is ever palpable. Occasionally it passes into the perineum after traversing the inguinal canal, to the upper part of the thigh via the crural ring, or to the root of the penis in front of the pubes.

In the various situations in which an undescended or ectopic testicle is placed it may be attacked by the several diseases which affect the normally placed organ, and thus give rise to pain; but in addition, owing to the effect of recurrent muscular strains and the comparative immobility of the organ, it is particularly liable to attacks of inflammation, especially when the testis is retained in the inguinal canal; in the intra-abdominal position it remains protected from muscular injury, while ectopic testicles have a greater range of mobility than has one that is retained in the inguinal canal and are thus especially prone to torsion. The inflammation of an undescended testicle may be so acute as to lead to gangrene of the organ, with or without torsion of the cord. The pain may be complained of first when the testes begin to enlarge at puberty, at which time an undescended right testicle may produce symptoms easily mistaken for appendicitis.

The diagnosis of undescended testicle rests upon the following points: the fact that one side of the scrotum is empty; the outline and situation of the swelling in the superficial inguinal region or elsewhere; the testicular sensation upon pressure; and the recurrent attacks of pain. An undescended testicle may give rise to acute pain from inflammatory lesions or from acute torsion of the organ, and may if it is in the inguinal canal give rise to symptoms suggesting a strangulated hernia. A partially descended testicle is often accompanied by an inguinal hernia. The misplaced testis is especially liable to become the seat of malignant disease.

It should be remembered that an imperfectly descended testis is a small and poorly developed organ and that spermatogenesis from the gland may be absent or only last for a short time after puberty.

V. TESTICULAR PAIN FROM LESIONS OTHER THAN IN THE TESTICLE

Complaint may be made of testicular pain when on clinical examination the testis is found to be normal. After an acute inflammation of the organ, even when no palpable nodule remains, the resulting cicatrization may cause aching in the organ, especially after *sexual excitement* or prolonged desire. Apart from former testicular disease pain may be felt in the organ if a *calculus* is present *in the pelvis of the kidney* or *upper ureter*, with a marked degree of *oxaluria*, or from stimulation of the peripheral nerves by *secondary deposits in the bodies of the lumbar vertebrae*, pressure from an *extramedullary intraspinal tumour* such as a neurofibroma, meningioma, or ependymoma, or the pressure of an *aneurysm* in this situation. Pain in the testicle is occasionally present in *appendiceal inflammation* when the appendix turns down into the pelvis. Finally when no organic cause of any sort is present the condition is usually called *neuralgia testis*; this is pain of an aching character which may occur in patients of a neurotic tendency.

Harold Ellis.

TESTICULAR ATROPHY

When one testis is smaller than the other, it is first necessary to determine which is the normal one; for when one is slightly enlarged it may be regarded erroneously as normal and the other as too small. Some inequality may be physiological, as is the case with paired organs generally. Physiological atrophy of the testes is apt to occur in advanced life; it may begin as early as 50, though many older men have testicles of normal size.

A testis in an abnormal position, in the inguinal canal or elsewhere, is subject not only to such causes of atrophy as may affect one normally situated, but may also be inhibited in growth from compression by surrounding parts.

The causes of atrophy of a normally situated testis may be grouped under three main headings as follows:

developed, and secondly the operative manœuvres necessary to put it in its place may, unless great care is exercised, damage its blood-supply.

Torsion as a cause of atrophy may give rise to confusion in that the textbook picture of sudden onset with severe constitutional signs reminiscent of a strangulated hernia is not by any means always the way in which these cases

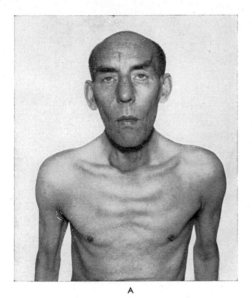
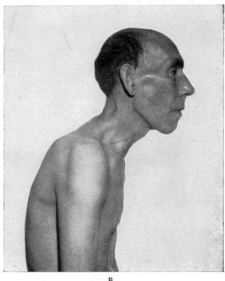

A   B

Fig. 766. Dystrophia myotonica, showing weakness and wasting of facial muscles.

1. Interference with the Blood-supply:

Compression of the spermatic cord, as by an inguinal hernia, a spermatocele, or an ill-fitting truss

Compression of the testicle by affections of the tunica vaginalis, such as hydrocele or haematocele

Venous stasis, the result of varicocele

As a sequel of operation in the region of the spermatic cord, e.g., for the cure of varicocele, spermatocele, or hernia

Elephantiasis

Torsion

Injury.

2. Atrophy after Orchitis or Epididymitis, due to such causes as:

Gonorrhoea

Tubercle

Mumps

X-rays

Typhoid fever

Klinefelter's syndrome

Syphilis.

3. Disturbance of the Endocrine System.

The cause in cases in Group 1 is generally obvious. Perhaps of all operations on the inguinal region the most likely to be followed by testicular atrophy is that for an ectopic, or imperfectly descended, testicle. The reason for this is twofold: in the first place the testicle, even before interference, is usually not very well

present. Not infrequently the condition is a subacute one, the testicle twisting a little way and then reverting to its natural state. This may be repeated on several occasions until finally the torsion becomes permanent. The diagnosis of an obscure 'orchitis' is often made in these cases, and the true nature of the condition never realized. In fact the syndrome may be so benign that, many years later, perhaps when the testicle becomes shrunken and fibrotic, the causative incident may have been forgotten.

Simple trauma to the testicle as from a blow with a cricket ball or from falling astride a fence or bar may cause a haematoma within the tunica albuginea, with pressure necrosis of the seminiferous tubules, and a gradual fibroblastic replacement which eventually leaves the testicle a small dense node of functionless fibrous tissue.

As regards Group 2, there may be a history of gonorrhoea, mumps, typhoid fever, or gout, in which case the diagnosis is clear. Mumps, however, is particularly likely to be overlooked, as orchitis may, on rare occasion, be the sole evidence of this complaint. Slight injury to the testicle, insufficient to damage a normal testicle, may cause a flare-up of the inflammation, particularly in old cases of gonococcal or tuberculous epididymitis.

X-rays are a possible cause of testicular atrophy, and users of X-rays are now careful to use a suitable protecting lead shield. That sterility can result from repeated applications of these rays is well known, and radium emanations may have a similar result.

Klinefelter's syndrome (seminiferous tubule dysgenesis) begins to become apparent about puberty, with a varying degree of eunuchoidism, gynaecomastia, azoospermia, and small testes. In most cases it is because of a developmental defect due to sex chromosomal abnormality. *Reifenstein's syndrome* is a hereditary disorder in which the patients resemble those with Klinefelter's syndrome but their chromosomal constitution is normal.

As regards Group 3, testicular atrophy may arise as the result of destruction, disease, or atrophy of the pituitary gland, especially its anterior lobe. In this class fall Simmonds's disease, progeria, and testicular atrophy following fracture of the base of the skull. Bilateral testicular atrophy is also a common feature of dystrophia myotonica (myotonica atrophica, *Fig. 766*). This disease is characterized by wasting of the sternomastoid and facial muscles, the muscles of mastication, of the forearms, the vasti, dorsiflexors of feet, and peronei. There is great difficulty in relaxing muscles once they have contracted, so that it may be impossible to drop an article which has been grasped. A smile tends to persist. Cataract, baldness, general loss of weight, and sexual impotence complete the picture. Atrophy also occurs in advanced hepatic cirrhosis and haemochromatosis.

R. G. Beard.

TENESMUS

Tenesmus signifies frequent and painful urge to go to stool, associated generally with straining and griping but with little evacuant result. A similar condition affecting the bladder is spoken of as *vesical tenesmus*, but for this a better-known term is STRANGURY (p. 764).

The most severe example of tenesmus is afforded by *acute dysentery*, in which after the onset of the disease loose faecal motions are passed, at first copious, then in smaller and smaller quantities until when there is practically nothing left to be expelled from the bowel the desire to defaecate urgently and repeatedly may still recur with painful straining but with the evacuation of only a little mucus or blood. The nature of the dysentery itself, whether due to *Entamoeba histolytica*, or to Shiga's or Flexner's or to other less well-known bacilli, is determined by bacteriological investigations of the stools.

Similar tenesmus may also occur in acute *cholera* when the stage of rice-water stools has been reached. Here again the diagnosis is suggested by the fact of residence in a locality where cholera is endemic or has recently broken out in epidemic form; it is confirmed by the discovery of the comma bacilli of cholera in the stools.

In Great Britain there are various types of *acute infective diarrhoea* which may simulate cholera.

In such cases tenesmus may be severe. Acute diarrhoea with much tenesmus may arise from the eating of unripe fruit; after a brief but acute illness rapid recovery is the rule. More serious are the acute attacks of vomiting and diarrhoea due to staphylococcal or other bacterial food contamination. Such cases may be sporadic, but epidemics may occur in the case of many persons eating contaminated food from a common source, some cases ending fatally. The bacteriology of the condition is complex; different micro-organisms are at the root of different outbreaks. The diarrhoea is at first painless, but severe tenesmus ensues after the bowel has become empty of everything but a little liquid together with mucus and exuded blood.

Chronic dysentery is less often responsible for tenesmus. The same applies to cases of *colitis* whether simple or ulcerative or associated with malignant disease of the bowel.

Intussusception causes tenesmus if the lower end of the intussusception has reached the pelvic colon or the anus. The symptoms will be those of intestinal obstruction, and when the intussusception is felt per rectum or seen protruding per anum there will be difficulty in distinguishing it from a polypus or prolapse of the rectum. The condition is commoner in infants about nine months old than in any other class of patient, and at this age tenesmus is not obvious. In older patients a subacute or chronic intussusception is comparatively rare; it is seldom diagnosed previous to operation.

Acute summer diarrhoea and vomiting of infants may be due to a number of different microorganisms.

Tenesmus may occur in cases of poisoning by *arsenic*. The diagnosis may be obvious when there is a history of the patient having taken the drug; choleraic diarrhoea and much tenesmus may come on subsequent to the initial vomiting and collapse, but there are circumstances when arsenic will only after a time be suspected as the cause of the symptoms. Accidental contamination of the water or of some food may have occurred, or some member of the household may be administering arsenic surreptitiously, perhaps in the form of weed-killer.

Other irritant drugs may produce tenesmus such as *cantharides, calomel, colocynth, croton oil, castor oil*, and in general most of the more powerful purgatives, now mostly dropped from the pharmacopoeia and no longer in general use.

Rectal Conditions. There remain for discussion the following local conditions of the rectum which produce painful and frequent but fruitless straining at stool, as the result of either irritation or obstruction:

1. CAUSES WITHIN THE LUMEN OF THE RECTUM:

Impacted faeces
A foreign body that has been inserted
Concretions
Worms.

2. CAUSES IN THE WALL OF THE RECTUM:

   Carcinoma
   Rectal prolapse
   Polypus or polypi
   Adenoma
   Haemorrhoids, especially if thrombosed
   Fissure
   Proctitis.

3. CAUSES OUTSIDE THE RECTUM:

   Periprostatic abscess
   Periproctal abscess
   Ischiorectal abscess
   Vesical calculus
   Retroverted gravid uterus
   Pelvic haematocele
   Ectopic gestation.

4. CAUSES OF NERVOUS ORIGIN:

   Rectal crises of tabes dorsalis
   Proctalgia fugax.

The diagnosis of all the above depends upon examination of the anal region, the rectum, and the vagina, by palpation with the finger or by inspection, direct or through a speculum, proctoscope, or sigmoidoscope.

Impacted faeces may simulate rectal carcinoma. But in the case of carcinoma of the rectum, one's finger when inserted seldom comes upon a mass of faeces, whereas with faecal impaction the mass is generally well within digital reach. The condition is not uncommon after middle age.

Rectal concretions differ from impacted faeces only in their composition. For instance, they may consist not of ordinary faecal material but of hard lumps of *barium, magnesium, chalk,* or other drug that has been given by mouth, or of the husks or products of some unusual meal—for example, a boy who had stolen a bundle of cinnamon sticks, chewed and swallowed them, and a day or two afterwards suffered from extreme tenesmus from the mass of undigested pieces that had become impacted in his rectum. *Hair balls* have caused similar trouble on very rare occasions.

Worms only cause tenesmus when infestation is very heavy. In trichuriasis (whipworm infestation) the so-called 'cocoanut cake rectum' is due to the congested prolapsed rectal mucosa and many small white worms.

All sorts of foreign bodies have been inserted in the rectum by perverts, or, when in a state of intoxication, by malicious companions.

Adenomata or long finger-shaped non-malignant polypi of the rectum sometimes produce an entanglement in which faeces become impacted higher up than the finger can reach and the patient may be thought to be suffering from carcinoma of the sigmoid or pelvic colon. Bleeding is unusual. The diagnosis depends on examination with the proctoscope or the sigmoidoscope.

Another condition which may simulate rectal carcinoma is *periproctal inflammation* followed by the formation of an abscess around the pelvic colon. The symptoms may be so severe that malignant disease may be suspected. The cause is generally some previous local inflammation in the rectum associated, it may be, with piles or a polypus which has hitherto produced no symptoms; in some cases carcinoma may produce such an abscess.

Proctitis may be part of a localized ulcerative colitis (granular or ulcerative proctitis) or due to gonococcal infection.

A *vesical calculus* is a rare cause of tenesmus. Such a calculus is generally one situated in a pocket of the bladder posteriorly. In such a case haematuria will, as a rule, have occurred.

The remaining conditions in the above list are diagnosed by rectal or vaginal examination or by a combination of the two.

The *rectal crises* of *tabes dorsalis* may be extremely painful. The patient complains of 'diarrhoea', but on inquiry it will be discovered that diarrhoea in the sense of fluid evacuation is less pronounced than is tenesmus—that is recurrent painful call to stool without material evacuation. Characteristically this symptom occurs in the early morning, to subside with comparative comfort for the rest of the day. Spontaneous remissions with ultimately complete cessation is the not unusual course. Supporting evidence may be afforded by the absence of knee-jerks and the existence of Argyll Robertson pupils, but visceral crises may be the only manifestation of tabes dorsalis.

Proctalgia fugax is another rather mysterious form of tenesmus. The subject experiences a cramp-like pain in the rectum usually soon after retiring to bed. The pain subsides spontaneously within a few minutes or at the most half an hour, although on occasion it may be extremely severe. No satisfactory explanation is forthcoming but from the description by sufferers, including a number of medical men, some nervous association seems responsible although which particular structure is to be incriminated is uncertain. Although many possible causes have been advanced, spasm of the sacro-coccygeus or of the levator ani is the most probable.

F. Dudley Hart.

THIRST, EXTREME

The most important of several stimuli which give rise to the sensation of thirst is an increase in the effective osmolality of body fluids, the volume of cells being diminished by a shift of water to the extracellular tissues.

Cases of extreme thirst may be subdivided into two main groups, those with and those without polyuria. With polyuria are identified such conditions as diabetes mellitus, diabetes insipidus, potassium depletion, hyperparathyroidism, and hysteria, which are discussed under POLYURIA (p. 650). In the other group of causes are included conditions and circumstances which are for the most part so obvious as to require no more than simple enumeration, for example:

1. Prolonged abstention from drinking, whether deliberate or the result of necessity.

2. Fevers and febrile states.

3. Excessive loss of fluid: (*a*) From the skin by profuse perspirations, natural or pathological; (*b*) From the stomach, from repeated vomiting; (*c*) From the bowel, diarrhoea; (*d*) Into serous membranes, as in acute peritonitis.

4. After severe haemorrhage: (*a*) External, e.g., postpartum, haematemesis, haemoptysis; (*b*) Internal, e.g., from duodenal ulcer, ruptured tubal gestation, leaking aneurysm.

5. Excessive use of diuretics.

6. Poisoning by drugs which dry up the secretions of the mouth, notably those of the belladonna group, or astringents such as alum, gallic acid, tannic acid, or perchloride of iron.

7. The taking of excess of certain salts, particularly sodium chloride.

F. Dudley Hart.

THROAT, SORE

Sore throat may be due to one or other of many different causes:

1. Affections of the Tonsils:

    a. ACUTE:

        Streptococcal or pneumococcal tonsillitis
        Quinsy
        Faucial diphtheria (*Fig.* 767)
        Anginose infectious mononucleosis
        Infection round foreign body, e.g. fish bone
        Agranulocytosis or granulocytopenia
        Syphilis, primary or secondary.

    b. CHRONIC:

        Chronic tonsillitis with intra-tonsillar retention of exudate
        Tonsillolith (rare)
        Tuberculosis
        Gumma
        Malignant disease (*Fig.* 768).

2. Affections of the Soft Palate, Faucial Pillars, and Pharyngeal Walls:

    a. ACUTE:

        Generalized pharyngitis due to virus and bacterial infections and associated with streptococcal tonsillitis, the exanthematous fevers, granulocytopenia.
        Retropharyngeal abscess
        Thrush
        Herpes
        Antibiotic and antiseptic lozenges used excessively
        Erythema multiforme, Behçet's and Stevens-Johnson syndrome, Reiter's disease
    Physical, chemical and thermal injury resulting for example from the passage of a swallowed bone, the swallowing of corrosives or the inhalation of toxic vapours or steam.

    b. CHRONIC:

        Chronic pharyngitis due to oral and gingival sepsis and the excessive consumption of alcohol and tobacco

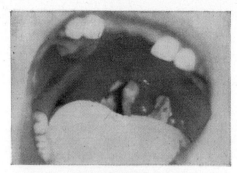

Fig. 767. Diphtheria.

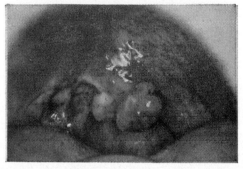

Fig. 768. Carcinoma of the tonsil.

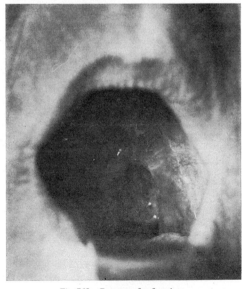

Fig. 769. Gumma of soft palate.

        Pharyngitis associated with nasal infection, e.g. chronic sinusitis
        Pharyngitis associated with mouth breathing secondary to nasal obstruction or caused by the inhalation of dry or impure air
        Chronic general disorders associated with anaemia and general debility
        Leukaemia
        Reticulosis

Malignant disease, locally
Gumma (*Fig*. 769)
Tuberculosis.

3. Affections of the Larynx:
Acute laryngitis
Tuberculosis
Malignant disease, in its later stages, or when associated with secondary infection
Trauma.

4. Acute and Subacute Adenitis of the cervical lymp-nodes.

5. Thyroiditis.

Notwithstanding the length of the above list the differential diagnosis of sore throat in most cases is not as a rule difficult. On the other hand, in certain cases and particularly when the complaint is of long-standing much investigation and circumspection may be necessary before a firm diagnosis is established.

Inquiry into the history is of the greatest importance and the area should be examined, preferably with a Lack's right-angled tongue depressor and powerful torch if a head-lamp or head-mirror is not available. Examination of the regional lymph-nodes is of course obligatory, and investigations include the examination of direct films and cultures from throat swabs and assessment of blood picture. In most cases of *acute* sore throat, and certainly where any suspicion of diphtheria or streptococcal tonsillitis is present, treatment must be begun without waiting the results of bacteriological investigations.

1. AFFECTIONS OF THE TONSIL

a. Acute. *Acute follicular tonsillitis* is usually caused by haemolytic streptococci and is characterized by white or yellow spots of debris which have been exuded by the crypts of the tonsil and stand out distinctly on the hyperaemic and, usually, swollen tonsils (*Fig*. 770). Later, as the spots become confluent a membrane may form. The patient is pyrexial (37·8–40° C) and has dysphagia and often foetor. There is enlargement of the cervical lymph-nodes which, particularly in children, may be enormous and very tender.

Quinsy or peritonsillar abscess is distinguished by the asymmetrical nature of the palatal swelling (*Fig*. 771) which pushes the corresponding tonsil downwards and towards the midline. The clinician should suspect quinsy if trismus is evident, rendering the examination difficult. The patient is indeed usually in a state of misery with severe pain, dysphagia, and cervical adenitis. The diagnosis is ultimately confirmed by the liberation of pus from the abscess.

Faucial diphtheria may be confused with acute membranous tonsillitis but in the former the onset is usually less acute and the constitutional symptoms and pyrexia at first less marked. The membrane in diphtheria is usually greyish in colour and adherent and spreads, involving several distinct anatomical regions, e.g., tonsils, faucial pillars, and pharyngeal wall. The diagnosis is confirmed by establishing the presence of Klebs-Löffler bacilli.

In *scarlet fever* the streptococcal tonsillitis is associated with an erythematous rash, circumoral pallor, and a 'strawberry tongue' and there may be more constitutional disturbance, e.g., nausea and vomiting, than is usually the case in uncomplicated tonsillitis.

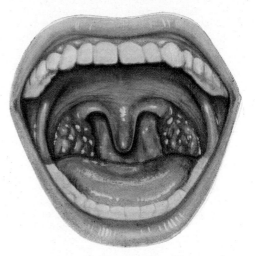

Fig. 770. Severe follicular tonsillitis. (*Illustration by Sylvia Treadgold.*)

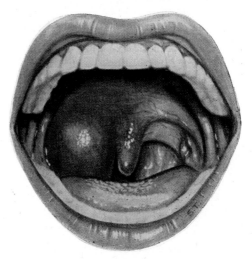

Fig. 771. Right-sided quinsy. (*Illustration by Sylvia Treadgold.*)

The *anginose form of glandular fever* often escapes diagnosis at first in favour of 'acute tonsillitis', and it may only be after a period of several days of malaise, prostration, headache, and lack of response to antibiotic treatment that the correct diagnosis is reached. In addition to the local, there is of course general involvement of lymph-nodes, and the spleen may be palpable. The tonsils, which can be so swollen as to be in danger of meeting in the midline, may be completely hidden by membrane and present a fearsome appearance. If the subject, usually a young adult, has previously undergone tonsillectomy, only those small lymphoid patches persisting in spite of the operation are inflamed. If there is any considerable mass of adenoid tissue, ulceration will produce a purulent bloodstained discharge from both anterior and posterior nares. The diagnosis is confirmed by the blood-picture which after an initial leucopenia shows an absolute lymphocytosis of up to 80 per cent, many of the monocytes and lymphocytes being atypical—the so-called 'glandular fever cells'. The Paul-Bunnell test which becomes positive at some stage of the disease in 90 per cent of cases may remain negative during the first few days of the infection, but a rising titre is significant.

Agranulocytic angina is characterized by necrotic or ulcerative lesions of the buccal mucosa, tonsils, fauces, oropharynx, and sometimes by lesions of other mucosal surfaces. The organisms are varied and culture of swabs does not assist the diagnosis, but the blood-picture shows granulocytopenia and the general condition of the patient steadily deteriorates. The causes are numerous and although some cases arise during the course of infections the majority are iatrogenic the cause being such drugs as the cytotoxic poisons, analgesics containing amidopyrine and certain antithyroid, antibacterial, and antirheumatic preparations.

In *Vincent's angina* the characteristic microorganisms are elongated fusiform bacilli and Vincent's spirochaetes. Vincent's ulceration of the fauces and tonsil may be extremely painful and is usually associated with gingivitis and foetor. The condition, sometimes known as 'trench mouth', tends to occur in crowded communities and particularly when standards of oral and dental hygiene are low. It responds slowly to treatment.

Syphilis may be seen in its primary form as a chancre of the tonsil when it occurs as an ulcer covered by slough and associated with massive cervical lymphatic enlargement. The diagnosis must be confirmed by the examination of a smear for *Treponema pallidum* under dark-ground illumination, as the serological reactions do not as a rule become positive for at least 4 weeks. In secondary syphilis there are 'mucous patches' or the so-called shallow 'snail-track' ulcers of the tonsils, fauces, and buccal mucosa together with the rash, lymphadenopathy, and other general manifestations of the condition. Again, *Treponema pallidum* will be found in the local lesions and the diagnosis can be further confirmed by serological tests.

b. Chronic. *Chronic tonsillitis* may be said to be present when recurrent attacks of acute tonsillitis occur with such frequency that the patient is scarcely ever free from symptoms and between attacks has a mild sore throat or a sensation of dryness and discomfort. Sometimes debris accumulates in one or more of the tonsillar crypts

and very rarely, as a result of the deposition of calcium salts, a tonsillolith or calculus of the tonsil may form. Its presence may be confirmed by probing and it is, of course, stony-hard to the touch.

There has always been a widespread fallacy, not only in non-medical but also in some medical sections of the community, that large tonsils are the result of chronic infection. This is not so, and in fact many tonsils which give rise to endless trouble are so small and buried as to be hidden by the anterior faucial pillar. There does exist one sign which is most significant and this is usually present—a flush or hyperaemia of the faucial mucosa in the immediate vicinity of the tonsil, often spreading to the soft palate and base of the uvula. Another though less constant sign is persistent enlargement of the cervical lymph-nodes.

Tuberculous ulceration may occur on the tonsils and fauces in the course of advanced pulmonary tuberculosis. The ulcers are shallow and one of their distinguishing features is that owing to the integrity of the sensory nerve endings they are exceedingly painful and associated with agonizing dysphagia.

Gummatous ulceration, on the other hand, is as a rule painless and the deep punched-out ulcer has to be distinguished from malignant disease. Serological tests must be carried out and usually biopsy in order to exclude dual pathology.

Malignant disease of the tonsil usually occurs as a deeply infiltrating ulcer but may be fungating or exophitic. If spreads slowly to the faucial pillars, palate, and buccal mucosa and the cervical lymph-nodes are usually involved early. Most of the neoplasms are squamous-celled carcinomas, but massive involvement of the tonsil, sometimes without ulceration, may occur in the reticuloses. The diagnosis is confirmed by biopsy.

2. AFFECTIONS OF THE SOFT PALATE, FAUCIAL PILLARS, AND PHARYNGEAL WALLS

Generalized acute pharyngitis is exceedingly common and occurs as one of the most striking manifestations of the adenovirus infections of the upper respiratory tract. It is thus seen in the common cold, in influenza, and in association with the exanthemas, streptococcal tonsillitis, sinusitis, and laryngitis. It also occurs in granulocytopenia and as a result of the excessive consumption of alcohol and tobacco.

The presenting symptom is of course 'sore throat' and it might be surmised that the pharyngeal and faucial mucosa should exhibit a raw, red beefy appearance. This indeed is often the case but the finding is by no means constant; in fact the throat may appear to be perfectly healthy.

Retropharyngeal abscess is a rare cause of acute dyspnoea and dysphagia rather than sore throat and is almost always confined to infancy. It is caused by abscess formation in the retropharyngeal lymph-nodes and on examination the posterior pharyngeal wall is pushed forward by a smooth swelling. Rarely, the retropharyngeal abscess caused by caries of the cervical vertebrae is seen and is confined to adults.

Oral or pharyngeal moniliasis (*thrush*), caused by *Candida albicans*, is seen as white patches affecting the pharyngeal and buccal mucosa and the surface of the tongue. The condition is seen commonly in infants, debilitated adults, and sometimes following antibiotic therapy. The yeasts and mycelia can be seen on direct examination of the smear and can also be cultured.

Herpetic ulceration of the nature of either *herpes simplex* or, on the other hand, *herpes zoster* of the glossopharyngeal nerve may occur on the buccal, palatal, or faucial mucous membrane. The ulcers have a yellow base, are surrounded by hyperaemia, and are painful.

Aphthous ulcers are common on the buccal mucosa, tongue, and floor of mouth and less common on the fauces, epiglottis, and lateral pharyngeal walls above the pyriform fossae, where they can only be seen in the laryngeal mirror. They are, however, an important entity in these latter sites as they are extremely painful and may escape notice. Usually the ulcers, with a whitish or yellow base, are not more than 3–4 mm. across but occasionally they are serpiginous in shape and cover a much larger area. The diagnosis is usually based on a history of such ulceration extending perhaps over a period of years.

Ulceration of the buccal and pharyngeal mucosa similar to the aphthous variety is also seen in *erythema multiforme* and in *Behçet's* and the *Stevens-Johnson syndromes*, when there is also ulceration of the external genitalia and the eyes. In Reiter's syndrome similar ulcers may occur and are associated with arthritis, urethrisis, and possibly ophthalmic manifestations.

Acute sore throat may be perpetuated by the continued use of *antibiotic and antiseptic lozenges*, and is probably partly the result of the destruction of the normal oropharyngeal flora. In the early stages the mucosa may appear hyperaemic and later monilial infection supervenes.

A more florid form of acute pharyngitis accompanies *physical*, *chemical*, or *thermal trauma* as from mouth breathing in a dry dusty atmosphere, the passage of rough unmasticated food or an actual foreign body, or the swallowing of corrosives or inhalation of toxic or hot vapours.

Chronic pharyngitis may be due to the excessive consumption of alcohol or tobacco or, commonly, both. It is also seen together with chronic laryngitis as a result of continued misuse of the voice, e.g., in street vendors and sergeant-majors. It may be associated with oral or gingival sepsis and with chronic nasal or sinus infection, in which case examination of the nose and nasopharynx and radiography of the paranasal sinuses will confirm the diagnosis. Obstruction of the nasal airways, from whatever cause, leads to mouth breathing and to the complaint of a dry, sore throat, particularly in the mornings on waking.

Careful examination of the pharynx in these cases of chronic pharyngitis will usually reveal generalized thickening and hyperaemia of the mucous membrane, and often aggregations of red or 'glassy' lymphoid tissue, particularly posterior to the faucial pillars when the appearance suggests a band of inflamed tissue on either side extending up into the nasopharynx—the so-called 'lateral-bands'.

Chronic sore throat associated with pharyngitis is common in general disorders including anaemias, and conditions associated with lowering of the general health, and when this symptom is present a full blood investigation together with any other appropriate tests are indicated.

Syphilis, tuberculosis, and malignant disease may also affect the faucial palatal and pharyngeal mucous membrane and have been described in the section on tonsillar disease.

3. LARYNGEAL CONDITIONS

Acute laryngitis may be due to the same microorganisms as acute tonsillitis or pharyngitis, and not infrequently follows a common cold or influenza, particularly if the voice is used to excess whilst the patient is suffering from an upper respiratory infection. The presenting symptom is loss of or huskiness of the voice, though usually there is sore throat and tenderness on compression of the larynx.

Acute epiglottis is of especial importance. In this condition the epiglottis is infected with *Haemophilus influenzae* causing, in adults, severe pain and dysphagia. It occurs in a more dramatic form in young children who may die from asphyxia within hours of the first complaint of 'sore throat'.

Laryngeal tuberculosis is now seldom seen owing to the advent of the antituberculous drugs. It may, however, occur during the course of untreated pulmonary tuberculosis in the form of ulceration of the posterior parts of the vocal cords. When the ulcers spread onto the arytenoids and ary-epiglottic folds, agonizing sore throat and dysphagia occur. The sputum contains tubercle bacilli.

Laryngeal syphilis may occur as a manifestation of the secondary or tertiary forms of the disease but is seldom painful unless complicated by secondary infection or perichondritis. The diagnosis is confirmed serologically.

Malignant disease of the larynx does not as a rule cause sore throat so long as the lesion is confined to the vocal cord. With spread to the arytenoids and ary-epiglottic folds the picture changes and painful dysphagia ensues. The diagnosis is confirmed by direct examination and biopsy.

Perichondritis of the laryngeal cartilages is indeed painful and occurs as a complication of laryngeal trauma, malignancy, or syphilis. The diagnosis may be considered if tenderness of the larynx is present in one of these conditions and is probably correct if there is an external sinus with offensive discharge. Tomography and direct laryngoscopy will confirm the diagnosis.

4. ACUTE ADENITIS OF THE CERVICAL LYMPHATIC NODES

This may produce marked soreness of the throat in addition to dysphagia, stiffness, discomfort, and pain. Mumps is not difficult to diagnose unless its possibility is forgotten, in which case it might be mistaken for oedema of the face or neck or other similar lesion. The way in which the swelling is located in the salivary glands, starting on one side and spreading to both, is often pathognomic. Cervical adenitis might simulate mumps, but careful palpation will generally enable one to determine that the swelling is in the lymphatic nodes. The reason for their involvement has then to be determined. This will probably have been from some inflammatory, ulcerative, or malignant focus in the head and neck, lungs, or breasts. The differential diagnosis will be based upon inspection and palpation, haematological, bacteriological, and radiological investigations, and in some cases examination of the nasopharynx, larynx, trachea, bronchi, and oesophagus under anaesthesia.

5. THYROIDITIS

Thyroiditis may cause the patient, very truly and very correctly, to complain of a sore throat, but the inflamed painful organ is here the thyroid.

Miles Foxen.

THYROID GLAND ENLARGEMENT

An enlarged thyroid gland gives rise to a swelling in the front of the neck, medial and deep to the sternomastoid muscles and medial to the carotid vessels, which, if the swelling is large enough, are displaced laterally. The gland is connected intimately with the larynx so that it rises and falls with the larynx and trachea during deglutition. This sign alone is generally sufficient to establish the diagnosis of enlarged thyroid gland, but there are two sources of fallacy: (1) A swelling not thyroid in origin but lying above it or in front of it, such as a subhyoid bursa or a suppurative perichondritis of the thyroid cartilage, may present the same sign: (2) A thyroid swelling, if fixed, as it may be by malignant growth, may not present it, although in this case the extent and degree of infiltration will render the reason for the lack of movement obvious and the diagnosis will not be affected. In almost every case, therefore, a swelling in the position of the thyroid gland which moves on deglutition indicates an enlargement of that gland.

Inspection with the patient at rest and on swallowing may alone be enough to render a diagnosis of thyroid swelling extremely likely.

Palpation will confirm this, and is usually best performed while standing behind the patient. The lateral lobes are palpated with the appropriate sternomastoid muscle relaxed, and, if the enlargement is only slight, help may be obtained by displacing the trachea towards the side being examined, when it is possible to introduce the fingers under the relaxed sternomastoid to feel the posterior border of the lobe. The trachea and larynx may of course already be the subject of pathological displacement by pressure of the enlarged gland and this should be determined at the time of palpation. The larynx should also be examined with a mirror for paralysis or asymmetry of the vocal cords. Vocal cord paresis will usually be accompanied by alteration in the voice and, if both cords are affected, possibly with dyspnoea and stridor as well.

The possibility of pressure effects always requires investigating, and these may be enumerated as follows:

Pressure on the trachea causing deviation or compression or both, with varying degrees of dyspnoea and stridor.

Pressure on the oesophagus causing dysphagia.

Pressure on nerves, usually the recurrent laryngeal nerves, producing various forms of vocal cord palsy with or without alteration in the voice, dyspnoea, stridor, and 'brassy' cough. The cervical sympathetic is occasionally involved, as shown by contracted pupil, ptosis, and enophthalmos.

Pressure on veins giving rise to engorgement and setting up of anastomotic channels.

Acute pressure symptoms may arise, or those already present may become acutely aggravated by haemorrhage into a cystic space in a goitre.

Retrosternal prolongation of the thyroid should not be forgotten, and may be recognized by dullness on percussion over the manubrium, but this sign is unreliable. When the patient is asked to swallow or cough it is sometimes possible to feel the lower limit of the gland as it rises; at the end of deglutition it slips back behind the sternum. The thyroid in the neck may occasionally appear of normal size in the presence of a retrosternal enlargement, and in a few rare cases the whole gland lies behind the sternum. Pressure symptoms are liable to be great when part or the whole of the gland is in this position, and sometimes the result of pressure on the great veins is seen in the presence of dilated anastomotic skin veins over the upper anterior part of the thorax.

Radiographic examination is a most useful adjunct in the diagnosis of thyroid enlargement, showing both the presence of retrosternal prolongation and tracheal displacement and compression. Other aids may be apparent with individual cases.

Varieties of Enlargement and their Differential Diagnosis:

PHYSIOLOGICAL ENLARGEMENT:
   Occurs at puberty and during menstruation and pregnancy, usually symptomless.

INFLAMMATORY ENLARGEMENT:
1. *Acute*: Acute thyroiditis, symptoms include the usual signs of acute inflammation; condition is rare.
2. *Chronic*: Tuberculosis, Syphilis, Riedel's disease, Lymphadenoid goitre (Hashimoto's disease).

SIMPLE GOITRE:
(Endemic and sporadic.) Parenchymatous goitre, Colloid goitre, Nodular goitre, Solitary (foetal) adenoma.

THYROTOXIC GOITRE:
Primary thyrotoxicosis (*Fig.* 772)
Secondary thyrotoxicosis.

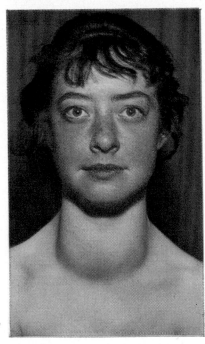

Fig. 772. Primary thyrotoxicosis. Note the even thyroid swelling, 'bright eyes', and exophthalmos. (*Courtesy of the Gordon Museum, Guy's Hospital.*)

GOITRE OF THYROID DEFICIENCY:
Cretinism
Myxoedema
Drugs, e.g., resorcinol, phenylbutazone.

MALIGNANT GOITRE:
Carcinoma.
Sarcoma (rare).

These conditions can be re-grouped for diagnostic purposes as follows:

THYROID ENLARGEMENT WITH THYROTOXICOSIS:
Primary Thyrotoxicosis (enlargement general).
Secondary Thyrotoxicosis:
Localized Enlargement—Toxic adenoma (rare).
Generalized Enlargement—Nodular goitre in which one nodule may be so large as to suggest a solitary adenoma, occasionally parenchymatous or even malignant goitre.

THYROID ENLARGEMENT WITH SIGNS OF DEFICIENT SECRETION:
Congenital—Cretinism.

Acquired—Myxoedema (mild deficiency may be exhibited by colloid or malignant goitre), Hashimoto's disease.

THYROID ENLARGEMENT UNCOMPLICATED:
Localized Enlargement—One large nodule in a small nodular goitre, Adenoma, Riedel's disease (early stages), Malignant disease (early stages).
Generalized Enlargement—Parenchymatous goitre, Colloid goitre, Nodular goitre, Lymphadenoid goitre, Riedel's disease (late stages), Malignant goitre (late stages).

The thyroid gland is in a continual state of fluctuating activity and the structure varies not only at different times but in different parts of the same gland. When enlarged, even more diversity of structure may be present. This may render clinical distinction of the various pathological types of simple goitre impossible. Parenchymatous, colloid, and diffuse nodular goitre will therefore be grouped together.

Thyroid Enlargement with Thyrotoxicosis. Primary thyrotoxicosis is characterized by the presence of toxic symptoms from the onset of the disease; in secondary thyrotoxicosis these symptoms develop after a simple goitre has been present for a variable period, often many years. The diagnostic points of each condition are tabulated below:

Various eye signs are described in connexion with exophthalmos, of which the following are the best known:

Von Graefe's sign—Lagging behind of the upper lid as the patient looks downward.
Dalrymple's sign—Retracted lids causing a wide palpebral opening.
Stellwag's sign—Diminished frequency of blinking.
Moebius' sign—Inability to maintain convergence for close vision.

Dalrymple's sign is fairly constantly present, but may be found in other conditions, while the other signs are neither constantly present nor confined to exophthalmic goitre.

Cretinism. Usually the thyroid is atrophic in this condition, but a goitre is occasionally present, especially in a long-standing case. An untreated patient is easily recognizable, but one seldom seen nowadays. Slow development, either physical or mental, should rouse a suspicion of thyroid deficiency, remembering other possible causes of backward development such as rickets, renal rickets, achondroplasia, etc. The diagnosis of cretinism will not be detailed more as it is barely relevant.

Myxoedema. As in cretinism, the thyroid is only occasionally enlarged, and here again a detailed account will not be given. The characteristic symptoms include slowed mentality, coarse features, dry skin, brittle nails and sparse coarse hair, and a gain in weight, often gross. (*See* THYROID FUNCTION, TESTS OF, p. 790.)

Certain drugs, e.g., resorcinol as an external application and phenylbutazone by mouth, may occasionally be associated with thyroid enlargement with signs of myxoedema reversible on stopping drug administration.

Lymphadenoid Goitre (Hashimoto's Disease). In this disorder the thyroid gland becomes infiltrated with lymphoid tissue possibly as a result of an auto-immune reaction. It is a disease occurring in women in middle life and usually produces a uniform, firm enlargement of the thyroid with evidence of hypothyroidism. The gland is often H-shaped. Laboratory tests for thyroid

determining this. *Nodular goitre* may give rise to a uniform enlargement, as also may *colloid goitre*. This last condition may present a smooth surface, as is usually the case in *parenchymatous* enlargement.

Malignant disease starts in one area and spreads to involve the whole gland, finally breaking through the capsule to invade surrounding

	PRIMARY THYROTOXICOSIS	SECONDARY THYROTOXICOSIS
Age of onset	Young	Middle aged
Onset	Acute	Insidious
Thyroid swelling	Not present before onset. Generalized soft elastic and vascular swelling, enlargement not gross. May harden if iodine has been given	Present before onset. Enlargement may be considerable; frequently nodular
		Rare, and if present slight
Exophthalmos	Generally present, often gross	Tachycardia. Cardiovascular
Heart	Tachycardia, but fibrillation and heart failure not common except in late or severe cases	degeneration most prominent symptom. Auricular fibrillation fairly common
Tremor and general excitability	Marked	Slight
B.M.R.	Markedly raised, often above 50 per cent	Raised, but not markedly, rarely above 50 per cent
Loss of weight	Marked	Present, not so marked
Increased perspiration	Marked	Present, not so marked
Results of iodine medication	Often striking improvement	Improvement, but of a lesser degree
Thyroid function tests	Raised	Raised
Radio-iodine uptake	Raised	Raised

function show low levels, increased serum cholesterol, a raised erythrocyte sedimentation rate, and auto-immune antibodies are present in the blood. Occasionally, lymph-adenomatous goitre will occur with normal thyroid function and, very exceptionally, with hyperthyroidism. In the past, diagnosis has often been made after operation as a result of histological section of the tissue removed, but with careful investigation this should not be necessary in a typical case.

Carcinoma of the thyroid may cause confusion, but this condition is practically never associated with hypothyroidism in an untreated case, and the serum proteins are undisturbed. Enlargement of the spleen and liver have been reported in conjunction with lymphadenomatous goitre and, if present, would serve to confirm the diagnosis.
Riedel's Disease is an interesting and rare condition where an intense sclerosing fibrosis starts in one area of the gland and spreads first to the whole gland and then to surrounding structures. The progress is slow as a rule, but gradually the trachea, the oesophagus, and the great vessels all suffer from constriction while the recurrent laryngeal nerves are affected early. The diagnosis from malignant disease is very difficult, but the condition should be suspected when an intensely hard goitre with pressure symptoms out of all proportion to its size is found in a young adult.
Uncomplicated Thyroid Enlargement. A true *foetal adenoma* is an uncommon condition, but a particularly large nodule in an otherwise small nodular goitre forming an asymmetrical swelling in the thyroid tissue is common. It may be cystic or solid but palpation is not always reliable in

structures. Movement on deglutition may be lost, the recurrent laryngeal nerve is involved early, and the growth tends to surround the carotid bundle rather than push it back, as is the case with large simple goitres, so that pulsation of these vessels may be impalpable in the middle of the neck. The sympathetic chain is often involved late in the disease. The swelling is usually hard, as in Riedel's disease, but tends to be much greater in size and more rapid in growth. Pressure symptoms are early and pain is often a marked feature, particularly on swallowing. Bone and lung metastases are not uncommon. One type of thyroid carcinoma, namely the papillary carcinoma, deserves special mention. This typically occurs in the fourth and fifth decades and metastasizes to the lymph-glands. The secondary deposits may be much larger than the primary which cannot be detected, so that these cases often present with soft lumps in the side of the neck which used to be called, erroneously, 'lateral aberrant thyroids'. Thyroid tissue so situated is always a secondary deposit from a small primary in the thyroid which has completely replaced the lymphoid tissue in which it germinated.

R. G. Beard.

THYROID, TESTS OF FUNCTION OF

Nearly all the circulating, organically bound iodine is normally incorporated in thyroxine (T_4). More than 99 per cent of this T_4 is bound to a specific thyroxine-binding globulin (TBG);

this bound T_4 is physiologically inactive. The protein-bound fraction is in equilibrium with the very small amount of free, physiologically active hormone. Tri-iodothyronine (T_3) accounts for the remaining small amount (about 1·5 per cent) of circulating organic iodine, and is bound to TBG in about the same proportion as T_4; on a molar basis free T_3 is physiologically more active than free T_4.

The binding protein is about a third saturated with hormone.

Circulating inorganic iodide is utilized by the thyroid gland to synthesize T_4 and T_3. It is taken up by, and concentrated in, the thyroid cells by an active transport process. Iodide is converted to iodine and is incorporated into tyrosine to form mono- and di-iodotyrosine. Condensation of two iodinated tyrosine molecules forms T_4 (two di-iodotyrosine) and T_3 (one mono- and one di-iodotyrosine), which are stored in the gland, bound to protein as thyroglobulin. This overall process may be affected in a variety of ways.

a. Antithyroid drugs inhibit hormone synthesis, but not uptake of iodide.

b. Inorganic, but not organic, iodide can be discharged from the gland by administration of perchlorate.

c. Any of the enzymes controlling these synthetic steps may be genetically deficient.

Uptake of iodide, conversion to iodine, and release of T_4 and T_3 from the gland into the circulation are all stimulated by thyrotrophic hormone (TSH). Release of TSH from the anterior pituitary gland is normally controlled by two factors.

1. It is *inhibited* by a rise in the circulating concentration of free thyroid hormone.

2. It is stimulated by the tripeptide, thyrotrophin-releasing hormone (TRH), which is synthesized in the hypothalamus and reaches the anterior pituitary gland by vessels in the pituitary stalk.

Assessment of Circulating Thyroid Hormone Level. As discussed below, *one* of the several tests for bound thyroid hormone concentration, when considered together with the clinical picture, is often adequate to diagnose thyroid disease. These tests, which all assume a normal TBG level, fall into two groups:

Estimates of bound thyroid hormone levels, either directly or by measurement of iodine content.

Indirect assessment of bound thyroid hormone levels by measuring the unoccupied sites on the TBG.

The bound hormone, making up 99 per cent or more of the total, can usually be assumed to be in equilibrium with the physiologically important free fraction in which we are interested, so that changes in one are reflected in changes in the other.

Estimates of Bound Thyroid Hormone. *Protein Bound Iodine (PBI).* Since circulating protein (TBG)-bound iodine is mostly in the form

of bound T_4, estimation of PBI is often used to assess the level of this hormone. Falsely high results are relatively common since contamination with iodide is difficult to avoid. Administration of some iodide-containing cough medicines, of drugs such as 'enterovioform', and of most radiological contrast media invalidates the results for weeks, months, or (for contrast media) sometimes years. *In vitro* contamination is also difficult to avoid. For this reason, low PBI results are more reliable than high ones. If other methods are available, this estimation should be abandoned.

Thyroxine (T_4). T_4 concentration may be assayed directly, and this is the estimation of choice. It has the advantage of being unaffected by iodine contamination.

Estimates of Unoccupied Binding Sites. If the concentration of TBG is normal, a reduction in the amount of hormone bound to it increases the number of unoccupied sites, whilst a raised hormone level reduces it. These sites may be measured directly by a T_3 uptake test, or indirectly by a resin uptake test. In both cases an excess of radioactivity labelled hormone (usually T_3) is added to the patient's serum under conditions in which the binding protein will combine avidly with it. The unbound radiohormone is then removed with a resin.

In the *T_3 uptake test* the amount remaining bound to the protein is estimated. The greater the number of unoccupied sites, the higher is the value, and, providing that the total TBG level is normal, the lower the amount of T_4 bound to it. Conversely, a low T_3 uptake indicates a reduced number of unoccupied sites, usually due to a high T_4 (hyperthyroidism).

In the *resin uptake test* the amount *not* bound to protein and removed on the resin is estimated. The less that binds to the protein, the more there is available to attach to the resin. Results are therefore opposite to those in the T_3 uptake test, being high if T_4 levels are high, and low if they are reduced.

Effect of Changes in Thyroxine-binding Globulin Levels on Assessment and of Thyroid Hormone. In all the tests discussed so far we have assumed a normal TBG concentration. In such a situation any one of them can be used to assess thyroid status. However, changes in the TBG level affect all these results. During the following discussion the reader should refer to *Fig. 773*.

Since, in the euthyroid subject, the *percentage* saturation of the protein with hormone tends to remain constant, a change of total TBG concentration alters both the amount of T_4 bound to it, and the number of unoccupied sites, in the same direction. The free hormone level, however, remains normal. Thus, a rise in TBG, by increasing the bound hormone elevates the PBI and total T_4, which do not now directly reflect the free T_4 level; on the basis of these results the patients might falsely be diagnosed as hyperthyroid. Since the number of unoccupied, as well as of occupied, binding sites is increased,

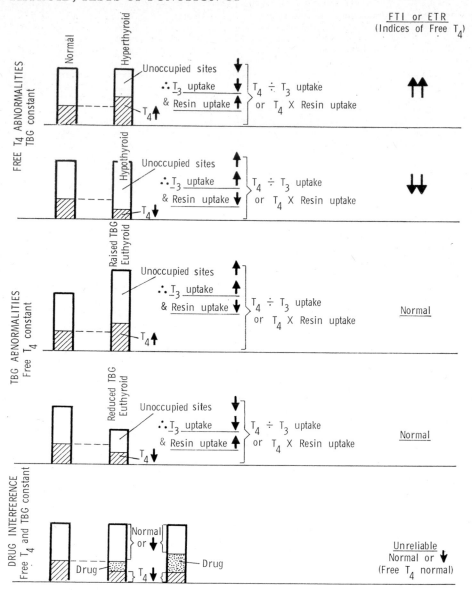

Fig. 773. Effect of changes in concentration of Thyroxine (T$_4$), Thyroxine Binding Globulin (TBG) and interfering drugs on tests for assessing thyroid hormone levels. FTI=Free Thyroxine Index. ETR=Effective Thyroxine Ratio. T$_3$=Tri-iodothyronine.

the T$_3$ uptake is raised and the resin uptake reduced; on the basis of these results the patient might falsely be diagnosed as hypothyroid. Conversely, patients with low levels of binding protein appear hypothyroid on the results of T$_4$ and PBI, and hyperthyroid on the T$_3$ and resin uptake test.

High TBG levels are common in pregnant women, newborn infants, patients on oestrogen therapy, and women taking oral contraceptive preparations. Low TBG levels are associated with protein-losing states, such as the nephrotic

syndrome. In any such subjects, and if the result of any of the above tests is equivocal, an attempt should be made to assess free hormone levels.

Assessment of Free Thyroid Hormone Levels. Direct methods for estimating free T$_4$ are not generally available. However, since rises in TBG concentration tend to overestimate free T$_4$ as assessed by bound T$_4$ or PBI, and underestimate it if unoccupied binding sites are measured, the latter can be used to correct the former. The value for total T$_4$ may be divided by the T$_3$ uptake, or multiplied by the resin uptake. The resulting figure may be called the *free thyroxine index (FTI)* or *effective thyroxine ration (ETR)* depending upon the method used.

Drug Interference with Assessment of Thyroid Hormone Levels. Many drugs compete with T_4 for binding sites on TBG, causing low T_4 levels, and sometimes reducing the unoccupied binding sites. In such circumstances even the FTI and ETR do not necessarily reflect free T_4 levels. The most common of such drugs are salicylates and diphenylhydantoin ('Epanutin'). This source of error should always be remembered if T_4 results are unexpectedly low.

The results are summarized in *Fig. 773*.

If the results of the above tests fall in the 'grey' area of overlap between normal and abnormal values, or if there is a question of drug interference, subsequent procedure differs depending whether hyperthyroidism or hypothyroidism is suspected.

Further Tests for Hyperthyroidism. Hyperthyroidism is almost always due to non-TSH dependent over-activity of the gland. The raised level of free thyroid hormones inhibits TSH secretion, and plasma TSH levels are usually undetectable. Unfortunately, the normal trophic hormone concentration is so low that measurement of basal levels is not useful as a test for hyperthyroidism. The aim is to demonstrate, indirectly, that pituitary TSH secretion is already maximally suppressed.

Thyroid Uptake of Radioiodide with T_3 Supression. This is probably still the most reliable test for confirming border-line hyperthyroidism. It cannot be used in patients taking antithyroid drugs or iodide-containing preparations (*see below*).

^{131}I or ^{132}I (both radioactive) are usually administered orally. Technetium (also radioactive) is handled by the gland in the same way, and may be given, by intravenous injection, instead of iodine. At a standard time after giving the isotope the proportion of administered activity in the gland is measured. If this is unequivocally high no further test is necessary.

In border-line cases the T_3 suppression test relies on the fact that, in normal subjects, TSH suppression by exogenous hormone impairs the thyroidal iodine uptake; however, the hyperthyroid gland is not under TSH control, and TSH is already suppressed. If after the first uptake test, tri-iodothyronine is administered for 6 days (120 µg./day), TSH will be cut off by feedback inhibition in the euthyroid subject and a further test will show a marked fall in neck uptake; in the hyperthyroid patient, because TSH is already maximally suppressed by high circulating hormone levels, the second test will show no change.

TRH Stimulation Test. As mentioned above, basal TSH measurement is not useful in diagnosing hyperthyroidism. Measurement of such levels after administration of TRH may be helpful. The test is based on the fact that in the normal subject TRH stimulates the output of TSH with a detectable rise in circulating levels.

If the pituitary is under strong negative feedback by high circulating levels of thyroid hormone TRH has less effect on plasma TSH levels. A normal rise in plasma TSH exlcudes hyperthyroidism, but there may sometimes be a 'flat' response in normal subjects. A similarly reduced response will, of course, occur in hypothyroidism secondary to pituitary disease; this is unlikely to pose diagnostic problems, since T_4 levels are low.

T_3 Thyrotoxicosis. Occasionally clinical hyperthyroidism may be associated with elevated T_3, but normal T_4, levels. In many of these cases T_4 levels rise later. T_3 may be assayed directly, but if this estimation is not available, such subjects will show failure of T_3 suppression of the neck uptake of iodine, and flat TRH response.

Further Tests for Hypothyroidism. Hypothyroidism may be due to primary failure of the thyroid gland, or may be secondary to impaired TSH secretion from the pituitary. In the latter condition other signs of hypopituitarism will be present.

Plasma TSH Levels. Plasma TSH concentration rises detectably in *primary hypothyroidism*. Its measurement is the most sensitive test for this condition.

In *hypopituitarism* low T_4 and low TSH levels coexist. There is a subnormal rise of TSH after TRH stimulation.

Thyroidal Uptake of Radioiodine and TSH Stimulation. This test is only necessary if TSH assay is unavailable. The thyroidal uptake of radioiodide is low, or low normal, in both primary hypothyroidism and in long-standing pituitary disease.

If exogenous TSH is injected, and the uptake is repeated, there is a marked rise in uptake in the normal subject. In *primary hypothyroidism* the rise is subnormal or fails to occur.

After prolonged *hypopituitarism*, with consequent TSH deficiency, some thyroid atrophy may occur and the response to exogenous TSH is also diminished. However, the condition is rapidly reversible, and a second dose of TSH will cause a further rise in uptake. In primary hypothyroidism there is no further response to a second dose. Prolonged administration of exogenous thyroid hormone, by suppressing pituitary TSH, causes a response similar to that in hypopituitarism.

Plasma Cholesterol. Levels of cholesterol are usually elevated in hypothyroidism. The finding, however, is so non-specific that it should not be used diagnostically if other tests are available.

Tests for the Cause of Thyroid Disorders

Circulating Thyroid Antibodies. These may occasionally be found in apparently normal subjects. They are most commonly associated with lymphocytic infiltration of the thyroid gland, such as occurs in Hashimoto's thyroiditis. Patients with such conditions may be hyper-, hypo-, or euthyroid.

Thyroid Scanning. A dose of radioiodide or technetium is administered, and the 'profile' of activity over the gland is mapped by a machine which moves a scintillation counter over the neck. 'Hot' areas indicate active nodules, while 'cold' ones are inactive. Retrosternal extension may also be detected by this method. The dose of radioactivity is larger than that given for an uptake test, which should be completed first.

Biopsy of the Thyroid Gland. This may be necessary to make a definite diagnosis, especially if malignant disease is suspected.

Potassium Perchlorate Discharge Test. In some of the very rare genetic disorders of thyroid hormone synthesis iodine can be concentrated in the cells of the gland, but incorporation into tyrosine is impaired. In the perchlorate discharge test radioiodide is administered, and the neck uptake measured as usual. Perchlorate is then given, and the neck uptake repeated. Abnormally high discharge of radioactivity from the gland indicates an excess of inorganic iodide in the gland, since organic iodine is not discharged by perchlorate.

Dissociated Neck Uptake and Circulating Thyroid Hormone Levels. High thyroidal radioiodide uptake is usually associated with high free T_4 levels, and low uptake with low hormone concentration. In three situations this may not be true.

    1. *Drugs may interfere with uptake*

    a. Administration of antithyroid drugs (such as thiouracil) which impair hormone synthesis, but not uptake of iodide by the gland. If peripheral T_4 levels fall, consequent increased TSH levels cause a high uptake.

    b. Iodide-containing compounds cause an apparently low uptake of radioiodide by the gland, since the radioactive compound is diluted by the large pool of stable iodide.

    2. *Thyroiditis.* At some stages of thyroiditis there may be dissociation between neck uptake and circulating T_4 levels. This may be either a high uptake with low T_4 or vice versa, depending on which stage of synthesis or discharge of hormone from the gland is affected.

    3. *Genetic defects of hormone synthesis.* In most of these conditions there is a defect in the synthetic pathway after the uptake of iodide by the gland and the picture is similar to that due to antithyroid drugs, with a high uptake and low T_4 levels.

Joan F. Zilva.

TINNITUS

Tinnitus is a term which denotes a ringing or whistling sound in the ears, but is customarily applied to other sounds such as hissing, throbbing, or roaring. It occurs both in cases of disease of the ear, and in cases in which there is no lesion of the auditory mechanism. The commonest causes of a hissing sound in the ears are wax in the external auditory canal or a blocked Eustachian tube. Tinnitus may be continuous or intermittent. Its intensity and character vary greatly in different patients; to some it is an intolerable annoyance, and occasionally has even

been the cause of suicide. The character of the sound may give some clue to the cause. Thus a pulsatile or rhythmical sound may be produced by the flow of blood through an atheromatous

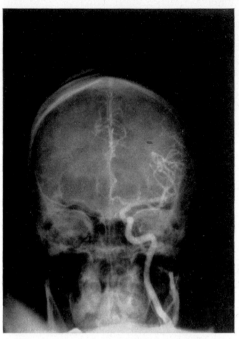

Fig. 774. Normal left-sided cerebral arteriogram; anterior view. (*Dr. R. D. Hoare.*)

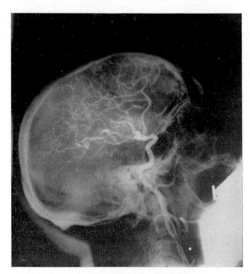

Fig. 775. Normal cerebral arteriogram: lateral view. (*Dr. R. D. Hoare.*)

internal carotid artery, which in its course through the carotid canal is separated from the tympanum only by a thin plate of bone. Internal carotid thrombosis should be suspected if the pulse in one carotid artery is absent or greatly diminished. The noise in the ear may be heard on the opposite side on account of compensatory dilatation. Other symptoms of this condition may be intermittent headache, often over one eye, transitory hemiparesis, transitory loss of vision in one eye, temporary aphasia, and fits. Digital compression of the carotid on the sound side may precipitate such phenomena, which also include hemiparaesthesia. A carotid arteriogram (*Figs.* 774–776) is diagnostic. Tinnitus is common in cases of arteriosclerosis, and conditions

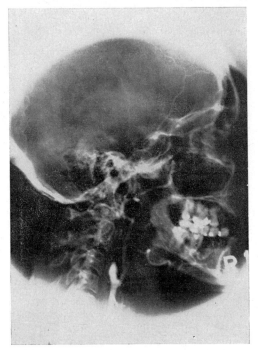

Fig. 776. Arteriogram showing occlusion of internal carotid artery. (*Dr. R. D. Hoare.*)

associated with high blood-pressure; it may also occur when there is severe anaemia; the noises heard may be variously described by patients as humming, hissing, rhythmic thumping, roaring, whistling, or musical. A crackling noise may be produced by cerumen, or a foreign body, in the external auditory canal. A bubbling noise may be due to catarrhal exudation in the middle ear. A crackling or clicking sound may be caused by spasmodic contraction of the dilator tubae and salpingo-pharyngeus muscles which are attached to the Eustachian tube. A clicking sound may be caused by intermittent contraction of the tensor tympani. In rare cases the tinnitus may be associated with an intracranial murmur, to be detected on examination of the head with the stethoscope.

A distinction must be made between tinnitus and hallucinations of hearing, the latter usually taking the form of hearing voices, and indicating psychosis. Tinnitus, however caused, is usually

influenced markedly by the general health and environment of the patient. Thus, sometimes the noises are less marked when the patient is in the open air, when his attention is occupied by other matters, or when the sense of hearing is occupied by listening to objective noises. Similarly, the trouble may be present only at night, but may appear in the day-time if the patient closes the external auditory meatus with his finger. Generally speaking, tinnitus becomes less marked and more bearable when the general health of the patient is good, and increases when the sufferer is out of heath, overworked, or unemployed, either mentally or physically. In women the trouble may be increased during pregnancy, menstruation, or the menopause.

Rapid changes of atmospheric pressure may cause various aural symptoms (barotrauma) including tinnitus—rising to heights, for instance in an aeroplane, or going to depths, as amongst miners or divers.

Though tinnitus is very common in diseases of the ear, yet serious lesions of the middle ear, internal ear, or auditory nerve may be present without this symptom. There is no constant relation between tinnitus and deafness. The former may be present with good hearing, but when long continued the hearing tends to become impaired. The sounds may persist when a patient has become totally deaf. The association of vertigo with tinnitus nearly always indicates labyrinthine disturbance secondary to vascular disease, e.g., arteriosclerosis or syphilis. Bouts of increasing deafness and tinnitus leading to sudden vertigo which is followed by a return of hearing (Lermoyez syndrome) are probably due to vascular spasm and allied to migraine.

Tinnitus may occur from the following diseases of the ear:

1. The presence of *cerumen, aural polypi,* or *a foreign body* in the external auditory meatus coming in contact with the drum. Removal of the offending body leads to the cessation of the tinnitus.

2. In any *inflammatory disease, acute or chronic, suppurative or non-suppurative, of the middle ear.* In catarrhal inflammation of the middle ear, the noise frequently has the character of bursting bubbles, and is due to movements of the viscid exudation in the ear itself. Chronic sinusitis may be the underlying cause. In *otosclerosis,* tinnitus is a very prominent and usually early symptom. It may occur before any alteration in hearing is present.

3. In diseases of the *internal ear* tinnitus may be severe and intractable; especially in *Ménière's disease, syphilitic disease* of the internal ear, and in those lesions of the internal ear which may arise in the course of *typhoid* and other *specific fevers. Extension of suppuration to the labyrinth* from the middle ear is also an important cause; and tinnitus, usually associated with deafness, may persist after *fracture of the base of the skull.*

Persistent unilateral tinnitus with progressive internal-ear deafness and vertigo raises suspicion of *acoustic nerve tumour.* Unilateral tinnitus with a ringing or bell-like quality and reduced hearing suggests cochlear involvement.

'Noises in the ears' are complained of in many general diseases with or without a lesion of the ear; thus, they are frequent in *anaemia, leukaemia*; some *cardiac lesion*, especially aortic regurgitation, may be found in the pulsatile variety of tinnitus. *Chronic nephritis, uraemia*, and *arteriosclerosis* with high blood-pressure may also be responsible for tinnitus, and it may occur during attacks of *neuralgia* or of *migraine*. Quinine, salicylates, and streptomycin may cause tinnitus.

Ian Mackenzie.
F. Dudley Hart.

TONGUE, PAIN IN

Pain in the tongue may be attributable to some obvious lesion, usually with breach of surface such as an epithelioma. Such conditions are discussed under the heading of TONGUE, ULCERA-TION OF (p. 779). On the other hand, pain in the tongue or soreness of the tongue may be an insistent complaint when there is no superficial evidence of abnormality. The conditions that have to be considered include the following:

1. *When the pain complained of is not on the dorsum, tip, or sides of the tongue but underneath or deeper*:

Injury to the fraenum linguae
Ranula
Calculus in the duct of a submandibular salivary gland
Foreign body in the tongue
Myositis
Trichinosis.

2. *When the pain complained of appears to be upon the surface of the tongue, even if it also affects the tongue as a whole*:

Bitten tongue
After an anaesthetic (mouth-gag)
Injury by tooth or dental plate
Smoking
The effects of over-hot beverages or foodstuffs
The effects of pungent condiments such as cayenne pepper
Antibiotic glossitis, associated with lichen planus, Behçet's disease, or pemphigus vulgaris
Moeller's glossitis
Glossitis of deficiency disease
Carcinoma.

The differential diagnosis depends upon the following considerations:

1. Pain Underneath the Tongue or Deeper

Injury to the fraenum linguae may cause visible abrasion or definite ulcer. The most injured spot is tender as well as painful, the diagnosis depending on careful attention to the appearances and to the site of greatest tenderness. The cause may be injury by a fish-bone or other sharp or puncturing object. In violent coughing bouts as in whooping-cough the protruded tongue may be forced against the lower incisor teeth with such violence that the fraenum becomes abraded, inflamed, or ulcerated.

Ranula is not painful unless it becomes inflamed. It is an asymmetrical red smooth swelling in the floor of the mouth under the tongue on one or other side of the fraenum. It may result from obstruction of the duct of one of the sublingual salivary glands but more often it is a retention cyst arising in one of the many mucous glands in the floor of the mouth.

Calculus in the duct of a submandibular salivary gland is not necessarily painful. It may produce discomfort or more or less severe pain recurrent or constant according to the degree of inflammation. The stone may be very small and difficult to detect either with a probe or by X-rays, but its existence may be suspected by the situation of the discomfort, or by the corresponding salivary gland swelling when the patient begins to eat, the stone interfering with the free passage of the increased flow of saliva. The calculus can frequently be palpated bimanually in the floor of the mouth and is occasionally seen to protrude through the duct orifice.

Foreign body in the tongue is uncommon, though a fish-bone may become impacted in it. More often the foreign body injures the tongue, itself escaping but leaving pain behind. The diagnosis depends on the accuracy of the story obtained or the discovery of the foreign body by palpation or by radiography.

Myositis of the tongue is seldom if ever a localized condition; it may, however, be a prominent feature in *polymyositis* or in *trichinosis*, in which the embryo trichinellae have a special predilection for the muscles at the base of the tongue which become stiff, painful, and tender. The diagnosis of trichinosis is difficult especially as it will hardly be thought of unless there is an epidemic at the time. The blood exhibits eosinophilia, but the only way of clinching the diagnosis is by demonstrating the trichinellae embryos microscopically in portions of the muscles excised.

2. Pain upon the Surface of the Tongue

Bitten tongue will usually present an obvious lesion but pain may persist after a tongue-bite even when no obvious bruising or breach of surface can be detected. The patient may be unaware of having accidentally inflicted the bite, if the accident occurred during sleep or during an epileptic seizure. Indeed, the occurrence of a local painful area in the tongue suggesting the effect of tongue-bite may be the first indication that the patient is an epileptic. In tetanus traumatic glossitis is common and may cause airways obstruction.

After general anaesthetics, patients often complain of soreness of the tongue resulting from the use of tongue forceps or of a mouth-gag.

Injury by a tooth or *dental plate* may cause a local painful place upon one side of the tongue often fairly far back, the pain being increased by movements of the tongue in speaking, eating, or swallowing. Fear of cancer is usual until the cause is found in the jagged edge of the adjacent tooth, or of the dental plate at the corresponding site. The condition needs to be watched carefully to be certain that the lesion disappears after the offending irritant is smoothed down or removed, and to allay any anxiety that the jagged tooth or plate may have initiated an epithelioma. Tuberculosis of the tongue, presenting as a painful deep persistent ulcer, is now rarely seen.

Antibiotic glossitis. A common cause of diffuse soreness of the tongue is the taking of antibiotics by mouth. The pain is sometimes due to infection with *Monilia albicans* which can be grown from the surface. Its preponderance is favoured by the wide-spectrum antibiotics. In other cases of antibiotic glossitis no such cause can be found and the change is attributed to vitamin deficiencies arising from suppression of normal gut flora. The tongue is clean, red, and very sensitive to heat (*Fig.* 777). Glossitis occurs in deficiency of vitamin B_{12}, and folic acid, in pellagra,

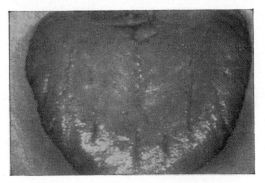

Fig. 777. Glossitis due to oral antibiotic.
(*Figs.* 777–780, *Professor Martin Rushton.*)

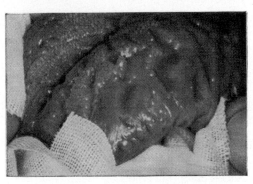

Fig. 778. Congenital fissuring of the tongue.

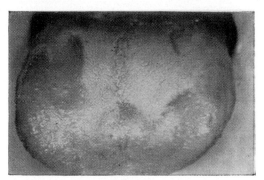

Fig. 779. Geographical tongue.

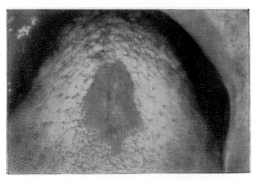

Fig. 780. Median rhomboid glossitis.

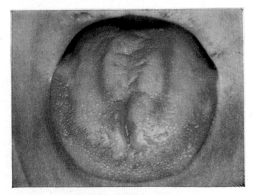

Fig. 781. Moeller's glossitis.

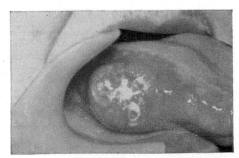

Fig. 782. Carcinoma of the tongue.

malabsorption syndrome, and the Plummer-Vinson syndrome, but seldom causes acute pain in these conditions.

Lichen planus affecting the tongue may be confused with monilia glossitis because both produce small whitish patches on the surface. The lichen tends to produce lines or a mesh of pearly dots and to favour the cheeks near the occlusal line of the molars.

The tongue may also become inflamed and painful in Behçet's disease, erythema multiforme, or pemphigus vulgaris.

Congenital fissured tongue (*Fig.* 778) or 'scrotal tongue' is thick, deeply fissured, and usually symptomless. If food particles lodge in the fissures infection may arise and thus cause pain.

Geographical tongue (*Fig.* 779) shows red denuded patches of irregular outline which often change their position. It causes anxiety rather than pain.

Median rhomboid glossitis (*Fig.* 780) is a rare congenital abnormality due to persistence of the tuberculum impar between the two halves of the tongue. It occupies the middle third of the dorsum and is smooth, shiny, and red. It carries no filiform papillae. Opalescent nodules may be scattered over the surface. The area may become inflamed and thus cause soreness and often unfounded fear of cancer.

Moeller's glossitis (*Fig.* 781), often confused with Hunter's glossitis of pernicious anaemia (q.v.), presents atrophic sharply defined red patches in the dorsum and sides: the atrophy in pernicious anaemia is evenly spread and the mucosa pale and dry. Spiced food causes pain. The condition may be met in allergic states, nutritional deficiencies, and with certain drug eruptions (e.g. reserpine).

Smoking and the effects of tea or other *hot liquid* or *food* may cause acute pain in the tongue lasting for days after the cause has ceased to act. *Pungent condiments* such as capsicum, cayenne pepper, ginger, and the like may similarly be responsible.

Minor viral diseases. Foot-and-mouth disease may rarely be contracted by humans from infected farm animals or consumed milk or milk products from infected herds, vesicles appearing in the mouth and on the tongue. In the so-called 'hand-foot-and-mouth disease', probably due to Coxsackie A viruses, children are affected. Vesicular stomatitis contracted from horses, cattle, and pigs occurs in North and South America.

Carcinoma of the tongue (*Fig.* 782) starts as a nodule, fissure, or ulcer, usually on the lateral border of the organ. At first painless, it becomes painful as it invades and becomes grossly septic. The pain often radiates to the ear, being referred from the lingual branch of the trigeminal nerve supplying the tongue along its auriculotemporal branch. Ulceration is accompanied by bleeding; hence the typical picture of late disease is an old man spitting blood into his handkerchief with a plug of cotton-wool in his ear.

Harold Ellis.

TONGUE, SWELLING OF

Swelling of the tongue is a condition the nature of which is generally obvious on inspection and palpation, if the history is taken into account at the same time. Many causes given in the following list need little detailed discussion:

1. Causes of Acute Swelling of the Tongue:

A bite or sting

Injury, for instance by a fish-bone, or by biting during an epileptic fit

Corrosives or acute irritant applications

Acute oedema, secondary to:
  a. Inflammatory conditions within the mouth—stomatitis (p. 661)
  b. The effects of certain drugs, e.g., mercury, rarely aspirin
  c. Erythema bullosum or pemphigus (p. 117)
  d. Variola
  e. Serum injections and other conditions liable to cause giant urticaria
  f. Angioneurotic oedema

Haemorrhage into the substance of the tongue, as in scurvy, leukaemia, and other haemorrhagic states.

2. Causes of Chronic or Persistent Swelling of the Tongue:

A. Where the Swelling is General:
  Macroglossia
  Cretinism
  Myxoedema
  Mongolism
  Acromegaly
  Primary amyloidosis

B. Where the Swelling is Local or Asymmetrical:
  Irritation by a dental plate or decayed tooth
  Epithelioma
  Gumma
  Leucoplakia (chronic superficial glossitis)
  Tuberculous infiltration
  Actinomycosis
  Ranula
  Calculus in a sublingual salivary gland
  Suprahyoid cyst
  Haemangioma or lymphangioma
  Sarcoma
  Lipoma.

If the nature of the tongue enlargement is not obvious from the history and simple inspection and palpation—as will probably be the case when it is due to a *bite, sting, injury, corrosive* or *irritant* application, after the use of *serum, mercury, aspirin,* or other drugs, *variola, pemphigus,* or *erythema multiforme* (*Fig.* 783)—it may be so from the concomitant symptoms, as in the case of *cretinism* (p. 223), *acromegaly* (p. 277), *mongolism* (p. 234), or *myxoedema.*

Simple *macroglossia* is rare; when it does occur the history is that it dates from youth or childhood, and the patient may otherwise be perfectly normal, unless he also has some other congenital peculiarity, such as macrocheilia (blubber-lips).

The chronic local lesions associated with swelling are in many cases accompanied by superficial ulceration, and the difficulties that may arise in distinguishing *simple, syphilitic,* and *epitheliomatous* trouble are discussed under TONGUE, ULCERATION OF (*below*). *Tuberculous* and *actinomycotic glossitis* are both rare, and may be mistaken for malignant or syphilitic disease. Tuberculous lesions are usually painful and this cause should always be thought of when considering the possible causes of a painful swollen tongue, particularly as the manifesta-

tongue, and *Ludwig's angina*. This is an acute inflammatory condition, often streptococcal in origin, affecting the floor of the mouth and tongue, and spreading rapidly through the deeper structures of the mouth, throat, and neck, and causing extreme swelling of all adjacent tissues.

Angioneurotic oedema of the tongue is rare, but it is important because it may, rarely, prove

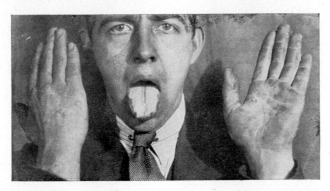

Fig. 783. Erythema multiforme bullosum affecting the tongue. (*Dr. S. Ernest Dore.*)

tions of tuberculosis of the tongue may assume unusual and bizarre forms. *Ranula* and *sublingual salivary gland calculus* or *cyst* both cause swellings that are beneath the front part of the tongue rather than in its substance, generally bulging up one side of the floor of the mouth near the fraenum linguae. A ranula is a distended mucous gland, and after enlarging slowly to perhaps the size of a chestnut, it often ceases to grow further; it does not fluctuate in its dimensions in relationship to meals as a salivary gland swelling often does. *Riga's disease*, allied to ranula, is a granuloma of the fraenum linguae resulting from infection behind the lower incisor teeth in a dirty mouth; it occurs mainly in children and may persist for months.

A *suprahyoid cyst* is situated in the root of the tongue posteriorly, where it arises from remains of the obsolete thyroglossal duct. It is seldom large; its nature is suggested by its situation.

An *angioma* of the tongue is rare; sometimes, however, after remaining latent for years, it grows with rapidity and necessitates an operation. The diagnosis may be suggested by the colour of the tumour, but histological examination subsequent to removal may be required before one can be sure whether the tumour is a simple angioma, an angiosarcoma, or a *sarcoma*.

A *lipoma* occurs not infrequently in the tongue and its lobulated form generally breaks surface and presents like a cluster of soft white cherries.

Haemorrhage into the substance of the tongue, with swelling and inability to speak or eat may result from certain blood disorders, such as acute leukaemia or primary or secondary thrombocytopenic purpura (*see* PURPURA, p. 669).

Acute oedema of the tongue may be due to *severe stomatitis, angioneurotic oedema of the*

fatal. As a rule there is a history of previous similar attacks in other parts of the body (*see* p. 589) and other members of the family may have had similar episodes. Tracheotomy may, though very rarely, be necessary as a life-saving measure, the diagnosis becoming clear only when the oedema of the tongue and adjacent parts subsides almost as rapidly as it came on, and the patient develops similar neurotic oedema, probably in other parts, on subsequent occasions.

R. G. Beard.

TONGUE, ULCERATION OF

To enable a good view to be obtained of the affected part the patient should be seated in a good light and the protruded tongue gently dried with a piece of soft linen. The presence of an ulcer being ascertained, its nature may be considered under the following heads: (1) *Carcinomatous*; (2) *Syphilitic*; (3) *Dental*; (4) *Tuberculous*; (5) *Ulcer in connexion with stomatitis*.

1. Carcinomatous Ulcer is much commoner in men than in women. It is practically unknown before the age of 30, and rarely starts before 45. The foul smell of the breath and the ill and wearied expression of the patient may awaken suspicion before the tongue is seen, for the sloughing ulcer is usually heavily infected, and the toxic absorption combined with pain and loss of sleep have a rapid and marked effect upon health. The tongue in a normal individual can be protruded from one to one and a half inches beyond the teeth; if the protrusion is limited, or if the tongue is not protruded straight, it can generally be inferred, except in cases of paralysis, that there is some tumour binding it down.

The position of the ulcer is to be studied and its relation to any sharp and carious tooth. An epithelioma is usually on the side of the tongue, but it may be anywhere on the upper, lateral, or under-surface or on the floor of the mouth, but is hardly ever exactly in the midline.

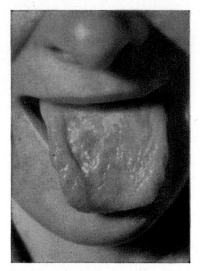

Fig. 784. Infiltrating surface epithelioma on dorsum of tongue. (*Mr. Grant Massie.*)

As regards the ulcer itself, the typical appearance when fairly developed may be described as irregular, deep, foul, sloughy, with raised nodular everted edges, and a surrounding area of induration. Other types associated with minimal ulceration of the mucous membrane are the scirrhus, where there is an excessive fibroblastic reaction, and the affected part of the tongue is shrivelled up as in the similar atrophic scirrhous cancer of the breast; and the nodular, where the lesion is mostly buried within the substance of the tongue and, like an iceberg, broaches the surface over a deceptively small area. In addition, the papilliferous type and multiple ulceration are not uncommon. Lastly there is the fissure carcinoma associated with leucoplakia (*Fig.* 785). Except in early cases some of the lymphatic glands are enlarged and hard, and they may be fixed. The submandibular group is generally the first affected, but the disease sometimes misses these and invades the carotid and even the supraclavicular glands. Examination, therefore, should not be concluded before the whole of the neck has been palpated. The diagnosis should have been made, however, before the disease has developed thus far; in its earliest stages an epithelioma may be represented by a superficial ulcer no more than a sixteenth of an inch in diameter, by a crack or a small lump, without any enlargement of the glands. In all these conditions, however, the ulcer is already hard and very resistant to any form of treatment. Any ulcer of the tongue occurring in a middle-aged man, and lasting for more than two or three weeks, should always awaken suspicion. (*Figs.* 784, 787.)

DIAGNOSIS FROM SYPHILITIC ULCER. This may be a very real difficulty, owing to the fact that the two conditions may exist side by side (*Fig.* 786), and that the syphilitic leucoplakia or leucomic

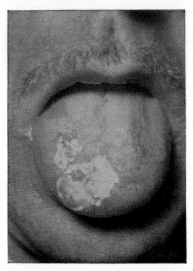

Fig. 785. Non-syphilitic leucoplakia of tongue.

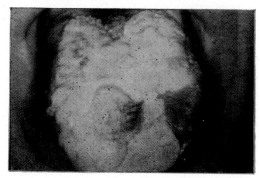

Fig. 786. Syphilitic leucoplakia of tongue with central epithelioma. (*Professor Martin Rushton.*)

wart may be the actual precursor of a cancer. Positive serological reactions, therefore, are not proof that an epithelioma is not present. If a well-formed gumma is present, antisyphilitic remedies soon make a great change in its appearance. Although a biopsy is necessary for a definite diagnosis, certain clinical criteria are characteristic and a putative diagnosis of gumma may be made when the ulcer is centrally situated, painless, serpiginous in outline, and has the steep-cut edges and wash-leather slough base typical of syphilitic ulcers elsewhere.

DIAGNOSIS FROM DENTAL ULCER. The ulcer in this case is caused by a carious or otherwise jagged tooth, and therefore is in a corresponding position on the tongue. Further, the ulcer is soft to the touch, and heals rapidly when the offending tooth is stopped or extracted. There is seldom difficulty in differentiation except when the ulcer is of very long standing.

2. Syphilitic Ulcer. This may be primary, secondary, or tertiary.

PRIMARY SYPHILIS or CHANCRE is certainly rare on the tongue, and, owing partly to its rarity and partly to the fact that it is unexpected, it is frequently missed. It is more common in men than in women, but it may occur even in children.

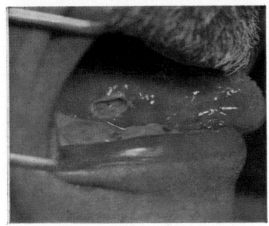

Fig. 787. Ulceration from epithelioma of the tongue. (Courtesy of the Gordon Museum, Guy's Hospital.)

It starts as a small pimple which ulcerates and becomes indurated, though the induration is not so marked as when it is situated on the glans penis. The appearance of a secondary rash with general enlargement of the lymphatic glands would indicate the true diagnosis. Further proof is supplied by positive serological tests, and the detection of spirochaetae in serum from the sore. Furthermore, the sore heals rapidly under the influence of treatment.

SECONDARY SYPHILIS manifests itself by the formation of mucous patches and superficial ulcers. The latter are almost always multiple, and situated along the edges and tip of the tongue, and with them are also found similar sores on the mucous membrane of the cheek, lips, palate, and tonsil, and at the edges of the mouth. The ulcers are small, round, painful, with sharply cut edges and a greyish floor. Other secondary symptoms will be present to make the diagnosis clear.

TERTIARY SYPHILIS or GUMMATOUS ULCERATIONS. These are divided into superficial and deep. *Superficial* gummata begin as small round-celled infiltrations in the mucous and submucous tissue. The ulcers are usually shallow, often irregular and associated with chronic glossitis, fissures, and leucoplakia. Though rare today they are extremely important, for they may be followed by epithelioma. The ulcers themselves are not at first indurated, but if surrounded by interstitial fibrosis may appear hard; a histological examination is essential if there is the

least doubt. A deep gumma starts as a hard swelling in the substance of the tongue. It is usually situated in the midline, and in the posterior half. Later it softens, breaks down, and shows itself as a deep cavity with irregular soft steep-cut walls, and a wash-leather-like slough at its base. It is not painful, and does not increase progressively in size. The important thing is to distinguish it from epithelioma and tuberculous disease. Unlike epithelioma it does not infiltrate widely or fix the tongue, its history is short, and it causes no pain. Furthermore, it yields rapidly to anti-syphilitic treatment.

3. Dental Ulcer is due to repeated small injuries from the sharp edge of a decayed tooth, and is situated opposite the tooth, generally on the side of the tongue. The ulcer is small, superficial, and not indurated unless it is of long standing. It is therefore not easily mistaken for any other kind of ulcer, or if doubt arises it is allayed by the healing of the ulcer on appropriate dental treatment: failure to heal within a fortnight suggests that it is an epithelioma.

There is a form of dental ulcer which is found on the fraenum of the tongue in children suffering from whooping-cough; during the violent expiratory spasms peculiar to the illness, the under-surface of the tongue may suffer from rubbing over the lower incisor teeth.

4. Tuberculous Ulcer of the Tongue is rare, but it occurs at that period of life during which tuberculous disease of the lung is common, between the ages of 15 and 35. It is due to infection with tubercle bacilli brought up into the mouth. The ulcer itself is usually on the tip of the tongue or the side in its anterior half and is generally painful, although sometimes entirely painless. The outline is irregular. The edges are usually thin and undermined, and the base is covered by pale granulations, or excavated clearly down to the underlying muscle-fibres; less commonly the edges are raised, though never everted or hard, and the base is nodular, sloughy, or caseous. It has often been mistaken for epithelioma or gumma. The fact that it is not hard, that it is usually painful, and that pulmonary tuberculosis is present should point to the true diagnosis. Negative serological tests exclude a syphilitic gumma, though histological proof may be necessary by biopsy, and cultures or animal tests for bacteriological confirmation. A further example of tuberculous ulceration is the so-called 'truncated tongue'. In this type there is an oedematous infiltration of the parenchyma of the tongue, causing it to become swollen and almost 'woody', and there is a shallow ulceration of the tip, giving an appearance as if part of the tongue had been amputated. In fact the clinical manifestations of tuberculosis of the tongue are so protean that this disease should always be suspected in unusual lesions, especially if associated with pain.

5. Ulcers in connexion with Stomatitis (Ulcerative Stomatitis). Septic infection of the mouth due to a variety of causes, such as irritation from

26

decayed teeth, alkalis, acids, or mercury, may be accompanied by the formation of small vesicles which, on bursting, give rise to superficial ulcers (*Fig.* 788). They are not limited to the tongue, but appear as well on the mucous membrane of the cheeks and gums. Aphthous stomatitis commonly occurs in conjunction with the febrile diseases of childhood. It is characterized by the formation of whitish spots on the buccal mucous membrane; and by the shedding of epithelium small superficial ulcers may be formed. The

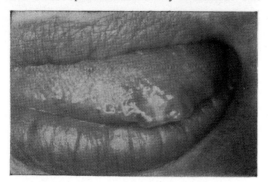

Fig. 788. Aphthous ulcer. (*Professor Martin Rushton.*)

ulcers of the tongue here occur in the course of a general inflammation of the mouth. One type that may be resistant to treatment is produced by Vincent's angina organisms; bacteriological tests give the diagnosis, but it may be suggested by the extreme foetor of the breath.

When ulceration of the tongue, and at the same time, very probably of the inside of the mouth generally, occurs in such conditions as *smallpox, chicken-pox, pemphigus, hydroa,* and other conditions that may affect the buccal mucosa as well as the skin, the diagnosis depends, not upon the appearances of the ulcers or the tongue, but upon the concomitant skin eruption.

R. G. Beard.

TRISMUS

Trismus, or lockjaw, signifies a maintained muscular spasm tending to closure of the jaws so that the mouth cannot be opened. The term does not include mechanical inability to open the jaws owing to such affections as mumps, alveolar abscess with surrounding inflammatory oedema, injury, Ludwig's angina, quinsy or severe tonsillitis, an odontoma, epithelioma of the mouth, myositis ossificans, and cervicofacial actinomycosis. There are two conditions which may not at first sight be obvious, but may lock the jaws together and simulate true trismus—*impaction of a wisdom tooth*, and *arthritic changes in the temporomandibular joint*. These are diagnosed by careful local examination of the teeth and of the joint respectively; in the latter case there may be arthritic changes in other joints

also. X-ray examination may be required to detect the joint changes or the impacted wisdom teeth (*Fig.* 789).

Circumstantial evidence will generally serve to distinguish trismus due to *hysteria* or to *facial neuralgia*; any doubt at first experienced is dispelled if the patient is watched for a while. Convulsive seizures in a hysterical patient with trismus can generally be distinguished from those due to tetanus or to strychnine poisoning by their polymorphous character, and by the fact that touching the patient, and other similar stimulation, does

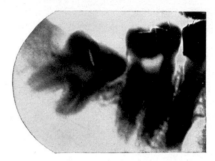

Fig. 789. Radiograph showing impacted third molar. (*Dr. Parker Tupling.*)

not bring them on so certainly as would be the case with strychnine or tetanus.

In fits, e.g., epilepsy, the trismus is of short duration and offers no difficulty in diagnosis.

Malingering may sometimes take the form of lockjaw, and it may be a little while before the fraud can be detected. In sleep the malingerer's muscles relax completely.

Catalepsy may include trismus amongst its varieties of maintained muscular contractions; the general mental symptoms will assist the diagnosis, and as a rule there are no convulsive seizures. Trismus may also occur in *Encephalitis*.

Trichiniasis is rare, but if infected pork is eaten raw, or insufficiently cooked, the larvae of the parasites find their way to many different muscles, and they show predilection for those of the tongue, mouth, and jaws. The resultant irritation, pain, and stiffness cause trismus, the origin of which may be difficult to determine unless the history points to pork. The patient is very ill in the earlier stages, with high fever, and the condition may be fatal. The malady may be epidemic. The blood exhibits eosinophilia. The final criterion of the diagnosis is the discovery of the typical parasites coiled up in their little oval cysts amongst the affected muscle-fibres.

Hydrophobia (Rabies) and **Tetany** seldom exhibit trismus as a prominent symptom. The former, though now almost unknown in Great Britain, would suggest itself if a convulsive illness developed after a bite by a dog, wolf, or other similar animal, particularly if the spasmodic muscular difficulty is markedly increased by efforts at swallowing. The symptoms may not develop for weeks or months after the bite, so that the patient may fall ill when he has come from a country overseas where rabies is endemic. *Tetany*, also rare, is at once distinguished by its typical carpopedal contractions; trismus, almost constant in tetanus, is nearly always absent in tetany.

Strychnine poisoning gives rise to generalized twitchings and convulsions long before trismus, the lateness of the development of the latter serving to distinguish it from tetanus. Furthermore there is complete muscular relaxation between spasms. There may be evidence of strychnine having been taken or administered, either by the mouth or hypodermically; the symptoms develop very acutely, and are often rapidly fatal.

Tetanus is the cause *par excellence* of trismus. The diagnosis is often obvious if the illness develops in an otherwise healthy person, with stiffness starting usually in the neck muscles, spreading to those of the face and jaw, and thence to the rest of the trunk and limbs, with extremely painful exacerbations on the slightest stimulation even by a stroke with a feather or the banging of a door; dysphagia; risus sardonicus (q.v.); opisthotonos; no complete relaxation of the stiff muscles unless an anaesthetic be given; a duration of days rather than hours; especially if all these things follow a few days, or a week or more, after a small penetrating wound which becomes septic. It may be possible to demonstrate the presence of the drum-stick bacilli in films prepared from the deeper parts of the wound. The chief difficulty arises when there is no clear history, or when the wound has been so small that it has healed or cannot be found; even then, most cases are so typical that they can be diagnosed as tetanus without difficulty. Unnecessary anxiety arises chiefly in cases of an impacted wisdom tooth, or of hysteria, where tetanus may be suspected at first; the subsequent course of the malady soon serves to exclude this. Involvement of the temporo-mandibular joint in a *serum reaction*, especially if prophylactic tetanus antitoxin has been given, may lead to the belief that tetanus has in fact set in.

Trismus may be simulated by *scleroderma* of the face. But here the condition is rather one of fixation of the skin than of the muscles; the skin becomes like parchment so that one cannot pick it up between the fingers, it feels firm or almost hard, and the patient becomes unable to open the mouth properly. The disease is of slow onset and gradual progress, so that there is seldom difficulty in diagnosis; but occasionally there are acute exacerbations in the scleroderma process, with rapid increase in the local pain and stiffness, but rarely is there difficulty in distinguishing it from true trismus.

Ian Mackenzie.

UMBILICAL REGION, PAIN IN

Pain felt by the patient at or near the navel may arise in the umbilicus itself, or may be referred to that region from some distant lesion.

Pain arising in the Umbilicus. If the pain is due to some cause in the umbilicus itself it will be accurately localized to the cicatrix. Movements of the abdominal wall will be restricted, and the umbilicus will be tender to palpation. Many abnormalities are found at this site, but they are usually painless unless infected.

UMBILICAL HERNIA. This is common in infants and in fat middle-aged people. The hernia of infants is a small spherical swelling, easily reducible and usually symptomless; indeed, in an infant the presence of a hernia should never be accepted as the cause of umbilical pain till more likely causes such as appendicitis and spinal caries have been eliminated. In old women the hernia is usually just above the umbilicus, and the umbilical scar is seen as a transverse slit just below the centre of the swelling. These herniae of adults give an impulse on coughing, but are rarely completely reducible. They are painless, unless something has gone wrong with their coverings or their contents. A localized throbbing pain, with redness and tenderness of the skin, but unaccompanied by colic or any feeling of illness, points to a local infection of the skin. More deep-seated pain suggests strangulation of the contents. If the swelling is irreducible and tender on compression, though the skin over it is normal, strangulation must be diagnosed; omentum alone may be involved, in which case the colic and vomiting of an intestinal obstruction are absent, but the distinction is unimportant, for immediate operation is required in either case.

ECZEMA AND SUPPURATION OF THE UMBILICAL SCAR. This is seen where owing to fat or an umbilical hernia the scar is deepened and leads to a retention of the secretions. The diagnosis is obvious.

EXTENSION OF ABDOMINAL LESIONS TO THE UMBILICUS. Chronic abdominal infections, such as tuberculous and pneumococcal peritonitis, and growths, particularly those of the stomach, may reach the umbilicus. The discovery of an abscess or a nodule in this situation may give the clue to some obscure abdominal pain, but the lump itself is usually painless.

Pain referred to the Umbilicus. Pain arising in any of the viscera supplied by sympathetic nerves is referred to an area roughly corresponding to the embryonic position of the viscus concerned. That due to stimulation of pain fibres in the spinal nerves, or in the tracts of the cord to which they lead, is felt in the segment supplied by those nerves. The 'visceral level' of the umbilicus is that part of the alimentary tract supplied by the superior mesenteric artery, that is, from the second part of the duodenum to the middle of the transverse colon; the segmental level is the 10th dorsal nerve and its corresponding cord segment. Visceral pain is often colicky and unpleasant, but described with difficulty in words; referred to a diffuse and indefinite area, usually accompanied at first by nausea or vomiting. Pain arising in spinal nerves is accurately localized, burning or aching in character, and often associated with muscular guarding or rigidity, and with hyperaesthesia in the skin of the part concerned.

PAIN ARISING IN THE AREA SUPPLIED BY THE VISCERAL NERVES. Appendicitis; Intestinal obstruction; Intestinal colic.

The commonest and by far the most important variety of pain in the umbilical region is a colic accompanied by nausea and vomiting. The three conditions mentioned above give an identical

and the unwillingness to bend should call attention to the spine. Localized tenderness will be found over one of the vertebrae, even in those rare cases where no deformity can yet be seen. A radiograph will confirm the diagnosis. Pains may also be referred from other spinal disorders such as crush fractures, neoplastic deposits, or ankylosing spondylitis.

Tabes Dorsalis. The only complaint of the patient may be of abdominal pain, often referred to the

DIFFERENTIAL DIAGNOSIS OF PAIN IN THE UMBILICAL REGION

	APPENDICITIS	INTESTINAL OBSTRUCTION	COLIC DUE TO IRRITANTS
History	Possibly previous attacks	Herniae. Previous operations or history of peritonitis. Swallowed foreign body in child or gall-stone in adult	Doubtful food. Others in family affected
Pain	Passes from colic at umbilicus to steady pain in right iliac fossa	Remains colicky and increases in severity	Remains colicky but relieved by vomiting or diarrhoea and tends to ease
Vomiting	Soon ceases, but may return if peritonitis extensive	Increases in frequency. Vomit becomes intestinal	Maximal at beginning and decreases
Bowels	Constipated, but enema produces action	Constipation absolute, even to flatus after the bowel distal to the obstruction has been evacuated	Diarrhoea soon appears unless forestalled by enemas
Temperature and pulse	Temperature 99°–102° F. Pulse raised moderately	Temperature normal or subnormal. Pulse mounting steadily	Temperature normal or subnormal. Pulse in ordinary case soon returns to normal
Abdominal wall	First slight tenderness over appendix. Later more marked tenderness and guarding	Usually no tenderness. Distension and peristalsis may be seen	No visible or palpable abnormality
Auscultation	Silence round caecum: normal sounds elsewhere	Increased peristaltic sounds	Increased peristaltic sounds
Rectal examination	Faeces. May be tender in peritoneum	No faeces. No tenderness	Faeces. No tenderness

clinical picture in the early stages, and it cannot be insisted too strongly that such a picture always calls for careful observation, and that an aperient or the use of morphine must be prohibited till the diagnosis is clear. The main points in differentiation are shown in the table above.

Other Visceral Pain referred to the Umbilicus. The pain of gall-stone colic, or the early pain of an acute pancreatitis, may be referred to the umbilicus, but is usually higher. Renal colic may exceptionally centre on the umbilicus. In each case the diagnosis is usually facilitated by other signs and symptoms implicating the organ concerned.

PAIN ARISING IN THE SPINAL NERVES AND SPINAL CORD

Chest Conditions. An early pleurisy may be characterized by sharp umbilical pain. The high temperature, rapid breathing, and working of the alae nasi will usually suggest that the lesion is above the diaphragm.

Spinal Caries. In children complaint of pain at the umbilicus may be the first symptom of tuberculous disease. The peculiar rigidity of the trunk

region of the umbilicus. The typical gastric crises may be replaced by a much more diffuse pain. A systematic examination of the central nervous system should be made in all cases.

Lead Poisoning. Severe attacks of cramp-like abdominal pains referred to the umbilicus may be the chief or even the only symptom. The patient's occupation may suggest the diagnosis, or a blue line may be seen on the gums during the routine examination. For other characteristic signs of plumbism *see* p. 53.

Tumour of the Spinal Column or *Cord,* and *Compression Myelitis.* Though a less common source of error, these must be borne in mind. The pain is usually of a girdle character, and some evidence of interference with the motor or sensory tracts supplying the lower limbs can be found.

R. G. Beard.

URETHRA, FAECES PASSED THROUGH

Faeces or faecal fluid are passed per urethram only when the bladder is in fistulous communication with some part of the bowel, or with an abscess infected with the *Escherichia coli*. PNEUMATURIA (p. 644) may occur at the same time. The chief causes are as follows:

Diverticular disease of the sigmoid colon with a fistula into the bladder (the commonest cause)

Carcinoma of the bladder opening into the rectum or into some loop of bowel which has become adherent to the bladder

Carcinoma of the rectum ⎫ opening into the blad-
Carcinoma of the sigmoid ⎪ der either directly or
colon ⎬ through the medium of
Carcinoma of the caecum ⎭ an intervening abscess

Carcinoma of the uterus opening both into the bladder and into the rectum

Crohn's disease of large or small bowel with vesical fistula

Prostatitis or prostatic abscess opening into the rectum

Rectovesical fistula from injury and sloughing, particularly after childbirth

Appendicular abscess opening into the bladder

Pelvic actinomycosis

The passage of faeces into the urine may be simulated by some cases of very foetid cystitis due to infection by *E. coli* especially in diabetic subjects.

If the symptom is due to carcinoma it matters little which viscus is the primary site by the time the growth has involved both bladder and bowel. The differentiation resolves itself, therefore, between malignant and non-malignant conditions. If malignant disease is not obvious it will nearly always be advisable to resort to surgical measures in the hope of discovering some curable primary condition—rectal, appendicular, prostatic, or otherwise. The diagnosis will be suggested by the history and confirmed by local examination or exploration.

Harold Ellis.

URETHRAL DISCHARGE

Causes:

1. Gonorrhoea
2. Non-specific urethritis
3. Trichomoniasis
4. Bacterial:
   Esch. coli
   Haemophilus
   Ducrey's bacillus
   Tuberculosis
5. Chemical
6. Traumatic:
   Instrumental
   Accidental
7. New growth
8. Foreign bodies

Any inflammatory process in the urethra causes a discharge. Although most commonly the result of infection by the *gonococcus*, by no means every urethritis is of this nature, and bacteriological examinations show that other organisms besides the gonococcus may produce a urethral discharge and the same symptoms as gonorrhoea. Further than this, a purulent discharge may occur in which no micro-organisms can be found; for instance, when the urethra has been injured or subjected to irritation by the injection of strong solutions, or when it contains a foreign body, such as a calculus or a retained catheter.

There is no doubt that an acute *non-specific* urethritis may be caused by other organisms than the gonococcus, and sometimes there is considerable trouble in completely curing it. These cases may cause complications in the genito-urinary organs similar to those due to the gonococcus, such as prostatitis, epididymitis, or cystitis. They may arise by the infection of the urethra by septic instrumentation, or after connexion with a woman with trichomoniasis. A careful bacteriological examination should always be made in order to determine the causative organism. An acute urethritis may accompany a haematogenous urinary infection; for instance, an acute infection of the upper-urinary tract due to *Bacillus coli* may be followed by acute cystitis, prostatitis, and urethritis, in which no other organism but *B. coli* can be found. *Non-specific (non-gonococcal) urethritis* is due to unknown infective agents. It is usually a venereal disease contracted in coitus. A watery, whitish penile discharge in males may be associated with mild dysuria and lower abdominal discomfort. The discharge may be so slight as to be overlooked, but there is a tendency for exacerbations and remissions to occur, and the urethral discharge is sometimes purulent, serous, or mucopurulent, often responding to tetracycline or tetracycline plus sulpha therapy. In Reiter's (Brodie's) disease there is arthritis and sometimes conjunctivitis in addition (*see* p. 463). In such cases although the urethritis may respond to tetracycline therapy, the arthritis does not. Reiter's disease, although commonly venereal in origin in Great Britain, may follow bacillary dysentery.

Gonorrhoeal Urethritis is due to the infection of the urethra by the gonococcus (*Neisseria gonorrhoeae*). The gonococcus is seen in a stained specimen to be *intracellular*, penetrating not only the leucocytes but also the epithelial cells found in a smear preparation, and, although the cocci may be found also between the cells, their appearance in the cells is strong evidence of their specific nature.

In any case presenting a purulent discharge from the urethra it is necessary, in order that appropriate treatment may be carried out, first to make a smear of the discharge for bacteriological examination, and secondly to make a culture of the discharge in order to determine drug sensitivity of the organisms, and also to confirm the smear test.

A gonococcal complement fixation test (G.C.F.T.) is not useful in diagnosis of early cases. It must be established that the pus comes from the urethra and not from beneath the prepuce. For the purposes of clinical investigation the urethra is divided into anterior and posterior portions, separated by the membranous urethra, the anterior comprising the bulbous and penile urethra, and the posterior the prostatic portion. A urethritis is also, according to its clinical aspect, acute or chronic, the acute form being characterized by a thick, creamy, purulent discharge, with pain, and the chronic by a thin, greyish, mucopurulent discharge. Acute gonorrhoea affects not only the superficial layers of the urethral mucous membrane, but also the subepithelial tissues and the glandular elements, causing a leucocytic infiltration. The tendency of the inflammation is to spread backwards along the canal so that the prostatic urethra may become infected even in the acute stage, though most frequently this occurs at a later period; the prostatic and the ejaculatory ducts may become infected, and the inflammation may spread to the seminal vesicles and epididymes. In the acute stages of the disease the infection of the anterior urethra is accompanied, as a rule, by redness of the external meatus, scalding pain during micturition, and painful emissions. These patients have described the pain on micturition as like passing red-hot fish-hooks through the urethra. Occasionally all pain is absent, especially in patients previously infected with gonorrhoea. If the anterior urethra alone is infected and the urine is passed into two glasses, the first portion will be turbid from admixture with the urethral discharge, whilst the second portion may remain clear.

When the posterior urethra becomes infected in the acute stages the symptoms are much more severe. Micturition is more painful and greatly increased in frequency, both by day and by night, the patient often being obliged to pass urine every half-hour. It may follow that prostatic abscess develops to complicate posterior urethritis, in which case micturition becomes very painful, or a painful retention of urine may occur. There is usually an associated high fever and a rigor. On rectal examination the prostate is found much swollen, hot to the touch, and extremely tender, while with an abscess a soft fluctuating area may be felt. An acute posterior gonorrhoea is only rarely accompanied by infection of the bladder, cystitis supervening on the urethritis.

The gonococcus is now usually insensitive to the sulphonamides. Current standard treatment comprises one intramuscular injection of 1·2 million units (1·2 g.) of procaine penicillin in the male or 3 daily injections at this dosage in the female. Some strains are relatively insensitive and, if cure is not obtained, culture and sensitivity of the organism are determined and appropriate treatment prescribed. This is usually Septrin (co-trimoxazole), 4 tablets twice daily for 2 days (each tablet contains trimethoprim 80 mg. and sulphamethoxazole 400 mg.).

In any case of chronic urethral discharge examination should be conducted to ascertain not only the seat of infection, but also the nature of the lesion promoting the discharge. For this purpose the patient is directed to pass urine into two separate glasses; if there is turbidity due to excess of phosphates this is cleared by the addition of acetic acid, when, if any threads or plugs of mucopus are present in the first specimen, they probably arise from the posterior urethra, whereas pus in, or turbidity of, the second shows that cystitis is present in addition. If threads are still present the test is carried out at weekly intervals until the urine is clear in both glasses. Follow-up tests are made by examining the urethral efflux following prostatic massage. If this test is normal a final test by passage of bougies and urethroscopy to eliminate presence of stricture, granulomatous areas, and polyps will complete the treatment and tests of cure. A precautionary serological test for syphilis should always be carried out 3 months after treatment with penicillin.

With successful treatment the purulent urethral discharge will disappear within 24 hours and the patient will be symptom-free in 2–3 days.

Since 1964 a fluorescent antibody test (Pariser, Farmer, and Marino) has been developed for the diagnosis of gonorrhoea in cases where the organism has escaped detection by smear or culture.

A urethral discharge may in rare cases be present in other conditions than that produced by gonorrhoea or non-specific urethritis, and as difficulty may arise if one of these cases is met with it is necessary to mention them.

Herpetic Urethritis. The mucous lining of the urethra may be affected by herpes in the same manner as other mucous membranes. There is irritation of the urethra during micturition, and a slight mucopurulent discharge from the meatus. The small vesicles may be seen by the endoscope, and may be associated with herpes of the prepuce or glans penis.

Soft Sores in the Urethra are distinctly uncommon. They occur in the terminal portion of the urethra, and cause painful micturition and a profuse, thin, purulent discharge, which contains no gonococci; Ducrey's bacillus may be found. There may be other sores on the glans penis, and an ulcerated surface will be seen on endoscopic examination. They occur within a few days of infection, and, if extensive, may produce narrowing of the urethra on healing. Lymph-nodes in the groins may be enlarged and tender.

Syphilis may affect the urethra either as a hard chancre or as a gumma.

The *chancre* occurs in the terminal inch of the urethra, forming a firm indurated mass which can be felt readily on external palpation. The meatus is oedematous and swollen, so that the introduction of an endoscopic tube is impossible; there is a thin, purulent, and often blood-stained discharge from the meatus. A urethral chancre must be diagnosed carefully from peri-urethral infiltration due to urethritis; the period of incubation from time of infection, the presence of small, hard inguinal glands, the occurrence of secondary lesions of syphilis, and positive serological tests will point to the diagnosis. The

Treponema pallidum (*Spirochaeta pallida*) may be found in the fluid expressed from the surface of the sore.

Gumma of the urethra is now extremely rare; it gives rise to a watery urethral discharge when it ulcerates. It may ulcerate through the canal and form fistulae, but may usually be recognized on careful examination.

Papillomata of the Urethra may occur either in the anterior or posterior portion, as small, pedunculated tumours in the canal, and frequently as a sequel to a chronic gonorrhoea. They may arise, however, in the urethra of a patient who has never had urethritis. They cause a thin, scanty discharge together with spontaneous urethral bleeding; they are seen readily through the endoscope and some are often visible when the lips of the meatus are retracted (*see Fig*. 373, p. 348).

Carcinoma of the urethra is very rare as a primary disease, and many of the cases recorded have been in association with stricture. It forms a tumour in the urethra palpable from the exterior, and causes painful micturition with a blood-stained discharge, and enlargement of the inguinal glands. Suspicion of carcinoma should arise if a hard, irregular tumour is felt in the course of the urethra, without gonorrhoeal infection, in an elderly patient. Carcinoma of the urethra may also occur as an extension from carcinoma of the bladder or prostate or as a malignant change in urethral papilloma; the papillary type will not be palpable from the exterior. The final diagnosis depends on histological examination of a portion of the growth, removed for biopsy through an endoscopic tube. An irrigating posterior urethroscope or panendoscope is the best instrument for this purpose.

Tuberculosis of the Urethra is always secondary to disease elsewhere in the genito-urinary tract, usually of the prostate or seminal vesicles; it is very rare. Tubercle bacilli may be found in the urethral smear.

Foreign Bodies in the Urethra may cause a purulent urethral discharge if they remain for any length of time. They may be introduced through the meatus by intent—matches, pins, etc.; or a piece may be detached from a damaged catheter; or a small calculus may come down from the bladder and be arrested; in the latter case the history is usually clear—sudden stoppage of the stream of urine during micturition, with penile pain; a calculus may be felt from the exterior or seen through the endoscope.

Harold Ellis.

URINE, ABNORMAL COLORATION OF

The normal amber colour of urine is due mainly to urochrome, a pigment of unknown constitution. The colour may be diminished, increased, or altered in character.

Pale urine is usually dilute, and associated with a diuresis. This is most commonly physiological, and is a normal response to a high fluid intake. It may be due to renal tubular failure (usually in the diuretic phase of acute oliguric renal failure), when water reabsorption from the glomerular filtrate is impaired. In this case the history usually points to the cause, and casts and protein are present in the urine. In all these cases the urinary osmolality and specific gravity are low. Osmotically active substances, such as glucose and mannitol, also impair water reabsorption, and the urine may be pale when there is much glycosuria, or when mannitol, or glucose and amino-acids are administered intravenously.

Dark urine of normal colour is usually concentrated with a high osmolality and specific gravity, and associated with oliguria. Dehydration from any cause is associated with increased reabsorption of water from the glomerular filtrate. Occasionally confusion may arise if there is mild bilirubinuria.

Orange Urines. A deep orange colour may be due to bile-pigments or to certain drugs, such as rhubarb and senna. In the former case the froth formed on shaking is yellow, and the appropriate tests are positive (*see* URINE, BILE IN, p. 809). In the latter the urine is usually alkaline and reverts to normal colour on acidification and no absorption bands are visible on spectroscopic examination.

Red Urines. A red colour in urine may be due to the presence of blood-pigments, porphyrin, uroerythrin, pyridium, beetroot, blackberries, etc., phenolphthalein in purgatives, and certain aniline dyes in sweets. Myoglobinuria may give a red- or brown-coloured urine (*see* p. 351). In the case of *porphyrinuria* (q.v.) the colour is typically 'port wine' in character, but may be pink or red. The blood-pigments are easily detected by 'Occultest' (Ames) tablets, which contain *o*-tolidine; this dye is oxidized to form a blue compound in the presence of haemoglobin, and by spectroscopic examination. The spectra of oxyhaemoglobin, reduced haemoglobin, methaemoglobin, or porphyrin may be seen (*see Fig*. 790 A–F). If much blood-pigment is present the colour may be brownish-black rather than red. The presence of intact red cells gives the urine a typical turbid or smoky appearance, whereas if the haemoglobin derivative is in solution in the urine the appearance may be that of a clear fluid (*see* HAEMOGLOBINURIA, p. 350; HAEMATURIA, p. 338). Urine containing porphyrin will also show typical absorption bands on spectroscopic examination. There may be either the acid porphyrin (*Fig*. 790 E) or those of the zinc porphyrin complex, which are very similar to those of oxyhaemoglobin. In the latter case the spectrum will revert to that of acid porphyrin on acidification with hydrochloric acid and the benzidine test will be negative. Uro-erythrin often contributes to the red colour of pathological urines but has no definite pathological significance. It is mainly seen adsorbed on deposit of urates (brick-dust deposit).

As regards the drugs mentioned, the colour due to pyramidone (amidopyrine) is not associated with a definite absorption band, and is discharged by the addition of either hydrochloric acid or sodium hydroxide. Phenolphthalein, on the other hand, gives an absorption band in the yellow-green region (556 mμ) and is decolorized by acidification. Eosin produces a pink urine with a green fluorescence. There is an absorption band in the green (520 mμ). The urine reverts to a normal colour when acidified with hydrochloric acid. The red colour due to beetroot,

before performing this test on the distillate. The untreated urine may give a purple colour with ferric chloride, but this test is not reliable. The patient may also have ochronosis, i.e., a tinting of the cartilages and conjunctivae with bluish-black phenolic oxidation products. Melanin (or melanogen) is found in the urine in cases of widely disseminated melanotic sarcoma, although it is not an invariable finding in this condition. In melanuria pigmented skin tumours will

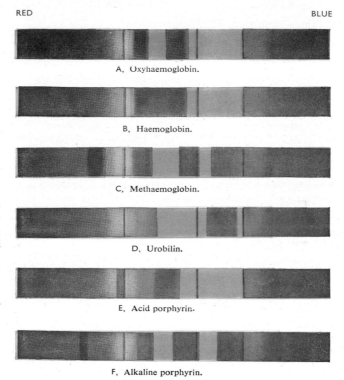

RED   BLUE

A, Oxyhaemoglobin.

B, Haemoglobin.

C, Methaemoglobin.

D, Urobilin.

E, Acid porphyrin.

F, Alkaline porphyrin.

Fig. 790. Spectral absorption bands.

blackberries, etc. (anthocyanuria) changes to yellow on making alkaline with sodium hydroxide. In cases of this type, it is usually a simple matter to find out what drug or article of diet has been given and to note the effect on the urine when it is discontinued.

Dark-brown or Black Urines. A dark-brown or black colour may be due to large amounts of methaemoglobin, to certain phenolic drugs such as phenol and cresol (carboluria), phenylhydrazine, to melanin, or rarely to the oxidation products of homogentisic acid in alkaptonuria. Even more rare is the excretion of *p*-hydroxyphenylpyruvic acid in tyrosinosis. In carboluria the colour may be greenish-brown and the urine will probably contain glycuronic acid, which will reduce Benedict's solution. Bromine water gives a white or yellow precipitate, but if protein is present the urine must be acidified and distilled

usually be present. A rare possibility is a primary melanoma in the eye with hepatic secondaries. The urine may be normal in colour when passed, but turns black on standing, from above downwards. The addition of oxidizing agents such as ferric chloride or nitric acid also produces a black colour. In the former case a browny-black precipitate of phosphates is formed. Thormählen's test, which is carried out as follows, is positive: to 5 ml of urine add a few drops of sodium nitro-prusside solution and 0·5 ml. of 40 per cent sodium hydroxide. After shaking, add sufficient glacial acetic acid to make the mixture strongly acid. A positive result is shown by a blue or blue-black colour. All these tests are tests for melanogen and are therefore not well shown by a stale urine in which the melanogen will have been converted to melanin.

In alkaptonuria the urine also darkens from above downwards or is black when passed or darkens when strong alkali is added. The metabolic congenital defect leads to accumulation and excessive excretion in the urine of homogentisic acid. The condition is present from birth and is usually noted by staining of napkins. Ochronosis may be present in later life. The urine will reduce Benedict's reagent and during this test the mixture will at once turn black if the urine was not black beforehand. It will also reduce silver nitrate solution in the cold. This is best demonstrated by adding 1 vol. of urine to 10 vol. of 3 per cent nitrate. The white precipitate of silver chloride turns grey or black in $\frac{1}{2}$–1 min. owing to reduction of the silver chloride to metallic silver. Addition of ferric chloride to the urine in alkaptonuria produces a transient green or blue colour. Homogentisic aciduria blackens undeveloped photographic films exposed to light. Its presence may be proved by chemical tests, chromatography, or specific enzyme assay.

Tyrosinosis is an even rarer inborn error of metabolism in which p-hydroxyphenyl-pyruvic acid is excreted. The urine darkens in air slowly if alkaline or after the addition of alkali, and causes some reduction of alkaline copper and ammoniacal silver nitrate solutions.

Green and Blue Urines. Such colours may be due to biliverdin, methylene blue, indigocarmine, indigo-blue, or to carbolic acid or flavine derivatives. Owing to the presence of urochrome, any blue compound in low concentration may produce a green colour. Biliverdin is an oxidation product of bilirubin and its presence in urine is usually seen in long-standing cases of obstructive jaundice. Methylene blue may be taken in proprietary pills or sweetmeats. It shows a typical absorption band in the red (668 mμ). It is partly removed from the urine by simple filtration, being adsorbed to filter-paper. It may be extracted from the urine by chloroform, and if the chloroform extract is washed with sodium hydroxide solution it is extracted in the aqueous layer, which assumes a pink colour. Indigocarmine is used as a test of renal function and its presence is therefore not as a rule unexpected. There is no absorption band and the urine is decolorized by boiling after the addition of a few drops of 10 per cent caustic soda. The substance may occasionally reach the urine from industrial dyestuffs. Flavine derivatives (acriflavine, 5-amino-acridine), which may be used as bladder wash-outs, produce a lemon-yellow urine with a green fluorescence, but no special test is usually required in this group. Indigo-blue is practically never seen in urine at the present time, but was at one time used in the treatment of epilepsy. With heavy indicanuria (q.v.) there may occasionally be sufficient oxidation of the indican to indigo-blue on standing to impart a blue tint to the phosphatic deposit.

Joan F. Zilva.

URINE, BILE IN

Bile constituents which may find their way into the urine include bilirubin, biliverdin, urobilinogen and urobilin, and bile-salts. Bilirubin imparts an orange tint but is often accompanied by its green oxidation product biliverdin. Urobilinogen is colourless but soon changes to the brown urobilin. This change may occur either before or after the urine is passed. Urine containing bile may therefore be orange, green, or brown in colour, but it is important to recognize that significant quantities of bile may be present without any colour change.

The following tests are recommended: gross amounts of *bilirubin* may be detected by shaking the urine and observing the colour of the froth, which is tinted yellow by bilirubin. Smaller but significant quantities of bilirubin will fail to give results with these tests and a more sensitive procedure (Harrison's test) is as follows: acidify 10 ml. of urine with one or two drops of dilute acetic acid and 1–2 ml. of 10 per cent barium chloride solution and filter. When the paper has drained dry spread it out and add to the precipitated barium salts one drop of dilute ferric chloride solution. A blue or green spot is a positive result. This test depends upon the conversion of bilirubin to biliverdin by ferric chloride. The tablet test ('Ictotest') employs the diazo reagent and is about as sensitive as Harrison's test.

Separate tests for *urobilin* and *urobilinogen* are not necessary as these two pigments have the same clinical significance. For preference, fresh urine should be tested for urobilinogen and for this purpose an afternoon specimen is better than one collected during the morning. One volume of urine is treated with one volume of Ehrlich's reagent (0·7 g. para-dimethyl-amino-benzaldehyde, 150 ml. conc. hydrochloric acid, and 100 ml. water) and, after shaking, two volumes of saturated sodium acetate solution are added. A deep red colour is a positive result. *Porphobilinogen* gives the same reaction but in this case, unlike that of urobilinogen, the red colour cannot be extracted by chloroform. Alternatively, the urine may be acidified by acetic acid, treated with one or two drops of iodine to convert urobilinogen to urobilin, and examined spectroscopically for an absorption band in the green-blue region (490 mμ). This mixture may also be treated with a saturated alcoholic zinc acetate suspension as in Schlesinger's test. It is then filtered and the filtrate shows a green fluorescence with excess of urobilin.

Tests for *bile-salts* have been largely abandoned as being of little diagnostic value.

Significance of Urinary Bile Tests. Bilirubin and urobilin(ogen), although frequently occurring together in the urine, do not have an identical significance in relation to liver dysfunction. The presence of bilirubin in the urine usually indicates an increase in the conjugated serum-bilirubin concentration and is therefore more or less equivalent to the demonstration of latent or overt jaundice. Since free bilirubin of serum has a much higher renal threshold than the conjugated variety bilirubinuria is rare in the purely haemolytic variety of jaundice. Occasional exceptions to this rule may occur if the liver is much damaged as a secondary result of anaemia or haemolysis. Bilirubinuria therefore usually signifies hepatocellular or obstructive jaundice.

Urobilin, on the other hand, is not directly related to jaundice and may frequently be present in its absence. Urobilinogen is formed from bilirubin by bacterial action in the intestine. It is reabsorbed into the blood-stream and excreted by the liver in the bile. Consequently urobilinuria signifies the presence of bile in the intestine. Excessive urobilinuria is therefore frequently found in the urine in haemolytic jaundice. As discussed on p. 511, it may also be present in excess in hepatocellular disease, but is of little diagnostic value for this condition. It will be absent from the urine if no bile is reaching the intestine at all as a result of complete biliary obstruction or occasionally from a complete failure of the liver to secrete bile. The latter event is uncommon in hepatitis and in such cases is said not to last more than one week.

Joan F. Zilva.

URINE, STRESS INCONTINENCE OF

The commonest variety of incontinence of urine in the female is the so-called 'stress incontinence'. In this condition coughing, sneezing, laughing, or any sudden strain leads to an involuntary escape of urine from the urethral orifice, the amount varying from a few drops to a few drachms. It is due to a weakening or relaxation of the sphincter mechanism at the neck of the bladder.

The condition is almost always due to obstetrical trauma, although not invariably so. The urethro-vesical junction has been dragged down and will be found to be lying at a lower level than normal. After an injection of an opaque medium into the bladder a radiograph will reveal the loss of the normal angle between the urethra and the bladder base. Usually a urethrocele is present and sometimes a cystocele in addition.

The condition may be first noticed in a young woman during the puerperium, following a prolonged labour where much stretching of the pelvic diaphragm has taken place. In the young, however, where the recovery of muscle tone is good, it is usually cured by the carrying out of postnatal exercises, designed to strengthen the pelvic muscles. Years later, however, due to ageing and weakening of the tissues, loss of tone in the pelvic muscles and increasing weight, the incontinence may reappear.

One must be careful to differentiate the condition from: (1) precipitancy of micturition, or so-called 'urge incontinence'; and from (2) true incontinence. In precipitancy of micturition or urge incontinence the involuntary loss of urine is preceded by an intense desire to void. The patient will frequently be unable to reach the lavatory in time to avoid wetting herself. In stress incontinence there is no such desire to pass urine at the time of the involuntary leakage. Urge incontinence is due to some lesion in the urinary tract causing bladder irritability or to some disturbance of its nerve-supply. Cystometry, measurement of pressures within the bladder and urethra at rest, during voiding and on straining and coughing, is helpful in deciding whether incontinence is due to excessive bladder tone from inflammation or to weakness of the urethral sphincter.

In true incontinence, due to a vesico-vaginal fistula, the leakage of urine is constant, though varying in amount from time to time. Methylene blue dye instilled into the bladder escapes into the vagina. In the case of a uretero-vaginal fistula there is a constant leakage of urine from one ureter, but the bladder fills from time to time from the other ureter and has to be emptied by voiding. Incontinence due to nervous system lesions must also be excluded.

T. L. T. Lewis.

URINE, URIC ACID AND URATES IN

The normal urinary excretion of uric acid and urate averages 0·5 g. per day, but may vary considerably according to the purine content of the diet. This is usually invisible, but visible deposits of uric acid and urates in the urine may occur and often have typical appearances. Thus uric acid resembles cayenne pepper, while urates usually form a fluffy deposit which is pink from adsorbed uro-erythrin ('brick dust').

Deposits of calcium, magnesium, and potassium urates are amorphous in character, whereas ammonium urate is crystalline and acid sodium urate may be either amorphous or crystalline. Ammonium urate may occur in urine of any reaction, whereas the others are always found in acid urine. Acid sodium urate is somewhat similar in appearance to leucine and also to the acetyl derivatives of sulphonamides. These substances, however, do not dissolve on warming. Urate deposits of crystals are easily identified by their solubility on warming and in excess of alkali. Uric acid, on the other hand, is always crystalline and occurs only in acid urine. The crystals are nearly always tinted brown from adsorbed urinary pigments. They may be partly aggregated together into larger particles to cause 'gravel'.

Both uric acid and urates tend to deposit chiefly in concentrated urines which are acid in reaction and may therefore be seen in any condition which produces a urine of this type. This would include dehydration from any cause, such as sweating, vomiting, or diarrhoea, any form of pyrexia, and heart failure. Non-opaque in straight X-rays, uric acid calculi are therefore more common a manifestation of gout in hot than in temperate climates. An increase in the total amount of urate produced per day is a contributory factor in *leukaemias* and in the presence of *large malignant tumours*, especially during the cell destruction following cytotoxic or radiotherapy. In these conditions there is a danger of renal failure due to urate precipitation in the kidney. Over-production is also a factor in most cases of *gout*. A proportion of patients with uric acid calculi excrete an abnormally acid urine, which favours urate precipitation at relatively low concentration. In most patients with primary gout there appears to be an isolated defect in the renal handling of urate, the main feature of which is that higher levels of plasma urate are needed to achieve the same values of urate clearance as in normal subjects.

The relation of the urate deposit to symptoms is important but difficult to define. The passage of 'gravel' may produce frequent and painful micturition, but large amounts of suspended urates or uric acid are frequently passed without symptoms. Similarly the passage of uric acid crystals gives no indication of the presence of a calculus, although it may suggest the nature of the calculus if one is known to be present. In such cases red cells are likely to be seen in the deposit in addition to the crystals. Needless to say, the deposition of crystals or deposit after the urine has been passed is a perfectly normal occurrence and does not in itself suggest any pathological lesion.

Joan F. Zilva.

VAGINA AND UTERUS, PROLAPSE OF

Prolapse is essentially a condition in which the supports of the vagina fail to hold it in place, with the result that it tends to turn inside out and to bulge externally at the vulva. Because the uterus is inserted into the vaginal vault, if the upper part of the vagina descends the uterus comes down with it as a uterine prolapse or vaginal vault prolapse. The vagina is normally held in place by the transverse cervical ligaments (of Mackenrodt), the pubo-cervical, and the utero-sacral ligaments. At a lower level the vagina is supported by the pelvic floor or levatores ani muscles. During pregnancy the supporting ligaments are softened and stretched and during childbirth the opening in the pelvic floor is enlarged. Prolapse therefore occurs mainly in women who have had children, but the vaginal vault may prolapse with projection of the cervix through the vulva in nulliparous women. Prolapse does not usually occur until the menopause and the patient complains of a swelling at the vulva giving rise to a feeling of bearing down and discomfort on walking or straining. The swelling and the symptoms disappear when the patient lies down. If the patient is examined in the left lateral or Sims' position, with a Sims' speculum holding back first the posterior and then the anterior vaginal wall, it is possible to determine which part of the vagina is prolapsing. Low down anteriorly is a *urethrocoele*, which is associated with stress incontinence of urine. At a higher level prolapse of the anterior vaginal wall contains the bladder to give rise to a cystocoele. Straining may cause kinking of the urethra with inability to micturate. The bladder does not empty completely and basal cystitis with urinary frequency is common. *Uterine (or vaginal vault) prolapse* occurs in three degrees. In the first degree the cervix descends to the vulva; in the second it protrudes through the vulva; and in the third, which is a *proccidentia*, the whole of the uterus is outside the vulva. Sometimes there is much elongation of the supravaginal portion of the cervix, the vagina is turned completely inside out, but the body of the uterus remains within the pelvis. If the vagina in relation to the posterior fornix prolapses it is related to the pouch of Douglas to give rise to an *enterocoele* containing loops of small gut or a *pouch of Douglas hernia*. Lower down the vagina posteriorly is the rectum and prolapse of this part gives rise to a *rectocoele*. It is possible to hook the finger into the rectocoele through the anus. Patients often find difficulty in emptying the rectum because the faeces tend to go forward into the pouch of rectocoele. Prolapse of the vaginal wall has to be differentiated from other swellings which protrude at the vulva. These include: a *fibroid polyp* which has a pedicle passing through the hard rim of the cervix into the uterine cavity where it is attached; *chronic inversion of the uterus*, a rare condition in which the uterus turns inside out, the fundus passing through the cervical rim leaving a cup-shaped depression where the uterine body should be; a long tongue-shaped *endometrial polyp*; a large *mucous polyp of the cervix*; a *vaginal cyst*; and a *malignant growth* of cervix or vagina.

T. L. T. Lewis.

VAGINAL DISCHARGE

The normal discharge from the vagina is a mixture of those from the uterine body, cervix, and vaginal wall; that from the uterine body is watery and small in amount; that from the cervix is thick and mucoid, but clear and transparent, like unboiled white of egg; that from the vagina is merely a transudation of plasma from the vessels, mixed with desquamated vaginal epithelium, and in virgins looks like unboiled starch mixed with water; it is small in amount. The bulk of the discharge found in the vagina comes from the cervix; there are more glands there than in any other part of the genital tract; there are no glands in the vagina. The cervical secretion is alkaline, consisting of mucus with a *p*H of 6·5. The secretion varies during the menstrual cycle, being abundant, clear, and almost free from leucocytes at the time of ovulation. At this time its elasticity is greater than one inch (*Spinbaarkeit*) and it is more easily penetrated by the spermatozoa. At other times of the month the cervical mucus is scanty, opaque, and tenacious. The secretion from Bartholin's gland, thin and mucoid, may be copious under sexual excitement, but under normal conditions it is scanty, and so does not contribute to a vaginal discharge. The vaginal mixed secretion is acid in reaction, owing to the presence of lactic acid produced by Doderlein's bacillus from the glycogen in the basal cells of the vaginal epithelium. This bacillus is normally found in the vagina from puberty to the menopause. The *p*H of the vagina is 4·5, the vaginal acidity being a bar to vaginal infection; unmixed uterine secretion is alkaline.

Normally, the amount of mixed vaginal discharge should do no more than just moisten the vaginal orifice; when the amount is so great as to moisten the vulva and consequently stain garments, the discharge is pathological. *Excess of the normal discharge* (*leucorrhoea*) may be due to (1) such conditions as anaemia, tuberculosis, chronic nephritis, indeed an debilitated state; (2) any condition causing increased pelvic congestion such as constipation, provoked but unsatisfied sexual desire, masturbation; (3) chronic passive congestion of heart disease or cirrhosis of the liver; (4) endocrine disorders resulting in hypersecretion of the cervical glands, the result of excessive oestrogen stimulation. This is not uncommonly found in those suffering from functional uterine bleeding; (5) no abnormality may be found. In many normal women a premenstrual mucoid discharge is seen, and in pregnant women leucorrhoea, the result of passive congestion or endocrine factors, is commonly encountered. Occasionally a congenital erosion may be responsible.

The composition of an abnormal discharge varies according to the source from which it comes and the acuteness of the inflammation; a frankly purulent discharge indicates acute inflammation, whereas a mucopurulent discharge indicates chronic inflammation involving the cervix.

1. The Mucopurulent Discharge. This, the commonest type, is a thick, white or yellow discharge. It contains much mucus, many leucocytes, masses of epithelium from the vagina (squames) and various bacteria: diphtheroids, streptococci, staphylococci, *Streptococcus faecalis*, *Bacillus coli*. Doderlein's bacillus will not be found. This discharge is typically produced by endocervicitis and cervical erosions. When endometritis is present as well, which is uncommon, the discharge becomes thinner and white, yellow, brown, or even blood-stained. Microscopically, the films made from the mixed cases show proportionally less mucus, but otherwise the constituents are the same.

2. The Frankly Purulent Discharge occurs in:

a. ACUTE CERVICITIS. Due to gonorrhoea or sometimes following puerperal or post-abortal infections; the cervix is red, swollen, and oedematous, being bathed in pus. There is nothing characteristic of gonorrhoeal discharges visible to the naked eye. The detection of the gonococcus can alone decide the question. This is often a matter of difficulty, because it is only in the few days immediately after infection that the organism can be found in the discharge. In chronic cases the gonococcus must be looked for in one of three places—in the interior of the cervical canal, in the urethra and Skene's tubules which open posterolaterally at the entrance to the urethra, or in discharge squeezed from the orifices of Bartholin's glands. Discharge from the cervical canal should be taken on a platinum loop after carefully wiping away discharge from the os uteri with sterile wool, using a vaginal speculum. This discharge should be spread on to two glass slides and put by to dry. Two other films should then be made by massaging the urethra from above downwards and collecting any discharge thus made to appear at the urinary meatus. It is important that micturition should not have taken place for several hours beforehand. Finally two films should be taken from the orifices of Bartholin's glands after squeezing the glands between the finger and thumb. After drying in the air the films should be fixed by passing through a flame and then stained by Gram's method, followed by neutral red as a counter stain. In films thus prepared gonococci are stained red (Gram-negative) while organisms which retain Gram's stain appear deep violet or black (Gram-positive). The gonococci are found as diplococci in the cytoplasm of the polymorphonuclear leucocytes and epithelial cells. Cultures of the discharge should also be taken and grown on a suitable medium such as Chocolate Agar.

b. GRANULAR VAGINITIS. The discharge is copious and purulent. It is associated with trauma of the vagina from the irritation of rubber, or bad fitting ring pessaries, or actual ulceration as in decubitus ulcers on prolapsed portions. Practically no mucus is found in such discharge unless the cervix shares in the inflammatory process.

c. TRICHOMONAS VAGINITIS. Due to a flagellate parasite, this produces a frothy purulent discharge causing local pain and soreness and being extremely irritating to the external genitalia. The discharge is green or greenish-yellow with small bubbles of gas in it and has a characteristic odour. The protozoon is to be found by diluting some of the vaginal discharge with normal warm saline and examining with a high-power lens, when the parasite, which is about the size of a leucocyte, will be found actively mobile, being propelled by its flagellae. The trichomonas lives in the vagina in symbiosis with the micrococcus *Aerogenes alcaligenes*, which organism forms the froth or bubbles so characteristic of the discharge. It is a Gram-negative micrococcus, smaller than the gonococcus. The

vaginal walls have a typical red stippled appearance.
d. MONILIA VAGINITIS. Common during pregnancy, giving rise to white patches of thrush on the vagina walls. It is a common cause of pruritus vulvae. It may complicate diabetes and the urine should always therefore be tested for sugar. If the white patches are scraped off the vaginal walls they leave raw bleeding areas. Vaginitis rarely exists alone, but when it does occur the discharge is thick and pasty if it is a simple catarrhal condition—pasty on account of the large admixture of vaginal squamous epithelium. Specimens of the discharge should be taken for recognition of the mycelium and spores in stained smears and for culture.

3. Offensive-smelling Vaginal Discharge is associated with decomposition; the discharge itself may decompose because it cannot escape fast enough from the passage, or the source of the discharge may be a decomposing substance like a *sloughing fibroid* or necrotic *carcinoma of the cervix*; in the two latter cases the discharge is copious, watery, and blood-stained, with a horribly fetid smell. When the discharge itself is decomposing it is usually thick and purulent, as when a retained foreign body such as a ring pessary, an internal tampon, or contraceptive cap is the cause. Infected retained gestation products, a faecal fistula, or a pelvic abscess rupturing into the vagina (*B. coli*) may occasionally be responsible. In old women a foul discharge may come from the interior of the uterus, a *pyometra*; in which case pus can be made to flow from the os uteri by squeezing the uterus or passing a sound; it is due to *senile endometritis*, or it may be associated with carcinoma of the uterine body or cervix.

4. Watery Blood-stained Discharge, not offensive, occurs with *carcinoma of the body of the uterus*, in early *carcinoma of the cervix*, with *mucous polypi, placental polypi, hydatidiform mole,* and *new growths of the Fallopian tubes.* Other causes such as endometrial hyperplasia, rupture of the membranes in early pregnancy, or an intermittent hydrosalpinx may be responsible. The differential diagnosis of these conditions cannot be made from the discharge alone, but must rest upon physical examination combined with the use of the microscope upon materials removed from the uterus. The use of vaginal smear tests (Papanicolaou) may help in the diagnosis, as in some cases cancer cells may be found in the discharge, but if malignancy is suspected reliance should not be placed on this test alone. Whenever there is any blood in the discharge the patient should be examined under anaesthesia and biopsies taken of the endometrium and cervix in case of malignancy.

Smears of the cervix and vagina may be taken with a wooden spatula (Ayre) for cytology. Malignant cells may be found in symptomless women with apparently normal cervices. Biopsy then reveals pre-invasive intra-epithelial carcinoma (*carcinoma-in-situ*). This condition is found in about 5 of every thousand women examined over the age of 30 years. Its discovery and removal from the population may lead to the reduction in incidence of invasive carcinoma of the cervix but the hoped-for abolition has not been realized due to the fact that only a small proportion of invasive growths seems to pass through a carcinoma-in-situ phase.

Vaginal casts may be composed of coagulated surface epithelium, the result of astringent injections or applications, and are recognized easily with the microscope. Membranous flakes may be passed with discharge in cases of *membranous vaginitis*; they consist of vaginal epithelium entangled in coagulated blood-plasma, and present quite a different appearance from casts of coagulated epithelial layers. These membranous masses may be seen lining the whole vagina, and are generally due to special organisms. The *diphtheria bacillus* has been found to be the causal agent in some; in others the *Bacillus coli communis.*

T. L. T. Lewis.

VAGINAL SWELLING

Inflammatory:

Gonorrhoeal
Non-specific: (*a*) Streptococcus; (*b*) staphylococcus; (*c*) *Bacillus coli*
Trichomonas
Monilia
Senile
Chemical.

New Growth:

1. Innocent:
   a. Cystic: (i) Cysts of Gartner's duct; (ii) implantation cysts; (iii) endometriomata
   b. Solid: (i) Fibroma; (ii) adenomyoma.
2. Malignant. Primary carcinoma, primary sarcoma, secondary carcinoma.

The vagina is resistant to infection because of its lining of stratified epithelium and the absence of glands; further protection is brought about by the action of Doderlein's bacillus on the glycogen in the vaginal cells, producing lactic acid which keeps the pH of the vagina at about 4·5. This acidity inhibits the growth of most organisms during the menstrual life of a woman; before puberty and after the menopause this protection is non-existent.

Trichomonas vaginitis is very common and gives rise to a typical red stippling of the vaginal walls, particularly in the fornices. The discharge is frothy, greenish-yellow in colour, and has a rather characteristic unpleasant smell. A discharge of sudden onset with soreness of the vulva is often due to trichomonas vaginitis.

Monilial infection may occur in the debilitated subject, but is most typically seen in diabetes. The discharge is thick, white, curdy, and adherent to the vaginal walls. An accompanying vulvitis that has the appearance of raw beef steak with a rather abrupt edge is characteristic; pruritus is the leading symptom.

Gonorrhoeal vaginitis is most frequently seen in the young child. It is not common in the adult because of the vaginal resistance to infection.

The non-specific forms of vaginitis, due to *B. coli, Staph. aureus*, and streptococci, are usually associated with the retention of some foreign body, such as tampons, or a ring pessary. It may also occur before puberty or following childbirth or abortion.

Chemical. Occasionally a too-hot vaginal douche or the use of strong chemicals, such as potassium permanganate, may be responsible. The characteristic signs of inflammation, with vaginal discharge, are present.

Senile Vaginitis. This is a common condition occurring after the menopause when the protective mechanism of the vagina is lost. The vaginal epithelium is thinned, and, in places, minute areas become completely denuded of epithelium, and appear as red points, giving a somewhat spotted appearance to the vagina. These areas may adhere and cause vaginal adhesions; they also cause a thin blood-stained watery discharge. On breaking down the adhesions with the finger, frank bleeding may take place. Senile vaginitis is most marked in the upper part of the vagina.

Cysts of Gartner's duct are cystic growths of the remains of the Wolffian duct, which has failed to be obliterated. They are always found in the anterolateral wall of the vagina. They may be small but sometimes grow to a large size, protruding outside the vaginal orifice and occluding the vaginal cavity. The characteristic position and cystic feel serve to differentiate them from the various types of vaginal prolapse. *Small implantation cysts* may be seen at the vaginal orifice posteriorly; they are small, and may follow operations on the perineum, or lacerations at childbirth. Occasionally an *endometrioma* may burrow through into the posterior vaginal fornix from the floor of the pouch of Douglas, forming nodular growths which tend to bleed at the time of menstruation. This condition may be confused with a primary carcinoma of the vagina, but it is not friable. Microscopic section will settle its nature.

Benign tumours. Sessile and pedunculated swellings arise in the vaginal wall which on histology are found to be papilloma, fibroma, or lipoma. They are uncommon.

Primary carcinoma of the vagina is rare. It occurs in the posterior fornix, often following the retention of a pessary which has been forgotten for a number of years. It usually takes the form of a typical epitheliomatous ulcer eventually producing a recto-vaginal fistula. Its friability and vascularity make the diagnosis clear, which should be confirmed by biopsy. A rare form of adenocarcinoma occurs in the vagina of teenage girls whose mothers took large doses of stilboestrol during their pregnancies. It has to be differentiated from benign adenosis vaginae in which there are numerous small swellings in the mucosa with a profuse discharge of mucus.

Secondary carcinoma usually spreads to the upper part of the vagina from the cervix. Occasionally metastases spread from carcinoma of the body of the uterus; they occur constantly at the lower end of the vagina in the midline anteriorly about half an inch behind the urethral meatus. Curettage reveals the uterine growth and biopsy the nature of the metastasis. Secondary growths have been described as occurring at the same site from primary carcinomata in the ovary and colon and also from hypernephroma of the kidney. They may ulcerate, causing bleeding. Microscopical examination will reveal their true nature.

Sarcoma of the vagina is rare, but occasionally the grape-like tumour (Sarcoma Botryoides or Mesodermal Mixed Tumour) may appear to originate in the vagina rather than in the cervix. It occurs in infants and young children and is one of the causes of vaginal bleeding before puberty. It has a characteristic appearance, like a bunch of grapes, and microscopic section proves its nature.

In the normal adult the healthy vaginal transudation will be found to contain many cornified cells and few, if any, leucocytes. This is due to the normal circulation of oestrogen. Excessive oestrogen stimulation leads to a multiplication of the layers of the vaginal epithelial cells with an increase in their glycogen content. At the menopause, due to lack of oestrogen stimulation, the transudation contains few cornified cells but many nucleated cells and leucocytes. It is thus possible, by examining a smear of vaginal cells obtained from the pool of discharge in the posterior vaginal fornix and rolled on to a slide with a swab-stick, to obtain some idea of the excess or deficiency of oestrogen. The healthy vaginal walls take on a deep brown colour if painted with Lugol's iodine solution, due to the abundance of glycogen in the vaginal cells. This is also an indication of oestrogen sufficiency.

As carcinoma is an exfoliative disease cancer cells can be found in preparations of vaginal and cervical smears in some cases of carcinoma of the cervix or corpus uteri. The taking of the smears is simple but the correct interpretation of the findings at present requires experience. It can be of the greatest use, however, as a positive smear test for cancer cells, in the absence of any symptoms or obvious signs of carcinoma of the uterus, calls for a thorough examination of the cervix by cone biopsy and the uterine cavity by curettage. In about 5 cases per thousand women examined the biopsy shows pre-invasive carcinoma-in-situ of the cervix. Invasive cancer can be prevented in these cases by the cone biopsy which usually removes all the abnormal epithelium. If the disease persists or recurs after cone biopsy positive smears are obtained and a hysterectomy can be done.

T. L. T. Lewis.

VEINS, VARICOSE ABDOMINAL

The point at which distension of veins becomes varicosity is arbitrary; most conditions that produce undoubted varicosity of the veins of the abdominal wall in some cases merely dilate them in others. When this dilatation is considerable

To test the direction of blood-flow, part of a vein should be chosen where there are no side branches, and the blood should be expressed from it by means of two fingers pressed gently down on the vein close together and then drawn apart whilst pressure over the vein is maintained by each; when a length of the distended

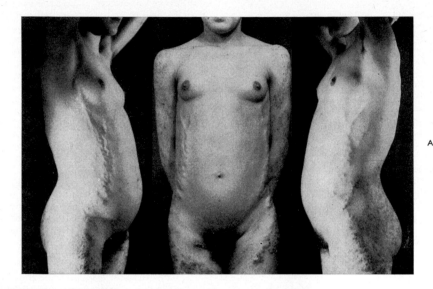

A

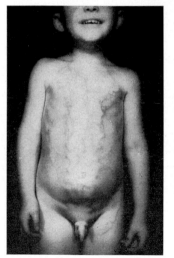

B

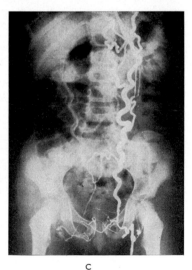

C

Fig. 791. Inferior vena caval obstruction showing greatly dilated collaterals by means of surface and infrared photography and by venography. (*Dr. R. G. Ollerenshaw, Manchester Royal Infirmary.*)

(*Fig.* 791) it nearly always has much diagnostic significance, particularly if the direction of blood-flow is reversed. Veins, however, may seem to be dilated when they are but unduly visible owing to wasting of the subcutaneous fat; or they may, in rare cases, be simply varicose, like veins in the leg, owing to idiosyncrasy or hereditary predisposition. In neither of these cases, however, is the blood-current in them reversed.

vein has been emptied in this way, one of the two fingers is taken off, and the time taken by the vein in refilling is noted. The procedure is repeated, the other finger being taken off this time; it is then generally easy to decide whether the vein fills from below upwards or from above downwards. Normally, the blood flows from above downwards in the veins of the lower two-thirds of the abdominal wall; when the blood-flow is from below upwards there is almost certainly obstruction to the inferior vena cava, the blood which is unable to return by it finding a collateral circulation via the abdominal parietes to the superior vena cava.

Obstruction to the inferior vena cava is due to one or other of three main groups of conditions, namely:

1. *Great general increase in the intra-abdominal tension*, owing to such conditions as: ascites; ovarian cyst; great splenic or hepatic enlargement.

2. *Thrombosis* without external obstruction.

3. *Obstruction by local compression*, especially by secondary growths in the retroperitoneal glands.

When the obstruction of the inferior vena cava is due not to the vein itself being thrombosed or invaded by new growth but to the *general intra-abdominal pressure* becoming so great that the vein is, so to speak, flattened out, the varicosity of the veins upon the abdominal wall is but a late symptom, and the diagnosis of the cause of the great abdominal distension, generally Ascites (p. 75) or a big tumour, will already have been made. If there is marked varicosity of the superficial veins early in a case of ascites the probability is that both are due to malignant disease.

When the inferior vena cava is obstructed by 'simple' thrombosis, the clotting will probably have started, not in the inferior vena cava itself, but below it, either in the legs or in the pelvis; oedema of the legs will be pronounced, and it may be ascertained that one leg became oedematous and painful before the other; when this is so it suggests thrombosis starting in the saphenous or femoral vein of one side, the other leg becoming affected later when the clot has spread up through the iliac veins of the one side to the inferior vena, and thence down the iliac veins of the other side. The higher the thrombosis extends the higher up the back will the oedema spread; and when the renal veins have been reached, albuminuria, with tube casts, haematuria, and ascites, may ensue, and acute nephritis may be simulated. Distension or varicosity of the veins of the abdominal wall assists in distinguishing such a case from one of acute or subacute nephritis; besides which there will be no oedema of the eyelids or face.

If there is no very tense distension of the abdomen; if the way the case began does not suggest thrombosis in one leg, or in the pelvis, extending upwards; and if, nevertheless, there is marked varicosity of the veins of the lower part of the abdominal wall, with the blood-flow in them reversed, so as to be from below upwards, the history being a relatively short one—the probability is that the inferior vena cava is being obstructed by something that is in immediate contact with it. There will very likely be symmetrical oedema of the legs, and possibly albuminuria and haematuria. It is remarkable how seldom an aortic aneurysm or other non-malignant mass obstructs a large vein sufficiently

to produce this collateral varicosity; hence, the presumption is that such varicosity indicates *malignant disease*. It is worthy of note that carcinoma of the kidney is prone to extend into the renal veins and thus into the inferior vena cava by direct extension—sometimes the malignant clot reaches as far as the right auricle, and may produce therein a pedunculated polypus. In such cases there has generally been haematuria or other renal symptom before evidence of inferior vena caval obstruction arises, whereby cases of growth in the kidney invading the inferior vena cava may be distinguished from cases of secondary growth in the retroperitoneal glands, which if they produced haematuria at all, would do so by first obstructing the inferior vena cava, and thence involving the renal veins. In such cases there are often other symptoms pointing to primary growth in some organ from which lymphatics drain into the retroperitoneal glands; the testes and ovaries should not be overlooked in this respect.

It is said that *cirrhosis of the liver* leads to varicosity of the veins around the umbilicus—the *caput medusae*; most cases of cirrhosis of the liver cause no distension of the superficial abdominal veins until the general intra-abdominal tension has been greatly increased by the tenseness of the ascites which occurs late. Not even the telangiectases that occur so commonly in men past middle age around the lower part of the chest, in a line with the attachments of the diaphragm, indicate cirrhosis; they are quite as common in cases of emphysema without cirrhosis.

Varicosity of the superficial abdominal veins generally indicates either thrombosis of the inferior vena cava, secondary to direct spread of thrombosis up to it from veins in the pelvis or in the leg, or else stenosis of the vena cava by secondary malignant disease.

R. G. Beard.

VEINS, VARICOSE THORACIC

Much of what has been said above about varicose abdominal veins applies also to those of the thorax. The veins on the chest wall may merely be unduly visible; but if they are really distended there is probably obstruction to one or other innominate vein or to the superior vena cava; the suspicion that this is so becomes a certainty if the blood current in the distended veins can be shown to be from above downwards instead of from below upwards. If the distension is bilateral, and associated with oedema of both arms and both sides of the neck, face, and head, it is the vena cava that is obstructed; if the distension is unilateral, with oedema of the corresponding arm, but little if any of the neck or face, the obstructed vessel is probably one innominate vein. The superficial varicosity may be only slight, but is sometimes extreme.

In arriving at a diagnosis of the cause of the venous obstruction, *malignant disease* within the thorax will be uppermost in one's mind—carcinoma of a bronchus with involvement of mediastinal glands is much the most common, though lymphoma, lymphosarcoma, and other tumours may be responsible. Less common is *thrombosis* extending to an innominate vein or to the superior vena cava from a whitlow, boil, or other inflammatory affection of the hand, arm, axilla, head, face, neck, shoulder, or front of chest; or *chronic fibrous mediastinitis*, resulting from repeated attacks of pericarditis and pleurisy, with matting together, not only of the pleurae to the diaphragm and pericardium, but also of all the structures in the superior, posterior, and anterior mediastina. The venous obstruction may be due to *aneurysm* of the thoracic aorta or a *non-malignant mediastinal tumour*, such as a hydatid cyst, a dermoid cyst, or a large congenital fibroma which may have been quiescent within the chest for years before starting to enlarge and obstruct structures in its neighbourhood. Although an aortic aneurysm does sometimes obstruct the superior vena cava sufficiently to cause distension or varicosity of the veins on the chest wall, such varicosity when the diagnosis lies between neoplasm and aneurysm indicates the former rather than the latter. Enlargement of the calcarine vein, a large vein running down the side of the chest wall in the mid-axillary line, and the vein liable to be injured when a horse is viciously spurred (hence the name), is indicative of portal obstruction of an intrahepatic type. This vein constitutes a collateral channel between the retrocolic veins (which are in communication with the portal system) and the intercostal veins.

R. G. Beard.

VERTIGO

The term 'vertigo' implies by derivation a subjective sense of rotation, either of one's self or of the surroundings, but it is helpful to include within the term simply a feeling of being off-balance, without any sense of rotation, which some patients with Ménière's disease experience between the more usual spinning attacks. Likewise the sensation which some people experience when looking down from a height or in the presence of diplopia might also be described as vertigo. It can then be concluded that vertigo, as more broadly defined, must always mean some involvement of the vestibular apparatus, either in its peripheral pathways or central connexions.

Vertigo due to affections of the *external auditory meatus* must be very rare, if indeed it occurs at all, but removal of wax is said to have cured vertigo on occasion. *Disease of the middle ear and blockage of the Eustachian tubes by catarrh or new growth* may be accompanied by vertigo but probably the labyrinth is affected too in all such cases. Thus otitis media can cause either a serous or a purulent labyrinthitis, and otosclerosis may spread to involve the inner ear. If infection has caused a fistula into the internal ear, vertigo can occur either spontaneously or by increasing the pressure in the external meatus (the fistula sign), or even by the pressure changes within the Eustachian tubes during swallowing. These conditions of the middle ear are usually accompanied by deafness and tinnitus, and by auriscopic evidence of disease.

Disease of the internal ear is the most common source of paroxysmal vertigo. Labyrinthine causes may be listed under six sub-headings:

1. *Spread of disease* from the middle ear as described above.

2. *Intoxications* such as salicylates, quinine, streptomycin, and acute alcoholism.

3. *Allergy* to foods, a very rare cause.

4. *Haemorrhage* into the semicircular canals, as in any disease accompanied by purpura or by a bleeding diathesis.

5. *Ménière's disease*: a common affection in the second half of life, due to degenerative changes in the membranous labyrinth with hydrops of the canals, and characterized by paroxysms of vertigo which last minutes or hours at a time and are often accompanied by pallor, prostration, vomiting, slight mental confusion, and pain behind the ear or a more generalized headache. Vestibular nystagmus occurs during the vertigo but is not present between attacks. Tinnitus and nerve deafness ultimately supervene but are often slight or absent in the early stages of the disease.

6. *Positional* vertigo, which may arise when the head is placed in a particular position, can result either from a peripheral or from a central lesion.

If peripheral, the condition is commonly attributed to disease of the otolith organ and severe vertigo is experienced when the head is lowered so that the affected otolith organ is undermost. The vertigo will eventually pass off if the head is maintained in this position and there will be increasingly less vertigo as the manœuvre of lowering the head with the affected otolith organ undermost is repeated. The vertigo may or may not be accompanied by nystagmus. This condition may develop after head injury, possibly as a result of nearby infection or for no apparent reason.

Positional vertigo may also arise, however, from central lesions such as disseminated sclerosis or cerebellar neoplasm, often metastatic, and in such cases there is no adaptation but the vertigo is present and persists for as long as the head is held in the critical position.

Affections of the vestibular component of the 8th nerve are an infrequent source of vertigo so far as is known at present. In *vestibular neuronitis* there are recurrent attacks of vertigo resembling those of Ménière's disease, but which differ from that disease in several respects—it occurs at a rather younger age, it is unassociated with deafness or tinnitus, the caloric responses are impaired in one or both ears, and the symptoms pass off in a matter of months or a year or two. In many cases there is evidence of infection in the nose, sinuses, or tonsils. There is no pathological evidence as to its nature, but the term 'vestibular neuronitis' serves as a convenient label pending further clarification of the subject. In some cases the discomfort falls short of obvious vertigo, amounting to no more than an intermittent sense of inequilibrium which is aggravated by moving the head or by walking.

Less common than the above are *gross lesions of the 8th nerve*, notably *acoustic tumours, syphilitic and other inflammatory affections of the cerebello-pontine recess, tumour of the petrous temporal bone, and gliomata and haemangioblastomata at the point where the nerve enters the pons*. The most important of these is the *neuroma*, a benign tumour which is easy to remove when small but which constitutes a formidable surgical hazard once it has grown large enough to produce the 'classic' signs—deafness, loss of the corneal reflex, facial weakness, homolateral cerebellar signs, and raised intracranial pressure with papilloedema. Fortunately, early diagnosis is now practicable in many cases at the stage of moderate deafness, with or without vertigo, and long before the facial or trigeminal nerves are affected, intracranial pressure is raised, or the internal auditory meatus is expanded by the growth. Tuning-fork tests give the same type of response when deafness is due to cochlear or 8th nerve disease: air conduction is better than bone conduction, and absolute bone conduction is diminished. But in cochlear lesions the deafness is characterized by the fact that once the threshold of hearing is reached, sounds are heard as well as in the normal ear—and may even appear louder. This phenomenon is called *recruitment* and it is absent in deafness due to affections of the nerve itself. That is to say, in an 8th nerve tumour the affected ear will hear less well than the normal side at all ranges of sound intensity. It is essential, therefore, to have audiometer tests carried out in all cases of vertigo and deafness for which no satisfactory explanation can be found.

Affections of the *medulla and lower pons* can cause vertigo. It may be paroxysmal or continuous, but generally speaking the diagnosis depends less upon the quality of the giddiness than on satellite symptoms and signs arising from simultaneous involvement of structures adjacent to the vestibular fibres and Deiter's vestibular nucleus. There is seldom tinnitus or deafness, because the auditory and vestibular pathways diverge after the 8th nerve enters the pons, but long tracts may be involved and nystagmus is present even when the patient is not actually feeling vertiginous; in labyrinthine and vestibular nerve lesions it usually ceases between attacks. Moreover, the nystagmus changes character: in labyrinthine and nerve lesions the quick component is always towards the affected side, whereas in central affections it is towards the left when the patient looks to the left and to the right when he looks to the right. (This is an oversimplification of a complicated subject, but it is

a useful working rule, valid for most cases.) The diseases which produce vertigo in this situation include *disseminated sclerosis*, thrombosis of the *posterior inferior cerebellar artery*, atheromatous *stenosis* of the basilar artery, *tumours*, and *syringobulbia*. A condition notable for its extreme rarity and for its popularity amongst collectors of the recondite is *cysticercosis of the fourth ventricle*, which has been known to cause vertigo when the head is moved.

Cerebellar disease and injury can give rise to vertigo, more especially if the lesion is acute, as in penetrating injuries and infarction, but generally speaking chronic lesions cause a sense of disequilibrium rather than a sense of movement. In the case of tumours, however, a true vertigo may occur either through direct pressure on the vestibular centre in the brain-stem, or from *a rise of intracranial pressure* (which is communicated to the labyrinth through the ductus endolymphaticus), or perhaps from traction on the 8th nerve. It is apposite to remark that *transient vertigo can be caused by any rise of intracranial pressure*, irrespective of the nature or position of the lesion.

Disease of the cerebral hemispheres seldom causes vertigo. It can occur as the aura of an *epileptic fit*, and is occasionally seen in *migraine*, but it is uncommon in supratentorial tumours unless the intracranial pressure is high.

The relationship between 'giddiness' and *head injuries* requires separate treatment, because it is seldom possible to ascertain the anatomical seat of the trouble. Following either minor or major cerebral contusion, the patient is apt to complain of dizziness on quick movements of the head or movements of the head in space. Occasionally it amounts to a true vertigo, but more often it falls short of this and is described as dizziness or giddiness. In a minority of cases there is evidence of damage to the labyrinth, or to the 8th nerve, but usually there is no such evidence and the patient comes to the doctor with complaints not only of dizzy spells but of nervousness, irritability, incapacity for mental and physical effort, and dislike of loud noises—a story liable to be mistaken for neurosis by the uninformed. There is evidence that such cases react abnormally to labyrinthine tests, but it is not clear whether the site of the damage is in the semicircular canals or in the afferent conducting system. The main interest of this work is to confirm what neurologists have believed for many years, viz., that there is an organic basis for 'dizziness' and vertigo after head injury. The fact that patients are sometimes encouraged by circumstances to prolong these symptoms for gain does not invalidate this view.

Vertigo also occurs in *anaemias*, in *hypertension*, and in *hypotensive states*. Anaemia, whether acute or chronic, can not only aggravate vertigo due to other processes but can also cause either lightheadedness or transient mild attacks of vertigo. With regard to hypertension, the position is confused by the circumstance that hypertension, atheroma, and labyrinthine disease are all found in the same age-group. While it is true that hypertensives sometimes complain of vertigo, there is no evidence that the raised blood-pressure is directly to blame and it is wiser to avoid this facile diagnostic alibi. The 'giddiness' of which so many hypertensives complain often resolves itself, on cross-examination, into a sense of confusion or faintness or lightheadedness rather than a true vertigo, and of those whose testimony survives interrogation some turn out to have labyrinthine disease and others are clearly suffering from focal or diffuse vascular lesions of the brain. In vertebral arteries atheromatous stenosis of the basilar artery is frequently accompanied by vertigo, presumably from reduction of blood-supply to the brain-stem. A further interesting cause of vertigo is the 'subclavian steal syndrome'. In this there is severe stenosis or occlusion of the subclavian artery before the origin of the vertebral artery and the blood-pressure in that arm is considerably reduced. Characteristically, when the arm is used the distal part of the subclavian artery is supplied by reverse flow by the vertebral artery, thus rendering the hindbrain ischaemic and causing vertigo. Vertigo induced by turning the head in a particular way, sometimes known as 'cervical vertigo', can occur in subjects suffering from atheromatous stenosis of the carotid artery, or a similar narrowing of the vertebral arteries. It is thought that the flow of blood to the brain is obstructed by the movement of the head, and there is some evidence that the vertebral artery may also be compressed within its bony canal by the bulging intervertebral disks of spondylosis. Unlike positional vertigo, it is a movement of the neck, and not the position of the head, which determines the symptoms. In place of vertigo there may be syncope or merely a feeling of lightheadedness. Hypertensive encephalopathy—cerebral symptoms of brief duration accompanying an exacerbation of an already high blood-pressure—is said to include vertigo amongst its protean manifestations; this may be so, but it is always difficult to be sure of this diagnosis. Any sudden fall of cardiac output, whether from a haemorrhage, cardiac infarction, cardiac arrhythmia, or a prolonged fit of coughing (laryngeal vertigo), can cause vertigo, either by itself or as a prelude to complete syncope. The common faint is often preceded by vertigo, but it is usually coupled with sensations of lightheadedness, nausea, and tinnitus.

Hypotensive drugs used in the treatment of hypertension may produce faintness and occasional vertigo, particularly after sudden changes of posture from recumbency to the erect position.

Finally, there is no evidence whatsoever that true vertigo, as defined here, can be 'psychogenic'. On the other hand, vertigo is a frightening and unsettling experience which, when persistent or recurrent, can cause anxiety and loss of morale even in the most stable of persons, and its effect on neurotic subjects can be cataclysmic. Indeed, the emotional and visceral disturbances may come in time to overshadow the organic nucleus of the illness.

Ian Mackenzie.

VESICLES

A vesicle is a circumscribed elevation of the skin varying in size from that of a pin's head to that of a small pea, containing serous fluid, which may be mixed with blood or become purulent. They may be of any shape, but are usually round.

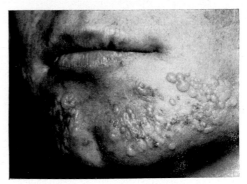

Fig. 792. Herpes simplex. (*Dr. Peter Hansell.*)

Larger serous elevations are classified as bullae (*see* p. 115).

Characteristic vesicular affections are herpes simplex and herpes zoster. *Simple herpes* (*Fig.* 792), which is caused by a virus, may occur anywhere on the body, but the face and the genitalia are mostly affected. While solitary attacks do occur, especially on the lips in the course of pyrexial diseases, it is much more common for it to recur at regular or irregular intervals, successive attacks appearing on the original site or close to it. At first there is a patch of erythema accompanied by burning or itching; on this vesicles rapidly form. These soon dry up and form yellowish crusts, which after a few days fall off leaving no scar. On the mucous membranes the course of the disease is slightly different; the vesicles become macerated and the top is rubbed off, leaving round excoriations or shallow ulcers. The commonest sites for *herpes genitalis* are the glans penis, the inner side of the prepuce, the labia, or the cervix uteri. Genital herpes cannot be mistaken if it is seen before rupture of the vesicles occurs. Occasionally the lesions of herpes genitalis become secondarily infected, when there will be enlargement of the inguinal glands, and if ulceration is considerable it may be mistaken for soft sore (*chancroid*). As a rule, however, the latter are multiple, have a foul base, excavate more deeply, and heal slowly. Soft sores are extremely painful. In some cases there may be doubt as between herpes genitalis and syphilitic chancre and it must be remembered that a herpetic lesion may be the site of inoculation of syphilis. Occasionally certain men, as the result of anxiety, develop genital herpes regularly after illicit sexual intercourse. The points of differentiation are, in herpes, the absence of induration, the less considerable and more transitory gland enlargement, the multiplicity, irregular

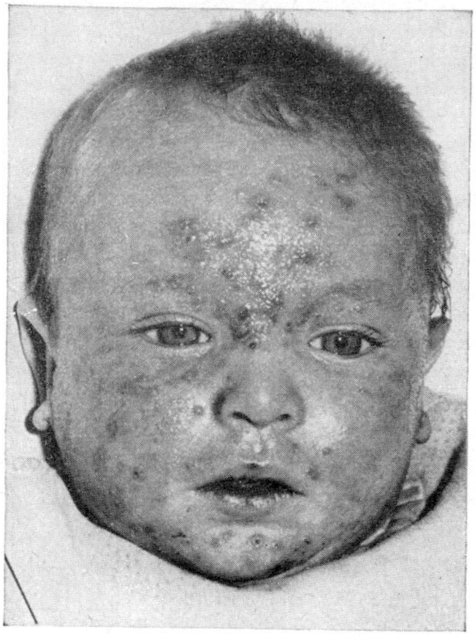

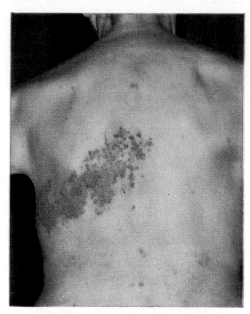

Fig. 793. Kaposi's acute varicelliform eruption. (*Dr. Peter Hansell.*)

form, and small size of the ulcers, and particularly the intense burning and itching, a chancre being absolutely painless.

In the crusted stage, *facial herpes* may resemble *impetigo*; but the rapid course it runs, its limited distribution, the fact that it is not auto-inoculable, and that in impetigo the lips are seldom attacked, should suffice to obviate confusion. It must be remembered, too, that impetigo can occur as a result of secondary infection of a herpetic lesion.

Kaposi's acute varicelliform eruption (*Fig.* 793) occurs in infants usually already suffering from a chronic skin disease such as infantile dermatitis. It is caused by the virus of herpes simplex and cases of contact with this disease have been proved. The lesions are vesicles of the chicken-pox type and are profuse, sometimes covering the whole body. The child becomes extremely ill with temperature up to 40° C. and a rapid pulse. Before the days of antibiotics which are used to control secondary infection there was a high mortality-rate. Very similar to this is *eczema vaccinatum* due to the vaccinia virus. Infants with eczema should not be vaccinated unless absolutely necessary.

In *herpes zoster* (zona, shingles) (*Figs.* 794, 795), which is a virus disease, clusters of vesicles on an erythematous base appear in the region of the skin distribution of one or more of the posterior spinal nerve-roots. This is preceded, accompanied, or followed by severe pain in the affected area. In rare instances the pain is slight and

transient. The number of vesicles on each patch varies considerably and sometimes they run together. In the majority of cases herpes zoster is unilateral. Occasionally there is enlargement

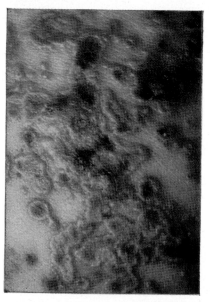

Fig. 794. Herpes zoster. (*Dr. Peter Hansell.*)

Fig. 795. Herpes zoster: close-up of vesicles. (*Dr. Peter Hansell.*)

of the lymphatic glands draining the area of skin involved. The limitation to one side of the body, the distribution in one or more nervous territories, and the pain usually suffice to distinguish herpes zoster from erythema multiforme and from dermatitis herpetiformis. In certain cases there is a history of association with varicella. These various characters serve to distinguish it also from herpes simplex. When the trunk is affected and the pain occurs first, it may be mistaken for that of pleurisy or some intra-abdominal condition. It should be added that in herpes zoster of the 5th nerve the conjunctiva and the eye may be attacked and sometimes the mouth, tongue, or palate.

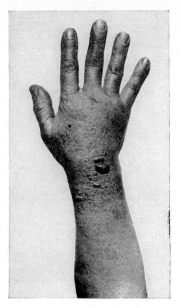

Fig. 796. Acute vesicular dermatitis. (*Dr. Peter Hansell.*)

The vesicle is a constant primary lesion in *dermatitis* (*Fig.* 796) or inflammation of the skin. Dermatitis may be exogenous or endogenous and acute or chronic. In some instances the vesicle is so minute as not to be obvious. The first sign is a patch of erythema accompanied by itching and burning; this is soon covered with numerous tiny vesicles. These enlarge and often coalesce; later they rupture, either spontaneously or by scratching, and a clear fluid exudes; the exudation continues once the surface of the skin has been broken and the exuded serum then dries to form crusts. The more acute the dermatitis the greater the degree of erythema and vesiculation. As the disease subsides there is less erythema and vesicle formation, and papules and scales begin to form. In mild cases the inflammation subsides rapidly, but much more frequently fresh crops of vesicles start up around the edge of the earlier patches, while new lesions are formed in other parts. Sometimes nearly the whole skin is involved. If the disease becomes chronic patches of lichenification (q.v.) due to long-continued scratching are formed. Thus the cardinal features of dermatitis, whatever the type and whatever the cause, are erythema, vesicle formation, rupture of the vesicles with

crusting from dried exudate, scale formation, and healing. Itching is a constant symptom and varies more with the temperament of the individual than with the stage of the disease.

Exogenous dermatitis, as its name implies, is inflammation of the skin from an external source and it may either be localized to a small area of skin or general in its distribution. It is acute, subacute, or chronic according to the intensity of the irritant factor. The symptoms are those of dermatitis in general, as described above. There are literally hundreds of substances that can produce dermatitis and they may act by direct irritation or by the affected individual having become sensitized to them, or be due to a personal idiosyncrasy.

Occupational or trade dermatitis: Dermatitis may occur in a great many occupations and is usually the result of continuous exposure to skin irritants, either from direct irritation or from an acquired sensitivity. There may, however, be an inherent idiosyncrasy; and it must be remembered that individuals with the seborrhoeic type of skin are more susceptible to skin irritants than others. It is also to be noted that in trade dermatitis it may be the method of cleaning the skin used by the workmen, i.e., strong soaps and cleansing solutions, rather than the materials used in the trade itself, that is responsible. In many trades, e.g., laundry work, the dermatitis may be due to the general conditions of a hot, steamy atmosphere rather than to any particular substance used; in gardeners it may be caused by irritation from plants as well as chemicals; in coal-miners working in deep, hot, damp pits, such as those in Kent, it is caused by friction of coal-dust on the moist and sweating skin, commonly on the legs.

The dermatitis may be acute or chronic, and once it has occurred there may be recurrences taking place over many years. Further, once dermatitis due to a particular substance has occurred recurrences may be produced by contact with other skin irritants. The picture may finally be complicated by the fact that in many instances what is originally a trade dermatitis may slowly and imperceptibly change to a chronic neurodermatitis, with powerful psychological factors playing a part in keeping it going. When this occurs the skin lesions may not show great change, but there may be more evidence of lichenification and scratching. It would be expected that in a trade dermatitis avoidance of the causal factor would be followed by a speedy cure. In many cases this is so, and when the disease persists for prolonged periods the supervention of neurodermatitis must always be considered. Further, the process may be complicated by the application of incorrect remedies. An extreme example of this would be a cement dermatitis becoming a penicillin or sulphonamide dermatitis and finally turning into a chronic and possibly incurable neurodermatitis. A valuable aid to diagnosis is the fact that this form of dermatitis usually begins on the sites in contact with the causative substance. A tremendous number of substances used in industry may cause dermatitis, ranging from common ones such as oil and grease, soda, and cement, to complicated chemicals employed in the manufacture of plastics and explosives.

In exogenous *dermatitis medicamentosa* it is drugs applied to the skin that cause the trouble.

or chronic. It may occur as a few localized patches, especially on the backs of the hands and feet, or it may be widespread (*Fig.* 797). The more localized forms are often described as *discoid or nummular eczema* (*Fig.* 798). Frequently there are large disk-shaped patches, and in the early stages the exudation and itching may be intense. It affects persons of all ages and may be

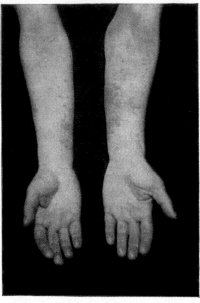

Fig. 797. Acute eczema. (*Dr. Peter Hansell.*)

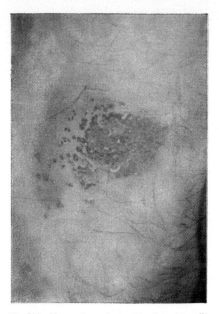

Fig. 798. Nummular eczema. (*Dr. Peter Hansell.*)

Constituents of many ointments and ointment bases may be the cause, e.g., lanoline, balsams, neomycin, and other antibacterial substances, anti-histamines, and local anaesthetics. Then there is dermatitis of the scalp, face, and neck produced by paraphenylendiamine hair dyes and dermatitis produced by the same chemical in dyed furs. Dyes are also responsible for many cases of clothing dermatitis (*Fig.* 269, p. 258), but in recent years free formalin has also been found to be an important cause as a result of some drip-dry processing. Plants and wood, especially the sawdust of certain woods, may produce dermatitis; and personal idiosyncrasy is an important factor in these cases, so that there is a great variety of causal substances.

Generally speaking, the diagnosis of exogenous dermatitis should be easy if its possibility is always borne in mind, for a history of contact with a noxious substance can always be elicited. Patch testing with the suspected materials (unless primary irritants, e.g., soaps) may be of great help in establishing the diagnosis.

Clinically, endogenous dermatitis differs in no way from exogenous dermatitis, and it is to this disorder that the term *eczema* is applied by some authorities. Endogenous dermatitis may be localized or generalized and acute, subacute,

very resistant to treatment. Endogenous dermatitis may rarely be caused by the ingestion of *drugs*, *chemicals*, and *foodstuffs*, usually the result of personal idiosyncrasy, but it may be due to an inherent instability of the skin or the presence of the seborrhoeic state. Dermatitis due to the parenteral administration of the arsphenamines and gold salts belongs to this category. Many cases of sudden spread of dermatitis are secondary to a small patch of dermatitis elsewhere on the body, especially a patch of varicose dermatitis on the legs. The mechanism is probably that of autosensitization.

Isolated localized patches of endogenous dermatitis may result from a rise in the blood uric acid (*gouty eczema*).

The distinction between dermatitis and *dermatitis herpetiformis* (*Fig.* 799) is usually simple. The earliest and most characteristic lesion of the latter disease is an eruption of crops of vesicles on an erythematous base. They tend to occur especially on the elbows, knees, base of spine, and in the scalp but may occur anywhere. The vesicles usually dry up and form scabs, but occasionally they coalesce to form bullae, which slowly shrink and finally shrivel up to a thick brown scab. Exudation is absent in dermatitis herpetiformis, and multiformity is a pronounced feature; erythematous, vesicular, pustular, papular, and urticarial elements being present in all stages of evolution. Eosinophilia is a constant feature of dermatitis herpetiformis and itching is intense. Histologically the vesicle is sub-epidermal as is the bulla in pemphigoid.

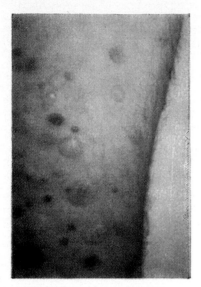

Fig. 799. Dermatitis herpetiformis.

Familial benign chronic pemphigus (Hailey and Hailey) is a familial disease in which there is a persistent recurrent vesicular dermatitis on the sides of the neck, in the axilla, groins (*Fig. 125*, p. 118), and sometimes other flexures. Occasionally there are bullae. The vesicles soon rupture leaving a crusted erosion resembling impetigo. The disease may die out in time.

Miliaria rubra (prickly heat) sometimes resembles the vesicular stage of dermatitis, but the vesicles remain discrete and do not coalesce; nor do they rupture, so that there is no exudation. Miliaria of all forms is a transitory affection and is associated with tingling rather than itching.

In *hydrocystoma*, which affects the face, small non-inflammatory vesicles appear in the substance of the skin grouped into patches which show no tendency to spontaneous involution or rupture. The vesicles are the result of dilatation of the coil gland ducts.

In *scabies* (*Figs.* 800, 801) a minute discrete vesicle is often present at one end of the burrow that is characteristic of the disease. All the other lesions are the result of scratching and may consist of papules, pustules, and crusts. Pustules are common on the hands, especially between the fingers. In dirty persons the burrows between the fingers and elsewhere which are characteristic of scabies are usually easy to identify. In clean people it is more difficult, but the distribution of the lesions should help, the parts most affected being those where the skin is thin—namely, the webs between the fingers, the front of the wrists,

on the lower abdomen, and a triangular area on the lower and inner part of each buttock. In men a solitary papule can usually be observed on the glans or shaft of the penis which is almost diagnostic in itself, and similar papules may be found on the breasts in women. The face is never affected except in infants in arms, who also usually exhibit burrows and papules on the inner sides of the soles of the feet. Nocturnal itching and a history of contact with a known case are important diagnostic features of the disease, and

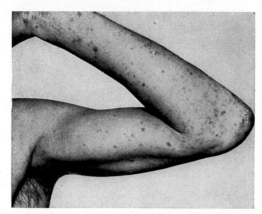

Fig. 800. Scabies: papules and pustules. (*Dr. Peter Hansell.*)

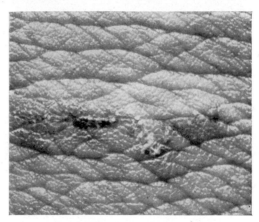

Fig. 801. Scabies: close-up of burrow on wrist. (*Dr. Peter Hansell.*)

an itching eruption affecting several members of the same family is most likely to be scabies. Once the technique has been learnt, it is comparatively easy to recover the *Acarus scabiei* from a burrow with the point of a pin and so confirm the diagnosis by observing the mite under a low-powered microscope.

In *pompholyx* (*Fig.* 802) (cheiropompholyx, dysidrosis) numerous minute vesicles are deeply embedded in the skin and show through the epidermis like boiled sago grains. It affects the palms and fingers symmetrically and also frequently the soles and toes. The general features of the affection, the limitation of the vesicles to the hands and feet, and their proneness to unite and form bullae which dry up, the tendency to recovery followed by repeated recurrence, are sufficiently distinctive, and the diagnosis is seldom in doubt. The affection may cause great irritation of the palms, and in a day or two the resultant

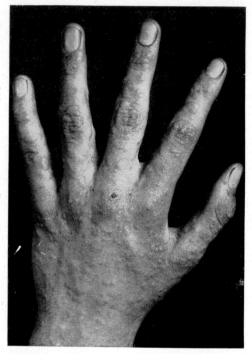

Fig. 802. Pompholyx. (*Dr. Peter Hansell.*)

scratching releases the retained fluid and the condition recovers rapidly, though there may be desquamation lasting for several days. In some slight cases there is a general resemblance to certain subacute and limited cases of dermatitis in which the lesions may present the sago-grain aspect; but instead of rupturing and weeping the vesicles in pompholyx tend to run together into bullae, which shrink and crust over. A *fungous infection of the feet* may resemble pompholyx, and in cases of doubt the presence of the causal fungus of ringworm will determine the diagnosis.

In *erythema multiforme* and *erythema iris* (*Figs.* 270, 271, p. 259) a small red spot appears upon which is formed a vesicle that is quickly surrounded by a zone of redness. When the central vesicle dries up it leaves a small scab, and a ring of secondary vesicles soon appears on the red zone. On the separation of the central scab the skin beneath has a blue congested appearance. The whole process may be repeated time after time until the concentric rings of vesicles and reddened skin look like a target. There is a

bullous form of this disease in which a large central bulla is encircled by vesicles of considerable size. The symptoms of erythema multiforme are so characteristic that the affection can scarcely be taken for anything else, but at times the bullous type may be extremely difficult to distinguish from pemphigoid and pemphigus.

Stevens-Johnson disease is regarded as a form of erythema multiforme. It occurs mostly in children and young men. It starts suddenly with malaise, headaches, and pyrexia, which may reach 40° C. There soon follows the eruption of vesicles on the lips, tongue, and buccal mucosa which may extend to the pharynx; later there is inflammation with vesicle formation of the conjunctivae and genitalia followed by erosions of the vagina or under the prepuce. Occasionally the nostrils and anus become involved. The lesions of vesicular or bullous erythema multiforme of the skin may or may not be present. The disease may prove fatal and blindness from scarring may occur.

In *hand, foot-and-mouth disease* (*see also under* ERYTHEMA, p. 257) small oval vesicles with an erythematous halo appear on the hands and feet and vesicles also occur in the mouth.

In *papular urticaria* vesicles sometimes appear on the top of the papules and the condition, which occurs mainly in children, may resemble scabies or varicella; but the burrows of scabies are absent and in varicella the vesicles are sparse, and there are no urticarial elements.

In *lymphangioma circumscriptum*, which affects the thighs, upper arms, genitalia, and buccal mucosa, there is an eruption of clusters of small deep-seated, thick-walled opalescent vesicles containing a milky fluid. The condition is due to cystic dilatation of lymph-vessels.

In *varicella* (chicken-pox) the main symptom is the eruption of vesicles; these only rarely become pustules. They are usually preceded by a faint macular erythema, and while they may arise anywhere on the body and mucosae, the commonest sites are the face, chest, back, and scalp, and the mucous membrane of the palate. After an incubation period of 2–3 weeks the rash develops within the first 24 hours and is accompanied by only the mildest constitutional disturbance. The rash appears in crops during the first 3 days and when some of the vesicles have already dried up to form crusts there are fresh ones appearing, so that there are lesions of various types present at the same time. Occasionally the vesicles pustulate, when there may be considerable general upset accompanied by high fever. A simple case of chicken-pox is easy to diagnose, but the severe pustular type has to be distinguished from smallpox.

In *variola* (smallpox) (*Fig.* 803) the pustules are usually multilocular; in chicken-pox, unilocular. In smallpox the preliminary vesicles are frequently umbilicated, in chicken-pox they are never umbilicated. In variola the rash is most abundant on the face and limbs, and least abundant on the chest and abdomen, and in varicella the rash is most profuse on the abdomen, chest, and face. There are, of course, exceptions to this in the case of both diseases. In varicella there are successive crops of vesicles and in smallpox there is only one set of lesions.

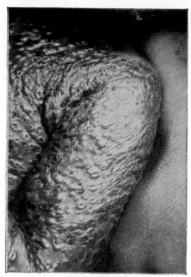

Fig. 803.—Variola.

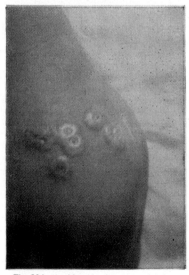

Fig. 804. Accidental primary vaccination.

A generalized vesicular or pustular eruption is a very rare sequel to *vaccination*. The rash appears on about the eighth day and may continue for several weeks. As a rule the eruption is a mild one, but a few fatal cases have been reported, especially in children.

The lesion of *primary vaccination* begins as a papule on an erythematous base which quickly becomes a vesicle and then a pustule. Later a crust forms which falls off to leave a small scar.

The vesicle usually appears in about 1 week and the crust falls off in 3–4 weeks. Occasionally primary vaccination is an accidental occurrence from contact with a recently vaccinated person (*Fig.* 804).

Vesicles sometimes are caused by the *bites* and *stings* of gnats, mosquitoes, and other insects, and should be recognizable from the history.

P. D. Samman.

VISION, DEFECTS OF

This subject may be considered in the following order: (I) *Normal vision*; (II) *Amblyopia*; (III) *Partial blindness*; (IV) *Complete blindness*; (V) *Defects in colour vision*; (VI) *Abnormal sensations of size*; (VII) *Night-blindness*.

I. NORMAL VISION

1. Visual Acuity. The act of vision comprises the perception of form, colour, and brightness; and the perception of space and distance. These faculties are possessed by all parts of the retina, though in varying degrees, and are of varying importance. One has to distinguish between peripheral and central vision; between merely seeing a thing and looking at it. An object is seen by any portion of the retina that has visual perception, but an object is only looked at when its image falls upon a particular portion of the retina, the macula, situated at the posterior pole of the globe to the outer side of the optic disk. The act of so directing the eye that the image of a given object falls upon the macula is termed 'fixation', vision obtained by the fixation of the eye is termed 'central vision', and owing to the anatomical structure of the retina at the macula, the vision here is the most acute of which the eye is capable, though its area is very limited. In the normal eye, central vision is capable of distinguishing two points or parallel lines which are separated by a space approximately subtending an angle of 1′—approximately the diameter of a small coin coin at 200 feet—and it is on this basis that ordinary test-types are constructed. Central vision, however, though acute, is very limited in extent; the field of acute vision is only about the size of the thumb-nail held at arm's length, all vision outside this area being comparatively blurred and indistinct. This limitation of the field of acute central vision is barely appreciated in ordinary circumstances, owing to the rapidity with which the retina receives consecutive visual impressions, and the constant movements of the eyes. Compared with the visual acuity of the central portion of the field of vision, peripheral vision is relatively poor, though it is of extreme value in a different way; to appreciate this it is only necessary to try to walk about looking through a roll of music; though central vision is unimpaired, and the smallest object can be seen distinctly, locomotion is almost impossible, owing to inability to see where one is going or to ascertain one's position in relation to surrounding objects, the peripheral portion of the field of vision being responsible for the automatic appreciation of these. On the other hand, a person deprived of central vision can see to get about quite well, and has useful vision for many purposes, though he is unable to read or write, recognize people when looking at them, or do any work in which fine vision is required.

2. Colour Vision. A person with normal colour vision can recognize six or seven distinct colours in the solar spectrum, and is able to appreciate many hundreds of varieties of colour caused by mixtures of them, and the colour perception of the normal person is most acute in the central portion of the field.

3. Brightness Perception. The central and peripheral portions of the field of vision vary much in their perception of brightness; in ordinary illumination the central portion of the field is the most efficient, but in a weak illumination the peripheral portion has a higher efficiency than the central part; in other words, there is in dim light a relative central scotoma or loss of vision. This fact has long been known to astronomers, who have found that in counting stars of low magnitudes, vision is much better if the particular constellation or group of stars is not looked at directly, the Pleiades being a well-known example; more of these stars can be counted when the vision is directed to a point to one side, and the same holds good of vision for any object in a dim light. Walking along a country road on a dark night, a footpath or track can be seen more easily if the gaze is directed forwards and not at the ground itself. These facts are correlated with the anatomical structure of the retina; in the region of the macula—the area of the retina endowed with acute vision—the cones are numerous, with few rods; towards the periphery of the retina the cones become fewer and the rods more numerous. The cones work in light of considerable brilliance, are capable of extremely acute vision for small objects, and are also concerned in the perception of colour. The rods, on the other hand, have no perception of colour; their perception of form is poor compared with that of the cones; but in very weak lights their visual acuity is greater than that of the cones, and the retinas of owls and nocturnal animals are more fully provided with rods than cones.

II. AMBLYOPIA

Amblyopia is the term applied to defective vision, and 'amaurosis' indicates blindness, in cases where there is little or no evidence of any ocular condition which might account for the visual defect. They are not, therefore, employed where there is any obvious intra-ocular or intra-cranial lesion. The commoner forms of amblyopia are:

1. Amblyopia ex Anopsia arises when an impediment to a clear retinal image prevents the development of full acuity. Thus in high refractive errors, especially high astigmatism and in those cases which have not been corrected in early life, it may be found that visual acuity is not normal even after correction of the refractive error, or that its return to normal is delayed. This is specially marked in the defective eye when one differs markedly from the other in refraction (anisometropia). In childhood squints there is usually some suppression of one retinal image, in order to avoid diplopia; and, if uncorrected (generally by occluding the master-eye) within a few years, this amblyopia becomes permanent ('strabismic amblyopia').

2. Toxic Amblyopia due to Lead, Alcohol, Tobacco, Quinine, Iodoform, Salicylates, Carbon Bisulphide, Filix mas, Antipyrin, etc. In tobacco amblyopia there is a central loss of vision for colours, green only in the earlier stages, subsequently green and red, and in extreme cases even a central scotoma for white. The patient may state that he sees better in a dull than in a bright light, and that he is incapable of reading or writing, or distinguishing silver from copper coins. In mild cases of toxic amblyopia the fundus appears normal; optic atrophy is evident if gross. In quinine amblyopia the retinal vessels also become constricted and the field of vision is diminished peripherally, though the blindness often precedes any ophthalmoscopic signs.

3. The Amblyopia of Migraine is usually transitory, and may occur either as a central scotoma, hemianopia, or monocular blindness; more rarely as a quadrantic hemianopia or a ring scotoma. The diagnosis is fairly easy, as the amblyopia seldom lasts more than a few minutes, and is followed usually by the characteristic headache and sickness of migraine, sometimes with fortification figures, flashes of light, and other subjective phenomena in the fields of vision.

4. Hysterical Amblyopia may, like other hysterical affections, take various forms such as loss of visual acuity, a loss of colour vision, or diminution in the visual field. The characteristic form of the visual field in hysteria is either a spiral contraction or an extreme concentric limitation. The symptoms, however, vary much at different examinations, a point of importance in diagnosis. In certain cases there may be a functional loss of vision in one or both eyes, which can be recognized as hysterical by the employment of Snellen's coloured types or some other device for deceiving the patient.

III. PARTIAL BLINDNESS

This may be: (*a*) *Hemianopia*; (*b*) *Central scotoma*; (*c*) *Peripheral constriction*; (*d*) *Quadrantic and asymmetrical defects.*

a. HEMIANOPIA. *See* p. 387.

b. CENTRAL SCOTOMA. A scotoma is a local defect in the visual field, and, from its position, may be either central or peripheral; it may also be negative or positive. A negative scotoma is one where the defect of vision exists, but where the patient is unaware of it. Sight is merely absent over that area. The best example of a negative scotoma is the blind spot in the field of vision caused by the exit of the optic nerve. This area is blind, but the individual is not conscious of any visual defects. Scotomata of this character exist where there is some injury of the visual layers of the retina itself, or of the optic nerve or tract.

A positive scotoma is one in which the visual defect is noticed as a black or coloured spot or cloud which obscures the vision in some part of the visual field. Such positive scotomata are usually due to opacities in front of the retina.

Scotomata frequently exist in the peripheral portion of the field of vision without being noticed, as they are of little importance in direct vision, and not discovered unless looked for carefully. A central scotoma, on the other hand, is noticed at once, however minute, because it affects direct vision and produces a considerable defect in the visual acuity. A central scotoma may be either relative or absolute, and may exist for colours only or for objects. Central loss of vision for colours, more particularly red and green, is associated with *tobacco* and *alcohol poisoning*. The colours cannot be recognized in small objects when looked at directly, though a red or green object in the peripheral portion of the field of vision will be recognized as such. This scotoma is associated with greater or less diminution of the general visual acuity, and vision in such cases is generally better in a dull than in a bright light. The scotoma is not always truly central, but may be paracentral or caeco-central, i.e., between the fixation point and the physiological blind spot.

Absolute central scotomata are met with in *disseminated sclerosis*, in certain forms of *hereditary optic atrophy* (Leber's atrophy), and may persist after *retrobulbar neuritis*. They are also sometimes found in the early stages of compression of the optic chiasma by a *pituitary tumour*. The central loss of vision known as eclipse blindness arises from an actual burn of the retina as a result of direct observation from the sun without protection. The effect is permanent and the lesion is visible ophthalmoscopically. In nearly 25 per cent of cases of disseminated sclerosis a central or paracentral scotoma exists, and the diagnosis in such a case will be confirmed by its association with the general symptoms of the disease, especially intention tremor, extensor plantar reflexes, exaggerated knee-jerks without sensory disorder, absent abdominal reflexes, and with other ocular symptoms, such as optic atrophy, paralysis of accommodation, paralysis of the extrinsic ocular movements, or nystagmus. There is usually some pallor of the optic disk, though this is no indication of the amount of visual defect. The diagnosis of a *hereditary optic atrophy* (Leber's atrophy) depends upon the history of a similar affection among family relations and its usual period of incidence, namely, early adult life. It is associated with either neuritis or, more commonly, atrophy of the optic disk. *Retrobulbar neuritis* usually occurs in young adults, commonly attacks one eye only, and is sudden in its onset, vision failing, even until there is no perception of light within a few hours; in most cases vision commences to return after a day or two, and is ultimately restored in a fortnight or three weeks; if any defect remains it is usually para-central, and is due to some injury to those axial fibres of the optic nerve which supply the macular region. Most cases of retrobulbar neuritis without apparent cause are due to disseminated sclerosis. Central scotomata after *migraine* are rare, but may be ascribed to that cause when there is a definite history of sudden loss of sight associated with the characteristic hemicrania and vomiting. Central scotomata are not always easy to map out on a chart, owing to the patient's loss of power of fixation; examination by an experienced observer is necessary. A small central scotoma may cause considerable failure of vision, even though it is too small to chart. Scotomata may also be *paracentral*, in the immediate neighbourhood of the fixation point, but not actually upon it, or may take an *annular* or *ring form* as in some cases of *choroiditis* or early *chronic glaucoma*, in which it may be the earliest and the most important sign.

c. PERIPHERAL CONSTRICTION. Peripheral constriction of the visual field occurs commonly in affections such as *glaucoma, optic atrophy, disseminated choroidoretinitis, retinitis pigmentosa*, and various *functional conditions*. The constriction of the visual field in *glaucoma* is usually most marked on the nasal side, and it may also be associated with atrophy and cupping of the optic disk (*Fig.* 624, p. 607). Central vision may remain good, even though the field of vision is extremely limited. The field of vision is, as a rule, most limited in *retinitis pigmentosa*, where the failure of sight will be found to be associated with night-blindness and characteristic ophthalmoscopic appearances, a small, ill-defined, waxy-looking disk, slender vessels, and diffuse superficial pigmentation of the equatorial zone of the retina in patches resembling Haversian bone corpuscles (*Fig.* 625, p. 607). This condition often occurs in two or more members of the same family, and may exist where the parents have been first cousins. A limitation of the field similar to that of retinitis pigmentosa is often met with in cases of *disseminated choroidoretinitis* and consequent optic atrophy; but may be distinguished from it by abundant evidence in the eye of deeper changes in the retina and choroid. Constriction of the field of vision may also occur in certain *functional states*, recognized by its variable character and the absence of all evidence of organic, ocular, or general nervous disease.

d. QUADRANTIC AND ASYMMETRICAL DEFECTS. A homonymous quadrantic defect is normally cortical in origin; unilateral and asymmetrical defects must be due to a cause situated in front of the chiasma.

IV. COMPLETE BLINDNESS

Total loss of vision, blindness, or amaurosis, may be: (1) *Bilateral*; (2) *Unilateral*.

1. Bilateral Blindness. Total blindness in both eyes may be congenital or acquired. Congenital blindness may be due either to absence of the eyes themselves, *congenital anophthalmos*, or to *congenital defects* in the development of the eyes.

Retrolental fibroplasia, in which a mass of whitish tissue is seen occupying the vitreous of an infant, was an increasingly common cause of blindness (usually bilateral) in infants, until it was shown to be the sequel to administration of oxygen (over 40 per cent), hence its frequency in premature babies. Since the cause was discovered (by Ashton in 1953) and the administration of oxygen to infants has been rigidly controlled the condition has virtually ceased to arise.

Total blindness may also be caused by *bilateral inflammatory affections* of the eyes, such as iritis with blockage of the pupils and consequent glaucoma, or ultimate shrinkage of the eyes, bilateral primary glaucoma, optic atrophy, or lesions of the optic chiasma. It is seldom due to lesions of the optic tracts, as this would only be caused by a bilateral lesion totally destroying the optic tract on both sides. An important form of sudden bilateral blindness is seen in *neuromyelitis optica* (Devic's disease). This malady is acutely febrile, and the loss of sight severe or complete, with symptoms of acute myelitis. The visual loss is usually the first symptom. If the patient survives, both aspects of the condition tend towards recovery.

The term 'amaurosis fugax' is applied to any condition causing loss of vision which recovers to leave no subjective disturbance. The causes are legion—inflammatory, toxic, nutritional, degenerative, hysterical, vascular, etc.

Another form of transient blindness is due to *spasm of the retinal arteries*. This may occur in cases of quinine or lead poisoning, in epilepsy, migraine, or eclampsia. Hypertensive patients are predisposed to this condition, as the result of endarteritis of the retinal arterioles. The loss of sight in a patient the subject of 'temporal arteritis' may be complete and permanent. Arterial spasm sometimes seems to occur in the absence of such causes in healthy young adults. In these cases the loss of vision may last only a few hours, and during its continuance it will be found that the retinal arteries are of a very slender calibre. It is to be noted that no cataract ever causes total blindness; provided that the rest of the eye is normal, a patient with the densest cataract can always perceive light, and also has the power of projection (the recognition of the direction from which the ray of light is coming).

2. Unilateral Blindness. Unilateral blindness is always due to some lesion in the eye itself, or to one between the eye and the optic chiasma. Lesions of the optic tract above the chiasma do not cause monocular blindness, but bilateral effects. Monocular blindness may be either sudden or gradual.

Gradual blindness may be due to any of the inflammatory affections of the eye mentioned above, or to such progressive diseases as optic atrophy or glaucoma.

Sudden blindness in one eye may be due to one of the following causes:

Detachment of the retina (*Fig.* 623, p. 606)
Embolism of the central retinal artery
Thrombosis of the central retinal vein (*Fig.* 620, p. 605)
Vitreous haemorrhage
Acute glaucoma (*Fig.* 624, p. 607)
Injury to the optic nerve due to an accident or fracture of the base of the skull
Compression of the optic nerve from haemorrhage, or dilatation of the nasal sinuses
Retrobulbar neuritis
Migraine
Hysteria.

The diagnosis of most of these causes is simple, owing to the characteristic ocular or ophthalmoscopic appearances. The only cases which present problems are those in which there is sudden loss of vision without visible ocular changes. These cases are usually due to retrobulbar neuritis, an acute affection of the optic nerve of obscure origin, characterized by rapid or even sudden loss of sight, with some pain and tenderness on movement of the eye. In most cases vision returns entirely; if there is permanent defect it takes the form of a central scotoma.

Monocular blindness may also occur in *migraine*, but in these cases it is of extremely short duration, seldom more than ten minutes or a quarter of an hour, and is followed by the characteristic headache, sickness, and fortification figures.

V. DEFECTS IN COLOUR VISION

Defects in colour vision may be either congenital or acquired; in congenital colour blindness there is inability to recognize in the spectrum one or more of the six or seven definitely distinct colours which may be apparent to a normal eye. The commoner cases of colour blindness are people who can see only three colours in varying shades, or those who can distinguish only two colours, the spectrum being made up of yellow and blue, the one gradually passing into the other.

Cases of congenital colour blindness can be recognized by examination with testing charts of 'pseudo-isochromatic' dots, or with more precision and certainty in a dark room by means of a lantern with properly coloured filters.

Acquired disturbances of colour vision are generally the sequel to damage to the retina and optic pathways by a wide variety of poisons. The rainbow-coloured haloes around lights are the classical feature of subacute glaucoma, associated with steaminess of the cornea, a shallow anterior chamber, dilatation of the pupil, and increased tension in the eyeball. Indefinite haloes may be produced by a film of mucus, from a conjunctivitis; but these disappear on winking. Haloes may also be due to the lens, but these are less bright and smaller than those of glaucoma.

VI. ABNORMAL SENSATIONS OF SIZE

Objects may appear to increase or diminish rapidly in size in the preliminary stages of an attack of epilepsy; and this variation in size of objects is occasionally noted by normal children, adult neurotics, and in the slight delirium of infantile febrile disorders. A tumour of the choroid which causes mechanical crowding or separation of the retinal elements may give rise to a corresponding abnormal sensation of size.

VII. NIGHT-BLINDNESS

Night-blindness, or *nyctalopia*, is commonly a congenital defect, having no organic ocular changes; it may also be associated with lack of vitamin A. It occurs most frequently in *retinitis pigmentosa*, diagnosable at once on ophthalmoscopic examination by reason of the pale optic disk, thin thready arteries and veins, and the characteristic spider-like pigment patches seen in the fundus.

P. Trevor-Roper.

VISION, SUBJECTIVE DISTURBANCES OF

There are a few common subjective disturbances of vision which have not been mentioned elsewhere.

The most dramatic are the flashes, sparks, colours, scotomas, and fortification spectra which are a frequent accompaniment of an attack of *migraine*. Occasionally (as 'phosphenes') they occur in healthy eyes after sudden movements, or as evidence of retinal traction (which may anticipate retinal detachment).

Spots before the Eyes. These may be considered under the headings of (1) Floating and (2) Fixed.

1. FLOATING SPOTS (MUSCAE VOLITANTES) are an almost universal symptom, although manifest only against a bright background; they often appear quite suddenly, and then very gradually fade away. They are probably due to condensations in the vitreous gel, in which even minor 'degenerative' changes, probably referable to physico-chemical change, may cause such symptoms. They may also be due to rupture of small retinal cysts; such an occurrence may rarely lead to peripheral detachment of the retina. The usual outcome is for them to break up and disappear or alternatively to sink and thus pass out of recognition. A far more serious cause of vitreous floaters is a uveitis, when the particles represent an inflammatory exudate, possibly with a cellular element. They are very common in high myopia, and represent part of the degenerative change characteristic of this condition. A rare cause of complaint of floating spots is the presence of small aggregations of mucus on the cornea, maybe in conjunctivitis but sometimes without apparent cause. Their movement or actual removal by the act of blinking reveals their origin. In all cases where floaters are complained of, careful examination is indicated in order to discover whether

they are symptomatic or have no real significance.

2. FIXED SPOTS may be due to one of a variety of causes. A lesion of the retina or choroid may be the cause; the limited central loss of vision caused by a macular lesion, especially the senile type, may be called a 'spot' by the patient. A fixed opacity in the vitreous may cast a shadow on the retina as may also, rarely, one in the lens or cornea. The paracentral scotoma of early chronic simple glaucoma must not be forgotten on account of its extreme importance. The larger scotomatous areas in the visual field caused by such conditions as detachment of the retina and neoplasm of the choroid are not properly described as spots except perhaps rarely in the very early stages.

Partial loss of field due to a central lesion, though hardly to be described as a 'spot', may also be so regarded and described by the patient. Sometimes a patient may become aware of the normal 'blind spot' which is due to the presence of the non-sensitive area where the optic nerve leaves the eye, especially if he be one-eyed, when the area is not covered in the binocular field by the corresponding sensitive area of the fellow eye. A reassurance that this is a normal phenomenon will put the complainant's mind at rest.

P. Trevor-Roper.

VOMITING

The term 'vomiting' implies the return and expulsion from the mouth of part or the whole of the stomach contents. There are conditions in which vomiting may be simulated although the vomited matter has never reached the stomach. It is convenient to deal with these before discussing the causes and differential diagnosis of true vomiting or gastric regurgitation.

In certain *diseases of the oesophagus* food may be swallowed and, after a varying interval of time, regurgitated. These conditions are:

Malignant disease
Fibrous stricture
Spasm
Pressure from without, as by aneurysm, new growth
'Idiopathic' dilatation or achalasia
Diverticula—'pressure' pouches.

If the obstruction be of long standing and near the lower end of the oesophagus, the interval between taking food and its regurgitation may be prolonged considerably, especially when the lumen has undergone much dilatation. This may occur with fibrous stricture, slowly growing carcinoma, or in the rarer cases known as 'idiopathic' dilatation of the oesophagus or achalasia.

Diverticula produced by a hernia-like protrusion of the mucous membrane through the muscular coats of the oesophagus become gradually filled, and, in addition to causing dysphagia by pressing on the oesophagus below, may simulate vomiting when its contents are voided. They occur immediately below the pharynx (Zenker's diverticulum), opposite the bifurcation of the trachea, or just above the diaphragm (epiphrenic).

The differential diagnosis of these oesophageal causes of vomiting, or rather regurgitation, is usually easy. The returned matter is undigested, alkaline or neutral in reaction, and generally diluted freely with mucus. Food may be retained for long periods in oesophageal pouches and returned unchanged. Confirmation of the diagnosis is by barium swallow and oesophagoscopy (*Figs.* 248, 249, 250, pp. 233, 235).

Certain persons may acquire the habit of voluntarily regurgitating portions of the stomach contents into the mouth, which may be ejected or again swallowed. There is no accompanying nausea. The condition is known as 'rumination' or 'merycism' (*see* p. 529).

The mechanism of deglutition may be deranged, and swallowing interfered with to such an extent that food or drink is returned. This may occur in cases of bulbar paralysis and myasthenia gravis. In diphtheritic paralysis the return of fluids through the nose owing to paralysis of the soft palate may be mistaken for vomiting. A similar mistake may occur in cases of bronchiectasis in which during the act of coughing quantities of pus have gushed up, not only from the mouth but also through the nose.

The regurgitation of milk in healthy infants after a hearty meal is often wrongly regarded as vomiting. It is due to simple overfilling, or sometimes to too rapid feeding; air that has been swallowed is belched up bringing some of the milk with it.

A brief account of the *mechanism of vomiting* will facilitate a classification of its causes. The parts concerned are the muscular coats of the stomach; the sphincter at the cardiac orifice; the diaphragm and the abdominal muscles; the vomiting centre and the chemoreceptor trigger zone situated in the medulla; the efferent nerve-fibres in the vagus supplying the musculature of the stomach, those in the phrenics the diaphragm, and those in the spinal nerves the abdominal muscles.

In the act of vomiting the walls of the stomach contract, the diaphragm is pushed violently downwards in full inspiratory position while powerful contractions of the abdominal muscles take place. The cardiac sphincter is simultaneously relaxed and the gastric contents are expelled, chiefly as the result of the pressure exerted on the stomach between the diaphragm and the abdominal muscles aided to some extent by reversed peristalsis. The pyloric sphincter is usually closed but it may become relaxed, in which case bile and intestinal contents may enter the stomach and appear in the vomit. The vomiting centre may be excited to action by stimuli reaching it from the stomach itself, by afferent fibres in the vagus, or from other parts by many different afferent channels. The centre may also be thrown into action by toxic substances acting on it directly, for instance by a subcutaneous injection of apomorphine.

In *retching*, forcible contraction of the stomach wall and of the diaphragm and abdominal muscles takes place as in vomiting, but there is no relaxation of the cardiac sphincter. In the condition known as *pyrosis* in which a quantity of burning fluid is brought up into the mouth the complete act of vomiting does not occur. Hiatus hernia is the usual cause.

The causes of vomiting fall into two main groups: (I) *Those acting directly on the vomiting centre*; (II) *Those acting reflexly on the centre.*

I. CENTRAL CAUSES

Certain drugs such as apomorphine, ergot alkaloids, and digitalis
Tobacco
Anaesthetics
Uraemia
Diabetes
Acute yellow atrophy of the liver (acute hepatic necrosis)
Addison's disease
Hypercalcaemia
Onset of acute infections, especially in children
Pregnancy
Recurrent, periodic, or cyclical vomiting in children.

There is some doubt whether or no Addison's disease, pregnancy, and recurrent vomiting should be included in this group. The vomiting of pregnancy may be partly reflex. The differential diagnosis of these conditions presents little difficulty. Examination of the urine will give evidence of the existence of renal disease in uraemic vomiting. The onset of drowsiness and coma in a diabetic patient may be attended by vomiting. Severe nausea and vomiting may occur in viral hepatitis, even before icterus appears, but persistent vomiting should arouse suspicion of acute hepatic necrosis.

Hypercalcaemia, whether due to hyperparathyroidism, sarcoidosis, metastatic bony malignant disease, or overdosage with vitamin D, may cause intractable vomiting. A similar syndrome may occur in rare cases of carcinoma without metastases.

Vomiting in Addison's disease is usually associated with abdominal pain, asthenia, characteristic pigmentation of skin (*Fig.* 729B, p. 729) and buccal mucosa (*Fig.* 536, p. 543), and a persistent low blood-pressure. The form of vomiting met with in young children, termed 'periodic', or 'cyclical', is very severe, and is accompanied by great wasting. The symptoms pass off after a few days, but tend to recur at intervals of months. The urine during the attacks contains acetone and diacetic acid. Vomiting, especially in children, is one of the earliest symptoms in specific fevers. The diagnosis rarely presents difficulty; the acute onset, general malaise, headache, pyrexia, sore throat, rash, etc., are substantially informative of the cause of the vomiting.

II. REFLEX VOMITING

1. Gastric Causes:

Irritating articles of food (hard, indigestible substances)

Emetics, such as zinc sulphate, mustard

Poisons:
Corrosives, irritants

Irritating drugs such as salicylates and alcohol

Gastritis:
Acute
Chronic

Pyloric obstruction:
Malignant disease
Fibrous stricture
'Hypertrophic stenosis' in infants
Pressure from without
Ectopic pancreas
Adult pyloric hypertrophy

Dilatation and 'hour-glass' contraction

Malignant disease

Ulcer

Venous congestion, as in conjestive cardiac failure, portal obstruction, cirrhosis of the liver.

2. Intestinal, Peritoneal, and General Visceral Causes:

Intestinal obstruction
Appendicitis
Intestinal worms
Following administration of enemata
Henoch's purpura
Peritonitis
Biliary colic
Renal colic
Acute pancreatitis
Certain conditions of the female genital organs:
Pregnancy
Ovarian disease
Extra-uterine gestation
Acute myocardial infarction
Pulmonary tuberculosis—vomiting may be of central origin or due to irritation of the bronchi
Irritation of the fauces or bronchi by direct stimulation, or by severe coughing:
Pertussis
Bronchiectasis
Pulmonary fibrosis
Shock:
Blows on the epigastrium, testicle, a kick on the knee, etc.

3. Affections of the Central Nervous System:

SPECIAL SENSES:
Offensive smells; tastes; repulsive sights.

BRAIN
Concussion
Cerebral tumour or abscess
Meningitis
Hydrocephaly
Cerebral haemorrhage
Thrombosis of cerebral sinuses
Middle-ear disease; Ménière's disease
Migraine
Epilepsy
Sea, train, motor-car, or aeroplane sickness
Emotional disturbances
Functional or hysterical vomiting
Radiation sickness.

SPINAL CORD
Gastric crises of tabes dorsalis.

Certain general principles may be laid down as important in the diagnosis of the cause of vomiting. Attention should be paid to its relation to food if any, and at what interval after a meal it occurs, whether or not preceded by pain, whether or not attended by nausea. The absence of nausea is a point of some significance; nausea is usually present in vomiting due to abnormal states of the alimentary tract or viscera, but is often absent in that due to concussion, cerebral tumour, meningitis, or other disease of the brain. But this feature must not be regarded as infallible in diagnosis. (*See also* NAUSEA, p. 565.)

The vomited matter should be inspected, and its quantity and general character noted. Alcohol and certain poisons such as carbolic acid and prussic acid may be recognized by their *smell*; a faecal odour may be detected in peritonitis and still more so in cases of intestinal obstruction as well as in the rare condition of gastrocolic fistula. *Blood* may be present, either dark or bright red, or dark brown and resembling coffee-grounds. (Coloured liquids and foodstuffs may be mistaken for blood.) Slight streaks of blood are common with severe vomiting, and are usually due to rupture of small vessels in the oesophagus or pharynx. In whooping-cough, blood is often mixed with mucus from the respiratory passages, and the contents of the stomach are ejected during the paroxysms. The *condition of the food remains* should be noted; the presence of substances, such as currants or seeds, taken it may be many hours or even days previously, would point to pyloric obstruction.

In any case of suspected poisoning the vomit should be kept for analysis. The *reaction* should be ascertained; in corrosive poisoning this may be strongly acid or alkaline according to the toxic agent. *Microscopical examination* may show sarcinae, yeast cells, or cell elements from a malignant growth. Intestinal contents may be mixed with the vomit. *Bile* is often present in any severe or protracted vomiting and is recognized readily by its colour and the usual tests.

1. Gastric Causes. Most *corrosive* and *irritant poisons* cause vomiting immediately after swallowing, accompanied by intense burning pain in the epigastrium. The vomit contains food, blood, mucus, and may have the characteristic odour of the poison. With some irritant poisons, e.g., arsenic or phosphorus, the vomiting may be delayed and resemble that of an acute gastritis. The diagnosis depends on chemical analysis of the vomit, as well as the associated signs and symptoms. Shreds of gastric mucosa may be seen or even a large portion of the mucosa forming a partial or complete cast of the interior of the stomach. Many drugs medicinally employed may cause vomiting if administered in excess, and, in the case of susceptible persons, even in ordinary pharmacopoeial doses, iron preparations being a good example.

In *acute gastritis* repeated vomiting is usually very severe and attended by abdominal pain. It occurs shortly after taking food and leads to some relief of pain. The vomited matter consists at first of food ingested, later of mucus and bile. There are often accompanying diarrhoea and febrile disturbances, especially in children.

Exceptionally the entire mucous membrane becomes detached, forming a cast of the stomach —*gastritis membranacea.*

In *chronic gastritis* pain is of variable degree. The vomited matter consists of partially digested food, mucus, and a considerable quantity of sour-smelling liquid. Hydrochloric acid is usually reduced, or entirely absent. When *dilatation* of the stomach is present, the quantity of liquid ejected is often very large; portions of food taken many hours previously may be recognized.

'*Hour-glass*' *contraction,* due to transverse constriction of the stomach by fibrous tissue, may be a cause of vomiting which resembles in most respects that associated with dilatation. Examination with a barium meal will generally establish the diagnosis (*Fig.* 353, p. 333).

In adults, the vomiting due to *pyloric obstruction* presents no characteristics other than those associated with the dilatation of the stomach which it usually produces. Evidence by X-rays that there is a large residuum in the stomach eight hours after the intake of the barium is the most direct method of demonstrating pyloric stenosis. The absence of free hydrochloric acid and the presence of blood in the vomit would favour the diagnosis of carcinoma. Persistent vomiting in young infants, especially if breast-fed, attended by wasting and constipation, arouses suspicion of *hypertrophic stenosis of the pylorus.* The vomiting in these cases is very forcible, the milk being pumped up violently, often very shortly after a feed. Visible gastric peristalsis and the presence of a small tumour in the epigastrium would complete the diagnosis. (*See also* p. 12.)

Vomiting is by no means universal in cases of non-malignant *gastric ulcer.* Pain as a rule occurs within an hour of taking food and is relieved by vomiting. The vomit consists of food more or less digested, a variable but generally at least normal quantity of free hydrochloric acid, and sometimes blood.

2. Intestinal, Peritoneal, and General Visceral Causes. In *intestinal obstruction* vomiting sets in after an interval the length of which may depend on the situation of the obstruction. The higher this is situated in the intestinal canal the earlier and more severe the vomiting. The contents of the stomach are returned first, and later, mucus, bile, and intestinal contents often of a dull brown colour and thin fluid consistence; obvious pieces of faecal matter are rarely distinguishable. Faecal vomiting should be recognizable by its odour.

Vomiting is an early symptom in *appendicitis* and may persist to resemble that met with in intestinal obstruction.

Intestinal worms may cause vomiting in children, probably owing to reflex irritation. A round-worm is sometimes found in the vomit.

Enemata induce vomiting in certain individuals and rare cases have been described when liquid injected per rectum has been returned by the mouth.

Vomiting is a common symptom in the condition known as *Henoch's purpura.* The vomit may contain blood from the mucous membrane of the stomach. It is usually accompanied by abdominal pain, sometimes of an acute and agonizing character closely simulating that occurring with intestinal obstruction, in consequence of haemorrhage into the intestinal wall or the mesentery, occasionally simulating or even giving rise to intussusception. Recurrent attacks of vomiting and abdominal pain associated with a purpuric eruption in a child would point to this not uncommon disease.

In *acute peritonitis*, vomiting is an early symptom; rarely the vomit may have a faecal odour. The history, together with the rigidity and immobility of the abdominal wall, generally indicates the need for early laparotomy.

In *biliary* and *renal colic* the vomiting accompanying the attacks of agonizing pain presents no special features. The pain in the upper right part of the abdomen and the onset of jaundice distinguish biliary colic from that due to renal calculus in which the pain is in the loin or the lower abdomen shooting down towards the groin and testicle and often followed by haematuria. Jaundice is absent if the gall-stone is in the cystic duct.

Acute pancreatitis may closely simulate intestinal obstruction in that it is attended by nausea and vomiting, constipation, and severe abdominal pain. The vomit is, however, not faecal in character; there is usually localized tenderness over the pancreas. There may be discoloration of the skin of the abdominal wall as described by Grey Turner. If laparotomy is performed (on account of the urgency of the symptoms), fat necrosis is usually found in the omentum and mesentery.

Severe nausea and vomiting may occur with acute myocardial infarction, especially of the posterior wall of the heart.

3. Affections of the Central Nervous System. In most of the preceding conditions nausea accompanies vomiting. In intracranial disease a special type of vomiting is met with generally known as 'cerebral vomiting'. In this, nausea is less conspicuous although not necessarily absent, vomiting occurs suddenly and often without warning and bears no relation to the ingestion of food. Vomiting of this type, especially if accompanied by headache, should arouse suspicion of organic cerebral disease—such as tumour, chronic subdural haematoma, abscess, meningitis, or sinus thrombosis. In all cases of vomiting with the least suspicion of an intracranial lesion a full examination of the central nervous system with X-ray of the skull must be carried out and the eyes should be examined with the ophthalmoscope, when papilloedema or optic atrophy may be identified (p. 607). Instances occur when attacks of vomiting may be the only symptom of an intracranial tumour long in advance of any other symptom or sign of increased intra-cranial pressure.

Cerebral haemorrhage may be attended by vomiting especially when the cerebellum is the part affected or when the harmorrhage is sub-arachnoid.

In *Menière's disease* vomiting may follow the attack of vertigo. Nausea and vomiting generally accompany the severe headache in attacks of *migraine*. In *epilepsy* vomiting is an occasional but unusual feature.

Functional or *hysterical vomiting* is not attended by nausea or pain, and although the vomiting may be a frequent occurrence the general state of nutrition often remains good. It is by no means unusual for a subject to vomit and return to complete a meal. Other hysterical manifestations are generally present in these patients and de-tailed interrogation may elicit a psychological cause to encourage the conclusion that the act symbolizes a (possibly subconscious) feeling of disgust. Some people are prone to vomit on the slightest psychological disturbance as a means of expressing their emotions.

The *gastric crises* in tabes are attacks of vomiting usually accompanied by severe epi-gastric pain. Occasionally, vomiting may be an isolated symptom. The attacks usually last for several days, and tend to recur at irregular intervals. During the intervals alimentary func-tions may be completely normal. The diagnosis would be supported by the characteristic Argyll Robertson pupil and the loss of the knee-jerks, but, in some cases, visceral crises are the only manifestation of tabes and a mistaken diagnosis of an abdominal catastrophe is by no means easily avoided. The absence of abdominal rigidity is an important feature.

Radiation Sickness. Attacks of vomiting not infrequently follow exposure to deep X-rays and similar forms of treatment.

C. Wastell.

VULVAL SWELLING

The differential diagnosis of vulval tumours includes not only true swellings of the vulva, but also swellings which appear at the vulva as a result of the displacement of other structures, as in cases of prolapse and cystocele, and lesions like kraurosis vulvae which are not strictly swell-ings at all. The lesions may be tabulated as follows:

Skin Lesions:

Dermatitis
Eczema, psoriasis
Vitiligo.

Inflammatory Lesions:

Vulvitis:
  Simple
  Diabetic
  Gonorrhoeal
Soft chancre
Papillomata

Granuloma inguinale
Syphilis:
  Hunterian chancre
  Condyloma
  Tertiary lesions
Tuberculosis
Furunculosis
Pseudo-elephantiasis
Lichenification
Primary atrophy
Lichen sclerosis
Leucoplakic vulvitis
Kraurosis vulvae
Lymphogranuloma venereum (esthiomène).

Cystic Swellings:

Hydrocele of the canal of Nuck
Bartholin's cyst
Sebaceous cyst
Mucous cyst
Implantation cyst
Dermoid cyst.

Blood Cysts:

Varicocele
Rupture of a varicose vein
Traumatic haematoma.

New Growths:

Caruncle
Fibroma
Lipoma
Angioma
Endometrioma
Neuroma
Fibromyoma of the round ligament
Endothelioma
Hydradenoma
Squamous-celled carcinoma (epithelioma)
Columnar-celled carcinoma
Sarcomata of various kinds
Chorionepithelioma
Melanoma.

Hernia:

Inguinal
Posterior labial
Perineal.

Displacement:

Prolapse of urethral mucous membrane
Prolapse of uterus
Cystocele
Rectocele
Inversion of the uterus
Fibromyoma of the vaginal wall.

Unclassified:

Simple anasarca.

Certain of these lesions stand out pre-eminently as presenting difficulties in diagnosis. The general principles by which solid tumours are distinguished from cystic, inflammatory swellings from new growths, new growths from herniae, need not be insisted upon here.

Skin lesions, i.e., dermatitis, eczema, psoriasis, occur as on other parts of the body. The white patches of vitiligo are not uncommon on the vulva. *Simple* or *erythematous vulvitis* may be the result of uncleanliness or the chafing of diapers, particulaly in the obese. It may be the result of an allergic response to nylon, to detergents used for washing underclothes, or to substances applied to the vulva as deodorants. The glycosuria of diabetes mellitus may produce considerable vulval irritation, and the urine should also be routinely tested for glucose in these cases. An extension of a monilial or trichomonas infection from the vagina to the vulva may cause vulvitis. Perhaps the commonest difficulties which arise in practice are the diagnosis of gonorrhoeal vulvitis from simple vulvitis, the venereal soft chancre from the syphilitic condyloma. In the acute stage of a *gonorrhoeal vulvitis* the gonococcus may be recognized in films made from the discharge. Acute gonorrhoeal vulvitis is uncommon in the adult. When it does occur its main clinical feature is its very acuteness. It is much commoner in infants and young children, when it may spread rapidly to other children in contact with them. Practically all acute forms of vulvitis appear alike clinically, so that detection of the gonococcus becomes a matter of importance. In chronic gonorrhoeal infections with vulval swelling as a rule the organism cannot be found in the general vulval discharge, but might be found in the urethra or in the cervix. A gonorrhoeal infection may be suspected if the patient gives a history of an acute onset, accompanied by scalding on micturition, and then there is redness of the orifices of Bartholin's glands and Skene's tubules, and much redness and swelling of the carunculae myrtiformes. Papillomata or warts of the vulva may occur also in chronic gonorrhoeal infections, and when due to a local virus infection, the warts being the only manifestation.

The *soft chancre*, from which Ducrey's bacillus (*Haemophilus ducreyi*) may be recovered bacteriologically, may be mistaken for the *condyloma of secondary syphilis*, but as a rule this difficulty should not occur. The soft chancre is a typical punched-out ulcer with a somewhat red base and clean edges, discharging pus. The condyloma, on the other hand, is a raised, flat-topped excrescence, with sodden, epithelium-covered surface. Soft chancres are not very numerous, as a rule, and are generally limited to the vulva. Condylomata are numerous, and may occur all over the labia, around the anus, and even on the skin of the thighs and gluteal region. Condylomata are from the start, or very soon after, accompanied by a sore throat and a typical papular skin rash, for they are secondary syphilitic lesions. Soft chancres clear up with antiseptics; condylomata persist for long periods, but clear up in two or three weeks as a rule under antisyphilitic treatment. Soft sores and condylomata may occur together, in which case the diagnosis may be still more difficult.

Differentiation between the *Hunterian chancre*, or primary syphilitic sore, and *squamous epithelioma* of the vulva is of vital importance to the patient if valuable time is not to be lost in the treatment of an epithelioma. The two lesions look much alike at first; they form a raised hard indurated mass in the skin, which may ulcerate

quickly as a result of superficial necrosis. Both give rise to a thin watery discharge, and to enlarged glands in the inguinal region which do not suppurate at first, but may do so later in the case of an epithelioma. It must not be forgotten that a primary chancre is seldom actually seen in women, while squamous epithelioma is directly visible. *Primary chancres* in the female may be multiple and then frequently do not show the typical hard induration as in the male. The chancre, left untreated, will be followed in due course by secondary lesions, but it is wrong to wait for these to appear. If there is the least suspicion of epithelioma the doubtful swelling should be excised and submitted to microscopical examination; a squamous epithelioma is detected easily in this manner in quite early stages, and does not in the least resemble a syphilitic lesion microscopically. The *Spirochaeta pallida* may be recognized by dark-ground illumination microscopy or in scrapings of a hard chancre by the Indian ink method, or when fixed and stained by Giemsa's or Levaditi's method. In sections, too, the spirochaete may be demonstrated, but for this purpose the excised growth *must* be fixed in 5 per cent formalin solution. Serological tests for syphilis, such as the Wassermann, Kahn, treponemal immobilization test (T.P.I.) and the Reiter protein complement-fixation test do not become positive until 6 or 8 weeks after the initial infection. If the lesion seems more likely to be chancre than epithelioma, antisyphilitic treatment would be adopted, and the diagnosis clinched by the rapid subsidence of the sore.

Tertiary syphilitic lesions are by no means common on the vulva. When they do occur they give rise to spreading ulceration with great destruction of tissue, and scarring in the older healed portions. The only lesions likely to be mistaken for them are some forms of epithelioma, and tuberculosis. Obviously, in such conditions the only reliable method of diagnosis is by excision of parts of the lesion and microscopical examination of sections made from them.

Granuloma inguinale is a chronic venereal infection with a tendency to ulceration and massive development of granulation tissue affecting the vulva and groins. It is transmitted by coitus. A similar condition can occur in the male. It starts as a raised papilloma which soon ulcerates, the ulcer having a typical serpiginous outline. The granuloma in the groin rarely suppurates. It heals in places and much scarring results. The condition is due to the Donovan body, a small encapsulated body with a curved rod-like nucleus. They are found in scrapings from the ulcers. The condition causes soreness and itching.

Lymphogranuloma venereum (esthiomène, or genito-anal scleroma): Initially a papule on the vulva, at the vagina orifice or on the cervix, which soon disappears to be followed by suppuration in the inguinal glands, and marked hypertrophy and ulceration of the affected parts, eventually leading to anal or rectal stricture if that region is affected. If the hypertrophy and ulceration are *pari passu* the condition is termed *esthiomène*; if hypertrophy predominates, genito-anal sclerosis, a form of elephantiasis, results. In the acute stage pyrexia may be present. It is due to a filterable virus. The diagnosis is made by the Frei test. It is found that a patient with the disease develops a cutaneous reaction following the intradermal injection of an antigen prepared from the virus. Both the latter diseases are uncommon in this country but are common among Negroes in America and elsewhere.

Tuberculous ulcers are very uncommon on the vulva. They are very indolent and can only be diagnosed with certainty in microscopical section.

Pseudo-elephantiasis of the vulva is usually a syphilitic affection of the labia minora, giving rise to great enlargement, with a rough and thickened appearance of the skin. It does not reach the dimensions of real elephantiasis due to lymphatic obstruction by the *Filaria sanguinis hominis*, a disease which is practically never seen in Britain.

Unilateral oedema of a labium minus is a fairly common condition, usually associated with an infected wound (furunculosis) or a primary syphilitic chancre. *Bilateral oedema* is almost always associated with general anasarca, the result of renal disease, pre-eclamptic toxaemia of pregnancy, cardiac disease, or pressure upon pelvic veins. It is not likely to be mistaken for any other disease.

Lichenification is the result of vulval dermatitis and mechanical irritation. The actual lesion is a prolongation of the dermal papillae, the result of oedema.

Primary Atrophy. Vulval atrophy causing dyspareunia occurs in elderly women as kraurosis vulvae. When it appears in younger women, at or before the menopause, it is referred to as primary atrophy.

Lichen Sclerosis. A condition of unknown aetiology. At first there are small, white, polygonal flat-topped papules, which tend to coalesce to form white plaques. Later atrophy occurs with stenosis of the introitus, a condition indistinguishable from kraurosis.

The essential lesion in all the above conditions is atrophic epithelium, resting on degenerate hyaline connective tissue in which there is inflammatory reaction. Any of these conditions may be followed by leucoplakia; dyspareunia may result.

Leucoplakia is a chronic inflammatory condition of the vulva associated with hyperkeratosis, parakeratosis, disappearance of the elastic tissue in the skin with round-celled infiltration and irregular enlargement of the inter-papillary downgrowths. The disease never involves the vestibule but occurs on the labia majora, parts of the minora, and hood of the clitoris. It may spread on to the perineum, thighs, and genito-femoral sulcus. It may occur at all ages but usually later in life. In its early stages there is redness and swelling of the affected parts. Later, in the hypertrophic stage the skin becomes thickened and white, sodden and hardened in places with shrinkage of the labia. Cracks and fissures may appear. In this stage the condition is precancerous. The fissured areas take on epitheliomatous changes. Leucoplakia gives rise to intense itching; occasionally a late atrophic stage develops, but keratinization is still pronounced.

Kraurosis vulvae is a condition only affecting the vestibule and vaginal orifice, and appears as an excessive shrinkage or atrophy of the vulval orifice associated with minute patches of dermatitis (red areas where the epithelium is denuded). It is a disease of post-menopausal life but may occur in the young if the ovaries have been removed. It is due to ovarian deficiency. It causes soreness and tenderness to touch, with severe dyspareunia. It does not cause pruritus vulvae.

Apart from a cyst developing in Bartholin's gland or duct, cystic swellings of the vulva are not common. A *Bartholin cyst* is recognized by its position on one side of the vaginal entrance, distending the posterior part of the conjoined labia, and also within the hymeneal ring. As a rule the orifice of the gland can be seen on the inner side of the cyst. The contents may be glairy mucoid fluid, or pus. A cyst of the duct of the gland will be felt as a more superficial swelling than the deeper cyst in the gland substance. A cyst may develop following a badly performed episiotomy. An abscess of the gland or cyst may form, the organism being either the gonococcus or skin organisms. Normally the gland is not palpable. If it can be felt it is either the seat of chronic inflammation or growth. As a rule a previous history of vulval inflammation or infection can be obtained. In practice, a Bartholin cyst is not likely to be mistaken for anything else; but it is wise to remember that *posterior labial hernia* occurs in the same situation, and that new growths of the vulva may occur there as elsewhere.

Varicocele of the vulva occurs practically only in connexion with pregnancy, and is unmistakable. It has the same 'bag of worms' feel as has a varicocele in a man, and as the veins are close to the skin a bluish colour is always to be noted. The patient is conscious of vulval swelling and discomfort, not amounting to pain, on standing. Although the veins look as if they might rupture during labour they seldom do.

Haematoma of the vulva is recognized as a blue or violet-coloured swelling covered by tense shiny skin, often spreading up into the pelvis by the side of the vagina. It arises soon after delivery but its appearance may be delayed some hours. The history alone will often decide the nature of the swelling, and its appearance is quite typical as a rule. Haematoma of the vulva may occur apart from pregnancy, and then is always traumatic.

Urethral caruncle and *prolapse of the urethral mucous membrane* may be mistaken for one another. The former, however, is always a pedunclated or sessile new formation, invari- ably springing from the posterior wall of the urethral orifice. It bleeds readily, is often, but not always, exquisitely painful, and is usually the result of infection. Prolapse, on the other hand, appears as a raised projection with rounded margins, and with the urethral canal in the centre as a dimple. The prolapsed portion may not necessarily include the whole ring of the mucous membrane. It may give rise to pain, and being always more or less strangulated, it is prone to bleed, much in the same way as a caruncle. It occurs as a result of some straining effort, or may accompany pelvic floor prolapse; it is not the result of infection.

The differential diagnosis of the new growths of the vulva presents no points of difference from their diagnosis in other parts of the body. The only common benign tumour is the *pedunculated fibroma*, while *squamous carcinoma* (*epithelioma*) is the only malignant growth which occurs at all frequently.

If the general characters of a *hernia* are borne in mind there should be no risk of overlooking or mistaking any of the varieties which occur in the vulva. The resonance on percussion if the hernia contains bowel, the reducibility of the contents, and the protrusion through a pre-existing open- ing, will usually suffice to distinguish herniae from other swellings. An obstructed or strangu- lated hernia is not so easy to recognize, but the accompanying acute symptoms and the history usually suffice to make the case clear, or at any rate to cause one to operate and arrive at the diagnosis thus.

Hydrocele of the canal of Nuck, an uncommon condition, may be mistaken for an inguinal hernia; but as a rule it is irreducible, circum- scribed, fluctuating, without any obvious neck running into the inguinal canal. When the canal of Nuck has a patent peritoneal communication the swelling disappears as the patient lies down, but it is not reducible in the characteristic man- ner of a hernia. The condition is rare.

The *displacements* included in the list above are dealt with under the heading of VAGINA AND UTERUS, PROLAPSE OF, p. 811.

Hydradenoma is an unusual tumour which arises from the sweat-glands on the labia. It presents as a solid nodule. The diagnosis is made on biopsy.

T. L. T. Lewis.

WEALS

Weals, the characteristic lesions of *urticaria* (*Fig.* 805), are flat-topped evanescent elevations of the skin, the result of local oedema of the dermis. They are the expression of an angio- neurotic excitation causing exudation of plasma. They are due to histamine release. Weals dis- appear rapidly as a rule without leaving any trace. They are usually pale in the centre, with a red periphery, but they may be uniformly rose- red or may have a whitish periphery, or rarely,

as the result of haemorrhage into them, they may be purplish. In size they vary from a pinhead upwards, and as a rule they are flat and slightly raised; generally round or oval, they are some- times irregular, or even linear, several inches in length; by running together they may form roughly circular plaques. They usually appear suddenly, last individually only a few hours, but may be succeeded by others in adjacent parts. They are always accompanied by itching or burning, which may be intense. The commonest cause of an acute attack of urticaria is dietetic,

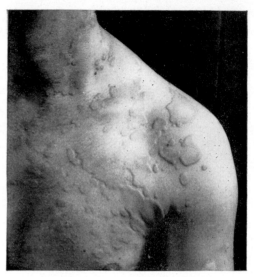

Fig. 805. Urticaria. (*Dr. Peter Hansell.*)

the affected person having apparently become hypersensitive to some foodstuff, the commonest being shell-fish or certain fruits such as the straw- berry. Almost any foodstuff may produce this effect in a given individual. Drugs may produce urticaria, common ones being penicillin, the sulphonamides, antipyrin, the barbiturates, aspirin, salicylates, iodides, bromides, morphine, antimony, neosalvarsan, and allied substances; various normal or antitoxic sera may have a similar effect, the urticarial eruption from serum injec- tions appearing usually after eight days. Among other possible causes intestinal parasites should be mentioned. The cause of urticaria in its com- mon recurrent form may be due to trigger factors such as preservatives or dyes (colouring matter) in foods which cause histamine release without being true allergens. In many cases, however, the cause cannot be found and some may be psychosomatic.

The sudden onset, the presence of the weals, the fugitive character of the eruption, the ir- regular distribution, and the severe itching, make the clinical picture of urticaria unmistakable. Very rarely the weal is surmounted by a blister (bullous urticaria) and the affection may be confused with pemphigus or with the erythematous stage of dermatitis herpetiformis; but its true nature is indicated by the history of the case, the course of the eruption, and the almost invariable presence at some points of typical lesions.

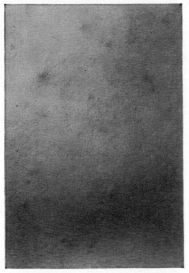

Fig. 806. Cholinergic urticaria. (*St. John's Hospital.*)

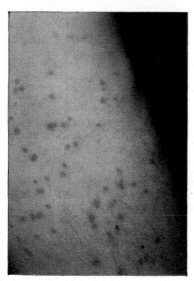

Fig. 807. Urticaria pigmentosa. (*St. John's Hospital.*)

Papular urticaria is distinguished by the presence of papules.

When weals are due to such local and accidental causes as the *bites of insects*, contact with the *stinging nettle*, or the after-effects of stinging by *jelly-fish*, the diagnosis is furnished by the history, and in insect-bites by the central punctum.

Some skins are so sensitive even in apparent health that weals rise upon the surface in response to *mechanical excitation*. For instance on writing with the finger-nail upon the skin, weal-like elevations may rise soon afterwards corresponding to the markings made (dermatographism or tache); the condition is an idiosyncrasy, not necessarily a disease or an indication of disease. A modified form of it is seen in the *tâche cérébrale of meningitis*. The weals that arise from external injury, for example from a whip-lash, cane, cat-o'-nine-tails, or from an accidental injury due to the effects of tree branches when passing through undergrowth, are self-evident.

In the uncommon *cholinergic urticaria* which is usually due to physical exercise the lesions are uniformly small and are surrounded by a distinct erythematous flare (*Fig.* 806).

In *urticaria pigmentosa* (*Fig.* 807) there are multiple small macular or papular lesions which urticate on scratching or when the patient is in a bath. The aetiology is unknown, but the lesions consist histologically of collections of mast cells. Rarely lesions occur in the internal organs, especially the bones. Occasionally also a single isolated lesion is found in young children and is then often surmounted by a bulla. When the condition begins in early childhood it usually clears spontaneously, but in most other cases it is permanent.

P. D. Samman.

WEIGHT, LOSS OF

Loss of weight is the result of inadequate alimentation whether from lack of food, poor appetite, or inability to swallow or to retain. It is important to distinguish between those patients who lose weight in spite of normal food intake and those whose calorie intake is diminishd. In children, the commonest causes are malnutrition from injudicious feeding and gastro-intestinal disease (*see* MARASMUS, p. 522); in adults, when loss of weight is considerable, with no definite physical signs and little relevant history, one thinks first of *malignant disease*, a chronic infection such as *tuberculosis, hyperthyroidism, diabetes mellitus, anorexia nervosa*, or some other *psychiatric disturbance*.

WEIGHT LOSS WITH ADEQUATE FOOD INTAKE

1. Increased Utilization
Hyperthyroidism
Chronic infections (e.g., pulmonary tuberculosis)
Anxiety states
Drugs: thyroid, amphetamine.

2. Diminished Absorption
Intestinal insufficiency states
Intestinal hypermotility states
Sprue: tropical and non-tropical
Chronic pancreatitis
Carcinoid
Short-circuit operations
Post-colectomy and post-gastrectomy states
Chronic hepatic disease
Dysphagia, e.g., scleroderma
Whipple's disease

Lymphatic obstruction
Drugs, purges.

3. Abnormal Calorie Loss
Diabetes mellitus
Fistulae
Intestinal parasites.

WEIGHT LOSS WITH DIMINISHED FOOD INTAKE

1. Psychogenic
Depression
Anorexia nervosa
Psychoses.

2. Gastro-intestinal
Peptic ulcer
Malignancy
Chronic colitis
Hepato-biliary disease
Intestinal insufficiency syndromes.

3. Malignant Growths
Lymphoma
Leukaemia

4. Uraemia

5. Chronic Infections

6. Chronic Non-infective Inflammatory Conditions
Rheumatoid arthritis
Systemic lupus erythematosus

7. Chronic Intoxications
Alcohol
Addictive drugs
Heavy smoking
Lead.

8. Advanced Crippling from any Cause

9. Endocrine Disease
Addison's disease and some cases of hypopituitarism (Simmond's disease).

10. Faulty Diet
Food faddism
Food intolerance.

11. Chronic Cardiac Conditions

Notwithstanding the most careful investigations, in not a few cases doubt as to the cause of loss of weight remains until, in the course of time, the patient either completely recovers, or else develops other signs or symptoms. Young persons may lose weight as the result of change of surroundings, for instance from active outdoor school life to work in a city office; care and anxiety, sorrow, disappointment in love, too strenuous a life of pleasure, irregularity of meals, over-long hours of work are familiar causes of what at the time may appear to be ominous loss of weight. In some cases an accompanying loss of appetite and inadequate food intake supply a plausible explanation. In other cases it appears that the nervous disturbance is in itself responsible, whether by interference with assimilation, by altering the metabolic rate, or by some more elusive mechanism. Many young girls taking up nursing lose weight initially, and regain it as they adapt to their new life.

Any affection of the alimentary tract interfering with proper digestion and absorption of food may produce loss of weight—gastric or duodenal ulcer, colitis in its many forms, such factors as too much smoking, excessive drinking, monotony of food or of circumstances, carious teeth, ill-fitting dental plates, pyorrhoea alveolaris, and the abuse of purgatives may contribute to the wasting. When gastric symptoms are prominent it may be difficult for the time being to tell whether the mischief is only functional ('nervous') dyspepsia or due to organic disease. Weight-loss also may occur after partial or total gastrectomy or colectomy, when a new 'normal' is created for the patient.

Any malady which produces *sleeplessness* or *persistent pain* may lead to serious loss of weight.

Chronic infections may not be obvious in themselves, and yet may produce loss of weight by interfering with general nutrition. One sees this in many who have returned from the tropics after infection by dysentery, yellow fever, malaria, dengue, hepatitis; chronic affections of the joints, the skin, or the alimentary tract, may produce loss of weight in a similar way. Particular mention should be made of chronic pyelonephritis, which, though a common malady, is often missed through neglect of bacteriological examination of the urine.

Liver affections exert a prominent influence upon general nutrition, and loss of weight exhibited by some sufferers from cirrhosis is familiar, though in the early stages the patient may be fat and towards the end loss of weight may be masked by deceptive increase due to ascites. In drug addiction weight-loss is often considerable.

The effect of *alcohol* upon body-weight is variable, some persons becoming stout, others thin, and others changing but little. This depends greatly on food (calorie) intake, beer-drinkers tending to become obese and pot-bellied. Broadly speaking it is heavy spirit drinkers who lose weight, and in some cases serious doubts may arise whether the loss in such a patient is due to alcoholic habits alone or whether there is not in addition some new growth or tuberculous affection. When alcoholism leads to peripheral neuritis there is often rapid and extreme loss of weight. In chronic crippling disorders such as rheumatoid arthritis, disseminated sclerosis, or hemiplegia marked loss of weight may occur, as it may in chronic congestive heart failure, where oedema may mask the wasting.

It is often far from easy to be sure whether the loss of weight that may occur in a patient of 70 or more years of age is merely the shrinking of *old age* and diminished appetite or due to underlying neoplasm or infection, such as tuberculosis.

Diabetes mellitus, especially in the young, may have loss of weight as its earliest symptom.

Addison's disease is another affection in which, besides the progressive asthenia, loss of weight may be marked. There may or may not have been attacks of syncope or of diarrhoea; the diagnosis is suggested by brown pigmentation of the skin, particularly in the flexures and groins, but also beneath the mucous membranes, particularly of the mouth (*Fig.* 808, *and see* p. 543), inside the lips, or within the cheeks where it is of

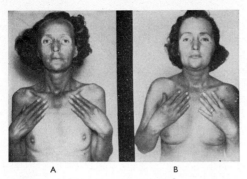

Fig. 808. Addison's disease before (**A**) and after (**B**), showing the effect of corticosteroid therapy, which has caused increased weight, well-being, and depigmentation of skin of face and body.

grey colour. The blood-pressure is usually very low.

Loss of weight is a prominent feature in cases of hyperthyroidism; it may be the first symptom to attract attention preceding tachycardia, nervousness, excessive perspiration, fine tremor of the outstretched fingers, exophthalmos, and symmetrical enlargement of the thyroid gland.

Anorexia nervosa is a condition in which wasting is the prominent symptom (*see* p. 75), but amenorrhoea often occurs very early in the disease.

F. Dudley Hart.

YAWNING

Yawning is such a commonplace physiological occurrence that very little is known about its aetiology. It is a reflex action whose pathways reach no higher in the central nervous system than the basal ganglia. The act itself consists of a tonic contraction of several muscle groups resulting in a deep inspiration, dilatation of the pharynx, and depression of the tongue and lower jaw. The physiological effects of the deep inspiration include an increase in venous return to the heart and, probably more significant, the opening of pulmonary alveoli which may have closed during a prolonged period of quiet breathing. If yawning is impossible, as in a patient on a ventilator, disseminated alveolar collapse may occur; this is the cause of the veno-arterial shunting and arterial hypoxaemia seen in this situation. The 'purpose' of the associated facial contortions is less easy to determine. It has also been noticed that the sense of smell is more acute during a yawn; this is probably as a result of a large bolus of air being brought into contact with an unusually exposed nasopharynx. The importance of an acute sense of smell for wild animals is clear and it has been postulated that this reflex may have had a survival value for primitive man.

The stretching of the arms, commonly associated with yawning, is known as 'pandiculation' and is also a reflex act. This information comes as a surprise to some but is conclusively proved by the fact that the paralysed arm in hemiparesis may demonstrate pandiculation even when no voluntary movement is possible.

It remains to give an account of the afferent side of this reflex arc. This can be based only on personal experience and everyday observations. Boredom and drowsiness certainly provoke yawning as does the sight or sound of someone else's yawn. This remarkable contagiousness of yawning is well known but no satisfactory explanation for it appears ever to have been offered.

Very occasionally yawning, especially when occurring very frequently, may be evidence of organic disease. It may be an epileptic phenomenon or occur following attacks of encephalitis along with other disturbances of respiration such as hyperventilation and Cheyne-Stokes breathing. Paroxysms of yawning may also be caused by cerebral tumours, especially those situated in the posterior fossa, and yawning can be regularly produced in an opiate addict by the injection of a narcotic antagonist.

P. R. Fleming.

INDEX

Berry aneurysm causing intracranial
 haemorrhage, 393
– – – optic tract lesion, 390
Berylliosis causing dyspnoea, 242
Beryllium disease, chronic, 156
Besnier's prurigo, 614
Bestiality, 62
Beta-blocking agents causing
 bradycardia, 112
Betazole hydrochloride in gastric
 secretion tests, 763
Bethanidine causing postural hypotension,
 283
Bicarbonate, depletion of, due to loss of
 intestinal secretions, 403
– excessive intake of, in metabolic
 acidosis, 404
– extracellular fluids as buffers in
 hydrogen ions, 401
Biceps, absence of, 557
– infective radiculitis affecting, 600
– jerk, depression of, due to disk
 prolapse, 501
– long head of, tendonitis of, causing arm
 pain, 501, 503
– reflex, depressed or lost, 694
– tendinitis causing shoulder pain, 724
Bicuspid aortic valve, bacterial infection
 of, 367
– – – stenosis of, 365
Biermer's anaemia (see Pernicious
 anaemia)
Biguanides, therapy with, hyperlactaemia
 with acidosis and, 403
Bilateral blindness, 827
– hilar lymphadenopathy of sarcoidosis
 causing cough, 191
– imperforate choanae in newborn
 causing nasal obstruction, 565
Bile, conjugated, failure of, to reach
 intestine, causing cholestasis, 443
– exclusion from intestine causing fatty
 faeces, 757
– and intestinal contents in vomit, 830
– leakage of, causing peritoneal
 adhesions, 446
– pigments causing dark faeces, 523
– porphyrin in, 655
– in urine (see also Biliuria), 809–10
– – tests for, 809
– vomit, 830
– vomiting in intestinal obstruction in
 newborn, 174
Bile-duct calculus, common, causing
 colic, 4
– – impacted in, causing jaundice, 476
– carcinoma of, causing jaundice, 443,
 445
– – common, causing colic, 4
– – simulating enlarged gall-bladder, 312
– common, accidental division of, causing
 jaundice, 443, 445
– – causes of jaundice within, 404,
 (Figs. 442–4) 444–5
– – compression of, 337
– – epithelial tumour of, 445
– – obstructed by duodenal
 diverticulum, 447
– – obstruction to, causing liver
 enlargement, 504, 506
– compression or invasion from outside
 causing jaundice, 443, (Fig. 445)
 446–7
– congenital obliteration of, causing
 jaundice, 443, 446
– dilatation, intrahepatic, in
 extrahepatic obstruction, 443
– dilated, in extrahepatic cholestasis, 443
– fibrosis, in primary sclerosing
 cholangitis, 443
– inflammation causing colic, 4
– intrahepatic, cancer involving, causing
 deepening jaundice, 507
– – carcinoma of, causing cholestasis,
 442, 443
– invasions by liver metastases due to
 raised serum bilirubin, 442
– involvement in pancreatitis causing
 jaundice, 757
– liver and, infections of, causing
 cholaemia, 206
– multiple hepatic abscesses connected
 with, 504
– obstruction causing cholangitis, 293
– – by stone causing enlarged
 gall-bladder, 312
– postoperative stricture of, causing
 sclerosing cholangitis, 443

Bile-duct, contd.
– rupture, of hydatid cyst into, jaundice
 due to, 10
– wall, causes of jaundice affecting, 443,
 445
Bile-pigments causing orange urine, 807,
 809
Bile-salts necessary for fat digestion, 756
– in urine, 809
Bilharzia eggs in urinary deposit, 92
– haematobia, 297
– – in bladder causing pyuria, 679, 687
– – causing blood per anum, 72
– – – penile pain, 636, (Fig. 652) 638
– – infestation, eosinophilia associated
 with, 254
– japonica causing liver enlargement, 510
– mansoni, 297
– – causing liver enlargement, 510
Bilharziasis causing blood per anum, 67,
 72
– – dysphoea, 243
– – haematuria, 339, (Fig. 368) 347
– – intestinal portal hypertension, 749
– – liver enlargement, 510
– – pyrexia, 288, 297, 300
– – pyuria, 680–90
– – strangury, 764
– – vesical colic, 4
– and cirrhosis of liver, 440
– intestinal, causing splenomegaly, 748,
 752
– pulmonary, causing pulmonary
 hypertension, 372
– spinal, cerebral and, cerebrospinal
 fluid in, 126
– vesical, haematuria due to, 92
Bili-Labstix, reaction of urine to, in
 obstructive jaundice, 444
Biliary calculus causing biliary cirrhosis,
 750
– cirrhosis causing arthropathy, 452
– – – finger clubbing, 301
– – – pyrexia, 295
– – – splenomegaly, 748, 750
– – and cholestasis, prolonged, 439, 441
– – – due to obstruction, 443
– – primary (see also Hanot's cirrhosis)
 441, 442–3
– – secondary, 441
– colic associated with jaundice and
 itching, 7
– – – pyrexia, 294
– – calculus causing, 4
– – causes of, 4
– – causing epigastric pain, 255
– – – hypochondriac pain, right, 408
– – – nocturnal pain, 408
– – – vomiting, 831, 832
– – constipation associated with, 176
– – preceding intestinal obstruction, 174
– – referred to pelvis, 630
– – shoulder tenderness in, 151
– disease, avoidance of food in, 75
– obstructive, 512
– fistula due to accidental division of
 bile-duct, 445
– inflammation causing rigors, 695
– obstruction causing fatty faeces, 757
– – – obstructive jaundice, 443
– – – steatorrhoea, 757
– – chronic, biliary cirrhosis secondary
 to, 441
– – distinguished from liver metastases,
 507
– – due to round-worms, 431, 445
– – extrahepatic, causing sclerosing
 cholangitis, 443
– – by hydatid daughter cysts, 10
– – intermittent, in chronic cholangitis,
 696
– – partial, urobilinuria in, 810
– tract enzyme tests to detect biliary
 disease, 512
Biliousness, migraine described as, 423
Bilirubin (see also Serum bilirubin)
– conjugated, (Fig. 441) 433
– excess in thalassaemia, 42
– in liver disease, 510
– obstructive biliary disease, 512
– transport into hepatic cell, failure of,
 436
– unconjugated, (Fig. 441) 433
– in urine, 807, 809
Bilirubinuria, due to infective hepatitis,
 437
– as indication of hyperbilirubinaemia,
 510

Bilirubinuria, contd.
– in relation to jaundice, 809–10
– signifying hepatocellular or obstructive
 jaundice, 810
Biliuria in diagnosis of abdominal pain, 7
– liver metastases, 508
Biliverdin causing green or blue urine,
 809
– in urine, 809
Bilocular hydrocele, 428
Bimanual examination in diagnosis of
 pelvic swelling, 627
– – – sterility, 758
– – of ovarian cyst, 77
– – pelvic organs in dysmenorrhoea, 230
– – recto-abdominal, in amenorrhoea, 19,
 20
– palpation in bearing-down pain, 93
– – of enlarged kidney, 471
– – – kidney causing pain, 417
– – – – tumour, left, 13
– – – – right, 13
– – – mobile kidney, 312
– – – perinephric abscess, 294
– – – renal calculus, 408
– rectal examination, position of patient
 for, 690
– – – of prostatic adenoma, 692
Bing-Siebenmann syndrome in familial
 deafness, 203
Binocular diplopia, 214
– vision, normal, 214
Biochemical picture of chronic active
 hepatitis, 440–41
Biopsy, bronchoscopic, of bronchial
 adenoma, 154, 354
– brush, 154
– of cervical neoplasm, 531
– in diagnosis of Bowen's disease, 732
– – epithelioma, 273, 731
– – gastric cancer, 423
– – Hodgkin's disease, 425
– – jaw epithelioma, 450
– – Kaposi sarcoma, 578
– – lymph-node abnormality, 157
– – lymphogranuloma inguinale, 633
– – lymphosarcoma, 425
– – mycosis fungoides, 733
– – nasal lupus, 564
– – tumour, 564
– – Paget's disease, 732
– – penile epithelioma, 634
– – polyarteritis nodosa, 466
– – popliteal swelling, 653
– – rectal carcinoma, 691
– – suppurating scrotal cyst, 710
– – tonsillar malignancy, 786
– – tuberculous pleural effusion, 148
– – vulval epithelioma, 834
– – – tertiary syphilis, 834
– in dysphagia due to laryngeal disease,
 236
– of endometrium and cervix in blood-
 stained vaginal discharge, 813
– gastroscopy with, in gastric ulcer, 255
– of hydradenoma, 836
– iliac crest, sampling of bone-marrow
 by, 37
– laryngoscopic, in diagnosis of laryngeal
 cancer, 400
– of lung, chest X-ray abnormality, 157,
 158
– needle, pleural, 148
– of orbital neoplasm, 263
– sigmoidoscopic, in diagnosis of colonic
 cancer, 412
– of supraclavicular lymphnode, 516
– tongue ulcer, 800
– tuberculosis of lymph-nodes, 514
– – tongue ulcer, 801
– urethral carcinoma, 807
– vaginal carcinoma, 814
Biot's breathing, 161
Biphasic basal temperature pattern
 characteristic of ovulation, 723
Bird-fancier's lung, 156, 241
– – finger clubbing rare in, 301
Bird-headed features in leprechaunism
 229
Birth, difficult (see Dystocia)
– injury to brachial plexus causing
 one-arm paralysis, 600
– – causing athetosis, 547
– – – cerebral paralysis, 164
– – – convulsions, 181, 182
– – – in infancy, 181
– – – hemiplegia, 392
– – – mental subnormality, 529

Cervicofacial actinomycosis causing
  inability to open mouth, 802
Cervix, acquired closure of, 20
– closure of, causing sterility, 758
– delayed dilatation of, 246, 248
– dilatation of, estimation of, 247
– imperforate, 20
– long conical, causing dysmenorrhoea,
  229
– malignant growth of, 811
– mucous polyp of, 811
– uteri, abnormal position of, causing
  sterility, 758
– – in gonorrhoeal cervicitis, 812
– – herpes on, 819
– – hypertrophy of, 811
– – lymphogranuloma venereum of, 834
– – primary chancre on, 617
– – rectal palpation of, 692
– – secretion from, 812
Chafing causing vulvitis, 833
Chagas disease, 752
– – myocarditis in, 378
Chalazion, 267
– granuloma of conjunctiva following, 172
Chalk forming rectal concretion, 783
Chancre associated with balanitis, 631
– – enlarged groin glands, 425
– – causing penile sore, (Fig. 647) 633
– – scrotal swelling, 710
– – vulval swelling, 833, 834
– distinguished from gummatous ulcer,
  634
– – – herpes genitalis, 819
– – – penile herpes, 632
– – – soft sore, 632, 633
– – – vulval epithelioma, 834
– extragenital, anthrax simulating, 678
– facial, 272–3
– finger, 303
– on lips, 273, 462
– lymph-node enlargement near, 513
– masked by inflamed prepuce, 632, 633
– penile epithelioma distinguished from,
  633
– perineum, 640
– primary, on cervix uteri, 618
– of scrotum, 709, 714
– simulating whitlow, 560
– superimposed on soft sore, 632, 633
– of tongue, 801
– urethral, 806
Chancroid (see Soft sore)
– causing leg ulcer, 492
Chapping of lips, 503
Charcoal biscuits causing dark faeces, 523
Charcot's disease causing bone swellings,
  100
– fever, 294
– hepatic intermittent fever, 695
– joints, 453, (Figs. 471–4) 468
– – due to congenital indifference to
  pain, 455
– – in Riley–Day syndrome, 455
Charcot–Leyden crystals in sputum, 754
Charcot–Marie–Tooth's disease (see
  Peroneal muscular atrophy)
Chediak–Higashi syndrome, functional
  leucocyte defects in, 496
Cheek(s), actinomycosis of, 288, 294, 324
– alveolar abscess pointing on, 448
– dilated venules on, in cirrhosis of liver,
  506
– in epiloia, adenoma sebaceum over, 182
– lesion of, causing cervical adenitis, 788
– perforation of, in cancrum oris, 324–5
– pigmentation of mucosa of, (Fig. 536)
  543
– swelling of, due to mercury poisoning,
  324
– telangiectases on, Fallot's tetralogy
  causing, 60
– ulcer associated with caecal
  actinomycosis, 416
Cheese-makers, lung disease in, 241
Cheilitis, 503
– due to vitamin-B₂ deficiency, 556
– exfoliativa, 503
Cheiropompholyx (see also Pompholyx)
– simulating ringworm of feet, 727
Chemical(s) agents associated with
  G-6-PD deficiency anaemia, 51
– – causing anaemia, 45
– burns causing gangrene, 313
– causes of local oedema, 587
– – vaginal swelling, 813
– causing acute hepatic necrosis, 337
– – bullae, 115

Chemical(s), contd.
– causing dermatitis, 821, 822
– – haemoglobinuria, 350, 351
– – haemolytic anaemia, 435
– and drugs, ataxia due to, 82
– poisons causing haemolytic anaemias,
  50, 52
– – and drugs, anaemia due to, 31
– purpuras associated with, 670
Chemosis, 268
Cherries causing dark faeces, 523
Cherry-red facies in carbon-monoxide
  poisoning, 169
Chesapeake haemoglobin causing
  polycythaemia, 650
Chest (see also Thoracic)
– abnormalities associated with yellow
  nail syndrome, 561
– acutely overdistended, in asthma, 189
– affections causing abdominal rigidity, 2
– barrel, 130
– bloody effusion in, 128
– conditions causing umbilical pain, 804
– contraction, unilateral, pleural
  thickening causing, (Fig. 135) 131
– crush injury to, causing diaphragmatic
  hernia, 211
– – – traumatic cyanosis following, 199
– deformity(ies), (Figs. 132–7) 129–33
– – congenital, (Fig. 134) 129
– – displacing liver downward, 504
– – due to rickets, 457
– – scoliosis, 739
– – in osteogenesis imperfecta, 456
– – resulting from disease, (Figs. 135–7
  130–3
– enlarged glands in, in Hodgkin's
  disease, 513
– examination following symptomless
  localized shadows in routine X-ray,
  154
– – in pertussis, 187
– funnel, 129
– normal configuration of,
  (Figs. 132, 133) 129
– pain, (Figs. 138–52) 133–43
– – in Asher's precordial catch, 612
– – central, (Figs. 139–50) 133–41
– – due to abdominal lesions, 140
– – – acute coronary insufficiency 133,
  (Fig. 142) 135
– – – angina, (Figs. 139–41) 133–5
– – – aortic aneurysm, (Fig. 152) 143
– – – Da Costa's syndrome, 141
– – – dissecting aneurysm, (Fig. 149) 139
– – – fibrosing alveolitis, 225, 241
– – – herpes zoster, (Fig. 138) 133
– – – intrathoracic malignant disease, 143
– – – mediastinal emphysema, 647
– – – musculo-skeletal causes, 140
– – – myocardial infarction, 133,
  (Figs. 143–9) 135
– – – – ischaemia, 133
– – – pericardial fat necrosis 139
– – – pericarditis, (Fig. 148) 137
– – – psychological conditions, 141
– – – pulmonary embolism, (Fig. 150)
  139
– – – – infarction, 149
– – – respiratory disease, 141
– – – spontaneous haemothorax, 128
– – – – pneumothorax, (Fig. 151) 142,
  225, 645, 647
– – – superficial lesions, (Fig. 138) 133
– – lateral, (Figs. 151, 152) 141
– – related to particular movements, 141
– – pus in (see also Empyema),
  (Figs. 153–5) 143–6
– radiograph in haemoptysis, 352
– – in sciatica, 498
– relative immobility of, in internal
  capsular lesion, 391
– right side, pain in, suggesting
  hepatoma of liver, 506
– serous effusion in (see also Pleural
  effusion), 128
– swelling due to tropical abscess, 505
– tactile hyperaesthesiae of, 151
– tenderness in (see also Tenderness in
  chest), 149–51
– wall, abscess arising in, lung abscess
  simulating, 151
– – air entering pleura through injury to,
  645
– – brawny induration of, actinomycotic
  empyema causing, 145
– – cold abscess of, 131
– – deformities due to scoliosis, 130

Chest wall, contd.
– – infection, empyema secondary to,
  145
– – lesions causing localized swellings,
  131
– – – – tenderness in chest, 150
– – localized changes in, 131
– – – shadows in X-ray, 152
– – lower tenderness along, 151
– – soft tissue tumours, 152
– – superficial tissues of, pain due to
  inflammation of, 133
– – swelling, fluctuating, empyema
  necessitas causing, 145
– – – intrathoracic disease causing, 131,
  132
– – tuberculosis of, 131
– – ulcer of, associated with ileocaecal
  actinomycosis, 416
– – unilateral contraction of,
  (Figs. 135–7) 131
– – – expansion of, 131
– X-ray abnormality in symptomless
  subjects, 151–60
– – in achalasia of the cardia, 159–60
– – adenocarcinoma, 156
– – adenoma, 153
– – allergic aspergillosis, 154
– – aneurysm of the aorta, 160
– – arteriovenous aneurysm of lung, 154
– – bilateral hilar lymph-node
  enlargement, (Fig. 164) 158
– – blood-borne metastases in lungs, 156
– – bronchial carcinoma, 153, 154
– – bronchiolo-alveolar cell carcinoma,
  154
– – central (mediastinal and
  paramediastinal) shadows, 157–8
– – chronic miliary tuberculosis, 156
– – coccidioidomycosis, 153
– – coin lesions, 153, 154
– – convulsions, 182
– – cryptococcal granuloma, 153
– – cryptogenic fibrosing alveolitis, 156,
  157
– – cysts, bronchogenic, (Fig. 167) 159
– – – dermoid, 158
– – – foregut, 158
– – – pleuropericardia, 160
– – – teratomas, 158
– – – in diaphragmatic hernias, 153
– – epithelioma, (Fig. 162) 153
– – extrinsic allergic alveolitis, 156, 157
– – haemosiderosis, secondary, 157
– – hamartoma, 153, 157
– – histiocytosis X, 156, 157
– – histoplasmosis, 153, 156
– – Hodgkin's disease, 158
– – in hydatid cyst, ruptured, 153
– – idiopathic pulmonary
  haemosiderosis, 156–7
– – intrathoracic goitre, 158
– – lymphoma of lung, 154, 158
– – mediastinal shadows, (Figs. 165–7)
  158
– – metastatic malignant disease, 158
– – necrobiotic nodules in lung, 154
– – oesophageal diverticulum, 160
– – physical examination, 153, 154, 157
– – pleural effusions, 152
– – – thickening, 152
– – – – exposure to asbestos, 153
– – pneumoconiosis, 155–6
– – pneumonia, 154
– – pulmonary alveolar microlithiasis, 156
– – – infarction, 154
– – sarcoidosis, 155, 157
– – silicosis, 155
– – solitary metastasis, 153
– – tuberculosis, 153, 154, 158
– – tumour, 158
– – – arising from ribs, 152
– – – – benign, 153
– – – neurogenic, 158–9
– – – soft tissue, 152
– – – thymic, 158
Cheyne–Stokes respiration,
  (Figs. 169, 170) 160–1
– – following encephalitis, 839
– – mechanism of, (Fig. 170) 160
– – precipitated by narcotics, 161
Chiasma, lesion at, causing bitemporal
  hemianopia, 387, 388
– pressure on, causing bitemporal
  hemianopia, 387, 388
Chick pea, ingestion of, causing
  lathyrism, 624
Chickens, psittacosis contracted from, 290

Dyspnoea, contd.
- on effort due to left ventricular failure, 369
- emphysema causing, (Fig. 256) 239
- excessive ventilation causing, 238–9
- exercise causing, 238
- on exertion in atrial septal defect, 373
- – Fallot's tetralogy, 374
- – fibrosing alveolitis causing, 241
- – in hypertensive heart disease, 95, 369
- – – methaemoglobinaemia causing, 199
- – with orthopnoea and nocturnal dyspnoea, 244
- extrinsic allergic alveolitis causing, 241
- factors combining to produce, in lung infections, 245
- heart-block causing, 114
- hypoventilation causing, 245
- increased ventilation causing, 237
- in infants, retropharyngeal abscess causing, 786
- iron-deficiency anaemia causing, 41
- laryngeal obstruction causing, 239
- left ventricular failure causing, 238, 246
- lung carcinoma causing, 238, 242
- mitral stenosis causing, 238, (Fig. 263) 246
- in newborn, 239
- obstructive airways disease causing, (Fig. 254) 237
- – lung disease causing, (Figs. 255–7) 239–40
- orthopnoea and nocturnal dyspnoea on exertion with, 244
- paroxysmal (see Paroxysmal dyspnoea)
- phaseochromocytoma causing, 98
- pneumoconiosis causing, (Fig. 259) 241
- pneumonia causing, 245
- progressive, due to ischaemic heart disease, 376
- psychogenic, 245
- pulmonary oedema causing, (Figs. 263, 264) 245
- – sarcoidosis causing, (Fig. 260) 242
- – tuberculosis causing, 240, 242
- – venous hypertension causing, 243
- on recumbency, 609
- reduced ventilating capacity causing, (Figs. 254–64) 237–45
- relieved by squatting in Fallot's tetralogy, 197
- in respiratory acidosis, (Table I) 404
- restrictive lung disease causing, (Fig. 254) 237, (Figs. 258–64) 240–5
- silicosis causing, (Fig. 259) 241–2
- tightness of chest in, angina simulated by, 141
- in uraemia, 63, 170
- with orthopnoea in aortic incompetence, 367
- – mitral stenosis, 371
- – wheezing expiration in obstructive lung disease, 239
Dyspnoeic index, 237, 245
Dysproteinaemias causing leg ulcer, 492
- – purpura, 670, 672
Dysrhythmias, cardiac, Cheyne–Stokes respiration complicated by, 161
- causing polyuria, 651
- complicating myocardial infarction, 136
- diagnosis of, 663
- due to myocardial infarction in elderly, 135–6
- paroxysmal, causing syncope, 284
- in post-pericardiotomy syndrome, 655
Dystocia, 246–97
- causes of, 246, 249
- prevention of, 246
- prolonged, causing paralysis, 498
- symptoms of exhaustion due to, 249
Dystonia musculorum deformans, athetoid movement, 547
Dystrophia adiposogenitalis (see also Fröhlich's syndrome), 580
- – in Hand–Schüller–Christian syndrome, 580
- – myotonia, 599
- – causing atrophy, 558
- – – dysarthria, 739
- – – gynaecomastia, 329
- – – testicular atrophy, (Fig. 766) 782
- – – depression or loss of tendon reflexes in, 693
- – fibrillation and fasciculation absent in, 551
- – gait in, 310

Dysuria due to amitriptyline, 543
- – pyelonephritis, 682
- in urinary-tract infection, 7

EALES'S disease, 608
Ear(s) abnormalities in mongolism, 278
- conditions, external, cough caused by, 186–7, 190, 192
- deformed, in Patau's syndrome, 219
- destruction of, in xeroderma pigmentosum, 733
- discharge (see also Otorrhoea)
- – meatal causes of, 609–10
- – middle-ear causes of, (Fig. 626) 609
- diseases causing scalp tenderness, 702
- – internal, causing tinnitus, 795
- examination of, in conductive deafness, 201
- external (see Auditory meatus; Auricle; External ear)
- foreign body in, causing tinnitus, 795
- gouty tophi in, (Fig. 466) 464
- infection causing meningitis, 359
- – – pneumonococcal meningitis, 360
- internal (see Inner ear)
- large, in leprechaunism, 229
- leakage of cerebrospinal fluid from, 169
- middle (see Middle ear)
- nervous pain in, 251
- nodules on, in sarcoidosis, 280
- noises in (see Tinnitus)
- pain around, due to venous sinus thrombosis, 696
- – behind, in Menière's disease, 817
- – due to glossopharyngeal neuralgia, 284
- – radiating to, in glaucoma, 266
- – redness and swelling behind, 292
- – of tongue carcinoma radiating to, 798
- pigmentation in ochronosis, 465
- polypus in, associated with otorrhoea, (Fig. 626 F) 610
- referred pain in, 251
- tophi in, (Fig. 466) 464
- wax in (see Wax in ear)
Earache, 249–52
- acute otitis media causing, 250
- boils in meatus causing, 249
- causes of local, 249
- in middle ear, 250
Eardrum (see Tympanum)
Early childhood, infancy and, diarrhoea in, 212
- diastolic murmur, 122
Eaton's agent causing arthropathy, 452
- – pneumonia due to, 143
Eau de Cologne causing pigmentation, 729
Ebstein's anomaly of tricuspid valve with reversed interatrial shunt, 197
- malformation of tricuspid valve, diastolic murmur in, 122
- syndrome, split first sound in, 383
Ecchymosis
- in nephritis with nitrogen retention, 45
- scurvy, 49
- skin pigmentation in, 730
Eccrine sweat-glands, affections of, 770
Echocardiography in prolapse of mitral valve cusp, associated with chest pain, 140
Echo-virus infection causing arthropathy, 452
Echolalia, 736
- in generalized convulsive tic, 551
Eclampsia causing haemolytic anaemia, 436
- – hypertensive encephalopathy, 171
- – cerebrospinal fluid pressure in, 124
- – – chyluria due to, 162
- – convulsions in, 181, 183
- – transient blindness in, 828
Eclipse blindness, 827
Ecstasy states in manic disorder, 262
Ecthyma, scab with areola in, 700
Ectodermal defect(s) causing alopecia, 15, 18
- – congenital, causing absence of shortness of nails, 559
- – – – anidrosis, 770
Ectomorphs, 580
Ectopia lentis (see Lens, dislocation of)
- vesicae causing urinary incontinence, (Fig. 534) 541
Ectopic beats causing irregular pulse, 663
- – with varying coupling intervals, (Fig. 672) 664–5

Ectopic, contd.
- bone formation in pseudohyperpara-thyroidism, 228
- focus, single, in mechanism of atrial fibrillation, 665
- gestation (see Extra-uterine gestation)
- – ruptured, Cullen's sign in, 4
- kidney in iliac fossa, 471
- pacemaker causing disordered impulse formation, 663
- pancreas causing vomiting, 831
- parathyroid, 308
- pregnancy, decidual cast of, 230
- rhythms causing rapid pulse, 771
- sinus tachycardia distinguished from, 613
- tachycardia, (Figs. 759–62) 771–3
- – hypotension due to, 100
- – rapid, angina associated with, 135
- testis (see Testis, ectopic)
- thyroid, scanning test over, 793
- ureter causing urinary incontinence, (Fig. 535) 541
Ectropion, 267
- atonic, causing epiphora, 256
- in Bell's palsy, 270
- cicatricial, 267
- – causing epiphora, 256
- following blepharitis, 267
Eczema, (Figs. 797–8) 822
- acute, in otorrhoea, 609
- associated with phenylketonuria, 643
- atopic, of napkin area, 562
- causing vulval swellings, 833
- eosinophilia in, 254
- gouty, 822
- mycosis fungoides simulating, 733
- and suppuration of umbilical scar, 803
- vaccinatum, 820
Edwards' syndrome causing dwarfism, 217, 219
Effort syncope, 284
- syndrome (see Da Costa's syndrome)
Effusion(s) associated with tuberculous pneumothorax, (Fig. 660) 648
- in chest, serous, (Figs. 156–8)146–9
- into joint in acute osteomyelitis, 103
- – – due to lymphogranuloma inguinale, 633
- – – recurrent, 460
- – – osteo-arthropathy, 302
- – pleural (see Pleural effusion)
Egg-shell crackling, (Fig. 209) 192, 194
- – due to bone erosion by aneurysm, 662
- – in jaw, 450
- – of medullary giant-cell tumour, 652
- – osteoclastoma, 107
- – periosteal sarcoma, 306
- – with pulsation due to osteosarcoma, 662
Egocentricity associated with epilepsy, 182
Egyptian splenomegaly, 752
Ehlers–Danlos syndrome, 452, 455
Ehrlich's reagent in testing urine for urobilinogen, 809
Eighth nerve affections causing vertigo, 817
- – neurofibroma causing facial palsy, 270
- – – compressing cerebellum, 546
- – neuroma causing vertigo, 818
Eisenmenger's complex, 374
- – causing cyanosis, 197
- syndrome, 374
- – pulmonary hypertension in, 140
Ejaculation, absence of, in impotency, 421
Ejection clicks, (Fig. 401) 383
- – aortic, 383
- – pulmonary, 383
- murmur, 120
- sound in aortic stenosis, 365, 368
- – Fallot's tetralogy, 374
- – pulmonary stenosis, 374
- – simulating presystolic murmur, 121
- systolic murmur, complete heart-block causing, 114
Elastic fibres in sputum, 755
- tissue, abiotrophy of, in pseudo-xanthoma elasticum, 334
Elbow(s) flexion in Parkinsonism, 310
- fracture near, causing Volkmann's contracture, 552
- and knees, lichen planus causing nodules on, 574
- pain in carpal tunnel syndrome, 601
- hypothermia in, 409
- papules in bend of, 614
- pulsatile swelling in front of, 662
- rheumatoid nodule in, (Fig. 585) 577
- ulnar nerve compression at, 603

Facies, contd.
- of dermatomyositis, 280
- encephalitis lethargica, 276
- exophthalmic goitre, (Fig. 294) 275–6
- gargoylism, 221, 455
- in hereditary osteoarthropathy, 302
- Hippocratic, 7
- – in peritonitis, 3, 8
- – in tympanites, 529
- of hypopituitarism, 275
- lenticular degeneration, (Fig. 300) 278
- mongolism, (Figs. 296–8) 278
- myasthenic, (Fig. 293) 275
- myopathic, 275
- of myxoedema, 49, (Fig. 290) 274–5, (Fig. 458) 458
- in Paget's disease, (Fig. 306) 282
- paralysis agitans, 276
- Parkinsonian, 276
- of pernicious anaemia, 280
- polycythaemia, (Fig. 303) 279
- in primary thyrotoxicosis, (Fig. 772) 789
- in rosacea, 304
- splenomegalic polycythaemia, (Fig. 303) 279
- of stupor, 766
- supravalvular aortic stenosis, (Fig. 331) 368
- tabes dorsalis, 277
- tabetic, 277
Facio-scapulo-humeral muscular dystrophy, 557, 626
Factitious hyperpyrexia, 405
- urticaria, (Fig. 758) 770–1
Factor I (*see* Fibrinogen)
- II (*see* Prothrombin)
- V, 671
- VII, 671
- – deficiency, congenital, 677
- VIII (antihaemophilic globulin), 670–2
- – deficiency causing haemophilia, 672, 676
- – – – von Willebrand's disease, 677
- IX (Christmas factor), 671
- – deficiency causing Christmas disease, 676
- X (Stuart-Prower factor), 671
- XI (plasma thromboplastin antecedent), 671
- XII (Hageman factor), 672
- XIII (fibrin-stabilizing factor), 672
Faecal accumulation causing hypochondriac pain, left, 407
- – – iliac swelling, left, 411
- – – in colon distinguished from splenomegaly, 746, 747–8
- – – distinguished from renal enlargement, 473
- – – due to colonic carcinoma, 473
- – – simulating caecal carcinoma, 416
- concretion causing appendicular colic, 4
- cultures in typhoid fever, 289
- discharge, umbilical, due to tuberculous peritonitis, 747
- fat estimation of stools in diarrhoea, 212
- – neutral or unsplit, 763
- – split, 763
- fistula, 804–5
- – causing offensive vaginal discharge, 813
- impaction causing colic, 5
- – – constipation, 174
- – – iliac pain, left, 410
- – – intestinal obstruction, 174
- – – of hepatic flexure, 12
- – in transverse colon, 12
- incontinence, 282
- – associated with anuria, 66
- masses above colonic carcinoma, 411
- – palpable ascending colon due to, 13
- – in pelvic colon, 14
- matter in urine due to spread of pelvic cancer, 349
- smell in fistula formation, 217
- – of vomit, 831, 832
- urobilinogen estimation, 510
- vomiting due to intestinal obstruction, 832
Faeces, abnormally hard, causing constipation, 178
- ankylostomata and ova in, 590
- Bilharzia ova in, 510
- blood mixed with, per anum, 68
- clay-coloured, due to pancreatic tumour, 12
- colonic accumulation of, causing abdominal swelling, 9

Faeces, contd.
- consistency of, and faecal incontinence, 283
- dark, simulating melaena, 523
- in dysentery, bacteriological examination of, 70
- – microscopical examination of, (Fig. 71) 70
- Entamoeba histolytica in, 70
- examination for Bilharzia ova, 72
- – in unexplained eosinophilia, 254
- – – weight-loss, 838
- fatty (*see* Fatty faeces)
- and gas, passage of, per urethram, 644–5
- in haemolytic anaemia, stercobilinogen in, 50
- hepatic pus in, 505
- impacted above colonic stricture, 177
- incontinence of (*see* Faecal incontinence)
- lead in, in lead poisoning, 324
- manual removal of, in dyschezia, 178
- microscopical examination of, for tape-worm ova, (Fig. 434) 430
- mucus in, 763
- occult blood in (*see* Occult blood in stools)
- pale and bulky, in obstructive jaundice, 443
- – due to cholestasis, 442, 443
- – or silvery, due to carcinoma of ampulla of Vater, 336
- passed through urethra, 804–5
- per urethram due to intestino-vesical fistula, 689
- porphyrin in, 653, 655
- pus in, 737
- thread-worms in, 431
- tubercle bacilli in, in ileocaecal tuberculosis, 416
- Vibrio cholerae in, 337
- white, in congenital obliteration of bile-ducts, 446
Faeculent vomiting associated with tympanites, 530
- – due to sigmoid volvulus, 410
- – – strangulated retroperitoneal hernia, 410
- – in intestinal obstruction, 174, 176
Fainting (*see also* Syncope), 283–5, 304
- fear of, anxiety causing, 73
- preceded by vertigo, 819
- spells due to cerebral arteriopathy, 208
- on standing, anaemia causing, 27
Faintness, anaemia causing, 27
- due to arsenic poisoning, 333
- – bleeding duodenal ulcer, 336
- – – gastric ulcer, 333
- – – peptic ulcer, 523
- – extra-uterine gestation, 534
- – phaeochromocytoma, 322
- – pulmonary embolism, 139
- suggesting haematemesis, 352
'Fainting lark', 285
Fallopian tubes (*see also* Tubal)
- – carcinoma of, causing metrorrhagia, 533
- – causes of pelvic swelling in, 627
- – closed, tests for, in sterility, (Figs. 750–2) 758
- – colic, 4
- – infection involving ovary, 699
- – neoplasm of, causing vaginal discharge, 873
- – rudimentary, causing sterility, 758
- – tumour causing hypogastric swelling, 13
- – – simulating enlarged kidney, 13
Fallot's tetralogy causing cyanosis, (Figs. 213, 214) 196
- – – dwarfism, 223
- – – dyspnoea, 238
- – – telangiectases on cheeks, 60
- – – ventricular enlargement, right, (Figs. 388–9) 374–5
- – continuous murmur in, 123
- – pulmonary second sound absent in, 383
- – syncope in, 284
- – systolic murmur in, 120
False image in diplopia, 215
- localizing sign in subdural haematoma, 169
- urinary incontinence, 539, 540
Falx cerebri, meningioma of, causing leg paralysis, 594

Familial acholuric jaundice (*see* Spherocytosis, hereditary)
- benign chronic pemphigus, (Fig. 125) 118, 823
- cardiomyopathy, 376
- cases of deafness, 203
- conditions causing paraplegia, 620
- congenital adiposa macrosomia, 582
- dysautonomia, 452, 455
- – hypertension due to, 99
- eosinophilia, 254
- hypertrophic polyneuritis, 556
- hypophosphataemia, 242
- lipochrome pigmentary arthritis, 453
- Mediterranean fever, joint manifestations, 452, 459
- myoclonic epilepsy, 549
Family causes of juvenile delinquency, 61
- history of allergy associated with eosinophilia, 254
- – in idiopathic epilepsy, 182
Famine fever (*see* Relapsing fever)
- oedema, 590
Fanconi syndrome, 23, 45, 488
- – in amnesia, 23
- – causing amino-aciduria, 23
- – diabetes insipidus in, 650
- – lowered renal threshold in, 321
Farber's disease, 453
Farmer's lung, 156, 241
- – finger clubbing rare in, 301
Fascia, deep, fixation of breast cancer to, 521
Fasciculation (*see* Fibrillation)
Fasciitis causing heel pain, 386, 387
Fasciola hepatica infestation causing hypochondriac pain, 409
Fat in abdominal wall in obesity, 9
- absorption, defect in, causing vitamin-K deficiency, 676
- – reduced, in obstructive jaundice, 444
- boy, 581
- causing turbid urine, 644
- embolism causing avascular necrosis, 465
- – following fracture causing cerebral embolism, 393
- intolerance in coeliac infantilism, 223
- introduced as lubricant, chyluria distinguished from, 162
- malabsorption of, causing marasmus, 522, 523
- – due to pancreatic steatorrhoea, 757
- metabolism excessive, causing ketosis, 470
- necrosis causing breast enlargement, 519, 520
- – due to pancreatitis, 832
- – in haemorrhagic pancreatitis, 255
- – pericardial, chest pain due to, 139
- in urine (*see* Chyluria)
Fatigability in Sydenham's chorea, 548
Fatigue, 285
- aggravating pseudonystagmus, 579
- – spasmodic torticollis, 552
- causing descent of shoulder girdle, 601
- – insomnia, 429
- – tremor, 544
- diplopia as manifestation of, 215
- due to cerebral arteriopathy, 208
- – Da Costa's syndrome, 141
- – heart-block causing, 114
- pernicious anaemia causing, 46
- phenomenon in myasthenia gravis, 625
- rapid, in myasthenia gravis, 310
- twitching of limb in, 549
Fatty acids in faeces, 763
- faeces (*see also* Steatorrhoea), 762–4
- – associated with pancreatic cancer, 747
- – in conditions of known aetiology, 762–4
- – due to pancreatic lesions, 725
- liver, 508
- masses, tenderness of, in panniculitis, 717
Fauces, inflamed, causing submaxillary lymph-node enlargement, 515
- irritation of, causing vomiting, 831–2
- mucous patches on, in syphilis, 633
Faucial diphtheria causing sore throat, 784, 785
- pillars, affections of, causing sore throat, 784, 786–7
Fava bean causing haemolysis in G-6-PD deficiency, 52
Favism causing anaemia, 52, 53
- – haemoglobinuria, 351
- – glucose-6-phosphate-dehydrogenase deficiency in, 351, 435

Infant(s), blindness in, due to retrolental fibroplasia, 828
- causes of intestinal obstruction in, 175
- or child(ren), blood and mucus per rectum in, due to intussusception, 176
- - gonorrhoeal vulvitis in, 834
- - sarcoma botryoides in, 814
- - stertor in, 760
- congenital hydrocele in, 428
- crepitus in skull bones of, 194
- Crigler–Najjar condition in, 436–7
- dyspnoea in, postpharyngeal abscess causing, 786
- Franconi syndrome in, 650
- frontal bone tumours in, 307
- galactosaemia in, 442
- galactosuria in, 320
- gastro-intestinal catarrh in, causing carpo-pedal spasms, 193
- hyperpyrexia in, environmental temperature causing, 405
- hypertrophic pyloric stenosis in, 832
- ileocaecal and ileocolic intussusception in, 13
- impetigo contagiosum of, 520
- influenzal meningitis in, 360
- intussusception in, 782
- Kaposi's eruption in, (Fig. 793) 820
- keratomalacia in, 186
- leucocyte count in, 36
- lymphocytosis in, 36
- male, intussusception in, 419
- meningococcal meningitis in, 360
- merycism in, 529
- methaemoglobinaemia, nitrate in drinking water causing, 199
- napkin-region eruptions in, 561
- Niemann–Pick disease in, 749
- normal chest of, 129
- pink disease in, 258, 556
- progressive emaciation in (see Marasmus)
- pulmonary hypertension in, 372
- purulent discharge from eyes of, 264
- rectal examination of intussusception in, 175–6
- regurgitation of milk by, 830
- rickets in, involuntary movements associated with, 545
- scabies affecting, 823
- subdural haematoma in, 169
- summer diarrhoea of, blood per anum due to, 67
- - - and vomiting of, 782
- umbilical hernia of, 803
- veno-occlusive disease of liver in, 506
- wind in, causing hiccup, 395
Infantile atrophy, 522
- coarctation of aorta, 98
- dermatitis, Besnier's prurigo following, 614
- - secondarily infected with herpes, 820
- encephalitis causing athetosis, 547
- febrile disorders, abnormal sensations of size in, 829
- gastro-enteritis causing diarrhoea, 212
- hemiplegia, athetosis associated with, 547
- hyperpyrexia, 405
- muscular dystrophy, 626
- palsy, leg ulcers due to, 491
- paralysis (anterior poliomyelitis) (see also Poliomyelitis)
- - talipes due to, 164, 166
- polycystic kidney, 66
- rickets causing dwarfism, 218, 222
- scurvy (see Scurvy, infantile)
- uterus causing amenorrhoea, 20
- - - sterility, 758
Infantilism associated with cirrhosis of liver, 223
- - dwarfism, 218, 222–3
- - gargoylism, (Fig. 235) 221
- coeliac, (Fig. 239) 223
- in cretinism, (Fig. 240) 223
- due to delayed adolescence, 217
- exclusion of syphilis in, 222
- hepatic, 223
- physical, due to congenital syphilis, 275
- pituitary (see Pituitary infantilism)
- renal, (Fig. 238) 222
Infarction causing neutrophilia, 493
- splenomegaly, 748, 750
- complicating meningitis, 359
- of lung in haemoptysis, 353, 355
- - septic, empyema secondary to, 145
- and perisplenitis in myeloid leukaemia, 55
- tissue, in sickle-cell disease, 51

Infection(s) of abrasion leading to leg ulcer, 491
- acute, causing liver enlargement, 504
- - - lymph-node enlargement, 515
- - - retrobulbar neuritis, 267
- - and chronic, axillary lymph-node enlargement due to, 84
- - leucocytosis in, 36
- - myelocytes in blood in, 37
- - systemic, in stiff neck, 568
- - alopecia secondary to, 15, 18
- - amyloidosis secondary to, 442
- - associated with cerebral lesion causing delirium, 205
- - purpuras, 670, (Figs. 678–9) 673
- - causing amnesia, 23
- - colic, 5
- - coma, 167
- - deafness, 203
- - diabetes insipidus, 650
- - gangrene, 313, 316
- - glycosuria, 322
- - haemolytic anaemia, 435
- - - - with jaundice, 436
- - headache, 804
- - jaundice due to hepatocellular damage, 437–8
- - leucopenia, 495
- - lymphocytosis in child, 59
- - mental subnormality, 529
- - neonatal jaundice, 436
- - neutrophilia, 493
- - normochromic normocytic anaemia, 43
- - paraplegia, 620, 621–2
- - polyneuritis and peripheral neuritis, 555
- - primitive leucocytes, 32
- - retroperitoneal fibrosis involving the ureters, 65
- chronic, anaemia associated with, 33
- - due to, 31, 39, 43
- - causing fatigue, 285
- - - marasmus, 522
- - - weight-loss, 838
- - plasma cells in marrow in, 37
- - sideroblastic anaemia complicating, 42
- convalescence from, lymphocytosis in, 36, 494
- dysmenorrhoea arising from, 229
- general, causing convulsions in infancy, 181
- - - urobilinuria, 810
- - delirium due to toxaemia from, 204–5
- - or local, intermittent bacteriuria indicating, 92
- - urine in, 92
- - and infestations causing eosinophilia, 254
- lassitude in, 489
- local, causing meningitis, 359
- long-standing, toxic granulation in, 495
- mild, causing transient pyrexia, 300
- of nervous system, delirium due to, 204, 205
- overwhelming, causing leucopenia, 496
- - leucocytosis diminishing in, 494
- - shock after, causing hypothermia, 410
- peripheral neuritis and, 555
- precipitating atrial fibrillation, 665–6
- proportion of mature to immature polymorphonuclear cells in, 495
- systemic, causing diarrhoea in infancy, 212
Infectious diseases, acute, causing menorrhagia, 525
- mononucleosis associated with sub-maxillary nodes, 575
- - - causing arthropathy, 452, 463
- - - epistaxis, 257
- - - jaundice, 437
- - - liver enlargement, 504
- - - lymph-node enlargement, 513
- - - meningitis, 361
- - - purpura, 670
- - - pyrexia, 287, 288, 300
- - - splenomegaly, 748, 752
- - cervical adenitis with sore throat in, 516
- - distinguished from acute leukaemia, 59
- - - lymphatic leukaemia, 58
- - lassitude in, 489
- - leukaemoid reaction in, 495
- - in lymph-node enlargement, 513
- - lymphocyte abnormalities in, 36, 37
- - lymphocytosis in, 36, 494
- - meningitis of, cerebrospinal fluid in, 126

Infective arthritis, acute, acute osteomyelitis distinguished from, 103
- - causing stiff neck, 566, 567
- - chronic, of sacro-iliac joint causing sciatica, 498
- - of lumbar spine causing iliac pain, 410, 413
- arthropathies, 452, 463
- causes of blood per anum, 67
- - dwarfism, 218, 222
- - facial palsy, 270
- - hemiplegia, 392, 394
- - hoarseness, 399
- - stiff neck, 566
- conditions of bones and joints, (Fig. 80) 88–9
- - - causing backache, 86, (Fig. 80) 89
- - - pyrexia, 288, (Fig. 309) 294–5, 300
- diarrhoea, acute, causing tenesmus, 782
- diseases causing dyspepsia, 4
- disorder, single rigor at outset of, 694
- endocarditis (see also Bacterial endocarditis), (Figs. 310–12) 291–2
- - colic associated with, 4
- - myocardial infarction associated with, 135
- fevers, acute, causing splenomegaly, 748, (Figs. 748–9) 751–2
- gangrene, 313, 316
- hepatitis, 437
- - acute hepatic necrosis following, 337
- - causing arthropathy, 452
- - - colic, 5
- - - liver enlargement, 504
- - - cerebrospinal fluid in, 125
- - virus, 437
- - hiccup, 395–96
- leg ulcers, 490, (Figs. 508–10) 491
- oedema, 587
- polyneuritis (see Polyneuritis of Guillain–Barré)
- radiculitis (see also Radiculitis, infective), 502
- sinus thrombosis, 695–6
- - - causing rigors, 695–6
Inferior oblique muscle, paralysis of, causing diplopia, (Fig. 230) 216
- vena cava, obstruction of, hepatic venous obstruction due to, 79
Infertility due to chronic salpingo-oophoritis, 629
- - tuberculous endometritis, 524
- factors, 757
Infestations and infections causing eosinophilia, 254
Inflammatory abdominal diseases requiring laparotomy, 5
- affections of eyes causing blindness, 828
- arthritis, 454
- arthropathies of spine, (Figs. 78, 79) 88
- causes of cervical gland enlargement, 516
- changes associated with eye pain, 266
- conditions causing pyrexia, 294–5
- diseases of kidney causing pyuria, 680–2
- facial swellings, 271
- infections, local, causing rigors, 694–5
- infiltration from lung causing arm pain, 501, 502
- lesions causing vulval swellings, 833
- muscular disease causing little atrophy, 557
- processes, bladder involvement in, causing pyuria, 679, 688
- swelling in abdominal wall, 9
- - of jaw, (Fig. 446) 448
- - - distinguished from tumours, 448
- - umbilicus in newborn, 9
- thyroid enlargement, 789
- vaginal swelling, 813
Influenza, bradycardia in convalescence from, 111
- causing arthropathy, 452
- - deafness, 203
- - delirium, 205
- - epididymitis, 775
- - epistaxis, 257
- - eye pain, 267
- - leucopenia, 496
- - menorrhagia, 525
- - orchitis, 775
- - retrobulbar neuritis, 267
- cerebral venous thrombosis following, 165
- lymphocytosis in, 494
- mucoid discharge in, 563
- nasal catarrh in, causing sneezing, 735

Mucosa in anaemia, colour of, 27
- erythema multiforme affecting, 325
- haemorrhagic erosions of, in lupus erythematosus, 260
- involved in small-pox rash, 678
- oozing of blood from, in thrombocytopenic purpura, 675
Mucosal bleeding in mercury poisoning, 324
- congestion causing antral pain, 451
- haemorrhages due to leukaemia, 695
- - in scurvy, 49
- involvement in acanthosis nigricans, 729
- irritability causing cough, 187
- pallor in diagnosis of dyspnoea due to anaemia, 246
- pigmentation in Addison's disease, 280, 729
- telangiectases, 60
Mucous casts of bowel, passage of, 763
- cyst causing vulval swelling, 833
- membrane involved in pemphigus vulgaris, 117
- - pemphigoid, 117, 118, 119
- nasal discharge, 563
- patches on lips, 503
- - of secondary syphilis, 617–18
- - in syphilis, 633
- - - of infancy, 102
- - on tongue, 801
- polypus causing metrorrhagia, 531, 533
- secretion, abnormality of, causing fibrocystic disease, 441
- tubercle of scrotum, 708–9
Mucoviscidosis (see Fibrocystic disease)
Mucus aggregation on conjunctiva causing muscae volitantes, 829
- in faeces (see also Blood and mucus in faeces), 763
- obstructing airways in bronchial asthma, 240
- passed with blood per anum (see Blood and mucus in stools)
- per anum due to pelvic abscess, 629
- per rectum due to villous tumour, 691
Mugging by drug addicts, 61
Mules, glanders contracted from, 678
Multicentric reticulohistiocytosis, 453, 465
Multifocal epilepsy due to cysticercosis, 183
Multilobed polymorphonuclear cells, 494
Multiloculated cystic disease of jaw, 450
Multiple abdominal masses, ascites accompanied by, 78
- cystic disease of breast, 521
- cysts of epididymis, 713
- exostoses, bone swelling due to, 100, (Fig. 98) 104
- myeloma (see Myelomatosis)
- polypi of rectum and colon, (Fig. 68) 68–9
Multiple sclerosis (see also Disseminated sclerosis)
- - causing micturition disorders, 538, 542
- skin lesions due to anthrax, 678
- staphylococcal folliculitis, 677
- swellings of breast, 519
Mumps causing arthropathy, 452
- - colic, 5
- - deafness, 203, 204
- - dysphagia, 236
- - epididymo-orchitis, 775
- - inability to open mouth, 802
- - parotid gland swelling, 697–8
- - scrotal swelling, 712
- - testicular swelling, 712
- cervical adenitis simulating, 788
- differential diagnosis of, in sore throat, 787
- encephalitis followed by obesity, 580
- facies of, 282
- hydrocele associated with, 779
- lymphocytosis in, 494
- meningitis, 358, 361
- meningo-encephalitis, cerebrospinal fluid in, 358
- orchitis causing gynaecomastia, 325, 327
- - - sterility, 758
- - - testicular atrophy, 775, 781
- testicular abscess complicating, 709
Munchausen syndrome in functional abdominal pain, 8
Munro-Kerr manoeuvre in diagnosis of disproportion, 247
Mural thrombus, myocardial, systemic embolism from, 136

Murmur(s), (Figs. 126–31) 119–23
- atrial systolic, 121
- blood-flow velocity causing, 119
- blowing, from orbital aneurysm, 263
- cardiorespiratory, 123
- continuous, (Fig. 131) 123
- - over pulmonary arteriovenous aneurysm, 198
- diastolic (see also Diastolic murmurs), (Figs. 129, 130) 121
- - delayed, 121
- - early, 121
- - immediate, 121
- distinguished from exo-cardiac sounds, 123
- ejection, 119
- Gibson, 123
- Graham Steell, 123
- and heart-sounds, documentation of, Wood (Paul) notation for, (Fig. 126) 120
- innocent, of childhood and adolescence, 121
- machinery, 123
- - in persistent ductus arteriosus, 370
- mid-diastolic (see Delayed diastolic murmur)
- mid-systolic (see Delayed systolic murmur)
- over interscapular collateral vessels, coarctation of aorta causing, 98
- palpable (see Thrill)
- pansystolic, 119–20
- subclavicular continuous, in pulmonary atresia, 197
- systolic (see Systolic murmurs)
Muscae volitantes, 74, 829
Muscarine causing jaundice, 437
- poisoning, Amanita mushrooms causing, 439
Muscle(s), affections of, causing paraplegia, (Fig. 646) 625, 626
- anaerobic, infection causing gas gangrene, 252
- balance, error of, causing eyestrain, 267
- biopsy in polyarteritis nodosa, 625
- calcification of, in myositis ossificans, 180
- congenital absence of, 557
- copper-coloured, in anaerobic streptococcal myositis, 252
- disease (see also Muscular disease)
- - causing loss of tendon reflexes, 693
- - - one-leg paralysis, 595
- fatigue affecting lumbar spine causing backache, 631
- inflammation about, causing contractures, 180
- metabolism, anaerobic, during exercise causing dyspnoea, 252
- pain associated with myoglobinuria, 351
- - due to benign myalgic encephalomyelitis, 619
- - - lymphocytic choriomeningitis, 361
- - - - St. Louis encephalitis, 361
- - and stiffness in McArdle's syndrome, 718
- - - and swelling in rat-bite fever, 696
- paralysed, of Cl. oedematiens infection, 252
- relaxation difficulty in myotonia congenita, 310
- rupture of, causing atrophy, 577
- - purpura, 670–7
- spasm due to tuberculous spine, 89
- - painful, in stiff-man syndrome, 760
- tenderness, 717
- - associated with sciatica, 497
- - in combined degeneration of cord, 622
- - due to infective radiculitis, 718
- - - spinal disease, 744
- - referred, 718
- tone, loss of, causing drop attack, 217
- - - in pink disease, 258
- tone, loss of, in pink disease, 258
- wasting associated with carcinoma, 720
- - due to amino acid malabsorption, 757
- - in sciatica, 497
- weakness associated with myoglobinuria, 351
- - due to hypercalcaemia, 88
- - - Morquio–Brailsford osteochondrodystrophy, 456
- wounds, contaminated, clostridial infections following, 252
Muscular atrophy, (Figs. 541–9) 552–8
- - in amyotonia congenita, 557
- - associated with hypertrophy, 557

Muscular atrophy, contd.
- - associated with paralytic scoliosis, 740
- - in Cushing's syndrome, (Fig. 594) 584
- - due to amyotonia congenita, 600
- - - peripheral nerve lesions, (Figs. 546–8) 552–7
- - in hand in shoulder–hand syndrome, 468
- - in hemiplegia, 391–2
- - of leg, claw-foot preceded by, 162
- - lower motor neuron lesions causing, (Figs. 541–8) 552–7
- - one-arm paralysis with, 599
- - one-leg paralysis with, 593–5
- - in polyarteritis nodosa, 556–7
- - progressive (see Progressive muscular atrophy)
- - spinal cord lesions causing, (Figs. 541–5) 552–3
- - in syringomyelia, 501
- causes of painful limp, 309
- contraction (see also Contractures), 178–81
- - due to fibrosis, 553
- - painful, in tetanus, 550
- - prolonged, after voluntary effort, 310
- - spasmodic, causing tinnitus, 795
- debility due to acromegaly, 450
- disease causing atrophy, (Fig. 549) 552, 556–7
- - - facial weakness, (Fig. 284) 270
- - - gait abnormalities, 310
- - - paraplegia, 618–20
- - or injury causing contractures, 178
- - primary, talipes due to, 164
- dystrophy(ies), (Fig. 549) 557–8
- - causing dyspnoea, 245
- - - kyphosis, 741
- - - lordosis, 743
- - - one-arm paralysis, 603
- - - scoliosis, 740
- - depression or loss of tendon reflexes in, 693–4
- - facio-scapulo-humeral, 557, 626
- - fibrillation and fasciculation absent in, 551
- - infantile, 626
- - juvenile, 626
- - Landouzy–Dejerine, 626
- - non-familial, simulating thyrotoxic myopathy, 558
- - primary, causing paraplegia, (Fig. 646) 625–6
- - talipes due to, 164, 167
- effort causing bone fracture, 307
- exercise, leucocytosis after, 493
- fatigability in myasthenia gravis, 558
- fatigue, tenderness of, 717–18
- fibrosis due to dermatomyositis, 557
- - talipes due to, 166
- flaccidity in icterus gravis neonatorum, 547
- guarding in spinal nerve pain, 803–4
- hyperplasia, pulmonary, causing dyspnoea, 243
- hypotonia in amyotonia congenita, 600
- - in tabes dorsalis, 277
- over-exertion causing cramp, 192
- paralysis causing lordosis, 743
- - local, causing shoulder pain, 723–4
- rheumatism (see also Fibrositis)
- - associated with referred pain, 718
- - due to appendicitis, 90
- - - manganese poisoning, 545
- - in epileptic fit, 500
- - icterus gravis neonatorum, 547
- - of neck, reflex, due to caries, 567–8
- - in paralysis agitans, (Fig. 537) 545
- - Parkinsonism, 545
- - - post-encephalitic, 545
- rigidity (see Rigidity, muscular)
- spasm, active, causing contracture in hysterical paralyses, 179
- - associated with spinal disease, 744
- - causing dysphagia, 234
- - dysphnoea, 234
- tenderness due to pink disease, 556
- tone, cerebellar regulation of, 81
- twitches due to aspirin poisoning, 169
- twitching, convulsive, uraemia causing, 63, 66
- weakness associated with spinal tenderness, 744
- - causing diffuse kyphosis, 741
- - - dysarthria, 739
- - - incoordination, 80
- - - lordosis, 743
- - due to Conn's syndrome, 98

Ossification of head, excessive, causing
  dystocia, 247
- of tendon insertion at knee, 652
Ossified or calcified subperiosteal
  haematoma, bone swelling due to, 105
- man, 181
- subperiosteal haematoma, calcified,
  bone swelling due to, 100
Osteitis, costal, tenderness in chest due to,
  150
- deformans (see Paget's disease)
- fibrosa in Albright's syndrome, 722
- - causing leontiasis ossea, 305
- - cystica, 88
- - generalized, causing jaw swelling,
  448, 450
- - localized, distinguished from
  adamantinoma, 450
- pubis, 453, 464
- - in post-prostatectomy syndrome, 464
- sternal, tenderness in chest due to, 150
- syphilitic, (Fig. 104 A) 107
Osteo-arthritic hip causing femoro-
  inguinal swelling, 287
- referred pain from, 498
Osteo-arthritis, acromegaly simulating, 458
- causing bone swelling, 100
- - crepitus, 194
- - painful limp, 309
- - stiff neck, 567
- of knee associated with lipomatous
  mass, 652
Osteo-arthropathy associated with
  gynaecomastia, 329
- hereditary, 301
- hypertrophic, 302
- pseudohypertrophic, (Fig. 468) 467
- - pulmonary, (Figs. 469–70) 453, 454,
  467
- - - hand in, 459
- pulmonary, due to pleural fibroma, 301
- - hypertrophic, 302
- - hypertrophic causing finger
  clubbing, 301
Osteo-arthrosis, (Fig. 452) 452, 453,
  (Figs. 456–7) 456–7
- associated with contractures, 180
- camptodactyly simulating, 455
- generalized, 456–7
- hands in, (Figs. 452, 457) 453, 456–7, 459
- Heberden's nodes in, 577
- hydrarthrosis in, 460
- rheumatoid arthritis distinguished from,
  456–7
- secondary to dysplasia epiphysialis
  multiplex, 455
- - traumatic, 455
- of shoulder causing pain, 724
- spondylitis causing kyphosis, 741, 742–3
Osteoblastic metastases of prostatic
  carcinoma, (Fig. 113) 111
Osteochondritis causing spinal tenderness,
  745
- dissecans, 452, 460
- - hydrarthrosis in, 460
- of ribs, due to typhoid, 132
Osteochondrodystrophy, Morquio–
  Brailsford, 452, 456
Osteochondroma, bone swelling due to,
  (Fig. 98) 100, 105
- of ribs, 132
- spinal, 90
Osteochondrosis, 452, 460
Osteoclastoma, bone swelling due to,
  (Figs. 105, 106) 100, 105, 107
- distinguished from osteogenic sarcoma,
  106
- - solitary bone cyst, 104
- - formation, bone cysts in von Recklinghausen disease, (Figs. 107, 108) 108
- of jaw, (Fig. 448) 449
- of long bone, egg-shell crackling over,
  (Fig. 209) 192
Osteodysplasty, joint affections in,
  452, 456
Osteogenesis imperfecta (see also
  Fragilitas ossium)
- - aortic incompetence in, 367
- - associated with scoliosis, 740
- - causing bone swelling, 100, 101
- - - dwarfism, (Fig. 236) 218, 221
- - joint affections in, 452, 456
Osteogenic sarcoma causing bone swelling,
  (Fig. 101) 100, 105–6
- - - popliteal swelling, 652
- - distinguished from Ewing's tumour,
  105
- - of jaw, 450

Osteogenic sarcoma, contd.
- - metastases to, causing pneumothorax,
  381
Osteoid osteoma, 467
- - arthropathy associated with, 453, 468
- - spinal, 90
Osteolytic sarcoma causing popliteal
  swelling, 652
Osteoma, bone swelling due to, 100, 105
- of jaw, 449
- maxillary antrum, 451
- osteoid, 467
- - spinal, 90
Osteomalacia causing arthropathy, 453
- - kyphosis, 742
- - spinal tenderness, 745
- - spontaneous fracture, 307, 308
- distinguished from osteoporosis, 88
- due to steatorrhoea, 756
- juvenile, 222
- skull softening in, basilar impression
  due to, 82
- with acidosis, 23
Osteomyelitis, acute, causing bone
  swelling, 100
- amyloid liver complicating, 509
- causing convulsions in infancy, 181
- - leg ulcer, 492
- - lung abscess, 187
- - oedema, local, 587, 588
- - pyrexia, 288
- - rigors, 695
- - sternal pain, 141
- cellulitis distinguished from, 588
- chronic, causing bone swelling,
  (Fig. 96) 100, 103
- endocarditis occurring in, 349
- neutrophilia in, 493
- non-tubercular, causing sciatica, 497
- of ribs or sternum causing chest-wall
  swelling, 132
- salmonella, in sickle-cell disease, 434
- of spine or pelvis in undulant fever, 90
Osteoperiostitis, syphilitic, of jaw, 448
Osteophytosis, cervical, causing shoulder
  pain, 724
Osteoporosis causing arthropathy, 453
- - crushed or wedged vertebrae, 87
- - fracture of vertebral body, 88
- - kyphosis, 739, 741, 742
- - scoliosis or kyphosis, 131
- - spinal tenderness, 745
- - spontaneous fracture, 307, 308
- in Cushing's syndrome, 584
- due to amino-acid malabsorption, 757
- - corticosteroids, (Fig. 83) 91, 469
- - gonadal dysgenesis, 219
- - hyperparathyroidism, high serum
  calcium in, 222
- osteomalacia distinguished from, 87
Osteosarcoma (see also Osteogenic
  sarcoma)
- egg-shell crackling with pulsation due
  to, 662
Osteosclerosis and fibrosis of marrow
  cavity in myelofibrosis, 749
Otalgia (see Earache)
Otitic barotrauma, 610
- hydrocephalus, 124
Otitis causing intracranial hypertension
  from dural sinus thrombosis, 124
- - meningitis, 359
- child with squint following, papilloedema in, 124
- externa, 201, 249, 250
- - serous discharge in, in otorrhoea,
  609
- media, acute, causing earache, 250
- - - in middle ear in otorrhoea, 609
- - causing cervical gland enlargement
  516
- - - convulsions in infancy, 181
- - - diarrhoea in infancy, 212
- - - headache, 363
- - - labyrinthitis, 203, 817
- - - - in child, 300
- - - scalp tenderness, 703
- - - stiff neck, 566
- - - tinnitus, 795
- - chronic suppurative,
  (Figs. 267, 626) 201, 204, 250, 609
- - - dural sinus thrombosis complicating,
  359
- - quiescent, 201
- - unilateral headache due to, 362
- neutrophilia in, 494
- secretory, 201, 204
- tympanic fluid in, 201

Otolith organ, disease of, causing vertigo,
  817
Otorrhoea, (Fig. 626) 609–10
- bloodstained, 250
- causing infective sinus thrombosis, 696
Otosclerosis causing deafness,
  (Fig. 219) 201
- - tinnitus, 201, 795
- conductive deafness in, (Fig. 219) 202
- involving inner ear, 817
Ovarian abscess causing pelvic pain, 630
- - - sterility, 758
- - - pyogenic organisms causing, 699
- activity, deficient, 22
- amenorrhoea, primary, 20
- biopsy, laparoscopy and, in amenorrhoea, 20
- carcinoma associated with dermatomyositis, 731
- - - neuropathy, 720
- - causing enlarged groin glands, 425
- - - lymph-node enlargement, 516
- - - metrorrhagia, 533
- - impacted in pelvis causing strangury,
  764
- - malignant deposits in pouch of
  Douglas from, 693
- - retroperitoneal secondaries of, 816
- - vaginal metastases of, 814
- - causes of colic, 5
- - hirsutism, 397
- chocolate cysts causing dysmenorrhoea,
  229, 230
- cyst(s), ascites distinguished from, 77,
  628
- - bladder distension mistaken for, 14
- - causing anuria, 65
- - - frequency of micturition, 537
- - - iliac swellings, 411, 418, 420
- - - pelvic swelling, 584–5
- - - sterility, 758
- - - vena caval obstruction, 591
- - colic due to torsion of, 5
- - distended bladder simulating, 627
- - distinguished from renal enlargement, 472
- - dullness in front and resonance in
  flanks in, 77
- - haemorrhagic, causing dysmenorrhoea, 230
- - impacted in pelvis causing strangury,
  764
- - infected, causing pelvic pain, 630
- - - - succussion sound, 767
- - malignant, ascites associated with, 77
- - obstructing inferior vena cava, 816
- - twisted, causing iliac pain, 410, 413,
  414
- - - simulating dysmenorrhoea, 231
- - pressure from, causing constipation,
  177
- - rectal palpation of, 693
- - renal cystic swelling simulating, 473
- - in right iliac fossa, 14
- - ruptured, causing pelvic pain, 630,
  631
- - - simulating dysmenorrhoea, 231
- - - simulating appendicitis, 414
- - suppurating, causing pyrexia, 288, 292
- - - distinguished from tubo-ovarian
  abscess, 699
- - twisted, causing abdominal rigidity, 3
- - - - pelvic pain, 630, 631
- - - - laparotomy required for, 6
- - - urachal cyst simulating, 630
- - uterine fibroid distinguished from,
  524, 627, 628
- - - - simulating, 628
- - with twisted pedicle, ascites with, 628
- cystadenoma, pseudomucinous,
  ruptured, pseudomyxoma peritonei
  due to, 77
- deficiency causing kraurosis vulvae, 835
- dermoid cyst causing pneumaturia, 645
- - - simulating bladder calculus, 478
- - - - gestation, 628
- - - - urachal cyst, 630
- destruction, bilateral, causing amenorrhoea, 20
- disease causing backache, 90
- - - vomiting, 831
- - pain referred to skin from, 630
- dysfunction causing dysmenorrhoea, 230
- dysgenesis causing amenorrhoea, 20
- endometriosis causing menorrhagia, 525
- - - pelvic pain, 631
- enlargement due to polycystic ovary
  syndrome, 398

Paralysis, contd.
- in muscular disease differentiated from
  lower motor neuron lesions, by
  electrodiagnosis, 252
- of one limb, lower, (Figs. 604–5) 593–6
- – – upper, (Fig. 606–8) 596–603
- of small muscles of foot, talipes due to,
  166
- soft palate, post-diphtheritic, 234
- spastic, associated with intermittent
  claudication, 193
- Todd's, 182
- transient, unilateral convulsion
  followed by, 182
- with wasting due to infective radiculitis,
  718
Paralytic brachial neuritis (see Radiculitis,
  infective)
- – radiculitis causing arm pain, 501, 502
- – ectropion, 267
- – ileus causing abdominal swelling, 9
- – – tympanites, 530
- – – loss of bowel-sounds in, 6
- – myoglobinuria, 351
- rabies, ascending paralysis in, 557
- – scoliosis, 130, 740
- – strabismus, 755
- – talipes, (Figs. 176–8) 165
Parametritic abscess causing pyrexia, 288,
  292
Parametritis causing pelvic pain, 630
- – pyrexia, 288, 294–5
- cervical erosion with, causing backache
  631
- dysmenorrhoea arising from, 229
- vesical colic associated with, 4
Paramyoclonus of Friedreich, 549
Paranasal sinuses, empyema of causing
  pyrexia, 293
Paranoid delusions, 206
- – in schizophrenia, 207
- – senile dementia, 208
- schizophrenia, confabulation simulated
  in, 172
- – delusions of, 207
- – violence of, 62
- trends in mental illnesses, 206
Para-oesophageal hernia, (Fig. 227) 212
- – causing anaemia, 40
Para-onychia (see Whitlow)
Paraparesis, spastic, syringomyelia
  causing, 163
Paraphenylendiamine hair dyes causing
  dermatitis, 822
Paraphimosis causing penile pain, 639
- due to balanitis, 631
Paraphysial cysts of third ventricle
  causing interruptions of consciousness,
  173
Paraplegia, (Figs. 642–6) 618–26
- affection of muscles causing, 620,
  (Fig. 646) 625–6
- causes of, 619–20
- causing foot ulcer, 304
- – micturition disorders, 539, 542
- cerebral, 624
- – talipes due to, (Fig. 177) 165
- congenital, 624
- – due to spinal cord defects, 623
- crural, due to cortical thrombosis, 394
- due to amyotrophic lateral sclerosis,
  620, 623
- – benign myalgic encephalomyelitis,
  619, 620
- – caisson disease, 171
- – combined degeneration of cord, 620,
  622
- – deficiency diseases, 620, 622
- – demyelinating diseases, 620
- – disseminated sclerosis, 620, 622, 624
- – encephalomyelitis, 620, 623
- – Friedreich's ataxia, 620, 623
- – infections, 620, 621–2
- – lower motor neuron lesions, 519,
  624–5
- – myelomatosis, 54
- – peroneal muscular atrophy, 625
- – poliomyelitis, acute anterior, 619,
  620, 624
- – polyneuritis, 624–5
- – pyramidal tract lesion, 618–19
- – Schilder's disease, 184
- – spinal cord compression, 619–20,
  (Figs. 642–5) 620–1
- – – – lesions, 618, (Figs. 642–5) 620–4
- – syringomyelia, 620, 623
- – upper motor neuron affections of
  brain, 620, 624

Paraplegia, contd.
- in extension, incomplete pyramidal tract
  severance causing, 618–19
- flexion due to complete pyramidal
  tract severance, 618–19
- – – spinal cord defect, 623
- – – – lesion, 550
- following meningococcal meningitis,
  359–60
- fracture-dislocation of spine with, 741
- hereditary, 620
- hysterical, 594, 626
- and impotence, 420
- necrotic myelitis, acute and subacute,
  causing, 620, 623
- spastic hereditary, 623
- syndrome, 453
- tonic spasms in, 549–50
- – flexor and extensor, 550
- traumatic, causing gynaecomastia, 325,
  328
- without sensory involvement, 619
Parapsoriasis, atrophic, (Fig. 709) 707
- en plâques, (Fig. 708) 707
- guttata, 707
Paraquat poisoning causing dyspnoea, 243
Parasagittal neoplasms causing paraplegia,
  620, 624
- region of motor cortex, injuries to,
  causing paraplegia, 620, 624
Parasellar tumours causing postural
  hypotension, 284
Parasite(s) bites causing enlarged groin
  glands, 424
- blood-borne, anaemia associated with,
  54
- causing blood per anum, 72
- – itching, 659
- – jaundice, 443, 445
- intestinal, associated with weight loss,
  838
- – increased appetite due to, 75
Parasitic diseases, eosinophil increase in,
  36
- infections associated with eosinophilia,
  54
- – causing haemolytic anaemia, 50
- – of nervous system, cerebrospinal
  fluid in, 125
- infestations associated with eosinophilia,
  254
- – causing marasmus, 522
- – in haemoptysis, 353, 356
Paraspinal disease causing head retraction,
  358
Parasternal impulse in mitral
  incompetence, 369
Parasystoles, (Fig. 672) 665
Parathormone-like substance, tumours
  secreting, causing polyuria, 651
Parathyroid adenoma causing osteitis
  fibrosa cystica, 88
- – – phalangeal cystic changes,
  (Fig. 503 B) 486
- – – skeletal rarefaction, 308
- – renal calculi associated with,
  (Fig. 503 A) 486
- ectopic, 308
- hyperplasia causing osteitis fibrosa
  cystica, 88
- overactivity causing osteitis fibrosa, 450
- tumour causing hyperparathyroidism,
  742
- – – spontaneous fracture, 307
Parathyroidectomy, tetany after, 193
Paratracheal node enlargement associated
  with sarcoidosis, (Fig. 164) 158
- – – in routine chest X-ray of
      symptomless subject, 158
Paratyphoid fever causing arthropathy,
  452
- – – bronchitis, 187
- – – leucopenia, 495
- – – pyrexia, 287
- – – splenomegaly, 748, 751
- – cervical arthritis following, 567
- – undulant, typhoid and, spinal
      symptoms delayed in, 89–90
Paratyphoidal appendicitis, 416
Paravertebral abscess causing pus in
  chest, 146
- – due to spinal caries, 741
- injection of anaesthetic to effect
  sympathetic block, 315
- muscles, tenderness referred to,
  posterior disk herniations causing, 86
Parenchymal lung disease causing
  dyspnoea, 238

Parenchymatous goitre, 789, 790
Parental behaviour in causation of
  anxiety state, 74
- – and delinquency in children, 61
Parietal bossing in rickets and congenital
  syphilis, 306
- and frontal bones in rickets, bossing of,
  101
- lesions causing agnosia or apraxia, 81
- lobe, right, post-Rolandic lesion of,
  painful aura due to, 83
- tumour causing amnesia, 24
Parieto-occipital cortex, destruction of,
  causing visual agnosia, 722
- – lesions of, causing amnesia, 24
- – – body agnosia in, 717
Parkinson's disease causing dysarthria, 739
- – – fatigue, 285
Parkinsonian facies, 274, 276
- gait, 310
- tremor, 545
Parkinsonism, 545
- causing apparent ptyalism, 661
- in hepatolenticular degeneration, 545,
  548
- post-encephalitic, 276, 545
- – causing dysarthria, 739
- – – localized sweating, 770
- simulating writer's cramp, 193
- tremor of, 544
Parorexia, 75
Parosmia, 735
Parotid enlargement associated with
  alcoholic cirrhosis, 440
- gland, chronic inflammation of, 697–9
- – inflammatory swellings of, 697
- – lesions, 699
- – surgery causing facial palsy, 270
- – swellings, position of, 271
- – – in uveoparotid polyneuritis, 270
- – swellings, aids to recognition of, 697
- tumours, 698–9
- – mixed, (Fig. 695) 699
Parotitis, alveolar inflammation
  simulating, 699
- in mumps meningitis, 361
- periostitis simulating, 448
Paroxysmal atrial fibrillation causing
  palpitations, 613
- cardiac dyspnoea, bronchial asthma
  distinguished from, 188, 189
- cold haemoglobinuria, 50, 350
- – – causing jaundice, 435
- coughing, 187, 190
- dyspnoea in aortic incompetence, 367
- – hypertensive heart disease, 95, 369
- dysrhythmias causing syncope, 284
- fibrillation causing convulsions, 181
- haemoglobinuria, 350
- – anaemia due to, 53
- headache, 362, 363
- – low cerebrospinal fluid pressure
      associated with, 123
- hypertension, 98
- – of phaeochromocytoma, bradycardia
      in, 111
- – spinal cord lesions causing, 99
- migrainous headache, 269
- myoglobinuria, 351
- nocturnal dyspnoea, hypertensive heart
  disease causing, 95
- – – in mitral stenosis, 371
- – haemoglobinuria, 50, 434–5
- – – anaemia due to, 31
- pain due to thalamic lesion, 716
- – of neuralgia, 364
- supraventricular tachycardia, 613
- tachycardia, 771–2
- – causing convulsions, 181, 183
- – due to phaeochromocytoma, 322
- – polyuria following attack of, 651
- – repetitive, 772
- vertigo, causes of, 817
- vomiting in gastric crises, 422
Paroxysms of pain in tabes dorsalis, 500
Parrot('s) nodes, 102
- – due to congenital syphilis, 522
- psittacosis contracted from, 290
Partial incontinence, post-prostatectomy,
  541
- pressures, method of measurement of,
  402
Parturition, leucocytosis during, 493
- mediastinal emphysema during, 647
- pressure on nasal septum during,
  causing nasal obstruction, 564
- sciatica during, 498
P.A.S. causing haemolysis, 435

Psychopath, aggressive, violent episodes of, 262
Psychopathic absence of feeling of guilt, 61
– personality, delinquency in, 60, 61
Psycho-sexual precocity due to testicular interstitial-cell tumour, 723
Psychosis associated with chronic liver disease, 170
– causing amnesia, 23, 25
– due to pellagra, 556
– organic, due to hepatic disease, 545
Psychosomatic upsets in childhood of anxious adult, 74
Psychotherapeutic agents causing postural hypotension, 284
Psychotic symptoms in cysticercosis, 183
P.T.A. deficiency causing haematuria, 339, 349
Pterygium, (Fig. 181) 172
Ptosis, (Figs. 666–7) 660–1
– associated with hand palsy, 596
– – migrainous headache, 269
– asymmetrical, due to botulism, 235
– due to botulism, 216
– – cervical sympathetic paralysis, 669
– – enlarged thyroid, 780
– – myasthenia gravis, 270
– – trachoma, 264
– hypotonic, in tabes, 277
– in pituitary exophthalmos, 215
– simulated in hysterical paralyses, 179
– of spleen, palpation in, 746
Ptyalism, 661
– in post-encephalitic Parkinsonism, 545
– with difficulty in swallowing, 661
Ptyalorrhœa, functional, 661
– hysterical, 661
Pubarché, premature, 722
Pubertal gynaecomastia, (Figs. 345 A, B, C) 325, 326
Puberty, acne vulgaris occurring at, 517
– breast pain due to onset of, 114
– delayed, causing temporary dwarfism, 218
– discharge from nipple at, 572
– enuresis disappearing at, 253
– epistaxis and sneezing at, 735
– irregular vaginal bleeding before, 531, 534, 535
– mastitis, 329
– menorrhagia of, 524, 525
– metrorrhagia occurring about, 533
– node, (Fig. 345 A) 325
– nodular plaques on breasts at, 519
– precocious (see Precocious puberty)
– thyroglossal cyst appearing at, 568
– thyroid enlargement at, 788
– unilateral breast enlargement at, 519
– vaginal bleeding before, 814
Pubes, urinary fistula above, due to gunshot injury, 542
Pubescent uterus causing sterility, 758
Pubic bone disease causing scrotal swelling, 714
– hair, diminished, in haemochromatosis, 507
– – lack of, in testicular feminization, (Fig. 346) 328
– – loss of, in hypopituitarism, 274
– – premature growth of, 722
– – reduced or absent, in haemochromatosis, 322
– – – in cirrhosis of liver, 507
– – scanty, in gonadal dysgenesis, (Fig. 231) 219
– 'sporran' masking normal genitalia in obesity, 229, 580, 582
Pubis, spine of, identification of, 285
Puerperal fever causing rigors, 695
– infection, cervicitis following, 812
– – septic infarction of lungs following, 145
– – – pelvic abscess due to, 629
– – septicaemia, anaemia due to, 43
– vaginitis, 814
Puerperium, haemoglobinuria during, 350
– pregnancy and, dural sinus thrombosis in, 124
– stress incontinence of urine appearing in, 810
Puffiness of face and ankles in acute nephritis, 66
Pulmonary(ies) actinomycosis causing empyema, 145
– alveolar microlithiasis in routine chest X-ray of symptomless subject, 156

Pulmonary(ies), alveolar, contd.
– – proteinosis, microscopy of sputum in, 755
– angiography, pulmonary embolism demonstrated by, (Fig. 150) 140
– arterial embolism causing lung abscess, 187
– – hypertension causing ventricular enlargement, right, 371
– – pressure, rising, due to obstructive lung disease, 239
– arteriovenous aneurysm causing finger clubbing, 301
– – – congenital, (Fig. 216) 198
– – fistula, continuous murmur due to, 123
– artery and aorta, transposition of, (Fig. 215) 197
– – branch of, murmur of stenosis of, 123
– – compression of, causing tricuspid incompetence, 376
– – dilated, in atrial septal defect, 373, 374
– – – in thrombo-embolic pulmonary hypertension, 372
– – peripheral, embolism in, pulmonary infarction due to, 148
– aspergillosis causing eosinophilia, 254
– atresia causing cyanosis, 197
– – continuous murmurs in, 123
– – and bronchial arterial anastomoses in pulmonary atresia, 197
– calcification, disseminated, due to systemic sclerosis, 243
– causes of cough, (Figs. 203–7) 191
– complications of psittacosis, 290
– congestion in heart disease, macrophages in sputum due to, 754
– – mitral stenosis causing cough, 192
– consolidation in pyaemia, 695
– – in Weil's disease, 438
– diastolic murmur after valvotomy for pulmonary stenosis, 122
– disease, abnormal exudates in, causing cough, 187
– – anxious facies of, 282
– – causing respiratory alkalosis, 405
– – cerebral embolism associated with, 168
– – chronic, anorexia in, 75
– – – causing cor pulmonale, 373
– – – exacerbated by infection, 188
– – – depression secondary to, 245
– – – gastritis associated with, 332
– – – polycythaemia secondary to, 276
– ejection click, 383
– – embolism causing cyanosis, 198
– – – dyspnoea, 238, 246
– – – syncope, 284
– – – transient atrial fibrillation, 665
– – – ventricular enlargement, right, 373
– – chest pain due to, (Fig. 150) 139
– – from phlebothrombosis of calf veins due to recumbency, 136
– – shock after, causing hypothermia, 410
– emphysema (see also Emphysema)
– – barrel chest of, 130
– eosinophilia, 254
– fibrosis associated with cystic fibrosis, 212–13
– – causing chest contraction, (Figs. 136, 137) 131
– – – cough, 191
– – – displaced heart, 381
– – – finger clubbing, 301
– – – vomiting, 831
– – in chronic active hepatitis, 440
– – diffuse, causing dyspnoea, 241
– – – cyanosis in, 195
– – – resulting from allergic alveolitis, 241
– – – in silicosis, 243
– – idiopathic, causing polycythaemia, 649
– – in miners, rheumatoid arthritis associated with, 459
– haemangioma in hereditary haemorrhagic telangiectasia, (Fig. 216) 198
– haemosiderosis, idiopathic, in routine chest X-ray of symptomless subject, 156–7
– – – sputum in, 754
– – hydatid(s) causing cough, 191
– hypertension associated with persistent ductus arteriosus, 122
– – causes of, 371–3
– – causing congestive heart failure, 196

Pulmonary(ies), hypertension, contd.
– – causing Graham Steell murmur, 122
– – – right ventricular hypertrophy, 382
– – – syncope, 284
– – – tricuspid incompetence, 375
– – – veno-arterial shunt, 374
– – – ventricular hypertrophy, right, 373
– – chronic, anginal pain in, 140
– – complicating 'maladie de Roger', 371
– – – transposition of great arteries, 197
– – developing on ventricular septal defect, mid-systolic murmur due to, 120
– – due to left ventricular failure, 371
– – in heart disease causing cyanosis, 196
– – 'passive', in mitral stenosis, 371
– – in persistent ductus arteriosus, 374
– – primary, 373
– – pulmonary ejection click in, 383
– – relieved by mitral valvotomy, 122
– – right atrial sound in, 384
– – shortening thrill of 'maladie de Roger', 656
– – splitting second sound in, 384
– – in systemic sclerosis, 243
– – thrombo-embolic, 372
– – in ventricular septal defect, 374
– – with reversed interventricular shunt, 197
– incompetence, Graham Steell murmur of, 371
– – immediate diastolic murmur in, 122
– infarct causing cerebral embolism, 168
– – – pleural effusion, 381
– – – pleurisy, 142
– – – due to embolism in peripheral pulmonary arteries, 148
– – post-pericardiotomy syndrome simulating, 656
– – secondary to thrombophlebitis, 148
– – serous effusion secondary to, 128
– – in sickle-cell disease, 434
– infection(s), acute, causing dyspnoea, 245
– – allergic alveolitis simulating, 241
– – chronic lung disease underlying, 246
– – in myelomatosis, 54
– – pleurisy due to, 142
– lesions in blastomycosis, 361
– – causing shoulder pain, 723
– manifestations of systemic lupus erythematosus, 243
– metastases causing pneumothorax, 380
– – of testicular tumour, 777
– muscular hyperplasia causing dyspnoea, 243
– mycoplasma infection, cold antibody complicating, 52
– oedema, acute, causing cyanosis, 196, 198
– – – X-ray appearances in, (Fig. 264) 245
– – in berylliosis, 242
– – cardiac causes of, 246
– – causes of, 245
– – causing cough, 192
– – – dyspnoea, (Figs. 263, 264) 243–5
– – – paroxysmal cardiac dyspnoea, 189
– – – respiratory alkalosis, 405
– – complicating myocardial infarction, 136
– – due to pulmonary venous hypertension, 245
– – frothy sputum of, 753
– – mitral regurgitation with, rupture of myocardial infarct causing, 136
– – precipitated by atrial fibrillation, (Fig. 673), 665–6
– – simulated in alveolar proteinosis, 243
– osteo-arthropathy (see Osteo-arthropathy, pulmonary)
– plethora in persistent ductus arteriosus, 370
– – ventricular septal defect, (Fig. 381) 371
– resection, extensive, causing dyspnoea, 240
– sarcoidosis causing dyspnoea, (Fig. 260) 242
– second sound, accentuation and diminution of, 382
– – – in mitral stenosis, 372
– secondary neoplasms causing cough, 191
– secretions, mechanisms for removal of, 186
– sepsis causing foul taste, 774
– – or putrefaction causing foul breath, 114

Rigor(s), contd.
- due to testicular abscess, 709
- - tropical abscess, 505
- - tularaemia, 290
- - yellow fever, 438
- initial, in malignant small-pox, 337
- in Lederer's anaemia, 53
- rare in typhoid, 289
- recurring, (Fig. 693) 694-6
- single, 694
- in typhus fever, 751
Riley–Day syndrome, 452, 455
- - hypertension due to, 99
Ring(s) scotoma, 827
- - in migraine amblyopia, 826
- sideroblasts, 43
- under eyes, 282
Ringworm (see also Tinea)
- of beard, 701
- black dot, of scalp, 701
- of body skin, (Fig. 722) 726
- - tropical, 727
- causing alopecia, (Fig. 7) 15, 16
- - scalp tenderness, 701
- of feet, conditions simulating, (Fig. 672) 677, (Fig. 698) 703, 727
- - simulating pompholyx, 824
- - and toes, (Fig. 724) 727
- groin (see also Tinea cruris), 562, 726
- interdigital, of toes, 561
- mange of dog or cat, 726
- of nails, (Fig. 550) 558, 561
- scalp, 701, 704
- - large-spored, 701
- simulating seborrhoeic dermatitis of scrotum, 714
- spreading to hands and body from feet, 727
- suppurating, causing lymph-node enlargement, 513, 515
- of toes, interdigital, (Fig. 724) 727
- X-ray treatment of, alopecia due to, (Fig. 14) 19
Rinne's test for hearing, 200
Rire en travers, 275
Risorius muscle, weakness of, in myasthenia, 275
Risus sardonicus, (Fig. 694) 697
- - due to tetanus, 550, 608, 803
Rituals, obsessional, 586
Rocky Mountain spotted fever causing purpura, 670, 674
- - - - - pyrexia, 287
- - - - - distinguished from typhus, 751
Rodent(s) causing rickettsial disorders, 289
- - tularaemia, 290
- ulcer, 573, 731
- - causing lymph-node enlargement, 515
- - of eyelid, 268, (Fig. 285) 271
- - face, (Figs. 285, 288) 271, 273
- - leg, (Fig. 512) 492
- - lupus vulgaris simulating, 574
- - molluscum sebaceum simulating, 573
- - in nasal vestibule, 564
- - seborrhoeic wart simulating, 615
- - superficial, 731
Rods and cones of retina, 826
Rolling hernia, (Fig. 227) 212
Romanowsky staining of bone-marrow aspirate, 37
Rombergism in sensory ataxia, 80
Root (see also Nerve-root)
- compression by neoplasm causing girdle pain, (Fig. 343) 319-20
- entry zone lesions, sensory loss due to, 720
- irritation causing iliac pain, 417
- lesion causing one-arm palsy, 596, 600
- - - one-leg paralysis, 594
- pain associated with spinal tenderness, 745
- - cervical, due to disk prolapse, 501
- - due to extramedullary tumours, 599
- - - myelomatosis, 54
- - - syphilitic pachymeningitis, 599
- - - felt in foot or leg, 309
- - - peripherally, 715
- - lumbar, extending to shin and foot, 498-9
- - thoracic, 319
- - unusual in foot, 498
- posterior (see Posterior root)
- tumours causing arm pain, 501
- - - paraplegia, 619
Rosacea causing erythema, 259
- lupus erythematosus simulating, 260
- papules of, (Fig. 637) 617

Rosacea, contd.
- post-prandial flushing of face in, 258
- simulating granulosis rubra nasi, 770
- telangiectasis associated with, 60
Rosaceous dermatitis, 259
Rose spots of typhoid fever, 289
Rose-Waaler test for rheumatoid arthritis, 577
- - in renal transplant arthropathy, 464-5
Roseolar rash of syphilis, 633
Rotation, subjective sense of, in vertigo, 817
Rothera's test for keto-acidosis, 470
Rothmund's syndrome, 728
Rotor syndrome causing jaundice, 442-3
Round ligament, fibromyoma of, causing vulval swelling, 833
- - tumour causing inguinal swelling, 427
- shoulders, 741
Round-worms, (Fig. 387) 392
- causing jaundice, 445
- increased appetite due to, 75
- in vomit, 832
Rub audible over hepatic carcinoma, 442
Rubber footwear, dermatitis due to, 115
Rubber-bleb naevus, blue, 59
Rubella arthritis, 452, 463
- causing erythema, 258
- - leucopenia, 495
- - lymph-node enlargement, 513, 514, 515
- - neonatal jaundice, 436, 438
- - purpura, 670
- lymphocytosis in, 37, 494
- maternal, causing deafness in child, 203
- plasma cells in blood in, 37
Rubin's test for tubal patency, 758
Rudimentary first rib, 601
Rumination, cud-chewing, 529, 830
- obsessional thinking, 586
Runners, long-distance, haematuria in, 349
- - haemoglobinuria in, 351
Rupia, papules of, 618
- scab of, 700
Rupture of aortic aneurysm, abdominal pain due to, 6
- hydatid cyst, 10
- - into peritoneal cavity, 10
- - myocardial infarct, 136
Ruptured ectopic gestation, Cullen's sign in, 4
- extra-uterine gestation, abdominal rigidity due to, 3
- - - laparotomy required for, 6
Russell bodies, 37
Rusty sputum in pneumonia, 187
RV (residual volume) measurement, 237

SABRE tibia, 104
Saccular aneurysm, rupture of, causing subarachnoid haemorrhage, 361
Sacral abscess, rectal palpation of, 692
- disease causing sciatica, 497
- nerves, pelvic tumour compressing, 631
- nerve-root lesions causing claw-foot, 162
- pain with haematuria, 340
- plexus, cervical cancer involving, 631
- - nerve trunks in, compression or injury of, talipes due to, 165-6
- root injury, sensory loss in, (Fig. 715) 718
- segments of spinal cord, claw-foot due to lesions of, 162
- tumour, rectal palpation of, 692
Sacralgia, 817
Sacro-iliac arthritis causing sciatica, 497, 498
- involvement in ankylosing spondylitis, 742
- joint(s) in ankylosing spondylitis, 453, 457, 459
- - bilateral involvement of, 89
- - changes in, in ankylosing spondylitis, (Fig. 79) 88
- - disease causing groin abscess, 425
- - - - iliac pain, 410, 413
- - - - sciatica, 498
- - involved in psoriatic arthropathy, 460-1
- - or spine, tuberculosis of, 89
- - strain causing backache, 631
- - subluxation causing sciatica, 497, 498
- - tenderness, 717
Sacro-ilitis causing backache, 631
- involving lumbosacral plexus, 718

Sacrum, fracture of, sensory loss due to, (Fig. 715) 718
- herpetic rash over, 540
- pain in pelvic organs felt over, 631
- rectal examination of, 692
Sagittal sinus, superior, thrombosis of, causing paraplegia, 620, 624
- - thrombosis causing hemiplegia, 392, 394
Sago-grain vesicles of pompholyx, 823-4
St. Gotthard tunnel workers, ankylostomiasis in, 72
- - - hookworm infestation in, 432
St. Louis encephalitis, 361
- - cerebrospinal fluid in, 125
Salazopyrin in ulcerative colitis, 71
Salicylate(s), affecting thyroid hormone assessment, 793
- amblyopia, 826
- causing headache, 364
- - purpura, 670
- - reducing substance in urine, 320
- - sweating, 770
- - urticaria, 836
- - vertigo, 817
- - vomiting, 831
- idiosyncrasy causing delirium, 205
- poisoning causing pulmonary oedema, 245
- therapy in rheumatic fever, 103
- in urine, test for, 320
Salicylazosulphapyridine in ulcerative colitis, 71
Salicylsylphonic acid (Ames) test for proteinuria, 657
- - - proteosuria, 657
Saline infusion, excessive, causing pulmonary oedema, 245
Saliva, difficulty in swallowing causing dribbling, 661
- excessive (see Ptyalism)
Salivary duct calculus causing tongue pain, 796
- - obstruction causing ranula, 796
- gland(s) enlargement in myeloblastic leukaemia, 58
- - - sarcoidosis, 242
- - submaxillary, swellings of, 571
- - swelling of, (Fig. 695) 699
- - - due to impacted calculus, 796
- - - position of, 271
Salivation associated with heartburn, 385
- due to mercury poisoning, 324
- in stomatitis, 324
- uncinate fit, 747
Salmonella causing chronic backache, 86
- - diarrhoea in infancy, 212
- - pyrexia, 287, 289
- food-poisoning causing diarrhoea, 213
- osteomyelitis in sickle-cell disease, 434
- typhi infection causing jaundice, 438
- typhimurium in typhoid disease, 289
Salpingitis, acute, causing abdominal rigidity, 3
- - - iliac pain, 410, 413, 415
- - causing colic, 4
- - - constipation, 176
- - - frequency of micturition, 537
- - - haematuria, 339, 350
- - - hypochondriac pain, right, 409
- - - iliac pyosalpinx, 14
- - - sterility, 758-9
- chronic interstital, causing pelvic pain, 630
- interstitial, chronic, causing menorrhagia, 525
- neutrophilia in, 494
Salpingo-oophoritis causing backache, 631
- - dyspareunia, 231
- - - pelvic abscess, 629
- - - pain, 630
- - - swelling, 626, 629
- - - tubal closure, 758
- - chronic, 699
- - causing menorrhagia, 525
- - dysmenorrhoea arising from, 229, 230
- - pelvic bone growths simulating, 630
- - tubal gestation simulating, 628
- - tuberculous, causing menorrhagia, 524
Sampling of bone-marrow, 38
Sand-fly fever causing leucopenia, 150
- in stiff neck, 568
Saphena varix causing femoral swelling, 286
- - distinguished from inguinal hernia, 426
Saphenous thrombosis spreading to vena cava, 816